Grace Burtis, PhD, RD

Judi Davis, MS, RD/LD

Sandra Martin, RN, MSN

Applied Nutrition and Diet Therapy

1988

W.B. SAUNDERS COMPANY

Harcourt Brace Jovanovich Inc.

Philadelphia   London   Toronto
Montreal   Sydney   Tokyo

W. B. SAUNDERS COMPANY
Harcourt Brace Jovanovich, Inc.

West Washington Square
Philadelphia, PA 19105

Library of Congress Cataloging-in-Publication Data

Burtis, Grace.
   Applied nutrition and diet therapy.

   Includes index.
   1. Diet therapy.   2. Nutrition.   I. Davis, Judi.   II. Martin, Sandra, 1945-   III. Title.
[DNLM: 1. Diet Therapy.   2. Nutrition.   WB 400 B973a]
RM216.B96   1988   615.8'54   87-9613
ISBN 0-7216-1282-2

Editor: Michael Brown
Designer: Terri Siegel
Production Manager: Bill Preston
Manuscript Editor: David Prout
Illustration Coordinator: Lisa Lambert
Page Layout Artist: Dorothy Chattin
Indexer: RoseMarie Klimowicz

Applied Nutrition and Diet Therapy   ISBN   0-7216-1282-2

Last digit is the print number: 9   8   7   6   5   4   3   2   1

Dedications

The task of writing a book places unbelievable demands upon the authors' families and friends, yet their support and love are fundamental to the effort.

To my remarkable husband, who is magnificent in brainstorming and providing the ideal growth environment with unconditional support, patient when necessary, and excellent in celebrating success.

—GB

To my husband and three children, who tolerated many frozen dinners while I was writing about how others should eat to improve their nutritional status.

—JRD

To my husband, Tom, and sons, Steven, Paul, and Jonathan.

—SWM

PREFACE

The study of nutrition can be an interesting and rewarding subject for nursing students not only for patient education but also for their own health. This book is designed to show nursing students how to apply sound nutrition principles in assessing, planning, implementing, and evaluating total patient care and to help the student contribute to the nutritional well-being of patients. A holistic approach to dietary management of a disease by the entire health care team is especially appropriate in order to coordinate totally integrated patient care.

Since the subject of nutrition is a top priority in today's society, the public faces the challenge of understanding nutritional information. Nurses should be able to discuss sound nutritional practices with their patients, clients, or the general public.

Nutritional information in this book is compiled clearly and concisely to give an understanding of the therapeutic value of foods in the normal diet. Using the behavioral objectives as a guide, both the student and instructor know the important information to be gained from each chapter. Questions at the end of each chapter help students determine their comprehension of the material. Learning is also challenged by case studies in many chapters. Throughout the text, specific suggestions are given for application of the material in *Clinical Implications*. *Focus On* boxes contain information that the student will not be expected to memorize but that may broaden the learning experience. *Fallacies and Facts* show how the newly learned material can be useful to evaluate harmful nutrition fads and misinformation. *Health Applications* encourage good nutrition for optimum health to avoid some degenerative diseases.

Section I of the book deals with basic principles of nutrition. An understanding of basic nutrition facts is required for the student to evaluate the flood of new information available and to make wise judgments about eating habits. This unit contains sections on how a vegetarian can obtain an adequate balance of nutrients, how to cope with lactose intolerance, the various caloric expenditures among physically handicapped persons, and carbohydrate loading for trained atheletes.

Problems specifically involved in application of basic nutrition principles through the lifespan and with ethnic groups are presented in Section II. Special considerations relevant for each group are discussed. Breast-feeding has been covered extensively to enable students to encourage this practice. Ethnic food patterns are presented so the nurse can recognize other dietary habits and incorporate any necessary modifications with sensitivity and respect.

Modifications of the diet that are essential to treat diseases are described in Section III. Pathological conditions affecting body systems are briefly examined; principles for the dietary treatment are emphasized. Pertinent nursing suggestions are cited. Integrated into the discussions are related laboratory findings and drug therapy. A specific chapter on nutritional assessments helps the student understand how to combine related observations with a physical assessment. The chapter on food and drug interactions will help the nurse to understand and to avoid potential iatrogenic conditions. Since the nurse is usually the health care team member most closely associated with intravenous and tube feedings, a thorough discussion of this subject is presented. Other subjects covered in this section in addition to diabetes mellitus, cardiovascular disease, and gastrointestinal problems are anemia, feeding techniques for handicapped persons, and controlling food allergies with a rotation diet.

The Appendix contains information for completing assignments and reference material. Food composition tables include the nutritive values of food from three sources: (1) the latest USDA Handbooks 8-1 through 8-14 that list dietary fiber, (2) items from fast food restaurants, and (3) supplementary and tube feedings. Tables that are important in nutritional assessments are included. The glossary includes many of the terms found at the beginning of each chapter as well as words not defined in the text to facilitate learning.

The nurse has considerable influence on the patient's food acceptance. With a better understanding of the importance of diet, the entire health care team can complement each other and ensure fast patient recovery. While specific amounts of nutrients are mentioned, much of this information is presented not so nurses can prescribe special diets but so they can recognize usual therapeutic measures for specific conditions and call any discrepancies to the attention of the physician or dietitian. This will also enable them to explain the reason for various treatments to the patient.

ACKNOWLEDGMENTS

When a book is started, it is impossible to imagine how many people with their different proficiencies will be necessary to complete the project. Whether the aid was constant, sporadic, or brief, each person's help is truly appreciated.

For consultation in specific areas, our gratitude is extended to Kennon Moffitt, R.D., L.D., Associate Director of Nutrition Services, St. Paul Hospital, Dallas, Texas (renal disease); Cheryl Henderson, R.D., Nutritionist, Department of Public Health and Preventive Medicine, Texas College of Osteopathic Medicine, Fort Worth (rotation diets); Barbara Clark, M.S., R.D., Director of Food Service, Arlington Independent School District, Arlington, Texas (school breakfast and lunch programs); Darrell Webb, R.Ph, Pharmacist, Long Term Care Unit, Texas Department of Health, Arlington (drugs); Judith Jamison, M.S., R.D., L.D., writer and consultant, Keene, Texas (nutritional assessments and enteral and parenteral feedings); Mary Evans, R.D., L.D., nutrition education specialist (retired), St. Paul Hospital, Dallas, Texas (diabetes mellitus); Joice Carter, M.S., R.D., L.D., Nutritionist, Mental Health and Retardation, Texas Department of Health, Arlington (government aging programs).

Grace Burtis would especially like to extend appreciation to Carol Bianchi, her steadfastly optimistic secretary, who continued to meet deadlines in spite of personal sacrifices. In addition, Laurie Miller and Kelly Steele are valued friends who kept her in touch with the current world.

Judi Davis would like to thank those who helped in the final organization of the book and when the going got tough: Janet Iania, her friend, and her mother, Margaret B. Ratliff, and her mother-in-law, Frances M. Davis.

Objective critiques from reviewers are invaluable to a good publication. We do appreciate the insight, perspective, words of encouragement, and valuable ideas of the following reviewers: Dr. Lavon Bartel of the University of Vermont; Carol Broxson of the University of Albuquerque; Teresa Giglio of the Albert Einstein Medical Center, Philadelphia; Dale J. Gordon of the Northern Maine Vocational Technical Institute; Carolyn Holbrook of the Medical College of South Carolina; Janette Jackson of Easley, South Carolina; Edna M. Jones of the Florida Junior College at Jacksonville; Joyce K. Keithley of the Rush–Presbyterian–St. Luke's Medical Center, Chicago; Debra Kirsh of Edison, New Jersey; Dr. Elizabeth Kunkel of Clemson University; Mary D. Kupper of Toledo, Ohio; Arlene Leonhard-Spark of Demarest, New Jersey; Mary Lucius of Beaver Creek, Ohio; Virginia Martin of the University of Southwestern Louisiana; Elizabeth Pinar of Arvada, Colorado; Valerie Reid of Santa Rosa Junior College; Dr. Jane Ross of the University of Vermont; Sandra Rothstein of Broward Community College, Fort Lauderdale; Elizabeth Skaggs of Bluefield State College, Bluefield, West Virginia; and Rosalie Utley of the University of North Dakota.

We also wish to thank the many persons at W. B. Saunders Company who worked so tirelessly in the various phases of planning and producing this book. We are especially grateful to Michael Brown, Dave Prout, Fran Mues, Bonnie Berry, and Pat Morrison, who were all available to provide assistance and encouragement whenever it was needed.

ABOUT THE AUTHORS

GRACE BURTIS, PH.D., R.D., received her B.S. in Home Economics from the University of Texas at Austin, and her M.S. and Ph.D. in Nutrition from Texas Woman's University in Denton. She has taught in the field of nutrition, serving on the faculty at California State Polytechnic University, San Luis Obispo, Hartnell Junior College, Salinas, California, Seattle University, and Texas Christian University in Fort Worth. She has served as a consultant for nursing homes and restaurants and as Home Service Director for Houston Natural Gas Corporation.

JUDI RATLIFF DAVIS, M.S., R.D./L.D., received her B.S. from the University of Texas at Austin, her M.S. in nutrition from Texas Woman's University in Denton, and completed a dietetic internship at Indiana University Medical Center in Indianapolis. She has worked in the field of nutrition for 15 years, having served as therapeutic dietitian at Rex Hospital in Raleigh, North Carolina, and Baptist Memorial Hospital in San Antonio, Texas, and consulted for nursing homes and mental health facilities in western Virginia, San Antonio, and the Dallas–Fort Worth area. She has also worked as a nutrition consultant for The Greenhouse, a health spa in Arlington, Texas, and for The Sugar Association. She has taught various nutrition and food service courses at Tarrant County Junior College in Fort Worth, Texas.

SANDRA WEBSTER MARTIN, R.N., M.S.N., obtained her B.S. in nursing at Texas Woman's University in Denton and her M.S. in Nursing at the University of Utah. She has worked as staff nurse, assistant head nurse, and head nurse at Parkland Memorial Hospital, Dallas, and University of Utah Medical Center in Salt Lake City, Utah, and as infection control nurse at Veteran's Administration Hospital in Dayton, Ohio. She has taught nursing students at Brigham Young University in Provo, Utah, and Texas Woman's University in Denton. She is presently a nursing instructor (generalist in care of adult patients) at the Dallas Center of Texas Woman's University.

TABLE OF CONTENTS

16
Dietary Management of Infancy, Childhood, and Adolescence

17
Maturity in the Life Span

18
Ethnic and Religious Influences

NUTRITION FOR OPTIMUM HEALTH

The "CCC" Crew: Collaboration— Coordination— Cooperation

1

THE STUDENT WILL BE ABLE TO:

- *Associate total health care of an individual with the combined cooperation of many specialized groups.*
- *Recognize that effective nutritional intervention is dependent on nursing care as well as collaboration with dietitians and the food service department.*
- *Identify the roles of nurses and dietitians in nutritional care.*

OBJECTIVES

Diagnosis-related groups (DRGs)
Dietetic assistant (D.A.)
Health
Holism
Registered dietitian (R.D.)
Registered dietetic assistant (D.A.)
Registered dietetic technician (D.T.R.)

TERMS TO KNOW

Never before has a society had so much information at its disposal to assure optimum health and well-being. Unfortunately, the wonderful utopia of having your own family doctor who comes into the home and knows all about you and your family *and* everything regarding health is gone. The sense of security that was part of yesterday has been replaced with vast technological and scientific discoveries that perform what would have been unimagined miracles among our ancestors. This sophisticated era requires specialists instead of general practitioners and even experts among the specialists.

With this boundless depth in each area, the specialist truly has more than enough to keep up with in his/her own narrow limits. No wonder a team approach is desirable! A single person could not possibly master all the available information.

The Holistic Team

Webster's New World Dictionary defines holism or wholism as a doctrine that "an integrated whole has a reality independent of and greater than the sum of their parts." When holism is applied to health, a physical ailment not only affects a specific area of the body but has other physiological effects as well as psychological, spiritual, social, and economic effects that frequently also affect other persons (family members or friends).

Optimum health care goals can be achieved best by a multidisciplinary team that extends beyond the physician and nurse. This team often includes a dietitian (and/or dietetic technician or assistant), laboratory technician, pharmacist, physical therapist, social worker, psychologist, dentist, and counselor. The patient, who is the focus of the team endeavor, must be included as an active and participating team member. When all available team members are not used, the rate and degree of recovery are often penalized. As Seigel (1974) so adeptly states:

What makes this group of people working together a team is that each member *needs* the other professional expert to provide . . . services. Because of the complexity of patient's problems, no one person has all of the skills and knowledge to manage these problems.

A health care plan is developed emphasizing the total person. Associated problems accompanying the illness need to be treated also (Carson, 1978). This new holistic philosophy of medicine, as compared to former medical procedures, can be seen in Table 1–1.

Health is a state of complete physical, mental, and social well-being and not merely the absence of disease or infirmity.
    —*World Health Organization*

Team membership in health care may vary and involve both "core members" and "consultants." Only the members of the team having skills to deal with that patient's care are actively

---

Table 1–1. *Changing Paradigms of Medicine*

Former Patterns of Medicine	New Directions in Medicine
Treatment is for specific symptoms and diseases (for example, prescribing aspirin for a headache).	The cause and impact of the symptoms or a disease are determined (for example, teaching a patient to react differently to stress in order to control tension headaches).
Drugs and surgery are the main treatments.	Diet, exercise, and the patient's attitudes are combined with other forms of medical treatment.
Patients are dependent on the knowledge and authority of the professional.	Patients are therapeutic partners at liberty to make their own decisions regarding their lives.
Physiological and psychological needs are separate entities (for example, the physician refers a patient to a psychiatrist in order to treat a psychosomatic ailment).	Physical and mental needs are interrelated (for example, although a specific food is not a physiological requirement, unfulfilled personal needs may complicate the healing process).
Prevention is viewed as immunization or refraining from smoking.	Medical problems are prevented through physical, spiritual, and mental well-being.
The professional is always calm and emotionally neutral.	Caring and understanding by the professional is a component of healing.

Table 1–2. Teamwork and Nutrition

Professional or Specialist	Nutritional Input
Physician	Makes the diagnosis. Reviews laboratory results for decisions about medications, diets, and other treatments. Discusses disease changes and implications of lifestyle on food intake.
Nurse	Assists patient eating. Documents food and fluid intake. Reports new diets or diet changes promptly. Assesses status and monitors patient progress in physical condition and eating behavior. Projects a positive attitude to the patient and family about food and the dietary department. Teaches and reinforces diet therapy instructions from other team members.
Dietitian	Reviews chart for relevant information. Assesses nutritional status. Plans nutritional care. Counsels patient, family, and staff.
Pharmacist	Offers information regarding drug-food interactions. Checks contraindications of drug content with patient's condition, i.e., sodium content.
Physical therapist	Helps patient with eating handicaps. Teaches appropriate exercises to strengthen problem areas and to improve total health. May teach calorie expenditures and activity costs.
Social worker	Finds assistance for nutrition problems, such as food stamps and meals on wheels.
Psychologist	Helps patient in adjusting to frustrations affecting needed changes in lifestyle. Leads discussion with staff about their own problems related to case work.

involved. Core members provide health care services needed by most patients in that given situation and develop the closest ongoing relationship with the patient. Consultants are called in when problems arise requiring additional expertise.

In health care, the physician is generally considered a core member or even the team leader. However, s/he is usually trained to diagnose and treat, rather than to deal with patient management and health maintenance, and to respond to acute problems, rather than problems of a chronic or psychosocial nature (Mason, 1977). A nurse, also a core member, is sometimes the team leader.

Teamwork is a close, cooperative effort to optimize the members' special skills and knowledge so the patient's needs can be met more efficiently and competently than would be possible by independent and individual action. In order for everyone's expertise to be fully utilized, the role of each team member needs to be defined and clarified (Benford, 1981). Table 1–2 lists a few contributions of various team members.

Frequently, roles overlap, but each member can have a different input regarding a nutrition issue. Since nurses have historically assumed considerable responsibility for the nutritional care of clients, sometimes these roles need to be clarified and emphasis placed on "support" rather than "competition". Whenever a dietitian is a member

of the staff, s/he will share in the nutritional assessment and in determining patients' nutritional needs. However, clinical nutrition is now so complicated that no single professional can handle all its ramifications.

When facilities do not have a dietitian, a nurse shares the responsibility with a physician for meeting the patient's nutritional needs and teaching him/her about the diet (Roe, 1979). S/He should be knowledgeable in basic nutrition but wise enough to know when the expertise of a consultant dietitian is needed.

Team members support one another not just to ask for help from others but to offer their advice and expertise. They must respect and understand each other's roles, abilities, and responsibilities. Teamwork relieves each individual from some of his/her responsibilities and stress.

The Patient

In a survey conducted by Lauer (1981), nurses were asked what they thought cancer patients were concerned about. Most replied, "Money to pay bills." In response to the same question, patients answered, "What can I expect? What is the exact stage of my illness? What can I do to help myself get well?"

The holistic health care team always includes the patient as an active member. This new sophisticated team helps patients see how they can advance their own cure. The most positive effect of this is that patients appreciate this and are more cooperative. Active participation can bring self-confidence. Energy and attention can go toward the positive roles of assisting this medical team.

Illness is not an end in itself but a creative opportunity for patients to learn more about themselves and their fundamental beliefs. In other words, clients can be helped to grow through a seeming tragic loss of role, self-esteem, body image, and/or body function.

Most patients fail to utilize all the possible types of self-help because they frequently do not know about them (Dodd, 1982). Alternative remedies, such as relaxation or stress control and exercise, can play significant roles in recovery (Cassileth, 1982). The holistic health care team cooperates and collaborates with patients to encourage them to assume increasing responsibility for their choices and to devise new approaches to health (Blattner, 1981).

DRGs and the Team

With the advent of diagnosis-related groups (DRGs) and less money available for health care costs, significant changes are occurring aimed at increasing the productivity of human and other resources and evaluating the usefulness of services provided. Health care is being challenged to make decisions on how to control costs while providing high-quality care within the new payment rates. The high cost of labor is being scrutinized, and any services not proven essential to better patient care are being eliminated. Currently, detailed criteria for nutritional care and food service (as well as all other disciplines for care) are being developed for each DRG. With the enactment of these defined standards, each institution needs to delegate which team members can best handle the tasks without overlapping duties.

The DRGs re-emphasize the necessity of efficient teamwork with each individual functioning at peak performance level, delegating as much work as possible to support personnel. The level of coordination among the disciplines may reflect

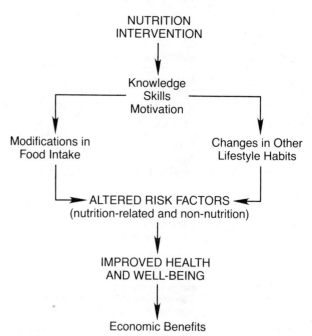

Figure 1–1. *Nutritional intervention. (Adapted from Mutch P: Cost-benefit and cost-effectiveness in dietetics. Presented to the Fort Worth Dietetic Association, 1984.)*

the quality of care provided. The involvement of all team members, including the patient, is necessary in order to control costs and decrease the length of stay in the hospital. Nutrition intervention can have economic benefits for the individual as well as the institution (Fig. 1–1).

The Nurse's Role

The nursing process is used to determine what the nurse can and should be doing for the client and the effects of those actions; it can also be used to determine areas where other team members are needed or can be helpful in the client's overall care. The nursing process provides nurses an orderly, systematic, and scientifically based approach to patient care. The process is analogous to a scientific or problem-solving process. Unlike these methods, it cannot be accomplished in a vacuum; its goal is to help the patient/client meet his/her biopsychosocial needs. By following this process, nurses can demonstrate accountability and evaluate the care they are providing (Fig. 1–2).

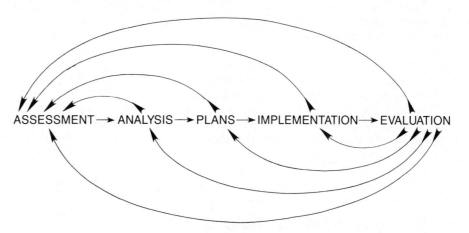

Figure 1–2. Throughout the nursing process, the patient is continually assessed. Each step is always re-evaluated. The process is homogenized; the steps are organized. (Adapted by permission from Griffith-Kenney, Janet W.; Christensen, Paula J., editors: Nursing Process: Application of Theories, Frameworks, and Models, 2nd ed. St. Louis, The C.V. Mosby Co, 1982. Developed by P. J. Christensen.)

ASSESSMENT → ANALYSIS → PLANS → IMPLEMENTATION → EVALUATION

Assessment. Although assessment is the first phase, it is continuous throughout the nursing process. Accurate assessment of clients leads to appropriate identification of their health status. During the data-gathering phase, information concerning the client's current nutritional status, interaction with others, health history, and environment are collected by the nurse. To be able to gather pertinent data about the client, the nurse must have a strong knowledge base reflecting information from different disciplines.

The nurse must be prepared to interact with clients in order to obtain subjective as well as objective data, which are gathered by observing the client and making specific measurements. Because the client's health is constantly changing, the subjective and objective data must reflect these changes.

As data are gathered and compared to accepted norms, relationships among the bits of information can be determined. Similarities in the data collected are noted and clustered to form patterns. The accuracy of the data gathering, in large part, determines the appropriateness of the total care plan.

Analysis. The analysis phase has three components: (1) interpretation of data, (2) identification of client needs, and (3) selection of the goals of care. Interpreting the pattern of these cues yields a nursing diagnosis. The American Nurses' Association defines a nursing diagnosis as a description of an actual or potential health problem that the nurse is educationally and legally capable of treating. Nursing diagnoses are composed of two components, the response statement and its inferred cause. The two components are joined by the expression "related to," for example, weight loss related to anorexia or obesity related to imbalance of intake versus activity expenditure. The

nursing diagnosis forms the basis for the design of the next three steps. Through the use of nursing diagnosis, nurses have a common language that can improve the quality of care.

Plans. Once the diagnosis has been established, client goals are then developed. Goals determine the direction for the alleviation or elimination of the response. These are broadly stated and reflect what the patient's condition or behavior will be at the outcome of nursing care. Achievement of these goals is dependent on the client's cooperation and must be developed collaboratively.

When the goal statements are in place, specific client behaviors, known as objectives, are then delineated. The objectives must be achievable by the client and should include time limits and a degree of accuracy; they should also be criterion-referenced.

In the planning phase, the nurse develops the strategies to achieve the objectives. Nursing interventions or actions are outlined to achieve the objectives and to eliminate the cause (the etiological statement). The actions of the nurse are not limited to direct care of the client, but also include collaboration and coordination with other team members.

Implementation. Implementation of the plan is the initiation and completion of actions necessary to accomplish the defined goals. The nurse is involved in the actual performance of the activities of daily living to assure the client's comfort and to maintain optimal functioning. S/He counsels clients about their health status and the correct principles, procedures, and techniques of health care. Nurses also monitor the work of staff members for whom they are responsible.

Evaluation. The fifth step of the nursing process is evaluation. In this step, the nurse determines the extent to which the goals of care have been achieved. S/He must recognize the effects of the measures used and the need to modify or change the goals established for client care. S/He must judge the accuracy of the implementation of measures and determine if a change in the environment, equipment, or procedure is necessary. The nurse must measure the impact of the goals by the degree of understanding the client has of the information or care given.

Role of Nutrition in Team Care

Nutrition can also be used as a self-help alternative measure for the patient. Foods can be chosen to help protect the body's immune system and to provide the energy and vitality for a high degree of wellness.

Diet is not always the cause or the only answer for an illness, but used in conjunction with other treatments, it may:
• Lessen the severity of symptoms.
• Decrease the need for medication.
• Delay the progression of disease.
• Increase stamina.
• Improve outlook.
Supplying nutritional needs is an essential part of providing total patient care.

Today, dietitians are the experts specifically trained in the role of nutrition and diet therapy, but they cannot do the job alone. A registered dietitian (R.D.) is best qualified to interpret nutritional information. An R.D. is registered with the American Dietetic Association (ADA) after completing at least four years of specialized academic study at an accredited college or university. Candidates must have some form of supervised work experience program (frequently called an internship) before taking an exam for initial qualification. Like other health professionals, dietitians must participate in continuing education to remain qualified. Education in the biological sciences, food science, behavioral sciences, and management systems is necessary to understand the relationship between food elements and the body's physical needs and why people choose the foods they habitually eat.

The dietitian can be supported or assisted by qualified paraprofessionals, such as a registered dietetic technician (D.T.R.) or dietetic assistant (D.A.). A D.T.R. has completed one of two ADA-approved associate degree programs in either nutrition care or food service management. The two-year program requires coordination of academic instruction along with clinical experiences. The D.T.R. in nutrition care is technically skilled to function as an assistant to the dietitian, while the D.T.R. in food service management can assume the role of technical assistant to the food service director. Dietetic technicians in nutrition care are often delegated the task of following patients on regular, soft, and liquid diets, while an R.D. provides nutrition services to patients on more complicated diets or patients with eating or feeding problems.

The D.A. performs assigned tasks in supervising food service, working under the guidance of a registered dietitian or a dietetic technician. A high school diploma or equivalent and the successful completion of a dietetic assistant program approved by the ADA are required. Normal and therapeutic diets as well as management and food preparation are surveyed in the programmed instruction.

The nurse's assistance to the dietitian is invaluable. The nurse, who has more "hands-on" time with patients than anyone else involved in their care, observes their physical and mental condition, listens to their problems, and fills most of their needs. Nurses are in a unique position to observe food intake, assess nutritional status, evaluate the response and attitudes of the patient to diet therapy and support the dietary teaching and regimen ordered for the patient. By communicating relevant information in the patient's chart, both the physician and dietitian will be aware of potential problems (Fig. 1–3).

Early recognition and referral of nutrition problems by the nurse may enhance the overall quality and scope of nutritional services. Subjective and objective data demonstrate nutritional status as well as medical status. A working knowledge of the relationships between diseases and dietary treatment helps the nurse in the prevention and treatment of disease. A basic knowledge of nutrition enables the nurse to make sound assessments and to know when to make appropriate referrals. The nurse is in a pivotal position.

Although the dietetic profession was developed in response to proliferation of nutritional knowledge and in order to relieve nurses of some of these duties, roles sometimes overlap. For instance, much of the data compiled for determining health status is the same as that necessary for nutritional assessments. By adding a few questions to the health workup form, nutritional status can be assessed, either by the nurse, dietitian, or

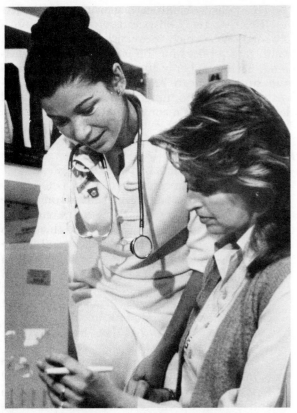

Figure 1–3. Charting is a good way of communicating pertinent information about the patient with other team members. (Courtesy of University of Arkansas Medical Sciences, Department of Nursing and Campus Media Services, Little Rock, Ark.)

• Understand the purpose of the diet and basic principles of modified diets.
• Be ready to informally discuss the diet with the patient when questions are asked.
• Praise and encourage patients to help them accept the food, even if it is not appetizing to you.
• Feed or assist the patient with foods, as necessary.
• Note what foods are disliked as well as favored and any eating difficulties. Relating this information both verbally and by charting is of vital importance.
• When food is not eaten, offer substitutions and notify the nutrition leader of the problems.
• Chart food intake with exact descriptions of food and beverages (also output, if requested), medications taken with food, and condition of the patient. In some cases, particularly diabetes mellitus, accurate charting is essential to prevent fatal consequences.
• Dietitians may also make notations in the patient's chart in order to communicate vital information with other team members. Do not neglect to read and communicate this information to all staff involved in the patient's dietary needs.
• The most effective preventive nutrition care is offered by health professionals with the most frequent contact with the public.
• Dietary instructions should be given to patients in easy-to-understand terms with admonitions of dangers if they are not followed.

dietetic technician. While some professionals feel nurses have no responsibilities regarding nutrition, delegation, teamwork, and collaborative relationships are key factors in this cost-control era. Some ways nurses can work cooperatively with the dietitian or dietary technician for the patient's benefit are cited in the following clinical implications.

Clinical Implications

• Health professionals with positive attitudes toward nutrition and diet are more likely to motivate patients to change or improve their eating habits.
• Be aware of the problems in the patient's home situation that may affect his/her adherence to the diet.
• Effective communication skills, such as active listening and observing, are essential to understand the patients' attitudes to the diet and their dietary needs. Report these findings to the team nutrition leader.

Teamwork with the Dietary Department

Problems encountered between departments can place the nurse in a difficult position between the patient and the dietary personnel. For organizational and cost-effectiveness, departments have policies and procedures to cover the needs of that institution most of the time. However, when working with different individuals and various situations, exceptions frequently arise. How well a department is able to adapt depends on a cooperative working relationship with other departments.

Frequent meetings between department heads to discuss and resolve problems can foster more understanding and awareness of each other's problems. Situations sometimes warrant exceptions to the rules, and occasionally policies need to be changed. Members of different staffs should become acquainted to enhance cooperation through better understanding of each other's policies.

Patients enter an institution unaware of its policies. Sometimes patients make demands without knowing that their requests are unusual. Explaining the situation may sometimes appease them. If possible, an employee from the dietary department can talk with patients and try to satisfy their needs. On the other hand, patients now are looking at the cost of their care and frequently feel that they should be entitled to whatever they want whenever they desire.

Summary

A holistic health care approach offers rewarding challenges to professionals and patients alike. A successful holistic health care team can accomplish many things.
- Learn what each member can do to assist the others.
- Share pertinent information with others through charting, talking, exchanging reports, and articles.
- Offer expertise when appropriate. Do not be embarrassed to ask questions of other professionals. The reassuring part of being a team member is that no one is supposed to know everything, and everyone can share what s/he does know.
- Meet together often to evaluate past results and plan future directions.
- For maximum results, call in others (maybe family, friends, trained volunteers, or other professionals such as a speech therapist) when trouble arises to strengthen the united approach.
- Clearly define roles for each staff person specifying what and how much is expected of him/her.
- Solicit the client to participate as a valuable member of this team.
- Be open-minded to alternative health care measures that support the orthodox medical program. At the same time, recognize and evaluate fraudulent and harmful procedures.
- Be sure each team member contributes and that one person does not try to do it all.
- Keep in mind the total well-being of the patient as well as the specific disease or illness presently being treated.

This holistic health care team might be called the "CCC" Crew (Collaboration—Coordination—Cooperation), which provides the ultimate in health care services for the patient's optimal well-being. Each member of the crew is essential. Optimum nutritional care requires that the dietary department, dietitians, nurses, and physicians work closely together on a continuing basis.

Review Questions

1. Mr. Evans, a cancer patient, was NPO (nothing by mouth) on Wednesday evening for tests on Thursday morning. After the tests, he had radiation treatment and was returned to his room at 11:15 AM. He states, "I really don't feel like eating much, but maybe a poached egg, grits, toast, and coffee would taste good." You know how important it is that he eat something, so you go ahead and call the dietary department.

   Dietary Policy: No hot breakfasts are served after 10:30 AM.

   Dietary Department Problem: The kitchen is in full swing loading lunch carts with cold foods; chefs are busy with lunch preparation and setting up cafeteria tray line when the nurse calls insisting on a hot breakfast for Mr. Evans.

   How should the situation be handled?
2. Sandra, a sickly child all her life, is in the hospital for surgery. Because of her health, her mother has catered to the child's demands in an effort to get her to eat. At home, she has been eating hamburgers, hot dogs, and french fries. In the hospital she refuses to eat, saying she doesn't like the foods. When you try to help her fill out her menu, she tells you she will eat a hamburger, french fries, and corn. None of these items is on the menu.

   Dietary Department Problem: Institutions buy foods packed in large quantities (A No. 10 can contains 25 servings; a package of frozen vegetables serves about 12). Small containers are not purchased because of their higher cost and the amount of storage space available. Whose problem is this? How should it be handled?
3. What suggestions can you offer to assure the patient's acceptance of food?
4. Name the main roles for each of these professionals that relate to food and nutrition: physician, nurse, pharmacist, dietitian, social worker, and counselor.

5. How could each of these people relate to the other team members to achieve an holistic program?
6. What are some questions the physician could ask each of the team members? What information can s/he give them to assure that they can perform their parts well?
7. What factors sometimes make it difficult for a nurse to cooperate with each of these fellow workers?
8. Why should the nurse know what diet the patient is receiving?
9. Why should nurses be informed about the types of food on a certain diet?
10. List five ways in which diet may affect a patient's well-being.
11. List some observations for the nurse to chart about food intake. Who will find this information particularly helpful?
12. Read over the policies and procedures for the dietary department in your hospital. If you do not understand why some are necessary, ask the dietitian. (The whys are usually not stated.)

Case Study: In 1976, Nadia Comaneci became the first woman in the history of Olympic gymnastics to make a perfect score, winning one bronze and three gold medals. When she came to the United States in 1979 to compete in the World Gymnastics Championships, everyone expected a brilliant and winning performance by Nadia. But after a couple of competitive performances, she was hospitalized with what was called a minor infection on her hand. In order for the Romanians to win, Nadia's participation was desperately needed. Healing did not take place as expected because Nadia's antibodies did not come to her defense as doctors anticipated. Upon further exploration, the *Fort Worth Star Telegram* (December 10, 1979) learned that Nadia had been eating only one full meal every two days and snacking on fruits and one or two vegetables in between in order to lose a few unwanted pounds.

With all the expertise it took to get her in this world-renowned position, was it possible that the Romanians didn't recognize the need for proper nutrition? Where was the breakdown? The entourage traveling with the gymnasts included not only coaches, but also a nutrition-doctor. But in this "team effort," the coaches and doctor were not always working as a team or concerned about the overall health of the gymnasts. The nutrition-doctor knew how the gymnasts should eat, but the coaches were concerned with body weight, long hours of practices, and quality workouts (which

meant no heavy foods during these times). Hence, Nadia got by with eating lightly and pleasing the coaches. Her body became so depleted that it was unable to fight off a simple infection. The malnourished body is susceptible to many infections because the immune defense system and the antibody response are decreased.

What could this team have done to work together better to assure Nadia's optimum health and brilliant performance?

REFERENCE LIST

Benford, RJ: Found: the key to excellent performance. *Personnel* 58(May–June):68, 1981.

Blattner, B: *Holistic Nursing.* Englewood Cliffs, NJ, Prentice-Hall, Inc, 1981.

Carson, JAS: Nutrition in a team approach to rehabilitation of the patient with cancer. *J Am Diet Assoc* 72(4):407, 1978.

Cassileth, BR: After laetril, what? *N Engl J Med* 306(24):1482, 1982.

Dodd, MJ: Assessing patient self-care for side effects of cancer chemotherapy. Part I. *Cancer Nurs* 5(6):447, 1982.

Lauer, P; Murphy, SP; Powers, M: Learning needs of cancer patients: a comparison of nurse and patient perceptions. *Nurs Res* 31(1):11, 1981.

Mason, M; Wenberg, BG; Welsch, PK: *The Dynamics of Clinical Dietetics.* New York, John Wiley & Sons, 1977.

Roe, D: *Clinical Nutrition for the Health Scientist.* Boca Raton, FL, CRC Press, 1979.

Seigel, B: Organization of the primary care team. *Ped Clin North Am* 21(2):341, 1974.

Further Study

Brill, NI: *Working with People; The Helping Process,* 3rd ed. White Plains, NY, Longman, Inc, 1984.

Carpenito, LJ: Diagnosing nutrition problems. *Am J Nurs* 85(5):584, 1985.

Gillick, MR: Common-sense models of health and disease. *N Engl J Med* 313(11):700, 1985.

Grimaldi, PL: Looking closely at nutritional assessment . . . Medicare payments. *Nurs Manage* 15(8):20, 1984.

Hoke, JL: Charting for dollars. *Am J Nurs* 85(6):658, 1985.

Hoppe, MC: Grow professionally in a growing field as a nutritional support nurse. *Nursing* 11(5):108, 1981.

Kast, FE; Rosenzweig, JE: General systems theory: Applications for organization and management. *J Nurs Adm* 11(7):32, 1981.

Korczowski, MM; Coevern, SV: Strengthen the nurse's role in nutritional counseling. *Nurs Health Care* 2(4):210, 1981.

Langford, TL: Collaborative relationships. In *Managing and Being Managed.* Englewood Cliffs, NJ, Prentice-Hall, Inc, 1981, p. 94.

McElroy, AM: Burnout—a review of the literature with application to cancer nursing. *Cancer Nurs* 5(3):211, 1982.

Morris, E: How does a nurse teach nutrition to patients? *Am J Nurs* 60(1):67, 1960.

Nugent, P: Management and modes of thought. *J. Nurs Adm* 12(2):19, 1982.

The World of Nutrition

2

THE STUDENT WILL BE ABLE TO:

- **Recognize and use nutritional terms.**
- **Identify the appearance and characteristics of well-nourished individuals.**
- **Point out why health quackery can be dangerous.**
- **Identify common themes of health quackery and why they are contrary to scientific information.**
- **Analyze health information for its scientific validity.**

OBJECTIVES

Appetite
Diet
Diet therapy
Dietary deficiency
Food
Food fad
Food quackery
Health foods
Hunger
Iatrogenic
Joule
Kilocalorie
Malnutrition
Natural food
Nutrients
Nutrition
Nutritional care
Nutritional deficiency
Nutritional status
Nutritionist
Organic

TERMS TO KNOW

For most of us, eating is not a difficult endeavor. Nutrition, on the other hand, involves the integration of physiological and biochemical reactions within the body as well as psychological and social factors that enter into the frequent decisions concerning food choices. The frequent use of chemical terms when nutrition is discussed prevents some individuals from learning more about the subject. Yet, we are constantly surrounded by chemistry. If you have ever made a cake, what happened if you left out the sucrose (sugar), the sodium bicarbonate and sodium aluminum sulfate (baking powder), or the sodium chloride (salt)? Mixing chemical ingredients in the recipe was not scary because of familiarity with the terminology, even though specific functions for each of the "chemicals" in the cake were unknown.

Basic Definitions

In this text, biochemical terms are used and explained so that the student gains a more thorough understanding of nutrition. It is not necessary that you be able to write any chemical formulas. The following words and their definitions are basic to your understanding of this subject.

Nutrition. Nutrition is the process by which living things utilize food for energy, growth and development, and maintenance. This includes eating foods to provide nutrients (1) necessary for body functions that cannot be synthesized and (2) utilized by the body to make essential compounds. Nutrition involves not only digesting food to make nutrients available but also absorbing and delivering nutrients to the cells where they are utilized and eliminating waste products.

Nutrients. Biochemical substances, or nutrients, are used by the body and must be supplied in adequate amounts from foods consumed. The six classes of nutrients obtained from foods are (1) water, (2) proteins, (3) carbohydrates, (4) fats, (5) minerals, and (6) vitamins.

Food. Food is any substance taken into the body to provide nutrients. All foods differ in the amount of nutrients they furnish. No single food contains all the essential nutrients in the amounts needed for optimum health. Any individual food can be compatible with good nutrition, provided "one knows the needs of the body, the composition of foods, and the appropriate role of foods in supporting life within the context of the total diet" (Deutsch, 1976).

Kilocalorie. The potential energy value of foods and the energy exchanges within the body are expressed in terms of the kilocalorie, which is a measurement of heat. A kilocalorie (kcal) is the amount of heat required to raise the temperature of 1 kg water 1°C. While a kilocalorie is the proper terminology and is being used more frequently, it has formerly been used interchangeably with Calorie or large calorie (abbreviated Cal). One kilocalorie is 1000 times larger than the small calorie (abbreviated cal) used in chemistry and physics.

Joule. The joule (J)—named for James P. Joule (1818–1889), an English physicist, who discovered the first law of thermodynamics—is the unit of energy used in the metric system and also for expressing energy values in nutrition. During this transition time of converting to the metric system, both the kcal and J are used. The following equivalents can be helpful:

$$1 \text{ kilocalorie} = 4.184 \text{ kilojoules (kJ)}$$

$$1 \text{ megajoule (MJ)} = 1000 \text{ kJ}$$

$$2500 \text{ kcal} = 10,450 \text{ kJ}$$

Nutritional Status. An individual's nutritional status is the condition of health as determined by the nutrients the body receives and utilizes. Food choices are critical in determining nutritional status. Table 2–1 notes clinical physiological characteristics of good and poor nutritional status. Although these signs take into consideration the total individual, most factors are subjective. None of these individual nutrition indicators can be used as the sole determinant of a person's status. Each of these signs should be scrutinized closely and correlated with information from a health history and examination, a dietary history, biochemical analysis (blood and urine tests), and anthropometric assessments (measurements of size, weight, and proportions of the human body). All of these together comprise a nutritional analysis or assessment, which is used to identify persons whose nutritional status could be improved.

The problem with most of these characteristics is that the signs are fairly vague, and when they do appear, they are not always the result of faulty eating habits but could be related to lack of sleep, heredity, or other non-nutritional factors. In today's society, clear-cut deficiency diseases are rare, and it is almost impossible for the average American to spot anything wrong with his nutritional status by physical appearance other than body weight and fat. However, since the state of health is affected by what a person eats, an evaluation of nutritional status is essential (Margen, 1979).

Table 2–1. *Physical Signs of a Normal Appearance or Suggestive of Malnutrition**

Body Area	Normal Appearance	Signs Associated with Malnutrition
Hair	Shiny; firm; not easily plucked.	Lack of natural shine; hair dull and dry; thin and sparse; hair fine, silky and straight; color changes (flag sign); can be easily plucked.
Face	Skin color uniform; smooth, pink, healthy appearance; not swollen.	Skin color loss (depigmentation); skin dark over cheeks and under eyes (malar and supra-orbital pigmentation); lumpiness or flakiness of skin of nose and mouth; swollen face; enlarged parotid glands; scaling of skin around nostrils (nasolabial seborrhea).
Eyes	Bright, clear, shiny; no sores at corners of eyelids; membranes a healthy pink and are moist. No prominent blood vessels or mound of tissue or sclera.	Eye membranes are pale (pale conjunctivae); redness of membranes (conjunctival injection); Bitot's spots; redness and fissuring of eyelid corners (angular palpebritis); dryness of eye membranes (conjunctival xerosis); cornea has dull appearance (corneal xerosis); cornea is soft (keratomalacia); scar on cornea; ring of fine blood vessels around corner (circumcorneal injection).
Lips	Smooth; not chapped or swollen.	Redness and swelling of mouth or lips (cheilosis); especially at corners of mouth (angular fissures and scars).
Tongue	Deep red in appearance; not swollen or smooth.	Swelling; scarlet and raw tongue; magenta (purplish color) of tongue; smooth tongue; swollen sores; hyperemic and hypertrophic papillae; and atrophic papillae.
Teeth	No cavities; no pain; bright.	May be missing or erupting abnormally; gray or black spots (fluorosis); cavities (caries).
Gums	Healthy; red; do not bleed; not swollen.	"Spongy" and bleed easily; recession of gums.
Glands	Face not swollen.	Thyroid enlargement (front of neck); parotid enlargement (cheeks become swollen).
Skin	No signs of rashes, swellings, dark or light spots.	Dryness of skin (xerosis); sandpaper feel of skin (follicular hyperkeratosis); flakiness of skin; skin swollen and dark; red swollen pigmentation of exposed areas (pellagrous dermatosis); excessive lightness or darkness of skin (dyspigmentation); black and blue marks due to skin bleeding (petechiae); lack of fat under skin.
Nails	Firm, pink.	Nails are spoon-shape (koilonychia); brittle, ridged nails.
Muscular and skeletal systems	Good muscle tone; some fat under skin; can walk or run without pain.	Muscles have "wasted" appearance; baby's skull bones are thin and soft (craniotabes); round swelling of front and side of head (frontal and parietal bossing); swelling of ends of bones (epiphyseal enlargement); small bumps on both sides of chest wall (on ribs)—beading of ribs; baby's soft spot on head does not harden at proper time (persistently open anterior fontanelle); knock-knees or bow-legs; bleeding into muscle (musculoskeletal hemorrhages); person cannot get up or walk properly.
Internal Systems:		
Cardiovascular	Normal heart rate and rhythm; no murmurs or abnormal rhythms; normal blood pressure for age.	Rapid heart rate (above 100, tachycardia); enlarged heart; abnormal rhythm; elevated blood pressure.
Gastrointestinal	No palpable organs or masses (in children, however, liver edge may be palpable).	Liver enlargement; enlargement of spleen (usually indicates other associated diseases).
Nervous	Psychological stability; normal reflexes.	Mental irritability and confusion; burning and tingling of hands and feet (paresthesia); loss of position and vibratory sense; weakness and tenderness of muscles (may result in inability to walk); decrease and loss of ankle and knee reflexes.

*From Christakis, G: *Nutrition Assessment in Health Programs.* Washington, DC, American Public Health Association, 1973.

Nutritional Deficiency. Deficiency symptoms appear to be caused by the lack of adequate amounts of an essential nutrient to support body functions. The person simply becomes sick for lack of an essential chemical. Inadequacies occur when the intake of nutrients is decreased by poor food choices, inadequate quantities of food eaten, or nutrients lost during processing, marketing, and storage of foods. Inadequate amounts are provided as a result of increased needs that could be attributed to healthy conditions (pregnancy, lactation, and growth periods); conditions in which metabolism is increased (fevers, injury, or surgery); decreased absorption (caused by vomiting and diarrhea or by intake of mineral oil); nutrient destruction or binding in the body; drug therapy that interferes with absorption or metabolism; and antibiotic therapy that alters the microorganisms of the intestinal tract so that essential vitamins are not synthesized.

Malnutrition. Malnutrition is faulty nourishment due to a deficiency, imbalance, or excess of nutrition. Nutritional deficiencies can be a deficit of energy and/or nutrients. Overnutrition is an excess of one or more nutrients (usually calories). Malnutrition can be present despite excessive nutrient and/or excessive caloric intake.

Diet. The kinds and amounts of foods and beverages available to and regularly chosen by an individual is his/her diet. Each person's diet is different because it has been influenced by his/her own opinions of food, family, customs, social patterns as well as physiological differences, emotions, and religious and cultural beliefs and patterns.

Dietary Deficiency. When an individual's diet does not supply the recommended amount of a nutrient, a dietary deficiency exists. This failure is not necessarily great enough to cause illness; the body may still be receiving enough of the nutrient to function, although not at optimum levels.

Diet Therapy. A diet prescription or diet therapy involves implementing a diet different from the person's normal way of eating. It may require certain foods in specific quantities at precise times.

Nutritional Care. Scientific knowledge used to help people choose foods that are nourishing to their body is nutritional care.

Hunger. Hunger is a physiologic need to provide the body with food. Weakness and the pain of starvation occur when hunger persists. Hunger may have a psychological impact interfering with that person's concentration on anything other than the need for food.

Appetite. The desire to eat is the individual's appetite. Since it is related to pleasurable sensations, appetite may function long after physiological need is met. Appetite is generally affected by cultural influences and meal habits.

Basic Concepts of Nutrition

1. The term "nutrition" applies to foods chosen, eaten, and utilized by the body.
2. Human beings require essential nutrients for each biochemical function. Nutrients are most effective physiologically when teamed with other nutrients. Many cannot be used unless the right combinations are present.
3. The nutrients necessary for life, growth, and health can be provided by foods. Note that the requirement is for nutrients, not for specific foods. However, people eat foods, and nutrient requirements and information must be interpreted into the "food" language people understand. The nutrients from food vary in usefulness, safety of use, and economy. Realistically, *no individual food is essential nor is any particular diet superior for everyone.*
4. The same kinds of nutrients are needed throughout life; only the amounts of nutrients change. The amount needed varies among individuals and at different ages throughout a person's life. These requirements change according to how well our bodies make use of the foods eaten and according to different stages of growth and development, sex, body size, weight, physical activity, and state of health.
5. The way food is handled affects the amounts of nutrients in the food as well as its safety, appearance, taste, and cost. This includes everything that happens to the food during growth, processing, storage, and preparation.
6. The body can convert some nutrients into other nutrients in order to meet its physiological needs. Because of the functional interrelationships of nutrients, study of their concerted actions as well as their individual actions is necessary (Callaway, 1981).
7. Nonessential nutrients can be utilized by the body, but are either not required or can be synthesized in adequate quantities from dietary precursors (Callaway, 1981). One such example is cholesterol.
8. Other than water, the nutrient of highest priority to the body is energy, which must be supplied from exogenous sources such as carbohydrates, fats, proteins, and alcohol or can be supplied in limited quantities from stores of these substances within the body (Callaway, 1981).
9. The human body has adaptive mechanisms that allow the individual to tolerate modest ranges in nutrient intakes. For instance, a decreased caloric intake is frequently accompanied by a decreased metabolic rate. Human life is astonishingly flexible. It can flourish on diets extremely high in fat (such as the Eskimo diet) to those very high in carbohydrates (such as Oriental diets) and from health food to fast food diets. It is the whole balance of the diet that matters, and the best balance incorporates a wide variety of foods.
10. The nutritive value of any specific food is relative—not absolute—and depends upon: (1) the content and amount of nutrients in the food the body can use, (2) the content and bi-

oavailability of nutrients in other foods in the individual's diet, and (3) the nutrient requirements for that individual. Thus, a specific food cannot be classified as "good" or "bad," but must be evaluated as part of total intake and requirements.

11. Increasing the variety of foods in the diet reduces the probability of developing isolated nutrient deficiencies, isolated nutrient excesses, and toxicity due to non-nutritive components or contaminants in any particular food (Callaway, 1981).

12. When the intake of any single nutrient is changed, the amounts of other nutrients in the diet are also altered. For instance, since red meats and eggs are excellent sources of iron, if cholesterol intake is decreased by less intake of these foods, the dietary intake of iron is usually decreased (Callaway, 1981).

13. In addition to the physical requirements met by food intake (already discussed), food meets many psychological needs, including personal, social, and cultural needs. For instance, a favorite food may not provide any specific physiological requirement, but if it is withheld, actual physical illness may result.

The premise of the science of nutrition is that, in any cultural circumstance or for any personal taste or preference, good nutrition is possible. The basis of nutrition is both individualized and generalized. It is in some ways always unique and in other ways always the same.

Food Fads and Misinformation

Nutrition is a very popular subject to the American public, but even with all the current knowledge, it is no easier to educate the public today than it was 50 years ago:

> More food notions flourish in the United States than in any other civilized country on earth, and most of them are wrong. They thrive in the minds of the same people who talk about their operations; and like all mythology, they are a blend of fear, coincidence, and advertising.
>
> *(Anonymous, 1938).*

Currently, nutrition is the biggest drawing card on the newsstands and, by some estimates, even more popular than sex (Deutsch, 1976). While the public is more food conscious, nutritional knowledge has shown little improvement. As the public's interest in nutrition increases, the myths surrounding nutrition continue to confuse, resulting in deteriorating eating habits. Purveyors of nutritional misinformation capitalize on people's fears and hopes by exaggeration and oversimplification through the health virtues or curative properties of foods. Too few people understand the effects of various nutrients upon the body and how the body uses these nutrients, thereby opening the door to food faddism or nutrition quackery.

Food fad is a catchall term covering all aspects of nutritional nonsense, characterized by exaggerated beliefs about the value of nutrition in health and disease. Food fads, like clothing fashions, are popular products or notions that many people follow enthusiastically for short periods. A food fad may be based upon a food fact or fallacy. People often begin a diet or believe claims for specific foods or supplements on the basis of something they read or hear without investigating its validity or effectiveness. Unfortunately, unscrupulous advertisers use the ignorance of the public and play on their fears to sell their products, sometimes distorting the truth.

While some fads are physically harmless, they may create an economic hardship for people of limited income because the foods or supplements may be expensive. Still others are nutritionally inadequate and could lead to serious deficiencies. A fad is frequently harmful because a person substitutes this therapy for the advice of a physician, thereby delaying medical treatment. As Jarvis (1984) states, "As important as nutrition is, it is never as important as the faddist claims."

Food superstitions, or irrational beliefs that have no scientific basis, are also common. An example of a food superstition is the belief that eating strawberries during pregnancy will give the infant a birthmark. Children tend to accept their parents' beliefs, which develop into established patterns that are very difficult to change in later years. Teenagers are most susceptible to food fads because of peer pressure. In order to be accepted socially, food choices are influenced by the current beliefs of the peer group.

Food quackery is the promotion of nutrition-related products or services having questionable safety and/or effectiveness for the claims made. These claims or promises may be due to ignorance, delusion, misconception, or intent to deceive.

The unknowns of medicine and disagreement among reputable scientists regarding interpretation of research findings foster nutritional misinformation. Magical solutions appeal to the anti-establishment, seekers of miracles and super-health, worriers, fashion followers, and those who distrust the medical profession. Given the right circumstances, such as confronting a chronic or incurable disease, potentially everyone is capable of exchanging sound judgment and common sense for miraculous cures. In this text, most chapters contain some fallacies and facts pertinent to the subject.

• FALLACIES and FACTS

Several prevalent themes are promoted by food quacks and should be discussed. Fake nutrition specialists may appear legitimate by their imposing titles, "advanced" degrees, and membership in organizations that allow anyone to join, regardless of qualifications (Herbert, 1981). Terms are frequently used to imply a meaning different from the officially accepted one, thus misleading individuals (Price, 1980).

FALLACY: Many arguments are presented about the need for dietary supplements.

• FACT: Certain disease states do create a need for supplementation, but a physician should diagnose these diseases through standard laboratory and clinical procedures and give supplements as indicated by standard medical protocols.

FALLACY: Food quacks claim that the modern doctor doesn't want patients to be healthy or that "doctors don't know any nutrition" (Herbert, 1981) in order to undermine faith in the physician.

• FACT: Although many medical schools do not offer specific courses in nutrition, more and more medical schools are including some nutrition curriculum (Dunfy & Bratton, 1980; Gallagher & Vivian, 1979). On the other hand, physicians have been well-trained in biochemistry and physiology and the role of nutrients in the body. In many medical schools, education stops short of interpreting this knowledge into food language, (or which foods contain specific nutrients), teaching basic nutritional concepts, and understanding how the body handles foods that are changed into nutrients in the digestive process (Stare, 1980).

Doctors have been swamped curing illnesses; thus, little time was allocated for teaching preventive health concepts. Preventive medicine to keep people well is a relatively new specialization. Due to the vast amount of information regarding total health care for which they are responsible, the complementary services of well-informed dietitians and nurses are usually welcomed.

FALLACY: The food quack often claims that produce grown in heavily fertilized soil lacks nutrients found in produce grown without the use of chemical fertilizers, or organically grown produce.

• FACT: "Organic," according to Webster's New Collegiate Dictionary, means "relating to, or dealt with by a branch of chemistry concerned with the carbon compounds of living beings and most other carbon compounds." All foods are organic because they are composed of organic compounds containing carbon. There is no advantage to eating an organic nutrient from one source as opposed to another, but fringe benefits may result from eating that nutrient in a natural food as opposed to a purified nutrient preparation.

Organically grown foods are allegedly grown without synthetic pesticides or fertilizers and processed without chemicals or additives. Once these organically grown foods are removed from the field, they cannot be identified from commercially fertilized plants (Barrett, 1980; Cornacchia & Barrett, 1980). "Plant roots absorb nutrients only in their inorganic form, regardless of whether the source is from manure, compost, or manufactured fertilizer. There is no scientific basis for claiming organic foods are more nutritious than conventional foods" (Stephenson, 1978). For instance, if there is enough usable phosphate in the soil for the plant to grow, it does. If phosphate is lacking, the plant will either not grow at all or not produce enough fruit for a good crop.

The mineral composition of a plant can be positively affected by fertilizer. For instance, iodine is a nutrient the plant will incorporate into its structure if present in the soil, but it can also grow well without it. If a soil is deficient in any mineral nutrient, the manure from animals fed plants from that soil will also be deficient in that nutrient. Soil analysis can determine what is missing so it can be included in the fertilization process (Barrett, 1980). Actually, "natural" foods contain pesticide residues just as often as conventional foods, but these residues in both cases are within federal tolerance levels (Stephenson, 1978).

FALLACY: *Food quacks also claim that today's foods are processed to the degree that all the nutrients are removed.*

• **FACT:** *"Natural" foods are understood by the scientific community to be produced with minimal processing and do not contain preservatives, additives, and other artificial ingredients (Cornacchia & Barrett, 1980). Food processing does not necessarily mean deterioration of quality (see Chapter 14).*

FALLACY: *The food faddist also presents specific foods as "miracle" or "health" foods.*

• **FACT:** *Magic foods are just as real as the pot of gold at the end of the rainbow. People who believe that they can live to be 100 if they ingest some expensive concoction probably also believe in the pot of gold. The fact is that thousands of delicious and wholesome foods are available, but there is no one magic or perfect food.*

Evaluating Health Foods. Usually all health, organic, and natural food products cost the consumer more than conventional foods. A survey conducted by the USDA indicated that organic foods cost approximately 1 1/2 times as much as regular foods (Cromwell, 1976). The price for comparable foods (sometimes even the same food) is normally the cheapest from the regular supermarket shelf, increasing somewhat in the health food section of the supermarket, and highest at the health food store (Lekon & Kris-Etherton, 1981; Stephenson, 1978).

Products sold both in health food and grocery stores labeled as health foods imply that all other foods are unhealthy, or are not as beneficial to health. A study of health food stores conducted by the New York City Department of Consumer Affairs concluded "no demonstrable health benefits are to be accrued from the consumption of 'health' instead of conventional foods" (Guordine et al, 1983). Despite many studies and reputable scientists who draw the same conclusion, health food sales continue to soar with astonishing predictions for growth (Fig. 2–1). Only by having a basic knowledge of nutritional concepts can health professionals be prepared to teach individuals the facts and thereby counteract this upward trend in health food sales.

The health food market is also attractive to supermarkets for several reasons: (1) It has a rapid growth rate, (2) the type of person who shops in health food stores generally has a higher income than other supermarket shoppers, and (3) higher gross profits accompany these specialty foods (Ruderman, 1982). The markup on health foods is 30 percent compared to 18 percent on regular supermarket items (Price, 1985). It is predicted that by 1990, "nutrition centers" will be located in 13,400 supermarkets (Sandlin, 1982).

How do quack health promoters get away with their lies and fake products? Strict laws protect consumers against false advertising and mislabeling as outlined in Table 2–2; but the health food rip-off is still big and dangerous business.

As active and conscientious as the government is in locating, pursuing, and cracking down on health swindlers, most of the enforcing agencies don't always have the staff or resources needed to handle all of the cases reported, let alone to find out about those products and ads not reported.
(USDHHS et al, 1980)

The First Amendment to the U.S. Constitution protects free speech and a free press; this also protects a person's right to dispense false, misleading, or deceptive health claims. If a food product makes false or misleading claims on the label, the Food and Drug Administration (FDA) can take action because of mislabeling. Until recently, manufacturers were only allowed to make nutritional claims on labels, such as "good source of vitamin C." Claims that the product might prevent, treat, or cure a disease were prohibited on the grounds that it was being marketed as an "unapproved drug," not as food. Within the past few years, a cereal manufacturer has challenged the FDA with advertisements stating that bran may prevent certain cancers. As a result, the FDA is expected to issue new guidelines soon to describe the conditions for similar health claims.

The Federal Trade Commission can take ac-

Table 2–2. Federal Laws to Protect Consumers

Laws	Enforcing Agency
Federal Food, Drug, and Cosmetic Act (1938)	Food and Drug Administration (FDA)
Truth in Advertising Act (1938)	Federal Trade Commission (FTC)
Mail Fraud and False Representation Statutes (1948)	U.S. Postal Service

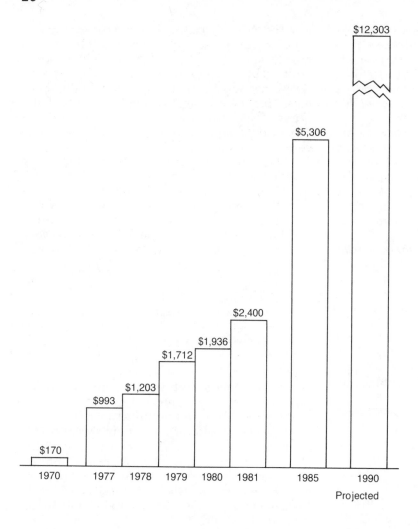

Figure 2–1. Trends in health food sales (in millions of dollars). (Data from Business Trend Analysts, Inc: Forecasts from Futures ... A Strategy Service 11(16), August 15, 1982, by permission.)

tion if false claims are made in advertising, so claims made on labels or in promotions are not usually false. Products can be legally promoted in books and magazine articles and on radio and television talk shows. Thus, these indirect promotions receive the protection of the First Amendment (Stephenson, 1978).

Evaluating Food Quackery. Evaluating nutritional information for quackery can be a tedious chore. One should begin by checking a person's credentials. Legitimate persons are usually affiliated with an established scientific facility and association. The information should be based on scientifically well-designed studies, preferably controlled, double-blind studies with a substantial number of subjects. Well-documented information usually has been reported in scientific journals. One should check that the substance being promoted has been proven safe and effective in the amounts prescribed by reviewing research studies. The questions in the *Focus on Scrutinizing*

Fraudulent Information can help to evaluate information for quackery. If the answer to several of these questions is yes, stop and investigate.

Evaluating Scientific Information. In addition to evaluating information for its nutritional validity, even scientific data needs evaluation before recommendations are made based on the conclusions. Both the strengths and weaknesses of the study design should be considered. A scientific study incorporates certain information that should be evaluated for its relevancy to the acceptance of the hypothesis. For instance, a study may not have used enough subjects to be indicative of the general population; the subjects may have cheated on the diet and not reported this; or the effects of nutrients in the body may differ when subjects are active or under stress, as compared to individuals maintained in a metabolic research unit. *Focus on Scrutinizing Scientific Research Information* will help one evaluate research studies with an intelligent skepticism.

FOCUS ON SCRUTINIZING FRAUDULENT INFORMATION

- Is the information based mainly on testimonials and case histories?
- Is the medical profession or a government agency prosecuting him/her because it does not accept the superior discovery?
- Are the claims extravagant or emotionally appealing, such as promises of youth, beauty, glamour, long life, or cure of disease?
- Are most diseases caused by a bad or faulty diet?
- Is there danger of being poisoned by food additives and preservatives?
- Are "natural" vitamins better than "synthetic" ones?
- Will the cure be quick, dramatic, or miraculous?
- Is the product good for a wide variety of ailments?
- Is the product or service being offered a "secret remedy" or a "recent discovery" not available from other resources?
- Is the remedy being sold door to door, by a self-styled "health advisor" or promoted by public lecture series or in a popular magazine?
- Are self-diagnosis and treatment being promoted?
- Is the claimant a credentialed member of a reputable organization such as the AMA?
- Is the claimant well trained but promoting something outside his/her realm of expertise?

The Role of Health Professionals. What role can the nurse play in combating nutrition fads and misinformation? Natalie Van Cleve stated in 1938 when times were different, but widespread misinformation on diet was just as prevalent as today:

> It is the duty of all professions active in the field of food and nutrition to cooperate in clarifying any misconceptions of the laity. "If the nurse does not know her vitamins, the patient will find a radio announcer who does."

The nurse is in a unique position to understand the causes of food faddism and to recognize their dangers. Understanding people and their love of "miracle" answers should help in recognizing the appeal of such misinformation. Secondly, a scientific background permits assessment of the potential effects of the uselessness of food

FOCUS ON SCRUTINIZING SCIENTIFIC RESEARCH INFORMATION

A well-written research paper probably contains reliable information of scientific value if the author has:
- Summarized and referenced other studies on the subject.
- Stated the hypothesis and purpose.
- Clearly outlined and described the procedures used.
- Presented data in a clear, concise, and systematic format.
- Provided tables and figures to show results.
- Discussed relationship of data to that done by others along with reasons for discrepancies.
- Supported conclusions by the results presented.

Some questions that the reader must consider in order to evaluate a study's relevancy include:
- Was it based on human or animal studies?
- Was this an appropriate sampling of the population?
- How many subjects were involved?
- Was there a control to determine effects of the change?
- How many factors in the study were changed, altered, or affected?
- Did the change affect anything else in the lifestyle that may have affected the outcome?
- Can the outcome of this study be duplicated by others?
- Is the length of time for the study long enough to allow the body to adapt to the change (as has been found with triglycerides)?

faddism. Nurses can provide patients with a clear understanding of the true essence of nutritional science—the process of nourishing or being nourished—rather than the polypharmacy of supernutrition and organic foods.

Doctors, nurses, and even dietitians have sometimes promoted nutritional misinformation by failing to apply their knowledge, from a lack of understanding of how the nutrients are utilized, or in search of fame and fortune.

Clinical Implications:

- Be aware that some health-trained colleagues have given and dispensed misinformation themselves.

- Speak out to protect the public from misinformation.
- Investigate the legitimacy of questionable information.
- Pay attention to your own nutrition habits.
- Know basic nutrition concepts and keep abreast of research so you can give patients positive advice based on a broad knowledge and understanding.
- Cultivate a professional relationship with one or more qualified dietitians or nutritionists to help you find valid reference books and answers to questionable ideas.
- Remember that health science is based on the axiom that no proposal or remedy is safe until demonstrated to be safe, nor is it effective unless demonstrated to be so.

Reliable Nutrition Expertise

Where should a nurse go for help to evaluate a nutritional claim? Many health organizations are available to help in scientifically looking at the information; some are listed in Appendix E-1 & E-2. Frequently, a physician may be able to help evaluate the information. Local universities or hospitals have dietary personnel (who should be team members) to either assist or refer one to the nearest group of dietitians. Food and nutrition computerized data bases monitor the literature on the subject and condense it into abstracts. Table 2–3 lists some resources for different types of food and nutrition questions.

The title **nutritionist** may or may not imply adequate training in the subject. If the nutritionist is also a registered dietitian, a professional credential is established. Sometimes, qualified dietitians, such as extension nutritionists and other nutrition majors with a master's or doctoral degree from an accredited school, may call themselves nutritionists, especially when their roles are related to teaching and research instead of the active participation of food service and diet therapy. However, in most states, anyone can identify himself or herself as a nutritionist because there is no accrediting agency to maintain standards. Therefore, many fraudulent people, with no formal training in health or nutrition will call themselves a nutritionist due to their interest in foods and health.

Summary

Nutrition not only involves eating but also includes why people make food choices, what happens to those foods in the body, and how the food affects a person's state of health. Certain basic concepts are fundamental to learning, understanding, and evaluating nutritional information. Misinformation regarding nutrition is abundant. There is an overwhelming amount of interest in the subject. Many persons are looking for an easy cure-all; many are looking for an easy buck. When the two meet, it is open season for nutrition quackery. Health professionals are qualified to fight this ever-increasing problem by using their scientific background to explain the foolishness of it all.

Review Questions

1. Compile a list of characteristics that describes a person who is in good nutritional status. How do you measure up to this?
2. Is there a problem of malnutrition in your community? What factors contribute to this problem?
3. How does nutritional status fit into a nursing assessment?
4. In your own words, define nutrition. Compare food and nutrition.

Table 2–3. Reliable Nutrition Resource Guide

Type of Information	Title	Resource
General food–nutrition question	Registered dietitian, nutritionist, home economist	Hospital; local or state health department; extension service of a land-grant university
More technical questions	Professor, registered dietitian	Nutrition or home economics department of a university or college
Questions on food preparation and preservation	Home economist	USDA-County Cooperative Extension Service; gas or electric company
Special diets	Registered dietitian	Hospital; local or state public health departments; volunteer health organization (e.g., a diabetes association)

5. How do diet and nutrition differ?
6. What physical criteria could a school nurse use in evaluating children who may need to be referred to a physician?
7. Discuss why persons in allied health professions should know the basic concepts of nutrition.
8. Compare the cost of three foods from a health food store with the cost of similar items in a supermarket. Which is more economical?
9. Find an advertisement in a popular magazine or newspaper for a health food product and list the merits of the product stated in the ad. Then list information about the product that might have been omitted or should be questioned.
10. What food superstitions are prevalent in your community? Do they result in any dietary problems?
11. According to an old saying, "Some people live to eat; others eat to live." Which statement identifies hunger? Appetite?

Case Study: As a nurse in an outpatient clinic, a slightly overweight lady comes in and is diagnosed with hypertension. She works as a maid for a lady who has told her that she must take large doses of natural vitamins and that, to control her blood pressure, she should be buying her food and vitamins at the health food store. Since you know she is having some financial problems in purchasing enough food for her family of six, how would you counsel her?

REFERENCE LIST

Anonymous, cited by Wilder, RM: Fads, fancies, and fallacies in adult diets. *Sigma Xi Q* 26:73, 1938.
Barrett, S: The genuine fakes. In *The Health Robbers,* 2nd ed. Edited by S Barrett and C Knight. Philadelphia, George F Stickley, 1980, p 231.
Callaway, CW: Bridging the gaps in human nutrition. *Nutr News* 44(4):5, 1981.
Cornacchia, HJ; Barrett, S: *Consumer Health. A Guide to Intelligent Decisions,* 2nd ed. St. Louis, C. V. Mosby Co, 1980, p 189.
Cromwell, C: Organic foods—an update. *Fam Econ Rev Summer* 1976, p 8.
Deutsch, RM: *Realities of Nutrition.* Palo Alto, CA, Bull Publishing Co, 1976.
Dunphy, MK; Bratton, B: Effective nutrition education program for medical students. *J Am Diet Assoc* 76(4):372, 1980.
Gallagher, CR; Vivian, VM: Nutrition concepts essential in the education of the medical student. *Am J Clin Nutr* 32(6):1330, 1979.
Guordine, SP; Traiger, WW; Cohen, DS: Health food stores investigation. *J Am Diet Assoc* 83(3):285, 1983.
Herbert, V: Will questionable nutrition overwhelm nutrition science? *Am J Clin Nutr* 34(12):2848, 1981.
Jarvis, WT: Combatting food faddism. *J Can Diet Assn* 45(3):202, 1984.

Lekon, BM; Kris-Etherton, PM: Meal cost analysis: health food store versus conventional food sources. *J Am Diet Assoc* 79(4):457, 1981.
Margen, S: Evaluation of nutritional status in the outpatient setting. *Med Clin North Am* 63(5):1095, 1979.
Price, CC: Natural foods. *Nat Food Rev* 11(summer):9, 1980.
Price, CC: Eating "natural" gains popularity. *Nat Food Rev* 28:14, 1985.
Ruderman, E: Focus on the food markets—health food labels. Cornell Univ Coop Ext, May 17, 1982.
Sandlin, S: Nutrient center gains tied to image and variety. *Supermarket News* May 17, 1982, p 46.
Stare, FJ: Nutrition—sense and nonsense. *Postgrad Med* 67(2):147, 1980.
Stephenson, M: The confusing world of health foods. *FDA Consumer* 12(6):18, 1978.
U.S. Department of Health and Human Services (USHHS); Public Health Service; Food and Drug Administration: *The Big Quack Attack: Medical Devices.* HHS Pub No. (FDA) 80-4022, January 1980.
Van Cleve, N: Food: facts, fad, and fancy. *Am J Nurs* 38(3):285, 1938.

Further Study

American Dietetic Association: Position paper on food and nutrition misinformation on selected topics. *J Am Diet Assoc* 66(3):277, 1975.
Barrett, S; Knight, G, (eds): *The Health Robbers,* 2nd ed. Philadelphia, George F. Stickley, 1980.
Council on Scientific Affairs: American Medical Association concepts of nutrition and health. *JAMA* 242(21):2335, 1979. *Consumer Reports:* 50(5):275, 276, 280, 282, 1985.
Cowart, V: Keeping foods safe and labels honest. *JAMA* 254(16):2228, 1985.
Editors of Consumer Reports: It's Natural! It's Organic! Or is it? *Cons Reports* 45(7):410, 1980.
Editors of Consumer Reports Books: *Health Quackery.* New York, Holt, Rinehart, and Winston, 1980.
Feldman EB; Kuske, TT: Food fads: in pursuit of the impossible dream. *Consultant* 22(6):262, 1982.
Grivetti, LE: Food fact, food myth—the scientific dilemma. *Food Tech* 38(8):14, 1984.
Guthrie, HA: "There's no such thing as junk food" . . . there are junk diets. *Health* 14(6):42, 1982.
Harper, AE: Science and the consumer. *J Nutr Ed* 11(4):171, 1979.
Herbert, V; Jarvis, WT; Monaco, GP: Obstacles to nutrition education. *Health Values* 7(2):38, 1983.
Herbert, V: Will questionable nutrition overwhelm nutrition science? *Am J Clin Nutr* 34(12):2848, 1981.
Herbert, V: Nutrition cultism. *West J Med* 135(3):252, 1981.
Herbert, V; Barrett, S: *Vitamins and "Health" Foods: The Great American Hustler.* Philadelphia, George F. Stickley, 1981.
Metress, SP: Food fads and the elderly. *J Nurs Care* 13(10):12, 1980.
Miller, RW: Critiquing quack ads. *FDA Consumer* 19(2):10, 1985.
National Dairy Council: Nutrition misinformation. *Dairy Council Digest* 52 (July–August), 1981.
Rynearson, EH: Americans love hogwash. *Nutr Reviews* 32(suppl):1, 1974.
Thompson, R: The sad allure of cancer quackery. *FDA Consumer* 19(4):36, 1985.
White PL; Selvey, N: Nutrition and the new health awareness. *JAMA* 247(21):2914, 1982.
Young, JH; Still, RS: Nutrition quackery: Upholding the right to criticize. *Food Tech* 35(12):42, 1981.

Food—The Magic Key

3

THE STUDENT WILL BE ABLE TO:

- **List the general physiological functions of the six nutrient classifications of foods.**
- **Name the basic food groups.**
- **Correctly categorize foods into the basic food groups.**
- **State the number of servings needed from each of the food groups.**
- **Identify significant nutrient contributions of each food group.**
- **Discuss factors that influence food habits.**
- **Assess dietary intake of an individual, using the basic food groups.**
- **Explain the different purposes of the RDA, basic food groups, and the U.S. RDA.**

Accessory foods
Calorie-dense
Enrichment
Essential foods
Fortified
Nutrient density
Recommended dietary allowances (RDAs)
U.S. recommended daily allowances (U.S. RDAs)

OBJECTIVES

TERMS TO KNOW

Foods are eaten for a variety of purposes. Not only is there a physiological purpose for eating, but food choices are influenced by one's tastes, budget, and cultural attitudes. Food grouping systems are used to translate technical nutritional needs into practical guidelines for food selections. Selecting a diet that provides physiological needs has enjoyable and healthful advantages. Guidelines that facilitate this process include the recommended dietary allowances, basic food groups, and nutrient labeling. Freedom of choice and variety in consumption are important components of individual and social life. In understanding why people choose the foods they eat, a knowledge of all these factors is necessary to appreciate others' food habits.

Physiological Functions of Nutrients

Physiologically, foods eaten are used for energy, building all tissues, and obtaining or producing numerous regulatory substances. The nutrients from food are divided into six major classes: carbohydrates, proteins, fats, vitamins, minerals, and water. Table 3–1 shows basic functions of the major nutrients; however, nutrients function interdependently, interacting in complex metabolic reactions, so the absence of adequate amounts of one nutrient can prevent the use of another even though it is present. Excesses of a nutrient can also interfere with other nutrients present.

Table 3–1. General Functions of Nutrient Classes

Physiological Function	Nutrients
Furnish energy	Carbohydrates Fats Proteins
Build and maintain body tissues	Proteins Minerals Water
Regulate body processes	Proteins Minerals Vitamins Water

Dietary Evaluations

Evaluations of dietary intake determine if adequate amounts of all required nutrients are being supplied by food intake. This is an important aspect of nutritional assessment; nevertheless, it is no easy task. Knowledge of an individual's ordinary food intake is a starting point for recommending changes. Diets are commonly evaluated by one of two guides: (1) recommended dietary allowances (RDAs), which assess nutrient intake, and (2) basic food groups, which categorize foods by nutrient content.

Recommended Dietary Allowances (RDAs)

RDAs identify nutritional needs in terms of specific amounts of nutrients that a healthy individual should receive every day to achieve his/her full growth and health potential (NRC, 1980). They are intended to be desirable daily amounts of nutrients to be consumed by groups of healthy people. A few points should be remembered about RDAs.

1. They are for healthy persons only; medical problems alter nutrient needs.
2. These are recommendations for optimal health, not minimum requirements to avoid deficiency symptoms. Healthy individuals often differ widely from one another in their nutrient requirements because of variations in body build, genetic makeup, etc. RDAs are set higher than the average known requirements (except the energy requirement), thereby allowing a margin of safety. Energy intake (or kilocalories) must match energy requirements within narrow limits, or undesirable changes in weight may result. As knowledge of toxicity and nutrient interactions have increased, many RDAs have been reduced.
3. RDAs are published by the government but are established by competent scientists and nutritionists who base their recommendations on evidence from epidemiological, physiological, clinical, and biochemical studies to insure optimal physiological functioning. RDAs are up-

dated about every five years, incorporating current scientific studies.

4. RDAs do not list all essential nutrients. Specifically, water, carbohydrates, essential fatty acids, and many trace elements are not included in the table. For example, the 1980 RDAs estimate "ranges" of safe and adequate daily intakes of three vitamins and nine minerals because of the limited amount of data available on which to base allowances. The assumption is that a varied diet providing recommended amounts of the listed nutrients will also furnish sufficient amounts of the omitted nutrients.

5. RDAs are used as a guide to (a) assess nutritional quality of diets, (b) evaluate the adequacy of food supplies in meeting nutritional needs of population groups, (c) establish standards for public assistance programs, (d) develop new food products, (e) establish guidelines for nutritional labeling of foods, and (f) develop nutritional education programs.

The proposed changes for the revised 1985 edition were rejected by the Food and Nutrition Board of the National Academy of Sciences. One reason given for the rejection was the alteration in the basic concepts of the RDAs. The RDA revisions committee, headed by Henry Kamin, Ph.D., felt that the intent of the RDAs—"to cover the nutritional needs of nearly all healthy people"— promised too much. A new definition was proposed: "to protect practically all healthy persons against nutritional deficiencies." According to this new concept, the RDAs for several of the nutrients decreased substantially. While the RDA levels for vitamins A, C, and B_6 and the minerals magnesium, iron, and zinc were all reduced, only the proposed levels for vitamins A and C met with opposition. (The proposed level for calcium for women was increased by 25 percent.)

Critics felt the changes would result in reductions in government-funded programs that are based on the RDAs (school lunches, food stamps, and institutional standards). So, even though the appointed committee thoroughly and objectively researched the scientific literature and made their recommendations, the 1980 RDAs are still in effect until a new committee is formed and can evaluate the new research.

To determine the nutritional quality of a diet (using the RDAs as a guideline), one must find the nutrient content of food (see Appendix A-1) and then tally the amount of individual nutrients for each item consumed during a 24-hour period. Totals are then compared to the RDAs for that particular person's age and sex, with adjustments being made for diverse weights and heights.

A diet that fails to meet the allowances could be adequate for a particular individual. Some people habitually consume less than the recommended allowances but still have an adequate diet, simply because the allowances are higher than the minimum requirements. The nutritional status of an individual cannot be evaluated from food intake records alone. These records are used to identify potential dietary problems or to confirm possible causes of problems detected during clinical and biochemical evaluations.

Unfortunately, there are no sure guidelines for establishing at what point diets become inadequate. The government generally considers a diet that provides two thirds of the RDAs adequate, whereas less than that is considered poor (Allen & Gadson, 1984). Dr. Guthrie (1985) states that a diet providing 100% of the RDAs would meet the needs of 97% of the U.S. population; at 90% of the RDAs, 66% of the population's needs would be met; and at 77% of the RDAs, 50% of the population's needs would be met.

Basic Food Groups

The basic food groups translate the recommended allowances for specific nutrients into a simple guide for meeting multiple nutrient needs by selecting from four basic categories of food. This guide can be adapted and modified imaginatively to meet the needs of individuals and families with different levels of income, cultural patterns, and lifestyles. Broad families of foods with similar kinds of nutrients are grouped together. The number of recommended servings differs according to the nutritional needs for various age groups and stages of life. Figure 3–1 shows approximate percentages of nutrients contributed by each of the essential food groups toward meeting the RDAs.

Four kinds of foods are considered basic to meeting nutritional needs: (1) milk and milk products, (2) meat or meat equivalents, (3) fruits and vegetables, and (4) grain (breads and cereals). These four food groups make specific nutrient contributions to the diet (Fig. 3–2). Other foods that contain mostly fats, sugars, unenriched or re-

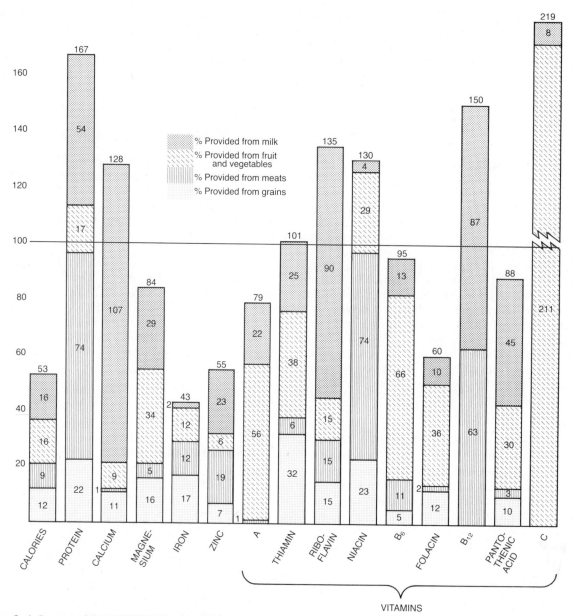

Figure 3–1. Percent of the 1980 RDA for an adult female contributed by meeting the basic food groups with the following foods: 2 oz. roast beef, 2 oz. tuna fish, 1½ cups 2% milk, 1 cup low-fat plain yogurt, 2 slices whole wheat bread, 2 slices enriched bread, 4 oz. orange juice, ½ cup broccoli, 1 medium banana, 1 medium baked potato. (Nutritive values and calculations from Nutritionist II software, Silverton, OR.)

fined cereal product, or alcohol have recently been introduced as a fifth group by the USDA; however, this has not been widely accepted.

Highlights of the daily food groups include:
- The groups are not applicable for infant feeding.
- The first four groups contain "essential" foods; another category contains "accessory" foods.
- Each category includes a variety of foods that contribute important and similar nutrients.

- No single food group furnishes all the nutrients; at least one essential nutrient is lacking in each food group.
- Within each group, individual food items have a unique nutritional profile.
- Variety from each category helps assure a desirable intake of nutrients.

Fruit and Vegetable Group. While foods in this group are valuable for their contribution of

CHECKING FOR VARIETY

Vegetable and Fruit Group

Provides:
Vitamin A
Vitamin C
Folic acid

Number of servings daily:
4 or more

Serving Size: 1/2 cup or 1 medium-sized

Lettuce	Beets
Cucumber	Grapes
†Cabbage	*Pumpkin
Mushrooms	Pineapple
Celery	*Peaches
‡Peppers	†Honeydew melons
*†Greens (all types)	*Apricots
‡Cauliflower	‡Orange juice
Bean sprouts	Sweet corn
Green beans	‡Orange
Spinach	*Winter squash
†Asparagus	*Cantaloupe
†Lemons	Apples
Plums	Pears
‡Broccoli	Bananas
†Tomato	Prunes
*Carrots	*Potato
‡Brussels sprouts	*Sweet potato
*†Papayas	Raisins
‡Strawberries	†Avocado
	Canned fruit (in syrup)

*Vitamin A
†Good source of vitamin C
‡Excellent source of vitamin C

Meat Group

Provides:
Protein
Niacin
Thiamin
Iron
Zinc
Vitamin B₁₂

Number of servings daily:
2 or more

Serving Size	
2 oz.	Chicken
2 oz.	Lean beef
2 oz.	Fish
1 oz.	Turkey
2 oz.	Lean pork chop
2 oz.	Ham
2	Eggs
1 cup	Dry beans and peas
2 oz.	Pork
2 oz.	Refried beans
2	Hot dogs
4 Tbsp.	Peanut butter
½ cup	Nuts

Milk Group

Provides:
Calcium
Protein
Riboflavin
Vitamin B₆
Vitamin B₁₂

Number of servings daily:
Child, 2–9 yr	2–3
Child, 9–12 yr	3 or more
Teenager	4 or more
Adult	2 or more
Pregnant or lactating woman	4 or more

Serving Size	
1 cup	Nonfat milk
1 cup	Buttermilk
1 cup	Low-fat milk
1 cup	Plain yogurt
1 cup	Whole milk
1½ oz.	Processed cheese
1½ oz.	Cheddar cheese
1 cup	Fruit-flavored yogurt
1 cup	Custard
1 cup	Milkshake
2 cups	Low-fat cottage cheese
1 cup	Pudding
1¾ cups	Ice cream
2 cups	Cottage cheese

Bread and Cereal Group

Provides:
Thiamin
Niacin
Iron
Protein

Number of servings daily:
4 or more

Serving Size	
1 slice	Whole-wheat bread
1 slice	Rye bread
½ bun	Hamburger or hot dog bun
½ cup	Grits
1	Tortilla
1 slice	White bread
5	Crackers
½ cup	Cooked cereals
½ cup	Rice
½	Bagel
½ cup	Brown rice
1 cup	Dry cereal
½ cup	Macaroni
½ cup	Spaghetti
1	Pancake
1	Biscuit
1	Muffin
1	Cornbread
1 cup	Presweetened cereal

Figure 3–2. The four food groups and their principal nutrient contributions to the diet.

29

fiber, vitamin C, and vitamin A, individual foods vary widely in their vitamin C and A content. It is important to know these variations and to understand the possibilities for choice within the group. This makes it possible to incorporate more foods with a high nutrient value and avoid poor choices. Figure 3–2 lists foods considered excellent sources of vitamin C (one serving recommended daily) and foods considered good sources (requiring two servings daily). Fruits and vegetables containing significant quantities of vitamin A are also noted.

Dark green vegetables also contribute calcium, iron, magnesium, riboflavin, and folic acid. Because of their high water and high fiber content, most fruits and vegetables are relatively low in calories.

Highlights of the fruit and vegetable group include:
- Using a variety of fruits and vegetables, four servings daily are recommended.
- At least one excellent or two good sources of vitamin C should be eaten every day (see Fig. 3–2).
- One excellent source of vitamin A should also be consumed daily or at least every other day (see Fig. 3–2).
- Choose fresh unpeeled fruits and vegetables and those with edible seeds, such as berries, for fiber.
- Foods in this group are relatively low in calories and fat (except for olives and avocados); no fruit or vegetable contains cholesterol.
- This is the only food group that contributes vitamin C to the diet.
- Foods rich in vitamins A and C may help lower the risk for cancers of the larynx, esophagus, and lungs (CDNC, 1982). (See Chapter 25.)
- Cruciferous vegetables—cabbage, broccoli, Brussels sprouts, and cauliflower—may help reduce cancer susceptibility (CDNC, 1982).

Grain Group. Also called the bread and cereal group, these foods are a dependable source of the B vitamins, iron, carbohydrates, and fiber. They provide some protein and are the major source of protein in vegetarian diets. All grain products are included in this group whether they are made from whole, refined and enriched, or fortified grains.

Whole grains (such as oats, rye, wheat, and corn) have three parts: the germ, endosperm, and bran. Each part varies in its nutrient content. Refining grain removes the germ and bran that cause it to spoil; however, the milled product is not as nutritious. Table 3–2 compares the nutrient content of rye and whole wheat breads with that of enriched white bread.

Iron, thiamin, riboflavin, and niacin are restored in the enrichment process approximately to their original levels. This process is federally controlled by the FDA, which establishes the quantity of nutrients that can be added (Friend, 1972). Whole-grain products contribute more fiber, magnesium, and folacin than do the enriched products.

Most breakfast cereals are fortified at nutrient levels higher than those occurring naturally in the grain, and even include some vitamins normally not present in the grain. Fortification has no legal standards and means that one or more nutrients that were not in the food naturally have been added to the product. Fortification can become dangerously high with regard to vitamins A and D if individuals eat large amounts of fortified foods.

Highlights of the bread and cereal group include:
- Four servings daily are recommended.
- The group is an important source of B vitamins naturally and of iron through fortification.
- Foods in this group are relatively inexpensive.
- Whole grain products are good sources of fiber.

Milk Group. Milk and cheese products are frequently relied upon to provide the calcium re-

Table 3–2. Comparison of Nutrient Values of Selected Whole Grain and Enriched Products*

Type of Bread	Protein (g)	Total Dietary Fiber (g)	Thiamin (mg)	Riboflavin (mg)	Niacin (mg)	Vitamin B₆ (mg)	Folacin (mcg)	Pantothenic Acid (mg)	Iron (mg)	Zinc (mg)	Calcium (mg)	Phosphorus (mg)	Magnesium (mg)
Whole wheat (28 g)	3	8.50	0.09	0.03	0.8	0.050	16	0.19	0.8	0.476	24	71	14.75
Rye (25 g)	2	—†	0.07	0.05	0.7	0.025	6	0.11	0.5	0.318	19	37	10.5
Enriched white (28 g)	2	2.72	0.11	0.06	0.8	0.011	10	0.11	0.6	0.188	21	24	5.25

*Nutrient data from Nutritionist II software, Silverton, OR.
†Not available.

quirement, but they also contribute significantly to the protein, phosphorus, riboflavin, and vitamins A, B_6, and B_{12} content of the diet. Fortified milk products are important sources of vitamin D; however, many milk substitutes (cheese and yogurt) are not fortified with vitamin D (unless made with fortified milk).

The milk group excludes high-fat dairy products such as butter and cream because they are not high in calcium, riboflavin, and protein. There is a large variation in the amount of calcium provided by the dairy products. To assure calcium requirements, the serving size is dependent on the amount of calcium in the food, i.e., 1 cup milk, 2 cups cottage cheese, or 1¾ cup ice cream all contain approximately the same amount of calcium.

Highlights for the milk group:
- Serving recommendations for this group are based on calcium requirements for various stages of life (see Fig. 3–2).
- Use of low-fat milk products can decrease calorie content significantly.
- Milk products are poor sources of iron and vitamin C.

Meat Group. Meat, poultry, fish, and beans are excellent sources of protein, phosphorus, and vitamins B_6 and B_{12}. This group, unlike the milk group, is an important source of iron, but a poor source of calcium. Choices within this group should include a variety, since each food has distinct nutritional advantages. Various meat choices are outstanding for their individual contributions (Table 3–3).

The new meat substitutes, or textured vegetables protein (TVP), are included in this group, but do not contain vitamin B_{12} naturally, since they are not derived from animal sources. Cholesterol occurs naturally in all foods of animal origin.

Highlights of the meat group include:
- Two servings daily (2 oz. each) are recommended.

Table 3–3. *Outstanding Contributions of Various Protein Foods*

Protein Food	Nutrient
Lean red meats	Iron B vitamins Zinc
Pork	Thiamin
Liver and egg yolks	Vitamin A Iron
Dry peas and beans, soybeans, and nuts	Magnesium Fiber
Fish and poultry	Low in calories and fat

- A variety of foods from this group should be used.

Accessory Foods. These calorie-dense foods are high in fats, sugar, or alcohol, providing mainly calories and few other nutrients. They are sometimes referred to as "empty calories."

Accesory foods contribute to palatability and make some nutritious foods more desirable. For instance, some persons may dislike milk but enjoy pudding or custard.

Fats and oils, while supplying twice as many calories per ounce as protein, sugars, or starches, result in a prolonged feeling of satiety. Margarine and butter are good sources of vitamin A. Vegetable oils are good sources of vitamin E and essential fatty acids, which are needed in the diet. Alcoholic beverages, such as wine, beer, and liquor, and unenriched refined bakery products are in this group because they contribute calories and few nutrients.

In general, the amounts of these foods to include in the diet depends on the amount of energy needed. When only the specified amounts of foods from each of the first four food groups are consumed, the caloric intake ranges from about 1100 to 1500 kcal—far below the caloric needs of a teenager.

Foods in this group, such as sugars and margarine or other fats, can be considered accessory foods and are used to (1) provide additional energy, (2) improve appetite appeal, and (3) enhance flavor (and therefore can be used to increase overall nutrient intake).

Highlight of the accessory food group includes:
- These high-energy, low-nutrient foods are intended to complement, not replace, foods from the other groups.

Problems with the Food Groups. The basic food groups are a useful tool; however, they cannot be relied upon to do the whole job. They have been severely criticized because of several limitations.

1. An individual can follow the daily food group pattern and still have an inadequate intake of iron, folic acid, B_6, vitamin E, magnesium, zinc, and possibly fiber, depending on the foods selected in each group (Guthrie & Scheer, 1981; King et al, 1978).
2. The food groups do not include enough of the foods that people regularly eat. When food mixtures or combinations are used, such as chicken potpie or lasagna, it is difficult to use the groupings. Also, assessing new food products and classifying them is difficult in this system (Light & Cronin, 1981).

3. Since the emphasis is on including foods rather than limiting them, using the food groups for dieting encourages overeating.

Summation Highlights:

• Select foods from the first four essential food groups carefully.
• Count only full servings. (The lettuce on a hamburger is only a fraction of a full serving.)
• Choose more than the minimum number of servings of the first four groups, especially increasing the number of servings of legumes and nuts from the meat group to increase the amount of iron, zinc, and fiber.
• Incorporate variety in meals for food value and enjoyment.
• Choose foods with fewer calories from each group. Figure 3–2 lists foods in each essential food group by placing those with lower caloric content first, so that a "calorie conscious" person would profit by choosing foods from the early part of the list most frequently.
• Encourage consumption of foods high in nutrient density.

Nutrient Density

Foods eaten to satisfy energy requirements must also satisfy the individual's allowances for all other nutrients. Nutrient density is the ratio between the calorie content and the nutrient composition in a food. In other words, it is a tool for determining the nutrient quality of a food. When foods are chosen that yield a high nutritive value for the energy they contain, they are considered to be nutrient-dense with respect to those nutrients. This information can be used especially to alter food intake within each of the four food groups when moderation in consuming accessory foods fails to reduce energy intake to a desired level.

Another Guide: Nutrition Labeling

To help the consumer make informed decisions about food choices in the supermarket, the government created a standard guideline for nutritional information on food labels. Nutrition labels on product packaging are based on the percentage of the U.S. Recommended Daily Allowances (U.S. RDAs) for each nutrient. Protein, vitamins A and C, thiamin, riboflavin, niacin, calcium, and iron are listed most frequently. The amounts represent the nutrients furnished by one serving of the food as determined by the manufacturer. Figure 3–3 is a sample of the nutrition label form and explains the type information displayed.

The U.S. RDAs are different from the RDAs previously discussed and should not be confused with them. The RDA tables were simplified; most of the U.S. RDA amounts are the highest requirements of the nutrients for individuals above four years of age. There are actually four sets of U.S. RDAs, with sets designed for special foods for infants, children under four, and pregnant or lactating women (see Appendix B-3).

For most individuals, the U.S. RDAs are not a satisfactory guide for assessing nutrient intake because some nutrient amounts are very high, yet many nutrients are totally ignored. As can be seen from Table 3–4, the U.S. RDA is double the RDA for vitamin B_{12} for a female 19 to 22 years of age. If the consumer tries to achieve 100 percent of the U.S. RDA for this nutrient, s/he may feel the need to rely on supplements or highly fortified foods. Fresh foods (fruits, vegetables, and meats) are not usually labeled. However, the U.S. RDAs are a useful tool to compare nutrient values of foods and to learn valuable sources of nutrients.

Computerized Dietary Analysis

Computerized dietary analysis is becoming increasingly popular among health professionals and consumers. Because of the speed and ease of calculation, nutritional care can be more individualized.

Problems do, however, exist with these analyses and they should be used with discretion. While errors frequently found in hand calculations are eliminated, the data provided are no more accurate than the food intake list being analyzed (what and how much the person says was eaten versus the actual intake) or the food composition information contained in the data bank. Several studies analyzing identical diets reveal large discrepancies in the results obtained using

NUTRITION LABELING LETS YOU IN ON WHAT'S INSIDE

Want to know what nutrients are in the food you eat?

It's simple. Just read the label on food packages and cans now on your supermarket shelves.

The Food and Drug Administration has developed a new labeling program to help you identify the nutrient content of the foods you buy. All labels with nutrition information must follow the same format. Any food to which a nutrient is added, or which makes a nutritional claim, must have a nutrition label. Nutrition labeling for other foods is optional.

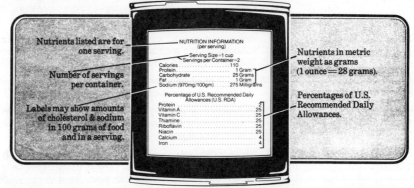

Figure 3–3. Explanation of nutritional information on food labels. (From U.S. Department of Health, Education, and Welfare, Public Health Service, Food and Drug Administration: Read the Label, Set a Better Table. DHEW Publication No. (FDA) 76-2049. Rockville, MD.)

The upper portion of the label shows you the number of calories in a serving of the food, and lists, in grams, the amount of protein, carbohydrate and fat. These are the three major nutrients that make up all the food we eat.

The lower portion of the label tells you the percentage of United States Recommended Daily Allowance (U.S. RDA) for protein and seven vitamins and minerals provided in one serving. Add percentages for each nutrient consumed throughout the day. When the daily total approaches 100, you are getting an ample supply of that nutrient.

The chart on the opposite side of this brochure shows what the U.S. RDA is for specific nutrients.

different software programs (Dwyer & Suitor, 1984; Adelman et al, 1983). Computers "know" only the information they have been given. If input information is incorrect, the computer cannot detect any errors, even large errors that may have been made by the programmer.

When the computer analysis determines an individual's intake of a nutrient to be low, a qualified person should investigate further to determine whether or not this is actually a problem. Proper interpretation of the findings is vitally important. For instance, a single day's diet can suggest a nutrient deficiency or excess, when this is not the person's habitual diet.

Some software programs have built-in standards for "satisfactory" intakes of some items, such as sugar or salt, for which no RDAs have been established. Instead, these items should be evaluated in the context of an individual's medical and physical condition. In summary, *computers cannot be used as substitutes for the human ability to think.*

Table 3–4. Comparison of the RDAs and the U.S. RDAs

Nutrients	U.S. RDA Adults and Children (over 4 yr old)	RDA Females (19–22 yr old)
Protein	45–65*	44 gm
Vitamin A	5000 IU	5000 IU
Vitamin C	60.0 mg	60.0 mg
Thiamin	1.1 mg	1.5 mg
Riboflavin	1.7 mg	1.3 mg
Niacin	20.0 mg	14.0 mg
Calcium	1.0 gm	800.0 mg
Iron	18.0 mg	18.0 mg
Vitamin B_6	2.0 mg	2.0 mg
Folic acid	0.4 mg	0.4 mg
Vitamin B_{12}	6.0 mcg	3.0 mcg

*45 gm if protein quality is equal to or greater than milk protein, or 65 gm if protein quality is less than milk protein.

Meal Planning

Use of the basic food groups facilitates meal planning and allows variations for individual preferences, cultural habits, and budgets. When planning a nutritionally balanced diet, several guidelines are important. A person should: (1) include recommended amounts of each of the basic food

Table 3–5. Guidelines for Meal Planning

Basic Considerations	Explanation
Food should be enjoyed.	Mealtimes should be pleasant and relaxed times. Eating is a social and psychological function as well as a physiological need. Taste preferences must be considered in addition to the ages of those eating. Relaxation aids digestion and improves the amount of nutrients absorbed.
Eat at least three meals a day.	Any menu pattern compatible with lifestyles and optimum performance of activities is acceptable, avoiding sluggishness from overeating or irritability caused by a lack of energy nutrients from the previous meal.
Breakfast is important.	Any nutritious food may be eaten. Food choices are limitless, but the biochemistry of the body and the mental and motor efficiency are all positively affected by the food intake at the first meal of the day.
Snacks do count.	Snacks can be important if they provide nutritious food absent from regular meals and if they do not result in overconsumption of calories.
Present attractive meals.	Appetite is affected by "eye appeal"; the colors of different foods in a meal should complement each other. (For example, spaghetti with tomato sauce, beets, and orange slices would not be appealing.)
Incorporate variety.	Variety stimulates appetites and helps improve food habits (Rolls, 1985). Combine foods of different textures (soft and crispy); different temperatures (some hot and some cold); contrasting flavors (sweet or sour, bland or spicy); different methods of food preparation (boiling, frying, using sauces, broiling); and different shapes or sizes. Do not repeat the same flavor in a meal (corn and cornbread).
Consider budget.	Family income and its size must be considered. Foods in season and those regionally available are usually less expensive and also have the highest nutrient content. Advertised specials can also save money. (See Chapter 14.)

groups, (2) utilize accessory foods to increase calories (if needed), and (3) consider foods or meals eaten outside the home. Some other important guidelines are listed in Table 3–5.

Clinical Implications:

- A flexible, sensitive attitude towards individual customs and practices is most effective in obtaining cooperation from patients or clients.
- If food habits of various cultures or socioeconomic groups are evaluated objectively, some of the practices will be determined to be beneficial and can be encouraged (see Chapter 18).

Health Application: Nutritional Counseling

The Counselor. Whereas in many situations, a dietitian or dietetic technician is available to offer nutritional counseling, in many outpatient and community clinical and home health care organizations, the nurse is given the responsibility of counseling clients regarding normal nutrition habits. Thorough knowledge of basic food and nutritional principles are prerequisites to satisfactory counseling. Interpretation of the principles of nutrition into practical terms for dietary change that the client can understand is a vital skill. (Instructing a client to increase the vitamin C content of his/her diet is not sufficient; instead, specific foods containing vitamin C that s/he likes and can afford and that are readily available must be discussed.)

An understanding of factors that influence food behaviors and techniques that help clients make appropriate changes is important. A good counselor establishes a rapport to make the client feel comfortable and does not use threats or commands. The counselor recognizes that dietary habits can be changed, but it is unrealistic to expect immediate and lasting change from a few counseling sessions.

The Client. Effective nutritional assistance reflects consideration of the client's environment, heritage, and individuality including social, economic, psychological, and clinical factors. Other factors, such as present and lifelong eating patterns, age, income, social status, education, activity, illnesses, handicaps, psychological problems, and degree of independence, all play an important part in the counseling process. Each individual has specific habits and unique problems, but clients are responsible for their own decisions about what changes to adopt. Although a spouse may provide support and be willing to help, only the client can effect the changes; therefore, it is essential that s/he be directly involved.

Counseling Techniques. Dietary counseling requires constant interaction with the client, not lecturing. The goal of dietary counseling is to produce a desirable change in food choices; this enhances the sense of well-being or may reduce the risk of an illness. Since each person is responsible for his/her own health, the individual must be an active participant throughout the counseling process. By providing information about food patterns and intake, listening to the counselor's evaluation and reasons for recommended changes, setting realistic goals, studying materials, and asking questions, the patient takes an active role in dietary counseling.

Through counseling, people receive information, clarify problems, and are encouraged to formulate plans for desirable and attainable changes. A counseling session is client-centered by eliciting the client's opinions and feelings about specific recommendations. Cues that indicate confusion, disinterest, or denial of the need to learn should be observed. Tactful inquiries are made to determine the client's understanding and learning. (Do not ask, "Do you understand?" but rather, "What other selections would you prefer if orange juice is not available?")

Ample time is allowed for the client to ask questions and to present problems and frustrations. Open-ended questions are asked in a nondirected way. (Rather than, "What did you eat for breakfast yesterday?" ask, "What time did you get up yesterday and when did you first eat?") After obtaining a dietary pattern, find some good things about the pattern and praise those things; negative and critical judgments about current practices are not helpful. As few changes as possible are made in habitual eating patterns.

Teaching techniques that involve more than one of the senses and seek the active participation of the client have more impact. Utilize slide or film presentations, food models, measuring cups, pictures, or nutrition labels to help in the learning process.

The Counseling Process. The counseling process is made up of four phases: assessment, planning, implementation, and evaluation. Collecting and evaluating information on dietary intake is the first phase. This includes information regarding social, medical, and dietary history.

From the assessment, realistic objectives are developed jointly by client and counselor. Short-range and long-range goals must be within the client's ability to implement them. The objectives are written down along with the counselor's suggestions about ways to implement them.

The food pattern obtained from the assessment may be critiqued by a dietary guide. The basic food groups are frequently utilized to evaluate food patterns quickly. A quick comparison of a previous day's intake and the basic food groups allows the client to recognize possible additions or modifications needed. Then, a plan can be discussed by which nutrients may best be obtained. The client can demonstrate modifications of the current menu pattern or meal plans by choosing food models or pictures to incorporate deficient nutrients.

The plan is only implemented by client compliance. S/He must be willing and be able to independently work toward the objectives. A basic understanding and a positive attitude are essential to enacting a plan. This would include planning menus, purchasing and preparing appropriate foods, and consuming the needed amounts.

Education is incomplete unless necessary changes are made; this is established by a follow-up evaluation. Progress is evaluated by both the client and the counselor to confirm success or to determine and reassess the initial plan.

• FALLACIES and FACTS

FALLACY: Milk is a perfect food.
  • **FACT:** Milk is definitely not a perfect food. In particular, all foods in the milk group are low in vitamin C, iron, and copper.

FALLACY: Milk is not necessary and can be omitted from the diet.
  • **FACT:** Milk must be eliminated from many individuals' diets because of an intolerance or an allergy. However, calcium is needed throughout life, with increased demands in elderly women to avoid osteoporosis. It is very difficult to plan menus adequate in calcium and riboflavin if milk and milk products are not included. Natural cheese and yogurt may be tolerated and offer needed nutrients, or calcium supplements may be needed (see Chapter 12).

FALLACY: Foods from the bread and cereal group are fattening.
  • **FACT:** Consumption from this group has been steadily declining while obesity has not. In comparison, one slice of bread has approximately 70 kcal; one egg or one apple has about the same caloric content. When breads and cereals are omitted, the B vitamins usually are inadequate, which in turn, affects the utilization of other nutrients.

FALLACY: Vegetable juices have magic healing qualities.

- **FACT:** *This is one of the many health food promotions. No vegetable or fruit or its juice has a specific disease-curing property.*
- **FALLACY:** *Vegetable juices are more nutritious than the vegetables themselves.*
- **FACT:** *The nutritive value of vegetables and their juices are approximately the same; however, the fiber has been removed from the juice.*
- **FALLACY:** *Beef should be eliminated from the diet due to its high caloric and cholesterol content.*
- **FACT:** *Beef is an important contributor of iron in the diet. Whereas iron is present in dark green leafy vegetables, the iron from red meat is more readily available and enhances the absorption of iron from other food sources eaten simultaneously. Variety is the key to any diet—not the total elimination of any particular food because of its imperfections.*

Summary

To make planning a well-balanced diet easier, guidelines have been formulated. Recommended dietary allowances indicate certain desirable levels of nutrient intake that are formulated for determining the adequacy of diets for different groups of people. Basic food groups categorize foods according to their nutrient content and determine the number of servings from each group to assure adequate nutrient intake. Problems are associated with each of these guidelines. Meal planning can be simplified by using the basic food groups; it is no easy task when attempting to satisfy individual persons with various preferences, needs, and problems.

Review Questions

1. What are the functions of foods in the body? List the nutrients necessary for each of the functions.
2. What is the purpose of dietary evaluations? What are three types of evaluations? What information would you learn from each?
3. Distinguish between recommendations and requirements.

4. Keep a record of all the foods you eat for 24 hours. Was it adequate, as evaluated by the basic food groups? Evaluate it in terms of the RDAs by adding the amounts of each nutrient for all foods eaten. Does your diet meet the RDA nutrient standards for your age and sex?
5. Collect nutrient labels for three similar products. Compare the nutrient values to determine which is a better souce of nutrients. Which is a better buy for the number of nutrients it contains?
6. Using Figure 3–2, list the number of times you eat each food in a week. Are the foods you eat most frequently towards the top or bottom of each group? Does this have any relationship to your weight?
7. Using nutrient labels, compare the nutrient density of chocolate milk, homogenized milk, and skim milk. Which has a higher nutrient density?
8. Plan attractive daily menus for one week using the basic food groups as a guideline, incorporating variety in types of foods, texture, temperature, flavors, and methods of preparation.

Case Study: Your client in the Women, Infants, and Children (WIC) health clinic is the single mother of three children (ages four years, two years, and six months). Her intake for yesterday included a sweet roll and Coke around 10 AM, a slice of cheese and crackers with iced tea about 12:30 PM, a midafternoon candy bar, fried chicken with fried potatoes and cornbread with margarine for dinner, popcorn and coke in the evening. From which of the basic four food groups is she lacking? Help her establish some goals for changing her eating patterns, remembering to set short-term, achievable goals initially.

REFERENCE LIST

Adelman, MO; Dwyer, JT; Woods, M; et al: Computerized dietary analysis systems: A comparative view. *J Am Diet Assoc* 83(4):421, 1983.

Allen, J; Gadson, K: Food consumption and nutritional status of low-income households. *Nat Food Review* 26:27, 1984.

Committee on Diet, Nutrition and Cancer, (CDNC), Assembly of Life Sciences, National Research Council: *Diet, Nutrition, and Cancer.* Washington, DC, National Academy Press, 1982.

Dwyer, J; Suitor, CW: Caveat emptor: Assessing needs, evaluating computer options. *J Am Diet Assoc* 84(3):302, 1984.

Friend, B: Enrichment and fortification of foods, 1961–70. *Nat Food Supply* 142(Nov):29, 1972.

Guthrie, HA: Application of the RDA. Presented at the American Dietetic Association's 68th Annual Meeting, October 10, 1985.

Guthrie, HA; Scheer, JC: Validity of a dietary score for assessing nutrient adequacy. *J Am Diet Assoc* 78(3):240, 1981.

King, JC; Cohenour, SH; Corruccini, CG; et al: Evaluation and modification of the basic four food guide. *J Nutr Ed* 10(1):27, 1978.

Light, L; Cronin, FJ: Food guidance revisted. *J Nutr Ed* 13(2):57, 1981.

National Research Council (NRC): *Recommended Dietary Allowances*, Washington, DC, National Academy of Sciences, 1980.

Rolls, BJ: Experimental analysis of the effects of variety in a meal on human feeding. *Am J Clin Nutr* 42(5 suppl):932, 1985.

Further Study

Anderson, JJB: Questions and answers about new recommended dietary allowances. *Consultant* 20(12):111, 1980.

Beare-Rogers, JL: Food and nutrition guidelines in Canada. *Prog Clin Biol Res* 67:481, 1981.

Dodds, JM: The handy five food guide. *J Nutr Ed* 13(2):50, 1981.

Nutrition labeling-terms you should know. *FDA Consumer Memo:* February 1976.

Food and Nutrition Board, National Research Council: Recommended Dietary Allowances: Scientific issues and process for the future. *J Nutr* 116(3):482, 1986.

Gillespie, AH; Roderuck, CE: Method for developing a nutrient guide. *Home Econ Res J* 11(1):21, 1982.

Guthrie, HA; Scheer, JC: Nutritional adequacy of self-selected diets that satisfy the four food groups guide. *J Nutr Ed* 13(2):46, 1981.

Guthrie, HA; Scheer, JC: Validity of a dietary score for assessing nutrient adequacy. *J Am Diet Assoc* 78(3):240, 1981.

Hansen, RG; Wyse, BW; Sorenson, AW: *Nutritional Quality Index of Foods*. Westport, CT, AVI Publishing Co, 1979.

Harper, AE: Recommended dietary allowances—1980. *Nutr Rev* 38(8):290, 1980.

Holder, JE: Don't just tell your patients—teach them. *RN* 48(7):29, 1985.

Lachance, PA: A suggestion on food guides and dietary guidelines. *J Nutr Ed* 13(2):56, 1981.

Lecos, C: RDAs: Key to nutrition. *FDA Consumer* 16(9):24, 1982.

National Dairy Council: The food group approach to good eating. *Dairy Council Digest* 52(6):30, 1981.

Nutrition Today: Nutrition's Mount Saint Helen's Eruption II. Special Report. Nutr Today 20(6): 4–23, 1986.

Peterkin, BB; Patterson, PC; Blum, AJ; et al: Changes in dietary patterns: one approach to meeting standards. *J Am Diet Assoc* 78(5):453, 1981.

Ruffalo, RL; Garabedian-Ruffalo, SM; Pawlson, LG: Patient compliance. *Am Fam Physician* 31(6):93, 1985.

Schucker, RE: Does nutrition labeling really affect food choices? *Nutr Today* 20(6):24, 1986.

Shell, ER: Why you always have room for dessert. *Am Health* 5(2):43, 1986.

Sources of error in reading food labels. *Patient Care* 20(11):90, 1986.

Vicker, CE; Hodges, PAM: Counseling strategies for dietary management: Expanded possibilities for effecting behavior change. *J Am Diet Assoc* 86(7):924, 1986.

Ward, DM: Why patient teaching fails. *RN* 49(1):45, 1986.

Zifferblatt, SM; Wilbur, CS: Dietary counseling: Some realistic expectations and guidelines. *J Am Diet Assoc* 70(6):591, 1977.

Resources

Recommended Dietary Allowances. Available from Office of Publications, National Academy of Sciences, 2101 Constitution Avenue, NW, Washington, DC 20418.

Food 2 . . . A Dieter's Guide and *Food 3 . . . Eating the Moderate Fat and Cholesterol Way.* Available from American Dietetic Association, P.O. Box 91403, Chicago, IL 60693.

Guide to Good Eating. Available from National Dairy Council, 630 North River Road, Rosemont, IL 60018.

Nutrition Labeling: How It Can Work for You. Available from The National Nutrition Consortium, Inc., 9650 Rockville Pike, Bethesda, MD 20014.

Read the Label, Set a Better Table. Available from the U.S. Department of Health, Education, and Welfare, Public Health Service, Food and Drug Administration, 5600 Fishers Lane, Rockville, MD 20852.

Digestion and Metabolism

THE STUDENT WILL BE ABLE TO:

- **Discuss factors that influence ingestion.**
- **Describe general functions of each digestive organ.**
- **Identify chemical secretions and their location necessary for digestion of energy nutrients.**
- **Name the energy nutrients and their end products of digestion that can be absorbed.**
- **Explain the role of gastrointestinal motility in the digestion and absorption process.**
- **State the purpose of the Krebs or TCA cycle in metabolism.**

OBJECTIVES

TERMS TO KNOW

Accessory organs
Alimentary canal
Anabolism
Apoenzyme
Bile
Bolus
Catabolism
Chyme
Chylomicron
Coefficient of digestibility
Coenzyme
Cofactor
Enzyme
Hydrolysis
Hyper- and hypogeusia
Lacteal
Lower esophageal
 sphincter (LES)
Lymphatic circulation
Metabolism
Microflora
Mitochondria
Olfactory nerves
Osmosis
Pepsin
Peristalsis
Pinocytosis
Pores
Portal circulation
Substrate
Villus

Physiologically, foods are eaten to nourish the body. Nevertheless, the foods we enjoy, such as hamburgers, are composed of large chemical molecules that cannot be utilized unless they are broken down to an absorbable form. The digestive system is designed to (1) ingest foods, (2) digest or break down the complex molecules into simple, soluble materials that can be absorbed (or pass through the gastrointestinal walls), and (3) eliminate unused residues. Only the three energy nutrients must be digested for absorption. Most vitamins, minerals, and water can be absorbed as eaten. If the alimentary tract is not functioning properly, the body may be unable to receive adequate amounts of nutrients.

Physiology of the Gastrointestinal Tract

The digestive system includes the alimentary canal and several accessory organs (Fig. 4–1). The alimentary canal is a tubular structure, extending from the mouth to the anus, with a length of about 30 feet (five times the height of an average man). It includes the mouth, pharynx, esophagus, stomach, small intestine (duodenum, jejunum, ileum), and the large intestine (cecum, colon, and rectum). The accessory organs include the salivary glands, liver, gallbladder, and pancreas.

Digestion involves two basic types of action on the food: (1) Mechanical activities—chewing and peristalsis—break up and mix foods permitting better chemical action, and (2) chemical activity from digestive juices throughout the tract (beginning with saliva) reduces foodstuffs to smaller molecules that can be absorbed.

Chemical Action

The process of digesting energy nutrients involves a chemical reaction called hydrolysis. In hydrolysis of nutrients, water is added to break a large molecule into smaller ones that are water-soluble and can be utilized by the cells of the body:

$$Protein + H_2O \rightarrow amino\ acids$$

$$Fat + H_2O \rightarrow fatty\ acids + glycerol$$

$$Carbohydrate + H_2O \rightarrow monosaccharides$$

These reactions do not proceed automatically. Enzymes are complex chemical agents that enable metabolic reactions to proceed at a faster rate without being consumed themselves. In the protein reaction (above), the protein is the substrate on which the enzyme would work and the amino acids are the product. The enzyme forms a temporary chemical compound with the substrate. When the reaction is completed, the complex breaks up, releasing the new chemical compound and the enzyme for its reuse.

Enzymes are proteins produced by cells from individual amino acids, utilizing a "template" or pattern to build the specific enzyme needed. Since the enzyme is reused, only small amounts are needed. Thousands of different reactions proceed in the body, each of which is controlled by different enzymes. Enzymes function somewhat like keys in that they are very specific and will work on only one substrate, similar to a key fitting one particular lock (Fig. 4–2). For instance, a digestive enzyme that aids in protein hydrolysis does not work on the peptide linkages present in hair protein because the enzymes do not fit. The name for some enzymes is derived from the name of the substrate on which it works, with the suffix "-ase", i.e., lactase is the enzyme produced to catalyze the breakdown of lactose.

Mechanical Action

The wall of the alimentary canal is the same from the esophagus to the rectum (Fig. 4–3). A circular layer of muscles encircle the tube, allowing the diameter of the tube to expand and contract. Food particles are therefore broken up and mixed by the churning action. The outer fibers of the muscular coat (longitudinal muscle) run lengthwise and are responsible for peristalsis. Involuntary rhythmic waves of contraction travel away from the mouth, carrying the food ahead of it the whole length of the alimentary tract; the process is assisted by muscular relaxation preceding it.

Valves, also called sphincter muscles, are door-like mechanisms between the digestive seg-

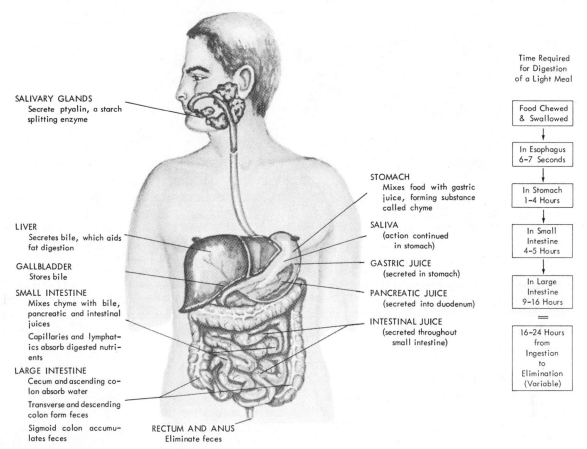

Figure 4–1. *The digestive process. (From* A Programmed Approach to Anatomy and Physiology: The Digestive System. *Washington, DC, Robert J. Brady Co, 1968, by permission.)*

ments. They are designed to (1) retain food in that segment until the work of the mechanical actions and digestive juices has been completed, (2) allow measured amounts of food to pass into the next segment, and (3) prevent food from "backing up" into the preceding area. The regulation of these valves is complex, involving muscular function and different pressures on each side.

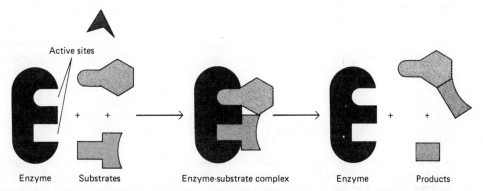

Figure 4–2. *Lock-and-key mechanism of enzyme action. The substrates fit the active sites much as keys fit locks. Note that when the products separate from the enzyme, the enzyme is free to catalyze production of additional products. The enzyme is not changed by the reaction. (From Solomon EP, Davis PW:* Human Anatomy and Physiology. *Philadelphia, W. B. Saunders Co, 1983, by permission.)*

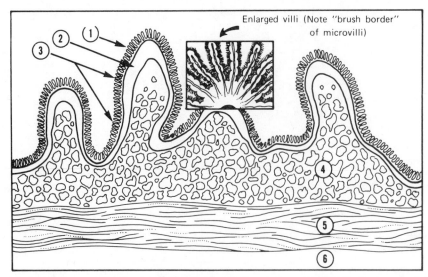

Figure 4–3. Layers of the digestive tract: (1) Mucosal folds, (2) muscularis mucosae, (3) villi, (4) circular muscle layer, (5) longitudinal muscle, and (6) outer serosa. (From Green ML, Harry J: Nutrition in Contemporary Nursing Practice. Copyright © 1981, John Wiley & Sons, Inc. Reprinted by permission of John Wiley & Sons, Inc.)

Clinical Implications:

- Disorders of motility in the esophagus produce painful swallowing or lodging of food so that less food is ingested, followed by weight loss (Iber, 1980).
- Loss of motility in the stomach and small intestine (seen in long-standing diabetics) results in impaired stomach and intestinal emptying. This allows excessive growth of bacteria, which may interfere with fat and vitamin absorption, and may injure the surface of the intestine (Iber, 1980).
- Gastrointestinal function can be assessed by auscultation. Gurgling, caused by air and fluid in the normal abdomen, indicates normal physiologic activity.

Mouth

Taste and Smell. Generally, food choices are influenced by the three senses of sight, smell, and taste. The presentation of food, its color or aroma, may be the basis for acceptance or rejection of the item. Visual aspects of eating were discussed briefly in Table 3–5. The combination of smell and taste preceeds the perception of flavor, each reinforcing one another.

The mouth plays an important role in the digestive system, not only because it is the "port of entry," but because of the presence of taste buds, the receptors for the sense of taste. Food stimulates the taste buds, and aromas stimulate the olfactory nerves (or sense of smell) (Bell et al, 1976). Satisfaction derived from food determines its acceptability. The basic taste sensations of sweet, sour, salty, and bitter are located on different parts of the tongue (Fig. 4–4). These four basic tastes reflect specific constituents of food (Table 4–1). In general, taste and smell are essential for influencing the intake to meet physiological needs, including the ingesting of food and salt. On the other hand, they are not infallible guides, as the chemical senses can be distorted by life experiences and disease states (Schiffman, 1983).

Toddlers have the largest number of taste buds (and a higher degree of taste sensitivity), resulting in an aversion for highly seasoned foods. The number of taste buds declines in later life, explaining the fact that elderly adults have a diminished taste sensitivity.

Foods are sometimes judged to be harmful or spoiled because of their odors, so the sense of smell is a protective mechanism. On the other hand, a person with a cold usually may lose his/her appetite because of a decreased sense of smell, which causes decreased palatability and enjoyment. Taste disorders are often the result of problems in smell rather than taste. When nutritional care is concerned, taste and smell abnor-

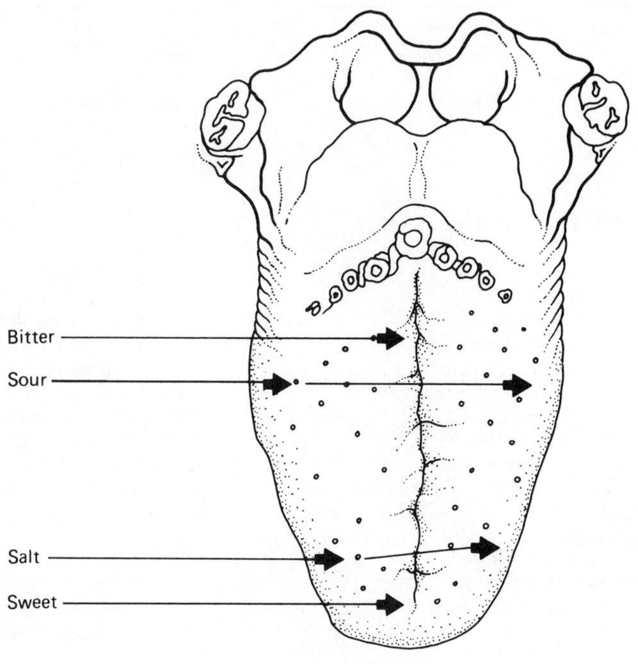

Figure 4–4. Regions of taste on the tongue. (From Green ML, Harry J: Nutrition in Contemporary Nursing Practice. Copyright © 1981, John Wiley & Sons, Inc. Reprinted by permission of John Wiley & Sons, Inc.)

malities must be considered. A loss of smell (anosmia), loss of taste (hypogeusia), or a heightened taste acuity (hypergeusia) is typical of some illnesses and drugs (Table 4–2), and will affect the individual's food intake.

Taste and smell disorders are not mere inconveniences or neurotic symptoms; they affect food choices and dietary habits, which can result in deterioration of an individual's general condition or nutritional status. Since taste stimulants affect salivary and pancreatic flow, gastic contractions and intestinal motility, taste disorders can also affect digestion (Schiffman, 1983).

Teeth. Another important role of the mouth in food digestion is the mechanical action of teeth, reducing the size of food particles. Digestion of food is facilitated by increasing its surface area.

Saliva. Some chemical action begins with secretions in the mouth. Saliva, secreted by the salivary glands, is mixed with the food particles. The functions of the different constituents in saliva are shown in Table 4–3.

Since food is normally in the mouth only briefly, salivary amylase just launches the digestion of starch. If a carbohydrate food, such as a cracker, is chewed and held in the mouth for a few seconds, it will begin to taste sweet, denoting the fact that some starch is being hydrolyzed to maltose.

Clinical Implications:

- A patient's appetite can be depressed by food that is served lukewarm or in large quantities, or that looks uninteresting or is tasteless.
- Smelling is an important component of flavor, and much of the pleasure of selecting and eating food is lost when the sense of smell is absent.
- Children who are fed crackers in an effort to decrease exposure to sugar between meals will "discover" the sweetness of crackers and may retain them in their mouth, thereby producing a cariogenic substance in the mouth.

Table 4–1. Basic Taste Sensations

Taste Sensation	Implication	Chemical Group
Sweet	Calories	Hydroxyl groups (-OH)
Sour	pH	Hydrogen ion (acids)
Salty	Electrolytes	Ionized salts
Bitter	Poison	Alkaloids and organic molecules

Table 4–2. Some Factors Affecting Taste and Smell*

Factor	Taste	Smell
DISORDERS		
Damage to chorda tympani	Absent/diminished	
Familial dysautonomia	Absent/diminished	
Head trauma	Absent/diminished	Absent/diminished
Cancer	Absent/diminished (sweet) Heightened (bitter)	
Chronic renal failure	Absent/diminished/distorted (sweet, salt, sour)	Absent/diminished
Cirrhosis	Absent/diminished	Absent/diminished
Niacin deficiency	Absent/diminished distorted	
Thermal burn	Absent/diminished/distorted	
Vitamin B$_{12}$ deficiency		Absent/diminished
Zinc deficiency	Absent/diminished	
Adrenal cortical insufficiency	Increased detection but decreased recognition	
Multiple sclerosis	Absent/diminished/distorted	Absent/diminished
Cushing's syndrome	Absent/diminished	Absent/diminished
Hypothyroidism	Absent/diminished/distorted	Absent/diminished/distorted
Diabetes mellitus	Absent/diminished (sweet)	Absent/diminished
Allergic rhinitis, nasal polyposis, sinusitis, bronchial asthma		Absent/diminished
Radiation therapy	Absent/diminished/distorted	
Cystic fibrosis	Individual variation, frequently increased	Individual variation, frequently increased
Hypertension	Absent/diminished (salt)	
DRUGS		
Dimercaprol, fluorouracil, lincomycin, griseofulvin	Altered/distorted	
Phenformin, lithium, metronidazole, disulfiram, sulfonylureas	Metallic taste	
Metaproterenol	Bad taste	
Amphetamines	Increased sensitivity (bitter)	
Furosemide	Peculiar sweet taste	

*Data from Schiffman, S: Taste and smell in disease. Reprinted by permission of *The New England Journal of Medicine* 308:1275, 1983.

Esophagus

The swallowing reflex moves a quantity of food called a bolus into the esophagus, which is transported to the stomach by peristalsis and gravity. The esophagus, a continuous tube about 10 inches long connecting the mouth with the stomach, penetrates the diaphragm through an opening called the esophageal hiatus. Just above the stomach, circular muscle fibers in the wall are slightly hypertrophied, to form the lower esophageal sphincter (LES). This strong muscle relaxes to permit food to enter the stomach, but contracts tightly to prevent the regurgitation or "backwashing" of the stomach contents.

Table 4–3. Digestive Functions of Saliva

Saliva Component	Classification	Function
Mucin	Glycoprotein	Lubricates food for easier passage (Mucin + water = mucus)
Amylase	Enzyme	Begins hydrolysis of starch to maltose
Lysozyme	Enzyme	Kills some ingested bacteria

Gastric Digestion

The bolus entering the stomach is mixed with gastric secretions by peristaltic contractions. Gastric secretions include mucus, hydrochloric acid, two enzymes, and a component called intrinsic factor. The mixture of food particles and gastric juices gradually becomes a semifluid paste called chyme.

Salivary amylase, which is active in a basic pH, continues its hydrolysis of carbohydrate until the acidity of the chyme is increased by hydrochloric acid (HCl) and it can no longer function. HCl is one of the most corrosive acids known, powerful enough to dissolve zinc (Ingelfinger, 1971). The low pH of the stomach contents (about 1.5 to 3.0) is beneficial for several reasons: (1) It kills or inhibits the growth of most food bacteria, (2) denatures proteins and makes them more easily hydrolyzed to amino acids, (3) activates gastric enzymes, (4) hydrolyzes some of the sugars, and (5) increases solubility and absorption of calcium and iron.

Two major enzymes are found in gastric juice—pepsin and lipase. Pepsin is capable of hydrolyzing large protein molecules to small polypeptide fragments, but not to individual amino acids. Pepsin is actually secreted in its inactive form, pepsinogen, but is converted to pepsin by HCl. Gastric lipase initiates fat digestion, mainly the short- and medium-chain triglycerides (emulsified and butter fats).

Mucus forms an alkaline coating on the lining of the stomach for protection against digestion of the stomach by pepsin. Intrinsic factor is essential for absorption of vitamin B_{12} in the small intestine.

Normal gastric secretion is regulated by nerve and hormonal stimuli. The senses to see, smell, and taste food stimulate the vagus nerve to increase gastric secretions. The vagus nerve also affects gastric secretions in response to emotions. Fear and depression are generally accompanied with decreased secretions; anger and hostility, with increased secretions.

The presence of food in the stomach will induce hormonal control of gastric secretions, with different foods eliciting differing secretion responses. Proteins, calcium, coffee, and alcohol are stimulants that increase the amount of HCl and pepsin in the stomach (Feldman et al, 1981). When chyme with a high fat content enters the intestine, a hormone (enterogastrone) is released to inhibit peristaltic action in the stomach.

In addition to foods, the stomach receives medications and other substances. Some of these substances are irritants to the stomach, making it subject to erosion, ulceration due to hypersecretions, and intolerances (Fein, 1980). Others that are not acted upon by the stomach are passed on unchanged.

The adult stomach has a capacity to hold 1 to 2 L and functions as a reservoir to hold an average meal from 3 to 4½ hours. The stomach empties at different rates depending on its size, the composition of the chyme, and to some extent, the size and energy density of the meal (Weiner et al, 1981) and contractions of the duodenum (Burks et al, 1985). The smaller the stomach capacity, the more rapidly it will empty. (This is exemplified in the infant or person with a partial gastrectomy who must be fed frequently.) Liquids pass through the stomach quite rapidly. Foods with a high carbohydrate content are generally the first to be released, followed by proteins, and lastly fat, which may remain in the stomach for three to six hours. Chyme is released from the stomach through the pyloric sphincter in small amounts to allow for adequate digestion and absorption in the small intestine (Weiner et al, 1981).

Gastric Absorption

Although some digestion of foods begins in the stomach, very few are completely hydrolyzed to nutrients the body can use at this stage. Therefore, very little absorption takes place in the stomach. Foods ingested in an absorbable form may be absorbed from the stomach in small amounts, including some water, alcohol, and a few water-soluble substances (sodium, potassium, amino acids, and glucose).

Clinical Implications:

- Since gravity facilitates the movement of food down the esophagus, patients who must remain horizontal have some difficulty swallowing. This is facilitated by the patient lying on the left side.
- Individuals with a lack of gastric HCl (achlorhydria) have excessive bacterial growth and putrefaction of the gastric contents.
- Achlorhydria is commonly associated with gastric cancer and pernicious anemia since the parietal cells of the gastric glands secrete both hydrochloric acid and intrinsic factor.
- Peptic ulcers are usually due to the digestive action of pepsin, when the hydrochloric acid somehow overwhelms the mucous protective coating of the stomach.
- Vomiting is one of the methods the body has of eliminating toxins in contaminated foods. Vomiting can also be stimulated by rapid changes in body motion or by drugs.

- Heartburn is the result of regurgitation of the stomach contents back into the esophagus. The acidic gastric secretions produce discomfort or pain, which may be relieved if the individual remains in an upright position after eating.
- A stomachache may be the result of eating more than the stomach can comfortably hold or eating too rapidly. The result may be "acid indigestion" followed by consumption of the highly advertised antacids. The stomach responds by secreting more acid to counteract the neutralizer so the digestive enzymes can do their work.

Small Intestine

Most of the energy nutrients are completely hydrolyzed in the small intestine, and their absorption as well as the absorption of most vitamins and minerals takes place in the small intestine. The small intestine is specially designed to perform these tasks with juices from the intestine and the accessory organs and its complex structure along the lumen walls. The small intestine is approximately 15 feet long, and foods are retained for three to ten hours.

Digestion. Throughout the walls of the small intestine are villi, or fingerlike projections rising out of the mucosa into the intestinal lumen (Fig. 4–3). These villi increase the surface area of this 24-foot tube to about 3000 square feet, all folded up to fit in the abdominal cavity (Pike & Brown, 1984). Each villus is also covered with a layer of epithelial cells containing microvilli that collectively form the brush border cells. This increases the surface area even further.

At the center of each villus is a lymphatic channel called a lacteal, which is important in the absorption of fats. A network of blood capillaries surrounds the lacteal. Nerve fibers in each villus act to stimulate or inhibit its activities (Fig. 4–5).

Many of the secretions in the small intestine are controlled by hormonal secretions. Acidic chyme entering the intestine stimulates the hormones secretin and pancreozymin to release bicarbonate ions and pancreatic juices, respectively, into the duodenum. Another hormone, cholecystokinin, responds to the presence of fat by stimulating the gallbladder to release bile. Therefore, chyme entering the small intestine through the pyloric valve is neutralized by mucus, pancreatic juices, and bile from the liver (pH 6 to 8).

Digestion of carbohydrates, proteins, and fats in the small intestine proceeds with secretions from the intestinal juices within the lumen, enzymes produced in the mucosa, pancreatic secretions, and bile, which is produced by the liver. These actions are summarized in Table 4–4.

Pancreatic juices enter the duodenum through the pancreatic duct and include enzymes for hydrolysis of carbohydrates, proteins, and fats. Pancreatic enzymes function best in the neutralized chyme. Although many bacteria are killed and digested in the acidic conditions of the stomach, some are retained in the intestine. Normal secretions and motility in the small intestine inhibit bacterial growth until the large intestine, where the pH and slower motility enhance bacterial growth.

The proteolytic enzymes are produced and stored in the pancreas in inactive form. Enterokinase, an intestinal enzyme, activates trypsinogen to its active form, precipitating a domino effect to activate the remaining proteolytic enzymes.

Approximately 1 L of bile is secreted daily by the liver. It is stored in the gallbladder, where the water is reabsorbed. Bile salts reduce surface tension of fat particles, as well as having an emulsifying effect, allowing greater exposure to intestinal and pancreatic lipases.

Specific digestive enzymes located within the microvilli are responsible for completing the digestive processes of carbohydrates, proteins, and fats. Not all the foods eaten can be completely digested. The human body does not have enzymes to digest cellulose, a carbohydrate found in plants.

Clinical Implications:

- An enzymatic deficiency in the gastrointestinal tract will result in some nutrients not being digested; therefore, they cannot be absorbed.
- The absence of bile leads to impaired digestion and absorption of fats and fat-soluble vitamins.

Absorption. The small intestine is the principal site for absorption (Fig. 4–6). Simple sugars, amino acids, glycerol, vitamins, electrolytes, and minerals (which are the end products of digestion) are absorbed principally in the duodenum and jejunum. Only after the nutrient is absorbed into the intestinal mucosa is it considered to be "in" the body (Pike & Brown, 1984).

The tremendous amount of surface area created by the villi makes absorption so efficient that very little absorbable substance reaches the large

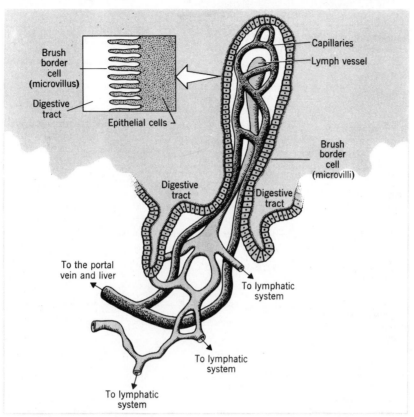

Figure 4–5. *A villus, the absorptive organ of the small intestine. (From Wilson ED, Fisher KH, Garcia PA:* Principles of Nutrition, *4th ed. Copyright © 1979, John Wiley & Sons. Reprinted by permission of John Wiley & Sons, Inc.)*

intestine. Villi are capable of movements, which facilitate absorption and stir up the chyme, exposing more surface area.

Absorbable nutrients pass through the microvilli and enter the portal or lymphatic circulation:

Water-soluble nutrients → portal circulation

Fat-soluble nutrients → lymphatic circulation

Mechanisms of Absorption. Substances pass through the intestinal wall in extremely complex processes. The most common routes of absorption occur through pores, carriers, and pumps (Fig. 4–7). A few substances may be absorbed by pinocytosis.

Pores. This process, also referred to as passive diffusion, is essentially osmosis, whereby a substance such as water or an electrolyte moves from a region of a higher concentration to one of a lower concentration.

Carriers or Pumps. Water-soluble molecules cannot penetrate the cell membrane because it has a high lipid content. Therefore, a carrier combines with the molecule, carries it through the cell wall, and releases it inside the cell. Additionally, when absorption is from a region of low concentration to higher concentration, cellular energy and a carrier are required. This method rapidly moves the nutrients into the cell and the blood supply.

Pinocytosis. Large molecules, such as whole proteins, may be absorbed in this manner. The process is described as a cell engulfing the molecule. Only small amounts of nutrients are absorbed in this manner, but intact proteins absorbed into the bloodstream in this manner may cause allergic reactions (Levinsky, 1981).

Absorption into the Portal Circulation. Monosaccharides, amino acids, glycerol, water-soluble vitamins, and minerals are absorbed from the small intestine through the mucosa into the portal circulation. They are transported through the portal vein directly to the liver, where metabolism begins. As a general rule, absorption of nutrients by passive diffusion occurs in the duodenum,

Table 4—4. Digestion in the Gastrointestinal Tract

Location	Secretion/Enzyme	Function	Nutrient Action
Mouth	Salivary amylase (ptyalin)		Hydrolyzes starch into disaccharides.
Stomach	Hydrochloric acid	Antibacterial. Activates pepsinogen, which is then called pepsin.	Converts Fe^{3+} to Fe^{2+} $Fe^{3+} \rightarrow Fe^{2+}$
	Pepsin		Hydrolyzes proteins into polypeptides.
	Gastric lipase		Hydrolyzes emulsified fats (butterfat) into glycerol and fatty acids.
	Intrinsic factor	Combines with vitamin B_{12}.	
	Mucin	Protects mucosa.	
Small intestine: Pancreatic juices	Trypsinogen		
	Trypsin	Converts chymotrypsinogen to chymotrypsin.	Hydrolyzes proteins and polypeptides into dipeptides.
	Chymotrypsinogen	Is converted to chymotrypsin.	
	Chymotrypsin		Hydrolyzes proteins and polypeptides into dipeptides.
	Procarboxypeptidase	Converts trypsin to carboxypeptidase.	
	Carboxypeptidase		Hydrolyzes polypeptides and dipeptides into amino acids.
	Pancreatic lipase (requires bile salts)		Hydrolyzes fats into glycerol, mono- and diglycerides and fatty acids.
	Pancreatic amylase		Hydrolyzes starch into maltose.
	Phospholipase		Converts lecithin into lysolecithin.
Intestinal juices (in microvilli)	Enterokinase	Activates trypsinogen, which is then called trypsin.	
	Aminopeptidase		Hydrolyzes polypeptides and dipeptides into amino acids.
	Dipeptidases		Hydrolyzes dipeptides into amino acids.
	Intestinal lipase		Hydrolyzes fats into glycerol and glycerides and fatty acids.
	Sucrase		Hydrolyzes sucrose into glucose and fructose.
	Maltase		Hydrolyzes maltose into glucose.
	Lactase		Hydrolyzes into glucose and galactose.
	Lecithinase		Hydrolyzes lecithin into fatty acids and glycerol and phosphoric acid.
	Bile	Accelerates action of pancreatic lipase. Emulsifies fats. Neutralizes chyme. Stabilizes emulsions.	
Large intestine	Mucus	Protects mucosa.	

whereas absorption by active transport mechanisms is prevalent in the ileum (Pike & Brown, 1984).

The end products of carbohydrate and protein digestion are monosaccharides and amino acids, respectively, and are usually absorbed in the lower duodenum and jejunum by active transport. Glycerol and medium- and short-chain fatty acids (10 or fewer carbon atoms) are water-soluble and enter the portal circulation like monosaccharides and amino acids.

All water-soluble vitamins except vitamin B_{12} are readily absorbed through the intestinal muco-sal cell via energy-dependent and carrier-mediated transport systems. Electrolytes are also absorbed by active transport into the intestinal villi. Sodium, potassium, chloride, nitrate, and bicarbonate are readily absorbed. Most of the polyvalent ions, especially calcium and iron, are poorly absorbed. Absorption can be affected by dietary conditions and is regulated by hormones in some instances.

Some water is absorbed from the stomach, but approximately 80 to 90 percent is absorbed in the small intestine by osmosis. Actually, water moves freely in both directions across the intesti-

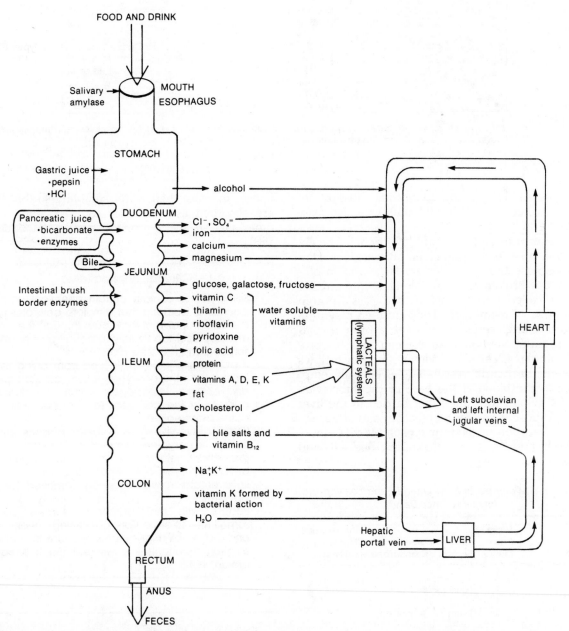

Figure 4–6. Sites of secretion and absorption in the gastrointestinal tract. (From Krause MV, Mahan LK: Food, Nutrition and Diet Therapy, 7th ed. Philadelphia, W. B. Saunders Co. 1984, by permission.)

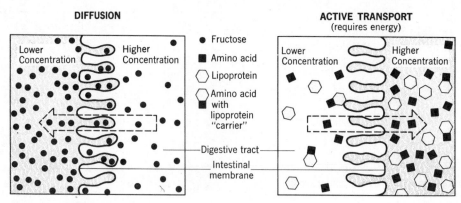

Figure 4–7. Absorption by diffusion and active transport. (From Wilson ED, Fisher KH, Garcia PA: Principles of Nutrition, 4th ed. Copyright © 1979 John Wiley & Sons. Reprinted by permission of John Wiley & Sons, Inc.)

nal mucosa. In addition to nutrient absorption, gastric secretions (totaling 9 L daily) are also reabsorbed (Table 4–5).

Absorption of Fat-Soluble Nutrients. The absorption process for long-chain fatty acids is complex because the molecules are large and insoluble. Fat is broken apart by bile salts into smaller entities called micelles, which can pass through the intestinal membrane. They are then resynthesized into triglycerides and given a protein coating, to enter the lymphatic system. This lipoprotein complex is called a chylomicron, which flows through the lymph vessels and eventually empties into the blood at the base of the subclavian vein. Chylomicrons are either carried to the liver or to adipose tissue for metabolism and storage.

Absorption of the four fat-soluble vitamins— A, D, E, and K—is not so complex. Bile salts and lipases increase their water solubility so that they are absorbed as a micellar complex along with other fats in the lymphatic system (Hollander, 1981).

Clinical Implications:

- Some foods contain certain chemical compounds or bacteria that stimulate peristalsis to the extent that materials pass through the alimentary tract too rapidly to permit proper absorption. This is called diarrhea.
- If pancreatic juice is blocked from being released from the pancreas, it may accumulate and activate trypsinogen, which can digest portions of the pancreas (a condition called acute pancreatitis).
- Unless preventive care is taken, persons with partial or complete removal of the stomach, duodenum, jejunum, or ileum may develop deficiency symptoms when digestive secretions or absorptive areas are removed (see Fig. 4–6).
- People with malabsorption disorders can sometimes tolerate fats containing medium- and short-chain triglycerides because their absorption mechanism is different (Bach & Babayan, 1982).

Table 4–5. Volumes of Fluid Entering and Leaving the Intestinal Tract Daily*

Fluid	Liters Into Lumen	GI Section	Liters Reabsorbed	Approximate "Efficiency" (Percent)
Diet	2	Jejunum	4–5 of 9	50
Saliva	1			
Gastric	2	Ileum	3–4 of 4–5	75
Bile	1			
Pancreatic	2	Colon	1–2 of 1–2	>90
Small intestine	1			
TOTAL	9	TOTAL†	8–9	

*From Weinsier, RL; Butterworth, CE, Jr: Handbook of Clinical Nutrition. St Louis, The C. V. Mosby Co, 1981, by permission.
†The stools normally contain 0.1 to 0.2 L of fluid daily. If they contain more than 0.3 L/day, diarrhea is usually present.

Large Intestine

Chyme remaining in the ileum is released through the ileocecal valve into the cecum in small amounts. Approximately 500 ml of chyme— only about 1/20 of the foods ingested and the secretions produced in the mouth, esophagus, stomach, and small intestines—arrives in the large intestine. For most adults, it takes between one and three days for foodstuffs to travel the full length of the gut.

Functions. The large intestine, so named because of its larger diameter, has little or no digestive function. Its main functions are to reabsorb water and electrolytes (mainly sodium and potassium) and to form and store the residue (feces) until defecation. Chyme entering the large intestine containing 500 to 1000 ml water is excreted as feces containing only 100 to 200 ml fluid (about 75 percent of the weight of the feces). Essentially, all absorption occurs in the proximal half of the colon.

The inner lining of the large intestine is relatively smooth, lacking the numerous villi found in the small intestine. The only important secretion is mucus, which protects the intestinal wall, aids in holding particles of fecal matter together, and helps to control the pH of the large intestine.

Undigested Residues. Material in the colon contains undigested residues, a few materials that could not be digested or absorbed, bile pigments, and water. Fiber, obtained from fruits and vegetables or whole-grain products, is part of the undigested residues that have a water-holding capacity and contribute to bulkier feces. The increased residue has a beneficial side effect of stimulating peristalsis, contributing to better muscle tone.

Microflora. Many bacteria, called microflora, have been identified in the large intestine, some performing important roles. Some of these organisms can break down substances that human enzymes are unable to digest; others synthesize vitamins needed by humans. Vitamin K, vitamin B_{12}, biotin, thiamin, and riboflavin are produced in this manner. Obtaining vitamin K is especially important in this way since quantities in the food supply are normally insufficient for adequate blood coagulation. The types of food eaten and medications taken influence the activity and relative numbers of bacteria. Bacterial activity produces various gases that contribute to flatus in the colon. Fecal odor is a result of the compounds produced by these bacteria.

Peristalsis. The large intestine is inactive for a large proportion of the time and the contents are moved at a very slow rate. After chyme enters the large intestine, it takes about 18 hours to reach the distal colon. The purpose of peristalsis in the large intestine is to force the feces into the rectum. These large waves occur only two to three times daily.

Clinical Implications:

- Feces retained in the large intestine too long allows more reabsorption of water and becomes hard and dry. Constipation can be treated by increasing the fluid intake or by increasing the nondigestible materials in the diet.
- The frequency of bowel movements is an individual matter, and patterns can vary from after each meal to once every two days.
- Antibiotic therapy normally kills the bacteria in the colon and inhibits bacterial production of vitamins.

Factors Affecting Digestion and Absorption

Digestibility. Ordinarily, when people talk about digestibility, they are referring to the comfort or ease of digestion, and how fast the food is removed from the intestine. However, digestibility also can mean the completeness of digestion. Some foods contain nutrients that cannot be digested and that pass through the gastrointestinal tract unabsorbed. Foods rich in fiber are digested more slowly and leave more residue than foods containing no fiber.

The coefficient of digestibility is a measure of food absorbed as compared to the amount consumed. (If the feces contains three percent protein, the coefficient of digestibility is 97 percent.) Approximately 92 to 97 percent of American diets is digested and absorbed (Table 4–6). Absorption for the energy nutrients is greater than that for the vitamins and minerals. If the nutrients are properly digested, absorption rates are as follows: carbohydrate, 97 percent; fat, 95 percent; and protein, 92 percent.

Usually, the process of cooking food makes food easier to digest. For instance, toasting bread begins the breakdown of the starch molecule. Cooking also enhances the digestibility of some foods, such as egg whites.

The rate of digestion is affected by how well the food is broken apart. If food is not well-chewed, it is more difficult to digest and consequently takes longer to pass through the intestinal tract. Liquid foods are absorbed faster than solid ones because digestive juices are rapidly mixed and can interact with all the molecules. Bowel habits, stress, exercise, colonic anatomy, and diet

Table 4—6. Percent Digestibility of Nutrients*

Food Group	Protein	Fat	Carbohydrate
Animal foods	97%	95%	98%
Cereals	85%	90%	98%
Legumes, dried	78%	90%	97%
Sugars and starches			98%
Vegetables	83%	90%	95%
Fruits	85%	90%	90%
Vegetable foods	84%	90%	97%
Total food†	92%	95%	97%

*From Merrill, AL; Watts, BK: *Energy Value of Foods—Basis and Derivation.* Washington, DC, U.S. Department of Agriculture, Handbook No. 74, 1955.
†Weighted by consumption statistics based on a survey of 185 dietaries.

(especially the amount of fiber) are different in each individual and are important factors that affect the rate of transit through the gut.

Other factors affecting digestion and absorption are as important to nutritional status as adequate intake: (1) The amount of the nutrient consumed; (2) physiological need; (3) the condition of the digestive tract, such as the amount of secretions, motility, and absorptive surface; (4) the level of circulating hormones; (5) the presence of other nutrients ingested at the same time that enhance or interfere with absorption; and (6) the presence of adequate amounts of digestive enzymes.

Psychological Influences. Not only is food selection affected by psychological factors, but also the utilization of nutrients is affected. Adequate production of digestive secretions is essential for hydrolysis of foods. Sadness, depression, fear, or pain may decrease gastric secretions; stress, anger, and aggression may increase them. If motility is increased, such as in diarrhea, nutrients are not exposed to digestive secretions and absorptive surfaces long enough for maximum absorption.

Physical Problems. Digestion and absorption are also affected by physical problems. For instance, a person who has lost his/her teeth is unable to chew foods properly and may avoid some foods completely. If a person has an inflamed or irritated mucosal surface, the absorptive area is decreased.

Metabolism

Metabolism can be defined as the continuous processes whereby living organisms and cells con-

vert nutrients into energy, body structure, and waste. In metabolic activity, the two major types of chemical reactions are catabolism and anabolism. Catabolism is the process in which complex substances are broken down into simpler substances. The phase of metabolism in which the absorbed products—glucose, amino acids, and fats—are oxidized to yield energy is called catabolism. Reactions in which the absorbed nutrients are used by the cell to build or synthesize more complex compounds is known as anabolism. These reactions require energy. Examples of this activity are building new muscle tissue, bone, or cellular secretions such as hormones.

Anabolism and catabolism are continuous reactions in the body. All cells in the epithelial lining of the gastrointestinal mucosa are replaced about every three to five days (Iber, 1980). In spite of this rapid turnover, the amount of catabolism is usually equal to the anabolism. This is referred to as dynamic equilibrium. During certain stages of life, such as growth periods or pregnancy, more anabolism is occurring than catabolism. When illness or stress occur, excessive catabolism is evident.

Other phases of metabolism include delivery of nutrients to the cells where they are needed and wastes to the sites where they can be excreted, respiration, utilization of the absorbed products by the cells, and excretion of wastes. The end products of catabolism of carbohydrates, proteins, and fats are carbon dioxide, water, and energy. (Nitrogen is an additional end product of protein.)

The Liver. The major distributing organ of foodstuffs to the body is the liver, which regulates the kinds and quantities of nutrients in the bloodstream. Substances absorbed from the intestines into the capillaries of the villi go directly to the liver (except for the fat-soluble substances, which go through the lymphatic system). The liver is a very complex chemical factory and a minor storage facility as well as a controller of nutrients in the circulating blood.

All monosaccharides are converted to glucose in the liver, because glucose is the major energy supply for cells. Glucose is maintained in the bloodstream at a certain level; the excess is stored as glycogen. Glycogen can be broken down to glucose and put into the circulating blood as needed.

Other end products of digestion may be either oxidized to provide energy, converted to glucose, protein, fat, or other substances, or released to circulate at prescribed levels in the blood to be used by cells throughout the body.

Within the cell, the energy-yielding products of digestion—glucose, fatty acids, and amino acids—can be utilized via a common pathway to yield energy called the Krebs or tricarboxylic acid (TCA) cycle (Fig. 4–8). The energy-releasing process is performed in the mitochondria of cells. Simple molecules are hydrolyzed into smaller pieces by a complex process that releases energy, which is stored in a high-energy molecule called adenosine triphosphate (ATP). ATP moves out of the mitochondria and becomes a ready supply of energy for the cell. Waste products—carbon dioxide and water—are removed from the body through the lungs and kidneys, respectively.

Absorbed vitamins and minerals are important for the reactions to proceed within the Krebs cycle and for other processes that allow the release of energy. In a sense, it can be said that metabolism of the energy nutrients is regulated and controlled by cellular enzymes and hormones.

The Krebs cycle, which converts carbohydrates, proteins, and fats to a utilizable form of energy, requires many enzymes. For the activity of some of these enzymes, an additional factor must be present. Some B vitamins function as coenzymes in the Krebs cycle. As such, it is a prosthetic group attached to the enzyme protein. The protein part of the enzyme is called the apoenzyme, and the nonprotein part (a vitamin in this instance) is called a coenzyme. An enzyme may also require a mineral or electrolyte, called a cofactor to function.

Anabolism involves utilizing carbohydrates, proteins, and fats to build the various substances that make up the body itself and the other substances necessary for the body. These nutrients are intertwined in this ability and frequently require the presence of vitamins and minerals. Ordinarily, amino acids are used to build proteins; still, some oxidative products of glucose can combine with amine groups to form amino acids. Fatty acids can be produced from glucose. To put it mildly, the body is a very complex system.

Kidney. The kidney performs an important metabolic task of removing waste products in the urine, and along with the liver, controls the amount of many nutrients in the circulating blood. Metabolic end products from the cells, unnecessary substances absorbed from the gastrointestinal tract, and potentially harmful compounds that have been detoxified by the liver are all excreted by the kidney.

The kidneys accomplish this by a process of filtration and reabsorption. Tubules in the kidneys are capable of conserving certain nutrients (glucose, amino acids, vitamins, and various min-

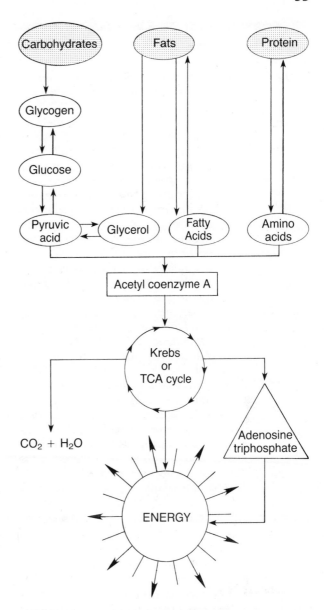

Figure 4–8. Central pathways of metabolism: How the body produces energy from the energy-containing nutrients using the Krebs or tricarboxylic acid (TCA) cycle.

eral ions) by reabsorbing them from the filtrate if they are needed or excreting them in the urine if they are not needed. In this way, kidneys help maintain a balance of the nutrients within the body.

Other routes of excretion of waste products are the bowel, which has already been discussed, the skin, which excretes water and electrolytes, and the lungs, which remove carbon dioxide and water.

• FALLACIES and FACTS

FALLACY: *Enzyme and hormone tablets can be taken as a supplement to replenish any deficiency.*

• **FACT:** *These substances are not absorbed intact from the intestinal tract. Enzymes and hormones are proteins built from amino acids. The process of digestion hydrolyzes the enzyme protein as it would any other protein. When gastrointestinal enzymes are needed (pancreatic insufficiency), enzymes are enterically coated so the contents are not released until they reach the intestine. Enzymes utilized by other parts of the body would be broken down to amino acids before absorption.*

FALLACY: *Foods that are fully digested do not cause weight gain. Enzymes cannot work simultaneously, causing undigested foods to accumulate and become fat.*

• **FACT:** *Enzymes present in the gastrointestinal tract must be able to work simultaneously for absorption. Otherwise, only nutritionally pure foods would be absorbed; few exist naturally. Foods not digested and absorbed are excreted in the stool, supplying no calories. Only digested foods have the potential of providing energy (Mirkin & Shore, 1981).*

Summary

The process of furnishing nutrients for utilization by the body first begins with the ingestion of foods, which can be physiologically affected by the senses of taste and smell. No matter how nutritious a food is, if it is not eaten, it cannot benefit the body.

The gastrointestinal tract is responsible for digesting the ingested foodstuffs into products the body can absorb and utilize. This can be accomplished by the mechanical actions and chemical secretions in the intestinal tract and accessory organs. Many factors, including psychological and hormonal factors, can affect how well the food is digested and absorbed.

The liver, the gatekeeper of metabolism, receives all the nutrients and oversees the transport of the nutrients to the cells where they are needed and of waste products to the organs where they can be excreted. The cells can metabolize the end products from the "energy nutrients" for the energy needed to perform their tasks, a process that requires the presence of certain vitamins and minerals.

Review Questions

1. Make a chart or diagram showing the gastrointestinal secretions, where they are produced, and their digestive actions on the nutrients present in milk. Homogenized milk contains the following: disaccharide, lactose, proteins, emulsified fats, calcium, riboflavin and vitamins A and D. Where would the end products be absorbed?
2. Define metabolism, catabolism, anabolism, enzyme, and coenzyme.
3. Your patient tells you "I just can't drink orange juice; it's too acid for my stomach." Knowing that the stomach has a pH of about 2, and the pH of orange juice is about 3.6, how would you handle the situation?
4. When bile production or secretion is decreased, which enzyme(s) are most affected?
5. If someone were feeling weak or faint from the lack of food, what types of food would you advise to quickly alleviate the symptoms?
6. If caloric intake were equal, which of the following breakfasts would probably postpone the feeling of hunger the longest?
    (1) Dry cereal with skim milk, toast with jelly, and coffee with sugar.
    (2) Egg with ham, toast with butter, and coffee with cream.
7. What are the absorbable products resulting from the digestion of carbohydrates, proteins, and fats?
8. Within what section of the alimentary canal does most of the digestion and absorption take place?

REFERENCE LIST

Bach, AC; Babayan, VK: Medium-chain triglycerides: an update. *Am J Clin Nutr* 36(5):950, 1982.
Bell, GH; Emslie-Smith, D; Paterson, CR: *Textbook of Physiology and Biochemistry*, 9th ed. New York, Churchill Livingstone, 1976.

Burks, TF; Galligan, JJ; Porreca, F; et al: Regulation of gastric emptying. *Fed Proc* 44(14):2897, 1985.

Fein, HD: Nutrition in diseases of the stomach. In *Modern Nutrition in Health and Disease*, 6th ed. Edited by RS Goodhart; ME Shils. Philadelphia, Lea & Febiger, 1980, p 892.

Feldman, EJ; Isenberg, JI; Grossman, MI: Gastric acid and gastrin response to decaffeinated coffee and a peptone meal. *JAMA* 246(3):248, 1981.

Hollander, D: Intestinal absorption of vitamins A, E, D, and K. *J Lab Clin Med* 97(4):449, 1981.

Iber, FL: The gastrointestinal tract: an overview of function. In *Modern Nutrition in Health and Disease*, 6th ed. Edited by RS Goodhart; ME Shils. Philadelphia, Lea & Febiger, 1980, p 35.

Ingelfinger, FJ: Gastric function. *Nutr Today* 6(5):2, 1971.

Levinsky, RJ: Food antigen handling by the gut. *J Trop Pediatr* 27(1):1, 1981.

Mirkin, GB; Shore, RN: The Beverly Hills diet. *JAMA* 246 (19):2235, 1981.

Pike, RL; Brown, ML: *Nutrition: An Integrated Approach*, 3rd ed. New York, J. Wiley & Sons, 1984.

Schiffman, SS: Taste and smell in disease (Part I). *N Engl J Med* 308(21):1275, 1983.

Weiner, K; Graham, LS; Reedy, T; et al: Simultaneous gastric emptying of two solid foods. *Gastroenterology* 81(2):257, 1981.

Further Study

Corman, ML; Veidenheimer, MC; Coller, JA: Cathartics. *Am J Nurs* 75(2):273, 1975.

Given, BA; Simmons, SJ: *Gastroenterology in Clinical Nursing*, 4th ed. St. Louis, The C.V. Mosby Co, 1984.

Hoppe, MC; Descalso, J; Kapp, SR: Gastrointestinal disease: nutritional implications. *Nurs Clin North Am* 18(1):47, 1983.

Ingelfinger, FJ: Gastrointestinal absorption. *Nutr Today* 2(1):2, 1967.

Ingelfinger, FJ: How to swallow and belch and cope with heartburn. *Nutr Today* 8(1):4, 1973.

McCormack, A; Itkin, J; Cloud, C: Correcting acid-base imbalance. *RN* 48(5):29, 1985.

Schiffman, SS: Taste and smell in disease. *N Engl J Med* 308 (22):1337, 1983.

Schiffman, SS: Recent findings about taste: important implications. *Cereal Foods World* 31(4):300, 1986.

Prerequisites: Fluid and Electrolyte Balance

5

OBJECTIVES

THE STUDENT WILL BE ABLE TO:

- **Recognize the importance of the nursing tasks in maintaining a patient's fluid balance.**
- **Explain water and electrolyte balance.**
- **List sources of fluids available to the body other than water.**
- **Describe how osmolality of a fluid can affect hydration status.**
- **Explain the fluid imbalances leading to edema and dehydration.**
- **Explain why foods are acid-forming or base-forming.**

TERMS TO KNOW

Acid ash
Acidosis
Aldosterone
Alkaline ash
Alkalosis
Anions
Buffer
Cations
Dehydration
Edema
Electrolyte
Extracellular fluid
Hypertonic
Hypotonic
Insensible perspiration
Interstitial fluid
Intracellular fluid
Intravascular fluid
Ions
Milliequivalents (mEq)
Milliosmole (mOsm)
Osmoreceptors
Osmotic pressure
pH
Rehydration
Water intoxication
Water of metabolism

Without water, life as we know it would not exist. It is essential in all biochemical processes. Water is a chief constituent of living cells, and survival requires a "sea" surrounding each cell. The body may survive for weeks without food; a few days without water can be fatal.

Information obtained from a physical history and examination (listed in *Focus on Assessing Hydration Status*) will help assess a patient's state of hydration or fluid balance. Nurses are continually performing many tasks to determine a patient's hydration status:

- Recording daily weight (240 cc water = ½ lb.).
- Recording fluid intake and output (urine, stool, vomitus, drainage).
- Monitoring laboratory values to confirm any abnormal signs evidenced in physical examination or records.

Functions of Water

Water is the most abundant component in the body; only with adequate water supplies does the body function at its optimal capacity. Its physiological roles consist of:

- Acting as a solvent for many chemicals in the body.
- Enabling chemical reactions to occur by actually entering into some reactions, such as hydrolysis.
- Maintaining the stability of all body fluids, being the main component and medium for fluids, secretions, and excretions—such as, blood, lymph, gastric secretions, urine, and perspiration.
- Enabling nutrients to be transported to the cells and providing a medium for excretion of waste products.
- Acting as a lubricant or buffer between cells to permit movement without friction.
- Regulating body temperature by evaporating perspiration from the skin.

DISTRIBUTION OF WATER

Water represents 50 to 60 percent of the total body weight in an adult; a healthy adult weighing 150 lbs. carries about 82 lbs. of water (or 10 gallons)! Body tissues contain various amounts of muscle tissue (80 percent), fat tissue (20 percent), and bone (25 percent).

FOCUS ON ASSESSING HYDRATION STATUS*

A. Medical History
   1. Certain diseases can disrupt fluid balance (diabetes mellitus, emphysema) and can determine the type of imbalance.
   2. Medications can disrupt fluid balance (steroids or diuretics).
   3. Abnormal losses of body fluids, such as:
      a. Diarrhea.
      b. Vomiting.
      c. Profuse sweating.
      d. Fever.
      e. Blood loss.
   4. Dietary restrictions can affect fluid losses (low sodium, low carbohydrate).
   5. Recent fluid and food intake.
   6. Fluid output in the last 24 hours (number of times voided, diarrheal episodes).
   7. Thirst (whether present or absent).
B. Clinical Observations
   1. Body temperature.
   2. Pulse rate.
   3. Respiration.
   4. Blood pressure.
   5. Skin and mucous membrane moisture.
   6. Edema.
   7. Weight loss or gain.

This information should be carefully considered along with certain laboratory data to determine the hydration status of a patient.

---

*Data from Metheny, NM; Snively, WD, Jr: *Nurses' Handbook of Fluid Balance*, 4th ed. Philadelphia, J. B. Lippincott Co, 1983.

Individuals with a higher percentage of muscle tissue (lean individuals) have a larger percent of body water. Thus, women with their larger fat stores have 50 to 54 percent body water, whereas men have 60 to 70 percent (Table 5–1). Since the storage of protein as muscle tissue is associated with water, when muscle tissue is being catabolized, it will be associated with rapid weight loss.

Infants have a much larger proportion of body water, about 75 percent. Because such a large percentage of the infant's body is water, fluid loss is more significant. Total body water decreases with age, as can be seen from Table 5–1. Due to the lack of water reserves in geriatric patients, close monitoring for signs of fluid loss is important.

Body fluids are distributed within two major

Table 5–1. Body Water as Percentage of Body Weight for Sex and Age

Age	Male	Female
Newborn*	77	77
6 months*	72	72
2 years*	60	60
10–18 years†	59	57
18–40 years†	61	51
40–60 years†	55	47
Over 60 years†	52	26

*Data from Sorensen, KC; Luckmann, J: *Basic Nursing: A Psychophysiologic Approach*, 2nd ed. Philadelphia, W. B. Saunders Co, 1986.
†Data from Edelman, IS; Leibman, J: Anatomy of body water and electrolytes. *American Journal of Medicine* 27(2):257, 1959.

compartments (Fig. 5–1). Fluids can move between compartments through semipermeable membranes. This movement is regulated so that the distribution remains stable.

Intracellular fluid is all the water within the cell, chiefly contained in muscle tissue. This represents at least one half of total body water. Extracellular fluid is all the water outside the cells, representing the body's transportation system.

Extracellular fluid can be subdivided into two categories: intravascular fluid is the water within the blood vessels, or plasma; interstitial fluid is the water in the tissues between the vascular spaces.

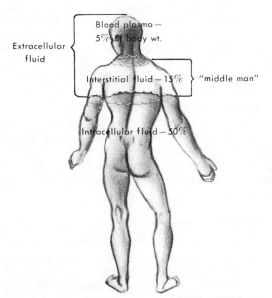

Figure 5–1. Fluid compartments of the body. (From Dienhart CM: Basic Human Anatomy and Physiology, 3rd ed. Philadelphia, W. B. Saunders Co, 1979, by permission.)

Clinical Implication:

- Rapid weight loss generally indicates loss of water rather than fatty tissue since 480 cc (2 cups) of fluid results in a weight loss of one pound.

FLUID INTAKE

Water must be supplied regularly for metabolic use and to compensate for body losses. The most obvious source of water for the body is the ingestion of liquids (Fig. 5–2). Since water is a constituent of all cells, solid foods also contribute a sizable amount of water. Surprisingly, some fruits and vegetables have a higher percentage of water than milk, and meats are more than half water. Table 5–2 shows percentages of water found in different foods.

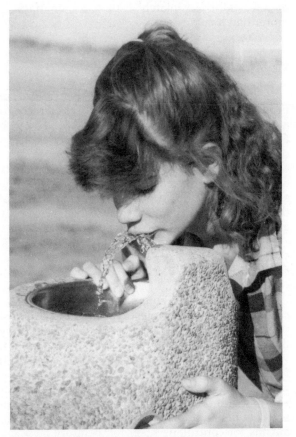

Figure 5–2. Fluid requirements rank second to our oxygen requirements. Water can provide some essential electrolytes and must be protected from environmental pollutants. (Courtesy of F. Davis, photographer.)

Table 5–2. Percentage of Water in Foods*

Food	Percent Water
Fruits and vegetables	70–99
Milk	88
Eggs	75
Cooked meats	50–70
Hard cheese	37–40
Bread	35
Margarine and butter	16
Nuts	5
Dry cereals and crackers	4
Shortening, oils, and sugar	0

*Data from Nutritive Value of Foods, *U.S. Department of Agriculture, Home Garden Bull No. 72*, Washington, DC, 1964.

Additionally, in the process of metabolism, some water is liberated and available to the body when solid foods are oxidized. This water, derived from foodstuffs, is called water of metabolism. The metabolism of fats produces approximately twice as much water as the metabolism of carbohydrates or proteins. Water supplied in this manner is approximately 300 to 350 ml/day, or more than a cup.

WATER ABSORPTION

No digestion is necessary for water absorption; it is transported freely in both directions across the intestinal mucosa by osmosis. As much as 1 L can be absorbed from the small intestine in one hour.

As mentioned in Chapter 4, approximately 8 L of digestive secretions are transferred into the alimentary canal daily. Normally, almost all of this plus the fluid intake is reabsorbed, with only about 100 ml being excreted in the feces daily.

NORMAL WATER LOSSES

Water normally enters the body only by absorption in the gastrointestinal tract, but it is lost through a variety of routes: (1) urine excreted by the kidneys, (2) perspiration from the skin, (3) water vapor in expired air from the lungs, and (4) feces from the bowel.

Insensible water loss is continuous and constant even though a person is not aware of it. Insensible perspiration is a part of the body's mechanisms for controlling body temperature.

Water losses in the form of sweat can vary greatly. An increase in body temperature is accompanied by increased sweating and loss of body heat. Strenuous exercise can greatly increase the amount of perspiration excreted, resulting in a fluid loss of up to 4 L per hour. Each liter of perspiration represents a heat loss of about 600 kcal. When large amounts of sweat are lost, the body compensates by producing less urine.

Water lost from the lungs is proportional to the rate of respiration. Strenuous exercise and fevers normally increase the rate of respiration and account for higher-than-normal water losses.

Losses from the urine and feces are more obvious. The amount of urine depends on the amount of fluid intake and the type of diet eaten. Waste products must be kept in solution, requiring a minimum of obligatory excretion of about 400 to 600 ml urine daily (Randall, 1980).

Protein metabolism produces larger quantities of waste products than other energy-yielding nutrients; a high-protein diet, which is popular for reducing and sports activities, increases the minimum amount of urine necessary to eliminate higher levels of waste products.

Beverages containing caffeine (coffee, tea, many cola drinks, and cocoa) increase urine production. An alcoholic beverage consisting of one ounce of pure alcohol requires eight ounces water for its metabolism. Therefore, alcohol will frequently cause a dehydration effect, usually resulting in increased thirst.

WATER BALANCE

Balance denotes a state of equilibrium, as when fluid intake is equal to the amount excreted. Figure 5–3 shows the average amounts of fluid intake required to balance the amounts excreted. Health and a feeling of well-being is dependent on water balance. Two mechanisms, the sensation of thirst and the role of the kidneys, ordinarily are able to maintain this equilibrium.

The amounts shown in the Figure 5–3 can be drastically changed in different climatic environments, with different levels of exercise, or with illnesses such as diarrhea or vomiting. The body cannot store water, so the amount lost must be replaced.

Clinical Implications:

- Water intake and loss are well-balanced by body mechanisms, and body weight fluctuates one to two percent on a daily weight basis (Randall, 1980).
- Inadequate water intake for optimal digestive functioning may result in constipation.

- One should be aware of clinical signs of a negative water balance to avoid the hazards associated with dehydration (especially decreased urinary output).
- Clinical manifestations of water balance are (1) normal serum sodium concentration, and (2) a 24-hour intake of 2500 cc balanced by an equal amount of output. These are notoriously inaccurate though, considering preformed metabolic sources of water and obligatory insensitive water losses. The 24-hour intake must provide for 500 cc urine excretion daily.
- Insensible water loss equals approximately 1000 ml/m² of body surface area daily for bedfast patients. This amount is higher if respiration is increased or when fever is present. If heavy perspiration losses necessitate clothing and bed linen changes, this information should be recorded in intake/output charting.

RECOMMENDED ALLOWANCE OF WATER

The adult requirement is about 1 ml/kcal. This requirement is based on the following favorable conditions: low-solute diet (not extremely high in salt or protein), minimum physical activity, and no obvious sweating. A diet of 2000 kcal would require 2000 ml, or at least 8 cups of fluid per day.

Infants require a greater proportion of water than adults. In addition to their greater body surface area, basal heat production per kilogram is twice as high in the infant as in the adult. Because of their greater metabolic rate, production of waste products and urine is larger. Therefore, the requirement for infants is about 150 ml/100 kcal. With fluid loss or insufficient intake, the infant becomes depleted more rapidly than an adult.

Electrolytes

Water balance cannot be complete without some knowledge of electrolytes, because the two are always interrelated. Compounds that dissociate in solution (become separate particles) are known as ions. Ions have either a positive or neg-

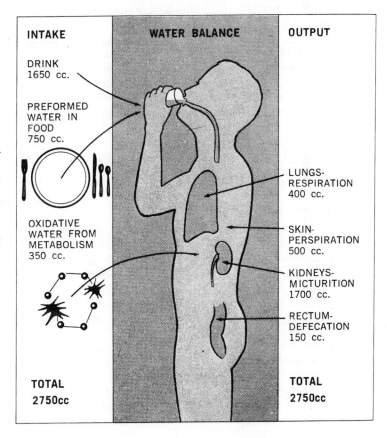

Figure 5–3. Man maintains the osmotic pressure of his body fluids at optimum level by adjusting his water intake and output. Most of his need of water comes from the liquid itself. Some he draws from the moisture in his food, and the remainder he manufactures himself. The importance of this "water of oxidation" varies according to species: the kangaroo rat, for example, drinks no water at all. His water need, proportionately the same as man's, is met by the moisture in his diet and that which he manufactures himself. (From Robinson JR: Water, the indispensable nutrient. Nutrition Today 5(spring):22, 1970. Reproduced with permission of Nutrition Today Magazine, P.O. Box 1829, Annapolis, MD 21404.)

INTAKE

DRINK 1650 cc.

PREFORMED WATER IN FOOD 750 cc.

OXIDATIVE WATER FROM METABOLISM 350 cc.

TOTAL 2750cc

WATER BALANCE

OUTPUT

LUNGS-RESPIRATION 400 cc.

SKIN-PERSPIRATION 500 cc.

KIDNEYS-MICTURITION 1700 cc.

RECTUM-DEFECATION 150 cc.

TOTAL 2750cc

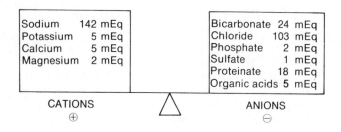

Sodium	142 mEq
Potassium	5 mEq
Calcium	5 mEq
Magnesium	2 mEq

Bicarbonate	24 mEq
Chloride	103 mEq
Phosphate	2 mEq
Sulfate	1 mEq
Proteinate	18 mEq
Organic acids	5 mEq

CATIONS ⊕   ANIONS ⊖

Figure 5–4. When their weights are written in milliequivalents, the cations and anions of extracellular fluid approximately balance each other. (From Sorensen KC, Luckmann J: Basic Nursing: A Psychophysiologic Approach. Philadelphia, W. B. Saunders Co, 1979, by permission.)

ative electrical charge and are known as electrolytes. Cations are positively charged (Na^+, K^+, Ca^{++}, Mg^{++}), and anions have a negative charge (Cl^-, HCO_3^-, HPO_4^{--}, SO_4^{--})

Water molecules, having both a positive and a negative side, orient themselves around ions, preventing the union of these oppositely charged particles. The number of cations present in a solution is equal to the number of anions. Electrolytes are important in both water balance and acid-base balance.

Electrolyte concentration in blood plasma is expressed in milliequivalents (mEq). Milliequivalents measure the chemical combining power of electrolytes in solution. For instance, potassium (K^+) can combine with one chloride (Cl^-) ion, or calcium (Ca^{++}) can combine with two chloride ions. When concentrations of ions in fluids are expressed in terms of milliequivalents per liter, the number of anions equals the number of cations (Fig. 5–4). In other words, milliequivalents measure the number of ionic charges present.

Since direct measurement of the total amount of body water is not possible, it is indirectly measured by serum concentrations of sodium. If body water is decreased, serum electrolytes will be elevated. This information must be interpreted by also looking at physiological and clinical signs, such as vomiting or decreased food intake.

ELECTROLYTES IN BODY FLUIDS

Normal electrolyte distribution is different in extracellular fluid than interstitial fluid (Fig. 5–5). Plasma and interstitial fluid electrolyte patterns are similar. Electrolyte concentrations, while quite different, are maintained within very narrow ranges. Changes in one compartment are reflected in changes in the other.

The principal cation in plasma and interstitial fluid is sodium; the principal anion is chloride. The principal cation in intracellular fluid is potassium; the principal anion is phosphate. The main difference between intravascular and interstitial fluids is the large amount of proteins in plasma.

OSMOTIC PRESSURE

As previously mentioned, cell walls in the body are semipermeable membranes. This allows water to flow into or out of the cell in order to equalize osmotic pressure or salt concentration of the intracellular and extracellular fluids. For instance, if the salt concentration on one side of the membrane is too concentrated, it is said to be hypertonic, and water is drawn from the area containing less salt to an area of higher concentration in order to equalize pressure on both sides of the semipermeable membrane (see Fig. 4–7). Osmotic pressure is directly proportional to the number of particles present. Therefore, the osmotic pressure of a solution can be calculated by adding up all the ions it contains.

Milliosmole. The milliosmole (mOsm) measures the osmotic activity of a solution, not the number of ionic charges. The milliosmole value for monovalent ions is the same as the milliequivalent value; the milliosmole value for multiple valence ions is the milliequivalent value divided by the valence number.

Substances that cannot easily pass through a cell membrane have the greatest influence on osmotic pressure. Proteins have an effect on osmotic pressure, but sodium and potassium electrolytes

Table 5–3. Plasma Chemical Constituents: Average Values in Health*

Constituent	Normal Range
Na^+	135–145 mEq/L
K^+	3.5–5.0 mEq/L
Ca^{++}	9–11 mg %
Mg^{++}	1.4–2.3 mEq/L
Cl^-	98–106 mEq/L
HCO_3^-	Adults: 25–29 mEq/L
	Children: 20–25 mEq/L
$HPO_4^=$	1.7–2.6 mEq/L
Protein	6–8 gm/100 ml
pH	7.35–7.45

*From Sorensen, KC; Luckmann, J: Basic Nursing: A Psychophysiologic Approach, 2nd ed. Philadelphia, W. B. Saunders Co, 1986, by permission.

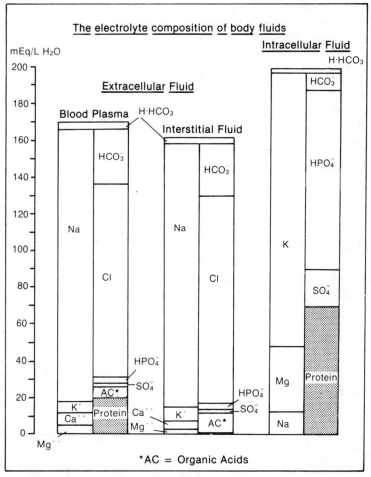

Figure 5–5. *A comparison of the electrolyte composition of the extracellular and intracellular fluid compartments. (From Sorensen KC, Luckmann J:* Basic Nursing: A Psychophysiologic Approach, *2nd ed. Philadelphia, W. B. Saunders Co, 1986. Adapted and reprinted by permission from Gamble JL:* Chemical Anatomy, Physiology and Pathology of Extracellular Fluid. *Cambridge, MA, Harvard University Press, 1947.)*

have the greatest control of body water volume and shifts of water into and out of cells.

Osmolality of body fluids is approximately 300 mOsm/L. Serum osmolality is another reliable measurement of hydration status. It usually increases with dehydration and decreases with water excess. Normal amounts of serum components that reflect hydration status are shown in Table 5–3. The body attempts to keep the contents of the gastrointestinal tract at this level also. Table 5–4 lists the osmolality of some common foodstuffs frequently given during gastrointestinal upsets or dehydration problems.

The *size* of the particle determines the *number* of particles present at a given concentration. For instance, a solution of disaccharides containing the same number of calories as a glucose solution

Table 5–4. *Approximate Osmolality of Some Common Foods**

Food	mOsm/L Water
Ginger ale	510
Gelatin dessert	535
Tomato juice	595
7-Up	640
Coca-Cola	680
Eggnog	695
Apple juice	870
Orange juice	935
Malted milk	940
Ice cream	1150
Grape juice	1170
Sherbet	1225

*From American Dietetic Association: *Handbook of Clinical Dietetics.* New Haven, Yale University Press, 1981.

would contain half as many particles. Hence, the solution with fewer particles (disaccharides) would have a lower osmotic pressure. Simple sugars are very small particles and increase the osmolality of a solution. Complex carbohydrates are larger and have a lower osmolality.

Most plasma osmolality is contributed by the ionized electrolytes Na^+, K^+, and Cl^-. Small particles (glucose, electrolytes, and free amino acids) contribute more to osmolality than do large particles (proteins, fats, or carbohydrates). Because of their insolubility in water, fats do not increase the osmolality of solutions. Proteins and all electrolytes, such as sodium and potassium, contribute significantly to the osmolality of a solution.

Clinical Implication:

- The osmolality of fluids has significant effects when enteral feedings or total parenteral feedings are utilized (see Chapter 21).

Regulation of Fluid and Electrolyte Balance

REGULATION OF WATER INTAKE

Thirst is the primary regulator of water intake. When as much as two percent of body water is lost, osmoreceptors, located in the hypothala-mus of the brain, are stimulated by increased osmotic pressure. Thirst is associated with decreased salivary flow and drying of the mouth; it creates a physiological desire to ingest liquids. This occurs when cells become dehydrated because of decreased extracellular fluid volume.

REGULATION OF WATER OUTPUT

Urinary excretion by the kidneys is dependent on the extracellular fluid concentration and volume of the interstitial fluid. The osmoreceptor system, especially sensitive to fluid volume, is activated by increased osmotic pressure in the body fluid, signaling the release of antidiuretic hormone (ADH) from the pituitary gland. Fluid output by the kidney is decreased by increasing water reabsorption, thereby conserving body fluids. Conversely, when ADH is not present because of adequate fluid intake, the tubule remains relatively impermeable to water and is excreted (Fig. 5–6).

In summation, when an individual works or exercises hard and consequently sweats a lot, s/he becomes thirsty and drinks liquids. A diet high in salty, dried foods, or concentrated sugars (candy) can also cause thirst. If excessive water or beverages are consumed, the kidney is fast to respond by increasing urinary volume.

Clinical Implications:

- Intravenous feedings (IVs) with electrolytes (see Chapter 21) are alternative therapies that are

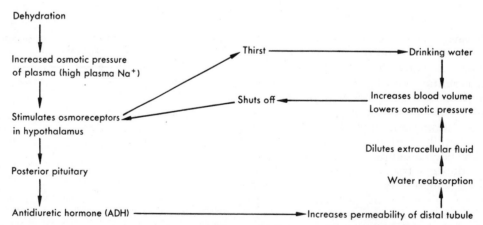

Figure 5–6. The regulation of water balance by thirst and antidiuretic hormone mechanisms. (Reprinted by permission of Macmillan Publishing Company from Normal and Therapeutic Nutrition, 16th ed. by E. R. Robinson and M. R. Lawler. Copyright © 1982 by Macmillan Publishing Co, Inc.)

frequently necessary for maintaining or correcting fluid and electrolyte imbalances.

- Antidiuretic hormone (ADH) deficiency may result from head trauma, surgery, or a tumor in the region of the hypothalamus and pituitary gland. Large volumes of diluted urine and great thirst accompanied by ingestion of large volumes of water may ensue.
- Insufficient water intake results when fluids are unavailable or when the individual cannot or does not respond to the thirst stimulus (due to some diseases and drugs). Individuals need to be encouraged to pay attention to the thirst mechanism.
- Comatose or confused patients may not be thirsty even when dehydrated.
- Dehydration is frequently observed in the elderly because their thirst mechanism may be depressed or absent and/or because the kidneys are unable to concentrate the urine.

ELECTROLYTE INTAKE AND ABSORPTION

Electrolytes (sodium and potassium) are naturally available from foods and fluids regularly ingested. Therefore, adequate intake is no problem unless requirements are increased, such as in diuretic therapy or heavy exercise. When body mechanisms are altered, intake must be decreased.

Because sodium and potassium are so plentiful, no RDAs have been established. The body requirement for sodium is between 500 to 1000 mg daily; estimated intake is about 2400 to 7200 mg sodium. Suggestions have been made that Americans should curtail their sodium intake (see Chapter 14). Table salt is 40 percent sodium and 60 percent chlorine. One teaspoon of salt contains approximately 2000 mg sodium. Body sodium levels are maintained at 144 mEq/L. Yet, serum sodium concentration is an index of water deficit or excess, not an index of sodium deficit or excess.

Some electrolytes are excreted from the body in the form of perspiration. Since sweat contains 50 to 100 mEq/L of sodium (half the amount found in blood), the Committee on Dietary Allowances recommends that salt intake be increased when sweat losses are more than 4 L. This would mean a weight loss of 8 lbs. The recommendation is two grams (less than a teaspoon) of table salt for each liter of sweat lost (or 2 pounds weight loss). Americans generally add this much to their food without having to take salt tablets. When a sodium deficit exists, the natural response is to desire salty foods or to salt foods more heavily than usual. Foods obviously high in salt are chips, salted popcorn and nuts, pickles, olives, steak sauce, mustard, soy sauce, bouillon, and canned soups.

The RDA committee has estimated the body's daily need for potassium to be about 2500 mg. Since usual intake is between 2000 and 4000 mg, intake of potassium is not a problem. The potassium content or oranges, bananas, dried fruits, fruit juices, potatoes, meats and nuts is high. However, high or low values of serum potassium are life-threatening and require immediate attention.

Monovalent electrolytes (sodium, potassium, chloride, nitrate, and bicarbonate) are absorbed more rapidly in the upper small intestine than in the distal portion. Sodium and potassium are absorbed regardless of the amount already in the body.

REGULATION OF ELECTROLYTE BALANCE

While some electrolytes are lost in perspiration, most are excreted in the urine. The regulation of the principal electrolyte in extracellular fluid (sodium) is controlled by the hormone aldosterone, which is secreted by the adrenal cortex when blood volume is decreased. The kidney tubules then reabsorb more sodium. When the sodium concentration in the blood deviates from normal, aldosterone secretion is inversely affected so that normal sodium serum levels are maintained by conservation or excretion of sodium in the urine (Fig. 5–7). If adequate amounts of water are ingested, it is difficult to overload the body with salt in healthy individuals.

Potassium, which is positively charged like sodium, is absorbed or excreted along with sodium ions. So, when large amounts of sodium are excreted, as with some types of diuretics, large amounts of potassium are also excreted. The body will retain sodium in an attempt to maintain fluid volume if excessive amounts are lost by routes other than the kidneys.

Clinical Implications:

- Few electrolytes are lost during imperceptible perspiration loss.
- When vomiting is persistent, water should be withheld because vomiting carries gastric secretions with it (Metheny & Snively, 1983).
- Without a physician's approval, water or ice chips are withheld from a patient receiving gastrointestinal suction. The water washes elec-

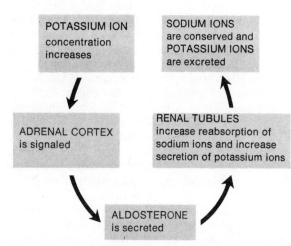

Figure 5–7. *If the concentration of sodium ions decreases, the kidneys act to conserve sodium ions. (From Hole John W Jr: Human Anatomy and Physiology, 3rd ed. © 1978, 1981, 1984, Wm. C. Brown Publishers, Dubuque, Iowa. All Rights Reserved Reprinted by permission.)*

trolytes from the stomach, leading to metabolic alkalosis (Metheny & Snively, 1983).

• Dietary carbohydrates can affect the sodium balance; carbohydrate overeating may result in acute sodium retention. Conversely, starvation and carbohydrate-free or low-carbohydrate diets increase sodium excretion.

• Starvation causes major changes in both water and electrolyte balance with initial weight loss principally caused by water and sodium excretion. This weight loss can be offset by small amounts of carbohydrate but not salt, protein, or fat (Randall, 1980).

Health Application: Water and Electrolyte Imbalances

Actually, the body's mechanisms for maintaining water-electrolyte balance perform remarkably well in spite of various intakes of these elements and ever-changing factors, such as temperature and exercise. Since electrolytes are in solution in the blood, anything that alters the amount of interstitial fluid likewise affects the electrolyte balance.

Dehydration. A reduced amount of interstitial fluid volume is referred to as dehydration. Fever, sweating, or insufficient intake can result in simple dehydration. During illness, the normal process of reabsorption is altered. This results in fluids being lost faster than their replacement; fluid and electrolyte imbalances may occur.

If fluid loss is slow or if water loss exceeds electrolyte loss, the first action within the body is the movement of water from within the cell to the hypertonic extracellular fluid in order to maintain osmotic pressure. The body compensates in this manner, while at the same time, the person experiences thirst and urinary volume decreases. If the body cannot maintain osmotic equilibrium, dehydration results. Dehydration is frequently encountered in health care facilities because illnesses can alter body mechanisms to maintain fluid balance. Dehydration is a serious problem demanding prompt attention. The stages of dehydration are shown in Figure 5–8; these signs are reflected in deviations from normal lab values (Table 5–5). A weight loss of 5 percent (10 percent in infants and small children) reflects moderate dehydration; 8 percent (15 to 20 percent in infants and small children) reflects severe dehydration. In replacing fluids (rehydration), considerations should be given to electrolytes lost along with fluid loss.

Clinical Implications:

• Dehydration may result in death, especially among children and geriatric patients, whose fluid intake is neglected.

• Extracellular dehydration is manifested by a weight loss of a half pound or more with 24 hours.

• Thirst can be indicative of extracellular dehydration, increased osmolality of body fluids, intracellular dehydration, decreased circulating blood volume, and dryness of the mouth (Fenton, 1969).

• Long-term use of laxatives and enemas can result in fluid-electrolyte disturbances (especially potassium). Advise patients to avoid using cathartics and enemas.

• To correct dehydration, carefully assess fluid intake and output. Encourage the conscious patient to drink plenty of fluids. Water and fluids containing electrolytes should be readily available (such as broth and fruit juices).

• An increase in body temperature can lead to a loss of total body fluid through increased respiration and through diaphoresis.

• If environmental temperature is elevated or if the patient is perspiring heavily, additional fluids containing electrolytes are needed to replace perspiration losses.

• The state of dehydration increases susceptibility to skin breakdown or pressure sores.

• There is no physiological reason to rest the bowel during diarrhea; oral fluids should be given, whenever possible. Absorption of most carbohydrates, amino acids, and electrolytes remains intact (Sack et al, 1978).

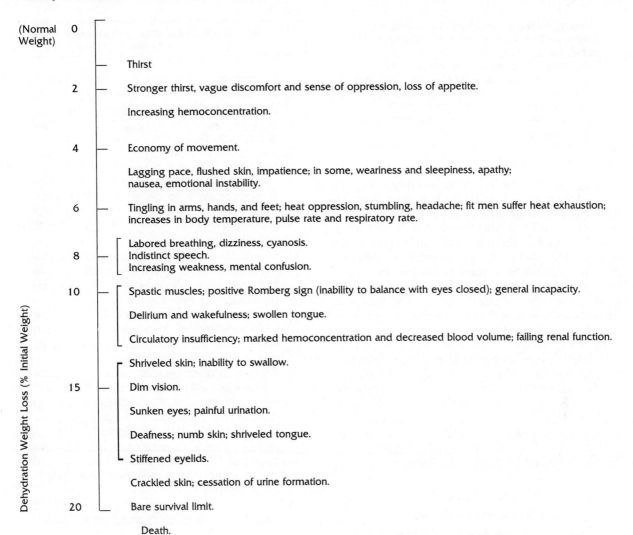

Figure 5–8. Spectrum of dehydration. (From Roth EM: Compendium of human responses to the aerospace environment, volume 3, section 15, NASA Contract No. NASr-115, 1967.)

Table 5–5. Dangerous High and Low Levels of Solutes in Plasma*

	Too High		Too Low	
	Mild to Moderate Symptoms	Severe Symptoms	Mild to Moderate Symptoms	Severe Symptoms
Sodium (mEq/L)	155–170	>170	120–130	<120
Potassium (mEq/L)	7–9	>9	2.2–3.0	<2.2
Calcium (mEq/L)	6–7	>7	3–4	<3
Magnesium (mEq/L)	>5	>10(?)	1 and below (?)	<1 (?)
Hydrogen ion, as pH	7.5–7.6	>7.6	7.0–7.5	<7.0
Glucose (mg/100 ml)	1000 or above (?)	—	40–60	<40
Protein (gm/100 ml)	—	—	3.4–5	<3

*From Keitel, HG: A primer for understanding and recognizing fluid and electrolyte imbalances. Consultant 3(2):42, 1963.

- When vomiting or diarrhea is present, the digestive secretions are also lost, enhancing the possibility of dehydration.
- Rehydration is safest with solutions of lower osmolality than plasma. A number of fluids, specially designed for patients recovering from surgery or rehydration after a sporting event, have an osmolality of 100, or one third of normal saline.

Edema. The state in which the body is in positive water balance (fluid intake is greater than excretion) is called edema. A large intake of water only temporarily dilutes blood volume. Excess water is stored in the interstitial fluid. If it is not accompanied by the correct amounts of electrolytes, the extracellular fluid is said to be hypotonic, and water enters the cells in an effort to equalize osmotic pressure. Excess fluid intake is normally excreted; however, edema results from abnormal amounts of body fluids in the interstitial space. This usually occurs when the kidney fails to excrete sodium properly. Edema frequently occurs in cirrhosis of the liver, congestive heart failure, and kidney diseases, which can cause excessive retention of salt and therefore water. Therapy for these conditions is discussed in Chapters 28, 32, and 33, respectively. Edema also occurs in protein-deficient diets because osmotic forces ordinarily exhibited by protein are lacking.

Clinical Implications:

- Edema of gradual onset is manifest by increased body weight. It is to be expected when there is a 24-hour weight gain of a half pound or more.
- Edema is not evident clinically until the interstitial fluid volume increases above 50 percent (Randall, 1980).

Water Intoxication. Excessive total body water accompanied by reduced electrolyte concentration is called water intoxication. It differs from edema in that it is an *intracellular* accumulation of fluid. Excess fluid entering the extracellular compartment lowers osmotic pressure. Water then enters the cells by osmosis. Some causes for this condition can be repeated tap water enemas, excess fluid intake (usually intravenously), or loss of electrolytes during gastric suction, vomiting, or diarrhea.

FOCUS ON *ENSURING FLUID BALANCE DURING EXCESSIVE SWEATING*

1. To prepare for sweat losses, particularly in hot weather, plenty of beverages should be taken before exercising. To ensure adequate hydration, 1 to 3 cups of water are adequate.
2. Avoidance of beverages containing alcohol and caffeine is advisable.
3. The best way to determine if fluid balance is maintained is to weigh prior to the activity or work and again afterwards. (If 3 lbs. are lost, then 6 cups of liquid should be drunk.)
4. To ensure electrolyte replacement, follow the guidelines stated in the electrolyte intake and absorption section. It is generally advisable for replacements to be made with food intake. Because salt tablets are so concentrated, large amounts of fluid are pulled into the gastrointestinal tract due to osmosis.
5. Patients should be encouraged to drink beverages with a lower osmolality than serum, so the osmotic forces causing the dilution of concentrated fluids do not create gastrointestinal discomfort or dehydration. (Fluids may contain 2.5 gm glucose per 100 ml of water and less than 10 mEq sodium and 5 mEq potassium per liter of water.)
6. Frequent breaks with small amounts of cool fluids (50 to 55°F) should be encouraged.

Health Application: Altered Requirements

Excessive Perspiration. Persons engaged in heavy work (especially in hot temperatures) and athletic activities have a critical need for increasing fluid intake. Evaporation of sweat from the skin is the major avenue of heat loss during exercise. It is necessary for body cooling. During periods of high humidity when sweat does not evaporate, a person's tolerance to heat is altered. Moisture in the air prevents dissipation of body heat.

The body must be in a positive state of hydration to have adequate amounts of body fluid for sweating. Fatigue is one of the first symptoms of mild dehydration. If fluid supplies are inadequate, blood volume drops, and the sweating mechanism ceases in order to maintain circulating blood. If this lasts for any length of time, body temperature will rise dramatically, which can result in brain damage, heart failure, kidney failure, and death.

Starting with a short daily exercise period and gradually increasing it will facilitate the body's tolerance for increased sweating. A positive fluid-electrolyte balance can be maintained from dietary intake, if food and drink are provided ad libitum and other precautions are followed, as outlined in *Focus on Ensuring Fluid Balance During Excessive Sweating*.

Fever. Metabolic rate increases about seven percent with each degree Fahrenheit rise in body temperature above normal (13 percent for each degree Celsius above 37°C). Prolonged high fever can easily lead to body fluid disturbances unless they are being replaced. Increased amounts of water and electrolytes are lost from the lungs, skin, and kidneys. The diminished appetite that normally accompanies fever makes it difficult to get adequate amounts of food and liquid into the patient to replace losses. Liquids need to be 3000 ml or more per day. Small, frequent amounts help avoid overtaxing the gastrointestinal tract. Frequently, the patient will be on a liquid diet, and emphasis must be placed on water and electrolyte intake to prevent severe depletion.

Restricted Intake of Water. Some physiological conditions require a restriction of fluid intake because of a patient's decreased ability to handle normal amounts of liquids. This occurs when cardiovascular conditions cause reduced circulation or when kidney function is impaired. Fluid may also be restricted in patients with intracranial pressure and cirrhosis. Thirst mechanisms are not altered, and the nurse must try to satisfy the patient's desire to drink with the limited fluid intake prescribed by the physician. A few tips in *Focus on Facilitating Fluid Intake Restrictions* can be helpful in making this restriction more tolerable for patients.

Acid-Base Balance

During healthy conditions, the acid-base balance is so well regulated that diet never has to be considered. The acidity or alkalinity of a solution is measured by pH, or the concentration of hydro-

---

FOCUS ON FACILITATING FLUID INTAKE RESTRICIONS*

1. Carefully limit fluids at mealtime.
2. Within dietary limitations, encourage plenty of fatty foods to help decrease the desire for fluid with the meal. (For instance, margarine may help a person to swallow a roll without having to "wash it down" with liquids.)
3. Encourage the dietitian to send moist foods. This would include raw vegetables and fruits. In contrast, mashed potatoes can be very dry. Gravies and sauces added to foods can help, if allowed on the diet.
4. Give small amounts of fluid at a time.
5. Eliminate salty foods and concentrated sweets such as candy, which produce thirst.
6. Give more and smaller medications at one time so that small amounts of total fluids are used in taking medications.
7. Give medications at mealtime.
8. Ice chips or ice cold water is sometimes more satisfying than water. Ice chips should be approved by the physician since they could be a hazard by changing the osmolality of the body fluid. Frozen electrolyte solutions may be better tolerated.
9. Gum chewing can stimulate salivary flow.
10. Keep the mouth clean by brushing the teeth frequently and rinsing the mouth.

---

*Data from Fenton, M: What to do about thirst. *Am J Nurs* 69 (5):1014, 1969.

---

gen ions (H+), which is expressed by pH values. A pH of 7 is neutral. Acids in solution lose hydrogen ions. When more hydrogen ions are present, the solution is acidic with a pH below 7. The lower the number, the stronger the acid or the more hydrogen ions it will release.

A base is a compound that accepts hydrogen ions in a solution. An alkaline solution has a pH above 7. The higher the number, the fewer number of hydrogen ions are released.

A buffer is a chemical that acts like a sponge by reacting with surplus hydrogen ions or releasing them. Buffers are very important in maintaining acid-base balance. Several buffer systems are active in the body. Blood buffers are bicarbonate, hemoglobin, and plasma proteins.

Extracellular fluids in the body are normally within the 7.35 to 7.45 pH, or slightly alkaline. When the pH is higher (7.46 to 7.8), the body is in a state of alkalosis; below the normal range (6.8 to 7.34) is a sign of acidosis. Life can exist between 6.8 and 7.8 pH.

pH OF FOODS.

Since acidity is a chemical measurement of the number of free hydrogen ions, it has nothing to do with taste sensations. If the metabolism of a food results in more cations (Ca^{++}, Mg^{++}, K^+, Na^+) than anions (Cl^-, S^{-6}, PO_4^{-3}), the food is said to be alkaline.

When some foods are eaten, such as lemons, they taste acidic because they contain some free organic acids. However, when orange juice with its acids is oxidized in the body, the result is carbon dioxide and water and a residue of potassium. Since potassium (the main end product of metabolism) is a cation, orange juice is a base-forming food. Vegetables, fruits, milk, and some nuts result in alkaline ash.

Protein foods, such as meat and eggs, leave residues of sulfur and phophorus or acid ash. Thus, acid-forming foods include meats, eggs, fish, and seafood. Fats, sugar, and starches contain no residue, and do not form excess cations or anions to affect the acid-base balance of the body (see Appendix D–6). (Fats and carbohydrates may indirectly affect acid-base balance in critically ill patients, as discussed in Chapter 26.) When a variety of foods is consumed from the food groups, the residue produced is reasonably balanced.

Plums, cranberries, and prunes contain an organic acid that the body cannot metabolize. Intake of these substances should slightly acidify the urine and are sometimes used to change the pH of the urinary tract. However, studies have shown that 4 L of cranberry cocktail are necessary to change urinary pH (Kahn et al, 1967; Bodel et al, 1959).

REGULATION OF ACID-BASE BALANCE

The metabolism of a normal mixed diet results in large amounts of carbon dioxide. This combines with water, resulting in carbonic acid which separates into a bicarbonate ion or an acid in the body. About 480 L of carbon dioxide is produced from an average daily diet. Therefore, the body has mechanisms to rapidly neutralize these acids produced. The body's buffering system, the lungs, and the kidneys all work efficiently together to maintain the proper pH in spite of the dietary composition.

While the composition of the diet influences the pH of the urine, assumptions for estimating the effects of diet on urine pH based on food composition tables are weak. The methods for such calculations are time-consuming and contain many errors. Dietary manipulations are definitely not precise but may provide information on the direction of change from one diet to another (Dwyer et al, 1985).

• FALLACIES and FACTS

FALLACY: Water is fattening.
- **FACT:** This is not true. Water is relatively heavy and makes up 60 percent of our body weight, but it cannot be metabolized to release calories and cannot be converted to fat.

FALLACY: Milk causes "cotton mouth" (dryness due to too little saliva).
- **FACT:** Saliva flow is related to the amount of perspiration and water content of the body, not by the types of foods eaten. Saliva flow may also be decreased for psychological reasons.

FALLACY: Water during an athletic event will cause stomach cramps.
- **FACT:** Drinking small amounts of water frequently during any period of increased exercise and heavy sweating is advisable. It combats the undesirable effect of dehydration and improves endurance.

FALLACY: Salt tablets should be taken anytime a person is profusely sweating.
- **FACT:** Although one needs to replace the sodium lost in perspiration, salt tablets are not advisable. Fluids are drawn from the body tissues to dilute the large amounts of salt in the stomach.

FALLACY: Water can be added to a solution to decrease the calories.
- **FACT:** The presence or absence of water in a solution contributes to its concentration. A beverage normally having 40 kcal in 4 oz. (10 kcal/oz.) can be diluted to have 40 kcal in 8 oz. or 40 kcal in a quart or in any volume you desire by adding water. The solution still has 40 kcal, but the calories per ounce decreases as water is added.

FALLACY: *Unless individuals choose their foods carefully, their body will become acidic, causing ulcers, pimples, and other illnesses.*

• **FACT:** *The body is well-adapted to handle large quantities of acid produced from foods. However, a wide variety of foods should be chosen to ensure adequate intake of nutrients.*

your fluid intake for one day. How do these compare?

4. What is obligatory water loss? What dietary factors affect minimum urine output?

5. What determines whether a food produces acid or alkaline ash? List five foods that result in acid ash and five foods that result in alkaline ash.

6. To what extent does the metabolism of a diet yielding principally acid ash or alkaline ash affect the acid-base balance? How can the acid- or base-forming foods be used beneficially?

Summary

All processes of life are dependent on an intricate balance of the chemicals dissolved in body fluids. Fluids are supplied from liquid intake, from water naturally present in food, and from metabolic processes. Fluid intake from ingested foods, fluids, and oxidation of foods must at least equal or exceed the losses from perspiration and respiration and in urine and feces. Accurate assessment of intake and output must include all sources of water gains and losses.

During normal healthy conditions, thirst is an adequate indicator for intake; the kidney adequately conserves or excretes fluids and electrolytes as necessary to maintain fluid electrolyte balance and to regulate acid-base balance. The nurse plays an important role in helping to maintain fluid-electrolyte balance when any of the body's mechanisms fail. It is more important to have an adequate intake of water than sufficient calories.

Review Questions

1. Define intracellular and extracellular fluid. What are the principal electrolytes found in each?

2. List sources of body fluids. Name the routes of fluid excretion from the body.

3. According to the RDAs, how many cups of liquid should you drink each day? Write down

REFERENCE LIST

Bodel, PT; Cotran, R; Kass, EH: Cranberry juice and the antibacterial action of hippuric acid. *J Lab Clin Med* 54(6):881, 1959.

Dwyer, J; Foulkes, E; Evans, M; et al: Acid/alkaline ash diets: time for assessment and change. *J Am Diet Assoc* 85(7):841, 1985.

Fenton, M: What to do about thirst. *Am J Nurs* 69(5):1014, 1969.

Kahn, HD; Panarietlo, VA; Saeli, J; et al: Effect of cranberry juice in urine. *J Am Diet Assoc* 51(3):251, 1967.

Metheny, NM; Snively, WD: *Nurses' Handbook of Fluid Balance*, 4th ed. Philadelphia, J. B. Lippincott Co, 1983.

Randall, HT: Water, electrolytes and acid-base balance. In *Modern Nutrition in Health and Disease*, 6th ed. Edited by RS Goodhart; ME Shils. Philadelphia, Lea & Febiger, 1980.

Sack, RB; Pierce, NF; Hirschhorn, N: The current status of oral therapy in the treatment of acute diarrheal illness. *Am J Clin Nutr* 31(12):2252, 1978.

Further Study

Burgess, RE: Fluids and electrolytes. *Am J Nurs* 65(10):90, 1965.

Del Bueno, DJ: Electrolyte imbalance. How to recognize and respond to it. Part I. *RN* 38(2):52, 1975.

Del Bueno, DJ: Electrolyte imbalance. How to recognize and respond to it. Part II. *RN* 38(3):54, 1975.

Garfinkel, HB: Gelfman, NA: Bicarbonate, not 'CO$_2$'. *Arch Int Med* 143(11):2063, 1983.

Goldberger, E: *A Primer of Water, Electrolyte and Acid-Base Syndromes*, 7th ed. Philadelphia, Lea & Febiger, 1986.

Kee, JL: Fluid imbalance in elderly patients. *Nursing* 3(4):40, 1973.

Metheny, NM; Snively, WD: *Nurse's Handbook of Fluid Balance*, 4th ed. Philadelphia, J. B. Lippincott Co, 1983.

Snively, WD: Roberts, KT: The clinical picture as an aid to understanding body fluid disturbances. *Nurs Forum* 12(2):133, 1973.

Protein: The Cellular Foundation

6

THE STUDENT WILL BE ABLE TO:

- *Describe protein digestion.*
- *List the possible fates of amino acids.*
- *Classify foods as sources of complete or incomplete proteins.*
- *Explain how proteins can be used to complement one another.*
- *Explain the relationship betweeen the nitrogenous substances in the body and protein nutriture.*
- *Plan menus to include the recommended protein level for a meat-containing diet and a vegetarian diet.*
- *Explain why various physiological states require different amounts of protein.*
- *State the problems associated with a protein deficiency or excess.*

Biological value
Deamination
Denaturation
Dynamic state
Essential amino acids
  (EAAs)
Kwashiorkor
Marasmus
Metabolic pool
Nitrogen balance
Nonessential amino acids
  (NEAAs)
Peptide linkage
Protein efficiency ratio
  (PER)
Transamination

OBJECTIVES

TERMS TO KNOW

Until the middle of the nineteenth century, many scientists thought that life was made from one basic chemical, which they named protein. It is true that protein is present in each living cell—nearly half of the dry weight of a cell is protein. Next to water, protein is the most plentiful substance in the body. No one will deny that proteins perform many important physiological functions. But it is not accurate to say that protein is more important than any other required nutrient, since protein cannot be fully utilized unless other nutrients are present. Protein is considered the main ingredient by most Americans who are frequently unable to plan a balanced meal without a meat entree, yet other essential nutrients frequently receive little or no attention.

Functions of Protein

Proteins are the principal source of nitrogen for the body. They are very large molecular structures, also containing the elements carbon, hydrogen, and oxygen and sometimes other elements such as sulfur and phosphorus.

As you learned in Chapter 2, proteins are necessary for growth, maintenance, and repair of body tissues and can provide energy. Some of the more familiar roles of protein are shown in Table 6–1. Actually, the functions of proteins fall into eight categories.

1. *Building new body tissues.* Since protein is a constituent of all cells, it is necessary for anabolism. During periods of increased growth (infancy, childhood, adolescence, and pregnancy), as well as in periods of wound healing or recovery (illness, surgery, burns, or fever), protein needs are increased for building new tissues.

2. *Repairing body tissues.* Due to continuous catabolism in all body proteins, new ones must be resynthesized from amino acids.

3. *Producing essential compounds.* Amino acids or proteins are constituents of the regulatory enzymes and hormones and other body secretions.

4. *Regulating water balance.* Plasma protein is another osmotically active substance in the maintenance of fluid-electrolyte balance. Protein dissolved in water forms a colloidal solution; in other words, it attracts water. Blood albumin (a protein) draws water from interstitial fluid or cells to maintain blood volume. During protein deficiency, a decreased amount of protein in the blood results in the appearance of edema because of a loss of osmotic balance.

5. *Regulating acid-base balance.* Plasma proteins are buffers that react with either acidic or alkaline substances to maintain the correct pH.

6. *Providing resistance to disease.* Antibodies or immunoglobulins, the body's main protection from disease, are proteins.

7. *Providing transport mechanisms.* Proteins enable insoluble lipid-substances to be transported through the blood.

8. *Providing energy.* After the nitrogen grouping has been removed, the remaining carbon skeleton can be used for energy, furnishing 4 kcal/gm. While this is not a main function for protein, it is utilized in this manner when (a) caloric intake from carbohydrate and fat is inadequate, (b) protein intake exceeds requirements, and (c) the essential amino acids are not available for synthesis of proteins.

Amino Acids

Amino acids are basic building blocks for proteins. About 22 different amino acids are present in proteins. All the billions of proteins associated with life are made from these amino acids. They can be compared to letters of the alphabet used in different sequences and different combinations to make billions of words. So it is with amino acids—only they can be combined not only in different sequential order but also in different geometric arrangements, because an amino acid is a three-dimensional structure, which may resemble a helix or spiral.

The number of various combinations of amino acids, their position in the molecule, and their spatial arrangement is very important, determining the function and character of the protein. For instance, the genetic problem in sickle cell anemia is that only one of the 500 amino acids in hemoglobin is incorrect.

INDIVIDUAL AMINO ACID STRUCTURE

The general design of amino acids is illustrated for better understanding in *Focus on the Structure of Amino Acids.* Thus, an amino acid contains a *basic* or amino grouping ($-NH_2$) and an *acidic* or carboxyl grouping ($-COOH$). This distinguishing structure allows the amino acid to act as a buffer by combining with either a base or an acid. The radical group is the part that varies to form 22 different amino acids.

Table 6–1. Classification of Protein by Function*

Classification	Body Location	Example	Function
Structural proteins	Skin, cartilage, bone	Collagen	Principal substance in connective tissue
Contractile proteins	Skeletal muscle	Actin, myosin	Muscle contraction
Antibodies	Blood plasma, spleen, lymphatic cells	Alpha globulins	Disease protection
Blood proteins	Blood plasma	Albumins	Control osmotic pressure of blood Maintain the buffering capacity of blood pH
	Blood	Fibrinogen	Blood clotting
	Blood	Hemoglobin	Transports oxygen from lungs to all parts of the body
Hormones	Endocrine or ductless glands (thyroid, pancreas, parathyroid, adrenals, pituitary)	Insulin	Regulates carbohydrate metabolism
		Growth hormone	Stimulates overall protein synthesis and growth
Enzymes	Throughout body—nearly 2000 different enzymes known; each highly specific in function		Biological catalysts; proteins which allow chemical reactions to proceed at their proper rate
	Stomach	Pepsin	Protein digestion
	Pancreas	Trypsin and chymotrypsin	Protein digestion
Nutrient proteins		Meat, fish, chicken, milk, cheese, eggs, peanut butter, nuts, soybeans, tofu, dried peas and beans	Sources of amino acids required by humans and other animals
Viruses	Microscopic infective agents	Smallpox, measles	Cause disease
Nucleoproteins	Cell nucleus	DNA	Determines and transmits hereditary characteristics; carries genetic (hereditary) code

*From Howard, RB; Herbold, NH: *Nutrition in Clinical Care,* 2nd ed. New York, McGraw-Hill Book Co., 1982. Reprinted by permission.

AMINO ACID CHAIN

Amino acids are able to combine with each other to make long chains. The carboxyl group of one amino acid attaches to the amino group of another amino acid and releases water in the process. The bond formed by amino acid linkages is called a peptide linkage. (See *Focus on Peptide Linkage*.) Two amino acids together form a dipeptide; several amino acids, a polypeptide. Foods and body proteins can be called polypeptides. The number of amino acids in a protein varies greatly (from 100 to 300), but it is specific for that protein.

DENATURATION

Proteins are very sensitive to heat, surface action, and extremes in pH, which results in alterations of their properties. These changes are called denaturation. Food preparation structurally alters protein molecules. For example, an egg white becomes white and fluffy when beaten; when subjected to heat, it becomes a solid or coagulates. When protein substances are subjected to the extremely acid medium in the stomach, they are denatured as the digestion process begins.

In most cases, digestibility and nutritional value are not affected by cooking procedures. Acids and heat coagulate proteins. Proper cooking sometimes facilitates digestion and utilization.

FOCUS ON THE STRUCTURE OF AMINO ACIDS

$$NH_2 \quad \text{(amino group)}$$
$$|$$
$$\text{Radical group} - C - COOH \text{ (acid group)}$$
$$|$$
$$H$$

FOCUS ON PEPTIDE LINKAGE

$$
\begin{array}{c}
\underset{H_2N-CH}{\overset{\overset{O}{\parallel}}{\underset{|}{C-OH}}} \\
\underset{Radical}{}
\end{array}
\;+\;
\begin{array}{c}
\underset{H-C-Radical}{\overset{\overset{H}{\underset{|}{H-N}}}{\underset{\underset{O}{\parallel}}{\underset{|}{C-OH}}}}
\end{array}
\xrightarrow{-H_2O}
\;Radical-\underset{H}{\overset{NH_2}{\underset{|}{C}}}-\overset{O}{\overset{\parallel}{C}}-NH-\underset{Radical}{\overset{H}{\underset{|}{C}}}-\overset{O}{\overset{\parallel}{C}}-OH
$$

For example, cooking makes egg albumin more readily digestible or cooking soybeans increases the amino acid bioavailability. On the other hand, processing affects proteins in cereal by binding lysine so it is not utilizable by the body.

CLASSIFICATION OF AMINO ACIDS

Amino acids can be classified according to their chemical nature—basic, acidic, or neutral (Table 6–2).

A very important classification of amino acids is whether they are required from food, or whether the body can make them in sufficient quantities to support growth. Nine essential amino acids (EAAs) are required in the diet (see Table 6–2). If any one of these is not present when the cell needs it for protein synthesis, the protein cannot be produced. Histidine is known to be essential for infants; recent evidence suggests it may also be essential for adults (Kopple & Swendseid, 1975).

Nonessential Amino Acids (NEAAs). These can be made by enzymes present in the body if a sufficient amount of protein is available to furnish the nitrogen needed. They are essential in protein formation but are not essential in the diet.

Protein Quality. The amounts of EAAs furnished by a food determine its ability to support growth, maintenance, and repair. Several methods of classification are used to evaluate a food's protein quality or its ability to support these functions.

Foods that supply adequate amounts of the nine essential amino acids to maintain nitrogen equilibrium and permit growth are known as *complete* protein or proteins of *high biological value*. These terms are synonymous. The biological value ranges from one to 100 with a higher score for proteins of higher quality. Foods of high biological value containing complete proteins are de-

rived from animal sources—egg, dairy products, meat, fish, and poultry. One exception is gelatin, which contains no tryptophan.

Proteins that do not contain EAAs in adequate amounts to support life have a low biological value and are called incomplete proteins. Vegetable and some grain proteins fall into this category; they contain all the essential amino acids but are incomplete because one or more EAAs are present in a low ratio, and the protein it furnishes is of fair or low biological value.

Most foods with protein content have all the EAAs, although the quantity of one or more of the EAAs may be insufficient. Proteins that support life but not normal growth are intermediate in biological value and are labeled partially incom-

Table 6–2. Classification of Amino Acids*

Classification	Essential Amino Acids	Nonessential Amino Acids
Neutral—one amino and one carboxyl group: Aliphatic.	Threonine Valine† Leucine† Isoleucine†	Glycine Alanine Serine
Aromatic—contains benzene ring.	Phenylalanine	Tyrosine‡
Heterocyclic.	Tryptophan	Proline Hydroxyproline
	Histidine	
Sulfur-containing.	Methionine	Cystine‡ Cysteine
Basic—two amino and one carboxyl group.	Lysine	Arginine Hydroxylysine
Acid—one amino and two carboxyl groups.		Aspartic acid Glutamic acid

*Adapted with permission of Macmillan Publishing Company from *Normal and Therapeutic Nutrition*, 15th ed, by C. R. Robinson and M. R. Lawler. Copyright © 1977, by Macmillan Publishing Co, Inc.
†Also called branched-chain amino acids (BCAA).
‡These amino acids are classed as semiessential.

Table 6–3. Limiting Amino Acids of Some Foods*

Food	Limiting Amino Acids
Cereal grains and millets	Lysine and threonine
Legumes (peas and beans)	Methionine, tryptophan
Soybeans, rice	Methionine
Sesame, sunflower seeds	Lysine
Peanuts	Methionine, lysine, threonine
Green leafy vegetables	Methionine

*From Deutsch, RM: *Realities of Nutrition*. Palo Alto, CA, Bull Publishing Co, 1976, by permission.

plete proteins. They contain all the EAAs, but the proportion of one or more of these amino acids is insufficient for optimum protein synthesis. This includes the proteins found in legumes, nuts, and grains. The amino acid in short supply relative to need is referred to as the limiting amino acid (Table 6–3).

Another measurement of the protein quality of a food is the protein efficiency ratio (PER). This measurement is used for nutrition labeling on food packaging in order to show a comparable measurement of protein. (One gram of protein from cornmeal is not equal to one gram of protein from chicken.) A high score (above or equal to 2.5) is given to foods of high biological value. Partially complete proteins have a score between 0.5 and 2.5.

Table 6–4. Special Functions of Amino Acids

Amino Acid	Functions
Tryptophan	Precursor of the vitamin niacin.
	Precursor of the neurotransmitter serotonin.
	Stimulates gastrointestinal activity.
Arginine, glycine, and methionine	Combine to form creatine.
Cystine	Component of bile acid.
Aspartic acid	Synthesis of asparagine.
Glycine	Combines with toxic substances for detoxification.
	Part of hemoglobin.
	Constituent of bile acid.
Glutamic acid, cysteine, and glycine	Synthesis of glutathione (for oxidation-reduction reactions).
Tyrosine	Synthesis of hormones epinephrine and thyroxine.
	Synthesis of the neurotransmitters dopamine and norepinephrine.
Histidine	Synthesis of histamine.
Phenylalanine	Precursor of tyrosine.
	Constituent of thyroxine and epinephrine.
Methionine	Donates methyl group (CH_3) for synthesis of compounds such as choline and creatine.

SPECIAL FUNCTIONS OF AMINO ACIDS

While all the amino acids are important, a few have special metabolic significance (Table 6–4). Recent research studies have linked several amino acids, especially tyrosine and tryptophan, with the production of neurotransmitters, which convey impulses between nerve cells in the brain causing motor responses. Tryptophan can raise the level of serotonin in the brain, which promotes sleep and lowers pain sensitivity. Tyrosine increases levels of dopamine, norepinephrine, and epinephrine. A high-protein meal results in increased brain tyrosine and has been used in treatment of depression and Parkinson's disease.

Digestion

Endogenous sources of protein, including products of catabolism within the gastrointestinal tract, are hydrolyzed and absorbed along with food proteins.

The process of protein digestion is summarized in Table 6–5. The chemical process begins in

Table 6–5. Enzyme Activity in Protein Digestion*

Enzyme and Its Location	Action
Stomach	
Pepsinogen	Activated to pepsin by hydrochloric acid.
Pepsin	Splits peptide chain where phenylalanine or tyrosine furnishes amino group.
Small intestine	
Trypsinogen†	Activated to trypsin by enterokinase.
Trypsin	Splits peptide chain where lysine or arginine furnishes carboxyl group.
Chymotrypsinogen†	Activated to chymotrypsin by trypsin.
Chymotrypsin	Splits peptide chain where carboxyl group is furnished by tryptophan, methionine, tyrosine, or phenylalanine.
Intestinal mucosa	
Aminopeptidase	Splits peptide linkage next to a terminal amino group.
Carboxypeptidase†	Splits peptide linkage next to a terminal carboxyl group.

*Reprinted with permission of Macmillan Publishing Company from *Normal and Therapeutic Nutrition*, 16th ed, by C. R. Robinson and M. R. Lawler. Copyright © 1982, by Macmillan Publishing Co, Inc.
†These enzymes are secreted by the pancreas.

the stomach. Hydrochloric acid activates the inactivated pepsinogen to pepsin. Pepsin is capable of digesting all types of proteins, even collagen (the connective tissue in meats). Pepsin initiates the hydrolysis of large protein molecules into simple forms called peptones and polypeptides. Hydrolysis of proteins occurs by splitting proteins between the amino acids at the peptide linkage. Pepsin does not usually complete hydrolysis to amino acids.

In the small intestine, enzymes continue the process of hydrolyzing protein intermediary products to amino acids. Each of these enzymes functions to break a specific type of peptide linkage in the amino acid chain. Enzymes in the intestinal epithelial cells are capable of finalizing the conversion to amino acids.

Absorption

Generally, all proteins are absorbed in the form of amino acids. But occasionally, a whole protein escapes digestion and is absorbed, probably by the process of pinocytosis. This may be an important factor in the development of immunity and allergic reactions caused by antigens.

The digestion of amino acids is very slow, but absorption is rapid. Approximately 90 to 95 percent of the ingested proteins is converted to amino acids and usually absorbed in the proximal part of the intestine. Absorption by active processes require energy, vitamin B_6, and manganese.

Protein hydrolysates (proteins predigested by enzymes) have been offered in weight reduction diets and postsurgical and gastrointestinal conditions where it was thought hydrolyzed substances would be more efficient. Free amino acid mixtures are not utilized with the same efficiency as equivalent amounts of protein (Adibi, 1976). When solutions of dipeptides are given, faster rates of absorption are observed than when free amino acid solutions are given (Silk, 1980). Even in extreme starvation, proteins can be digested as long as food can be swallowed.

Metabolism

Amino acids pass through the portal vein into the liver. The liver is an "aminostat," monitoring the intake and breakdown of all amino acids, except the branched-chain amino acids (BCAA), which are metabolized in the muscle (Jeejeebhoy, 1981). The liver allows individual amino acids to enter the general circulation only at specific levels, so each amino acid is available as needed by the cells to synthesize each individual protein. Amino acids transported in the blood are rapidly removed for use by the cells. If individual amino acids rise above the prescribed level in the blood, they are removed and oxidized for energy. The normal level of amino acid nitrogen (or amino nitrogen) in the blood ranges from 4 to 6 mg/dl. This level is a balance among amino acid absorption, formation (intake and endogenous production), and utilization.

Protein metabolism is always in a constant dynamic state with continuous catabolism and anabolism to replace worn-out proteins. Even during growth (a period normally considered as an anabolic period), muscle catabolism is elevated as the cell remodels the highly organized tissue (Ballard & Gunn, 1982).

In addition to the exogenous sources of protein from foods, endogenous sources from tissue catabolism releases additional amino acids that

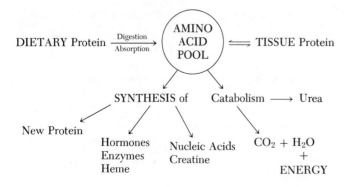

Figure 6–1. Amino acids from food and body tissues enter a common pool, which is drawn upon for synthesis of protein and other compounds or from which amino acids are degraded for energy needs. The word "pool" refers to the total amount of a substance present in the body. "Pool" is a concept, rather than a delineated location, mass, or compartment. (From Routh JI, Eyeman DP, Burton DJ: Essentials of General, Organic and Biochemistry, 3rd ed. Philadelphia, W. B. Saunders Co, 1977, by permission.)

can be used in anabolic reactions. This reservoir of amino acids is called the amino acid metabolic pool. As shown in Figure 6–1, these reserves are available to maintain the dynamic state of equilibrium.

This metabolic pool (70 gm of amino acids) could hardly be classified as a large storage of protein. Increasing muscle size is considered an increase in body mass, not protein storage. It is evident that to maintain a satisfactory state of protein nutrition, a daily supply of EAAs is necessary. The synthesis of proteins is very sensitive to food intake.

Anabolism-Catabolism Balance

Anabolic and catabolic processes, which utilize amino acids from the metabolic pool and absorption, are controlled by hormones. The liver is the major organ of regulation.

ANABOLISM

In addition to the influence of hormones, anabolism is dependent on the presence of all EAAs. Protein synthesis is also affected by caloric intake. If calories are below energy needs, tissue proteins are used for energy, resulting in increased nitrogen excretion. Production of nonessential amino acids in the liver is an anabolic process called transamination. The amino group is simply transferred from one compound to a new carbon skeleton forming a new amino acid. This process requires pyridoxal phosphate (vitamin B_6).

SYNTHESIS OF PROTEINS

Proteins are synthesized by individual cells for their own use. Cells are unable to make proteins used by different types of cells. All the EAAs must be available simultaneously. It is not a stepwise process where a protein can be started and then completed by waiting until the needed amino acid appears.

Deoxyribonucleic acid (DNA), a nucleotide present in the nucleus, is the template and controls protein synthesis. The messenger ribonucleic acid (mRNA) copies the pattern from DNA in the nucleus and carries it to the ribosomes in the cytoplasm (Fig. 6–2). Transfer RNAs (tRNAs) form a complex with each individual amino acid, directing it to its proper position in the chain. The RNA–amino acid complex moves to the mRNA where enzymes are present to promote peptide linkage (Fig. 6–3). Upon completion of synthesis, the protein is released from the ribosome to serve its specific function in the cell.

CATABOLISM

Amino acids are catabolized principally in the liver but, to some extent, in the kidney. Catabolism begins with the nitrogen grouping being removed from the amino acid, resulting in a carbon skeleton and ammonia. This process, known as deamination, requires the B vitamins pyridoxine and riboflavin.

The carbon skeletons (keto acids) can be used to (1) make nonessential amino acids, (2) produce energy via the Krebs cycle, or (3) be converted to fats and stored as fatty tissue. Most of the protein consumed yields amino acids that are glucogenic, i.e., they are potential sources of glucose for the body. The remainder are ketogenic and synthesized into fat. When amino acids are not needed

Table 6–6. Hormonal Influences in Protein Metabolism

Hormone	Effect	Mechanism
Pituitary growth hormone	Anabolic	Stimulates extra tissue synthesis during infancy and childhood.
Androgen and testosterone	Anabolic	Stimulate extra tissue synthesis during preadolescence and adolescence.
Adrenocortical hormones	Catabolic	Stimulate increased nitrogen excretion.
Insulin	Anabolic	Facilitates the entry of amino acids into the cells.
Thyroid		
Normal amounts	Anabolic	Regulates basal metabolic rate.
Excessive amounts	Catabolic	Increases basal metabolic rate.
Glucagon	Catabolic	Stimulates gluconeogenesis and ketogenesis from proteins.

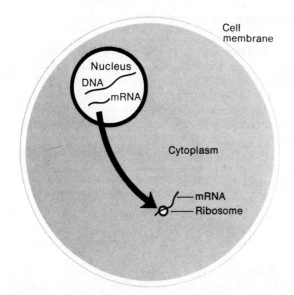

Figure 6–2. *After copying a section of DNA information, a messenger RNA molecule (mRNA) moves out of the nucleus and enters the cytoplasm. There it becomes associated with a ribosome. (From Hole John W, Jr: Human Anatomy and Physiology, 3rd ed. © 1978, 1981, 1984, Wm. C. Brown Publishers, Dubuque, Iowa. All Rights Reserved. Reprinted by permission.)*

for protein anabolism and energy is not needed, they are converted to fat and stored in the body.

Nitrogen Balance and Blood Serum Levels

Since nitrogen is a unique characteristic of protein metabolism, measurements of nitrogen and nitrogenous constituents in the blood and urine assess protein equilibrium in the body. Nitrogen balance refers to the anabolic and catabolic reactions involving protein substances. While nitrogen balance means that the output is equal to input, nitrogen atoms that are excreted are usually not the same as those ingested. For an individual to be in nitrogen equilibrium, not only must the diet contain required amounts of protein, but caloric intake must also be adequate or else protein will be used for energy. During cer-

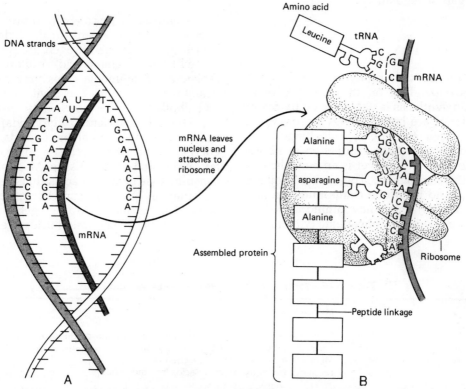

Figure 6–3. *Protein synthesis. A) mRNA formation. The DNA strands separate in one area; a strand of RNA is built up as shown and then leaves the nucleus. B) The mRNA becomes associated with ribosomes. Then tRNA molecules are assembled on the mRNA strand in a sequence complementary to it. Each tRNA bears an amino acid. In this way, the amino acid sequence of the finished protein is determined. (From Solomon EP, Davis PW: Human Anatomy and Physiology, 2nd ed. Philadelphia, W. B. Saunders Co, 1983.)*

Table 6–7. Nitrogen Balance

N balance: body protein constant
N intake = N excretion
Positive N balance: increase in body protein
N intake > N excretion
Negative N balance: decrease in body protein
N excretion > N intake

Positive N Balance	Negative N Balance
Growth	Inadequate intake of protein (fasting, gastrointestinal tract diseases).
Pregnancy	Inadequate caloric intake.
Convalescent periods	Illnesses, such as fevers, trauma, infections, or wasting diseases.
Athletic training	Injury or immobilization.
	Deficiency of essential amino acids.
	Accelerated protein loss (albuminuria, protein-losing gastroenteropathy).
	Burns.
	Increased secretion of thyroxine and glucocorticoids.

tain stages of life, the body is in positive nitrogen balance, while other states indicate negative balance (Table 6–7).

In nutritional assessments, in addition to blood and urine tests, anthropometric measurements such as muscle mass or midde upper arm circumference are used to determine protein nutriture.

NITROGEN INTAKE AND EXCRETION

Nitrogen intake can be measured by the amount of protein ingested. Protein is 16 percent nitrogen; each gram of nitrogen represents 6.25 gm of protein. (See *Focus on Protein-Nitrogen Conversions*.)

Nitrogen is excreted principally in the urine, but small amounts are lost in feces, sweat, vomitus, skin, menstrual fluid, and hair.

SERUM AND URINE NITROGEN

Protein status is indicated by several blood serum and urine measurements containing nitrogen, which is the result of protein metabolism (Table 6–8).

The urine urea nitrogen rate or urea production rate is normally used as an index of protein breakdown and indicates nutritional adequacy. Urea is the major waste product of protein catabolism. Ammonia, a toxic substance, is transformed

---

FOCUS ON PROTEIN-NITROGEN CONVERSIONS

To determine the amount of nitrogen consumed from food, multiply the grams of dietary protein by 0.16.

To determine the amount of muscle wastage (grams of protein lost), multiply the grams of nitrogen excreted by 6.25.

to urea in the liver and excreted by the kidneys. An average adult excretes 13 gm daily. Urea and ammonia vary directly with dietary protein levels (Latner, 1975). Approximately 75 percent of the ingested nitrogen is excreted.

Creatine and creatinine are also end products of protein metabolism. Creatine is found chiefly in muscles or in the blood in route to the muscles for the synthesis of phosphocreatine. Creatine in the urine indicates the breakdown of muscle tissue, as during fevers and starvation.

Urinary creatinine, a waste product from creatine, is normally constant in any given individual and is indicative of muscle mass in the body. During calorie deprivation or when inadequate amounts of essential amino acids are consumed, muscle is catabolized for fuel and creatinine excre-

Table 6–8. Hematologic Values and Urine Measurements Affected by the State of Nitrogen Balance

Test	Normal Values
Serum nonprotein nitrogen (NPN)	15–35 mg/dl
Serum urea	20–45 mg/dl
Urinary urea nitrogen	9–20 mg/dl (30 gm/24 hr)
Urinary urea nitrogen (pregnancy)	5–12 mg/dl
Urinary ammonia nitrogen	0.5–1.2 gm
Uric acid	
males	3.8–7.1 mg/dl
females	2.6–5.6 mg/dl
children	2.0–5.5 mg/dl
Creatinine (serum)	1.0–1.5 mg/dl
Urinary creatinine	
males	1–2 gm/24 hr
females	0.8–1.8 gm/24 hr
Creatinine coefficient (mg creatine nitrogen/kg/24 hr)	
Serum transferrin or total iron-binding capacity (TIBC)	250–450 mg/dl
Serum albumin	3.5–5.0 gm/dl or above
males	7.5–10
females	5–8

tion falls. Creatinine measurements assume that there are no significant dietary sources of creatinine (Munro & Crim, 1980).

Uric acid is an end product of purine (a protein) catabolism. The amount of uric acid excreted is indicative of the amount of dietary purines found in organ meats and meat extracts (bouillon and gravies).

Plasma proteins are a source of protein available for the tissues. During protein deprivation, the level of plasma proteins remains normal despite protein losses from the tissues. Studies show that a 1 gm decrease in total circulating plasma protein due to protein deprivation represents a concomitant loss of 30 gm of tissue protein (Latner, 1975).

Clinical Implications:

- Increasing protein intake does not necessarily increase muscle tissue.
- Amino acids are used for energy if not needed for growth and repairs of the body or if caloric intake is inadequate for energy requirements.
- The catabolization of amino acids results in the waste product urea.
- Serum albumin is more indicative of protein intake than plasma albumin.
- Protein deprivation causing a decrease in albumin results in edema, and a decrease in globulins results in impaired resistance to infections.

Requirements for Protein and Amino Acids

The quantity of protein the body needs is based on the size and rate of growth. (The body needs more protein for a growth state or maintenance and repair of a larger body mass.) Protein requirements involve an interrelationship between protein quality, quantity, and the amount of calories in the diet. To a certain extent, the better the quality of protein, the less quantity is required. The required amounts of the EAAs along with the criteria for determination of high-quality proteins are listed in Table 6–9. Requirements for protein are based on the assumption that EAAs and calories are provided in adequate amounts.

The RDAs for protein are based on an individual's age and *desirable* body weight. The requirement is based on the amount of nitrogen needed for nitrogen balance allowing for amounts lost by the body through ordinary routes. Using data from many nitrogen balance studies, the National Research Council (1980) has determined the *minimum* requirement of protein for adults to maintain nitrogen equilibrium is about 0.47 gm/kg. Using the 0.47 gm/kg, a person weighing 120 lbs. (54.5 kg), would require 25.6 gm of protein.

Since the RDAs provide a margin of safety,

Table 6–9. Estimated Amino Acid Requirements in Humans*

Amino Acid	Requirement, mg/kg body weight/day			Amino Acid Pattern for High-Quality Proteins, mg/gm of protein
	Infant (4–6 months)	Child (10–12 years)	Adult	
Histidine	33	?	?	17
Isoleucine	83	28	12	42
Leucine	135	42	16	70
Lysine	99	44	12	51
Total S-containing amino acids (methionine and cystine)	49	22	10	26
Total aromatic amino acids (phenylalanine and tyrosine)	141	22	16	73
Threonine	68	28	8	35
Tryptophan	21	4	3	11
Valine	92	25	14	48

*Two grams per kilogram of body weight per day of protein of the quality listed in column 4 would meet the amino acid needs of the infant.

From Food and Nutrition Board, National Research Council: *Improvement of Protein Nutriture.* Washington, DC, National Academy of Sciences, 1975.

the National Research Council (1980) states, ''The allowance for the mixed proteins of the United States diet becomes 0.8 gm/kg of body weight per day.'' With this standard, a person weighing 120 lbs. (54.5 kg) requires 44 gm of protein.

When any condition of health or disease puts the body in negative nitrogen balance, an increased protein intake (above the RDAs) avoids catabolism of tissue and plasma proteins. The RDAs are proportionately higher for different ages and stages of life to adjust for the increased anabolism. One rule of thumb is that protein should never exceed 15 to 20 percent of caloric intake.

Other disease states, illnesses, or surgery, increase protein requirements; however, RDAs have not been set for these conditions. Supplementation with foods of high biological value can help prevent protein malnutrition and shorten recovery periods. Individual balance studies that measure nitrogen intake and urinary excretion can be used to calculate the amount of protein needed to establish equilibrium.

While Americans commonly ingest more protein than recommended, ordinarily it is only necessary to limit dietary protein in some physiologi-

cal disease states affecting the liver and kidney. Since these organs are heavily involved in protein metabolism and excretion of protein waste products (see Chapters 28 and 33, respectively), if they are diseased, excessive amounts of protein cannot be properly handled.

Food Sources

PROTEIN CONTENT OF FOODS

Foods with high protein content are readily available in the United States. The average protein content of a few foods is shown in Table 6–10. The food supply available for consumption in the United States furnishes 99 gm protein per person daily, much above the recommended allowance.

The protein contribution from each of the basic food groups is shown in Figure 6–4. This adequately meets the needs of all groups of people except pregnant women. The recommendation of

Table 6–10. Average Protein Content of Foods in Four Food Groups*

Food	Average Serving	Protein gm	Protein Quality Limiting Amino Acids
Milk Group			
Milk, whole or skim	1 cup	9	Complete
Nonfat dry milk	7/8 oz. (3–5 Tbsp.)	9	Complete
Cottage cheese	2 oz.	10	Complete
American cheese	1 oz.	7	Complete
Ice cream	1/8 qt.	3	Complete
Meat Group			
Meat, fish, poultry	3 oz., cooked	15–25	Complete: higher protein for lean cuts
Egg	1 whole	6	Complete
Dried beans or peas	1/2 cup, cooked	7–8	Incomplete: methionine
Peanut butter	1 Tbsp.	4	Incomplete: several amino acids borderline
Vegetable-Fruit Group			
Vegetables	1/2 cup	1–3	Incomplete
Fruits	1/2 cup	1–2	Incomplete
Bread-Cereals Group			
Breakfast cereals, wheat	1/2 cup, cooked 3/4 cup, dry	2–3	Incomplete: lysine
Bread, wheat	1 slice	2–3	Incomplete: lysine
Macaroni, noodles, spaghetti	1/2 cup, cooked	2	Incomplete: lysine
Rice	1/2 cup, cooked	2	Incomplete: lysine and threonine
Cornmeal and cereals	1/2 cup, cooked	2	Incomplete: lysine and tryptophan

*Reprinted with permission of Macmillan Publishing Company from *Normal and Therapeutic Nutrition*, 16th ed, by C. R. Robinson and M. R. Lawler. Copyright © 1982, by Macmillan Publishing Co, Inc.

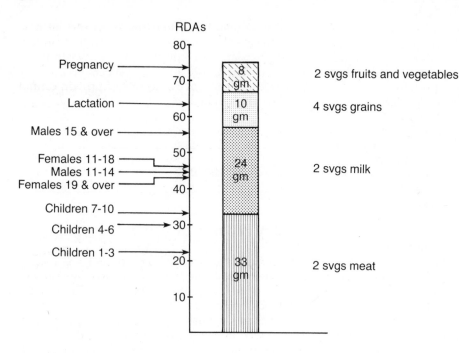

Figure 6–4. Protein contribution of the basic food groups as compared to the RDA for different ages, sexes, and stages of life. Grams of protein contributed by meeting the basic food groups with the following foods: 2 oz. roast beef, 2 oz. tuna fish, 1½ cups 2% milk, 1 cup low-fat plain yogurt, 2 slices whole wheat bread, 2 slices enriched bread, 4 oz. orange juice, ½ cup broccoli, 1 medium banana, 1 medium baked potato.

3 cups of milk for pregnancy increases the protein content of the diet to meet recommended levels.

AMINO ACID CONTENT OF FOODS

The food supply in the United States furnishes 64 gm of protein from meats and milk products, or complete proteins. Table 6–11 lists the amounts of amino acids furnished by some complete and incomplete protein foods as compared to the requirements for a human being. In spite of the fact that amino acids are not limited in the food supply, some people choose plant sources of protein for economic reasons or out of individual convictions. The essential amino acids can be supplied by plants but relatively large amounts of these individual foods must be consumed to match the protein obtained from animal sources.

These EAAs that are low in grains are abundant in other plants such as legumes. As you can see in Table 6–3, beans are low in methionine and tryptophan, and corn is low in lysine and threo-

Table 6–11. Comparison of Amino Acid Content of Various Foods with Requirements*

Amino Acids	Hamburger	Egg	Dried Beans (cooked)	Brown Rice (cooked)	Adult Male Need
Isoleucine	1.3	0.85	0.45	0.12	0.84 gm
Leucine	2.0	1.10	0.67	0.22	1.12 gm
Lysine	2.2	0.82	0.58	0.10	0.84 gm
Methionine	0.62	0.40	0.08	0.05	0.70 gm
Phenylalanine	1.0	0.75	0.43	0.13	1.12 gm
Threonine	1.1	0.64	0.34	0.10	0.56 gm
Tryptophan	0.56	0.21	0.07	0.03	0.21 gm
Valine	0.29	0.95	0.48	0.18	0.96 gm
Histidine	(unknown, but not of concern generally)				(unknown)
Total Essential Amino Acids†	9.91	5.7	3.1	1.83	
Total Protein	25.0	12.9	7.8	2.55	
Calories in 100 grams	(257)	(162)	(118)	(119)	

*From Deutsch, RM: *Realities of Nutrition.* Palo Alto, CA, Bull Publishing Co, 1976.
†Plus histidine values.

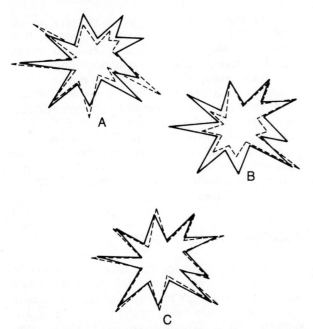

Figure 6–5. Complementing protein: The bold line represents the "ideal" amino acid pattern or a high-quality protein. A) The dotted line in this star represents the amino acid pattern in a peanut. B) The dotted line in this star represents the amino acid pattern in a sunflower seed. C) Together, the peanut and the sunflower seed supply more than the necessary amount of all nine amino acids. (From Pemberton C: Creative Eater's Handbook: Better Nutrition Through Vegetarian Eating. Oakland, CA, American Heart Association, Alameda County Chapter, by permission.)

nine. When both are eaten together at the same meal, as in pinto beans and cornbread, they are said to be complementary to each other. Thus, an adequate quantity of amino acids can be provided by eating two incomplete proteins in which different EAAs are missing (Fig. 6–5). The deficiencies of one are offset by the adequacy of another. When plant sources are planned to complement each other, less volume is required. Complementary combinations include foods having different limiting amino acids. Additionally, small amounts of complete proteins can be combined with plant foods, such as in macaroni and cheese, to provide adequate amounts of EAAs.

Clinical Implications:

- Protein requirements should be met by foods from several sources (even with animal protein foods) because of other nutrients that accompany the protein. For example, pork is an excellent source of thiamin; red meats furnish a significant amount of iron. In contrast, too many eggs in the diet would contribute excessive cholesterol.
- One should be especially alert to the variety and timing of protein sources when requirements are being met by plant sources.
- Healthy individuals will be in nitrogen balance appropriate for their stage of life if their diet contains adequate calories with the recommended number of servings from all four of the basic food groups.
- Too much emphasis on high-protein foods may result in inadequate amounts of other nutrients in the U.S. diet, especially when the food budget is low.
- Protein sources are generally the most expensive foods. When patients have limited finances, counsel them to (1) eat protein in adequate but not excessive amounts, (2) use complementary sources of protein so less expensive foods can be purchased, and (3) purchase less expensive kinds of protein foods (see Chapter 14).

Effects of Deficient and Excessive Protein Intakes

PROTEIN DEFICIENCY

While protein supplies in the United States are plentiful and drastic protein deficiency is not common, several groups of people are susceptible to insufficient intakes: (1) elderly persons who are unable to prepare nutritious meals or uninspired to eat, (2) low-income groups, (3) strict vegetarians, (4) those with a lack of education or who are unwilling to shop wisely, and (5) chronically ill and hospitalized patients.

While protein-energy malnutrition (PEM) is uncommon in the United States, given the above conditions, malnutrition frequently lurks behind closed doors. Certain physiological conditions, listed in Table 6–12, may also precipitate PEM. An insufficient intake of protein causes a negative nitrogen balance. Tissues are depleted of reserves, blood protein levels are lowered, and resistance to infections is lowered. Also, the ability to withstand the stresses of injury or surgery are lowered with increased recovery periods.

Because of insufficient quantity of high-quality proteins and calories in other areas of the world, PEM is commonly seen. Kwashiorkor de-

Table 6–12. Causes of Protein-Energy Malnutrition*

1. Impaired intake of dietary protein
   a. Insufficient quantity or quality.
   b. Impaired intake due to systemic disease, e.g., cerebrovascular accident or chronic infections.
   c. Impaired intake due to localized gastrointestinal disease, e.g., benign or malignant esophageal stricture.
2. Impaired digestion and/or absorption
   a. Selective enzyme defect, e.g., enterokinase or trypsinogen deficiency.
   b. Generalized enzyme defect, e.g., pancreatic exocrine insufficiency.
   c. Impaired small intestinal assimilation, e.g., celiac sprue, short bowel syndrome.
3. Excessive enteric protein loss
   a. Gastric or intestinal mucosal disease, e.g., Menetrier's disease, intestinal lymphangiectasia.
   b. Extraintestinal disease, e.g., constrictive pericarditis, thoracic or abdominal lymphatic blockade, i.e., lymphoma.
4. Disorders with multiple causes
   a. Advanced malignancy.
   b. Chronic renal failure with uremia.
   c. Other chronic debilitating diseases.

*From Freeman, HJ; Young, S. K.: Digestion and absorption of protein. *Annual Review of Medicine* 29(12):99, 1978.

velops when young children receive adequate calories, but not enough high-quality protein (Fig. 6–6). It usually appears after the child has been weaned from breast milk. Marasmus is also seen in infants when there is a deficiency of both protein and calories (see Chapter 20).

Kwashiorkor and marasmus are very serious health problems, which have been given much attention by the United Nations and the World Health Organization. Supplementations have been made in the form of skim-milk powder, Incaparina (a food powder made from corn, cottonseed, and sorghum with mineral and vitamin supplements), and the addition of lysine to cereal products. However, most of these efforts to improve the status of world nutrition have not been well accepted for various reasons, and the protein-energy problems of the world still exist (Behar, 1979; McLaren, 1974).

EXCESSIVE PROTEIN INTAKE

An upper limit for safe levels of protein intake has not been determined. Most Americans give proteins a high priority and feel there is no such thing as too much protein in the diet. Frequently, 150 to 200 percent of the RDAs is eaten. However, too much protein can result in some of it being stored as fat, possibly resulting in obesity. A recent study concluded that rats fed high levels of protein conserved energy more efficiently than when less protein was fed (Donald et al, 1981).

Another concern regarding high-protein intake is its effect on calcium balance. The RDAs in the United States for calcium are double the al-

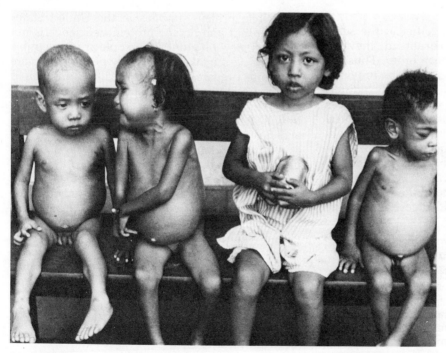

Figure 6–6. One child in this picture is healthy; the other three, all from the same community and of about the same age, are victims of the deficiency disease, kwashiorkor. Note that the faces and abdomens of the two on the left look quite full, due to the accumulation of water as edema. The fact that the children are in reality pitifully thin is apparent from looking at the arms. (Courtesy of World Health Organization, photo by H. Oomen.)

lowances established for most other nations because of the large amounts of protein consumed. An oversupply of any nutrient has an impact on the rest of the diet. Calcium accompanies protein wastes as they are excreted because there is less reabsorption of calcium in the renal tubules. Modest increases (about 30 gm) in dietary protein do not affect calcium balance (Mahalko et al, 1983), but a high-protein diet increases urinary calcium, (Hegsted & Linkswiler, 1981; Linkswiler et al, 1981). This may have detrimental effects especially in patients with osteoporosis (Licata et al, 1981).

A concern especially in infant nutrition is fluid imbalances due to excessive protein. The metabolism of 100 calories of protein requires 350 gm of water, compared with 50 gm of water for a similar amount of carbohydrates or fats. Therefore, water requirements are increased and the end products of protein metabolism in the bloodstream are increased.

Health Application: Vegetarianism

More and more, vegetarianism is becoming a way of life for many Americans. While vegetarianism is not new and has been documented back to biblical times, no society has ever been discovered that is exclusively vegetarian (Farb & Armelagos, 1980). Basically, a vegetarian diet consists of no meat, poultry, or fish. With careful planning, it can provide a very healthy, balanced diet. Four types of vegetarian diets differ in the types of foods included or excluded.

Vegan or Strict Vegetarian Diet. This diet contains only food from plants, including vegetables, fruits, and grains. No foods of animal origin are allowed (meat, milk, cheese, eggs, butter). This is the strictest type diet and requires the most cautious planning to achieve combinations that provide the necessary amounts of amino acids. The use of complementary proteins provides proper quantities of EAAs.

Lactovegetarian Diet. In addition to foods from plants, dairy products are included. ("Lacto-" comes from the Latin word, for milk, *lactis*.) Meat, poultry, fish, and eggs are excluded. Milk and cheese products complement plant products and enhance the amino acid content.

Ovolactovegetarian Diet. This vegetable diet is supplemented with milk, cheese, and eggs. ("Ovo-" comes from the Latin word for egg, *ovum*.) Only meat, poultry, and fish are excluded. If adequate quantities of eggs, milk, and milk products are consumed, all nutrients will be provided in sufficient quantities. Strict supervision is not warranted unless serum cholesterol levels require dietary fat restrictions. If salt restriction is necessary, most cheeses should be avoided and fresh rather than canned vegetables should be used.

Ovovegetarian Diet. This diet consists of foods from plants with the addition of eggs. Meat, poultry, fish, and dairy products are excluded.

Advantages and Problems. Much can be said of the healthy aspects of the vegetarian diets. There is no reason why an adequate diet cannot be obtained (with the exception of the strict vegan diet) even though it requires more planning and knowledge of the amino acid content of various foods. As shown in Table 6–13, the only food group changed is the protein or meat group. Various combinations of protein-containing foods are used to complement or supplement one another (Table 6–14).

As you will note from Table 6–3, methionine (a sulfur-containing amino acid) is limited in many of the vegetarian foods and is the most difficult to obtain. Cystine (another sulfur-containing amino acid), which can be made from methionine in the body, is available from nuts and soybeans. It is important to stress that all the essential amino acids must be present in the diet daily.

Some groups, especially the Seventh-Day Adventists, have supplemented protein intake with many textured vegetable protein (TVP) products. These are meat analogs produced from vegetable proteins, usually soybeans. The protein in these products is of good biological value; however, they also have a high sodium content.

Since vitamin B_{12} is only available from meat and animal products, vitamin B_{12} supplements are necessary for vegans. It may take years to deplete an adult's body stores of vitamin B_{12} and to develop deficiency symptoms. Brewer's yeast, soy-fermented tempeh, or fortified breakfast cereals can be used as sources of vitamin B_{12}. Direct vitamin supplementation is also a possibility.

Strict vegetarians and lactovegetarians are also at risk of iron deficiency. Iron-rich vegetables accompanied by good sources of vitamin C are encouraged for optimum absorption. Additionally, iron-enriched foods or iron supplementation (20 mg daily) can be used. Iron supplementation is mandatory during pregnancy, early childhood, and adolescence and after any major loss of blood. The use of eggs in the ovolactovegetarian diet increases iron intake.

While calcium intake is low because of the lack of milk products in the vegan diet, the low intake of phosphorus and protein makes absorption of calcium from vegetables more efficient. However, calcium supplementation is recommended during pregnancy and lactation when requirements are high.

Of primary concern is the lactating female who strictly adheres to the vegan diet, thus affecting the nutritional quality of breast milk and increasing the chances that the baby may fail to thrive. Additionally the weaned child is prone to protein deficiency; cases of PEM in vegans have been documented in the United States. Soy-based milk products can be used to complement other plant proteins eaten. The use of peanut butter is also encouraged. The rate of growth of vegan children should be carefully monitored.

The Zen macrobiotic diet has been proven "to cause irreversible damage to health and ultimately lead to death" (CFN, 1971). The diet is composed of natural foods, predominantly vegetarian. Initially, the diet consists of grains, vegetables, fruits, and approximately 10 percent animal products. One gradually works through 10 stages of eliminating certain foods until the last stage, consisting of just rice and herb tea, is reached. As a result of several deaths and nutritional deficiencies, the American Medical Association's Council on Foods and Nutrition has condemned this diet as a threat to human health.

Clinical Implications:

- The limitations of the vegetarian diet should be recognized during periods of positive nitrogen balance (such as infancy or growth) or during periods of increased catabolism (such as stress, surgery, and illness) in which nitrogen requirements are increased.
- Minerals most likely to be inadequate and needing special emphasis in the vegetarian diet include calcium, iron, and zinc (see Chapter 12).
- Benefits of the vegetarian diet include better weight control and less constipation, diverticular disease, and colon cancer (Dwyer, 1983); a lower incidence of gallstones (Pixley et al, 1985); less breast cancer (Goldin et al, 1982); lower blood pressure (Ophir et al, 1983; Armstrong et al, 1979); less osteoporosis (Marsh et al, 1983; 1980); and a decreased rate of coronary artery disease (Phillips et al, 1978).
- When working with vegetarians, keep lines of communication open by respecting the individual's decision, unless eating habits are clearly potentially harmful.
- Low-energy intake is a common problem of vegetarians. During pregnancy, this results in inadequate weight gains. High-energy, nutrient-dense foods are recommended to increase energy intake.
- When energy intakes are adequate, protein intakes are usually satisfactory, especially among ovolacto vegetarians.

Table 6–13. *Vegetarian Food Guide**

Food Group	Standard Serving	Number of Servings (by Age)			
		1–3 Years	4–6 Years	7–12 Years	Adult
Milk and Milk Products†	1 cup	2–3	2–3	3–4	2
Vegetable Protein Foods					
1. Legumes	1 cup	1/4	1/2	1/2	1‡
Textured vegetable protein	20–30 gm, dry				
Meat analogs	2–3 oz.				
2. Nuts and seeds	1 1/2 Tbsp.	1/4	1/2	3/4	1
Peanut butter	4 Tbsp.				
Fruits and Vegetables					
Total daily	1/2 cup cooked 1 cup raw 1/2 cup juice	2–3	3–4	4–5	4§
Green leafy	daily	1	1	1	1
Vitamin C rich	daily	1	1	1	1
Breads and Cereals**					
Whole-wheat bread	1 slice	3	3–4	4–5	4
Cooked cereal	1/2–3/4 cup				
Other					
Eggs	1	1	1	1	3–4/week
Fats	1 tsp.	1–3	2–3	2–3	3

*Adapted from Vyhmeister, IB; Register, UD; Sonnenberg, LM: Safe vegetarian diets for children. *Pediatric Clinics of North America* 24(1):207, 1977.
†Soy milk fortified with vitamin B_{12} may be used if desired.
‡Include 1 cup dark greens to help meet the adult female iron requirement.
§To help meet the female adult requirement for iron, 2 cups legumes should be included.
**Include a variety of yeast-raised, whole-grain breads, and a serving of whole-grain cereal. (Yeast breads contain more nutrients than quick breads when made with the same ingredients.)

Table 6–14. *Guidelines and Examples for Complementary Proteins*

1. Combine legumes (dried beans, peas, lentils, soybeans, soybean curd (tofu), mung beans, split peas, garbanzos) with grains (barley, millet, rice, oats, rye, brown rice, cornmeal, bulgur, and wheat).
2. Combine legumes with nuts and seeds (almond, cashew, pecan, brazil nuts, walnut, peanut, pumpkin, sesame, sunflower).
3. Combine grains with nuts and seeds (Only a few combinations achieve a "complete protein." Foods from another group might also be included.)
4. Combine vegetables with legumes, grains or corn, or potatoes.
5. Combine eggs or dairy products with any vegetable protein source.

Grains and Legumes: Rice and beans, wheat-soy bread, corn-soy bread, cornbread and black-eyed peas, corn tortillas and beans, lentil soup and rye crackers, baked beans with brown bread, beans in a tostada, or brown rice and peas.

Legumes and Nuts/Seeds: Roasted soybean snacks with bean dip, raw peanuts and sunflower seeds, stir fry tofu with slivered almonds and broccoli, seed bread with split-pea soup.

Grains and Nuts/Seeds: Rice and sesame seeds, wheat germ and peanuts, rice and cashews, peanut butter on wheat bread, or noodles and cashews.

Vegetables and Legumes, Grains or Corn, or Potatoes: Dark green leafy vegetables with pinto beans, stir-fried vegetables with kidney beans, steamed broccoli and corn over brown rice, fresh lima beans and corn, corn and potato casserole, spinach-potato salad, or gumbo with okra, corn, and lima beans.

Grains and Milk Products: Cottage-cheese salad with sesame seeds and garbanzos, milk in legume soup, cheese sauce for beans, or vegetable quiche with peanut-butter muffins.

• FALLACIES and FACTS

FALLACY: *Eating a lot of foods high in DNA and RNA (nucleic acids) is the key for staying young because they decrease with increasing age.*

• **FACT:** *These chromosomal strands naturally present in foods are the blueprint that makes food what it is. (Without that blueprint, the strawberry could have developed into a cherry.) Cells replace themselves using the DNA template. If cells were able to utilize the DNA from other cells or organisms, cells in the liver might start producing urine.*

FALLACY: *Brown eggs are more nutritious than white.*

• **FACT:** *The color of the eggshell is not related to its nutritional value. The breed of hen determines the color of the eggshell.*

FALLACY: *Gelatin is a good source of protein and helps to build strong fingernails.*

• **FACT:** *While gelatin is pure protein, it does not contain all the essential amino acids for growth, repair, and maintenance of the body. Whether protein improves fingernail formation is questionable. Fingernail formation can be influenced by the state of nutrition, endocrine system and disease as well as the environment.*

FALLACY: *Fertilized eggs are more nutritious than unfertilized ones.*

• **FACT:** *The presence of one additional cell in the egg hardly seems significant to its nutritional value.*

FALLACY: *Elderly persons require less protein than younger adults.*

• **FACT:** *Because of the dynamic state of the body, there is always a need to replace tissue protein. Protein requirement of the elderly is at least equal to that of the young adult or may be increased (NRC, 1980).*

FALLACY: *Meat burns its own calories.*

• **FACT:** *The calories from meat are the same as the calories from any other food source—protein, carbohydrates, or fat. While the digestion process requires energy, the amount required is much less than the amount produced in the metabolism of these energy-yielding nutrients.*

FALLACY: *In the United States, breads and cereals should be supplemented with the amino acid lysine since natural lysine is unavailable.*

• **FACT:** *Lysine fortification is beneficial in countries where proteins are in short supply. Breads and cereals are not heavily relied upon for their protein content in the United States and therefore do not need to be fortified with lysine.*

FALLACY: *A diet high in protein causes drowsiness.*

• **FACT:** *A high-protein diet does not raise tryptophan levels in the blood. Other amino acids that accompany the high protein intake compete with the brain's uptake of tryptophan. Therefore, the greater the percentage of protein intake, the less tendency of serotonin levels in the brain to increase. Foods containing 40 to 45 percent protein may actually decrease brain serotonin (Wurtman & Fernstrom, 1974), whereas a meal principally composed of carbohydrate plus a tryptophan supplement results in higher serotonin levels (Ashley et al, 1982).*

FALLACY: *Vegetarian children do not achieve potential growth.*

- **FACT:** *The heights of children and adults in a Seventh-Day Adventist group who have eaten vegetarian diets all their lives are similar to norms for nonvegetarians. While their growth rate was slower, the children reached optimal anthropometric measurements. However, growth curves of vegetarian children from nontraditional philosophical and religious groups (such as macrobiotics and the International Society for Krishna Consciousness) were lower in weight and height depending on age, sex, and diet than for nonvegetarian children. Height was more affected than weight. Energy intakes of vegetarians were below recommended levels, whereas protein intakes were adequate (Dwyer et al, 1983).*

FALLACY: *Lysine inhibits the growth of the herpes virus.*

- **FACT:** *Some early and uncontrolled studies seemed to support this, but double-blind placebo-controlled studies found no effect on the appearance or rate of healing of herpetic lesions (Milman et al, 1980; 1978). Since large intakes of a single amino acid may interfere with absorption of other amino acids, this long-term practice could lead to amino acid imbalances.*

FALLACY: *An increased protein intake is advised for a weight reduction diet because protein delays the onset of hunger.*

- **FACT:** *No evidence has proven that protein substituted for the same amount of calories from carbohydrate or fat has a greater satiating effect (Sunkin & Garrow, 1982). In fact, fat results in a greater satiety because it is digested more slowly than protein or carbohydrate.*

Summary

Proteins, made up of amino acids, are required in sufficient quantities for replacement of body tissues that are constantly in a dynamic state. Additional amounts are needed to support growth. Protein can also be a source of energy for the body. If insufficient quantities of calories are available for energy requirements, protein will be used for its caloric contribution—4 kcal/gm. Excess protein consumed can be used for energy or stored as fat.

Essential amino acids are not made in the body and must be provided by the diet. Animal proteins contain the essential amino acids in balanced proportions and are considered complete. Plant foods contain protein; however, the amino acid content is not in the proper proportions for human needs. They can be combined to complement one another to provide the required quantities of amino acids.

Blood serum levels and urine excretion of nitrogenous products are used to determine a person's protein nutriture, or nitrogen balance.

The required amount of protein necessary for most individuals can be supplied by 2 cups of milk; two 2-oz. portions of meat, fish, or poultry; and small amounts of protein furnished by the grain and the fruit and vegetable group.

Review Questions

1. Define amino acid, essential amino acid, nitrogen balance, and complementary proteins.
2. Name the functions of proteins.
3. Using your desirable weight, how many grams protein should you consume?
4. Given an individual weighing 150 lbs. who has a caloric intake of 2500 kcal, if the diet averages 15 percent protein, how many calories are provided by proteins? How many grams of protein is this? How does this fit into the RDA allowance for this individual?
5. What would you tell strict vegetarian parents about feeding their infant?
6. What are the effects of too much protein in the diet? Too little?
7. Explain the relationship between calories and protein.
8. What are two methods of obtaining the EAAs from vegetarian foods? List two food combinations for each that would provide adequate amounts of EAA.
9. Why does the infant need more protein per unit of weight than the adult?
10. If a person eats more protein than his/her body needs, what happens to the excess protein?
11. Evaluate the protein quality of the following meals: (1) Cooked bulgur wheat with honey, oatmeal toast with margarine, fresh grape-

fruit, and herb tea; (2) Peanut butter on whole-wheat bread, split-pea soup, a fresh peach, and soy milk; (3) Lentils and rice, cooked Brussels sprouts, carrot-raisin salad, whole-wheat bread with margarine, an apple, and herb tea.

REFERENCE LIST

Adibi, SA: Intestinal phase of protein assimilation in man. *Am J Clin Nutr* 29(2):205, 1976.

Armstrong, B; Clarke, H; Martin, C; et al: Urinary sodium and blood pressure in vegetarians. *Am J Clin Nutr* 32(12):2472, 1979.

Ashley, DV; Barclay, DV; Chaufford, FA; et al: Plasma amino acid responses in humans to evening meals of differing nutritional composition. *Am J Clin Nutr* 36(1):143, 1982.

Ballard, FJ; Gunn, JM; Nutritional and hormonal effects on intracellular protein catabolism. *Nutr Rev* 40(2):33, 1982.

Behar, M: Vegetable proteins in human nutrition. *Biblthca Nutr Dieta* 28:40, 1979.

Council on Foods and Nutrition (CFN): Zen macrobiotic diets. *JAMA* 218(3):397, 1971.

Donald, P; Pitts, GC; Pohl, SL: Body weight and composition in laboratory rats. Effects of diets with high or low protein concentrations. *Science* 211(4478):181, 1981.

Dwyer, J: Health implications of vegetarian diets. *Compr Therapy* 9(4):23, 1983.

Dwyer, JT; Andrew, EM; Berkey, C; et al: Growth in "new" vegetarians' preschool children using the Jenss-Bayley curve fitting technique. *Am J Clin Nutr* 37(5):815, 1983.

Farb, P; Armelagos, G: *Consuming Passions: The Anthropology of Eating.* Boston, Houghton Mifflin Company, 1980.

Goldin, BR; Adlercreutz, H; Gorbach, SL; et al: Estrogen excretion patterns and plasma levels in vegetarian and omnivorous women. *N Engl J Med* 307(25):1542, 1982.

Hegsted, M; Linkswiler, HM: Long-term effects of level of protein intake on calcium metabolism in young women. *J Nutr* 111(2):244, 1981.

Jeejeebhoy, KN: Protein nutrition in clinical practice. *Br Med Bull* 38(1):11, 1981.

Kopple, JD; Swendseid, ME: Evidence that histidine is an essential amino acid in normal and chronically uremic men, *J Clin Invest* 55:881, 1975.

Latner, AL: *Cantarow and Trumper Clinical Biochemistry,* 7th ed. Philadelphia, W. B. Saunders Co, 1975.

Licata, AA; Bou, E; Bartter, FC; et al: Acute effects of dietary protein on calcium metabolism in patients with osteoporosis. *J Gerontol* 36(1):14, 1981.

Linkswiler, HM; Zemel, MB; Hegsted, M; et al: Protein-induced hypercalciuria. *Fed Proc* 40(9):2429, 1981.

McLaren, DS: The great protein fiasco. *Lancet* 2(July 13):93, 1974.

Mahalko, JR; Sanstead, HH; Johnson, LK; et al: Effect of a moderate increase in dietary protein on the retention and excretion of Ca, Cu, Fe, Mg, P, and Zn by adult males. *Am J Clin Nutr* 37(1):8, 1983.

Marsh, AG; Sanchez, TV; Chaffee, FL; et al: Bone mineral mass in adult lacto-ovo-vegetarian and omnivorous males. *Am J Clin Nutr* 37(3):453, 1983.

Marsh, AG; Sanchez, TV; Mickelsen, O; et al: Cortical bone density of adult lacto-ovo-vegetarian and omnivorous women. *J Am Diet Assoc* 76(2):148, 1980.

Milman, N; Scheibel, J; Jessen, O: Lysine prophylaxis in recurrent herpes simplex labiales: a double-blind, controlled crossover study. *Acta Dermatovenerologica* 60(1):85, 1980.

Milman, N; Scheibel, J; Jessen, O: Failure of lysine treatment in recurrent herpes simplex labialis (letter). *Lancet* 2(Oct 28):942, 1978.

Munro, HN; Crim, MC: The proteins and amino acids. In *Modern Nutrition in Health and Disease,* 6th ed. Edited by RS Goodhart; ME Shils. Philadelphia, Lea & Febiger, 1980, p 51.

National Research Council: *Recommended Dietary Allowances.* Washington, DC, National Academy of Sciences, 1980.

Ophir, O; Peer, G; Gilad, J; et al: Low blood pressure in vegetarians: the possible role of potassium. *Am J Clin Nutr* 37(5):755, 1983.

Phillips, RL; Lemon, FR; Berson, WL; et al: Coronary heart disease mortality among Seventh-Day Adventists with differing dietary habits: A preliminary report. *Am J Clin Nutr* 31(10 suppl):S191, 1978.

Pixley, F; Wilson, D; McPherson, K; et al: Effect of vegetarianism on development of gallstones in women. *Br Med J* 291(July 6):11, 1985.

Silk, DBA: Digestion and absorption of dietary protein in man. *Proc Nutr Soc* 39(1):61, 1980.

Sunkin, S; Garrow, JS: The satiety value of protein. *Hum Nutr Appl Nutr* 36A(3):197, 1982.

Wurtman, RJ; Fernstrom, JD: Effects of the diet on brain neurotransmitters. *Nutr Rev* 32(7):193, 1974.

Further Study

American Dietetic Association: Position paper on the vegetarian approach to eating. *J Am Diet Assoc* 77(1):61, 1980.

Breeling, JL: Marketing protein for the world's poor. *Today's Health* 47(2):42, 1969.

Christoffel, K: A pediatric perspective on vegetarian nutrition. *Clin Pediatr* 20(9):632, 1981.

Dwyer, JT; Kandel, RF; Mayer, L; et al: The "new" vegetarians. *J Am Diet Assoc* 64(4):376, 1974.

Dwyer, JT; Mayer, L; Dowd, K; et al: The "new" vegetarians: the natural high? *J Am Diet Assoc* 65(5):529, 1974.

Hillman, H: Vegetarianism: an alternative diet or a crazy fad? *Nurs Times* 77(11):444, 1981.

Johnston, PK: Getting enough to grow on. *Am J Nurs* 84(3):336, 1984.

Lappe, FM: *Diet for a Small Planet,* 10th ed. New York, Ballantine Books, 1982. (A *must* for anyone planning vegetarian menus.)

Miller, RW: There's something to be said for never saying 'please pass the meat'. *FDA Consumer* 15(1):24, 1981.

National Academy of Sciences: *Alternative Dietary Practices and Nutritional Abuse in Pregnancy,* 1982. (Available from Food and Nutrition Board, 2102 Constitution Avenue, N.W., Washington, DC 20418.)

Protein content of selected plant foods. *Patient Care* 20(11):50, 1986.

Ross, T: The vegetarian diet: Animal, vegetable, mineral? *Nurs Mirror* 151(2):22, 1980.

Sanders, TAB: Vegetarian diets. *Nurs Times* 77(11):446, 1981.

Truesdell, DD; Acosta, PB: Feeding the vegan infant and child. *J Am Diet Assoc* 85(7):837, 1985.

Williams, ER: Making vegetarian diets nutritious. *Am J Nurs* 75(12):2168, 1975.

Carbohydrate: The Efficient Fuel

7

OBJECTIVES

THE STUDENT WILL BE ABLE TO:

- *Identify the major carbohydrates in foods and the body.*
- *Describe the digestion of carbohydrates in the stomach and small intestine.*
- *Identify normal body mechanisms that decrease and elevate blood glucose levels.*
- *List the ways glucose can be used by the body.*
- *State the functions of dietary carbohydrate.*
- *State why carbohydrate should be included in the diet.*
- *Identify dietary sources of lactose, other sugars, and starches.*
- *State the role and sources of dietary fiber.*
- *State the number of calories provided per gram of carbohydrate.*

TERMS TO KNOW

Cariogenic
Cellulose
Fiber
Gel
Gluconeogenesis
Glucosuria
Glycogenesis
Glycogenolysis
Glycolysis
Hemicellulose
Hydrophilic
Hyper- and hypoglycemia
Ketosis
Lignin
Mono-, di-, and
  polysaccharide
Protein-sparing

During the 1950s, carbohydrates somehow acquired a bad reputation in the United States. Statements have been made in best-selling books to the effect that we are the victims of "carbohydrate poisoning." Indeed, these unscientific rumors have affected food patterns.

In 1983, total calorie consumption was approximately the same as in 1909. By contrast, the total amount of carbohydrate in the U.S. food supply available for use declined about 20 percent (Marston & Raper, 1985). Carbohydrates supplied from starches (primarily grain products) declined sharply from 335 gm to approximately 190 gm/day (Marston & Welsh, 1984).

Despite these trends in the United States and Great Britain, carbohydrate has been the major source of energy in the human diet since the dawn of history (Connor & Connor, 1976). Worldwide, carbohydrates are the most important course of energy, furnishing up to 90 percent of the calories for many African nations.

Carbohydrates are the most economical form of energy. More energy can be produced per acre of land from plant foods because animals must first convert energy from plants into proteins and fats. Additionally, the inclusion of dietary carbohydrate adds variety and palatability to the diet.

Carbohydrates are made by all plants from carbon, hydrogen, and oxygen. In the process of photosynthesis, the carbon is combined with a molecule of water, such as $C—H_2O$. As Deutsch (1976) states, "A hydrated carbon is a carbohydrate."

Classification

Carbohydrates are not just $C—H_2O$, but different numbers of hydrated carbons in different structural formations. Generally, the chemical structure is in these proportions: $C_n(H_2O)_n$. Hence, empiric formulas such as $C_6H_{12}O_6$; or $C_{12}H_{22}O_{11}$ could readily be identified as carbohydrate. (When two monosaccharides join together, one molecule of water is liberated.) The number of carbon atoms in the molecule is used to classify carbohydrates; monosaccharides or simple sugars contain two to six carbon atoms, disaccharides are double sugars, containing 12 carbon atoms; polysaccharides contain over 12 carbon atoms.

Mono- and disaccharides are sugars that contribute to the palatability of a food because of their sweetness. Temperature, pH, and the presence of other substances influence the sweetness of a food. Relative sweetness of sugars is measured by subjective sensory tasting; sucrose is used as the standard of comparison and is given a value of 100 (Table 7–1).

MONOSACCHARIDES

The simplest carbohydrates are monosaccharides; they are absorbed without further digestion. The monosaccharides of greatest significance in foods and in body metabolism are the hexoses—glucose, fructose, galactose, and mannose. These are all six-carbon sugars, having the same empiric formula, $C_6H_{12}O_6$. Their structure is different, which affects their physical properties, including solubility and sweetness. *Focus on the Chemical Structure of Monosaccharides* shows the slight differences between six-carbon sugars having the same empiric formula.

Glucose. Also called dextrose, grape sugar, and corn sugar, glucose is naturally abundant in many fruits, such as grapes, oranges, dates, and in some vegetables, including fresh corn and carrots. It is prepared commercially as corn syrup or by special processing of starch. Intravenous fluids are normally dextrose solutions with some electrolytes added.

Glucose is the principal product formed by the digestion of di- and polysaccharides. It is the form of carbohydrate circulating in the blood, utilized by cells for energy.

Sorbitol. Sorbitol is a sweetening product (called a sugar alcohol), derived from glucose. For a given quantity, it adds about the same amount of sweetness as dextrose; it also furnishes the same amount of calories. The benefit of sorbitol is that it is absorbed slowly.

Fructose. This sugar (also known as levulose) is found naturally in honey and fruits. It is the sweetest of the monosaccharides (see Table 7–1) and a product of the digestion of sucrose. Fructose can be manufactured from glucose, meaning that a fructose-containing product may have been produced from a grain product.

Galactose. Another six-carbon sugar is galactose, which is not found in a free state in nature, but is a product of lactose digestion (milk sugar). While the primary source of galactose is milk, legumes also contain some galactose. Physiologically, it is a constituent of nerve tissue and produced from glucose during lactation in the synthesis of lactose.

FOCUS ON THE CHEMICAL STRUCTURE OF MONOSACCHARIDES*

Glucose	Galactose	Mannose	Fructose
$(C_6H_{12}O_6)$	$(C_6H_{12}O_6)$	$(C_6H_{12}O_6)$	$(C_6H_{12}O_6)$

*Monosaccharides, or hexoses, are represented as straight chains called stick formulas. The chemical formula is the same, but the atoms are arranged differently, as shown by the encircled grouping.

Mannose. This sugar is not found in a free state in foods but is derived from some legumes. Mannitol, derived from mannose, is found in foods. Because of advances in technology, *mannitol* is a caloric sweetner obtained from specially processed invert sugar syrup (see sucrose). It is expensive to produce; excessive consumption may have a laxative effect.

Xylitol. Xylitol is a sweetener with approximately the same perceived sweetness and caloric value as sugar. It is found in its natural state in fruits and vegetables (lettuce, carrots, and strawberries). Poor absorption causes a laxative effect.

Table 7–1. *Relative Sweetness of Sugars and Sweeteners**

Sugar or Sugar Product	Sweetness Value
Levulose	173
Invert sugar	130
Sucrose	100
Dextrose	74
Sorbitol	60
Mannitol	50
Galactose	32
Maltose	32
Lactose	16

*From Freed, M: Fructose—the extraordinary sweetener. *Food Product Development* 4(February-March):38, 1978, by permission.

Pentoses. Five-carbon sugars, called pentoses, include ribose, xylose, and arabinose. Ingested pentoses are not utilized but eliminated in the urine and feces. The body synthesizes pentose sugars from other carbohydrates, as needed in the cell. Physiologically, ribose is important as a constituent of ribonucleic acid (RNA), deoxyribonucleic acid (DNA), and the B vitamin riboflavin.

Other Sugars. Raffinose, a trisaccharide, and stachyose, a tetrasaccharide, cannot be hydrolyzed by humans. Their presence in dry beans may cause flatulence.

DISACCHARIDES

Two hexose sugars joined together are called a disaccharide. They are not important in human metabolism because they contribute to body function only after they have been digested. All are hydrolyzed during digestion to their constituent monosaccharides for absorption:

Sucrose = glucose + fructose

Maltose = glucose + glucose

Lactose = glucose + galactose

Sucrose. Granulated table sugar is refined from sugar cane and sugar beets to separate the sucrose from the indigestible parts of the plants. It is also found in molasses, maple syrup, and maple sugar. Some fruits and vegetables (apricots, peaches, plums, raspberries, honeydew, muskmelons, beets, carrots, parsnips, winter squash, peas, corn, and sweet potatoes) naturally contain larger amounts of sucrose than glucose or fructose.

Sucrose can be processed to produce a 50:50 ratio of its monosaccharides glucose and fructose. This liquid sugar is known as invert sugar. It has the advantage of tasting sweeter than comparable amounts of sucrose.

Lactose. The sugar found in milk is lactose, which contains two monosaccharides, glucose and galactose. Lactose is unique to mammals, comprising 4.5 percent of cow's milk and 7.5 percent of human milk. In the fermentation of milk, some of the lactose is converted to lactic acid, giving buttermilk and yogurt their characteristic flavors.

Maltose. Also called malt sugar, maltose does not occur naturally. It is produced by fermenting grains and is present in beer and some processed cereals and baby foods. It is also combined with dextrins in infant formulas. Maltose is hydrolyzed to two molecules of glucose before absorption.

Clinical Implications:

- Individuals should limit their intake of hard candies containing sugar alcohols (mannitol, sorbitol) to 3 to 4 pieces spread throughout the day to prevent gastric cramping.
- Galactose, found in some legumes, would not be well-tolerated by persons with the genetic disorder galactosemia.
- Mannitol, which is a derivative of a six-carbon sugar, has been used as a diuretic agent for elimination of drugs in the urine, to reduce intracranial pressure, and to correct hyponatremic overhydration (Ginn, 1974).
- Some sweeteners produced from corn, especially high fructose corn syrup, may not be tolerated by persons allergic to the parent grain.

POLYSACCHARIDES

Complex carbohydrates, also called polysaccharides, are composed of many monosaccharides. These chains are very large, sometimes containing as many as 1500 or more simple sugars.

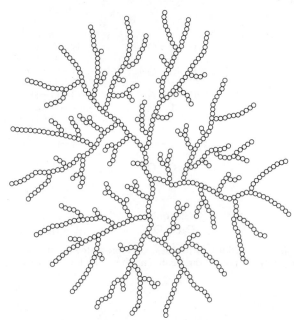

*(From McGilvery RW: *Biochemistry: A Functional Approach*, 3rd ed. Philadelphia, W. B. Saunders Co., 1983, by permission.)

The chains have different structures and can be branched or straight. One example, glycogen, can be seen in *Focus on the Structure of Glycogen.*

Some polysaccharides have a role in energy storage and are digestible; the second group, largely indigestible by human intestinal enzymes, is called dietary fiber (Fig. 7–1).

Starch. Energy for the plant is compactly stored as starch. Most complex carbohydrates in the diet are in the form of starch, which is found in cereal grains, roots, vegetables, and legumes.

The amount of starch present in a vegetable increases with its maturity, as it stores up energy for the new plants to survive until it can produce leaves and photosynthesize its own energy. Freshly picked corn tastes much sweeter than after it has been picked for several days, i.e., simple sugars continue to develop into starch. The amount of starch in a fruit decreases as it ripens, i.e., the complex carbohydrates are broken down in the ripening process into simple sugars.

Starch granules are insoluble in cold water. Starches are encased in a cell wall called cellulose. Cooking facilitates the digestive process by causing the granules to swell, rupturing the cell wall

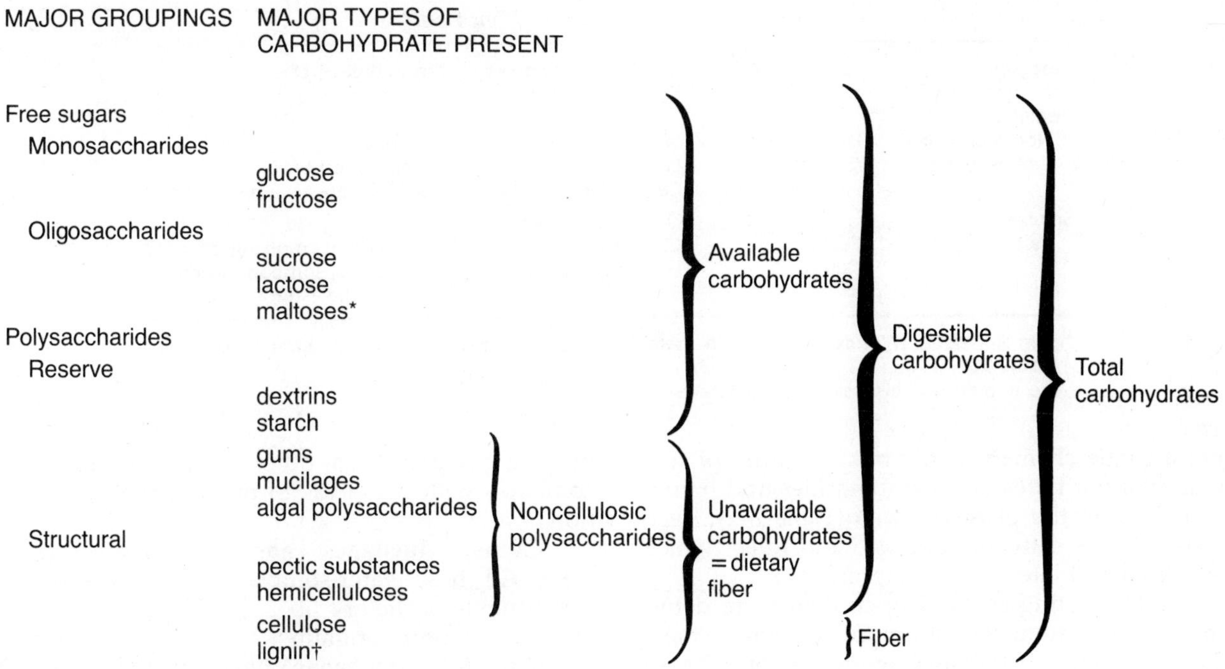

MAJOR GROUPINGS	MAJOR TYPES OF CARBOHYDRATE PRESENT				
Free sugars					
Monosaccharides					
	glucose				
	fructose				
Oligosaccharides			Available carbohydrates		
	sucrose				
	lactose			Digestible carbohydrates	
	maltoses*				Total carbohydrates
Polysaccharides					
Reserve					
	dextrins				
	starch				
	gums				
	mucilages	Noncellulosic polysaccharides	Unavailable carbohydrates = dietary fiber		
	algal polysaccharides				
Structural					
	pectic substances				
	hemicelluloses				
	cellulose		Fiber		
	lignin†				

*Including maltotriose, maltotetrose, etc., from glucose syrups.

†Not a carbohydrate but an aromatic polymer.

Figure 7–1. *Nutritional classification of the carbohydrates in the diet. (From Southgate DAT, Bailey B, Collinson E, et al: A guide to calculating intakes of dietary fiber. Journal of Human Nutrition 30:303, 1976. Reprinted courtesy of John Libbey & Company, Ltd.)*

so that digestive enzymes have access to the starch inside the cell. In cooking, this swelling is referred to as thickening. Industrially, food starch is modified by chemicals to produce a better thickening agent.

Dextrins. Intermediate products of the digestive enzymes on the starch molecule are as follows:

Starch → dextrins → maltose → glucose

Dextrins are also produced when starch is subjected to dry heat (e.g., toasting bread).

Glucose Polymers. Industrially-produced carbohydrate supplements are composed of glucose, maltose, and dextrins. They are used to increase the calorie intake of individuals who have increased calorie requirements or who are unable to ingest adequate amounts of calories from their regular diet. They are well-suited for clear-liquid diets or protein-, fat-, or electrolyte-restricted diets. These products can be mixed easily with most foods and beverages without making them excessively sweet. The glucose is readily absorbed and utilized, providing 4 kcal/gm like other carbohydrate products. Their low osmolality minimizes the occurrence of osmotic diarrhea. These products include Polycose (Ross), Moducal (Mead Johnson), and Summacal (Biosearch).

Glycogen. Energy in humans and animals is stored as a very large branched-chain polysaccharide called glycogen (see *Focus on the Structure of Glycogen*). Stored in the muscle and liver, it is readily available as a source of glucose and energy. Carbohydrates are frequently consumed in excess of immediate energy needs. Excess glucose is converted to glycogen until the limited glycogen storage capacity is filled; simultaneously and even after glycogen stores are filled, glucose is also converted into fats and stored as adipose tissue. Glycogen is of little importance as a dietary source of carbohydrate because it is rapidly degraded to lactic acid when animals are slaughtered.

Structural Polysaccharides. Dietary constituents that contribute to dietary fiber cannot be digested by humsn gastrointestinal enzymes. These structural polysaccharides, or dietary fiber, are

Table 7–2. Classification of Plant Fiber*

Category	Component	Major Food Sources	Physiological Effects
Insoluble			
Noncarbohydrate	Lignin	Vegetables	Uncertain
Carbohydrate	Cellulose	Wheat	Increase fecal bulk
	Hemicelluloses[†]	Cereals, vegetables	Decrease intestinal transit time
Soluble			
Carbohydrate	Pectin	Citrus fruit	Delay gastric emptying, slow
	Gums	Legumes, oats, barley	glucose absorption, lower
			serum cholesterol

*From Anderson, JW: Physiological and metabolic effects of dietary fiber. *Federation Proceedings* 44(14):2902, 1985.
[†]Also termed noncellulosic polysaccharides.

not a single chemical entity but a mixture of several different types of polysaccharides and lignin, combined in the plant cell wall (Table 7–2). Each type exhibits different physiological roles, which are discussed later in the chapter.

Tables listing crude fiber content were determined by antiquated procedures, which measured mainly cellulose and lignin fractions. These are being updated, reflecting higher dietary fiber amounts than crude fiber tables (Lanza & Butrum, 1986). Product labels may list the amounts of fiber in one serving, but one should be certain that this is dietary fiber, not crude fiber.

Although much research is being conducted, the physiological properties of each component in fiber have not been fully identified. This has been a very complex and confusing task because the composition of the cell walls in the plant and its physical properties vary with the plant's age and maturity as well as its growing conditions.

Cellulose. The most plentiful polysaccharide found in plants is cellulose. While it is not digested by human digestive enzymes, it serves as a substrate for microbial fermentation and has a hydrophilic ability to attract water, promoting efficient intestinal function.

Hemicellulose. Another important food fiber, hemicellulose, is actually composed of various sugars, including xylose, glucose, and mannose. Hemicelluloses absorb and retain water in the gut but have little effect on stool size. Gastrointestinal bacteria can digest much of the hemicelluloses.

Pectin. Pectins are nondigestible polysaccharides that form a gel with water. They are used in the preparation of fruit jams and jellies to form a gel water in an interconnecting network.

Lignin. Lignin is a woody substance, closely associated with cellulose in plants. While it is the only noncarbohydrate fiber, it is grouped with the polysaccharides. Lignified fibers are less digestible

by gut bacteria than other polysaccharides. It combines with bile acids to prevent their absorption.

Gums, Mucilages, and Algal Polysaccharides. All these water-soluble polysaccharides are components of dietary fiber. Mucilages are found in the endosperm of grains. Algal polysaccharides (alginate and carrageenan) have the ability to absorb water, thicken, and emulsify. All these products are frequently used as additives, especially in milk products such as ice cream.

Ingestion Through Absorption

INTAKE

Carbohydrates, including starches but especially sugars, add palatability to the diet. Limited research has been conducted on the importance of taste to nutrition. Pleasant taste stimuli favorably affect the activity of the digestive system (Kare, 1975). The desire for sweetness is not considered an acquired taste since newborn infants exhibit a preference for it.

DIGESTION

Carbohydrate is the only nutrient that starts breaking down chemically in the mouth. Saliva secretions are stimulated by the presence of food in the mouth, or even the thought, smell, or sight of foods. Ptyalin, or salivary amylase, begins the process of hydrolyzing starch to dextrins and

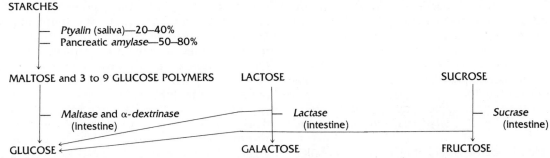

Figure 7–2. Digestion of carbohydrates. (From Guyton AC: Textbook of Medical Physiology, 7th ed. Philadelphia, W. B. Saunders Co, 1986, by permission.)

maltose. The action of salivary amylase continues until the chyme is acidified, which usually takes more than 30 minutes, resulting in at least one third of the starch being hydrolyzed to maltose. If the starch remained in the stomach for a long enough period of time, the acid in the stomach could hydrolyze it to monosaccharides.

Chyme entering the small intestine contains some starch, maltose, lactose, sucrose, and other disaccharides and monosaccharides from the ingested foods. Intestinal and pancreatic juices complete the digestion to monosaccharides. As disaccharides come into contact with the brush border cells, they are hydrolyzed by their enzymes into glucose, fructose, and galactose. Of the disaccharides, hydrolysis of lactose is the slowest. Sucrase and, to some extent, lactase activity is somewhat affected by levels of these sugars in the diet (Rosenweig, 1974); in other words, if the intake of these sugars is routinely low, the amount of their respective enzymes will be decreased. A synopsis of carbohydrate digestion is shown in Figure 7–2.

ABSORPTION

The digestion process is completed faster than the monosaccharides can be absorbed, except for lactose. Absorption occurs mainly in the lower duodenum and jejunum, but some may be absorbed in the ileum.

Factors influencing the amount of time for digestion and absorption of a monosaccharide depend on how fast it is released into the small intestine and the mixture of foods already present in the intestine. The condition of the mucous membrane, hormones, and the adequacy of vitamin intake also affect absorption rates (Latner, 1975). Undigested disaccharides can be absorbed as such but are usually excreted in the urine.

Clinical Implications:

- Abnormal carbohydrate absorption is typical in enteritis.
- Pancreatic amylase is present in sufficient quantities to hydrolyze starches even in patients with severe pancreatic disease. Starches are an important source of calories for these patients (Gray & Fogel, 1980).

Metabolism

BLOOD SUGAR LEVEL

Monosaccharides are transported through the portal vein to the liver where fructose, galactose, sorbitol, and xylitol are converted to glycogen (Pike & Brown, 1984).

Glucose is the most common circulating sugar in the blood; it is the main energy source for cells. The level of circulating glucose is closely monitored by the liver, constantly maintained at a level between 80 and 90 mg/dl. After a meal, blood sugar levels will increase to 120 to 130 mg/dl because only 10 percent is taken up by the liver on the first pass (Crapo, 1981). However, it returns to normal within two to three hours. A newborn's blood sugar level is low—30 mg/dl—and falls faster and to a greater degree than in fasting adults. During a prolonged fast with regular amounts of activity, blood sugar falls after two days and reaches a minimal level after four to six days (a drop of 15 to 30 mg/dl). With continued fasting, the blood sugar rises during the second week to approximately the original level.

This consistent blood sugar level is significant, indicating the necessity for a certain amount of sugar in the blood for normal functioning of body tissues. The level is constant between meals and rarely falls below 70 mg/dl. When the blood sugar level exceeds 160 to 180 mg/dl, some glucose will exceed the renal threshold and is excreted in the urine (glucosuria). The blood sugar level is so closely regulated that glucosuria is infrequent.

A blood glucose level below 60 mg/dl is called hypoglycemia; a blood level above 120 mg/dl is hyperglycemia. Both symptoms are very serious and the precipitating cause should be identified. (Chapters 29 and 30 discuss these metabolic problems and therapeutic diets for them.) The fasting blood glucose level is the best indicator of overall glucose homeostasis and requires eight hours of fasting prior to the test. The normal range for fasting blood sugar is 45 to 95 mg/dl. When fasting blood sugar is elevated, a glucose tolerance test is in order.

Glucose tolerance tests (Fig. 7–3) reflect the metabolic response to a carbohydrate challenge following 12 hours of fasting. Glucose response is somewhat affected by the type of diet (Fig. 7–4). For accurate measurements, the individual must be on a well-rounded diet for three to seven days prior to the test to have full glycogen storage. After starvation or a low carbohydrate diet, tolerance is diminished and a person will normally have a very high blood sugar peak.

In the past, it was assumed that all mono- or disaccharides (sugars) produced a higher glucose response than starches. Dr. J. A. Jenkins and colleagues have challenged this, comparing the hyperglycemic response of individual foods with a reference food. Indeed beans and fructose yield much flatter glycemic response curves than glucose and potatoes. In other words, differences in blood glucose response to different foods cannot be accurately predicted from tables of food composition (Jenkins et al, 1983).

This research reveals a myriad of biological responses to different carbohydrate foods. Based on these findings, foods have been classified for their glycemic index, using white wheat bread as the reference standard (Table 7–3). Factors affecting the glycemic response include dietary fiber, the form of the food (e.g., wheat flour induces a

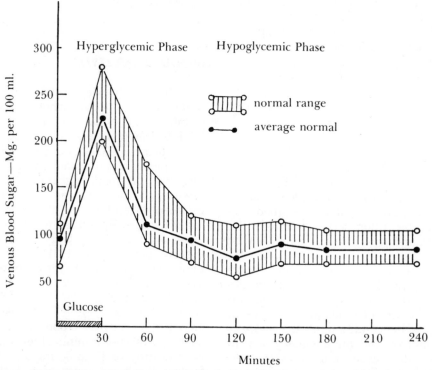

Figure 7–3. *Intravenous glucose tolerance test. (From Latner AL: Cantarow and Trumper Clinical Biochemistry, 7th ed. Philadelphia, W. B. Saunders Co, 1975, with permission.)*

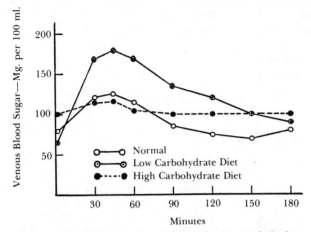

Figure 7–4. Effect of previously high and low carbohydrate diets on oral glucose tolerance test. (From Latner AL: Cantarow and Trumper Clinical Biochemistry, 7th ed. Philadelphia, W. B. Saunders Co, 1975, with permission.)

greater response than wheat noodles), digestibility, cooking, the presence of antinutrients (enzyme inhibitors, phytates), starch-protein or starch-lipid interaction, carbohydrate content of previous meals, and other causes.

A complex hormonal system maintains a constant blood sugar. These include insulin, glucagon, thyroxin, the adrenocorticoids, and the catecholamines. The hormone that lowers the blood sugar level is insulin. Beta cells within the islets of Langerhans in the pancreas produce insulin. When hyperglycemia occurs, insulin is secreted to lower blood sugar levels by several methods; conversely, hypoglycemia will elicit the secretion of several hormones that increase blood glucose (Fig. 7–5).

The process by which sugars are stored as glycogen is called glycogenesis. The glycogen can be broken down by the liver to maintain constant sugar levels, referred to as glycogenolysis.

Muscle tissue is also able to store carbohydrates as glycogen; however, the enzymes necessary for glycogenolysis are lacking. Glycogen in muscle tissue is broken down to lactic acid, a process referred to as glycolysis, which also releases energy for the cells. Glycolysis is an anaerobic process involving the production of lactic acid or pyruvic acid from glucose or glycogen. Ordinarily, lactic acid is oxidized by oxygen (aerobically) to yield (via the Krebs cycle) carbon dioxide, water, and energy, which is stored as ATP (adenosine triphosphate). Production of too much lactic acid results in its being released into the blood to be converted to glucose.

Table 7–3. Glycemic Index of Foods*

Food	Glycemic Index
Grain and Cereal Products	
White bread	100
Whole-wheat bread	99
Brown rice	96
White rice	83
White spaghetti	66
Whole-wheat spaghetti	61
Rye bread	58
Breakfast Cereals	
Cornflakes	119
Weetabix	109
Shredded Wheat	97
All Bran	73
Oatmeal	85
Fruits	
Raisins	93
Banana	79
Orange juice	67
Orange	66
Grapes	62
Apple	53
Pear	47
Peach	40
Grapefruit	36
Plum	34
Vegetables	
Baked potato	135
Instant potatoes	116
New potatoes	81
Yams	74
Frozen peas	74
Sweet potato	70
Dried Legumes	
Canned baked beans	60
Kidney beans	54
Butter beans	52
Chickpeas	49
Lentils	43
Soybeans	20
Dairy Products	
Ice cream	52
Yogurt	52
Whole milk	49
Skim milk	46
Sweeteners	
Maltose	152
Glucose	138
Honey	126
Sucrose	86
Fructose	30

*Adapted from Jenkins, DJA; Wolever, TMS; Jenkins, AL; et al: The glycaemic response to carbohydrate foods. *Lancet* 2(August 18):388, 1984.

Another method by which blood sugar level can be increased is the conversion of noncarbohydrate substances, especially amino acids and glycerol, to glucose, a process called gluconeogenesis.

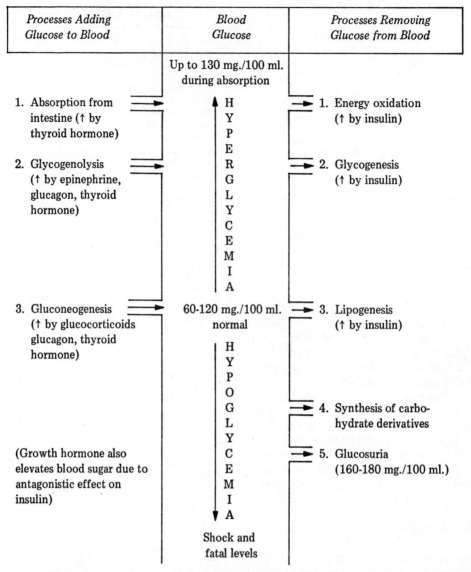

Figure 7–5. Maintaining blood glucose levels. (Adapted by Lewis C: Nutrition and Diet Therapy: Proteins and Carbohydrate. Philadelphia, F. A. Davis, 1976. Reprinted with permission of Macmillan Publishing Company from Textbook of Biochemistry, 4th ed, by E. S. West, W. R. Todd, H. S. Mason, and J. T. Van Bruggen. Copyright © 1966 by Macmillan Publishing Co, Inc.)

Carbohydrate metabolism is dependent on an adequate supply of B vitamins and two minerals, phosphorus and magnesium. The amount of carbohydrate eaten affects the requirement for B vitamins. Carbohydrate metabolism is summarized in Figure 7–6.

FUNCTIONS OF SUGAR

The absorbed sugars can be used in one of six ways.

1. Source of energy. The principal role of the absorbed sugars is to provide energy for the body and heat to maintain body temperature. The central nervous system and the lens of the eye can only use glucose for energy, while other tissues can also use fats. From the glycolysis process, each gram of carbohydrate—whether it was originally from a sugar or a starch—provides 4 kcal.

2. Stored as glycogen. Glycogen is another way absorbed monosaccharides furnish energy when the body needs it. Excess glucose is converted to glycogen, stored in the muscles, and released as

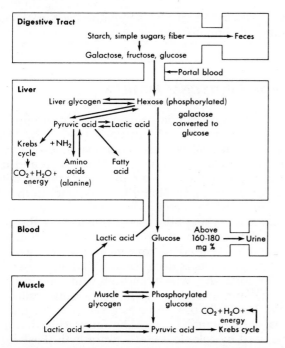

Figure 7–6. Pathways of carbohydrate metabolism. (Reprinted with permission of Macmillan Publishing Company from Normal and Therapeutic Nutrition, 16th ed, by C. R. Robinson and M. R. Lawler. Copyright © 1982 by Macmillan Publishing Co, Inc.)

energy when needed. It may also be stored in the liver and released to maintain blood sugar level. There is no form of energy storage in the brain.

Glycogenesis in the liver is partly dependent on the diet. In a fasting state, the liver contains little glycogen; after a meal, four to five percent of the weight of the liver is glycogen. The total amount is actually relatively small—only enough to meet energy demands for less than a day.

3. Converted to triglycerides and stored as fat. This process, called lipogenesis, occurs when large quantities of carbohydrates are eaten. Blood sugars ensure replenishing of glycogen stores; however, excessive amounts result in less fat being oxidized and in carbohydrate being converted to fat and stored in fatty tissue.

4. Converted to other necessary carbohydrates. Monosaccharides are important constituents of many compounds that regulate metabolism (Table 7–4).

5. Converted to nonessential amino acids. The liver can utilize the carbon framework from the sugar molecule and the amine group contributed by the breakdown of an amino acid to produce nonessential amino acids needed in the body.

6. Eliminated in the urine. When blood glucose levels exceed 160 to 190 mg/dl, the kidney cannot reabsorb it all, and it is eliminated via the urine. This is called the renal threshold. Normally, urine glucose contains 1 to 15 mg/dl.

Clinical Implications:

- High carbohydrate diets lead to a general increase in insulin's ability to promote glucose removal from plasma (Kolterman et al, 1979).
- Pain and emotional excitement (fear, anxiety, apprehension) accelerate hepatic glycogenolysis because of increased epinephrine and glucocorticoid secretion.

Table 7–4. Some Body Compounds Containing Carbohydrate

Compound	Function
Glucuronic acid	Combines with toxic chemicals and bacterial by-products in the liver, functioning as a detoxifying agent.
Heparin	Prevents blood clotting.
Chondroitin sulfates	Found in connective tissue, cartilage, and heart valves. Capable of binding water.
Immunopolysaccharides	Part of infection-resistant mechanism.
Deoxyribonucleic acid (DNA) and ribonucleic acid (RNA)	Compounds responsible for the genetic material and cell duplication.
Galactolipins	Constituents of nervous tissue.
Glycosides	Components of steroid and adrenal hormones.
Keratan sulfate	In connective tissue.
Hyaluronic acid	Component of intercellular material and synovial fluids. Can bind a large amount of water.
Dermatan sulfate	Present in tissues rich in collagen, especially in the skin.

- Blood glucose concentrations are increased only slightly when fructose, sorbitol, or xylitol are given (Forster, 1974); less insulin is required for their metabolism (Crapo & Kolterman, 1984).

Other Functions of Dietary Carbohydrates

Previously discussed were the roles of carbohydrates: (1) as an energy source, (2) as a constituent of many body compounds, and (3) as a constituent of nonessential amino acids. In addition, carbohydrates have an important role in: (4) normal fat metabolism, (5) sparing protein, (6) increased growth of intestinal bacteria, (7) maintaining gastrointestinal motility, and (8) increasing the dietary intake of protein, minerals, and B vitamins.

NORMAL FAT METABOLISM

The oxidation of fats requires the presence of some carbohydrates. When the intake of carbohydrates is low, the body relies on energy from larger amounts of fats. Fats are metabolized faster than the body can oxidize the resulting intermediate products called ketone bodies. Ketosis is the accumulation of incompletely oxidized fatty products. It can be prevented with 50 gm intake of carbohydrates.

PROTEIN-SPARERS

Carbohydrates, by furnishing energy in the diet, are said to be protein-sparing. Energy is a number one need of the body. With insufficient carbohydrate intake, the body burns protein for fuel. When carbohydrate intake is sufficient, protein can be used to build and repair tissue. Carbohydrate and protein intake at the same meal increases protein utilization.

INTESTINAL BACTERIA

Lactose, by remaining in the gastrointestinal tract longer than other disaccharides, encourages the growth of bacteria that synthesize certain vitamins (B-complex and vitamin K).

GASTROINTESTINAL MOTILITY

The contribution of fiber in the gastrointestinal tract has several functions (Fig. 7–7). Fiber tends to normalize intestinal transit time—increasing it in persons with slow transit time and decreasing it in those with rapid transit time (Spiller & Amen, 1975). Its ability to bind water in the intestine and to increase bulk from nondigestible substances causes decreased transit time through the alimentary tract. Thus, the length of time tissues are exposed to cancer-causing nitrogenous waste products is decreased. An added benefit is stool softening, which helps prevent constipation.

Water-insoluble fibers, especially cellulose and hemicellulose, serve as a substrate for microbial fermentation, producing fatty acids that can be used by colonic bacteria for growth (Eastwood & Passmore, 1983). These fibers increase stool bulk, exercising the digestive tract muscles by increasing the radius of the colon and preventing the muscle from being chronically contracted. Therefore, muscle tone is maintained, colonic pressure is diminished, and the gut is able to resist bulging out into the pouches frequently seen in diverticulosis.

Water-soluble fibers such as pectins, gums, mucilages, and algal polysaccharides are physiologically important for their gel-forming ability. Pectin increases the viscosity of chyme in the gut, thereby delaying the absorption of glucose and other nutrients. These can also bind bile acids and are classified as being hypocholesteremic. Lignin is able to bind bile, electrolytes, and many drugs. Another benefit is that fiber-rich foods are not calorie-dense and may help an individual to fill up on a fewer number of calories (Anderson, 1985; Eastwood & Passmore, 1983; Gray & Fogel, 1980).

OTHER NUTRIENTS

Carbohydrates are normally accompanied by other nutrients. Starches are especially important for their contribution of protein, minerals, and B vitamins. Whole-grain products are superior because of their fiber plus other nutrients; enriched products should always be used as opposed to those processed but not enriched.

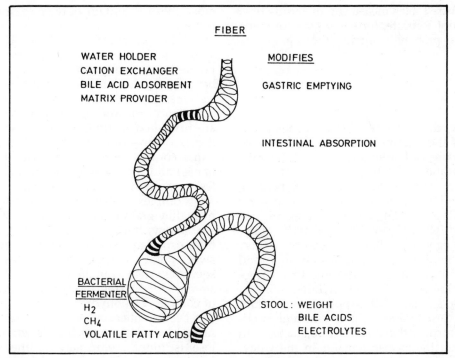

Figure 7–7. *Physiology and function of fiber along the gut. (From Eastwood MA, Passmore R: A new look at dietary fiber.* Nutrition Today *19(5):6, 1984.)*

Clinical Implications:

- Ketosis frequently occurs in uncontrolled diabetes mellitus or in persons who are not eating (because of illness or dieting) because they are burning fat rather than carbohydrate.
- Adequate nutrition that increases glycogen stores will facilitate the elimination of poisonous materials such as carbon tetrachloride, alcohol, and arsenic (Levine, 1976).
- Glycogen stores in the heart are critical for continuous functioning of the cardiac muscle.
- The best source of fiber to relieve constipation is bran.
- Some vegetables and fruits (bananas, white potatoes, and apples) are high in pectins, which bind water. They are frequently used to check diarrhea but can also help relieve constipation by softening the stool.
- Pectin is used in combination with an absorbent, kaolin, to treat diarrhea (Kaopectate).
- Enthusiastic individuals who eat excessive amounts of bran gain no benefit from the surplus and expose themselves unnecessarily to known hazards, such as decreased mineral absorption, and perhaps unknown hazards, too.

Dietary Requirements

Since humans can convert amino acids and a part of the fat molecule to glucose, a specific requirement for carbohydrate has not been established by the National Research Council. People can be adequately nourished at extremely high or low levels of carbohydrate intake, provided their energy, protein, and other nutritional needs have been met. A reasonable proportion of the caloric intake should consist of carbohydrates (50 to 100 gm digestible carbohydrate) with the emphasis on complex carbohydrates to avoid ketosis, excessive breakdown of protein, loss of electrolytes, and involuntary dehydration. A diet high in carbohydrate will maintain glycogen reserves, whereas a diet high in fat and low in carbohydrate and protein results in poor glycogen reserves.

Although dietary fiber is important, a specific RDA has not been made. Approximately 40 gm of dietary fiber daily has been suggested for a high-fiber intake (Dietary recommendations, 1986). Currently the American diet provides less than 20 mg dietary fiber. Tables measuring the crude fiber in foods are not accurate; for every gram of crude fiber, the food probably contains 2 or 3 gm of dietary fiber.

SOURCES

Presently, the American diet furnishes about 45 percent of the calories from carbohydrates, or almost 400 grams carbohydrate daily. Of this total intake, fruits and vegetables represent about 17 percent; grains and legumes, about 38 percent; and sugars and sweeteners, also about 38 percent (Marston & Raper, 1985). Carbohydrates are furnished by the following food groups: milk, grain, fruits and vegetables, and "accessory foods" (which includes sweeteners, jellies, syrups, and many desserts). A few food items and their carbohydrate contribution are shown in Table 7–5.

The only animal food supplying significant quantities of carbohydrate is milk and milk products, which furnish the disaccharide, lactose. In cheese-making, the lactose remains in the whey, which is removed as a by-product. Consequently, most cheeses contain only trace amounts of lactose.

Other sugars are furnished by table sugar, syrups, jellies, jams, and honey. Sugars are incorporated into many popular foods (e.g., candy, beverages, cakes and desserts, chewing gum, and ice cream) which accounts for their widespread acceptance. Sugars, mainly glucose and fructose, are furnished in fruits and vegetables in varying degrees depending on their maturity (ripe bananas contain more simple sugars than green bananas) and their water content (spinach contains less carbohydrate than potatoes).

Complex carbohydrates or starches are furnished by grain products—wheat, corn, rice, oats, rye, barley, buckwheat, and millet. Some vegetables, especially root and seed varieties (potatoes, sweet potatoes, beets, carrots, peas, and winter squashes) also contain considerable amounts of starch. Dried beans and peas are excellent sources of complex carbohydrates.

Dietary fiber, especially hemicellulose, is furnished by whole-grain breads and cereals. Cellulose is found principally in the stems, roots, leaves, and seed coverings of plants; raw fruits

Table 7–5. Common Carbohydrates in Foods per 100 gm of Edible Portion

Food Item	Monosaccharides and Reducing Sugars* (gm)	Lactose* (gm)	Sucrose* (gm)	Starch* (gm)	Total Dietary Fiber[†] (gm)	Noncellulose Polysaccharides[†] (gm)	Cellulose[†] (gm)	Lignin[†] (gm)
Apple (flesh only)	15.0	—	3.1	0.6	1.42	0.94	0.48	0.01
Banana	8.4	—	8.9	1.9	1.75	1.12	0.37	0.26
Grapefruit	3.2	—	2.9	—	0.44	0.34	0.04	0.55
Peaches	6.2	—	6.6	—	2.28	1.46	0.20	0.62
Strawberries	4.9	—	1.4	—	2.12	0.98	0.33	0.81
Broccoli tops	—	—	—	1.3	4.10	2.92	0.85	0.03
Brussels sprouts	—	—	—	—	2.86	1.99	0.80	0.07
Cauliflower (boiled)	—	—	—	—	1.80	0.67	1.13	trace
Lettuce	1.4	—	0.2	—	1.53	0.47	1.06	trace
Onions, raw	5.4	—	2.9	—	2.10	1.55	0.55	trace
White potatoes	1.0	—	—	17.0	3.51	2.49	1.02	trace
Ice cream (14.5% cream)	—	3.6	16.6	—	—	—	—	—
Whole milk	—	4.9	—	—	—	—	—	—
Yogurt	—	3.8	—	—	—	—	—	—
Peanuts	0.2	—	4.5	4.0	9.30	6.40	1.69	1.21
Peanut butter	0.9	—	5.9	—	7.55	5.64	1.91	trace
Wheat flour (patent)	2.0	—	—	68.8	3.15	2.52	0.60	0.03
Brown flour				N/A	7.87	5.70	1.42	0.75

*Data from Hardinge, MG: Carbohydrates in foods. *Journal of the American Dietetic Association* 46(3):197, 1965.
[†]Data from Southgate, DAT; Bailey, B; Collinson, E; et al: A guide to calculating intakes of dietary fibre. *Journal of Human Nutrition* 30:303, 1976.

Table 7–6. Dietary Fiber in Flours, Breads, and Breakfast Cereals*

	Total Dietary Fiber	Noncellulose Polysaccharides	Cellulose	Lignin
White flour	3.15†	2.52	0.60	0.03
Brown flour	7.87	5.70	1.42	0.75
White bread	2.72	2.01	0.71	trace
Brown bread	5.11	3.63	1.33	0.15
All Bran	26.70	17.82	6.01	2.88
Cornflakes	11.00	7.26	2.42	1.32
Grapenuts	7.00	5.14	1.28	0.58
Rice Krispies	4.47	3.47	0.78	0.22
Shredded Wheat	12.26	8.79	2.63	0.84
Special K	5.45	3.68	0.72	1.05

*Data from Southgate, DAT; Bailey, B; Collinson, E: et al: A guide to calculating intake of dietary fibre. *Journal of Human Nutrition* 30:303, 1976.
†All values shown are grams per 100 gram serving.

and leafy vegetables are good sources. Legumes are also a good source of dietary fiber. The pectin contributed by fruits and vegetables is an important source of fiber. The fiber content of foods is decreased by most refining processes, as shown in Table 7–6. The effect of cooking on fiber is not clear.

CARBOHYDRATE AND LACTOSE INTOLERANCE

Some people are unable to handle specific carbohydrates because of insufficient amounts of disaccharide enzymes. When that carbohydrate is eaten, the sugar is fermented by intestinal bacteria. This results in malabsorption of the disaccharide, accompanied by diarrhea, abdominal cramps, and flatulence.

The most common carbohydrate malabsorption syndrome, lactose intolerance, is so prevalent among adults of several ethnic groups, it is considered normal (Fig. 7–8). Lactase deficiency is determined by a biopsy of the intestinal mucosa or by indirect methods such as the lactose tolerance test or breath hydrogen test (Newcomer & McGill, 1984).

Three types of lactase deficiency have been identified. Congenital lactase deficiency is a rare condition, which may be present at birth due to an inborn error of metabolism. The most common problem is lactase deficiency. About 70 percent of American black adults and over 90 percent of the Oriental adults suffer from primary adult lactase deficiency. This is possibly an inherited problem, as evidenced by its frequency within various cul-

tures. There is a normal developmental age-related decrease in lactase activity. Finally, low lactase activity, called secondary lactase deficiency, may be temporary as a result of gastrointestinal diseases or damage to the intestinal mucosa, such as in sprue, regional enteritis, and bacterial infections.

Treatment of lactase deficiency is simple. Since the ability to tolerate lactose is not an all-or-nothing phenomenon, the amount of dairy products is reduced to the tolerance level. Milk is tolerated better when taken with a meal. Whole milk is tolerated better than skim milk (Newcomer & McGill, 1984). Fermented dairy products—especially yogurt but also cottage cheese, buttermilk, sour cream and cheeses—are often better tolerated by lactase-deficient individuals because they contain a bacteria that breaks down the lactose. Savaiano and colleagues (1984) have observed that the bacteria in unpasteurized yogurt digest the lactose in the gastrointestinal tract. LactAid is a commercially available enzyme that "digests" some of the lactose in milk.

When milk intake is curtailed, the missing nutrients should be somehow supplemented, either by intake of other high-calcium foods or calcium supplements. Lactose malabsorption does not seem to have any significant effect on the absorption of protein, fat, or calcium (Newcomer & McGill, 1984).

Clinical Implications:

- Lactase deficiency is increased in patients with osteoporosis, possibly secondary to diminished

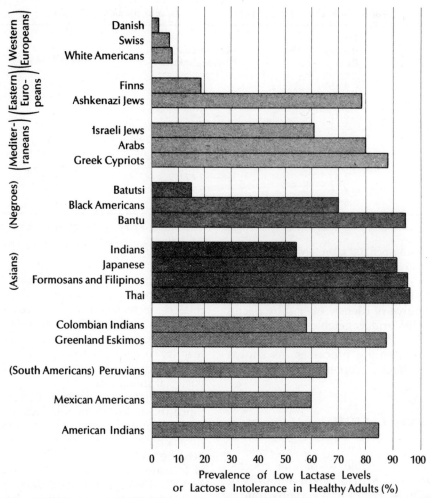

Figure 7–8. Among the population groups sampled thus far, almost all with a high prevalence of lactose intolerance (or low lactase level) are those in which dairying and milk drinking have been traditionally minimal or absent; conversely, lactose intolerance has been relatively rare in traditional dairying and milk-drinking populations. (From Bayless TM: Recognition of lactose intolerance. Hospital Practice 11(10):100, 1976. Illustration by Albert Miller.)

absorption of calcium from milk or the reduced intake of milk (Newcomer & McGill, 1984).

• Limited quantities of milk (up to 1 pint per day) are tolerated well by some patients with lactase deficiency.

• Lactose is added to some drugs and food products as a filler or carrier; patients should be taught to scrutinize labels.

• Unpasteurized yogurt, which is better tolerated by lactose-intolerant individuals, provides the individual with the nutrients lacking from the omission of all milk products (Savaiano et al, 1984).

Health Application: Current Issues Involving Carbohydrates

Carbohydrates are an important part of the body's metabolic processes. Sugars are also important, whether they originated from the glycerol portion of fat, degradation of a protein, table sugar, or dextrose intravenous feeding. Normal physiological conditions and disease states affect carbohydrate metabolism, which is reflected in serum glucose levels. Some conditions, especially diabetes mellitus, require dietary regulation of carbohydrate (see Chapter 29).

Sugar and Nutritional Adequacy. Sugar contributes carbohydrates and calories. A marked increase in soft drink consumption from 13.6 gallons in 1962 to 38 gallons per person in 1981 (Bunch & Kurland, 1984) could account for the decreased consumption of milk, which contains many other essential nutrients. A diet high in sugar from too many pastries and candies is less likely to be adequate in other nutrients. Scientific studies do not support the claim that sugars interfere with the bioavailability of vitamins, minerals, or trace nutrients or the notion that dietary imbalances are preferentially caused by increased sugar consumption (Sugars Task Force, 1986).

On the other hand, sugar increases palatability and may induce people to eat certain foods otherwise disliked. Combining sugar with other nutritious foods, as in milk pudding, may increase the variety of foods consumed and enjoyed.

Starches and Nutritional Adequacy. Frequently, individuals eliminate complex carbohydrates in the belief that they are fattening. This can result in an insufficient intake of B vitamins, iron, and fiber. The use of wholesome, unprocessed grains, fruit and vegetables is to be encouraged. Fiber content of the diet should be increased gradually so the gastrointestinal tract can adjust to the change.

Carbohydrates and Dental Caries. Tooth decay is affected by many factors. Carbohydrates (including sugars and starches that are hydrolyzed by amylase) can be digested by bacteria in the mouth, leaving plaque and acids that lead to tooth decay.

When a cariogenic food is eaten, the pH of the plaque is lowered by the bacterial fermentation of the carbohydrate. A pH below 5.5 will dissolve tooth enamel. Adequate amounts of saliva flow increase the clearance of the food and bacterial substrate from the mouth. Generally, the pH remains low for at least 30 minutes following the intake of a food.

Some foods, such as milk and aged cheese, actually protect the teeth by inhibiting acid production (White-Graves & Schiller, 1986). Bibby and colleagues (1986) found that some foods high in sugar were removed quicker and did not lower the pH of plaque as much as starchy foods with less sugar.

Total carbohydrate or sucrose content of the diet is not as important as the type of food and frequency of consumption. Sticky foods and those that remain in the mouth for a longer time are more cariogenic than liquid foods. Frequent snacks provide more opportunities for bacterial growth. Two good ideas are to always brush after eating and to offer sweets as part of the meal instead of as snacks.

Carbohydrates and Obesity. There is no evidence that carbohydrates or sugars are a cause of obesity (Danowski et al, 1975). Excessive caloric intake—whether of carbohydrates, proteins, fats, and alcohol—leads to obesity. Even when reducing, it is important to consume some carbohydrates, especially vegetables, fruits, whole-grain breads and cereals, to prevent ketosis and to provide vital nutrients. While excessive calories from sugar intake could lead to obesity, epidemiological studies and several individual studies have shown that obese individuals actually consume less sugar than thin individuals (Gonzalez, 1983; Nuttal & Gannon, 1981; Bierman, 1979).

Dietary Fiber and Health. Claims have been made that the lack of dietary fiber is the cause of many Western diseases—diverticulitis, appendicitis, constipation, cancer of the colon, hyperlipoproteinemia, and diabetes. The subject is being extensively researched. Increasing dietary fiber by increasing the intake of unprocessed sources of complex carbohydrate is beneficial for reasons cited earlier.

However, just increasing fiber intake is not a cure-all for these diseases. Brans and wood cellulose added to high-fiber products are not utilized by gut bacteria (Van Soest, 1978). The addition of large amounts of purified fiber such as lignin and bran is not advised because many minerals—especially calcium, iron, and zinc—are bound by the fiber and possibly excreted (Kelsay, 1982; Fernandez & Phillips, 1982; Oku et al, 1982).

· FALLACIES and FACTS

FALLACY: *Home-ground flour is nutritionally superior to commercially ground.*

· **FACT:** *Whole-grain flours are superior to white bleached flours; however, grinding one's own flour cannot be justified. The use of whole-grain flours or products made with whole grains will improve the nutritional content of fiber, some vitamins, and minerals in the diet. Flours that have not been bleached are nutritionally superior to bleached flours. However, some brown breads, labeled as "wheat bread," can be deceiving because of added color. These may be made from white flour that has not even been enriched. High-fiber breads* frequently have added wood pulp. This increases the fiber of the diet, but it is not as effective as the natural fiber from whole grains. Read ingredient labels to determine if the product warrants its additional cost.

FALLACY: Sugar in the raw (or turbinado sugar) is nutritionally superior to white sugar.

• **FACT:** Raw sugar is a tannish, coarse, granulated solid obtained from the evaporation of sugar cane juice that has been extracted from cane. The U.S. Food and Drug Administration has labeled raw sugar as "unfit for direct use as food or as a food ingredient because of the impurities it ordinarily contains."

Turbinado sugar, sold in health food stores, is raw sugar that has been partially refined by washing. It contains some of the original mineral matter from the cane sugar. As far as either of these sugars providing some of the minerals and vitamins lacking in the refined product, raw sugar contains less than half a percent (0.49 percent) of mineral-containing ash. The remaining 99.51 percent is sugar. Raw sugar hardly seems to be a good source for anything except carbohydrate.

FALLACY: Blackstrap molasses is good for anemia and rheumatism.

• **FACT:** Blackstrap molasses (not to be confused with unsulfured molasses found in grocery stores) does contain a few minerals and vitamins (especially iron, potassium, and thiamin); however, it would take 6 Tbsp. of blackstrap molasses to provide the daily iron requirement for a woman's calorie intake of 258 kcal. Needless to say, many other foods are much better sources of iron and other nutrients.

FALLACY: Honey is good for you.

• **FACT:** Honey is formed by bees from the nectar they gather. It varies in composition and flavor, depending on the source of the nectar. A tablespoon of honey has more calories than a tablespoon of table sugar. Its high fructose content causes it to taste sweeter than sucrose. Honey contains minimal amounts of thiamin, riboflavin, and ascorbic acid. If one prefers the taste of honey to sucrose, fine; however, it is also a sweetener that

should only be relied upon for its carbohydrate content.

FALLACY: Some individuals are addicted to sugar.

• **FACT:** There is no scientific evidence that sugar is addictive. However, some individuals overindulge in sweets. Dr. Wurtman (1984) has shown in several studies that carbohydrate-rich foods increase the synthesis and release of the brain neurotransmitter serotonin. Serotonin causes a calm, relaxed feeling, decreasing sensitivity to pain. The increased serotonin level curtails the need and desire for carbohydrate; less carbohydrate is consumed at the following meal. Carbohydrate snacking seems to be related to a physiological need to increase the level of brain serotonin. This physiological desire for sweets and starches cannot be satisfied by any other food, but can be controlled by a drug, fenfluramine.

FALLACY: Refined carbohydrates, especially sugar, cause hyperactivity, criminal behavior, and a lot of other behavioral problems.

• **FACT:** While it is a commonly accepted belief among lay people that sugar causes hyperactivity in children, scientific studies have not supported this (Position paper, 1985; Statement, 1984). While a few studies testing the effect of sugar on hyperactive behavior have found a positive correlation, most have found no correlation (Gross, 1984; Rapoport, 1982/83) or observed a calming effect (Rapoport, 1986; Behar et al, 1984).

Dietary substances such as carbohydrates may affect levels of brain neurotransmitters that control nervous system activity and may consequently affect behavior. The intake of carbohydrate elicits the production of insulin, which causes the removal of amino acids except tryptophan out of the bloodstream (Wurtman, 1983). Increased serotonin levels are linked to several behaviors such as sleep patterns (Hartmann, 1986; Yogman & Zeisel, 1983), mood swings, depression, aggression, mental alertness, and motor activity (Brewerton et al, 1986; Spring et al, 1986; Young, 1986; Wurtman, 1986, 1983; Rapoport, 1982/83). However, evidence of an association be-

tween diet and behavior is considered weak, and it is important to be critical of scientific claims regarding diet and behavior (Diet and behavior, 1986).

As for a link between diet and crime, proponents fail to agree upon a single mechanism by which diet would cause such abnormal behavior. Several hypotheses include reactive hypoglycemia, excess sugar, food additives, food allergies, vitamin and mineral deficiencies and excesses, and neurotransmitter imbalances (Gray, 1986).

FALLACY: *Sugar found in candies is "bad"; and sugar from fruit is "good."*

• **FACT:** *Sugar is sugar. Wherever it originated, the products that are absorbed—glucose and fructose—are chemically and biologically the same. As a rule, one would expect the fruit to contain more vitamins and minerals than candy, but that is not always true.*

Summary

Carbohydrates supply 40 to 80 percent of the calorie requirements of diets around the world. A well-balanced diet can be planned that is low or high in carbohydrate content. Carbohydrates include simple carbohydrates, or sugars, and polysaccharides (starches and dietary fiber).

All dietary carbohydrates are broken down to monosaccharides (glucose, fructose, and galactose) in the gastrointestinal tract. Most are converted in the liver to glucose, which is transported to and utilizable by the cells. Fructose is commonly found in fruits; galactose is not found free in nature, but is a constituent of the disaccharide lactose.

Each of the disaccharides is glucose paired with another monosaccharide, fructose, glucose, or galactose. The two disaccharides of dietary significance are sucrose and lactose. Sucrose (table sugar) as well as monosaccharides are concentrated sources of energy and enhance the palatability of many foods. They should not be used to replace essential foods that provide other nutrients but can be used with discretion to enhance intake of some nutrients.

Two polysaccharides, starch and cellulose, make important contributions in the diet. Starch is found predominantly in grains and starchy vegetables, which also contain protein, minerals, and vitamins. Dietary fiber includes cellulose, pectin, hemicellulose, and lignin. It is found in fruits, vegetables, and whole-grain breads and cereals and is important in maintaining gastrointestinal functions.

Carbohydrate is stored in small amounts in the body in the form of glycogen. This is used for cellular energy and to maintain blood glucose, which is essential for the central nervous system. While there is no recommended dietary allowance for carbohydrate, it should be supplied in the diet daily to prevent ketosis and muscle wasting.

Review Questions

1. Differentiate between the three classes of carbohydrates.
2. Trace the route of carbohydrate from ingestion to its metabolism, including the enzymes, the site of the activity and the absorbable products.
3. What are the main sources of fiber in the American diet? What are the main sources of starch in the American diet? List three of your favorite foods high in sugar.
4. What is the carbohydrate circulating in the blood? What is the normal concentration? How is this maintained if too little carbohydrate is eaten? If very large amounts are eaten?
5. What are the functions of sugars in the diet? What are the functions of dietary fiber?

Case Study: Your patient has been on a clear-liquid diet for three days. She refuses to eat Jell-O and has taken very little bouillon. Today, the only intake she had was the following: 6 oz. pineapple juice (26 gm carbohydrate), 4 oz. cranberry juice (21 gm carbohydrate), 10 oz. orange juice (36 gm carbohydrate), and 2 cups hot tea with 2 tsp. sugar (8 gm carbohydrate). How many calories did she consume?

REFERENCE LIST

Anderson, JW: Physiological and metabolic effect of dietary fiber. *Fed Proc* 44(14):2902, 1985.

Behar, D; Rapoport, JL; Adams, AJ; et al: Sugar challenge testing with children considered behaviorally "sugar reactive." *Nutr Behavior* 1:277, 1984.

Bibby, BG; Mundorff, SA; Zero, DT; et al: Oral food clearance and the pH of plaque and saliva. *J Am Dental Assoc* 111(3):333, 1986.

Bierman, EL: Carbohydrates, sucrose and human disease. *Am J Clin Nutr* 32(12 suppl):2712, 1979.

Brewerton, TD; Heffernan, MM; Rosenthal, NE: Psychiatric aspects of the relationship between eating and mood. *Nutr Rev* 44(5 suppl):78, 1986.

Bunch, K; Kurland, J: How America quenches its thirst. *Nat Food Review* 27:14, 1984.

Connor, WE; Connor, SL: Sucrose and carbohydrate. In *Nutrition Reviews' Present Knowledge in Nutrition.* New York, The Nutrition Foundation, Inc., 1976, p 33.

Crapo, PA: Sugar and sugar alcohols. *Contemporary Nutrition* 7(12), 1981.

Crapo, PA; Kolterman, OG: The metabolic effects of a 2-week fructose feeding in normal subjects. *Am J Clin Nutr* 39(4):525, 1984.

Danowski, TS; Nolan, S; Stephen, T: Obesity. *World Rev Nutr Diet* 22:270, 1975.

Deutsch, RM: *Realities of Nutrition.* Palo Alto, CA, Bull Publishing Co, 1976.

Diet and behavior symposium proceedings: Summary. *Nutr Rev* 44(5 suppl):252, 1986.

Dietary recommendations for chronic diverticulosis. *Nutr & the MD* 12(2):4, 1986.

Eastwood, MA; Passmore, R: Dietary fibre. *Lancet* 2(July 22):202, 1983.

Fernandez, R; Phillips, SF: Components of fiber impair iron absorption in dogs. *Am J Clin Nutr* 35(1):107, 1982.

Forster, H: Comparative metabolism of xylitol, sorbitol, and fructose. In *Sugars in Nutrition.* Edited by HL Sipple; KW McNutt. New York, Academic Press, 1974, p 259.

Ginn, HE: The renal metabolism and uses of mannitol. In *Sugars in Nutrition.* Edited by HL Sipple; KW McNutt. New York, Academic Press, 1974, p 607.

Gonzalez, ER: Studies show obese may prefer fats to sweets. *JAMA* 250(5):579, 1983.

Gray, GE: Diet, crime and delinquency: A critique. *Nutr Rev* 44(5 suppl):89 1986.

Gray, GM; Fogel, MR: Nutritional aspects of dietary carbohydrate. In *Modern Nutrition in Health and Disease.* Edited by RS Goodhart; ME Shils. Philadelphia, Lea & Febiger, 1980, p 99.

Gross, MD: Effect of sucrose on hyperkinetic children. *Pediatrics* 74(5):876, 1984.

Hartman, EL: Effect of L-tryptophan and other amino acids on sleep. *Nutr Rev* 44(5 suppl):70, 1986.

Jenkins, DJA; Wolever, TMS; Jenkins, AL; et al: The glycaemic index of foods tested in diabetic patients: New basis for carbohydrate exchange favouring the use of legumes. *Diabetologia* 24(4):257, 1983.

Kare, MR: Monellin. In *Sweeteners: Issues and Uncertainties.* Washington, DC, National Academy of Sciences, 1975.

Kelsay, JL: Effects of fiber on mineral and vitamin bioavailability. In *Dietary Fiber in Health and Disease.* Edited by GV Vahouny; D Kritchevsky. New York, Plenum Press, 1982, p 91.

Kolterman, OG; Greenfield, M; Reaven, GM; et al: Effect of a high carbohyydrate diet on insulin binding to adipocytes and on insulin action in vivo in man. *Diabetes* 28(8):731, 1979.

Lanza, E; Butrum, RR: A critical review of food fiber analysis and data. *J Am Diet Assoc* 86(6):732, 1986.

Latner, AL: *Cantarow and Trumper Clinical Biochemistry*, 7th ed. Philadelphia, W. B. Saunders Co, 1975.

Levine, R: Carbohydrates. In *Modern Nutrition in Health and Disease*, 5th ed. Edited by RS Goodhart; ME Shils. Philadelphia, Lea & Febiger, 1976, p 99.

Marston, RM; Raper, NR: The nutrient content of the food supply. *Nat Food Review* 29(winter-spring):5, 1985.

Marston, RM; Welsh, SO: Nutrient content of the United States food supply, 1982. *Nat Food Review* 25(winter):7, 1984.

Newcomer, AD; McGill, DB: Clinical consequences of lactase deficiency. *Clin Nutr* 3(2):53, 1984.

Nuttal, FQ; Gannon, MC: Sucrose and disease. *Diab Care* 4(2):305, 1981.

Oku, T; Konishi, F; Hosoya, N: Mechanism of inhibitory effect of unavailable carbohydrate on intestinal calcium absorption. *J Nutr* 112(3):410, 1982.

Pike, RL; Brown, ML: *Nutrition: An Integrated Approach*, 3rd ed. New York, John Wiley & Sons, Inc, 1984.

Position paper of the American Dietetic Association on diet and criminal behavior. *J Am Diet Assoc* 85(3):361, 1985.

Rapoport, JL: Effects of dietary substances in children. *J Psychiatr Res* 17(2):187, 1982/83.

Rapoport, JL: Diet and hyperactivity. *Nutr Rev* 44(5 suppl):158, 1986.

Rosensweig, NS: Adaptive effects of dietary sugars on intestinal disaccharidase activity in man. In *Sugars in Nutrition.* Edited by HL Sipple; KW McNutt. New York, Academic Press, 1974, p 174.

Savaiano, DA; El Anouar, AA; Smith, DE; et al: Lactose malabsorption from yogurt, pasteurized yogurt, sweet acidophilus milk, and cultured milk in lactase-deficient individuals. *Am J Clin Nutr* 40(6):1219, 1984.

Spiller, GA: Amen, RJ: Dietary fiber in human nutrition. *CRC Crit Rev Food Sci Nutr* 7(1):39, 1975.

Spring, BJ; Lieberman, HR; Swope, G; et al: Effects of carbohydrates on mood and behavior. *Nutr Rev* 44(5 suppl):51, 1986.

Statement of the Resource Conference on Diet and Behavior. *Nutr Rev* 42(5):200, 1984.

Sugars Task Force: Evaluation of health aspects of sugars contained in carbohydrate sweeteners. Division of Nutrition and Toxicology, Center for Food Safety and Applied Nutrition, FDA, 1986.

Van Soest, PJ: Dietary fibers: Their definition and nutritional properties. *Am J Clin Nutr* 31(suppl):S12, 1978.

White-Graves, MV; Schiller, MR: History of foods in the caries process. *J Am Diet Assoc* 86(2):241, 1986.

Wurtman, JJ: The involvement of brain serotonin in excessive carbohydrate snacking by obese carbohydrate cravers. *J Am Diet Assoc* 84(9):1004, 1984.

Wurtman, RJ: Behavioural effects of nutrients. *Lancet* 1(May 21):1145, 1983.

Wurtman, RJ: Ways that foods can affect the brain. *Nutr Rev* 44(5 suppl):2, 1986.

Yogman, MW; Zeisel, SH: Diet and sleep patterns in newborn infants. *N Engl J Med* 309(19):1147, 1983.

Young, SN: The effect of aggression and mood of altering tryptophan levels. *Nutr Rev* 44(5 suppl):112, 1986.

Further Study

Crapo, PA: Theory versus fact: The glycemic response to foods. *Nutr Today* 19(2):6, 1984.

Eastwood, MA; Passmore, R: A new look at dietary fiber. *Nutr Today* 19(5):6, 1984.

Englert, DM; Guillory, JA: For want of lactase. *Am J Nursing* 86(8):902, 1986.

Fielden, H: When roughage is the fibre of health. *Nurs Mirror* 151(6):32, 1980.

Glinsmann, WH; Irausquin, H; Park, YK: *Evaluation of Health Aspects of Sugars Contained in Carbohydrate Sweeteners.*

Washington, DC, Food and Drug Administration, 1986.

Hardinge, MG: Carbohydrates in foods. *J Am Diet Assoc* 46 (3):197, 1965.

Harland, B; Hecht, A: Grandma called it roughage. *FDA Consumer* 11(6):18, 1977.

Heaton, KW: The real value of fiber . . . dietary fiber. *Consultant* 19 (8):23, 1979.

Jenkins, DJA; Jenkins, AL; Wolever, TMS: Simple and complex carbohydrates. *Nutr Rev* 44(2):44, 1986.

Kolata, G; Goldfarm, T: In praise of pasta and beans. *Am Health* 2(3):50, 1983.

Leaves, A: Hospital diets: A question of fibre. *Nurs Mirror* 154(1):43, 1982.

Lecos, CW: Sugar: How sweet it is—and isn't. *FDA Consumer* 14(1):21, 1980.

National Dairy Council: Nutrition update: Sugar. *Dairy Council Digest* 55(4):21, 1984.

Potter, JD: Fibre in the prevention and management of chronic disease. *Aust Fam Physician* 11(4):292, 1982.

Skinner, S; Martens, RA: *The Milk Sugar Dilemma: Living with Lactose Intolerance,* 1985. (Available from Lactose Intolerance, P.O. Box 957, East Lansing, MI 48823.)

Stephen, AM: Should we eat more fibre? *J Human Nutr* 33(6):403, 1981.

Stephenson, M: Fiber: Something healthy to chew on. *FDA Consumer* 19(5):30, 1985.

Taylor, DL: Hyperglycemia: Physiology, signs, and symptoms. *Nursing* 83(2):52, 1983.

Taylor, DL: Hypoglycemia: Physiology, signs, and symptoms. *Nursing* 83(3):44, 1983.

Wahlqvist, ML: Sugar and human health. *Aust Fam Physician* 10(10):818, 1981.

Yen, PK: Nutrition: Carbohydrate is not a villain. *Geriatr Nurs* 3(5):334, 1982.

Lipids: The Condensed Energy

8

THE STUDENT WILL BE ABLE TO:

- *Identify the basic structural units of dietary lipids.*
- *Describe how fatty acids affect the properties of fat.*
- *Identify the secretions and processes involved in triglyceride digestion and absorption.*
- *Name the essential fatty acid and some of its functions.*
- *Describe the metabolism of fatty acids in cells.*
- *Describe metabolic events leading to ketosis and the role of the diet.*
- *List the functions of fats in the diet.*
- *List the functions of fats in the body.*
- *List dietary sources for saturated and polyunsaturated fatty acids, and cholesterol.*
- *Distinguish between chylomicrons and other lipoproteins.*
- *State the effect of polyunsaturated fatty acids on serum cholesterol.*
- *Identify the number of calories provided per gram of fat.*

Cholesterol
Eicosapentaenoic acid
Fatty acid
Ketone bodies
Linoleic acid
Lipolysis
Lipogenesis
Lipoproteins
Micelles
Mono- and
  polyunsaturated fatty
  acids
Omega-3 fatty acids
P/S ratio
Saponification
Saturated/unsaturated
Steatorrhea
Triglyceride
Wetting agent

OBJECTIVES

TERMS TO KNOW

Unsweetened coconut, mayonnaise, blue cheese salad dressing, almonds, pecans, sausage—what do all these things have in common? Each of these food items is more than half fat . . . a vital constituent of our diet. Other foods that are principally fat include butter, margarine, shortening, lard, vegetable oils, salad dressings, visible meat fats, and poultry skin. Foods containing less fat (much of which is invisible) are cream, homogenized milk (and products made from it), egg yolks, meat, fish, olives, nuts, avocados, and whole-grain cereal products. The percentage of fat in many foods is listed in Table 8–1.

The level of fat in the United States food supply from about 1911 to 1984 has steadily increased 34 percent (Marston & Raper, 1986), with the proportion of calories provided by fat increasing from 32 to 42 percent (Fig. 8–1). Fat from animal sources has declined slightly during the past few years, with more fats coming from vegetable sources. Currently, 57 percent of the fat intake is from animal sources (Marston & Welsh, 1984).

Classification and Characteristics

Fats in the diet should actually be called *lipids* in order to include the structural and functional lipids discussed in this chapter. Lipids are similar to carbohydrates and contain the same three elements—carbon, hydrogen, and oxygen. However, lipids contain less oxygen in proportion to hydrogen and carbon. Because of their structure, their metabolism utilizes more oxygen and releases more energy than either carbohydrates or amino acids. Their structure also allows them to be stored compactly with little or no water. Generally, proteins and carbohydrates require more space for storing the same number of calories. If the body were unable to store fats, we would be much bigger and heavier.

Clinical Implication:

• Foods having higher fat content are more calorie-dense; those with a lower fat content are bulkier. A ¼ cup of peanuts and seven whole carrots have the same number of calories

Table 8–1. Percentage of Fat in Foods*

Percent Fat	Food
90–100	Salad and cooking oils and fats, lard.
80–90	Butter, margarine.
70–80	Mayonnaise, pecans, macadamia nuts.
50–70	Walnuts, dried unsweetened coconut meat, almonds, bacon, baking chocolate.
30–50	Broiled choice T-bone and porterhouse steaks, spareribs, broiled pork chop, goose, cheddar and cream cheeses, potato chips, French dressing, chocolate candy.
20–30	Choice beef pot roast, broiled choice lamb chop, frankfurters, ground beef, chocolate chip cookies.
10–20	Broiled choice round steak, broiled veal chop, roast turkey, eggs, avocado, olives, chocolate cake with icing, french-fried potatoes, ice cream, apple pie.
1–10	Pork and beans, broiled cod, halibut, haddock, and many other fish, broiled chicken, crabmeat, cottage cheese, beef liver, milk, creamed soups, sherbet, most breakfast cereals.
<1	Baked potato, most vegetables and fruits, egg whites, chicken consommé.

*From FDA Consumer: *Primer on Three Nutrients.* HHS Publication No. (FDA) 81-2026, revised January 1981.

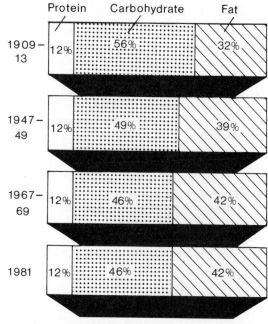

Figure 8–1. Sources of energy in the U.S. food supply. (From Marston SM, Welsh SO: Nutrient content of the national food supply, 1981. National Food Review 21 (winter):17, 1983.)

(210), but the carrots have only a trace of fat, 7 gm of protein, and 49 gm of carbohydrate. The peanuts have only 7 gm of carbohydrate, 9 gm of protein, and 18 gm of fat.

While lipids are a heterogeneous group of chemical types, lipids can be distinguished by their insolubility in water and solubility in organic solvents such as ether and chloroform. They generally contain a fatty acid or a fatty acid derivative.

Lipids can be divided into two classes: (1) the fats that occur both in foods and in the body, and (2) structural or complex lipids that are produced in the body to form part of the membrane structure, to transport fat, or to synthesize key lipid hormones or catalysts. Fats contained in foods that the body can utilize are triglycerides, fatty acids, phospholipids, and cholesterol. Lipids found solely in the body include lipoproteins and glycolipids.

CHEMICAL STRUCTURE

Triglycerides, also called neutral fats, are the most common fat found in foods (of both animal and plant origin). The basic structural unit of fats (Fig. 8–2) is three (tri-) fatty acids attached to one molecule of glycerol (glycer-). A mono- or diglyceride is one or two fatty acids attached to the glycerol molecule. Mono- and diglycerides are found in the small intestine and result from hydrolysis of triglycerides during digestion. Each of the three fatty acids in a triglyceride can be different—long or short, saturated or unsaturated. Their physical

properties are affected by about 20 different fatty acids frequently found in foods. The fatty acid is a straight chain of any number of carbon atoms (generally a multiple of two). Short-chain fatty acids contain 4 to 6 carbons; medium-chain fatty acids, 8 to 12 carbons; and long-chain fatty acids, more than 12 carbons. While medium-chain and short-chain fatty acids are easier to digest and absorb, most fats from foods (especially vegetable fats), contain predominantly long-chain fatty acids (16 to 18 carbon atoms). Saturation of a fatty acid depends on the number of hydrogen atoms attached to the carbon (Fig. 8–3). Long-chain fatty acids are classified according to their degree of saturation.

Saturated Fatty Acids. Bonding between carbon atoms determines the saturation of a fat. Saturated fatty acids contain single bonds exclusively, each carbon atom having two hydrogen atoms attached to it. Palmitic and stearic acids are the most prevalent saturated fatty acids, which are found in animal fats, cheese, butter, coconut oil, and chocolate.

Monounsaturated Fatty Acids. When two adjacent carbon atoms are joined by a double bond because two hydrogen atoms are lacking, the fatty acid is monounsaturated, i.e., only one double bond exists. The most abundant monounsaturated fatty acid is oleic acid, which is found in olive and peanut oils.

Polyunsaturated Fatty Acids. When two or more carbons are connected by double bonds (Fig. 8–3), the fatty acid is polyunsaturated; four or more hydrogen atoms are lacking. Plant fats are predominantly polyunsaturated fatty acids (PUFAs). Linoleic, linolenic, and arachidonic acids all contain 18 carbon atoms and are polyunsatu-

Figure 8–2. Chemical structure of a triglyceride.

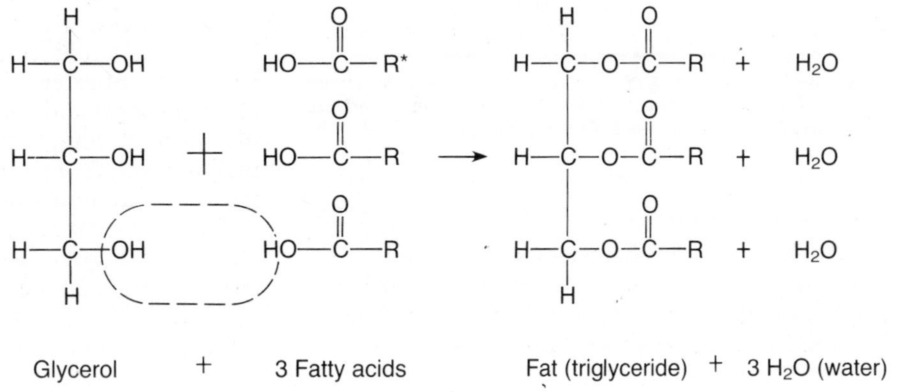

Glycerol + 3 Fatty acids → Fat (triglyceride) + 3 H₂O (water)

1 Carbon has a valence of four, which means that in a chemical reaction four atoms may attach to the carbon atom to form a compound.

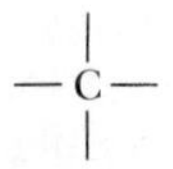

$$-\overset{|}{\underset{|}{C}}-$$

2 During a chemical reaction in which all the valence bonds of a fatty acid become filled with hydrogen, the compound formed is referred to as *saturated*, that is, *"saturated with hydrogen."*

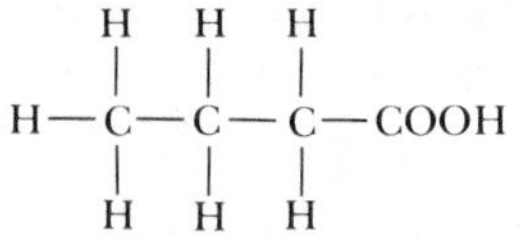

$$H-\overset{\overset{H}{|}}{\underset{\underset{H}{|}}{C}}-\overset{\overset{H}{|}}{\underset{\underset{H}{|}}{C}}-\overset{\overset{H}{|}}{\underset{\underset{H}{|}}{C}}-COOH$$

Saturated fat, butyric acid ($C_4 : O$)
(4 carbon atoms, no double bond,
found in butter)

3 In the carbon chain of the fatty acid, when there are two less hydrogen atoms attached to the carbon atom, the carbon atoms join their two available valence bonds and make a *mutual bond*. Adding this new mutual bond to an existing bond forms a *double bond*, thereby creating a state of *unsaturation*, which provides room for more hydrogen. It is the number of double bonds present along the carbon chain of the fatty acid that determines the degree of saturation. When there are many double bonds present in a fatty acid, there is more space available to combine hydrogen, and the fatty acid is known as *polyunsaturated*. When there is only one double bond in the fatty acid, it is known as *monounsaturated*.

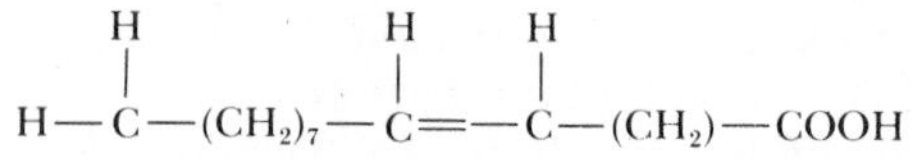

$$H-\overset{\overset{H}{|}}{\underset{\underset{H}{|}}{C}}-(CH_2)_7-\overset{\overset{H}{|}}{C}=\overset{\overset{H}{|}}{C}-(CH_2)-COOH$$

Monounsaturated, oleic acid ($C_{18} : 1$)
(18 carbon atoms, 1 double bond
found in olive oil)

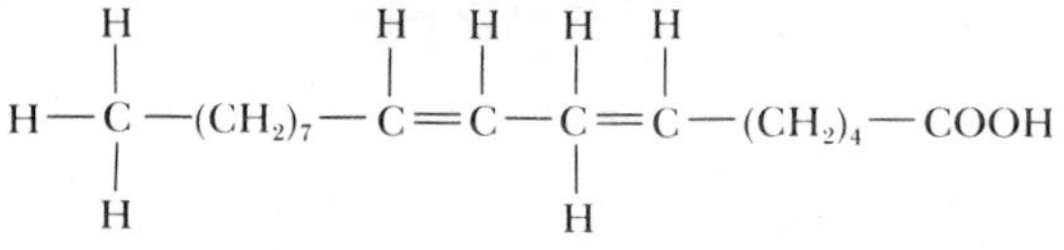

$$H-\overset{\overset{H}{|}}{\underset{\underset{H}{|}}{C}}-(CH_2)_7-\overset{\overset{H}{|}}{C}=\overset{\overset{H}{|}}{C}-\overset{\overset{H}{|}}{C}=\overset{\overset{H}{|}}{C}-(CH_2)_4-COOH$$

Polyunsaturated, linoleic acid ($C_{18} : 2$)
(18 carbon atoms, 2 double bonds
found in vegetable oils)

Figure 8–3. *The process of saturation of a fatty acid. (From Howard RB, Herbold NH: Nutrition in Clinical Care, 2nd ed. New York, McGraw-Hill, 1982. Reprinted by permission.)*

rated. They differ in their degree of saturation. Linoleic acid is the most prevalent PUFA and is the predominant fatty acid in safflower, sunflower, corn, cottonseed, soybean, and sesame oils. It is

essential nutritionally because the body is unable to manufacture it.

Omega-6 fatty acids, e.g., linoleic and arachidonic acids present in most vegetable oils, have their first double bond on the sixth carbon from the omega (terminal) end of the molecule. Omega-3 fatty acids, eicosapentaenoic acid (EPA) and docosahexaenoic acid (DHA), are unique in that the first double bond is located three carbons from the omega end of the molecule. These omega-3 fatty acids, which are contained in fish oils, appear to have many health benefits. Although the body can convert linolenic acid (an omega-3 fatty acid) into both EPA and DHA, the process is very slow, especially in the presence of large amounts of linoleic acid (Tinoco et al, 1979).

P/S Ratio. The amount of PUFAs is compared with the amount of saturated fatty acids to determine its P/S ratio. Triglycerides have mixed fatty acids, but foods containing predominantly saturated fats are called saturated. If PUFAs exceed saturated fatty acids, the food is classified as polyunsaturated. No triglyceride occurring naturally is totally saturated or unsaturated. While monounsaturated fats have been demonstrated to have a lipid-lowering effect (Grundy, 1986), their effects on health have not been conclusively proven.

Nutrition labeling permits labels to state in addition to the grams of fat in the food the grams of polyunsaturated and saturated fats, which can be used to determine the P/S ratio. For example, 6 gm of PUFA and 2 gm of saturated fatty acids give a P/S ratio of three to one. While margarines and oils can have a P/S ratio of three to one, the overall ratio of a prudent diet is one or 1½ to one.

Characteristics of Fatty Acids

Carbon chain length and the degree of saturation determine various properties of fats, including the melting point, flavor, and hardness.

Hardness. The temperature at which the fat becomes a liquid (melting point) determines its hardness. Shorter-chain fatty acids (12 carbon atoms or less) and unsaturated fatty acids are liquids at room temperature and are called oils. Animal fats contain mostly saturated fats and are solids at room temperature. Generally, the fat of herbivora is harder than carnivora, that of land animals is harder than aquatic animals, and the fat of lamb and beef is harder than pork and chicken. Milk fat contains a large amount of saturated fatty acids, but many are short-chain fats.

Hydrogenation. Hydrogen can be added to a fat at the double bonds in the presence of a catalyst to convert a polyunsaturated vegetable oil to a saturated fat, raising its melting point. This is done commercially to produce solid margarines and vegetable shortenings. The process increases the proportion of saturated fatty acids and also reduces the amount of linoleic acid.

Hydrogenation can be controlled so that "tub" or "soft" margarines are available from oils with different proportions of PUFA, depending on the amount of hydrogenation. Vegetable oils are hydrogenated to make shortening, which results in a better cake texture. During hydrogenation, the shape of the fatty acid is altered. PUFAs naturally occur in what is called the "cis" (i.e., on the same side) configuration; the carbon chain bends so that hydrogens stick out on the same side of the molecule. During processing, the groups may rotate so they are on opposite sides of the bond, in the "trans" position. Although the long-term health effects of this change are unknown, an essential fatty acid, linoleic acid, is ineffective when modified in this way.

Rancidity. When fats are exposed to air and light, they become rancid. High temperatures increase this oxidative process. Fats with a high proportion of unsaturated fatty acids are more susceptible because oxygen can attack the double bonds. The peroxides formed may be toxic in large amounts. However, unpalatable flavors and odors generally prevent the person from eating it.

Vitamin E, a fat-soluble vitamin, is an antioxidant and, to some degree, protects the oil. But, when used as an antioxidant, it is inactivated as a vitamin for the body. Antioxidants, e.g., butylated hydroxyanisole (BHA) and butylated hydroxytoluene (BHT), are added to commercially processed fats and oils to prevent their spoilage.

Saponification. When fatty acids are separated from the glycerol molecule, the free fatty acid can combine with an electrolyte, such as calcium, to form an insoluble "soap." When this saponification occurs in the intestine, the "soap" is excreted in the feces, a condition called *steatorrhea*.

Clinical Implication:

- Saponification occurs in diseases characterized by poor fat absorption (such as sprue) and inflammatory conditions (such as pancreatitis). Calcium loss can be significant.

GLYCEROL

When fatty acids are removed from the triglyceride, the remaining alcohol fragment is glycerol. It is water-soluble and can be used by the body to make glucose.

COMPOUND LIPIDS

Glycerol and fatty acids combined with carbohydrate, phosphate, and/or nitrogenous compounds are called compound lipids (e.g., phospholipids, glycolipids, and lipoproteins). They are found in foods and are produced by the body.

Phospholipids. In addition to fatty acids and alcohol, phospholipids contain phosphorus and a nitrogenous base. They are generally present in the invisible fats found in both plant and animal foods. Commercially, phospholipids are used as additives in products to aid in emulsification.

Lipoprotein. Lipoproteins contain various amounts of triglycerides, phospholipids, and cholesterol combined with protein. They are produced in the liver and intestinal mucosa to transport insoluble fats. Several types are present in the body: high-density lipoproteins (HDLs), low-density lipoproteins (LDLs), and very low-density lipoproteins (VLDLs). Their role in heart disease is discussed in Chapter 32.

Chylomicrons, formed for the absorption of lipids, are the least dense. They are the transport mechanism of fats through the lymph system and contain small amounts of protein but large amounts of triglycerides. They are considered a borderline group of lipoprotein (Alfin-Slater & Aftergood, 1980).

CHOLESTEROL

Cholesterol is a fat-related lipid with a complex ring structure called a sterol (Fig. 8–4). It is found *only* in animal tissues, such as egg yolk, milk fat, and meats. The liver and intestines can synthesize all the cholesterol the body needs without intake (1 gm), but the average diet contains 479 mg/day (Marston & Welsh, 1984).

SYNTHETIC FATS

Medium-chain triglycerides (MCTs) do not occur naturally and contain eight to ten carbon atoms in each fatty acid. They are easily digested and are produced commercially for individuals with fat malabsorption problems.

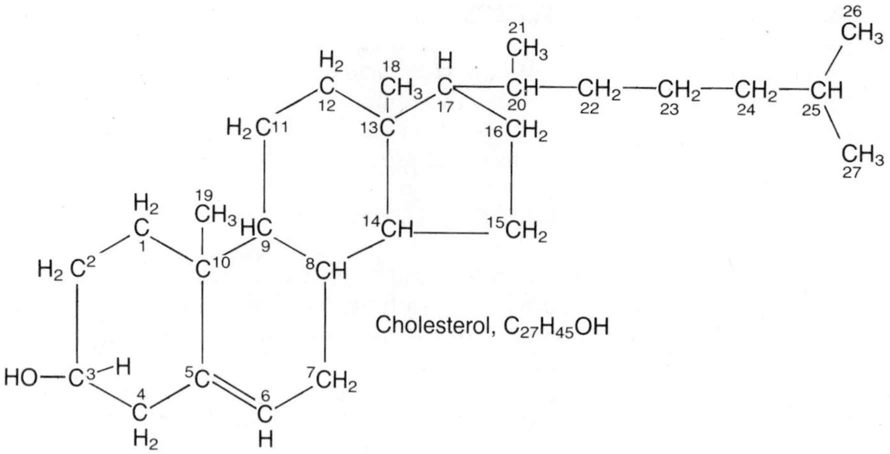

Cholesterol, $C_{27}H_{45}OH$

Figure 8–4. *Chemical structure of cholesterol.*

Sucrose polyester is a synthetic fat that resembles conventional dietary fats and can be substituted in many foods, but it is not absorbed. Presently, its potential is still being investigated as a substitute for dietary fat in weight control (Glueck et al, 1982) and for reducing serum cholesterol and LDL levels (Mellies et al, 1985; Glueck et al, 1979).

Digestion

Most fats in the diet are in the form of triglycerides, or neutral fats. Additionally, they contain varying amounts of phospholipids and cholesterol. Of course, the first action on fats is the chewing process, which helps to physically break apart the fats and to warm them.

Gastric lipase in the stomach begins the chemical hydrolysis of fats. Due to the insolubility of fats in the watery solution (they rise to the top), gastric lipase is not able to act on them. Only the fats that are already emulsified, e.g., milk fat and egg yolk, receive any attention from this enzyme. However, gastric lipase plays a more important role in the newborn and premature infant and possibly in individuals with cystic fibrosis, all of whom have low levels of pancreatic lipase and bile salts (Hamosh et al, 1981).

Glycerol and medium- and short-chain fatty acids (10 or fewer carbon atoms) are water-soluble and can be digested as other water-soluble molecules entering the portal circulation. These fatty acids are transported to the liver bound to albumin.

The presence of fat in chyme stimulates the release of cholecystokinin, which causes the gallbladder to contract and release its bile. Bile salts are very important to emulsify and reduce surface tension of fats and thereby allow large insoluble molecules to be divided into smaller particles. Bile, secreted by the liver at a rate of about 1 L/day, is stored in the gallbladder, where it is concentrated by reabsorption of water, until it is needed to facilitate digestion. Peristalsis facilitates the mixing and emulsification process by bile.

Lipases in the pancreatic and intestinal secretions are able to hydrolyze triglycerides to fatty acids and glycerol.

Absorption of Fat-Soluble Nutrients

Fatty acids that have chains of 12 or more carbon atoms are insoluble in water and must enter the bloodstream via the lymphatic system. These large molecules can be absorbed by the lacteals of the villi. The mechanism for absorption of these fatty acids is a complicated procedure of three stages (Fig. 8–5).

1. Bile salts are wetting agents that make fatty acids more water-soluble. Bile salts combine with products of fat digestion and disperse them into tiny units called micelles. These can pass through the intestinal membrane. Bile salts are

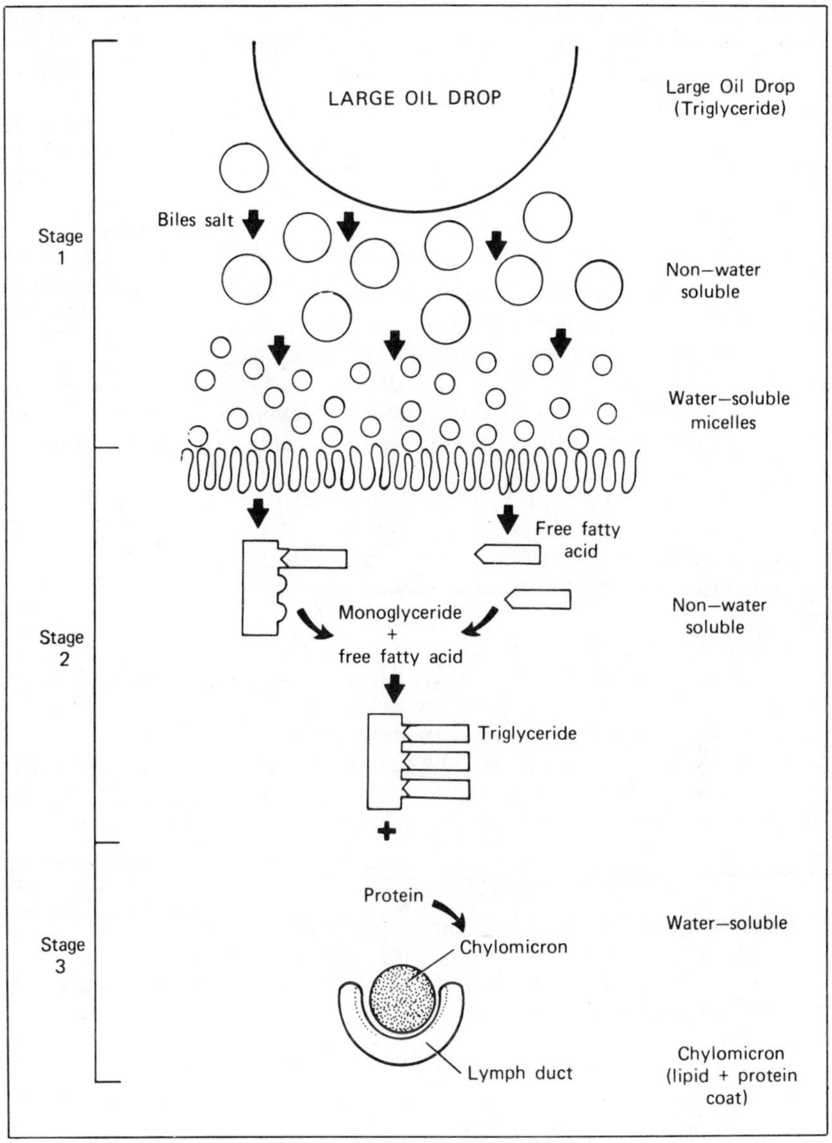

Figure 8–5. *Absorption of fats. (From Green ML, Harry J: Nutrition in Contemporary Nursing Practice. Copyright © 1981, John Wiley & Sons, Inc. Reprinted by permission of John Wiley & Sons, Inc.)*

separated from the fat products after they pass through the intestinal wall to be reused again.

2. In the intestinal mucosa, the digestion of the mono- and diglycerides may be completed by the action of the enzyme intestinal lipase. All the available fatty acids and glycerol molecules are synthesized into new triglycerides.

3. In the final stage, the new triglyceride is enclosed with a protein coating. This lipoprotein complex is called a chylomicron and can at last enter the lymphatic system. These chylomicrons are carried through the lymph system to the thoracic duct to enter the bloodstream at the subclavian vein. The chylomicrons are then transported to the liver and adipose tissue for metabolism and storage.

Bile salts, reabsorbed in the ileum, are recirculated through the liver, and again stored in the gallbladder. When an abundance of bile is present, approximately 97 percent of the fat is absorbed; the absence of bile results in up to 40 percent of the fat being excreted in the feces (Guyton, 1986). A large amount of fat in the feces is called steatorrhea.

The percentage of cholesterol absorbed is highly variable, being influenced by the amount of cholesterol fed at one time, presence of bile, frequency of ingestion, type of dietary fats, and other factors. About half of the dietary cholesterol is absorbed.

Digestibility

Digestion of high-fat meals is slower than for other energy-containing nutrients, resulting in such phrases as "high satiety value" or "sticks to the ribs." The higher the fat content of a meal, the longer the food remains in the stomach. Nevertheless, about 95 percent of the ingested fats is absorbed.

Soft fats that are liquids at body temperature (like margarine) are more easily digested than hard fats, such as meat fats. Fried foods are digested more slowly than foods cooked by other methods.

Hydrocarbons, such as motor oil and mineral oil, cannot be utilized by the body. They actually are not even classified as fats. However, in the past, mineral oil has been used in food preparation for calorie-restricted diets. The use of mineral oil is not advisable because its laxative effect reduces absorption of fat-soluble vitamins.

Clinical Implications:

- Infants, young children, and some older adults may experience discomfort after high-fat meals. Softer, more emulsified fats, such as those in milk and eggs, may be better tolerated.
- Foods fried in low temperatures absorb excessive amounts of fats, while those fried in very high temperatures result in decomposition of some fats, which can be irritating to the intestine.
- Lipid malabsorption occurs most frequently when bile salts and/or pancreatic lipase are not available or when mucosal cells are damaged (as in celiac disease), resulting in steatorrhea.
- Medium-chain triglycerides (MCTs) may be digested and absorbed in patients with digestive or absorptive disorders affecting utilization of long-chain triglycerides (Bach & Babayan, 1982).
- When appreciable amounts of MCTs are supplied in the diet, they are rapidly oxidized, rendering many ketone bodies. Thus, they are not advised for patients with diabetes (Bach & Babayan, 1982).

Plasma Lipids and Fat Metabolism

Chylomicrons being transported to the liver via the lymphatic system result in a cloudy or milky appearance of the blood. Plasma triglycerides are extremely variable, ranging between 10 to 200 mg/dl. Most of the triglycerides are transported in the blood as LDLs and VLDLs.

FAT METABOLISM

The liver is the principal regulator of fat metabolism (Fig. 8–6). Hormones involved in carbo-

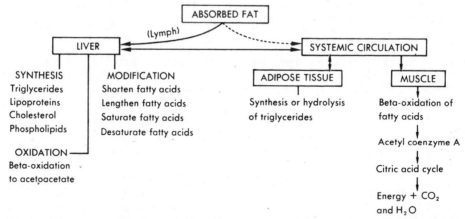

Figure 8–6. The liver and adipose tissue are principal organs of fat metabolism. (Reprinted with permission of Macmillan Publishing Company from Normal and Therapeutic Nutrition, 16th ed, by C. R. Robinson and M. R. Lawler. Copyright © 1982 by Macmillan Publishing Co, Inc.)

Table 8–2. *Hormonal Role in Fat Metabolism*

Hormone	Effect	Action
Insulin		Activates lipoprotein lipase.
Lack	Decreases lipogenesis; increases lipolysis.	
Excess	Increases lipolysis; inhibits fat utilization.	
Thyroxin	Increases lipolysis.	Increases rate of energy metabolism.
Glucocorticoids	Increase lipolysis.	Increase fat-cell membrane permeability.
Adrenocorticoids	Increase lipolysis.	Stimulate secretion of glucocorticoids.
Epinephrine and norepinephrine	Increase lipolysis.	Increase the release of free fatty acids from fat cells.

hydrate metabolism also control fat metabolism (Table 8–2). In the liver, fatty acids can be hydrolyzed or modified by shortening or lengthening or by adding double bonds prior to their release into the circulation. The liver is the sole source of lipoprotein synthesis, releasing or removing them from the bloodstream, thus regulating blood lipid levels.

The liver also regulates the circulating blood cholesterol by controlling the amount of cholesterol produced, removing cholesterol from the blood, producing bile acids from cholesterol, and excreting bile acids via the bile into the intestine. Cholesterol is present in the blood primarily in LDLs and HDLs. Normally, total serum cholesterol in men ranges from 140 to 260 mg/dl.

Lipotropic substances present in the liver prevent fat accumulation in the liver. These include choline, vitamin B_{12}, and possibly inositol. Fatty livers can be the result of starvation, diabetes mellitus, deficiency of lipotropic substances, poisons, drugs, and excessive alcohol intake.

Metabolism of chylomicrons in the liver results in triglycerides being transported to the tissues for energy or other uses, or carried to adipose tissue to be stored. Fats in the blood are the result of not only absorption from foods but also the conversion of carbohydrates and proteins into fats. Plasma-free fatty acids range between 0.3 to 0.5 mEq/L. The higher values occur when more lipolysis is taking place.

If the triglycerides produced during the absorption process are to be used for energy, they must be broken down again to glycerol and fatty acids. The glycerol is usually converted to glucose or used to make new triglycerides.

OXIDATION OF FATTY ACIDS

In a process called beta oxidation, triglycerides are broken down into two carbon entities, which enter the same Krebs cycle as glucose to yield energy. When the body oxidizes one pound of fat, 3500 kcal are released for energy. (This is more than most people use in a 24-hour period).

When excessive amounts of fats or proteins are oxidized for energy, the liver is overwhelmed, and ketone bodies are formed. Ketone bodies are not oxidized in the liver but are carried to the skeletal and cardiac muscles where they are rapidly metabolized under normal circumstances.

The capacity of the tissues to utilize ketone bodies may be exceeded when the glucose supply is reduced. Ketones accumulate in the blood (ketosis) and spill over into the urine (ketonuria). This condition can occur in starvation, in diabetes mellitus, or on very-low-carbohydrate reduction diets. Even during ketosis, ketone bodies are being oxidized normally in the tissues.

Ketosis can be a dangerous condition for several reasons. These strong acids must be neutralized by alkali to maintain the acid-base balance in the blood. Thus, they are generally carried through the blood and into the urine with sodium. If the condition continues, acidosis may result. In addition to the loss of sodium ions, large amounts of water are lost, which can lead to dehydration (or rapid weight loss for the dieter). Elevated blood ketones promote hyperuricemia (elevated uric acid). When the glucose blood levels remain low for several days, the brain and nerve cells will adapt to utilize some ketones for fuel.

In promoting high-protein, low-carbohydrate diets, ketonuria has been suggested as an effective way of excreting calories to lose weight. However, at most, about 20 gm/day of ketones may be excreted in the urine, or less than 100 kcal/day.

FAT SYNTHESIS

Triglycerides can be synthesized in the intestinal mucosa, in adipose tissue, and in the liver. Fat synthesis (lipogenesis) and breakdown (lipolysis) are continual processes, which are in equilibrium when the energy needs of the body are balanced.

Clinical Implications:

- Ketosis does not occur just because of rapid breakdown of adipose tissue, but when accompanied by carbohydrate deprivation.
- Ketosis should be avoided during pregnancy because ketone bodies cross the placenta and may negatively affect the fetus's cerebral development (Pitkin, 1979).
- High ketone levels result in an unusual breath odor, similar to acetone or nail polish remover.
- High ketone levels, associated with starvation or high-protein, low-carbohydrate, low-calorie diets, result in decreased appetite and occasionally nausea.

Metabolic Interrelationships

As you may have observed, a discussion of the metabolism of the energy-containing nutrients cannot be isolated from the others because of their many points of interaction. Lipids do not contribute significantly to the synthesis of amino acids, but glycerol from triglycerides can be used for synthesis of carbohydrates. Even though fats are a good source of energy, carbohydrate is the preferred fuel. The body cannot metabolize excessive quantities of fat without some side effects, namely ketosis, hyperlipemia, and fatty liver. Carbohydrates also provide oxaloacetate for lipids to enter the Krebs cycle and can form the carbon skeletons of nonessential amino acids. Fatty acids and the carbon skeletons of certain amino acids can be converted to glucose. Proteins contribute to the synthesis of some lipids, for example, lipoproteins.

Catabolism from all classes of foodstuffs involves oxidation through the Krebs cycle to produce energy. A sufficient quantity of calories in the diet from carbohydrate or lipids influences protein metabolism. In some situations, one nutrient can be substituted for another because of the interrelationships. For example, a decrease in carbohydrate increases lipolysis; a protein excess can be used for energy.

Not only are these three nutrients necessary; vitamins and minerals are essential for their digestion, absorption, and metabolism (in the Krebs cycle). While they are not required in large quantities, as are the energy nutrients, their presence is just as important. When there is a deficiency, reactions cannot proceed. For example, even though protein may be consumed alone (as in liquid protein supplements), many other nutrients, including vitamins and minerals, must be present for the protein to be utilized by the cells. While each nutrient has its specific function, all the nutrients must be present simultaneously for optimal benefits.

Metabolic interrelationships are complex and cannot be fully covered in this text. These interrelationships are important, and for optimal utilization of nutrients, food sources for all the nutrients should be incorporated into every diet. The easiest way to accomplish this is to include a variety of foods from all the food groups.

Role of Fats in the Diet

Fats have many important roles in the diet, and a moderate amount should be included.

CONCENTRATED ENERGY

Fats in the diet are a concentrated source of energy for the body, furnishing 9 kcal/gm. Foods high in fats are generally referred to as "calorie dense," which to a certain extent has its merits. It is not necessary to consume large volumes of food to furnish the energy requirements.

PROTEIN AND THIAMIN SPARERS

As an energy source, fats are also referred to as "protein sparing," since they allow protein to be used for the important functions of building and repairing rather than for calories. Fats are thiamin-sparing when they are utilized for energy, as compared with carbohydrates, which require thiamin.

SATIETY VALUE

Fats are important in the diet for their high satiety value. Since they depress gastric secretions and retard emptying time of the stomach, they delay the rapid development of hunger frequently observed after high-carbohydrate meals.

PALATABILITY

Fats contribute to palatability and flavor of foods. Their use in cooking improves the texture. The flavors of fruits and vegetables are generally droplets of oil. Only a drop of peppermint oil will produce a minty-tasting product. The characteristic pungent flavor of vinegar is a fatty acid, acetic acid.

OTHER NUTRIENTS

Fats are important because they furnish essential nutrients such as linoleic acid. Fat-soluble vitamins are generally found in foods containing fat. The absorption of these vitamins is facilitated by the presence of fats in the intestinal tract.

Importance of Fats as Constituents of Body Compounds

FAT STORAGE

Adipose tissue has several roles: It is a concentrated energy source, protects internal organs, and maintains body temperature.

Energy. Excess carbohydrates and protein are converted to fat and stored in adipose tissue. Adipose tissue is a form of stored energy. Fatty acids can be utilized as an energy source by all cells except erythrocytes and those of the central nervous system. Lipids can be stored in almost unlimited amounts. Individuals have been known to survive total starvation for 30 to 40 days. In the past, when food supplies were unpredictable, heavier persons were respected and admired more.

Protection of Organs. Fatty tissue surrounds vital organs and provides a cushion for them,

thereby protecting them from traumatic injury and shock.

Insulation. The subcutaneous layer of fat functions as an insulator that preserves body heat and maintains body temperature. Excessive layers of fat can also deter heat loss during warm weather.

Two types of fat are present in the body—white and brown. The fat in subcutaneous tissue, abdominal cavity, and intramuscular fat is known as white fat. Up to 95 percent of these fat cells are triglycerides stored in liquid form. Brown fat has a different role than energy storage. It is located particularly in the interscapular region and the back of the neck. Instead of releasing fatty acids into the blood as an energy source, the fatty acids in these cells are oxidized for production of heat. Energy is not collected and stored as ATP but dissipates as heat to warm the body. The role of brown fat is unknown, but it may account for the variability in energy requirements of individuals.

ESSENTIAL FATTY ACIDS

Linoleic acid (18-carbon chain with two double bonds) is an essential fatty acid (EFA). It cannot be synthesized by the body and must be supplied from dietary sources. Arachidonic acid (18-carbon chain with four double bonds) is also an EFA, but the body can produce it from sufficient quantities of linoleic acid. These EFAs are required for proper growth and healthy skin. Deficiency results in poor growth, dermatitis (Fig. 8–7), lowered resistance to infection, and poor reproductive capacity. Linolenic and linoleic acid compete for the same enzymes in the body. Omega-6 and omega-3 fatty acids are not interconvertible in the body's metabolic pathways, so a dietary source of each may be necessary (Tinoco et al, 1979).

Cholesterol Metabolism. The presence of EFAs affects cholesterol metabolism. Serum cholesterol can be lowered by diets high in the EFAs or PUFAs.

Phospholipids. Also called phosphatides, phospholipids are produced from EFAs. They are formed in essentially all cells and are the second most prevalent form of fat in the body. They are key components of cellular membranes. Because of their strong affinity for water-soluble and fat-soluble substances in the molecule, phospholipids

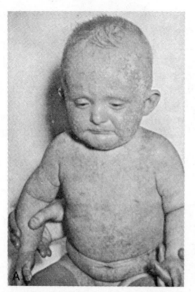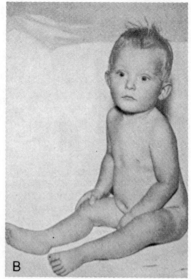

Figure 8–7. *The first symptoms identified specifically as being due to essential fatty acid (EFA) deficiency were skin lesions in rats. Similar lesions were seen in infants given formulas devoid of EFA. This research was carried out before the critical nature of EFAs was known. Ethical considerations would prohibit such research today. A) Six-month-old infant with very resistant eczema appearing at 2½ months of age. B) The same child six months later after a source of linoleic acid had been included in the diet. (Courtesy of the late Dr. A. E. Hansen.)*

are a part of the lipoprotein molecule important in fat absorption and in the transport of fats in the blood.

Phospholipids include lecithin, cephalin, and sphingomyelins. *Lecithin*, the most widely distributed phospholipid, is a component of the erythrocyte plasma membrane and is present in all cells. *Cephalin* is present in thromboplastin, necessary for blood clotting. *Sphingomyelins* are important constituents of brain tissue and of the myelin sheath around nerve fibers.

Prostaglandins. Prostaglandins are a group of hormone-like compounds important in smooth muscle contraction, gastric secretion, pancreatic function, and lowering of blood pressure. These are synthesized in the body from arachidonic acid. Prostaglandins are 20-carbon unsaturated fatty acids (Fig. 8–8), like arachidonic acid. They

PGE_1

PGF_{1a}

Figure 8–8. *Two representative prostaglandins. (From Ternay AL Jr: Contemporary Organic Chemistry, 2nd ed. Philadelphia, W. B. Saunders Co, 1979.)*

are the most potent biologically active substances yet discovered; very small amounts are present.

Omega-3 Fatty Acids. These are mainly found in fish and have different metabolic effects than linoleic acid. Omega-3 fatty acids can alter the synthesis of prostaglandins and appear to affect diseases such as atherosclerosis by inhibiting hepatic triglycerides. Bleeding time is increased and platelet adhesiveness is decreased by larger dietary amounts of these fatty acids (Phillipson et al, 1985).

CHOLESTEROL

Although cholesterol is not a dietary requirement, it has important functions as a constituent of brain and nervous tissues, a precursor of vitamin D and steroid hormones, a constituent of bile salts, and a structural component of cell membranes.

GLYCOLIPIDS

Glycolipids are produced from fatty acids, carbohydrate, and nitrogen. Cerebrosides and gangliosides are included in this classification. Structurally, they are components of brain and nerve tissue and certain cell membranes, where they function in cell permeability for fats.

Clinical Implication:

• Essential fatty acid deficiency has been observed in adults given long-term, fat-free intravenous feedings.

Dietary Requirement of Fat

Linoleic acid is the only dietary requirement for fat. The American Academy of Pediatrics (1976) recommends three percent of the calories in infant formulas be EFAs.

The requirement for adults is lower, about one to two percent of the calorie intake (15 to 25

gm of fat). Linoleic acid is stored in the tissues of adults when dietary intake is high. Excessive amounts of PUFAs increase vitamin E requirements. Without adequate vitamin E, encephalomalacia and sterility may occur. Fortunately, vegetable oils containing linoleic acid also have large amounts of vitamin E. The USDA estimates that about 25 gm of linoleic acid per capita per day is available in the U.S. food supply (Marston & Welsh, 1984).

In addition to being an important energy source, dietary fat is a carrier for fat-soluble vitamins. These needs can also be met by a diet containing 15 to 25 gm of dietary fat (NRC, 1980). However, 43 percent of the calories or 166 gm/day in the typical American diet is fat (Marston & Raper, 1986) (see Chapter 14).

Sources

People frequently consume more fat than they realize because of the "invisible" fats in the milk and meat groups.

Foods high in saturated, monounsaturated, and polyunsaturated fatty acids are itemized in Table 8–3. Percentages of PUFAs are shown in

Table 8–3. Fats in Foods

Saturated
  High Fat Content: Beef, lamb, luncheon meats (cold cuts, frankfurters, etc.), pork (including ham and salt pork), hard yellow cheeses, sweet cream, sour cream.
  Low Fat Content: Veal, organ meats, whole and part-skim milk, yogurt, cottage cheese.

Monounsaturated
  High Fat Content: Duck, goose, eggs.
  Low Fat Content: Chicken, turkey.

Polyunsaturated
  Low Fat Content: Fish, shellfish, salmon, tuna.

Fats and Oils
  Saturated: Butter, lard, coconut oil, palm oil, hydrogenated or "hardened" vegetable oils, regular margarine.
  Monounsaturated: Olive oil, peanut oil.
  Polyunsaturated: Safflower oil, corn oil, cottonseed oil, sesame oil, soybean oil, sunflower oil, salad dressings from these oils, special margarines listing liquid oil first.

COMPARISON OF DIETARY FATS

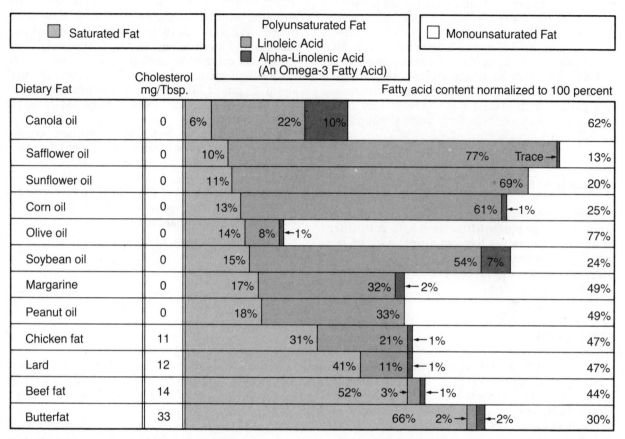

Figure 8–9. *Percentage of polyunsaturated fats in foods. (From* Fats, Cholesterol and the Family Diet. *University of California Agricultural Extension Service, Publication HXT-51, June 1963.)*

Figure 8–9. The fat composition and P/S ratio of various foods are shown in Table 8–4.

Linolenic acid is present in linseed oil (not available in the U.S.), canola oil (Puritan), soybean oil, and small amounts in green leafy vegetables and meat fats. EPA and DHA are found in fish, the amount of which varies depending on species, sex, age, season, and food supply. Plankton is an excellent source of linolenic acid.

Cholesterol is found only in animal products; it is not found in egg whites or plant foods. It is highest in egg yolk, liver and other organ meats.

Health Application: Current Issues Involving Fats

The following conditions involve excess body lipid concentrations and require alteration of the amount and/or type of fat in the diet: obesity, gallbladder disease, diabetes mellitus, fatty infiltration of the liver, and hyperlipidemia. Lipids may also play a role in cancer. Dietary fat is modified in malabsorption syndromes, such as cystic fibrosis. Fats may be poorly tolerated in

Table 8—4. Cholesterol, Fat, and Fatty Acid Composition of Various Foodstuffs*

	Cholesterol	Fat	Saturated Fat	P/S[a]
	mg/100 gm of food	gm/100 gm of food		
I. Eggs, meat, fish, and poultry				
Egg				
Yolk[b]	1200	34	10.1	0.4
White	0	0		
Beef (average)[c]	69	10–15	5–7	0.04
Pork and ham[c]				
Average	63	10–15	4–5	0.3
Bacon fat	104	100	32	0.3
Bacon, cooked	22	52	17	0.3
Sausage	65	26	9	0.3
Lard	17	100	38	0.3
Lamb (average)[c]	74	10–15	6–8	0.1
Veal (average)[c]	71	10	5	0.04
Poultry (chicken and turkey)				
Average (no skin)[c]	67	5	2	0.7
Turkey skin	110	42	12	0.7
Fish (average)	59	3	0.06	3.8
Shellfish				
Clams, oysters, and scallops[d]	53	2	<0.4	4.0
Shrimp, lobster, crab, and abalone	121	1	<0.2	4.0
Variety (organ) meats	300–2000	1–20		
II. Dairy products				
Butter	228	80	49.8	0.1
Milk				
Skim (0.1% fat)	2	0.2	0.1	0.1
Fortified skim (0.5% fat)	3	0.5	0.3	0.1
Buttermilk	4	0.7	0.4	0.1
2% milk (2.0% fat)	8	2.0	1.3	0.1
Whole milk (4% fat)	13	3.5	2.2	0.1
Cream				
Heavy or whipping	137	37.9	23.6	0.1
Sour	45	18.5	11.5	0.1
Thin cream (Half & half)	40	11.7	7.3	0.1
Ice cream, vanilla	44	12.4	7.6	0.1
Ice milk, vanilla	13	5.0	1.0	0.1
Sherbet	4	1.3	0.7	0.1
III. Cheeses				
Up to 10% fat				
Count-down	5	1.0	0.6	0.1
Cottage, rinsed or dry	1	0.5	0.3	0.1
Cottage, low-fat (2%)	6	1.4	0.9	0.1
Cottage, regular (4% fat)	14	4.0	2.5	0.1
Ricotta, part skim	30	8.5	5.3	0.1
10–20% fat				
Ricotta, whole milk, and mozzarella, part skim	51	14.6	9.2	0.1
20–30% fat				
Camembert, Edam, blue, Parmesan, provolone, Swiss (pasteurized process), Swiss, processed cheddar, cheese food (cheddar), Neufchatel, mozzarella (low-moisture), American pasteurized process, brick	79	26.9	15.5	0.1

*From Connor, WE: U.S. Dietary goals; a pro view, with special emphasis upon the etiological relationships of dietary factors to coronary heart disease. In *Human Nutrition—Clinical and Biochemical Aspects*. Edited by PJ Garry. Washington, DC, American Association for Clinical Nutrition, 1981. Reprinted with permission from *Clinical Chemistry*.

Note: 100 g = 3.3 oz. raw weight or 2.5–3.0 oz. cooked weight

[a]P/S, ratio of polyunsaturated to saturated fats.

[b]One yolk = 20 g = 240 mg of cholesterol.

[c]Average values for meat are on the basis of lean, well-trimmed meat (10–15% fat).

[d]These shellfish also contain other sterols (24-methylenecholesterol, brassicasterol, and 22-dehydrocholesterol) whose effects upon plasma cholesterol are not known.

Table 8–4. Cholesterol, Fat, and Fatty Acid Composition of Various Foodstuffs (Continued)

	Cholesterol	Fat	Saturated Fat	P/S[a]
	mg/100 gm of food	gm/100 gm of food		
30–40% fat				
Cheddar (mild and sharp), colby, cream, Muenster, Limburger, Roquefort	95	31.9	17.1	0.1
IV. Fats				
Vegetable oils (average)[e]	0	100	16.1	3.3
Vegetable shortenings (average)	0	100	27.3	0.8
Vegetable margarines, soft stick and tub (average)	0	80	14.1	1.9
Peanut butter (average)	0	50	10.6	1.4
Non-dairy creamers[f]				
Poly-perx	0	10	1.7	2.2

[e]Excluding cocoa butter, coconut oil, and palm oil.
[f]Excluding non-dairy creamers containing coconut oil.

gallbladder and pancreatic diseases (see Chapter 28). Fat intake is increased for those who need to gain weight or for inducing ketosis in seizure patients. Lands (1986) has suggested that many diseases are related to an excess of omega-6 fatty acids (which inhibit omega-3 fatty acids). New research efforts are implying that these fatty acids are linked to heart disease, strokes, allergies, and cancer.

Obesity. Excess storage of fat is a common disorder in the United States. While the cause is overconsumption, calories from fat are so concentrated that relatively small quantities may rapidly increase caloric intake.

Blood Lipid Levels. Elevated blood lipids are related to diet, although not directly. Hyperlipidemia is associated with heart disease (Consensus Conference, 1985). While many factors can affect blood lipid levels (Consensus Conference, 1984), much research has been conducted to determine these dietary effects. Elevated serum cholesterol and triglyceride levels may be lowered by dietary manipulations (see Chapter 32).

Cancer. Fats have been implicated in colonic and breast cancers even though findings are inconsistent. Research has shown that lipids play a role in controlling immune function. Although it has never been shown that excessive or deficient amounts of nutrients cause cancer, carcinogenesis can be promoted by diet. During a period of increasing cancer incidence, consumption of PUFAs from vegetable oils also increased while consumption of saturated fatty acids decreased. While adequate amounts of EFAs are critical for immune response, excessive amounts of PUFAs are immunosuppressive and promote tumorigenesis (Carroll, 1984; Chandra, 1983; Beisel, 1982; Vitale & Broitman, 1981).

Some research has shown that the processing of vegetable oils, which slightly alters the chemical structure of fatty acids, could be involved in carcinogenesis, but more evidence is needed (Enig et al, 1978).

Alcohol Metabolism

While alcohol is considered by some to be a drug, it is utilized by the body for calories. Ethyl alcohol does not have as much oxygen as carbohydrates—it contains more hydrogen, similar to fats; therefore, its caloric value is between the two (7 kcal/gm). Calorie content of alcoholic beverages can be calculated by using Table 8–5.

Since no digestion is required, alcohol is rapidly absorbed from the stomach and small intestine. Most of the metabolism of alcohol takes place in the liver. The large percentage of hydrogen from alcohol unbalances the liver cell chemistry.

Normally, fat would be oxidized to produce energy. The alcohol provides an alternate fuel that is oxidized instead of fat. Since alcohol metabolism is substituted for fat metabolism, a side effect of large amounts of alcohol will cause lipids to accumulate, leading to fatty liver. Very little alcohol

Table 8–5. Calculation of Caloric Content of Liquor*

To calculate the kilocaloric content of an amount of liquor the following equation can be used:

$$0.8 \text{ kcal/proof/oz.} \times \text{proof} \times \text{ounces} = \text{kcal}$$

0.8 kcal/proof/oz. = the factor necessary to account for the kilocaloric density of alcohol (7 kcal/gm) and the fact that not all of the alcohol in liquor is available for energy.

proof = 2 × the percentage of alcohol in the liquor and is necessary because not all of the liquor is alcohol.

ounces = the amount of liquor consumed.

For example, to calculate the kilocaloric content of two 4-oz. glasses of wine (12% alcohol):

$$0.8 \text{ kcal/proof/oz.} \times 24 \text{ proof} \times 8 \text{ oz.} = 154 \text{ kcal}$$

*From Krause, MV; Mahan, LK: *Food, Nutrition and Diet Therapy,* 7th ed. Philadelphia, W.B. Saunders Co., 1984. As adapted from Gastineau, CF: Alcohol and calories. *Mayo Clinic Proceedings* 51(2):88, 1976.

is excreted in the urine or through the lungs; the body has no storage mechanism for it; therefore, it must all be metabolized, predominantly by the liver. There are no feedback controls to limit the rate of its oxidation (Lieber, 1976). When large quantities of ethanol must be oxidized, several metabolic problems may develop (Lieber, 1975) including hyperlactacidemia and hyperuricemia, enchanced production of lipids and lipoproteins, decreased lipid oxidation and steatosis, reduced gluconeogenesis and hypoglycemia, and inhibition of drug metabolism. Alcohol can affect nutrition in several ways (see Chapter 28).

Clinical Implication:

- The body can metabolize small, frequent amounts of alcohol better than a large amount over a short period of time. About 14 gm/hr (70 kg) is the maximal rate of alcohol metabolism; higher intakes could be fatal.

• FALLACIES and FACTS

FALLACY: *Fried foods are not well digested.*
- **FACT:** *While the digestion of fried foods takes longer, digestion is as complete as for other foods in most persons if the proper frying temperature is used.*

FALLACY: *Vegetable oils without additives are better for you than those preserved with an antioxidant.*

- **FACT:** *When antioxidants are not present, vegetable oils are rapidly oxidized and become rancid. Vitamin E is one of the most effective antioxidants and, if it has not been oxidized, can function in the body in normal vitamin E metabolism.*

FALLACY: *Bananas and avocados are loaded with cholesterol and fat and should be avoided by persons trying to lose weight or lower blood cholesterol.*

- **FACT:** *Cholesterol is found only in animal products. Bananas contain a trace of fat; avocados are 16 percent fat, 20 percent of this is saturated fatty acids. Both are good sources of several vitamins and minerals.*

FALLACY: *Oils are less fattening than solid fats.*
- **FACT:** *All fats yield 9 kcal/gm; therefore, oils and fats have the same amount of calories.*

FALLACY: *Lecithin lowers blood cholesterol.*
- **FACT:** *Lecithin is readily manufactured by the liver to meet the metabolic needs of the body. Unless the lecithin is specially processed, lecithinase in the intestine will hydrolyze lecithin so that it is not absorbed as such. Lecithin supplements lower serum cholesterol in some individuals, but in other studies, lecithin lowers the blood cholesterol only transiently. It is not lowered in individuals with Type II hyperlipidemia (Wood & Allison, 1982).*

Summary

Lipids are important sources of energy in the diet and are the body's principal form of energy storage. They furnish more than twice as many calories (9 kcal/gm) as proteins or carbohydrates. When more calories are consumed than the body needs, it is stored as adipose tissue (3500 kcal = 1 lb. of fat); this adipose tissue will be oxidized for energy when the diet is deficient in calories.

Lipids, being insoluble, must be emulsified in order to be digested or carried in the bloodstream. Fats in the gastrointestinal tract are emulsified by bile and transported to the liver as chylomicrons via the lymphatic system. Fats transported in the blood are complexed with protein, called lipoproteins.

The essential fatty acid required in the diet is linoleic acid, supplied by safflower, corn, soybean, and cottonseed oils and nuts such as almonds and walnuts. From this, the body can make other fatty acids it needs—linolenic and arachidonic acids. Cholesterol is produced by the body and is not a necessary constituent of the diet. It is, however, an essential constituent of all cells.

Lecithin and other phospholipids play important roles in nervous tissue and in the transport of fats. The body can also make these; therefore, they are not necessary dietary constituents.

Fats are furnished in the diet mainly from meat, whole milk products, and added fats, such as margarine and salad dressings. Polyunsaturated fats are supplied from vegetable oils. Cholesterol is supplied from animal products, especially organ meats, shellfish, and eggs. Cholesterol is not found in any plant product.

Review Questions

1. Define lipid, hydrogenation, triglyceride, lipoprotein.
2. How do polyunsaturated fats and saturated fats differ chemically?
3. In observing physical properties of fats, how could you make an intelligent guess about the polyunsaturated and saturated fat content of a food?
4. What unsaturated fatty acid is essential in the diet? What are the functions of unsaturated fatty acids in the body?
5. Compare the labels of three brands of stick margarine, three brands of tub margarine, and two brands of diet margarine. How do they differ in their P/S ratio?
6. List the functions of fat in the diet.
7. What is ketosis? Why does it occur?
8. Describe the role of cholesterol in the body.
9. Calculate the caloric value of the following items:
   - 2 slices bacon (8 gm fat, 4 gm protein)
   - 1 Tbsp. margarine (12 gm fat)
   - 1 Tbsp. whipped margarine (8 gm fat)
   - 1 Tbsp. mayonnaise (6 gm fat)
   - 1 Tbsp. lard (13 gm fat)
10. If one pound of body fat is equal to 3500 calories, is it possible to lose or gain one pound of body fat per day?

REFERENCE LIST

American Academy of Pediatrics, Committee on Nutrition: Commentary on breast-feeding and infant formulas, including standards for formulas. *Pediatrics* 57(2):278, 1976.

Alfin-Slater, R; Aftergood, L: Lipids. In *Modern Nutrition in Health and Disease*. Edited by RS Goodhart; ME Shils. Philadelphia, Lea & Febiger, 1980, p 113.

Bach, AC; Babayan, VK: Medium-chain triglycerides: An update. *Am J Clin Nutr* 36(5):950, 1982.

Beisel, WR: Single nutrients and immunity. *Am J Clin Nutr* 35(suppl):417, 1982.

Carroll, KK: Role of lipids in tumorigenesis. *J Am Oil Chem Soc* 61(12):1888, 1984.

Chandra, RK: Nutrition, immunity and infection: Present knowledge and future directions. *Lancet* 1(March 26):688, 1983.

Consensus Conference: Treatment of hypertriglyceridemia. *JAMA* 251(9):1196, 1984.

Consensus Conference: Lowering blood cholesterol to prevent heart disease. *JAMA* 253(14):2080, 1985.

Enig, MG; Munn, RJ; Keeney, M: Dietary fat and cancer trends: A critique. *Fed Proc* 37:2215, 1978.

Glueck, CJ; Hastings, MM; Allen, C; et al: Sucrose polyester and covert caloric dilution. *Am J Clin Nutr* 35(6):1352, 1982.

Glueck, CJ; Mattson, FH; Jandacek, RJ: The lowering of plasma cholesterol by sucrose polyester in subjects consuming diets with 800, 300, or less than 50 mg of cholesterol per day. *Am J Clin Nutr* 32(8):1636, 1979.

Grundy, SM: Comparison of monounsaturated fatty acids and carbohydrates for lowering plasma cholesterol. *N Engl J Med* 314(12):745, 1986.

Guyton, AC: *Textbook of Medical Physiology*, 7th ed. Philadelphia, WB Saunders, 1986.

Hamosh, M; Scanlon, JW; Ganot, P, et al: Fat digestion in the newborn. *J Clin Invest* 67(3):838, 1981.

Lands, WEM: *Fish and Human Health*. Orlando, FL, Academic Press, 1986.

Lieber, CS: The metabolism of alcohol. *Sci Am* 234(3):25, 1976.

Lieber, CS: Liver disease of the alcoholic: Pathogenesis and metabolic complications. *Ala J Med Sci* 12(4):355, 1975.

Marston, RM; Raper, NR: Nutrient content of the food supply. *Nat Food Review* 32(winter):6, 1986.

Marston, RM; Welsh, SO: Nutrient content of the U.S. food supply, 1982. *Nat Food Review* 25(winter):7, 1984.

Mellies, MJ; Vitale, C; Jandacek, RJ; et al: The substitution of sucrose polyester for dietary fat in obese hypercholesteremic outpatients. *Am J Clin Nutr* 41(1):1, 1985.

National Research Council (NRC): Recommended Dietary Allowances. Washington, D.C., National Academy of Sciences, 1980.

Phillipson, BE; Rothrock, DW; Conner, WE; et al: Reduction of plasma lipids, lipoproteins, and apoproteins by dietary fish oils in patients with hypertriglyceridemia. *N Engl J Med* 312(19):1210, 1985.

Pitkin, RM: What's new in maternal nutrition? *Nutr News* 42(2):5, 1979.

Tinoco, J; Babcock, R; Hincenbergs, I: Linoleic acid deficiency. *Lipids* 14(2):166, 1979.

Vitale, JJ; Broitman, SA: Lipids and immune function. *Cancer Res* 41(9):3706, 1981.

Wood, JL; Allison, RG: Effects of consumption of choline and lecithin on neurological and cardiovascular systems. *Fed Proc* 41(14):3015, 1982.

Further Study

Burr, GO; Burr, MM: A new deficiency disease produced by the rigid exclusion of fat from the diet. *Nutr Rev* 31(8):248, 1973.

Crocker, KS; Gerber, F; Shearer, J: Metabolism of carbohydrate, protein, and fat. *Nurs Clin North Am* 18(1):3, 1983.

Feeley, RM: Cholesterol content of foods. *J Am Diet Assoc* 61(2):134, 1972.

Grande, F: The role of fat in child nutrition. *Nutr Metab* 24(suppl 1):147, 1980.

Holt, PR: Fats and bile salts. 1. Physiologic considerations. *J Am Diet Assoc* 60(6):491, 1972.

Holt, PR: Fats and bile salts. II. Pathologic considerations. *J Am Diet Assoc* 60(6):495, 1972.

McCulloch, J: Biochemistry 2. Build up to an attack. *Nurs Mirror* 154(5):34, 1982.

National Dairy Council: Nutrition update: Fat/cholesterol. *Dairy Council Digest* 55(5), 1984.

National Dairy Council: Nutrition and the immune response. *Dairy Council Digest* 56(2), 1985.

Shaw, S; Lieber, CS: Nutrition and alcoholic liver disease. In *Nutrition in Disease*. Columbus, OH, Ross Laboratories, 1978.

Ten Hoor, F: Cardiovascular effects of dietary linoleic acid, *Nutr Metab* 24(suppl 1):162, 1980.

Truswell, AS: Diet and plasma lipids—a reappraisal. *Am J Clin Nutr* 31(6):977, 1978.

Energy Requirements: Normal, Physically Challenged, and Athletic

9

THE STUDENT WILL BE ABLE TO:

- **Calculate energy needs according to the individual's weight and activities.**
- **Explain the sources of energy.**
- **Identify factors affecting metabolism.**

TERMS TO KNOW

Aerobic
Aerobic work capacity
Adenosine triphosphate (ATP)
Anaerobic
Basal energy expenditure (BEE)
Basal metabolism rate (BMR)
Bomb calorimeter
Carbohydrate loading
Circadian rhythm
Energy
Glycogen
Lactic acid
Law of conservation of energy
Lean body mass (LBM)
Photosynthesis
Room calorimeter
Specific dynamic action (SDA)

Without energy from chemical reactions, a person could not bat an eye, wiggle a toe, or think a thought. Energy from food is converted into forms of energy the body can use: electrical for the brain and nerves, mechanical for muscles, thermal for body heat, and chemical for synthesis of new compounds.

Energy

Energy is the ability, or power, to do work. The law of conservation of energy states that energy can be neither created nor destroyed. Even though the form of energy may change, it does not disappear or go away.

Photosynthesis. The origin of energy formation is the sun's radiant energy on green plants. Chlorophyll and carotenes from plants use this energy to convert carbon dioxide and water to glucose, releasing oxygen as a by-product, which is known as photosynthesis. Then, the animals that consume plants can create more complex forms of carbohydrate for the other organic nutrients.

Energy Production. After foods are chewed and digested, the energy nutrients (carbohydrates, protein, fat and alcohol) are converted to glucose, fatty acids, and amino acids. These basic nutrient units are delivered to cells where, at the direction of specific enzymes and various cofactors, they are reduced for use. The simplest process by which food energy is made available for use by the cell is glycolysis. This process is anaerobic (occurring without oxygen), and only carbohydrates are metabolized in this manner. However, this is an inefficient method of energy production.

The more complex and efficient way to produce energy requires respiration of oxygen from the atmosphere. Aerobic oxidation occurs through the Krebs cycle within the mitochondria (known as the powerhouse of the cell). These chemical reactions constitute the energy cycle causing organic

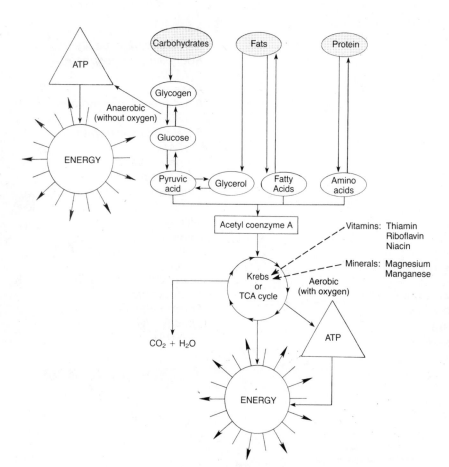

Figure 9–1. Simplified version of energy production in the body. Potential energy from the storage of glycogen is dependent upon the increased intake of carbohydrates. Since this pathway is anaerobic (without oxygen), it can be used immediately without delay. The major pathway of energy production is through the Krebs cycle, which is dependent upon adequate coenzymes of certain vitamins and minerals plus oxygen (aerobic).

nutrients to be catabolized into the carbon dioxide and water from which they were originally formed. This process releases the energy that held these constituents together (Fig. 9–1). These reactions may be simply seen as:

$$\text{carbon dioxide} + \text{water} + \text{sunlight (energy)} \rightarrow \text{glucose} + \text{oxygen}$$

followed by the reverse:

$$\text{glucose} + \text{oxygen} \rightarrow \text{carbon dioxide} + \text{water} + \text{energy}$$

Enzymes act as catalysts to speed up the reactions of energy production without being changed themselves. Coenzymes differ from enzymes since they must be continually replaced from food intake. The main coenzymes—thiamin, niacin, and riboflavin—are indispensable throughout the energy-releasing pathway. Carbohydrate metabolism is highly dependent on the presence of thiamin, which is a part of the coenzyme required in the transitional step between the anaerobic and aerobic phases. Since thiamin and niacin are particularly essential in many reactions to release energy, the RDAs for these B vitamins are based upon the number of kilocalories consumed. Other cofactors essential for energy release include magnesium and potassium.

STORAGE OF ENERGY

Whether excessive food intakes are in the form of proteins, carbohydrates, alcohol, and/or fats, they are all stored as adipose tissue.

Energy for the brain is dependent upon carbohydrates. Because thiamin is essential for carbohydrate metabolism, a thiamin deficiency is closely linked to aberrations of brain function. One safety reaction synthesizes glycogen from the deaminated portions of some amino acids to provide the necessary carbohydrate for the nourishment of the brain. Maintaining adequate liver glycogen stores is the preferred source of glucose for the brain.

Energy Sources

Glucose can be converted to glycogen and stored as a ready source of energy. The metabolism of the basic nutrients can result in the release of energy, which the body stores as adenosine triphosphate (ATP). ATP is an instant source of cellular energy for mechanical work, transport of nutrients and waste products, and synthesis of chemical compounds.

ATP units often are called the currency or "money" the body uses as the need arises. Since ATP can be metabolized without oxygen, the reaction is classified as anaerobic. The body must always have a supply of ATP, and several systems within the body insure a constant supply.

Another storage form of energy in the muscle cells is phosphocreatine (PC), which can almost instantaneously provide the energy required to regenerate ATP. Within a few minutes of vigorous exercise, the small stores of ATP and PC are depleted; therefore, the body relies on glycogen as a secondary source of energy, which recharges the ATP-PC system within the muscle cells. Glycogen is converted to ATP in the mitochondria.

In the postabsorptive state, approximately 500 gm of glycogen are stored in the body—400 gm in muscle and 100 gm in the liver. This amount of glycogen is equivalent to 2000 kcal or one day's energy supply (Cahill, 1986).

The amount of glycogen stores varies greatly and is dependent on the amount of carbohydrate in the diet, not the number or frequency of feedings. Glycogen stores are depleted with a carbohydrate-poor diet even when high levels of fat and protein are eaten. (Costill et al., 1981).

LACTIC ACID

Muscle glycogen does not form blood glucose, but instead forms lactic acid irreversibly. Formation of lactic acid is one of the important steps to prevent the instantaneous release of the total energy present. Since oxygen is required, the speed of conversion to ATP is reduced.

Because lactic acid is a fairly strong acid, the appearance of large quantities in the bloodstream tends to reduce the alkaline reserves and cause acidosis (which the buffer systems try to prevent). This in itself is an automatic stimulus to increase the respiration rate so that more oxygen facilitates oxidation of the lactic acid. Also, as the intensity of the work increases, the faster a person exhales in order to remove the excess carbon dioxide formed from the oxidation of the lactic acid. Logically, the body is limited in its ability to inhale enough oxygen to oxidize the lactic acid as quickly as it is formed (i.e., the limit is a function of the efficiency of the circulatory system). Prolonged strenuous exercise produces fatigue as the lactic acid momentarily accumulates faster than the body can supply oxygen to oxidize it, resulting in a temporary acidemia and insufficiency of ATP to activate the muscle.

AEROBIC WORK CAPACITY

Maximal oxygen uptake can be about 35 to 40 ml/kg of body weight per minute for an average middle-aged man or as much as 70 ml/kg/minute in a well-trained, young athlete. Work at low intensity, such as a brisk walk using about 1 L of oxygen, is the limit of aerobic work capacity, or work that does not build up lactic acid in tissues.

Steady state indicates work at or below the aerobic capacity because it can be maintained for a long time without fatigue. However, intense work continued for a long period depletes glycogen stores with the accumulation of lactic acid. After the work is finished, continued heavy breathing maintains larger oxygen supplies until the lactic acid is completely metabolized and tissue stores are replenished.

For maximum work output, it is best to alternate periods of intense work with short rest periods, such as 10 minutes of intense work and five minutes of rest. A slowed pace prevents an expenditure rate that exceeds aerobic capacity. The trained athlete is capable of longer periods of sustained work before becoming fatigued and accumulating an oxygen debt.

THE ROLE OF CARBOHYDRATES

Dietary carbohydrates assure optimal glycogen stores and are digested easier and faster than other energy nutrients. Since carbohydrates require less oxygen for their metabolism, diets with little or no carbohydrate are not as effective in supporting exertion. However, calories from carbohydrates alone will not produce optimum energy without adequate protein intake (Barac-Nieto et al., 1980). Higher kilocalorie intake when protein is inadequate is useless. Energy utilization is remarkably sensitive to both the quantity and quality of dietary protein (MacLean & Graham, 1979). Restricted protein and/or limited energy from fats and carbohydrates can be equally harmful.

THE ROLE OF FATS

While carbohydrate plays a dominant role in heavy exercise when the muscle's oxygen supply is limited, fat provides about half the energy during steady-state work. Although fats can be stored in body depots in virtually inexhaustible amounts (providing more than twice as many calories per gram as glycogen or tissue protein), their slower rate of metabolism makes them a less efficient source of quick energy. When energy demands require protein to be used, then the requirement for protein is increased to meet the body's specific needs for protein, i.e., growth and repair of tissue.

While alive, humans never cease to need energy. Even during sleep, the body requires energy for the obvious minimum tasks of respiration and circulation as well as many intricate activities within each cell.

Basal Metabolism

Basal metabolism is the energy required for the involuntary work of the body to maintain life including respiration, circulation, and maintenance of muscle tone and body temperature. Basal metabolism is lowest when the person is lying down, awake, rested, and relaxed in a comfortable environment, not having eaten for 12 to 15 hours. Since digestion and absorption require energy, the basal metabolism rate is the amount of energy required when the body is in a postabsorptive state (the period after all the digestive and absorptive processes have been completed). Unless physical activity is above average, the basal metabolic rate represents the largest proportion of an individual's energy requirement.

FACTORS AFFECTING THE BASAL METABOLISM RATE (BMR)

Various factors can increase or decrease the BMR, which determines the caloric needs.

1. Sleep: The Ebb of Life. After a few hours of sleep when the metabolism rate is lowest, muscles are more relaxed. About 10 percent less energy is needed for the BMR during the relaxed state of sleep.

Respiratory or cardiac arrests are more frequent during the "ebb of life" period, which is from about 2 till 6 o'clock. A circadian rhythm in the timing of death for both surgical and nonsurgical patients has been documented (Moore-Ede et al., September 1983). Respiratory or cardiac arrests in patients are more frequent during this time, and many clinical indexes will vary, such as temperature, blood, and urine constituents, or there may be increased or decreased effects of drugs (which may result in toxicity for borderline medications).

Meditation (such as transcendental meditation) is another factor that may lower the BMR further, as much as twice the magnitude of the decline after several hours of sleep (Wallace & Benson, 1972).

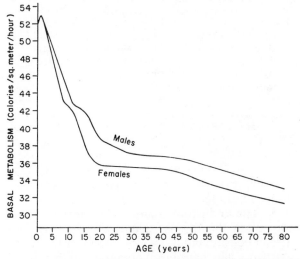

Figure 9–2. Normal basal metabolic rates at different ages for each sex. (From Guyton AC: Textbook of Medical Physiology, 7th ed. Philadelphia, W. B. Saunders Co, 1986, by permission.)

Clinical Implications:

- This circadian rhythm (24-hour periodicity) of the decreased BMR has a specific meaning for the nurse who does not work the regular day shift. Night-shift workers are often plagued by insomnia and fatigue and are the first to leave the nursing profession. Since it takes 7 to 14 days for the body to adjust to a new sleep pattern, a nurse who alternates days and nights can expect to have trouble sleeping two weeks a month and can also expect to be less efficient during the "ebb of life" period.
- Persons alternating day and night shifts have serious sleep disruption, increased levels of cardiovascular risk factors, gastrointestinal disorders, emotional disturbances, and impaired coordination (Moore-Ede et al., September 1983).
- Recommendations to minimize these circadian effects include:
  1. Choose a diet high in carbohydrate, low in protein for optimum energy;
  2. Avoid caffeine and alcohol; drink at least 6 to 8 glasses of water or other fluids per day;
  3. Do not exercise vigorously before bedtime;
  4. Avoid frequent work schedule shifts (TV, Congress study problems, 1983).

2. Age. From birth till age two, growth results in the highest BMR, which decreases until the puberty growth spurt, and is followed by a gradual decline for the rest of the life cycle (Fig. 9–2). This is one reason why children do not feel as cold as their parents under the same weather conditions. Since the BMR decreases about two percent every 10 years after age 25, many people who maintain their previous eating habits without increasing activity gain weight.

3. Pregnancy and Lactation. Growth during the last trimester of pregnancy raises the BMR about 15 to 30 percent. The amount of energy necessary to produce milk for lactation increases the BMR as much as 40 percent.

4. Surface Area. The more surface exposed, the greater the BMR. Because of greater surface area, a tall, thin person would require more energy than a short, heavy one of similar weight.

5. State of Health. Certain illnesses and diseases may increase or decrease the BMR. Individuals recovering from a wasting illness require extra energy to build new tissue. Additionally, the activity level may be influenced by such conditions as lack of sleep or exhaustion, tenseness, fatigue, or depression.

6. Types of Body Tissue. In adulthood, the lean body mass (LBM) is the best single predictor of the BMR (Cunningham, 1980). Because cells in muscles and glands are more active than those in bone and fat, body build influences the BMR.

While muscle tone is an important factor in metabolism, the state of tension or relaxation has an effect, too. Athletes, who have better muscle tone than sedentary people, require more calories than the nonathletic person of similar size and shape. Therefore, more food may be eaten by athletes without weight gain.

Clinical Implication:

- During environmentally high temperatures, obese persons (with their extra layers of insulation) should be careful to avoid heat stroke, even though others around them are not suffering similar conditions.

---

7. Sex. Sex hormones indirectly influence BMR. Girls generally use less energy than boys (Spady, 1980). As adults, the amount of lean body tissue versus fat tissue is a distinguishing factor—normally, women have more fat tissue and use fewer kilocalories.

8. The Endocrine Glands: Chemical Messengers. Often the thyroid gland is blamed as the cause of obesity, but these cases occur only rarely. Thyroxine, the hormone containing iodine from the thyroid gland, has a greater influence on the rate of internal processes than the secretions from any other gland.

The BMR almost doubles in hyperthyroidism, or Graves' disease, in which too much thyroxine is secreted. The BMR may also be too slow (30 to 50 percent of normal) when too little thyroxine is secreted, as in hypothyroidism, which may result in myxedema or even cretinism (see Chapter 30).

Adrenal glands affect metabolism to a lesser degree. Stimulations by fright, excitement, or even joy can cause a temporary rise in the BMR by releasing catecholamines, particularly epinephrine. The pituitary gland accounts for about 15 to 20 percent increase in the BMR during growth for children and adolescents.

Clinical Implication:

- Increased thyroxine activity can cause vitamin deficiencies because the quantity of many of the different enzymes is increased; vitamins are essential parts of some of these enzymes or coenzymes. Without supplementation, thiamin and vitamins B_{12} and C may become deficient. Porous bones may result from greater losses of calcium and phosphorus caused by increased thryoxine activity (Guyton, 1986).

---

9. Temperature

Climate. For those who live in colder climates, the BMR will be slightly higher in order to maintain normal body temperature. However, even in Antarctica, the BMR fluctuates seasonally, peaking in the autumn and spring and decreasing during the dark winter months (Campbell, 1982).

Body Temperature. For each 1°F rise above body temperature, the BMR increases 7 percent.

Clinical Implications:

- Because of accelerated BMR, a fever will increase energy requirements as much as 100 to 125 kcal/day for each 1°F above normal body temperature for an average-sized person. Drinking cool liquids not only helps lower the internal temperature but also helps prevent dehydration.
- Shivering is the body's way of asking for more energy or heat. Extra clothing or a warmer room environment can be useful, or a warm snack at any time, particularly before bedtime, can be helpful.

---

10. Fasting and Starvation. Persons who are undernourished or fasting for long periods of time have a lower than normal BMR. This is a result of decreased muscle mass as well as an adaptative body process to conserve energy.

Energy Measurement

Carbohydrates, fat, protein, and even alcohol are chemical sources of energy for humans. (Vitamins and minerals are not energy sources but catalysts for energy-producing reactions.)

POTENTIAL ENERGY

The amount of energy, or kilocalories, available in a food may be precisely calculated by placing a weighed amount of food inside a bomb calorimeter (Fig. 9–3). As it is burned, the increase in water temperature indicates the heat given off or the potential (free) energy of that food.

PHYSIOLOGICAL FUEL VALUE

Not all the free energy is available to the body. Certain small amounts of energy are used in digestion so that it is necessary to reduce the values obtained in the bomb calorimeter to those that are physiologically available, which is also called the coefficient of digestibility.

The physiological fuel values commonly used are: 4 kcal per gram of carbohydrate, 9 kcal per gram of fat, 4 kcal per gram of protein, and 7 kcal per gram of alcohol.

DETERMINATION OF ENERGY REQUIREMENTS

The energy required by the body is expressed in units of kilocalories (see Chapter 2).

Basal Metabolic Rate. There are several methods of determining the BMR. Since the exact BMR is still difficult to determine, one general guideline recommends using 1 kcal/kg body weight per hour for men and 0.95 kcal/kg body weight per hour for women (2.2 kg=1 lb.), as shown in *Focus on the Calculation of the Basal Metabolism Rate.*

The BMRs of healthy men usually range about 1600 to 1800 kcal (6500 to 7500 kJ) daily and 1200 to 1450 kcal (5000 to 6000 kJ) for women.

Basal Energy Expenditure. Another method that may be used for determining the basal energy expenditure (BEE) is a formula devised by Harris and Benedict.

$$\text{BEE for a female} = 65.096 + 9.563 \text{ (wt. in kg)} + 1.85 \text{ (ht. in cm)} - 4.676 \text{ (age in years)}$$

$$\text{BEE for a male} = 66.473 + 13.752 \text{ (wt. in kg)} + 5.003 \text{ (ht. in cm)} - 6.755 \text{ (age in years)}$$

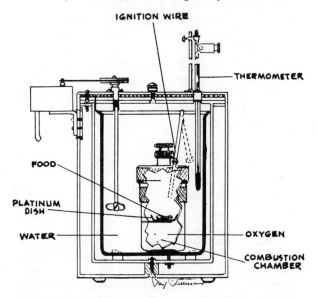

Figure 9-3. Bomb calorimeter. (From Nizel AE: Nutrition in Preventive Dentistry Science and Practice, 2nd ed. Philadelphia, W. B. Saunders Co, 1981, by permission.)

FOCUS ON *Calculation of the Basal Metabolism Rate*

1 kcal/kg of body weight × 24 hrs = basal metabolism rate for males (kcal)

or

0.95 kcal/kg of body weight × 24 hrs = basal metabolism rate for females (kcal)

A man weighing 185 lbs. has 84 kg body weight (185 lbs. ÷ 2.2 kg):

1 kcal × 84 kg × 24 hrs = 2016 kcal

A woman weighing 120 lbs. has 54.5 or 55 kg of body weight:

0.95 kcal × 55 kg × 24 hrs = 1254 kcal

The Harris-Benedict equation predicts the BEE in healthy, nourished individuals but is unreliable in the malnourished patient (Roza & Shizgal, 1984). Nomograms also have been devised to measure the BMR. Nomograms are graphic methods that include more variables. For example, height and weight might be included instead of weight alone, as in the BMR and BEE.

Other Energy Requirements

Voluntary Work and Play. The most variable factor affecting total energy needs is muscle activity, which is influenced by the activity level. Body size affects the amount of kilocalories required to do any one activity. The intensity of the work or play also affects the amount of energy used.

The tired feeling after a period of mental work usually is due to tension rather than use of stored energy. Mental activity uses almost no extra energy (about 50 to 80 kcal/hr). Half of a glass of skimmed milk or an apple furnishes the amount of energy required for an hour of mental activity. The best criterion to evaluate energy expenditures is based on body weight, the amount of time involved, and the degree of strenuousness of the activity.

FOCUS ON *Calculation of Total Energy Needs*

Determine ideal body weight (IBW) = 55 kg (see Appendix)

Basal metabolism needs = 0.95 kcal/kg IBW/hr (Female)

Basal metabolism needs:
Female, 165 cm tall, 55 kg IBW

$$0.95 \text{ kcal} \times 55 \text{ kg} \times 24 \text{ hrs} = 1254 \text{ kcal}$$

Minus sleep: (Subtract 0.1 kcal/kg of IBW/hours of sleep)

$$0.1 \text{ kcal} \times$$
$$55 \text{ kg} \times 8 \text{ hours of sleep} = \quad \begin{array}{r} 1254 \text{ kcal} \\ - \ 44 \text{ kcal} \\ \hline 1210 \text{ kcal} \end{array}$$

SDA = 10% (Basal + activity allowance − sleep allowance)

Cost of activities above the BMR expenditures:

Sedentary	30%	
Light	50%	(Sitting, walking, standing)
Moderate	75%	(Standing, walking)
Very active	100%	(Strenuous or heavy work, constantly active)

Total kilocalorie requirements for a female with light activities would be:

1254 (basal) − 44 (sleep) + 625 (light activity) = 1835 kcal
SDA (10% × 1835 = 183.5 or
      184.) = +184

Total requirements   2019 kcal daily

Although the thermogenic effects of a training period may persist after the exercise session, the absolute increase in calories expended after physical exertion is small. However, those who begin an exercise program often report increased vigor and physical exertion in other aspects of their daily routines resulting in more energy expenditures (Elliot & Goldberg, 1985).

Specific Dynamic Action. Food digestion, like other body functions, requires energy. The specific dynamic action (SDA) or the calorigenic (thermogenic) effect of food refers to the increased heat production resulting from the metabolism of food. While each nutrient when eaten separately has its own specific effect, the SDA of a mixed diet is estimated to be about 10 percent of the energy required for basal metabolism and activity combined.

Total Energy Requirements. To figure the total energy expenditures, (1) calculate the basal metabolism, (2) add the energy costs of the voluntary and involuntary activities, then (3) add the 10 percent for the SDA. An example is shown in *Focus on the Calculation of Total Energy Needs*.

The latest live-in calorie counter, a 10′ × 12′ room calorimeter, is being developed by USDA (Fig. 9–4). Computers record the amount of energy supplied by foods and how an individual makes use of the energy. Heat sensors in the unit's walls measure how many calories are expended by an individual while living in the chamber for periods up to six days (Goins, 1986).

SPECIAL CONDITIONS

Estimating the energy needs of a hospitalized patient is a time-consuming and inexact process; many larger institutions have purchased portable metabolic carts specifically for this function. The metabolic cart (Fig. 9–5) is an indirect calorimeter using a computer programmed to calculate the exact needs of a patient. The patient inhales air from the room through one valve and exhales into the computer through the second valve. By measuring the amount of oxygen consumed and the amount of carbon dioxide exhaled, the number of calories utilized daily is determined.

This new device is especially effective for patients with severe burns or trauma that cause hypermetabolism (elevated metabolic rate). If calories are underestimated, the body must utilize stored energy (fat and protein), making the individual more susceptible to infection. If too many calories are given, the body has to work harder to convert excess calories to fat.

Energy Balance

The proper energy balance for a stable weight is maintained when the caloric intake from food equals the amount of energy in the form of heat needed for body processes and physical activities (Fig. 9–6). When more calories are consumed than the body needs, the excess is stored as fat, resulting in weight gain. A negative energy balance will result in weight loss.

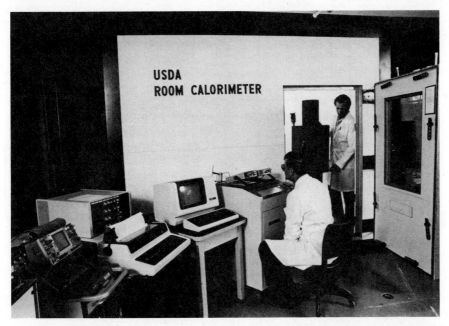

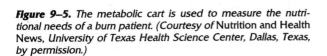

Figure 9–4. *One of six in the world, USDA's room calorimeter, when complete, will measure heat given off (calories used) by human subjects. In testing the calorimeter, one researcher steps inside while another reviews the computer output. (Courtesy of USDA's* Food News for Consumers, *3(2):5 summer 1986.)*

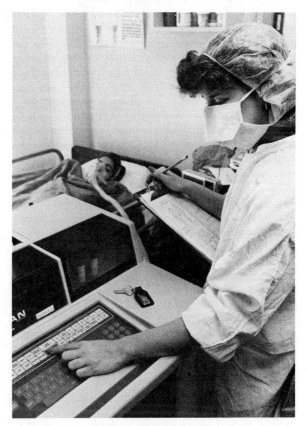

Figure 9–5. *The metabolic cart is used to measure the nutritional needs of a burn patient. (Courtesy of* Nutrition and Health News, *University of Texas Health Science Center, Dallas, Texas, by permission.)*

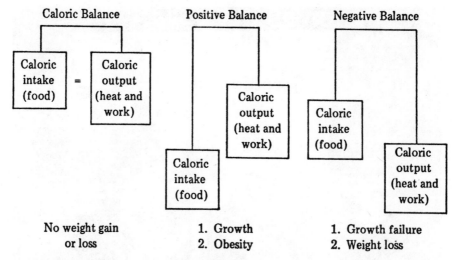

Figure 9—6. Caloric balance. (From Lewis C: Nutrition and Diet Therapy: Girth Control. *Philadelphia, F. A. Davis, 1976, by permission.)*

One pound of body fat is equivalent to 3500 kcal. To gain one pound of fat, a person must consume 3500 kcal more than s/he uses; a positive energy balance is desirable during periods of growth. To lose one pound of body weight, energy intake must be 3500 kcal less than the number of calories used.

Many healthy adults are able to control energy intake to balance energy output with little effort; their appetite controls food intake to balance energy expenditure. However, how the appetite controls the intake is poorly understood.

On the other hand, overweight people have a very difficult time losing extra pounds and maintaining their energy balance to keep off unwanted pounds. Weight control can be approached by one of two methods: The number of calories consumed can be decreased, or physical activities can be increased. Generally, a combination of both is most effective (see Chapter 24).

Energy Needs of the Physically Challenged

Extra energy costs result from various deformities of the joints of the trunk and lower extremities. Since more energy is required, hemiplegics or amputees decrease walking speed to a point at which the energy demands are tolerable. Their movement at 1 to 2 miles/hr requires almost the same amount of energy as normal subjects walking at 3 miles/hr.

Energy costs vary with the efficiency of the prosthetic design and weight as well as with the age of the amputee. Wheelchair ambulation by amputees requires no more energy than normal walking at the same speed. For the paraplegic using crutches, the expenditure is two to four times greater than that of a normal person walking at the same speed and increases rapidly with small increases in speed (Shils, 1980).

Clinical Implication:

- One of the major problems for the physically challenged is excessive body weight. Three ways to combat this problem include:
  1. Encourage mobility by increasing familiar activities and offering suggestions to initiate appropriate new activities.
  2. Explain the various kilocalorie levels of different foods and kilocalories utilized so the client understands precisely how weight is controlled.
  3. Plan meals and snacks together for optimum nutrients within the kilocalorie limit for weight maintenance.

Athletic Competition

Athletic competition places unusual and unique demands upon the body for energy. Various activities have particular requirements. The most potentially exhausting events are marathons and triathalons.

An ideal training diet should maintain energy balance and provide 10 to 15 percent of energy as protein, 30 percent as fat and 55 to 60 percent as carbohydrate (Brotherhood, 1984). This protein allowance provides 1.5 to 2.0 gm/kg/day for a 70 kg person. If weight loss is desired, fat should be reduced instead of carbohydrates or proteins.

PROTEIN

Slightly higher protein needs are more important for the athlete than the sedentary person, but these are easily met. Most athletes consume more protein than they need. A modest 10 percent protein intake for a 3000 kcal diet offers a 70 kg man 1.1 gm of protein/kg of body weight. During the early stages of training, an increased intake of protein (1.2 gm/kg body weight per day) is recommended to support an increased synthesis of muscle mass. However, this is usually automatically met with increased energy intake.

Weight lifters, body builders, and those involved in intensive strength training need a minimum protein intake of 2.0 gm/kg body weight daily. More than that amount is available with the diets consumed, so this 10 percent of total kilocalories is sufficient; no protein supplementation is required (Kris-Etherton, 1985).

Protein is especially useful in providing iron and some of the B vitamins. Iron anemia frequently occurs in athletes (see Chapter 34). This is not fully understood but may be due to inadequate protein intake.

Clinical Implications:

- Excessive protein intake exceeding 2.0 gm/kg/-day has several disadvantages such as displacing carbohydrate intake, increasing undesirable animal fat if from animal sources; and increasing excess nitrogenous breakdown products that require extra water for urinary excretion imposing further water stress (Brotherhood, 1984).

- Iron intake and laboratory values should be monitored regularly for optimal energy as well as prevention of anemia.

ENERGY BALANCE

Though the athlete may be heavier than his/her "ideal" or "functional" body weight, s/he will not be considered obese. Most male and female athletes compete best if their body fat is between 8 to 10 percent and 12 to 14 percent, respectively. Normal, well-nourished men and women average 15 and 26 percent body fat, respectively (Kris-Etherton, 1985).

Extreme fluctuations in weight should be avoided. In order to qualify for some events, not only food, but water is too severely restricted. Some wrestlers, for example, gain 4 to 8 lbs. after weigh-in and before the match or even as much as 17 lbs. the morning after the match (Short & Short, 1983).

Food intakes may or may not meet the athlete's energy requirements. One of the highest reported intakes for one day is 14,000 kcal for a football player. Gymnastic and wrestling teams report the lowest intake of 400 kcal, which cannot possibly meet their optimal energy needs or basic nutritional demands (Fig. 9–7). Identification of the athletic sport and ideal body weight for the sport are necessary to determine and provide information regarding each group's special needs (Short & Short, 1983).

When more than 4000 kcal are required for athletes, the bulk of complex carbohydrates may be intolerable for some people. They may have to eat larger amounts of energy-dense foods such as sugar and fat in order to gain sufficient energy. Endurance athletes exhibit enhanced glucose tolerance and "ideal" serum lipid profiles, so these increases pose no threat to their health (Costill & Miller, 1980).

Time limitations become a factor when athletes try to consume enough energy for their events. Probably at least five hours a day are spent practicing, several hours for school, and about 12 hours for sleeping. With intense training and high rates of energy expenditure, the need for sleep increases. If the activity requires 6000 kcal or more (and if s/he is still growing), consuming enough food is indeed challenging. Basic kilocalorie costs of some athletic events are shown in Table 9–1.

Lack of calories can result in amenorrhea, or loss of menstruation, among competitive women

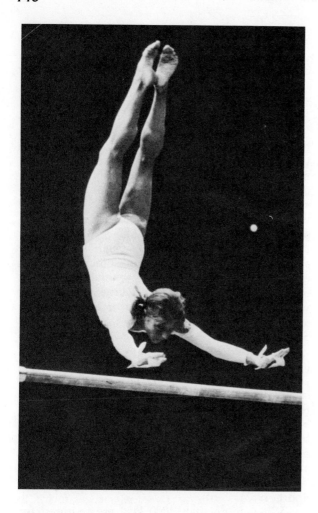

Figure 9–7. *A picture of health—the Soviet gymnast Olga Korbut in action. (Photo courtesy of SHO/Novosti.)*

athletes. This delayed puberty occurs in up to 50 percent of competitive runners and ballet dancers, 25 percent of noncompetitive joggers and 12 percent of swimmers and cyclists as opposed to the 3 to 5 percent of women in the general population (Mayer & Goldberg, 1986).

A serious side effect of amenorrhea is a lower bone density than normal with an increased inci-

Table 9–1. *Energy Needs for Athletic Events**

3000–4000 kcal		3000–5000 kcal	3000–6000 kcal	4000–6000 kcal
Discus	Hurdles	880-yd. run	Football	Cross-country running
Hammer throw	Long jump	1- & 2-mile runs	Basketball	6-mile run
Shot-put	Hop, step, jump	Swimming events	Ice hockey	Marathon running
Javelin	Pole vault	over 100 yd.	Lacrosse	Soccer
High jump	Long horse vault	Wrestling	Tennis	Cross-country skiing
Diving	Swimming events	Most gymnastic events	Gymnastic all-around	
Ski jumping	50- & 100-yd.	Downhill, slalom skiing	Fencing	
440-yd. dash	Baseball		3-mile run	
	Golf			

*From Buskirk, ER: Some nutritional considerations in the conditioning of athletes. *Annual Review of Nutrition* 1:319, 1981, with permission.

Note: Table assumes that body weight and size are similar among participants of the sport. The kilocalorie cost of the activities listed would be approximately 10% less for females.

dence of stress fractures and curvature of the spine. Ordinarily, exercise is conducive to maintaining bone density, but reduced caloric intake resulting in weight loss during puberty lowers estrogen levels, which results in reduced bone density. Therefore, amenorrhea should be a sign to increase caloric intake to avoid penalizing the lifelong integrity of the bones (Mayer & Goldberg, 1986).

OTHER NUTRIENTS

The foundation for athletic needs is an adequate diet providing the RDAs for all nutrients. Increased nutrient intake is not necessary during athletic events as long as additional kilocalories are provided for the extra demands and the proportions of nutrients maintain the desired balance (Houston, 1979). An exception, however, is that, along with increased energy requirements, there are increased requirements for thiamin (0.5 mg/1000 kcal with a minimum of 1.0 mg for any intake between 1000 and 2000 kcal), riboflavin (0.6 mg/1000 kcal), and niacin (6.6 mg/1000 kcal or not less than 13 niacin equivalents for intakes of less than 2000 kcal). This is consistent with the RDAs since the requirements for these B vitamins are based upon 1000 kcal of food intake. However, repeated studies show that young women require more riboflavin to achieve biochemical normality than the RDAs indicate. Exercise increases this requirement to at least 1.25 mg/1000 kcal (Belko et al., 1983). Without sufficient quantities of these vitamins, other food cannot be completely metabolized by the Krebs cycle for its available energy.

Vitamin A is the one nutrient reported to be low among both men and women athletes (Short & Short, 1983). More attention should be given to fruits and vegetables. This would help protect against potassium depletion, also frequently found to be low. No other exceptional changes in quantities of normal nutrients are involved with athletic performance.

Clinical Implications:

- If the individual is not gaining strength as expected, a detailed look at total food intake must be part of the overall assessment, e.g., adequate rest and mental and physical condition.
- Be aware of the signs of compulsion and obsession in athletes. These include running while ill or in pain, incidence of injuries, negative feelings when unable to run, neglect of a conscious cool-down period, low weight levels, and a tendency to increase workouts following perceived dietary indiscretions. Too much emphasis on leanness and strict weight control require nutritional counseling (Walsh, 1985).

Serum testosterone levels are significantly lower with low body fat, large loss of body fat, and large weight loss. As a result, occasionally, wrestlers have reported decreased sex drive as well as decreased strength and endurance when undergoing rigid dietary restriction for weight loss (Strauss et al., 1985).

BEVERAGES

Nutrition during athletic events has two goals: first, to maintain an adequate level of hydration and, second, to provide energy to delay the onset of fatigue.

Fluid and Electrolyte Replacement. Beverages should minimize physiological imbalances that occur during exercise and prevent injury and/or enhance performance. Water intake before exercise of moderate intensity seems to be beneficial in terms of temperature regulation and cardiovascular homeostasis (Lamb & Brodowicz, 1986). Approximately 8 to 16 oz. of cold water should be taken by the athlete 10 to 15 minutes before exercise to hyperhydrate the body.

The athlete should take 8 to 16 oz. of fluid every 10 to 15 minutes during exercise. Sufficient water replacement is the most critical factor in athletic events since as little as two to three percent of body weight loss through sweating can cause measurable impairments in circulatory and thermal regulatory function (Grandjean, 1985). Further loss can cause a decrease in strength and endurance and a reduction in aerobic work capacity (Williams, 1985). Many athletes routinely lose more than five percent of their body weight in water. When the body cannot be cooled through sweat, heat stroke and death are likely possibilities.

Thirst cannot be regarded as an indicator for water replacement. A sweat loss of one pound (2.2 kg) of body weight is equal to two cups (480 ml) of water. Fluid loss for temperature regulation during vigorous excercise can be over 2 L/hr (Elliot & Goldberg, 1985). Weighing nude before and after events to determine fluid needs is the most accurate method of adequate water replacement.

Electrolytes rarely require replacement unless the event is of long duration. Sodium and potassium are lost in very small quantities; they can be maintained or replaced easily by foods or beverages high in these electrolytes before and after events. Low concentrations of sodium increase gastric emptying and fluid absorption from the intestine (Kris-Etherton, 1985). Drinks for sports events should contain less than 10 mEq/L of sodium and less than 5 mEq/L of potassium. Commercial drinks, such as Gatorade and Quickick, contain twice this amount of sodium (Coleman, 1986). Salted water should contain no more than one level tablespoon of salt per gallon (Grandjean, 1985).

Marathon runners particularly must protect themselves from too much as well as too little fluid. Water intoxication and dilutional hyponatremia are possible in duration events with intakes of large quantities of free water. Recommendations for runners are 100 to 200 ml of water every 2 to 3 km, or 3 to 8 L of fluid during an 80-km race, and 3 to 10 L for a 100-km race. (Hyponatremia, 1986). Cold fluids empty more rapidly than warm (Brotherhood, 1984). Sodium may be replaced in these events by soups, stews, or sports drinks.

Sugar Content. Carbohydrate ingestion during most athletic events is unnecessary. However, beverages containing some carbohydrate can minimize disturbances in temperature regulation and cardiovascular function as well as water. Additionally, these beverages can maintain serum glucose during prolonged exercise, slow the depletion of muscle glycogen, and enhance athletic performance better than water (Coleman, 1986). On the other hand, a moderate amount of sugar intake before exercise may cause an insulin response with subsequent accelerated glycogen depletion and hypoglycemia.

Instead of providing quick energy, the sugar content of commercial sports beverages may actually interfere with performance. Sugar has a greater impact on gastric emptying rate than volume or temperature. Since the foremost goal is replenishment of fluids, a rapid gastric emptying rate is best for preventing dehydration. If the sugar content is too concentrated, water is drawn from the plasma into the intestinal tract, thereby compounding the problem.

Glucose polymer sports drinks are available, such as Bodyfuel 450 (Vitex Foods), Exceed (Ross), and MAX (Coca-Cola). These glucose polymer solutions have lower osmolality than solutions of glucose, fructose, or sucrose; therefore, equivalent amounts of carbohydrate do not cause the fluid imbalance that results in gastrointestinal distress. Beverages containing 5 to 10 percent glucose or sucrose, or 5 to 20 percent glucose poly-

mers can be consumed every 15 to 20 minutes with no harmful side effects (Lamb, 1986). If the beverage is palatable to the athlete, it is more likely that enough fluid will be consumed to maintain performance.

Clinical Implications:

- Children have reduced ability to endure exercise in extreme heat. Fluid intake should be closely monitored.
- Children acclimate to exercise in the heat more gradually than do adults (Grandjean, 1985).

Alcohol. Consumption of alcohol within two hours of participation in mild exercise in a cold environment results in greater heat loss and lower blood glucose levels. Moderate levels of blood alcohol can impair thermoregulation, thus alcohol ingestion prior to any activity in a cold environment is contraindicated (Graham, 1981).

CURRENT POPULAR THEORY: CARBOHYDRATE LOADING

A high-carbohydrate diet for three days preceding strenuous activity was recommended as long ago as 1940. Increased glycogen stores can affect endurance performances lasting 60 minutes or longer.

Composition of the meals before competition affects performance. After eating a normal mixed diet, a person on a cycle ergometer could continue for 85 to 145 minutes. After a fat/protein diet, they were exhausted in less than 60 minutes, but when the period of glycogen depletion was followed by a diet rich in carbohydrate, the work time was at least 180 minutes. Not only could they perform longer but they could go faster (Brotherhood, 1984). Figure 9–8 shows the ability of a carbohydrate diet compared with a protein and fat diet to replace glycogen stores after exhaustive exercise.

Astrand (1968) has been a leading advocate of carbohydrate loading. His research shows almost double the energy is available through optimum muscle glycogen stores. More than 4 gm/100 mg of muscle, or as high as 700 gm (about 2800 kcal), can be obtained by three days of low-carbohydrate intake followed by three days of high-carbohydrate intake before the event.

The classic glycogen-loading regimen produces muscle glycogen depletion by exercising nearly to exhaustion with a carbohydrate starvation phase of a low-intake (50 to 75 gm daily or 10

GLYCOGEN REPLACEMENT

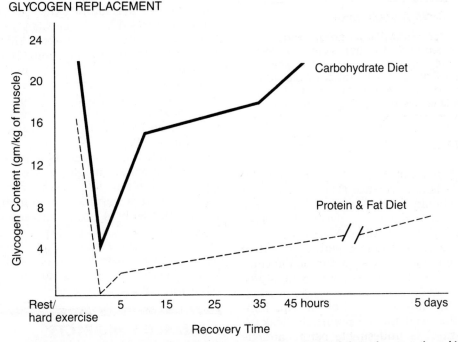

Figure 9–8. Glycogen replacement: After performing exhaustive exercise that depleted their glycogen, the subjects ate either a high-carbohydrate diet, which refilled the glycogen in two days, or a high-protein, high-fat diet, which left the glycogen stores unfilled, even after five days. (From Bergstrom, J: Hermansen L; Hultman, E; et al: Diet, muscle glycogen and physical performance. Acta Physiologica Scandinavica 71:140, 1967, by permission.)

percent of one's kilocalories), high-protein, high-fat diet for three days. The following three days consist of little or no exercise to permit muscle glycogen storage with a high carbohydrate diet (70 percent).

Side effects accompany the extra glycogen storage with this extreme regimen. Hypoglycemia and ketosis with nausea, dizziness, irritability, fatigue, a diminished exercise capacity, and the possibility of an exercise-induced injury may be expected with the low-carbohydrate diet (Kris-Etherton, 1985).

To avoid these side effects, a modified carbohydrate loading regimen is now recommended, which begins one week prior to the event. On days one to three, 300 to 350 gm of carbohydrate are eaten with tapering of exercise (90 minutes on day one, 40 minutes on days two and three). Then on days four to six, 500 to 600 gm carbohydrate are given with only 20 minutes of exercise on days four and five and rest on day six. This results in a muscle glycogen level 2.5 times above normal (Sherman et al, 1981).

Athletes participating in stop-start sports should consume 500 to 600 gm of carbohydrates per day for adequate glycogen stores (Costill et al., 1981). A carbohydrate intake of 60 percent of total calories should be the goal for the small gymnasts who must limit calories to 1200 to 1500 daily to maintain desired weight (Grandjean, 1985).

Complex carbohydrates should be chosen to achieve more glycogen storage. Simple carbohydrates such as sugar near the beginning of the event result in the opposite effect—a brief rise in energy but a dramatic drop soon after. Fatigue results from the hypoglycemia, and less muscle glycogen is available.

Glycogen storage can be an expensive handicap to the athletes who need no extra weight to perform their short-term activities. Excess storage of glycogen can be detrimental since each molecule of glycogen contains between 2 to 4 gm of water (Cahill, 1986). Sprinters and jumpers may in fact gain an advantage from reducing their carbohydrate intake moderately 24 hours prior to competition (Brotherhood, 1984).

Clinical Implication:

- Complaints of having "no energy" may be due to inadequate glycogen stores. Women especially who are on severe diet regimens may be omitting as much carbohydrate from their menus as possible and may exist for long periods of time with depleted glycogen stores.

PREGAME MEALS

The composition of the meal before a competitive event affects performance. The stomach and upper bowel should be empty to prevent gastric distress; the liver and muscle glycogen reserves should be as high as possible. Maximum workload can be maintained longer with a period of glycogen depletion followed by a diet rich in complex carbohydrates to increase glycogen stores (Brotherhood, 1984).

Probably the most hallowed of the time-honored fads is the need for the prematch steak. A high-protein meal is undesirable before athletic events because of the slow digestive process required; it should be eaten at least four hours before the event, making another small meal or snack necessary to prevent hunger. If the protein from the steak is needed for energy, it must be converted to carbohydrates. Protein conversions produce the by-product urea, a toxin that is removed from the body through urination. Exercise produces similar toxins, so the combined effect of removing these waste products is excessive and places unnecessary strain on the excretory mechanism plus increased dehydration (Parish, 1979). Fatty foods should be minimized because of their prolonged digestion times.

The American Alliance for Health, Physical Education and Recreation (1971) suggests that the pregame meal (three to four hours before competition) include: one serving of roasted or broiled meat or poultry; one serving of mashed potatoes or a baked potato or 1/2 cup of macaroni, rice, or pasta; one serving of vegetables; one cup of skim milk; one teaspoon of fat; two teaspoons of jelly or other sweets; one serving of fruit or juice; one serving of sugar cookies or plain cake. One should also take one or two cups of additional beverages and salt the food well.

LIQUID MEALS

As coaches have faced the problems of lowered performance caused by pregame nausea, muscle and leg cramps, and depleted glycogen stores, they have found that liquid meals relieve these problems. Liquid meals, e.g., Ensure (Ross), Meritene (Sandoz), and Sustacal (Mead Johnson), may be taken up to one hour before an event without harmful effects. These do not replace the fluid benefits of plain water. If any extra supplements are taken with these liquid meals to give extra protein or carbohydrate, the higher concentrations can backfire to cause cramping and diarrhea (Smith, 1976).

A serious problem exists when young hockey players participate in games too frequently; the glycogen stores in leg muscles are not replaced rapidly enough resulting in diminished performance. But with 24 hours between games plus a high carbohydrate diet (60 percent), muscle glycogen stores can be restored. In addition, liquid meals in these cases can be beneficial one to two hours before the games to minimize fatigue (Houston, 1979).

• FALLACIES and FACTS

FALLACY: *Eat spinach for extra muscular strength.*
- **FACT:** *Spinach is high in iron, which is necessary for optimal physical performance because without adequate iron the oxygen-carrying capacity of the blood is reduced. Still, many other sources such as liver and red meats are comparable in the quantity of iron and result in more absorption of the iron.*

FALLACY: *Because of excessive sweating, athletes lose zinc and should take zinc supplements.*
- **FACT:** *Zinc is a part of perspiration, but it is needed only in trace amounts that can easily come from an adequate diet that contains good sources of zinc, such as poultry and eggs.*

FALLACY: *Eat a candy bar for quick energy.*
- **FACT:** *Even though candy mainly contains carbohydrates, it still requires too much time to digest to provide an immediate energy boost (Diet myths, 1984). Glucose ingestion (40 to 80 gm/hr) prevents hypoglycemia, but hypoglycemia fails to affect endurance, and its prevention does not delay exhaustion (Felig et al., 1982). Preplanning before the event for optimum glycogen stores, repeated water intake to prevent dehydration, and a simple fruit beverage, such as orange juice, can be the most useful regimen.*

FALLACY: *Salt tablets may be taken when heavy sweating occurs.*

- **FACT:** *Although one needs to replace the sodium lost in perspiration, salt tablets are not advisable. Fluid is drawn into the gastrointestinal tract from body tissues to dilute the large amounts of salt in the stomach, which causes cramping, nausea, vomiting, and dehydration. The normal diet can replace the salt lost in sweat more satisfactorily (Kris-Etherton, 1985).*

FALLACY: *Red meat is needed to build muscle and blood and for optimum physical strength.*

- **FACT:** *The iron found in meat does contribute to normal levels of hemoglobin, and its protein helps build and restore muscle as well as all body tissues. However, other iron and protein sources can do the same. It is not necessary to eat meat for muscles any more than to drink blood to build blood. Actually, after the normal protein needs are met, carbohydrate gives more energy for physical activities than the protein of meat.*

FALLACY: *Steak dinners are the ultimate celebration after an athletic event.*

- **FACT:** *Athletic performance depletes glycogen stores demanding carbohydrate intake to replace those depleted amounts. Without carbohydrates, glycogen levels can remain exhausted as long as five days.*

FALLACY: *Since coffee contains caffeine, three or four large mugs should make an athlete alert and quick. Caffeine can improve energy supply by causing the glycogen supply to last longer.*

- **FACT:** *Several studies have demonstrated that 250 to 330 mg of caffeine (2 to 2 1/2 cups of coffee) ingested one hour before exercise stimulates the release of free fatty acids to spare glycogen, increases energy, and minimizes feelings of exertion (Costill et al, 1978; 1979). However, others do not support this theory. Carbohydrate furnishes about 90 percent of the energy initially and fat, about 10 percent. Later, most of the energy is derived from free fatty acids. For most people, one to two cups of coffee probably has no harmful effects, but some persons are more sensitive than others to caffeine. With increased coffee intake, the effects on the central nervous system and circulatory system may cause insomnia, excitement, restlessness, ringing in the ears, tachycardia, premature contractions of the heart, and quickened respiration. Often gastric irritation and muscle tension occur. Losses of important body fluids can be accentuated by diuresis (ADA, 1980).*

Summary

Human beings use fats, carbohydrates, protein, and even alcohol as fuel for the chemical, mechanical, electrical, and thermal energy necessary to maintain life. As these nutrient intakes are increased for higher energy production, thiamin, niacin, and riboflavin must also be consumed in larger amounts. Otherwise, the larger food intake cannot be metabolized for its intended purposes of extra energy and body repairs.

Adenosine triphosphate (ATP) is an instant source of cellular energy. Phosphocreatinine (PC) also provides quick energy. Follow-up energy comes from glycogen stores in muscle tissues, which can almost be doubled by a high dietary intake of complex carbohydrates.

The final assessment of achieving desired energy levels may be determined by a fully energized body for athletic or work performance and the maintenance of normal body weights.

Review Questions

1. Define the following: carbohydrate loading, circadian rhythm, and specific dynamic action.
2. Figure your total caloric needs for one day (basal metabolic rate plus estimated voluntary energy expenditures plus SDA).
3. What activities could you do to lose one pound per week?
4. Is the basal metabolic rate higher or lower in:
   a. Men or women?
   b. An athlete or a sedentary person of the same sex, weight, and age?
   c. A person 40 years old or one who is 20 years old?
   d. A woman who is not pregnant or one who is pregnant?
   e. A man six feet tall or one 5½ feet tall (if they both weigh the same amount)?

5. How many kilocalories of protein, fat, and carbohydrate are in 1 cup of fresh whole milk that contains:

8.5 gm protein, 8.5 gm fat, and 12.0 gm carbohydrate?

6. Muhammed Ali achieved a dramatic weight loss of about 18 kg (39.6 lb.) in about 60 days. A strict diet, heavy exercise, thyroid supplements, and a diuretic drug produced his large weight loss. When he was defeated in a boxing match for the heavyweight championship, some of his fans were shocked. What happened to his physical condition? (Buskirk, 1981).

Case Study: Jay G. is a 16-year-old high school athlete. He is on the football and baseball teams. He has been told by his classmates that he needs to eat a high-protein, low-carbohydrate diet. His mother is concerned about this approach to diet and contacts her best friend who is a nurse.

1. How many additional grams of protein does an athlete need each day above the recommended allowances? Is there a difference when the athlete is a body-builder?
2. For increased energy expenditures, what should be the primary source of nutrients?
3. What is the effect of a high-protein intake?
4. What is the desirable percent of body fat for a male athlete? A female athlete?
5. Which vitamins are important in the production of energy?

REFERENCE LIST

American Alliance for Health, Physical Education, and Recreation: *Nutrition for Athletes: A Handbook for Coaches.* Washington, DC, 1971.

American College Sports Medicine: Position statement on heat injuries. *Med Sci Sports* 7:7, 1975.

American Dietetic Association (ADA): Nutrition and physical fitness, an ADA statement. *J Am Diet Assoc* 76(5):437, 1980.

Astrand, PO: Diet and athletic performance. *Nutr Today* 3(2):9, 1968.

Barac-Nieto, M; Surr, GB; Dahners, HW; et al: Aerobic work capacity and endurance during nutritional repletions of severely undernourished men. *Am J Clin Nutr* 33(11):2268, 1980.

Belko, AZ; Obarzanek, E; Kalkwarf, HF; et al: Effects of exercise on riboflavin requirements of young women. *Amer J Clin Nutr* 37:509, April 1983.

Brotherhood, JR: Nutrition and sports performance. *Sports Med* 1(5):350, 1984.

Buskirk, BR: Some nutritional considerations in the conditioning of athletes. In *Annual Review of Nutrition.* Edited by WJ Darby. Palo Alto, CA, Annual Reviews Inc, 1981.

Cahill, GF: The future of carbohydrates in human nutrition. *Nutr Rev* 44(2):40, 1986.

Campbell, IT: Nutrition in adverse environments. 2. Energy balance under polar conditions. *Hum Nutr Appl Nutr* 36A(3):165, 1982.

Coleman, E: Fluid replacement drinks. *Sports Medicine Digest* 8(7):6, 1986.

Costill, DL; Dalsky, GP; Fink, WJ: Effects of caffeine ingestion on metabolism and exercise performance. *Med Sci Sports Exerc* 10:155, 1978.

Costill, DL; Fink, WJ; Lower, RW: Influence of caffeine and carbohydrate feeding on endurance performance. *Med Sci Sports Exerc* 11:6, 1979.

Costill, DL; Miller, JM: Nutrition for endurance sport: Carbohydrate and fluid balance. *Int J Sports Med* 1:2, 1980.

Costill, DL; Sherman, WM; Fink, WJ; et al: The role of dietary carbohydrates in muscle glycogen resynthesis after strenuous running. *Am J Clin Nutr* 34(9):1831, 1981.

Cunningham, JJ: A reanalysis of the factors influencing basal metabolism in normal adults. *Am J Clin Nutr* 33(11):2372, 1980.

Diet myths. *Am Fam Physician* 29(1):364, 1984.

Elliot, DL; Goldberg, L: Nutrition and exercise. *Med Clin North Am* 69(1):71, 1985.

Felig, P; Cherif, A; Minagawa, A; et al: Hypoglycemia during prolonged exercise in normal men. *N Engl J Med* 306(15):895, 1982.

Goins, I: The latest line-in calorie counter. Food News for Consumers. *USDA* 3(2):4, 1986.

Graham, T: Alcohol ingestion and man's ability to adapt to exercise in a cold environment. *Can J Appl Sport Sci* 6(1):26, 1981.

Grandjean, AC: Nutritional aspects of athletic performance. *Cereal Foods World* 30(12):848, 1985.

Guyton, AC: *Textbook of Medical Physiology,* 7th ed. Philadelphia, W.B. Saunders Co, 1986.

Houston, ME: Nutrition and ice hockey performance. *Can J Appl Sport Sci* 4(1):98, 1979.

Hyponatremia associated with ultramarathon running. *Sports Medicine Digest,* 1986.

Kris-Etherton, PM: Sports nutrition: nutrition, exercise and athletic performance. *Food Nutrition News* (National Live Stock and Meat Board) 57(3), 1985.

Lamb, DR; Brodowicz, GR: Optimal use of fluids of varying formulations to minimize exercise-induced disturbances in homeostasis. *Sports Medicine* 3(4):247, 1986.

MacLean, WC Jr; Graham, GG: The effect of level of protein intake in isoenergetic diets on energy utilization. *Am J Clin Nutr* 32(7):1381, 1979.

Mayer, J; Goldberg, J: Exercise without the fear of fragile bones. *Fort Worth Star-Telegram,* July 16–17:10AA, 1986.

Moore-Ede, MC; Czeisler, CA; Richardson, GS: Circadian timekeeping in health and disease. Part 1. Basic properties of circadian pacemakers. *N Engl J Med* 309(8):469, 1983.

Moore-Ede, MC; Czeisler, CA; Richardson, GS: Circadian timekeeping in health and disease. Part 2. Clinical implications of circadian rhythmicity. *N Engl J Med* 309(9):530, 1983.

O'Neil, FT; Hynak-Hankinson, MT; Gorman, J: Research and application of current topics in sports nutrition. *J Am Diet Assoc* 86(8):1007, 1986.

Paish, W: *Diet in Sport.* London, E P Publishing Ltd, 1979.

Roza, AM; Shizgal, HM: The Harris Benedict equation reevaluated: Resting energy requirements and the body cell mass. *Am J Clin Nutr* 40(1):168, 1984.

Sherman, WM; Costill, DL; Fink, WJ; et al: Effect of exercise-diet manipulation on muscle glycogen and its subsequent utilization during performance. *Int J Sports Med* 2:114, 1981.

WM; Costill, DL: The marathon dietary manipulation to optimize performance. *Am J Sports Med* 12(1):44, 1984.

Strauss, RH; Lanese, RLR; Malarkey, WB: Weight loss in amateur wrestlers and its effect on serum testosterone levels. *JAMA* 254:3337, 1985.

TV, Congress study problems of shift rotation. *Am J Nurs 83* (8):1121, 1983.

Wallace, RK; Benson, H: The physiology of meditation. *Sci Amer* 226(2):84, 1972.

Walsh, VR: Health beliefs and practices of runners versus nonrunners. *Nursing Research* 34:353, 1985.

Williams, MH: *Nutritional Aspects of Human Physical and Athletic Performance*, 2nd ed. Springfield, IL: Charles C Thomas, 1985.

Further Study

Beaton, GH: Energy in human nutrition. *Nutr Today* 18(5):6, 1983.

Burke, LM: Nutrition for the footballer. *Aust Fam Physician* 13(8):625, 1984.

Calloway, DH: Zanni, E: Energy requirements and energy expenditure of elderly men. *Am J Clin Nutr* 33(10):2088, 1980.

Clark, N: *The Athlete's Kitchen*. Boston, CBI Publishing Co, 1981.

Cunningham, JJ: An individualization of dietary requirements for energy in adults. *J Am Diet Assoc* (80(4):335, 1982.

Energy requirements. How much is enough? *Nutr Rev* 38(10):337, 1980.

Evans, WJ: Hughes, VA: Dietary carbohydrates and endurance exercise. *Am J Clin Nutr* 41(5):1146, 1985.

Fogoros, RN: "Runner's trots": gastrointestinal disturbances in runners. *JAMA* 243(17):1743, 1980.

Horton, ES: Effects of low energy diets on work performance. *Am J Clin Nutr* 35(5):1228, 1982.

Hursh, LM: Practical hints about feeding athletes. *Nutr Today* 14(6):18, 1979.

Keren, G; Epstein, Y: The effect of high dosage vitamin C intake on aerobic and anaerobic capacity. *J Sports Med* 20(2):145, 1980.

Saltin, B; Rowell, LB: Functional adaptations to physical activity and inactivity. *Fed Proc* 39(5):1506, 1980.

Tufto, D; Hefnawy, M: Pasta vs Gatorade. *Food Eng* 54(7):10, 1982.

Resources

Product information is available from:

Bodyfuel 450:   Vitex Foods, Inc.
1821 East 38th Place
Los Angeles, CA 90058

Exceed: Exceed/TMD
4921 Para Drive
Cincinnati, OH 45237
800/543-0281

MAX: Coca-Cola Foods
P.O. Box 2079
Houston, TX 77001
800/2-GET-MAX

The Miracle Workers: Fat-Soluble Vitamins

10

OBJECTIVES

THE STUDENT WILL BE ABLE TO:

- *Define and describe the fat-soluble vitamins.*
- *Identify deficiencies of each.*
- *Select food sources to meet the recommended daily allowances for an adult for each vitamin.*
- *Compare and contrast the functions, sources, and deficiencies of each of the fat-soluble vitamins.*

TERMS TO KNOW

Antioxidant
Biological activity
Carotene
Follicular hyperkeratosis
Hemorrhagic disease
  of the newborn
Hypervitaminosis
Hypovitaminosis
International Unit (IU)
Keratinization
Keratomalacia
Nyctalopia
Osteomalacia
Pityriasis rosea
Precursor
Prothrombin
Prothrombin index
Retinoid
Retinol
Retinol-binding protein
  (RBP)
Retrolental fibroplasia
Rickets
Tocopherol
Vitamin
Vitamin megadose
Xeroderma
Xerophthalmia
Xerosis

Vitamins, the miracle workers, are the catalysts for all reactions required to utilize proteins, fats, and carbohydrates for energy, growth, and cell maintenance. A well-chosen adequate diet contains all of these nutrients.

Vitamins are not foods but chemicals contained in food. They furnish no energy or building materials for the body. We would starve to death on vitamins alone, yet they cause the reactions that release energy from foods and participate in vital processes for health and normal body functions. Therefore, vitamins are not a magical cure for vague disorders, or, even worse, *all* disorders, as some swindlers pretend.

While no vitamin contains kilocalories, some vitamins, especially water-soluble thiamin and niacin, are essential to the production of energy through the Krebs cycle. So, they are closely associated with energy requirements. In other words, eating fats, carbohydrates, and proteins without enough of these two B vitamins means the energy could not be utilized. The opposite is also true. Megadoses of these vitamins cannot be used without an adequate supply of fats, carbohydrates, proteins, and even minerals. No single nutrient can work alone. They never work single-handedly but in partnership with each other as well as hormones, enzymes, fats, carbohydrates, and proteins. A vitamin is a general term for a number of unrelated organic substances present in foods in small amounts that are necessary for normal metabolic and physiological functions.

Most vitamins come in several forms with only one form performing one task, making them even more difficult to identify. As organic substances, they are easily destroyed by heat, oxidation, and chemical processes used in their extraction.

REQUIREMENTS

While vitamins are vital to life, they are required in minute amounts. Vitamins are similar to metal trace elements because so little is required, and they are like hormones because of their potent effects, but they must come from an outside source because they cannot be produced by the body. Each vitamin is essential even though the amount may vary from 2 to 4 mcg for vitamin B_{12} to as much as 45 to 60 mg/day of vitamin C, or a 10,000-fold difference.

Nutrition is a very young science. Several scientists who discovered specific vitamins, for example, are still alive. A reminder of the infancy of nutritional science is that previous research has been based on deficiency symptoms. Interactions among nutrients, optimal doses, toxicity doses, and many other facets still need to be studied. Nutritional information is like the tip of an iceberg with unlimited potential research, including information regarding the effects of megadoses of one vitamin on other nutrients, optimal amounts to prevent diseases, and interrelationships of drugs and nutrients.

During periods of stress (such as periods of unusually rapid growth, pregnancy, lactation, fever, accidents, disease, surgery, or burns), higher demands are made upon the body. Requirements for most of the vitamins, especially the water-soluble ones, are increased.

MEGADOSES

Large doses of vitamins are sometimes advocated with intakes of 20 to 600 times the RDAs. A vitamin megadose is at least 10 times greater than the RDA. A megavitamin is actually a misnomer because the amounts are so high that the particular vitamin functions as a drug rather than as a nutrient. A well-established principle of pharmacologic therapy is that all substances are potentially toxic if the dose is large enough.

Searching for the best possible health or attempting to cure diseases or to compensate for their poor eating habits, Americans spend over $1.5 billion annually on food supplements. Estimates suggest that 50 percent of adults in the United States use vitamin supplements regularly (Scala, 1980). Usually, physicians are not consulted. By taking advice given in health food stores to use vitamin supplements for various health problems, individuals become their own diagnosticians and may delay seeking competent medical attention.

No single class of drugs is the target of as much quackery, misunderstanding, misrepresentation, and misuse as vitamins. Many people consider vitamins safe to take in any amount, but each year, thousands of vitamin poisoning cases occur; the majority are children. Vitamins A, C, and E are most likely to be taken in excessive doses (Dubick & Rucker, 1983). Many different symptoms may result from the toxicity of vitamin megadoses.

Similarities of Fat-Soluble Vitamins

Although the four fat-soluble vitamins (A, D, E, and K) differ in function, utilization, and sources, they have several similar characteristics: (1) they are soluble in fat or fat solvents, (2) they are fairly stable to heat, as in cooking, (3) they do not contain nitrogen, (4) they are absorbed in the intestine along with fats and lipids in foods, and (5) they require bile for absorption.

Fat-soluble vitamins are different from water-soluble vitamins mainly because they are stored in the body longer. Since vitamins A and D are stored for long periods of time, minor shortages may not be identified until drastic depletion has occurred. For example, enough vitamin A can be stored in the liver to meet the basic needs for about a year or longer; less than optimal amounts may be present for some time before the shortage is obvious.

MEASUREMENTS

International Units (IU), based upon absorption rates in animal studies, have been used to measure fat-soluble vitamins A, D, and E. Still, these rates do not always represent the absorption rates of humans. Presently, conversions are being made to the weight measurements in micrograms or milligrams.

Vitamin D potency, like that of vitamin A, is expressed in International Units or in United States Pharmacopeia (USP) units, (which are equal). A similar change is under way for vitamin E with the IU expression being replaced with milligrams of alpha-tocopherol equivalents. At the present time, all of these terms may be used.

Vitamin A

Retinol is the dietary source of vitamin A from animal sources, and beta-carotene is a provitamin present in vegetables. About 1 mg (3000 IU) of vitamin A per day is required to produce a normal vitamin A serum level between 15 and 60 mg/dl (Bushnell et al, 1984).

Previously, vitamin A has been measured in International Units (IU). One IU is equivalent to the biologic activity of 0.6 mcg of pure beta-carotene or 0.3 mcg of retinol. However, the term "International Unit" is being replaced by retinol equivalents (RE) since it is more accurate. One RE equals 3.33 IU or 1 mcg retinol or 6 mcg of beta-carotene.

PHYSIOLOGICAL ROLES

Vitamin A has many roles in the body, but the main functions relate to the health and integrity of the body orifices and their linings. It is also required for normal bone growth and development.

DEFICIENCIES

Changes in the eyes are usually one of the first signs of vitamin A deficiency, but skin changes also may be present. Even mild vitamin A deficiency is directly associated with at least 16 percent of all deaths in children one to six years of age in Asia. Vitamin A deficiency interferes with the normal immune responses (Gunby, 1984).

Growth of Bones. Cessation of bone growth may result in overcrowding of the brain and central nervous system within the skull and spinal column, causing paralysis from cranial pressure and consequent brain and nerve injury. In some instances, a pinched optic nerve results in blindness.

Epithelial Cells. One of the most important functions of vitamin A is to maintain the integrity of the epithelial cells. Deterioration of epithelial tissues incurs damage to mucous membranes and loss of cilia, which constantly help keep membrane surfaces clean. As a result, surfaces of the skin and membranes lining all passages that open to the exterior of the body as well as the glands and their ducts are susceptible to disease. Early signs of vitamin A deficiency include sinus trouble, sore throat, and abscesses in the ears, mouth, or salivary glands due to infections along the deteriorated linings.

Keratinization. Later, the epithelial cell degeneration of the linings in the body results in dry and scaly skin with plugs of hornlike material. This is referred to as keratinization. Keratin is a protein that forms dry, scale-like tissue such as hair and nails. Keratomalacia is the term used for the similar condition of the eyes that begins with xerotic spots (Bitot's spots) on the conjunctiva, while the cornea becomes xerotic and insensitive (xerotic keratitis). The haze increases until finally the entire cornea becomes soft and colliquative necrosis occurs.

Xeroderma. Dryness of the skin is one of the first clinical symptoms of vitamin A deficiency. It is followed by follicular hyperkeratosis in which the skin is like goose flesh on the buttocks and arms. The next step is xeroderma in which skin becomes scaly. It can progress till the whole body is covered with scaly skin that is flaky and similar to dandruff.

Night Blindness. Although it is not an infallible sign, night blindness (nyctalopia) frequently indicates a deficiency in retinol. Visual perceptions in dim light are altered, as when automobile headlights are dimmed, which can be extremely dangerous. In the early depletion stages, administration of vitamin A can promptly relieve these symptoms. However, color blindness and other

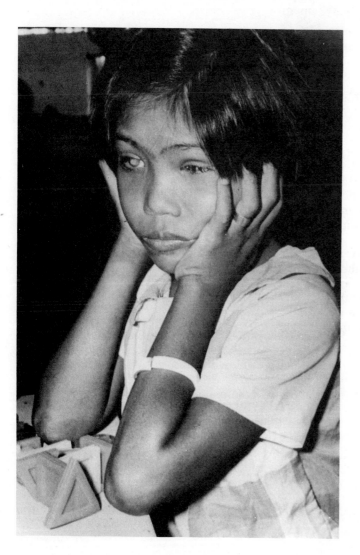

Figure 10–1. *Blindness from xerophthalmia. If this girl had been given food containing vitamin A, she need not have lost her sight. (Photo courtesy of WHO/Helen Keller International.)*

visual disorders cannot be corrected with vitamin A.

Xerophthalmia. Degeneration of epithelial cells in the eye occurs, secretion of tears ceases, lids are swollen and sticky with pus, and eyes are sensitive to light in xerophthalmia. Ulcers of the eye may occur and, without treatment, result in blindness (Fig. 10–1).

Health Application: The Role of Vitamin A

Cancer. Carotene has consistently been associated with cancer prevention because of its importance to the integrity of cells. The intake of green and yellow vegetables is believed to reduce the relative risk of cancer mortality (Colditz et al, 1985). Apparently, vitamin A stimulates the host immunity defenses (Shekelle et al, 1981; Thatcher et al, 1980).

Vitamin A has also been used beneficially topically and intralesionally for skin malignancy (Sporn & Newton, 1979).

Vitamin A has a chemopreventive role for patients with benign breast disease who are at high risk for developing breast cancer. Oral doses of 150,000 IU/day of vitamin A for three months can reduce pain and breast masses in patients with benign breast disease (Band et al, 1984).

Skin Disorders. Synthetic retinoids have been developed to inhibit carcinogen-induced neoplasia, which requires higher concentration of vitamin A. One of the synthetic retinoids, also known as isotretinoin (Accutane), has been proven effective in the treatment of severe recalcitrant cystic and conglobate acne. Usually, four months of therapy clears the disease with long-term remissions. Some major toxic side effects similar to those seen with chronic hypervitaminosis (cheilitis, xerosis, pruritus, dry mouth, conjunctivitis, epistaxis, nausea, vomiting, and bone and joint pain) have been reported, but they cease upon discontinuance of therapy (Bushnell et al, 1984). Conception is not advisable for at least one month to avoid the potent teratogenic effects and major fetal abnormalities and risk of spontaneous abortion (Bushnell et al, 1984; Hall & Goodman, 1984).

Currently, vitamin A supplementation is premature and not advisable; however, including daily food sources high in carotene and preformed vitamin A is recommended.

SOURCES

Vitamin A, as preformed retinol, is found in milk fat and butter (it is often added to skim milk and margarines), cod liver oil, and liver. It is also present as carotene or provitamin A in yellow, orange, and green leafy vegetables.

Carotene is deep red in pure form and derives its name from carrots, from which it was first isolated. Chlorophyll covers up the carotenoids in green vegetables. This does not mean that all foods with similar colors are high in this vitamin. However, most fruits and vegetables with these colors are high in carotene or vitamin A content. The deeper the color, the more vitamin A activity.

Vegetables and fruits in season—at their peak of production and lowest in price—are the most flavorful and highest in nutrient value in most cases (Johnson et al, 1985). Examples are shown in *Focus on Food Combinations That Provide the RDA of Total Vitamin A for an Adult.*

ABSORPTION AND UTILIZATION

The average American diet derives about half of its vitamin A activity from the active form with the remainder from the provitamin A or carotene. Vitamin A is better utilized by the body from animal sources, e.g., liver and beef. Absorption and utilization of vitamin A depends upon the amount of fat in the diet, the method of food preparation, and the rate and completeness of digestion. Absorption is optimal when body stores are depleted and when optimal amounts of other interrelated nutrients are present. For example, retinol-binding protein (RBP) is a carrier for vitamin A. Zinc deficiency appears to interfere with normal RBP metabolism. The presence of vitamin E and the hormone thyroxine also enhances the use of vitamin A. Thus, simply taking vitamin pills cannot ensure good health.

TOXICITY

Certainly, there are more dangers than advantages from taking megadoses of the fat-soluble vitamins. This is especially true for vitamins A and D, which are more readily stored than vitamins E and K.

An overdose of vitamin A seldom occurs from eating foods, but vitamin A intoxication is possible from an excessive intake from food sources. Pseudotumor cerebri (PTC) is a syndrome of elevated intracranial pressure characterized by headache and papilledema that results from excessive vitamin A intake. Patients eating beef liver one or two times a week have been observed with PTC (Selhorst et al, 1984). The toxic effects of hypervitaminosis A have been reported in men (as well as dogs) who ate polar bear liver, which contains 13,000 to18,000 IU/gm. Fortunately, such dietary circumstances are rare.

Hypercarotenemia is accompanied by yellow pigmentation of the skin occurring first on the palms and the soles and then the nasolabial folds. It may be distinguished from jaundice by the fact that the scleras retain their normal white color. Excessive intake of foods high in carotene, e.g., 4 lbs. of carrots per day or 1200 oranges within six weeks (Sharman, 1985), and other bizarre diets must also have a counterproductive effect upon other nutrients.

Overzealous mothers can unintentionally induce vitamin A toxicity in their children. Toxicity has been reported in infants less than one year old (Stimson, 1961). Symptoms for children three months to three years of age include severe headache, weakness, loss of appetite, itchy rash, pain in the long bones, enlargement of the liver and spleen, hypoplastic anemia, leukopenia, precocious skeletal development, clubbing of the fingers, and sparse coarse hair (Horrobin, 1971). One of the peculiarities of vitamins is that the symptoms of an overdose frequently resemble those caused by a deficiency. For vitamin A, these include:

> Anorexia, headache, blurred vision, irritability, hair loss, muscle soreness after exercise, general drying and flaking of the skin, maculoerythematous eruptions of the shoulders and back, cracking and bleeding of lips, reddened gingiva, and nosebleeds (NNC, 1978).

The symptoms frequently include painful subcutaneous swelling occurring in the areas of muscle attachments on the long bones. The liver and spleen may be perceptibly enlarged and anemia may be present.

VITAMIN A SUMMARY

Vitamin Names: Retinol, provitamin A (carotene) and anti-infective vitamin.

Daily Allowances: 1000 mcg RE* (5000 IU) for men, 800 mcg RE (4000 IU) for women, 1000 mcg RE (5000 IU) for pregnant women, 1200 mcg RE (6000 IU) for lactating women, and 400 to 700 mcg RE (2000 to 4000 IU) for children.

Important Sources: Liver; egg yolk; green, yellow, or orange vegetables and fruits; whole

*RE = retinol equivalents.

milk; whole-milk cheese; butter; cream; and fortified margarines.

Physiological Functions:
1. Production of rhodopsin (visual purple).
2. Forms and maintains the integrity of mucosal epithelium to ensure healthy functioning of eyes, skin, hair, teeth, gums, various glands, and mucous membranes.
3. Synthesizes glycoprotein.

Deficiency Symptoms: Night blindness, keratinization of epithelium, follicular hyperkeratosis, keratomalacia, faulty bone and tooth development, skin and mucous membrane infections, xerophthalmia, blindness, and death.

Contraindications:
1. Impairment of wound healing in patients receiving topical vitamin A.
2. Corticosteroids may inhibit anti-inflammatory effect.
3. Oral contraceptives cause significant amounts of vitamin A in plasma.
4. Mineral oil interferes with absorption of all fat-soluble vitamins.

Hypervitaminosis A Symptoms: Headaches, pseudotumor cerebri, irritability, miosis, anorexia, loss of hair, dry skin, pruritus, tender extremities, hepatomegaly and splenomegaly, roentgenographic evidence of elevation of the periosteum of the long bones, high serum vitamin A levels, increased serum lipids, hypoplastic anemia, leukopenia, clubbing of the fingers, and advanced skeletal development (Loebl & Spratto, 1980).

Proposed Toxicity Level: 50,000 IU/day for adults is maximum (Stimson, 1961).

Clinical Implications:

- Explain to patients that vitamin prescriptions should be followed explicitly; toxicity can result from increasing the amounts.
- Learn the signs of deficiencies of vitamins; observe patients, especially the young and the elderly, for these indications. When in doubt, consult with the physician and/or dietitian.
- Recommend storing vitamins in a cool, dark place to prevent deterioration.
- Jaundice or celiac disease or any disorder that affects fat absorption will also affect fat-soluble vitamin absorption.
- The alcoholic or alcoholic-cirrhotic patient may be deficient in vitamin A and/or zinc because both of these nutrients are affected by ethanol and by a diseased liver. Ethanol intake can cause abnormal adaptation to the dark. Therefore, abnormal adaptation to the dark or impaired taste and smell may indicate alcoholism or cirrhosis (Russell, 1980).

FOCUS ON	FOOD COMBINATIONS THAT PROVIDE THE RDA OF TOTAL VITAMIN A FOR AN ADULT

Food	IU	Food	IU	Food	IU
½ Pink grapefruit	540	Orange juice, 1 cup	270	Tomato juice, 1 cup	1,940
1 Egg	260				
Margarine, 1 Tbsp	470	Margarine, 1 Tbsp	470	Chicken, 3 oz.	200
Green beans, ½ cup	390	Carrots, 2 whole	15,860	Spinach salad, ½ cup	510
Corn, ¼ cup	145	½ Avocado	310	Apple	120
Margarine, 1 Tbsp	470	Banana	230	Margarine, 1 Tbsp	470
Skim milk, 2 cups	1,000	Skim milk, 2 cups	1,000	Skim milk, 2 cups	1,000
	3275*		18,140*		4240**

*RDA for men 51 years old is 2400 calories and 5000 IU of vitamin A. RDA for women 51 years old is 1800 calories and 4000 IU of vitamin A.

**For the three days the amount of vitamin A is an average of 8,551 IU/day. The total amount for the week can be used for vitamin A since it is stored for long periods. Notice how easy it is to meet the RDA with some facts about food sources. An extremely high source like carrots, apricots, liver, or spinach can assure the average intake is adequate. On the other hand, one tablespoon of parsley (300 mg) or the green tops of onions (240 mg) can be a helpful boost.

- Vitamin A toxicity can be masked, especially when protein-energy malnutrition (PEM) is present. Retinol-binding protein (RBP) and vitamin A excretions are reduced, which occurs when the liver is not healthy. In such cases, a high-protein (120 gm/day), high-kilocalorie, low–vitamin A (4000 IU/day) diet may be prescribed (Masked hypervitaminosis, 1982).
- The only unequivocal therapeutic use for vitamin A is for the treatment of hypovitaminosis A in night blindness and the milder conjunctival changes. Corneal damage must be treated as an emergency; a dose causing a rapid increase in the level of vitamin A in the blood plasma may be necessary.
- Prescriptions should never be shared with friends, especially high-dose vitamin A analogues for acne.
- A poor vitamin A status is one of the features associated with a higher prevalence of prematurity and intrauterine growth retardation found in poorly nourished mothers (Shah & Rajalakshmi, 1984).
- Patients with primary biliary cirrhosis usually have a high incidence of vitamin A deficiency; however, they should not be given vitamin supplementation unless dark adaptometry or electro-oculography is abnormal. A serum albumin concentration of 35 gm/L is a level below which ocular evaluation should be considered to assess the need for vitamin A supplementation (Shepherd et al, 1984).
- While oral contraceptive agents (OCAs) may deplete some vitamins, they increase plasma vitamin A, yet lower carotene levels. Present research indicates that women using OCAs may take a multivitamin pill with the usual 5000 IU of vitamin A without harmful effects (Thorp, 1980).
- For the alcoholic, the beneficial range of vitamin A supplementation is probably narrower than for the average individual, because alcohol enhances the vitamin A present. Just as vitamin A deficiency may adversely affect the liver, an excess of vitamin A is also known to be hepatotoxic (Leo & Lieber, 1982).

Vitamin D

PHYSIOLOGICAL ROLE

Vitamin D is intricately related to calcium and phosphorus, each being required for optimal utilization of the other. The primary role of vitamin D is for the mineralization of bones and teeth and regulation of blood calcium levels.

DEFICIENCIES

A vitamin D deficiency affects the skeletal structure in both children and adults. Blood analyses showing serum calcium or phosphorus above or below normal values, the failure of bones to grow properly in length, or x-rays show-

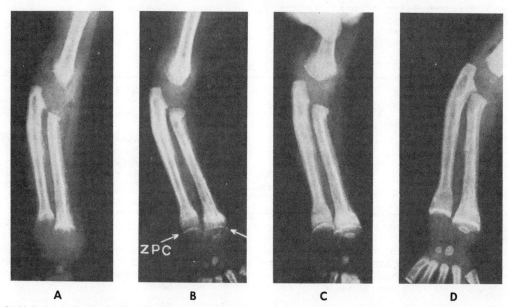

A   **B**   **C**   **D**

Figure 10–2. A) Active rickets; cupping and fraying of distal ends of radius and ulna; double contour along lateral outline of radius (periosteal osteoid). The two dense zones in the shaft of the ulna are calluses of greenstick fractures. B) Healing rickets after 12 days of treatment with vitamin D. Zones of preparatory calcification; above them in the rachitic metaphyses, there is beginning calcification. C) Healing rickets after 18 days of treatment. The zones of preparatory calcification are well defined, and the rachitic metaphyses appear well calcified. The epiphysis of the radius has become visible. D) Healing rickets after 29 days of treatment. Zones of preparatory calcification, rachitic metaphyses, and shafts have become united. (Reprinted, with permission, from Behrman RE, Vaughan VC: Nelson Textbook of Pediatrics, 13th ed. Philadelphia, W. B. Saunders Co, 1987.)

ing abnormal epiphyses of the bones indicate deficiencies (Fig. 10–2). Since vitamin D is intricately related to calcium and phosphorus functions, a change in any one of these three nutrients affects the others.

Rickets. As early as 500 B.C. deficiency symptoms now called "rickets" were observed. Later, it was called the "English disease" because of its prevalence among many children working in industry and living in crowded slums in England. The name rickets came from the word "wrikken," meaning to bend or twist.

Rickets is characterized by weak bones that become curved or misshapen from bearing the weight of the body. Rachitic deformities develop such as bowlegs or knock-knees (Fig. 10–3). When

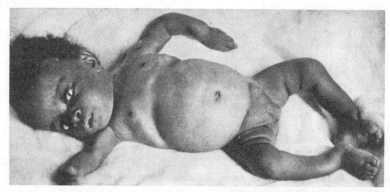

Figure 10–3. Deformities in rickets, showing curvature of the limbs, potbelly, and Harrison groove. (Reprinted with permission from Behrman RE, Vaughan VC: Nelson Textbook of Pediatrics, 13th ed. Philadelphia, W. B. Saunders Co, 1987.)

rickets develops in children, the epiphyses (growing points) of bones do not develop normally, so bones are twisted and warped. Other bone changes include a row of beadlike protuberances on each side of the narrow, distorted chest (pigeon breast) at the juncture of the ribs and costal cartilage (rachitic rosary), which predispose the person to lung diseases (Fig. 10–4). A narrow pelvis is also observed, making childbearing difficult in women.

Rickets usually occurs in children between one to three years of age, a time of extremely rapid growth with only a brief period to acquire adequate vitamin D stores. For this reason, pregnant and lactating women and infants usually receive a supplement. This vitamin can be passed from the mother to the infant before birth and in breast milk. The RDA is 400 IU/day for infants, children, and pregnant or lactating women.

Osteomalacia. Vitamin D deficiency in adults is called osteomalacia; it is also intricately related to calcium intake. Adult rickets or osteomalacia is a condition of decreased bone mineralization or softening of the bones, which may lead to deformities of the limbs, spine, thorax, and pelvis. The main symptoms are skeletal pain (as in arthritis) and muscle weakness resulting in an uneven gait or kyphosis. The condition is more prevalent in women of child-bearing age with calcium depletion due to multiple pregnancies or inadequate intake, or in women who have little exposure to the sun.

SOURCES

Vitamin D is unusual because of the body's ability to convert vitamin D precursors to their active form upon exposure to sunshine and its availability from foodstuffs.

Sunshine. The body can produce enough vitamin D (sometimes called the sunshine vitamin) from sunlight in order to prevent rickets. This is one reason that sunshine has been known as a source of health. The bright sunlight between 10 AM and 2 PM offers the most conversion. As little as 10 to 15 minutes in the sun is a significant length of time. Most subjects experience an increase in vitamin D during the summer months with a lower amount during the winter months because of less sun exposure (Savolainen et al, 1980). Even though the dietary intake of vitamin D is low in some populations, rickets does not appear in children when they are exposed to adequate amounts of sunshine, as shown in a recent study in Finland (Lamberg-Allardt et al., 1984).

Individuals who cover their bodies almost completely, e.g., nuns, business people in suits with little time outdoors, or those who live in areas with heavy smog or little sunshine, are unable to utilize sunshine as a source of vitamin D. A heavily pigmented child is also more susceptible to rickets. Osteomalacia is also commonly found in elderly persons consuming inadequate diets with little exposure to sunshine.

The two significant forms of vitamin D for

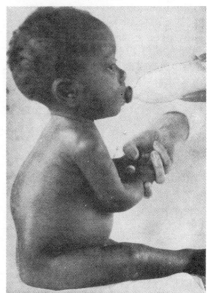

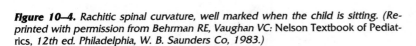

Figure 10–4. Rachitic spinal curvature, well marked when the child is sitting. (Reprinted with permission from Behrman RE, Vaughan VC: Nelson Textbook of Pediatrics, 12th ed. Philadelphia, W. B. Saunders Co, 1983.)

humans are vitamins D_2 (ergocalciferol) and D_3 (cholecalciferol). With adequate exposure to sunlight, vitamin D_3 is synthesized in the epidermis (Fig. 10–5).

Food. The fact that vitamin D is limited in foods is not of great concern since it can be produced from the ultraviolet rays of the sun reaching the skin. For this reason, many scientists think of this vitamin more as a hormone than a vitamin. It is indeed a steroid, so its actions are similar to hormones. Even though adequate quantities of this vitamin may be derived from exposure to sunlight, an additional food source is necessary in most cases.

Without fortification, the dietary intake is small and variable. It is estimated that a diet made up of the best (unfortified) food sources of vita-min D would supply only about 100 to 150 IU/day. Since the recommended intake for normal adults is 400 IU/day of vitamin D, adults usually require some fortified foods.

Foods are not legally required to be fortified, but fortification of milk is prevalent because of its popular consumption among children and because other nutrients present meet their growing skeletal needs. The contents of calcium and phosphorus in milk are beneficial in absorption and utilization of vitamin D. Other foods such as margarines, infant cereals, prepared breakfast cereals, chocolate beverage mixes and cocoa have been fortified; however, there is a danger of toxicity from excessive intakes if several foods are fortified.

Vitamin D deficiency is most frequently seen

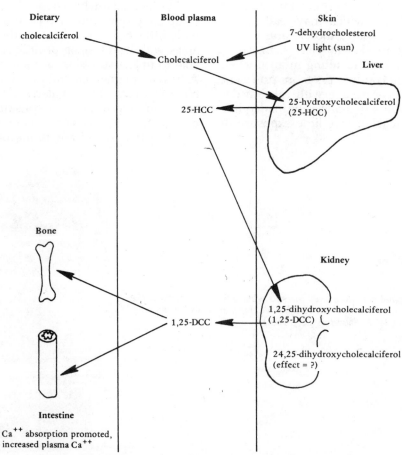

Figure 10–5. Vitamin D metabolism. (From Anderson CE: Vitamins, in Schneider HA; Anderson, CE; Coursin, DB: Nutritional Support of Medical Practice 2nd ed. Philadelphia, Harper & Row, 1983, p. 44).

in children and the elderly. Plasma vitamin D is significantly lower in older individuals than in a younger population, but it is consistently higher for men than women among the elderly (Omdahl et al, 1982). When supplementation is recommended, care must be used to prevent toxic overdoses.

As with all nutrients, optimal absorption occurs when all closely interrelated nutrients (particularly calcium) are present in sufficient quantities. Conversely, diets high in fiber can result in less absorption of vitamins D and E (Omaye et al, 1983).

PRESERVATION

Storage in cool, dark places (freezer or refrigerator) helps preserve vitamin D content. Fish liver oils are packaged in dark glass.

TOXICITY

Vitamin D can be toxic if too much is ingested. Early symptoms of calciferol poisoning are listed in a later section; detection of these symptoms and reducing dosage immediately is imperative. The high potency of this vitamin makes it important for consumers to understand the importance of taking or giving the exact prescribed dose to avoid toxicity. For example, toxicity from excessive vitamin D may arise when the mother of an infant mistakenly gives some concentrated calciferol preparation by the teaspoonful, believing that it is similar to cod-liver oil and not realizing that it may be 50 times more potent.

Caution must be exercised when feeding infants. An infant on an evaporated milk formula with a vitamin supplement can easily ingest two to four times the RDA of vitamin D; 800 to 1600 IU vitamin D is added to most commercial milk and infant formulas. In the United States, milk is commonly fortified with 5000 IU/qt. and margarine with 15,000 IU/lb. However, since fortification is optional (only 93 percent is fortified), it cannot be taken for granted. By totaling the daily intake from the nutrition labels, parents can determine the amount of vitamin D the child (or adult) is receiving. This information plus the amount of exposure to sunlight must be considered before giving vitamin D supplements.

VITAMIN D SUMMARY

Vitamin Names: Calciferol, vitamin D_2 (ergocalciferol), vitamin D_3 (cholecalciferol), antirachitic factor.

Daily Allowances: 5 to 10 mcg (200 to 400 IU) of cholecalciferol for adults (less with age), 10 to 12.5 mcg (400 to 500 IU) for pregnant and lactating women (depending on age), and 10 mcg (400 IU) for children.

Important Sources: Fortified or irradiated milk (main source), fish oils, liver, butter, and egg yolks. Synthesized in skin by activity of ultraviolet light.

Physiological Functions: Absorption of calcium and phosphorus.

Deficiency Symptoms:
1. In children, rickets—soft and fragile bones, enlarged joints, bowed legs, and deformities of the chest, spine, and pelvis.
2. In infants, tetany.
3. In adults, osteomalacia (soft bones).

Contraindications:
1. Cholestyramine—absorption of calcitrol from intestine.
2. Digitalis—chance of cardiac arrhythmias due to hypercalcemia.
3. Magnesium-containing antacids—chance of hypermagnesemia.
4. Thiazide diuretics—hypoparathyroidism and hypercalcemia.

Hypervitaminosis D Symptoms: Early symptoms include loss of appetite, nausea, vomiting, diarrhea, bloody stools, polyuria, muscular weakness, lassitude, and headaches. More serious symptoms are anorexia, renal failure, and metastatic calcification.

Proposed Toxicity Levels: Excessive doses (150,000 to 300,000 IU/day) over prolonged periods of time may lead to hypervitaminosis D, which may result in a mobilization of calcium from bone tissue, which in turn, leads to osteoporosis and pathological calcification of the soft tissues such as the kidney (Loebl & Spratto, 1980).

Clinical Implications:

- Conditions that may lead to vitamin D deficiency include any abnormalities that interfere with intestinal absorption (e.g., diarrhea, steatorrhea, celiac disease, and biliary obstruction) or possible degenerative changes in activity of the parathyroid or thyroid glands.

- Some infants and children have unusually low tolerances for vitamin D.
- Vitamin D supplements should be given only in prescribed dosage since the amount for each patient is highly individualized.
- Patients on prolonged, high-dosage vitamin D therapy should have regular tests, such as the Sulkowitch test for urinary excretion of calcium (Loebl & Spratto, 1980).
- One should observe the urine for cloudiness and a red color, which indicate toxicity, when massive doses of vitamin D are used (Loebl & Spratto, 1980).
- Lead absorption decreases vitamin D concentrations in children, so that the possibility of increased lead absorption should be considered in children with reduced serum vitamin D concentrations (Rosen et al, 1980).
- Vitamin D–deficient rickets has been reported in the United States among blacks, especially Black Muslims because of total dietary restrictions of animal-derived products, including milk and eggs (Vitamin D, 1980).
- Anticonvulsant drugs, such as phenytoin and phenobarbital, stimulate the inactivation of vitamin D, directly affecting skeletal and intestinal mineral metabolism to cause osteomalacia (Livingston & Bone, 1983).
- Mortality rates from colon cancer in the United States are the highest in populations exposed to the least amount of natural sunlight. Research indicates that the differences in vitamin D production and calcium absorption have an influence upon this condition (Garland et al, 1985).
- In case of a vitamin D overdose, one should immediately discontinue calcitriol therapy, start a low-calcium diet, and withdraw all calcium supplements. In an acute, accidental overdose, induction of emesis or gastric lavage is beneficial if the overdose is discovered within a short time. Administration of mineral oil may increase fecal excretion.
- An overdose of vitamin D is potentially lethal. Early signs of toxicity include hypercalcemia, fall in serum alkaline phosphatase, nausea, vomiting, metallic taste, dry mouth, weakness, headache, and muscle or bone pain.
- Vitamin D_3 must be metabolically altered first in the liver and then in the kidney to function. Because it is formed in the kidney and activates serum calcium and phosphate concentrations, it is sometimes considered a hormone (DeLuca, 1975). When chronic renal failure occurs, bone disease (such as osteomalacia) in adults or rickets in children frequently results.
- Persons who have no exposure to sunlight need a diet that is closely monitored for sufficient vitamin D and/or supplementation to maintain adequate stores of vitamin D (Newton et al, 1985).
- There is more danger of individuals obtaining too much vitamin D rather than too little. Supplementation should be carefully and cautiously selected with consideration for exposure to sunlight and food (Holmes & Kummerow, 1983).

Vitamin E

DISCOVERY

As late as 1922, Dr. Herbert Evans, a scientist, and Dr. Katherine Bishop, a physician, discovered vitamin E (isolated from lettuce and wheat germ) was necessary for successful reproduction in rats.

This vitamin activity was named tocopherol from the Greek *tokos*, childbirth, and *pherein*, to bear, plus the chemical suffix *-ol*, signifying an alcohol. Actually, there are many tocopherols, which are collectively called vitamin E. The biological activity of the tocopherols varies; the alpha structure is the most potent.

FALSE HOPES

In 1922, vitamin E was known as the "antisterility factor." Although closely related to fertility and successful ovulation and fertilization in rats, it is useless in the treatment of sterility in humans. Vitamin E does not prevent habitual abortions or cure toxemias in human pregnancies. It is a misnomer to call vitamin E the "reproduction vitamin" since all vitamins are necessary for reproduction.

Even though few of the exalted claims about this vitamin are true, many health hustlers are making a fortune from them. To date, however, it has not been proven that vitamin E can improve sexual potency, eliminate heart disease, prevent baldness, improve athletic performance, prevent muscular dystrophy, or increase longevity. Yet, it is highly efficient in preventing cell membrane damage from naturally occurring peroxides or substances that have been suggested as playing a role in the aging process. Due to the complexity of the aging process, vitamin E is not the sole answer.

PHYSIOLOGICAL ROLE: ANTIOXIDANT

Vitamin E protects vitamin A and unsaturated fatty acids because it can accept oxygen, therefore acting as an antioxidant. Thus, it protects the integrity of normal cell membranes and assists in prevention of hemolysis of red blood cells.

Tocopherols are the main natural antioxidants that prevent fats and oils from becoming rancid. The action is similar to that of many preservatives used by the food industry to prevent fats from becoming rancid. This partially explains why an increased intake of the polyunsaturated fats increases the demand for more vitamin E intake.

EFFECT OF POLYUNSATURATED FATS

Enthusiasm for discoveries can lead to mismanagement of a new concept. When the suggestion was made to modify the diet from highly saturated fats to more polyunsaturated fats (PUFAs), it was discovered excessive intakes of PUFAs destroyed vitamin E. Consequently, higher intakes of linoleic acid or other PUFAs increase the requirement for vitamin E. Most of the polyunsaturated oils also contain vitamin E, but when stores are low or when chemical processes have destroyed vitamin E, the requirement increases more than for similar amounts of saturated fats in the diet. Table 10–1 shows the amounts of vitamin E and linoleic acid in some foods. Ideally, both of these nutrients would be available in similar amounts.

INTERRELATIONSHIPS OF VITAMIN E

There are many interrelationships between nutrients. For optimum utilization of available vitamin E from food intake, adequate amounts of vitamins A and C as well as selenium must be present (McKay, 1985). Vitamin E and selenium function together in a complex system that protects cells from the detrimental effects of oxygen radicals. Evidently, selenium has a sparing action on vitamin E but cannot replace it.

PRESERVATION

Vitamin E is fat-soluble, stable to heat, but readily destroyed by oxidation and ultraviolet light. Normal cooking temperatures are not destructive, but some is lost in freezing and processing. (This is unusual; most nutrients are preserved by freezing.) Frying results in vitamin E losses.

Table 10–1. Food Sources of Vitamin E

	Vitamin E (mg)	Unsaturated Fat (gm)	Linoleic Acid (gm)
Vegetable oil (1 Tbsp.)			
Corn	11.3	12.2	7.2
Safflower	5.2	12.5	9.8
Soybean	12.5	11.6	7.1
Nuts (¼ cup)			
Almonds, dry-roasted	8.3	16.5	3.8
Peanuts, roasted	6.7	13.5	5.2
Pecans	5.9	18.0	3.8
Sunflower seeds	12.3	15.1	10.8
Walnuts	5.9	15.5	12.8

Data from: *The Food Processor* (computer software), ESHA Research Corporation, P.O. Box 13028, Salem, OR 97309; Agricultural Research Services: *Nutritive Value of American Foods in Common Units*, Agriculture Handbook No. 456, U.S. Department of Agriculture, 1975; and Consumer and Food Economics Institute, Agricultural Research Services: *Nutritive Values of Foods*, Home and Garden Bulletin No. 72, U.S. Department of Agriculture, 1970.

Health Application: The Role of Vitamin E

Retrolental fibroplasia (RLF). RLF occurs in about 11 percent of all preterm infants weighing less than 1500 gm. A quarter of these become blind; however, oxygen toxicity and RLF sequelae may be suppressed or eliminated by early nontoxic prophylactic therapy with vitamin E (Diplock, 1982).

DEFICIENCIES

Since vitamin E is widely distributed in foods, dietary deficiencies seldom occur if a well-balanced, varied diet is consumed. Still, some premature infants born with inadequate reserves develop an anemia that requires treatment with iron, folic acid, and tocopherol.

TOXICITY

Lack of research on excessive amounts of vitamin E prevents prediction of toxic levels; however, sound reasons exist to question the prevailing concept that large amounts of vitamin E (more than 50 times the RDA) can be safely ingested over prolonged periods of time without medical monitoring. It is prudent to recommend that the level of daily intake of vitamin E for therapeutic purposes not exceed 150 mg, or 10 times the RDA (Witting, 1972). Again, interrelationships become important as the unbalanced ratio between vitamins E and K may lead to impaired blood coagulation (Loebl & Spratto, 1980). The best recommendation at this time is to use polyunsaturated oils that are high in vitamin E along with a well-balanced diet without further supplementation.

Vitamin E *may* have a role in preventing a large number of degenerative disorders, although present evidence does not support this view. Surely no other vitamin has such a rapt audience awaiting new research releases.

VITAMIN E SUMMARY

Vitamin Names: Tocopherol; alpha-, beta-, and gamma-tocopherol; antisterility vitamin.

Daily Allowances: 10 mg for men, 8 mg for 11- to 14-year-old boys, 8 mg for women and girls age 11 and older, 10 mg for pregnant women, 11 mg for lactating women, 3 to 4 mg for infants, and 5 to 7 mg for children one to ten years old.

Important Sources: Vegetable oils, whole grains, wheat germ, leafy vegetables, egg yolk, and legumes.

Physiological Functions: Intracellular antioxidant, protects fat in the body's tissue from abnormal breakdown, stability of biological membranes, hemopoiesis, and reproduction (in animals).

Deficiency Symptoms: RBC hemolysis, creatinuria, ceroid deposits in muscle, and abnormal fat deposits. Deficiency is unlikely. In premature infants, anemia may occur, which requires iron, folic acid, and tocopherol. Sterility in male rats and resorption of fetus in female rats as well as muscular dystrophies have been observed in animals but not in humans.

Contraindications: Vitamin E decreases the response to iron therapy.

Hypervitaminosis E: Large doses over prolonged periods may cause skeletal muscle weakness, disturbances of reproductive functions, and gastrointestinal upset (Loebl & Spratto, 1980).

Proposed Toxicity Levels: Potencies of products differ widely, so dosage should be based on International Units.

Clinical Implications:

- The incidence and severity of retrolental fibroplasia (to which low birth weight (LBW) infants are prone) are significantly reduced when daily doses of vitamin E are given (Hittner et al, 1981).
- Plasma vitamin E concentration in a newborn infant is about one third of an adult's, and that of an LBW infant is even lower. Plasma vitamin E concentration rises more rapidly in breast-fed infants than in those fed cows' milk (NRC, 1980).
- Since chronic fat malabsorption reduces the absorption of fat-soluble vitamins, vitamin E particularly should be administered early to provide the most benefit (Harding et al, 1985).

Vitamin K

DISCOVERY

In 1934, Henrik Dam in Copenhagen discovered a severe hemorrhagic disease in newly hatched chickens on a ration adequate in all known vitamins and dietary essentials. By giving hog liver fat or alfalfa, normal clotting time was restored. Dam named the antihemorrhage factor vitamin K from the Danish, *koagulation*. In 1939, vitamin K was isolated, and a few months later, it was synthesized.

FORMS

At least three forms of vitamin K have been identified, all belonging to a group of chemical compounds known as quinones. The naturally occurring vitamins are K_1 (phylloquinone), which occurs in green plants, and K_2 (menaquinone), which is formed by *Escherichia coli* bacteria in the large intestine. Water-soluble forms of K_1 and K_2 are available for use by individuals unable to absorb the fat-soluble form. The fat-soluble synthetic compound menadione (K_3) is two to three times as potent as the natural vitamin.

PHYSIOLOGICAL ROLE

The main function of vitamin K is the coagulation of blood. Several steps in the blood-clotting process depend upon vitamin K. However, the identification in 1974 of a vitamin K–dependent protein in bone suggests a more complex role (National Dairy Council, 1982).

DEFICIENCIES

Primary vitamin K deficiency is uncommon, but disease or drug therapy may cause deficiencies. Even though limited amounts of vitamin K are stored in the body, a shortage of vitamin K is unlikely since it is derived from both food and the microflora of the gut. Green, leafy vegetables are high in vitamin K, fruits and cereals are low, and meats and dairy products are intermediate in concentration.

A deficiency may occur in the following situations: (1) immediately after birth because bacteria are not present in the gastrointestinal tract, (2) when the absorption of fatty substances is abnormal, (3) after sterilization of the bowel by antibiotics, (4) when drugs have been used to prevent blood clotting, and (5) severe liver disease.

Malabsorption. Any condition of the biliary tract affecting the flow of bile prevents the proper absorption of vitamin K. Since vitamin K is a fat-soluble material, bile is necessary for its absorption. Bleeding tendencies would be increased by obstruction of the bile ducts, jaundice, or gallbladder disease.

In the past, severe bleeding during or after an operation for obstruction of the bile duct was a complication of great concern to surgeons. Today, it is recognized that this danger can be circumvented by an injection of vitamin K before the operation.

Vitamin K deficiency is common in celiac disease and sprue (which affect the absorbing mucosa of the small intestine), or other diarrheal diseases (such as ulcerative colitis), which cause rapid loss of intestinal contents (Intestinal microflora, 1980). Intravenous administration of vitamin K may be indicated.

Anticoagulant Therapy. Dicumarol is an anticoagulant often used to treat coronary thrombosis. With a molecular structure similar to that of vitamin K, it acts as an antimetabolite or antagonist to vitamin K in the enzymatic process. Dicumarol fits into vitamin K's spot in the enzyme-substrate complex, thereby preventing normal blood clotting. This discovery opened a new area in the treatment of arterial or venous thrombosis using heparin or dicumarol for anticoagulant therapy. Anticoagulant therapy carries the risk of hemorrhage, but even this has been applied to beneficial products such as warfarin, which exterminates rats by bleeding them to death.

Newborn Infants. Newborn infants may develop hemorrhagic disease due to vitamin K deficiency because (1) the gut is sterile during the first few days after birth, and (2) food sources must contain adequate amounts to increase the newborn's supply (Olson, 1984). In about one of every 800 infants born (between the second and fifth days of life) bleeding occurs in the skin, nervous system, peritoneal cavity, or alimentary tract (melena neonatorum). Premature infants, anoxic infants, and infants of mothers taking anticoagulants are most susceptible to development of hemorrhagic disease of the newborn because of poor placental transfer of vitamin K, failure to establish vitamin K–producing intestinal flora, or trauma at birth. The concentrations of prothrombin and other clotting factors are low for approximately one week after birth, and newborn infants are often given a single dose of vitamin K intramuscularly immediately after birth to prevent hemorrhage (AAP, 1971).

Breast milk and commercial infant formulas normally contain vitamin K in sufficient quantity to prevent deficiency.

PROTHROMBIN INDEX

In vitamin K deficiency, blood clotting time is prolonged. The amount of prothrombin in the blood can be roughly gauged by measuring plasma clotting time under standard conditions, which is called the prothrombin index or prothrombin time.

VITAMIN K SUMMARY

Vitamin Names: K = menadione, K_1 = phylloquinone (food sources), K_2 = menaquinone, (synthesized in intestinal tract), K_3 = synthetic menadione (water-soluble and requires no bile salts for absorption). Also called the coagulation factor and antihemorrhagic vitamin.

Daily Allowances: Not established—oral dose of 1 to 2 mg considered adequate for healthy persons.

Important Food Sources: Lettuce, spinach, kale, cauliflower, cabbage, egg yolk, soybean oil, and liver.

Physiological Functions: Production of pro-thrombin, a compound required for normal clotting of blood.

Deficiency Symptoms: Hypoprothrombinemia and prolonged blood clotting times, hemorrhagic disease of the newborn, and hemorrhages. Deficiency rarely occurs.

Contraindications: Vitamin K should not be taken either alone or in a general vitamin preparation if the patient is on anticoagulant therapy. Deficiencies in intestinal malabsorption (e.g., sprue, celiac disease, or colitis) are other contraindications. Sulfa drugs with antibiotics interfere with absorption.

Hypervitaminosis K Symptoms: Kernicterus.

Proposed Toxicity Levels: Vitamin K_1 administered orally is much less toxic in large amounts than the water-soluble derivatives of a menadione (Owen, 1971).

Clinical Implications:

- Dosage of vitamin K_3 (menadione) for infants is critical since an overdose may cause irreversible brain damage (Loebl & Spratto, 1980).
- Intravenous administration of vitamin K may cause severe or even fatal reactions including transient flushing of the face, sweating, a sense of constriction of the chest, and weakness. Cramps, weak and rapid pulse, convulsive movements, chills and fever, hypotension, cyanosis, or hemoglobinuria has been occasionally reported. Shock or even cardiac and respiratory failure has also been observed.
- Injectable or colloidal solutions should be stored in a cool (5 to 15°C or 41 to 59°F) dark place. They should not be frozen.
- Since light destroys vitamin K, protect intravenous feedings from exposure to light and complete the feeding within two to three hours, not faster than 10 ml/minute (Loebl & Spratto, 1980).
- Prolonged use of antibiotics may adversely affect the normal bacterial flora of the intestine so that vitamin K deficiency occurs.
- Patients receiving coumarin drugs to maintain vitamin K–dependent coagulation factors at tolerable levels for atherosclerotic heart disease may develop even lower levels resulting in serious hemorrhaging problems if high intakes of vitamin E are taken simultaneously (Vitamin K, 1982).
- Vitamin K deficiency frequently occurs in patients with Crohn's disease, ulcerative colitis, or certain chronic forms of gastrointestinal disorders treated with sulfasalazines or antibiotics. Plasma vitamin E also is reduced in patients

with vitamin K deficiency. Vitamin K treatment is recommended (Krasinski et al, 1985).
- Excessive amounts of vitamin A and/or vitamin E have an antagonizing effect on vitamin K and may result in a deficiency of vitamin K (Olson, 1984).

• FALLACIES and FACTS

FALLACY: *Vitamin pills containing 10 times the RDA are a better buy.*
- **FACT:** *Only the recommended daily allowances (RDAs) should be used unless special conditions exist that require prescribed modifications. No vitamins should be routinely taken without carefully scrutinizing the dose and food intake.*

FALLACY: *Better to be safe than sorry. Everyone should take vitamin pills!*
- **FACT:** *Healthy individuals do not need vitamin supplements if they eat a well-balanced diet from the basic food groups.*

FALLACY: *Expensive vitamins provide superior nutrients resulting in better health.*
- **FACT:** *Higher prices of vitamin pills are related to the advertising and sales promotion budgets. The cost of the chemicals in the vitamin pills is minimal. Price has nothing to do with nutrient value. At all times, the goal of the wise customer is to buy the amount and type of pill desired, which can be established by reading the label, not by seeing the television commercial.*

FALLACY: *Only "natural" vitamins should be taken.*
- **FACT:** *Vitamins are chemical substances naturally occurring in foods, but the same chemical compound may be formed synthetically to perform in exactly the same way as the natural food source vitamin. The chemical structures have been identified and are identical. One advantage to a synthetic vitamin is that it is usually more compact and smaller in size. In some cases, the natural form of a vitamin is less potent (folic acid) or more susceptible to degradation (vitamin E). The forms of niacin and vitamin B_6 in supplements and additives are more efficiently utilized than the forms found in whole-grain cereals.*

FALLACY: *A tired feeling without as much energy as desired implicates the need for vitamin supplementation.*

• **FACT:** *There are many nutrients that produce energy. In fact, almost all known nutrients have at least an indirect, if not a direct, influence on how much pep a person has. Even those that are identified as direct energy producers, such as iron, B vitamins (especially thiamin and niacin), and carbohydrates, cannot be used by the body without many other nutrients. A strange phenomenon can occur with megadoses. Excessive intakes of many vitamins can result in symptoms similar to deficiency states, which means that fatigue can be caused by a self-medicated overdose. The wisest advice for fatigue is to be sure that a well-balanced diet is eaten leisurely without stress, outdoor exercise is a regular practice, and rest is adequate. If fatigue continues, laboratory assessments should be ordered.*

FALLACY: *"My favorite movie star claims this particular vitamin supplement is the reason for his good health."*

• **FACT:** *This may or may not be true. Just because someone you like and admire promotes a product does not make it true. Anecdotal accounts are what an individual believes. Only valid tests among large enough populations can be used as conclusive evidence.*

FALLACY: *Vitamin Q is required for normal blood clotting.*

• **FACT:** *Dr. Armand Quick found a substance in soybeans which he named after himself. This aids coagulation, but no scientific investigation has proven it essential or required from a source outside the body (Briggs & Calloway, 1984).*

Summary

Vitamins function primarily in enzyme systems that facilitate the metabolism of amino acids, fats, and carbohydrates. All of the nutrients—fats, carbohydrates, proteins, minerals, and vitamins—are interdependent, which means they must have enough of each of these other nutrients present in the body at the same time in order to function properly. They are intricately interrelated, and overdosing of any one nutrient is just as harmful as being deficient in any one.

It is important that no one be misled into believing that vitamins are cure-alls. Only persons with pathological conditions under continuous medical supervision are candidates for supplementary intakes in excess of the RDAs. Megadoses (more than 10 times the RDA) may be considered drugs instead of vitamins and may have harmful effects.

The fat-soluble vitamins are unique because they are stored in the body for long periods of time. However, this increases the chances of toxicity particularly from overdoses of vitamins A and D.

Main functions of these vitamins include: (1) vitamin A for the maintenance of the integrity of orifices and their linings, (2) vitamin D for strength of bones and teeth, (3) vitamin E as an antioxidant to protect cells; and 4) vitamin K for blood clotting. Each vitamin has its own specificity to and interrelationship with each other. All are enhanced by the ideal amount of the other nutrients.

Review Questions

1. Which fat-soluble vitamins are the most toxic? What are the symptoms of toxicity? What treatment is recommended for each?
2. Why is food fortified with vitamin D?
3. What would be adequate food intake for one day to meet the RDA for vitamin A?
4. Janie is excited about vitamin E. She wants to be sure her intake is generous, so she bought a vitamin E supplement. When she discovers that you are studying nutrition, she starts to brag about her plan. How would you respond?
5. Keep a record of your food intake for one day. Use the table of nutrient values of foods in the Appendix for the amounts of vitamin A. Was your diet adequate? What are some food choices you could make for improvement?

Case Study: Mr. A.C. comes to the local health clinic complaining of headaches, nausea, and constipation for the past six weeks. As the nurse gathers assessment data, she learns that Mr. A.C. sustained a tibial fracture 12 months prior to this visit. Following the fracture, the patient attempted to enhance the healing process by increasing his intake of vitamin D and calcium. Lab data reveal a serum calcium of 12.8 mg/dl. Further questioning also reveals polydipsia and polyuria for the past three weeks.

1. What is the normal range for serum calcium?
2. What is the RDA for vitamin D?
3. What foods are good sources of vitamin D?
4. What are the sequelae of an elevated serum calcium?
5. What nursing diagnoses might be derived from the assessment data?
6. What would be the effect of administering phosphate?

REFERENCE LIST

American Academy of Pediatrics (AAP) Committee on Nutrition: Vitamin K supplementation for infants receiving milk substitute infant formulas and for those with fat malabsorption. *Pediatrics* 48(3):483, 1971.

Band, PR; Deschamps, M; Falardeau, M; et al: Treatment of benign breast disease with vitamin A. *Prev Med* 12(9):549, 1984.

Briggs, GM; Calloway, DH: *Nutrition and Physical Fitness*, 11th ed. New York, Holt, Rinehart & Winston, 1984.

Bushnell, DE; Billstein, S; Schwartz, RA; et al: The retinoids in acne. *Am Fam Physician* 30(3):221, 1984.

Colditz, GA; Branch, LG; Lipnick, RJ; et al: Increased green and yellow vegetable intake and lowered cancer deaths in an elderly population. *Am J Clin Nutr* 41(1):32, 1985.

DeLuca, F: The kidney as an endocrine organ involved in the function of vitamin D. *Am J Med* 58(1):39, 1975.

Diplock, AT: Vitamin E, selenium and free radicals. *Med Biol* 62(2):78, 1982.

Dubick, MA; Rucker, RB: Dietary supplements and health aids—a critical evaluation. Part 1—vitamins and minerals. *J Nutr Ed* 15(2):47, 1983.

Garland, C; Shekelle, RB; Barrett-Connor, E; et al: Dietary vitamin D and calcium and risk of colorectal cancer. *Lancet* 1(February 2):307, 1985.

Gunby, P: 'Mild' vitamin A deficiency now major world problem? *JAMA* 252(22):3086, 1980.

Hall, JG; Goodman, DS: Vitamin A teratogenicity. *N Engl J Med* 311(12):797, 1984.

Harding, AE; Matthews, S; Jones, S; et al: Spinocerebellar degeneration associated with a selective defect of vitamin E absorption. *N Engl J Med* 313(1):32, 1985.

Hittner, HM; Godio, LB; Rudolph, AJ; et al: Retrolental fibroplasia: Efficacy of vitamin E in a double-blind clinical study of preterm infants. *N Engl J Med* 305(23):1365, 1981.

Holmes, RP; Kummerow, FA: The relationship of adequate and excessive intake of Vitamin D to health and disease. *J Am Coll Nutr* 2(2):173, 1983.

Horrobin, DF: *Biochemistry, Endocrinology ,and Nutrition*. New York, GP Putnam's Sons, 1971.

Intestinal microflora, injury and vitamin K deficiency. *Nutr Rev* 38(10):341, 1980.

Johnson, CD; Eitenmiller, RR; Lillard, DA; et al: Vitamin A activity of selected fruits. *J Am Diet Assoc* 85(12):1627, 1985.

Krasinski, SD; Russell, RM; Furie, BC; et al: The prevalence of vitamin K deficiency in chronic gastrointestinal disorders. *Am J Clin Nutr* 41(3):639, 1985.

Lamberg-Allardt, C; Ojaniemi, R; Ahola, M; et al: The vitamin D intake of children and adolescents in Finland. *Hum Nutr Appl Nutr* 38A(5):377, 1984.

Leo, MA; Lieber, CS: Hepatic vitamin A depletion in alcoholic liver injury. *N Engl J Med* 307(10):597, 1982.

Livingston, S; Bone, HG: Long-term anticonvulsant therapy and vitamin D metabolism. *JAMA* 249(7):939, 1983.

Loebl, S; Spratto, G: *The Nurse's Drug Handbook*, 2nd ed. New York, Wiley Medical Publications, 1980.

Masked hypervitaminosis A and liver injury. *Nutr Rev* 40(10):303, 1982.

McCay, PB: Vitamin E: Interactions with free radicals and ascorbate. *Ann Rev Nutr* 5:323, 1985.

Miller, BF; Keane, CB: *Encyclopedia and Dictionary of Medicine, Nursing, and Allied Health*, 3rd ed. Philadelphia, W.B. Saunders Co, 1983.

National Dairy Council: Fat soluble vitamins. *Dairy Council Digest* 53(3), 1982.

National Nutrition Consortium, Inc.: *Vitamin-mineral safety, Toxicity and Misuse*. Chicago, IL, American Dietetic Association, 1978.

National Research Council (NRC): *Recommended Dietary Allowances*. Washington, DC, National Academy of Sciences, 1980.

Newton, HMV; Sheltawy, M; Hay, AWM; et al: The relations between vitamin D_2 and D_3 in the diet and plasma 25–OH D_2 and 25–OH D_3 in elderly women in Great Britain. *Am J Clin Nutr* 41(4):760, 1985.

Olson, RE: The function and metabolism of vitamin K. *Ann Rev Nutr* 4:281, 1984.

Omaye, ST; Chow, FI; Betschart, AA: In vitro interactions between dietary fiber and C–vitamin D and C–vitamin E. *J Food Sci* 48(1):260, 1983.

Omdahl, JL; Garry, PF; Hansaker, LA; et al: Nutritional status in a healthy elderly population. *Am J Clin Nutr* 36(6):1225, 1982.

Owen, CA Jr: Vitamin K group. *Pharmacol Toxicol* XI:492, 1971.

Rosen, JF; Chesney, RW; Hamstra, A; et al: Reduction in 1,15-dihydroxyvitamin D in children with increased lead absorption. *N Engl J Med* 302(20):1128, 1980.

Russell, RM: Vitamin A and zinc metabolism in alcoholism. *Am J Clin Nutr* 33(12):2741, 1980.

Salonen, JT; Salonen, R; Lappetelainen, R; et al: Risk of cancer in relation to serum concentrations of selenium and vitamins A and E: Matched case-control analysis of prospective data. *Br Med J* 290(February 9):417, 1985.

Savolainen, K; Maenpaa, PH; Alhava, EM; et al: A seasonal difference in serum 25–hydroxyvitamin D_3 in a Finnish population. *Med Biol* 58(February):49, 1980.

Scala, J: Are food supplements necessary? *Nutr Today* 15(5):25, 1980.

Selhorst, JB; Waybright, EA; Jennings, S; et al: Liver lovers' headaches: Pseudotumor cerebri and vitamin A intoxication. *JAMA* 252(24):3365, 1984.

Shah, RS; Rajalakshmi, R: Vitamin A status of the newborn in relation to gestational age, body weight, and maternal nutritional status. *Am J Clin Nutr* 40(4):794, 1984.

Sharman, IM: Hypercarotenaemia. *Br Med J* 290(January 12):95, 1985.

Shekelle, RB; Liu, S; Raynor, WJ Jr; et al: Dietary vitamin A and risk of cancer in the Western Electric Study. *Lancet* 2(November 28):1185, 1981.

Shepherd, AN; Bedford, GJ; Hill, A; et al: Primary biliary cirrhosis, dark adaptometry, electrooculography, and vitamin A state. *Br Med J* 289(December 1):1484, 1984.

Sporn, MB; Newton, DL: Chemoprevention of cancer with retinoids. *Fed Proc* 38(11):2528, 1979.

Stimson, WH: Vitamin A intoxication in adults: Report of a case with a summary of the literature. *N Engl J Med* 265(8):369, 1961.

Thatcher, N; Blackledge, G; Crowther, D: Advanced recurrent squamous cell carcinoma of the head and neck. *Cancer* 46(6):1324, 1980.

Thorp, VJ: Effect of oral contraceptive agents on vitamin and mineral requirements. *J Am Diet Assoc* 76(6):581, 1980.

Vitamin D deficiency rickets, revisited. *Nutr Rev* 38(3):116, 1980.

Vitamin K, vitamin E, and the coumarin drugs. *Nutr Rev* 40(6):180, 1982.

Witting, LA: Recommended dietary allowance for vitamin E. *Am J Clin Nutr* 25(3):257, 1972.

Further Study

Almquist, HJ: The early history of vitamin K. *Am J Clin Nutr* 28(6):656, 1975.

Bowerman, SJA; Harrill, I: Nutrient consumption of individuals taking or not taking nutrient supplements. *J Am Diet Assoc* 83(3):298, 1983.

Breskin, MW; Trahms, CM; Worthington-Roberts, B; et al: Supplement use: Vitamin intakes and biochemical indexes in 40 to 108 month-old children. *J Am Diet Assoc* 85(1):49, 1985.

Cirrhosis, abnormal dark adaptation, and vitamin A. *Nutr Rev* 37(3):73, 1979.

Gonzalez, ER: Vitamin E relieves most cystic breast disease; may alter lipids, hormones. *Med News* 244(September 5):1077, 1980.

Haddad, E; Blankenship, JW; Register, UD: Short term effect of a low fat diet on plasma retinol and alpha-tocopherol and red cell alpha-tocopherol levels in hyperlipidemic men. *Am J Clin Nutr* 41(3):599, 1985.

Herbert, V: The vitamin craze. *Arch Intern Med* 140(2):173, 1980.

International Vitamin A Consultive Group: *Guidelines for the Eradication of Vitamin A Deficiency and Xerophthalmia.* New York, Nutrition Foundation, Inc, 1977.

Livingston, S; Bone, HG III: Long-term anticonvulsant therapy and vitamin D metabolism. *JAMA* 249(7):939, 1983.

McCollum EV: Dean of nutrition science. *Nutr Rev* 37(3):65, 1979.

McCollum EV: *From Kansas Farm Boy to Scientist.* Lawrence, KS, University of Kansas Press, 1964.

Metabolism of vitamin D in lead poisoning. *Nutr Rev* 39(10):372, 1981.

Mobarhan, S; Russell, RM; Underwood, BA; et al: Evaluation of the relative dose response test for vitamin A nutriture in cirrhotics. *Am J Clin Nutr* 34(10):2264, 1981.

Moss, BK: Using vitamin and mineral supplements. *Patient Care* 18(16):81, 1984.

Ott, DB; Lachance, PA: Retinoic acid—a review. *Am J Clin Nutr* 32(11):2522, 1979.

Smith, R: Rickets and osteomalacia. *Hum Nutr Clin Nutr* 36C(2):115, 1982.

Sutker, LR; Dirskell, JA: Vitamin E status of adolescent girls. *Research* 83(6):678, 1983.

The vitamin pushers. *Consumer Reports* 51(3):170, 1986.

White, JM: Vitamin A-induced anaemia. *Lancet* 2(August 25):573, 1984.

Why vitamin fortification? *Food Eng* 57(2):96, 1985.

Witting, LA; Lee, L: Dietary levels of vitamin E and polyunsaturated fatty acids and plasma vitamin E. *Am J Clin Nutr* 28(6):571, 1975.

More Miracle Workers: Water-Soluble Vitamins

11

THE STUDENT WILL BE ABLE TO:

- *Compare the characteristics of water-soluble vitamins with those of fat-soluble vitamins.*
- *Discuss the pros and cons of vitamin supplementation.*
- *Identify deficiency signs for each vitamin.*
- *Differentiate between scientific facts versus food fads concerning vitamins.*
- *Select foods to meet the daily RDAs for vitamin C and thiamin.*
- *Discuss the role and sources of vitamin B_{12} for vegetarians.*

TERMS TO KNOW

Antagonist
Antivitamin
Ariboflavinosis
Avitaminosis
Beriberi
Cheilosis
Extrinsic factor
Flavin adenine
   dinucleotide (FAD)
Flavin mononucleotide
   (FMN)
Flavoprotein
Inositol
Intrinsic factor
Lipoic acid
Megavitamins
Niacin equivalent
Para-aminobenzoic acid
   (PABA)
Pellagra
Polyneuritis
Scurvy

The Mystery of Discovery

Nutrition is a fascinating subject with all the intrigue and challenge found in mysteries. It is as unlimited in scope as the best science fiction. Have you ever wondered how scientists discovered facts about nutrition?

In southern Europe, particularly Italy and Spain, epidemics were recorded in the 1800s. Thousands of people had rough, red skin with open sores on their hands, neck, and face. They also had bright red tongues, infected eyes, peculiar reflexes, difficulty in walking, swollen or emaciated legs, and paranoid disorders. For many, the eventual outcome was death.

There was no limit to the holistic team member approach at that time. Many questions were asked by everyone. Is this condition contagious? Do health care workers develop these same symptoms while caring for these patients? Should these people be isolated to prevent harmful exposure to others? Is the water pure to drink? Is the air contaminated? Could there be a toxin in the food? Is the disease transmitted or caused by insects?

In spite of the efforts of many persons, this condition was not understood until Joseph Goldberger, a public health physician in the United States, stumbled upon the first clue in 1927. While working in an orphanage among children with these symptoms, he noted a few healthy children. Upon investigation, they were discovered to be sneaking down to the kitchen to steal extra servings of bread, milk, and leftover food.

Goldberger called this nutritive factor the pellagra-preventing (P-P) factor. Finally, the main vitamin responsible for pellagra (niacin) was discovered by Conrad Elvehjem, a scientist at the University of Wisconsin, in 1937 (McCollum, 1957).

Many years later, this group of vitamins was called the vitamin B complex. Not until 1948 was the last B vitamin, B_{12} or cobalamin, discovered.

Characteristics of Water-Soluble Vitamins

Water-soluble vitamins have their own unique set of characteristics. Each of the B vitamins contain nitrogen, which is lacking in vitamin C and the fat-soluble vitamins. As vital coenzymes, B vitamins are required for normal growth, nerve and brain function, reproduction, and almost every cellular reaction in the body.

Since they are not stored in the body for more than a few days, frequent or daily consumption is imperative. Procedures to retain the vitamins during cooking and handling are given in Chapter 14.

INFLUENTIAL FACTORS

Even though the RDAs list the amounts of vitamins for various ages and both sexes, many factors modify an individual's requirements. One of the first components is the previous intake of a vitamin. For example, a person taking twice the RDA for vitamin C requires an adjustment period when levels are decreased.

Other factors that influence individual requirements include smoking, alcohol, caffeine, drugs, and stress. Periods of unusually rapid growth, pregnancy or lactation, fever, and recovering from accidents, disease, surgery or burns are all considered stressful. Diet composition also affects some nutrient levels, e.g., a protein-rich diet or a diet high in carbohydrates or energy.

DEFICIENCIES

Frequently, blood serum levels of water-soluble vitamins are low without apparent clinical symptoms. Rarely will only one of the B vitamins be deficient; at least two or three are usually significantly low as well as protein. Research in one large hospital revealed the daily intake for thiamin, riboflavin, pyridoxine, and ascorbic acid was lower than the RDAs (Lemoine et al, 1980). In conjunction with the increased requirement necessary for healing, these vitamins should be given special attention.

Clinical Implication:

- Oral contraceptives apparently increase the need for folate, ascorbic acid, riboflavin, and pyridoxine (Massey and Davison, 1979). Nutritional assessment is advised.

Thiamin

DISCOVERY

In 1890, Eijkman, a Dutch physician, and Grijns noticed a type of polyneuritis in chickens fed leftovers from a prison hospital kitchen in Java where patients had beriberi. Changing from polished to whole-grain brown rice reversed these symptoms. When this substance was chemically identified in 1937, it was called thiamin (from *thio*, sulfur-containing and *amine*, nitrogen, but later the *e* was dropped).

PHYSIOLOGICAL ROLES

Thiamin functions in the metabolism of carbohydrates, fats and proteins. However, the main effects of thiamin deficiency are disturbances of carbohydrate metabolism, which is impossible without thiamin. Thiamin triggers the various steps in the Krebs cycle to release energy. It is also crucial for normal functioning of the brain, nerves, muscles, and heart.

REQUIREMENT

Since thiamin is a coenzyme in the Krebs cycle, the requirement is based upon the number of kilocalories eaten. Those engaged in rigorous physical activity burn more energy, so more thiamin is required. Focus on Daily Intakes of Thiamin gives examples of how to meet the RDA. Information about all the water-soluble vitamins is summarized in Table 11–1.

DEFICIENCIES

Since thiamin is required for the metabolism of fats, proteins, and carbohydrates, a wide range of symptoms develops with insufficient intakes.

Beriberi. Individuals with beriberi cannot move easily as the condition progresses. Centuries ago the Singhalese called the condition beriberi, which means "I cannot."

Beriberi affects the nerves, gastrointestinal tract, and heart. Deep muscle pain in the calf is indicative of thiamin deficiency, which results from degeneration of myelin sheaths of nerve fibers in the central nervous system and peripheral nerves. A flex in the knee and a drop in the muscles supporting the toes and feet cause the high-

---

FOCUS ON DAILY INTAKES OF THIAMIN

RDA: Male, 51 years old, 2400 calories: 1.2 mg

Female, 51 years old, 1800 calories: 1.0 mg

½ cup Tomato juice	0.06	½ cup Orange juice	0.11	½ cup Grapefruit juice	0.05
2 slices Rye bread	0.10	½ cup Oatmeal	0.10	3 slices Wheat bread	0.27
3 oz. Pork	0.78	1 Egg	0.04	½ cup Bran flakes	0.29
2 cups Skim milk	0.20	2 slices Wheat bread	0.18	3 oz. Turkey	0.04
½ cup Peas	0.21	3½ oz. Tuna	0.04	½ cup Green beans	0.04
1 Tbsp. Sunflower seeds	0.18	½ cup Zucchini	0.04	½ cup Brown rice	0.09
2 Carrots	0.12	¼ cup Bulgur	0.10	½ cup Lima beans	0.06
		½ cup Black-eyed peas	0.25	2 cups Skim milk	0.20
		2 cups Skim milk	0.20	1 Apple	0.06
Totals*	1.65		1.06		1.10

*Thiamin can be stored in the body for about 10 days; average for these 3 days = 1.27 mg.

From U.S. Department of Agriculture: *Nutritive Value of American Foods in Common Units.* Agriculture Handbook No. 456, Agriculture Research Service, 1975.

Table 11–1. *Summary of Water-Soluble Vitamins* (Continued)*

Recommended Daily Allowances of Vitamins	Important Sources	Physiological Roles	Hypovitaminosis or Deficiency Symptoms
Thiamin (B₁) 0.5 mg/1000 kcal Males (23–50): 1.4 mg (51 +): 1.2 mg Females: 1.0 mg Pregnancy: 1.3–1.4 mg Lactation: 1.5 mg Infants: 0.3–0.5 mg Children (under 10): 0.7–1.2 mg Boys (11–22): 1.4–1.5 mg Girls (11–22): 1.1 mg	Pork, liver, chicken, fish, beef, whole grains, wheat germ, dried yeast, enriched cereal products, nuts, lentils, and potatoes.	Energy and integrity of central nervous system.	Poor appetite, constipation, fatigue, depression, apathy, neuritis in legs, cardiac failure, Wernicke-Korsakoff syndrome, and wet and dry beriberi.
Riboflavin (B₂) 0.6 mg/1000 kcal Males (11–50): 1.6–1.7 mg (51 +): 1.4 mg Females (11–22): 1.3 mg (23 +): 1.2 mg Pregnancy: +0.3 mg Lactation: +0.5 mg Infants: 0.4–0.6 mg Children (1–10): 0.8–1.4 mg.	Milk, liver, meat, fish, eggs, enriched cereal products, green leafy vegetables	Protein metabolism and healthy eyes.	Dermatitis, photophobia, glossitis, and cheilosis.
Niacin *(tryptophan is precursor; also called nicotinic acid, nicotinamide, and niacinamide)* Men and women: 14–20 niacin equivalents or 6.6 mg/1000 kcal Males (11–18): 18 mg (19–22): 19 mg (23–50): 18 mg (15 +): 16 mg Females (11–14): 15 mg (15–22): 14 mg (23 +): 13 mg Pregnancy: + 2 mg Lactation: + 5 mg Infants: 6–8 mg Children (1–10): 9–16 mg.	Liver, poultry, meat, fish, eggs, whole grains, enriched cereal products, legumes (e.g., peanuts), and mushrooms.	Energy and integrity of central nervous system.	Dermatitis, decreased energy, weakness, apathy, mental confusion, anorexia, and pellagra (dermatitis, diarrhea, depression or dementia, and death).
Pyridoxine (B₆), pyridoxal, and pyridoxamine 2 mg Males: 2.2 mg Females: 1.8–2.0 mg Pregnancy: +0.6 mg Lactation: 0.3–0.6 mg Children (1–10): 0.9–1.6 mg (11–18): 1.8–2.0 mg.	Pork, organ meats, meat, poultry, fish, corn, legumes, seeds, grains, wheat, potatoes, bananas, green leafy vegetables, and green beans.	Protein metabolism (several roles), converts tryptophan to niacin, hemoglobin synthesis, and integrity of central nervous system.	Nervous irritability, seborrhea-like skin lesions, weakness, anemias (hypochromic, microcytic, and of pregnancy), chemical dependencies, and convulsions (in infants).

*All vitamins are essential for normal growth.

stepping gait of beriberi patients. Paralysis and muscle atrophy follow.

Later, body tissues become swollen as fluid accumulates in the cells. This condition is called wet beriberi and appears first in the legs and thighs of the patient (Fig. 11–1). Emaciation, which may occur instead, is called dry beriberi.

Because the beriberi sufferer breathes with great difficulty, s/he develops an enlarged heart that beats rapidly. Death is usually caused by car-

Table 11–1. Summary of Water-Soluble Vitamins (Continued)

Recommended Daily Allowances of Vitamins	Important Sources	Physiological Roles	Hypovitaminosis or Deficiency Symptoms
Pantothenic Acid Not yet determined but probably 5–10 mg is adequate. Supplied in normal diet.	Present in all plant and animal foods. Eggs, kidney, liver, salmon and yeast are best sources.	Energy Formation of some hormones, hemoglobin, and nerve regulating substances.	Deficiency seen only with severe multiple B-complex deficits.
Biotin Not known but probably 0.03 mg.	Liver, meat, eggs, legumes, nuts, milk, most vegetables, grapefruit, tomato, watermelon, and strawberries.	Energy and synthesis of fatty acids and amino acids. (Closely related to folic acid and pantothenic acid, biotin is synthesized in intestinal tract.)	Depression and anorexia.

Folic acid, folate, folacin, and tetrahydrofolic acid
    0.4 mg
    Adults: 400 mcg
    Pregnancy: 800 mcg
    Lactation: 500 mcg
    Infants: 30–45 mcg
    Children (1–10): 100–300 mcg
    Boys and girls (11–23): 400 mcg
	Green leafy vegetables, liver, beef, fish, dry beans, lentils, whole grains, asparagus, and broccoli.	Red blood cell maturation. (Folic acid is synthesized in intestinal tract.)	Treatment for tropical sprue, pancytopenia, and various anemias (macrocytic, of pregnancy, and megaloblastic). There may be blood cell regeneration in pernicious anemia but no control of neurological problems.

PABA (part of folic acid).	Same as folic acid.	Treatment of rickettsial diseases.	Same as folic acid.

Vitamin B_{12}, cyanocobalamin, and hydroxycobalamin
    3.0 mcg
    Adults: 3 mcg
    Pregnancy: 4 mcg
    Lactation: 4 mcg
    Infants: 0.5–1.5 mcg
    Children: (1–6): 2.0–3.0 mcg
    Boys and girls (7–18): 3 mcg
	Only in animal foods: liver, meat, salt-water fish, oysters, milk, and eggs.	Red blood cell maturation and essential for normal function of all body cells.	Neurological degeneration and macrocytic or pernicious anemia.

Vitamin C or ascorbic acid
    60 mcg
    Adolescents
        (15+–Adults: 60 mg
    Pregnancy: 80 mg
    Lactation: 100 mg
    Infants: 35 mg
    Children (1–10): 45 mg
    Boys and Girls (11–14): 50 mg
	Citrus fruits, strawberries, cantaloup, tomatoes, sweet peppers, cabbage, potatoes, kale, parsley, turnip greens, and broccoli	Maintains integrity of capillaries, promotes healing of wounds and fractures, aids tooth and bone formation, increases iron absorption and protects folic acid, and helps form collagen for healthy connective tissue.	Bruise and hemorrhage easily, incomplete or slow wound healing, gingivitis (loose teeth, gums that bleed easily, and sore mouth), anemia, scurvy.

diac impairments. This condition is the only heart disease attributable to the deficiency of a single dietary constituent; it is fully preventable and usually curable.

Thiamin has a pivotal role in a wide spectrum of disorders. One of the later findings is thiamin anemia. Thiamin-responsive anemia syndrome includes anemia with diabetes mellitus and sensori-

neural deafness. This is alleviated with large doses of thiamin (Mandel et al, 1984).

Morale Vitamin. Thiamin is called the morale vitamin because, within 10 days of deficiency, persons become depressed and irritable, are unable to concentrate, lose interest in their work, and experience fatigue and loss of stamina. The brain and central nervous system, almost entirely

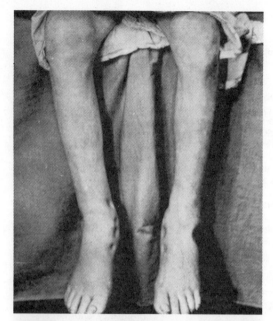

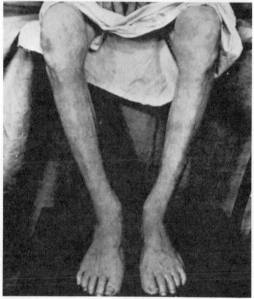

Figure 11–1. Patient before and after treatment for vitamin B_1 deficiency (so-called "wet" beriberi). A) Swelling of the legs and marked pitting edema in the ankle region. B) Ten days after initiation of thiamin therapy; during which the patient lost 40 pounds. Presumably this weight loss was due to the loss of fluid because the general nutritive state was greatly improved. (From Spies: Rehabilitation Through Better Nutrition. Philadelphia, W. B. Saunders Co, 1947, by permission.)

dependent upon glucose for energy, are seriously impaired when thiamin is not present. Although thiamin is not a cure for mental disorders, mental patients whose intake is restricted may manifest an intensification of their psychiatric symptoms.

Wernicke-Korsakoff Syndrome. In 1881, Wernicke described a neurological disorder characterized by jerky, rhythmical movements of the eyes (nystagmus), weakness of eye muscles, an unsteady, staggering gait (ataxia), disorientation, and apathy.

A few years later, Korsakoff described a psychosis, also occurring in alcoholics, characterized by a severe defect in memory and learning with confabulation usually present. Past events can be remembered with verifiable accuracy, but more recent events from earlier in the day are forgotten. The patient tends to provide a superficially convincing tale rather than saying, "I don't remember."

In 1971, it was concluded that Wernicke's disease and Korsakoff's psychosis are manifestations of the same pathological process and are attributable to thiamin deficiency. Early diagnosis is essential so that thiamin therapy is initiated early in the course of the disease and in the same large doses as for wet beriberi. Clinical features usually suggest the syndrome, but because of its rarity in many communities, it may easily be overlooked. A quick response to thiamin therapy confirms the diagnosis. The syndrome usually occurs in alcoholics, because alcoholic intake increases the thiamin requirement. However, it may arise secondary to any disorder that seriously impairs nutrition.

Clinical Implications:

- A careful dietary history, including alcohol consumption along with detailed physical assessment of the cardiovascular and neurological systems, will help clarify the early stages of thiamin deficiency.
- Although immediate clinical response to thiamin therapy is often dramatic, ultimate recovery may be incomplete and relapses may occur, especially if the precipitating factors persist. Recovery is usually extremely slow after prolonged paralysis.
- Mercurial diuretics increase urinary loss of thiamin. Mercury toxicity closely resembles symptoms of thiamin deficiency. To verify mercury contamination, thiamin levels must also be known (Farkas, 1979).
- Beriberi heart failure occurs especially in patients who continue hard physical work, maintaining a high cardiac work load; however, heart failure is rare in patients with severe peripheral neuritis with adequate bedrest.
- Oral anticoagulants may interact with B complex vitamins and cause hemorrhage.
- Raw fish contains an active enzyme, thiaminase, which destroys thiamin.
- Thiamin deficiency is often an unsuspected cause of lactic acidosis; treatment with thiamin should be promptly initiated (Campbell, 1984).

Riboflavin

DISCOVERY

As early as 1879, a yellow-green fluorescent pigment was seen in various laboratory experiments, but riboflavin was not isolated from milk until 1933, when it was shown to be an important vitamin and coenzyme.

Riboflavin was first called the "old yellow enzyme." Pigments that possess these fluorescent properties were designated as flavins. German chemists found that rats grew faster when given a dietary source of a yellow compound called "ovoflavin," which they isolated from egg (*flavus* is Latin for yellow). Later, it was found to be composed of ribitol (similar to the sugar ribose) and attached to a flavin-like compound, hence the name riboflavin.

PHYSIOLOGICAL ROLES

Riboflavin functions in the metabolism of carbohydrates, proteins, and fats to release cellular energy in coenzyme forms of flavin mononucleotide (FMN) and flavin-adenine dinucleotide (FAD). Closely related to the metabolism of protein, all conditions requiring increases in protein (e.g., burns or growth spurts) lead to additional riboflavin requirements. Riboflavin is also essential for healthy eyes, as a part of an enzyme in tissue reproduction, and in hydrogen transport.

BODY STORES

The body guards its stores of riboflavin carefully; even in severe deficiency as much as one third of the normal amount is present in the liver, kidney, and heart. Factors other than dietary intake affect riboflavin body stores. Thyroid and adrenal hormones control the enzymatic conversion of riboflavin into its active coenzyme derivatives. A mixed diet that contains a pint of milk and a portion of meat products daily assures an adequate riboflavin supply.

DEFICIENCIES

Ariboflavinosis is one of the most common deficiency diseases. Rarely does an individual seek medical advice for it, but it may accompany other deficiencies, especially those of the B vitamins. Riboflavin deficiency affects the eyes like vitamin A but in different ways. Ocular symptoms appear consistently on a low-riboflavin diet and may precede all other manifestations. Eyestrain, fatigue, itching, burning, sensitivity to light, and frontal headaches are the most frequent complaints. Cheilosis, another main symptom, results in cracks and sores around the corners of the mouth; the skin is scaly and has red sores.

While clinical ariboflavinosis may be absent, biochemical ariboflavinosis is widespread. Dietary supplementation for teenagers is frequently necessary to insure adequate riboflavin nutrition during growth and associated stress. In fact, supplementation must be above the RDA to be effective. Less animal protein and marginal riboflavin intake also contribute to ariboflavinosis (Ajayi & James, 1984).

Clinical Implications:

- The sensitivity of riboflavin to light may result in decomposition of the vitamin during phototherapy of hyperbilirubinemic infants (Rivlin, 1979).
- Hyperthyroidism, fevers, the added stress of injuries or surgery, and malabsorption syndromes are factors that increase riboflavin requirements.

Niacin

DISCOVERY

After an extensive search for over 20 years, the "pellagra-preventing factor" was identified as a B vitamin. Nicotinic acid from tobacco was isolated as a chemical compound in 1867, long before scientists discovered that it was a vitamin that prevents pellagra. In 1922, Goldberger concluded that blacktongue in dogs was similar to pellagra in humans, a disease he had cured by diet modifications (McCollum, 1957). The beneficial vitamin nicotinic acid became known as niacin, so it would not be confused with nicotine.

NIACIN EQUIVALENTS

The body obtains niacin not only directly from the diet but indirectly from the conversion of an amino acid, tryptophan, and possibly also from that synthesized by intestinal microorganisms. Allowances are now given in terms of niacin equivalents that include dietary sources of niacin plus its precursor tryptophan. Approximately 1 mg of niacin may be formed from 60 mg of tryptophan in the diet.

Tryptophan is found mainly in milk, eggs, and meats. With foods high in niacin plus those having tryptophan, it is easy to meet the dietary requirement for niacin equivalents in the United States.

PHYSIOLOGICAL ROLES

Niacin is crucial in the production of energy (ATP) in the coenzyme forms of nicotinamide-adenine dinucleotide (NAD) and nicotinamide-adenine dinucleotide phosphate (NADP). Other roles include glycolysis, fat synthesis, and tissue respiration.

DEFICIENCY

Pellagra has been referred to as "the three D's—dermatitis, diarrhea, and depression or dementia." Some add another D—death. Tissues that show damage as a result of niacin deficiency are chiefly the skin, gastrointestinal tract, and nervous tissues. The most striking and characteristic symptom of pellagra is a reddish skin rash especially on the face, hands, or feet that always appears on both sides of the body at the same time—i.e., it is bilaterally symmetrical. When exposed to sunlight, the skin becomes dark. Casal's necklace or collar extends in a fairly broad band entirely around the neck. If the band is incomplete, the lesions are striking in their symmetry. In many instances, the necklace continues down the neckline like a broad cravat.

Backs of the hands are an even more frequent site of these lesions. Here, the lesions may extend up the arm to form the glove or gauntlet of pellagra (Fig. 11–2). Pellagra means "rough skin," and the skin may look like goose flesh. When the deficiency state is advanced, the skin becomes progressively harder, drier, more cracked and covered with scales and blackish crusts due to hemorrhages.

Pellagra is usually associated with a maize (corn) diet. Much of the niacin is lost in milling or is in an unavailable form unless the food is prepared with alkali, as in corn tortillas. Corn products are relatively deficient in tryptophan.

VITAMIN MEGADOSES

The safe and recommended daily intake of niacin is 13 mg for most women and 18 mg for men.

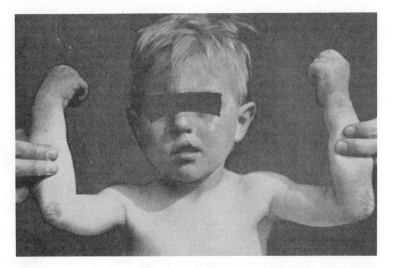

Figure 11–2. Pellagra in a three-year-old boy, showing lesions on the hands and elbows and an early lesion over the nose and malar eminences. (From Behrman, RE; Vaughan, VC: Nelson Textbook of Pediatrics, 13th ed. Philadelphia, W. B. Saunders Co, 1987, with permission.)

Niacin is one of the first vitamins used in very large doses in the regimen called orthomolecular psychiatry to treat schizophrenia. Orthomolecular pertains to the theory that certain diseases are associated with biochemical abnormalities resulting in increased needs for certain nutrients, e.g., vitamins, and can be treated by administration of large doses of these substances (Miller & Keane, 1983). Some mental disturbances seen in pellagra also resemble those found in schizophrenia, although scientific documentation cannot link the two.

Another effect of megadoses of niacin (3 to 6 gm/day) relates to its ability to lower both serum cholesterol and triglyceride. However, the benefits of long-term niacin therapy, in light of its side effects and toxicity, are questionable. Flushing and itching are common after large doses of niacin, and more toxic side effects may include nausea, hypotension, tachycardia, fainting, and hypoglycemia.

Researchers have tested the effect of niacin in dilating blood vessels to prevent a second incidence of myocardial infarction in patients with coronary heart disease. Though the incidence of a second nonfatal infarction was reduced, several kinds of arrhythmias outweighed potential benefits. The most common serious side effect caused by toxic doses of niacin is liver damage.

Clinical Implications:

- Niacin and thiamin are particularly related to a normal appetite; however, weight-conscious people should not avoid these vitamins.
- Patients should understand that flushing is a frequent side effect after a therapeutic dose of niacin. Patients who feel weak and dizzy after taking niacin should lie down until they recover and then inform their physician.
- Since riboflavin deficiency often accompanies pellagra, supplemental riboflavin should accompany niacin treatment.

Vitamin B_6

Vitamin B_6 is the term commonly used for this group of three vitamins—pyridoxine, pyridoxal, and pyridoxamine. Pyridoxal phosphate, the coenzyme form of vitamin B_6, is closely involved with the synthesis and metabolism of amino acids. Vitamin B_6 enhances the formation of niacin and improves folic acid metabolism.

Vitamin B_6 differs from other B complex vitamins. Body stores are small but repletion is gradual, which is not the case with other B vitamins (Tarr et al, 1981). This indicates the importance of maintaining an adequate intake.

PHYSIOLOGICAL ROLES

Several essential roles for vitamin B_6 have been identified: (1) as a coenzyme in protein metabolism, (2) in the conversion of tryptophan to niacin, (3) in hemoglobin synthesis, (4) in synthesizing unsaturated fatty acids from essential fatty acids, (5) in producing energy from glycogen, and

(6) in proper function of the nervous system including brain cells.

DEFICIENCY

Even though deficiency states are rare, several symptoms have been observed: sideroblastic anemia, oxalate stone formation, and central nervous system abnormalities.

A few years ago, infants developed seizures after being fed a commercial infant formula in which vitamin B$_6$ was destroyed during processing and storage (Ink & Henderson, 1984).

Breast-fed infants may have plasma B$_6$ levels as low as 1/10 of those of formula-fed infants (Ink & Henderson, 1984). More than four weeks of lactation may be required to reach adequate plasma concentrations of vitamin B$_6$. Therefore, these infants may be at risk for vitamin B$_6$ deficiency (Kirksey et al, 1981).

The mother's body stores of vitamin B$_6$ are critical to the well-being of the newborn infant (Ejderhamn & Hamfelt, 1980). Oral contraceptives taken for more than 30 months prior to pregnancy have been reported to result in low vitamin B$_6$ concentrations in maternal plasma at five months of pregnancy, at delivery, and in the milk (Roepke & Kirksey, 1979). Since women taking oral contraceptives appear to have an increased requirement, a daily intake of 2 mg of vitamin B$_6$ is recommended.

Health Application: Therapeutic Uses of Vitamin B$_6$

Even though vitamin B$_6$ has been used for a number of years by obstetricians for the control of nausea and vomiting of pregnancy, its effectiveness has not been proved in controlled studies (Sauberlich & Canham, 1980).

Vitamin B$_6$ has been used with varying degrees of success to treat premenstrual syndrome (PMS), schizophrenia, and autism (Crawford, 1984). However, the normal recommended daily intake is 2 to 4 mg; the prescription for megadoses of 2 to 6 gm/day may cause sensory neuropathy (Schaumburg et al, 1983).

Doses as high as 250 to 500 mg/day have been effective in patients who have kidney stones secondary to hyperoxaluria (Balcke et al, 1983). Several groups of physicians have prescribed pyridoxine in such doses for as long as six years for various conditions without ill effects (Mitwalli et al, 1984).

On the other hand, one patient developed typical pyridoxine-induced sensory ataxia while taking a 500 mg capsule daily for over two years. Symptoms included the sensation of electric shocks shooting down the spine upon neck flexion, progressive gait unsteadiness ascending to the hips, numbness in the hands, lips, and left cheek, absent tendon reflexes, and flexor plantar responses. The patient was unable to walk without assistance. A diagnosis of multiple sclerosis was proposed, but these symptoms improved immediately when vitamin B$_6$ supplementation stopped (Berger & Schaumburg, 1984).

Clinical Implications:

- Any infant with intractable seizures should be diagnostically considered for vitamin B$_6$ dependency. Even though it is rare, an increased requirement of this vitamin within the central nervous system can cause such seizures (Crowell & Roach, 1983).
- Some persons apparently have a higher requirement for pyridoxal phosphate. Despite normal serum levels, oral lesions around the mouth respond to treatment with pyridoxine (Bamji & Laxmi, 1979).
- Other drugs that have antivitamin B$_6$ properties, such as penicillamine (used to treat Wilson's disease), may require pyridoxine supplements (Sauberlich & Canham, 1980).
- Excessive pyridoxine can reduce clinical benefits of levodopa therapy in Parkinson's disease (Sauberlich & Canham, 1980).
- Large doses (10 to 25 mg/day) of vitamin B$_6$ are helpful in the treatment of seizures and resulting neurologic damage (Ink & Henderson, 1984).

Pantothenic Acid

Pantothenic acid is similar to the other B vitamins in its metabolic roles. Pantothenic is from the Greek word meaning "from everywhere," and indeed, distribution of this vitamin is widespread. Since it is water-soluble and extremely fragile, large losses during the processing and preparation of foods occur.

PHYSIOLOGICAL ROLES

Pantothenic acid is involved in the Krebs cycle with carbohydrates, fat, and protein metabolism in the form of coenzyme A. Additionally, it is important in the formation of certain hormones, nerve-regulating substances, and hemoglobin.

FOOD SOURCES

Individuals on a low-energy diet need to make a careful selection of foods for pantothenic acid content. Food tables often list inaccurate dietary intakes of pantothenic acid in processed and prepared foods since estimates are usually based on the raw-food values, which are not necessarily consistent with cooked-food values (Walsh et al, 1981). Table 11–1 shows the best sources for pantothenic acid.

Biotin

One of the most potent vitamins known is biotin. Because of its widespread distribution in foods, human deficiency is rare. Lately, however, pediatricians have diagnosed nutritional biotin deficiency resulting in skin rashes (Tanaka, 1981).

PHYSIOLOGICAL ROLES

Biotin is a coenzyme in the synthesis of fatty acids and amino acids. Its role involves formation of energy from the metabolism of glucoses.

Clinical Implication:

- Avidin, a protein in raw egg white, interferes with absorption of biotin.

Folic Acid

Folic acid (also called folacin) is found mainly in dark-green leafy vegetables (its name is derived from the Latin word for leaf, *folium*). Folacin was first used clinically in 1945 by Spies, who demonstrated its effectiveness in the treatment of macrocytic anemias of pregnancy and tropical sprue. This vitamin and iron are universal supplements during pregnancy (see Chapters 15 and 34.)

PHYSIOLOGICAL ROLES

Most of the attention for folate deficiency has been focused on pregnant women. Increased folate requirements are necessary during pregnancy for DNA formulation. Another primary function is in the formation of heme, the iron-containing part of hemoglobin. Factors that increase metabolic rate, such as infection and hyperthyroidism, or increased cell turnover such as hemolytic anemia, rapid tissue growth in a fetus, or malignant tumor, cause increased need for folate. Alcohol consumption, oral contraceptives, and other drugs may interfere with absorption to increase requirements.

Folacin (also called pteroylglutamic acid or PGA) is transformed within the living organism to a biologically active form called folinic acid. This transformation of folacin to folinic acid requires ascorbic acid. Folic acid is interrelated with vitamin B_{12}, which is required for choline synthesis, DNA synthesis, maintenance of normal levels of mature red cells (erythropoiesis), and synthesis of purines and pyrimidines.

FOOD SOURCES

Raw foods are the best sources of folic acid because it is extremely easy to destroy by heat. Sources other than green leafy vegetables are listed in Table 11–1.

DEFICIENCIES

Anemia from folic acid deficiency usually is called megaloblastic anemia or megalocytic anemia (see Chapter 34). Red blood cells do not develop normally; they become extremely large yet cannot transport oxygen to the cells. Gastrointestinal and neurological disorders occur. In fact, folic acid is used successfully to treat sprue, a gastrointestinal disease.

Growth is abnormal with folic acid deficiency. A conspectus of the research is this area citing over 800 references is available in Rodriguez (1978).

Clinical Implications:

- High concentrations of folic acid can have a convulsant effect (Herbert et al, 1980).
- Alcohol intake interferes with folate absorption, causing deficiencies (Rosenberg et al, 1982).

Vitamin B₁₂

The oral effectiveness of vitamin B_{12} is dependent upon the intrinsic factor found in normal gastric juice for its absorption. In fact, rarely is a deficiency of vitamin B_{12} caused by insufficient dietary sources (unless vegetarian diets are followed), but lack of intrinsic factor is the cause.

PHYSIOLOGICAL ROLES

Both vitamin B_{12} and folate are required for DNA synthesis. Vitamin B_{12} is essential for normal functioning of all body cells as well as the central nervous system and for hematopoiesis and nucleoprotein and myelin synthesis. Most importantly, it is related to certain anemias especially in the prevention of pernicious anemia (see Chapter 34).

SOURCES

Vitamin B_{12} is not found in plants unless they are contaminated by microorganisms (legumes and root vegetables). Ordinarily, dietary sources are meats and animal products.

Clinical Implications:

- A high vitamin B_{12} intake will result in accumulation in the liver with increasing age (McLaren, 1981).
- High intakes of certain fibers can aggravate a precarious vitamin B_{12} balance in individuals with a poor dietary intake (Dietary fiber, 1979).
- Patients who have had permanent gastric surgery or ileal damage must receive monthly injections of vitamin B_{12} for life (Herbert et al, 1980).
- Concomitant ingestion of megadoses of ascorbic acid via foods or tablets can destroy substantial amounts of vitamin B_{12} (Herbert, 1979).
- Because vitamin B_{12} is found only in meat products, vegans (i.e., strict vegetarian) require a daily supplement of 1 mcg (Herbert et al, 1980).

Vitamin C

Centuries ago, sailors quickly learned that scurvy would affect most of them on long voyages and cause many deaths. Even a few vegetables such as acidified cabbage (kraut) and some fruit (especially limes), could prevent this awful scourge. Vitamin C still remained unidentified until 1928, when Szent-Györgyi, a Hungarian scientist living in the United States, first isolated it.

PHYSIOLOGICAL ROLES

Some of the extensive functions of vitamin C include:
1. Healing of wounds and fractures.
2. Reduced liability to infections.
3. Production of collagen, (the basic protein substance of connective tissue that helps support body structures such as skin, bones, and tendons).
4. Maintenance of intracellular cement substance with preservation of capillary integrity.
5. Facilitation of iron absorption and utilization.
6. Participation in tooth and bone formation.
7. Prevention of folacin oxidation and conversion of folinic acid.
8. Possible coenzymatic function in the metabolism of amino acids.
9. Biosynthesis of steroid hormones.

Health Application: Therapeutic Use of Vitamin C

Important indirect evidence indicates ascorbic acid consumption is associated with a lower risk of gastric and esophageal cancer. Such assumptions are based upon the consumption of fruits and vegetables high in vitamin C. While limited direct evidence exists today for the role of vitamin C in cancer prevention, early studies also implicate vitamin C in the reversion of transformed cells (CDNC, 1982).

DEFICIENCIES

Scorbutic patients are often extensively evaluated for other disorders. Instead of scurvy, more

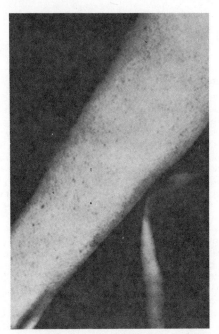

Figure 11–3. Perifollicular hemorrhages on the leg of a 16-year-old boy with scurvy. (From Nizel AE: Nutrition in Preventive Dentistry Science and Practice, 2nd ed. Philadelphia, W. B. Saunders Co, 1981, by permission.)

serious disorders such as deep vein thrombosis, vasculitis, and systemic bleeding are suspected. Scurvy can mimic these conditions. Symptoms may develop within 60 to 90 days with total elimination of vitamin C from the diet (Fig. 11–3).

The requirement for vitamin C is increased under many situations in which it is directly involved (e.g., healing and fighting infections), and it is detrimentally affected by many drugs (e.g., tobacco and aspirin).

Elderly persons, especially those who live alone or who avoid acidic foods to control esophageal reflux, and patients undergoing peritoneal dialysis or hemodialysis are at greatest risk to become scorbutic. Daily supplementation of 300 mg vitamin C replenishes the total body pool in as little as five days (Reuler et al, 1985).

FOOD SOURCES AND REQUIREMENTS

Table 11–1 shows food sources of vitamin C. *Focus on Daily Intakes of Vitamin C* shows examples of how to meet the RDA. Since this vitamin is easily destroyed and is only stored for short periods, the inclusion of some food sources at most meals and snacks becomes an ideal choice, just as the time-released vitamin C pill is better utilized.

Storage also plays a part in the vitamin's preservation. Fruit juices kept in an air-tight container that fits the amount stored will retain more vitamin C. A pint of juice in a pint container with an airtight lid protects the vitamin C content better than a pint of juice in a gallon container. Table 11–2 summarizes the debate over vitamin C supplementation.

Clinical Implication:

- Since vitamin C enhances the absorption of iron, particular attention should be given to avoid routine use of intravenous fluids containing the usual 3 gm of ascorbic acid for a daily intravenous injection in iron-overloaded patients, such as alcoholics (Herbert et al, 1981).

FOCUS ON	DAILY INTAKES OF VITAMIN C

RDA: Male,   51 years old, 2400 calories: 45 mg
Female, 51 years old, 1800 calories: 45 mg

½ cup Tomato juice	20	½ cup Grapefruit	47	½ cup Orange juice	60
¼ cup Broccoli		½ cup Green peas	10	1 Baked potato	20
Totals	35		57		80
	55				

From U.S. Department of Agriculture: *Nutritive Value of American Foods in Common Units.* Agriculture Handbook No. 456, Agriculture Research Service, 1975.

Table 11–2. The Great Vitamin C Debate.
Should megadoses of vitamin C (ascorbic acid) be the regular daily intake?

Pro	Con
1. Vitamin C can be used to cure a cold.	
• Dr. Linus Pauling, who received the Nobel Prize in Chemistry as well as the Peace Prize, recommends 1 to 5 gm/day vitamin C daily to reduce incidence and severity of the symptoms of colds (Pauling, 1970).	• Although Dr. Pauling is a brilliant and outstanding scientist, one should realize that the same studies he interpreted one way were disputed by other well-qualified nutrition scientists. His theories command attention, but further research is needed to prove the validity of this assertion or to find new and unanticipated answers. One of the greatest contributions any scientist can make (other than discovery itself) is to ask probing questions. • A study among Marine recruits for 8 weeks did not conclusively prove vitamin C benefits for colds. Even though the ascorbic acid group *claimed* to have less discomfort, no difference was reflected in obvious symptoms, sick-call visits, or training days lost (Pitt & Costrini, 1979). • A small beneficial effect of vitamin C megadoses was found in some other studies related to colds that were repeated in different daily doses of vitamin C (250, 1000, and 2000 for prophylaxis and 4000 to 8000 mg for therapy). The incidence of illnesses was not decreased, and only small and questionable prophylactic and therapeutic effects were shown. A significant fact is that the smallest dose was as effective as the largest dose (Hodges, 1980). • No therapeutic benefit was seen (Creagan & Moertel, 1979).
2. Vitamin C megadoses are important in cellular immune function (or immunocompetence).	
• Pauling says that vitamin C is essential to maintain the integrity of the cell, to resist malignant invasive growth, and to activate the immune mechanism, which may be its principal means of protection from cancer. Pauling claims that if patients with cancer had not received chemotherapy, the high doses of ascorbic acid would have cured them (Creagen & Moertel, 1979).	• Unfortunately, no properly designed, randomized, controlled studies have been able to support (or validate) this claim. Available evidence makes it unconscionable to withhold chemotherapy and to give the cancer patient large amounts of ascorbic acid instead (Creagen & Moertel, 1979).
3. Large amounts of vitamin C are needed for tissue saturation.	
• Albert Szent-Györgyi, who won the Nobel Prize for discovering vitamin C, admonishes, "Stop thinking of ascorbic acid as a vitamin. Go beyond the molecular level—gaze at the intense activity constantly taking place at the electronic level of the life of the cell." He explains that ascorbic acid is the force that removes an electon from a cell, which throws the entire, quiet intracellular system out of balance. This instability can mean the difference between life and inertness, between the cell dividing and reassembling into two healthy cells or becoming abnormal and possibly cancerous (Szent-Györgyi et al, 1979).	• The amount of intake for tissue saturation is the debatable question. Excess ascorbic acid is believed to be excreted through the urine. If a habitual intake of vitamin C (80 to 100 mg daily) keeps a person in a state of saturation, what is the justification for megadoses? The important point to remember is that, if 100 mg is the amount required for saturation, megadoses should be in time-released form, or they will go through the body without the desired effect. • A normal total body pool of vitamin C is approximately 1500 mg. When the pool drops below 350 mg, clinical manifestations of scurvy appear; however, an intake of only 10 mg/day maintains a pool size of about 350 mg (Reuler et al, 1985). • Dependency occurs very quickly when megadoses of vitamin C are taken. Individuals may have problems adjusting to smaller doses (Irwin and Hutchins, 1976).
4. Vitamin C blocks carcinogenic nitrosamine formation.	
• This supposedly occurs through direct reaction with nitrous acid derived from dietary nitrite, medication-derived nitrite, or nitrite formed within the gut.	• Since this reaction has not been repeatedly confirmed, suggestions have been made that ascorbate treatment might be effectively applied to foods containing added nitrite or that food sources high in vitamin C could be eaten at the same time.
5. Vitamin C megadoses improve athletic performance.	
• Some coaches have believed that vitamin C megadoses improve athletic performance.	• Studies show that athletic performance does not improve after massive doses of vitamin C.

Table 11–2. The Great Vitamin C Debate.
Should megadoses of vitamin C (ascorbic acid) be the regular daily intake? (Continued)

Pro	Con
6. Vitamin C prevents atherosclerosis.	
• For quite some time, claims have been made that vitamin C might be useful in the prevention or cure of atherosclerosis.	• These claims have not had conclusive results to verify them—more research is required (Ramirez & Flowers, 1980).
7. Vitamin C is essential to optimum wound healing.	
• Limitless claims have been made declaring vitamin C will cure various diseases and symptoms.	• This is a fact. Vitamin C is essential to aid healing, but it is not the cure by itself. The questionable part is how much. A diet rich in vitamin C sources may be able to satisfy ascorbic acid needs in many cases. Daily consumption of 500 mg of ascorbic acid can be accomplished in a number of ways through appropriate food selection, but providing 1000 mg vitamin C daily through food sources alone is much more difficult and is rarely achieved by a sensible diet.
8. Ascorbic acid improves the ability to maintain attention at a dull and monotonous task and improves memory.	
• Many claims have been made that short- and long-term memory can be improved by vitamin C intake.	• No improvement in memory, alertness, concentration, or mood was identified by higher ascorbic acid intakes (Adam, 1981).
9. Generous doses of ascorbic acid (1 gm/day or more) will lessen musculoskeletal symptoms.	
• Pain in muscles and bone joints can be cured by high vitamin C intake.	• Large doses frequently produce diarrhea, the source of which is unrecognized (Hoyt, 1980). Megadoses also often cause side effects such as nausea and abdominal cramps (Dubick & Rucker, 1983). No valid studies have proven that musculoskeletal symptoms disappear.
10. Smokers require larger amounts of vitamin C.	
• Smokers have a higher metabolic turnover rate for vitamin C than nonsmokers. At least 140 mg ascorbic acid are required for smokers to reach steady-state concentrations and total body pools compared to those of nonsmokers (Kalimer et al, 1981).	• Vitamin C in the amount of 140 mg/day can easily be obtained from foods. If the turnover rate is higher for smokers, frequent intakes are as important as amounts.
11. Increased amounts of vitamin C are needed for stress and trauma.	
• Dr. Pauling claims four times the regular intake (at least 240 mg/daily) is required for stress and trauma (Enloe & Hartley, 1978).	• Large amounts of vitamin C are lost during sucn periods, but the question is how much to ingest and what other affects these amounts have. • Large doses of vitamin C can interfere with vitamin B_{12} absorption and metabolism, and this problem may not be overcome by vitamin B_{12} supplementation (Herbert & Jacob, 1974). • A false-positive result from a urinary glucose test may be obtained if ascorbic acid megadoses are being taken (because of structural similarity to glucose). In patients taking vitamin C supplements who are monitored for urinary glucose, a specific test for glucose, like chromatography, should be used to determine urine or blood glucose levels. • Most of the testing for harmful effects has been done for short periods.

Both sides have legitimate theories. Until more research can be conducted, the soundest advice is to eat foods rich in vitamin C daily and preferably with every meal. Since this vitamin is easily destroyed, raw vegetables and fruits are advisable. Self-medication of ascorbic acid megadoses may cause undesirable side effects.

Pseudovitamins

Other substances that resemble the B vitamins are sometimes touted as important. No deficiencies of these substances have been observed in humans, and no recommendations for intakes have been advised since they exist abundantly in foods and/or are formed within the body. But they have been identified as specific agents in various reactions within the body.

VITAMIN B₁₅

Also called pangamic acid, vitamin B_{15} is a substance that has been isolated but does not fit the prerequisites of a vitamin.

CARNITINE

Like choline, carnitine has been identified in fat metabolism (Bray & Briggs, 1980) but can also be synthesized by the body. Diseases have been associated with carnitine deficiency but are genetic rather than the result of dietary deficiencies.

PARA-AMINOBENZOIC ACID (PABA)

PABA is not a specific vitamin but rather a part of folate. Other than its vitamin activity, it is best known as a sunscreen to prevent skin damage.

CHOLINE AND INOSITOL

These two substances sometimes are called B vitamins. They work as coenzymes in metabolism, but no deficiencies have been observed (Appel & Briggs, 1980).

Choline is listed as the ninth B vitamin by some; others group it with the pseudovitamins. Infants may be vulnerable to choline deficiency, so the recommendation has been made to include 7 mg/100 kcal in milk-based formulas. It has been labeled as lipotropic. Vitamin B_{12} and folacin are involved in the biosynthesis of choline and methionine. Therefore, adequate intakes of these vitamins must be considered in relationship to any experiments with possible choline deficiency.

BIOFLAVONOIDS

This term refers to flavonoids that have biological activity. They have been shown to act as antioxidants, protecting ascorbic acid and other components from oxidation (Park et al, 1983). Most flavonoids are located in the skin or peel of many fruits and vegetables. In 1936, Szent-Györgyi found that red-pepper extract or lemon juice was effective in certain pathological conditions characterized by increased permeability of the capillary wall. They are not considered vitamins, however, because they have not been proven to be essential in the diet (Weininger & Briggs, 1980). These substances were called vitamin P until 1950 when this term was discontinued in favor of the more descriptive bioflavonoids.

LIPOIC ACID AND UBIQUINONE (COENZYME Q)

Also included in the list of pseudovitamins are substances such as lipoic acid and ubiquinone that have been identified but not classified as vitamins.

• FALLACIES AND FACTS

FALLACY: *Pantothenic acid prevents gray hair, relieves postoperative paralytic ileus, and helps heal burns and skin lesions.*

• **FACT:** *These claims have not been verified. A deficiency of pantothenic acid is usually accompanied by graying of the hair, but megadoses cannot prevent this natural process.*

FALLACY: *Natural vitamins, such as vitamin C from rose hips, are better than man-made vitamins.*

• **FACT:** *For the amount of vitamin C usually listed on the label, it would be impossible to get enough rose hips into the bottle. Other sources have been added to increase the content. Not only do synthetic vitamins have exactly the same formula as those from food sources, but there is at least one example of a man-made vitamin that is better than the naturally occurring one. Man-made folic acid is utilized about twice as well as the one found in nature, which is bound in a form that is not readily assimilated (Jukes, 1974).*

FALLACY: *Bioflavonoids should be used in therapeutic roles for vascular purpura, hypertension, degenerative vascular disease, rheumatic fever, arthritis, and cancer.*

• **FACT:** *At this date, no conclusive evidence demonstrates that bioflavonoids are effective in preventing or treating any human disease (Weininger & Briggs, 1980).*

FALLACY: *Hyperactive children should be given megavitamins as used in orthomolecular treatments.*

• **FACT:** *Results show that megadoses of niacin, ascorbic acid, pyridoxine, and pantothenate have no beneficial effect on hyperactivity and may be associated with gastrointestinal complaints and hepatotoxicity (Megavitamins, 1985).*

Summary

Water-soluble vitamins are fragile, cannot be stored in the body for long periods of time, and are absolutely crucial for optimum health. Not only do all of the food groups need to be included in the daily intake, but variety from each food group is equally important.

Vitamin supplements are not necessary for optimum health and can be devastating in megadoses. Learning about food sources for nutrients is the best way to ensure the proper amount of all nutrients. If supplements are taken, not more than the RDA should be taken unless prescribed by a physician. This amount can be excessively high if vitamin-rich foods are eaten also (see Table 11–1).

Sharing information about nutrition, especially vitamins, might be welcomed among associates. The medical team approach offers many personal bonuses to the health care professional as well as to the patient.

Review Questions

1. Which two water-soluble vitamins are most involved in the metabolism of fats, proteins, and carbohydrates to form energy (ATP) through the Krebs cycle?

2. Name the deficiency conditions associated with thiamin, riboflavin, niacin, vitamin B_{12}, and ascorbic acid.
3. How do water-soluble vitamins differ from fat-soluble ones? What do these differences mean as you choose foods for your own menu?
4. What are the disadvantages of taking vitamin megadoses? Advantages?
5. Name three foods that are excellent sources for each of these vitamins; thiamin, riboflavin, and vitamins C and B_{12}?
6. What should vegetarians know about vitamin B_{12}?

Case Study: Mr. A.K. has been diagnosed to have pernicious anemia. His red blood cells are macrocytic and normochromic, and he shows evidence of nervous system damage with impaired judgment, hallucinations and decreased reflexes. He has started on vitamin B_{12} injections and has been informed that these will have to be continued indefinitely. After discharge, Mr. A.K. discontinues the injections for which he has to travel to the clinic, and he uses high-dose supplements of multivitamins.

1. Why were the vitamin B_{12} injections originally prescribed?
2. Will the multivitamins provide the needed nutrient?
3. What is the possible outcome of Mr. A.K.'s self-medication attempts?
4. Develop a tentative nursing diagnosis from this history and at least one goal.
5. Why are patients who have had a gastrectomy at risk to develop pernicious anemia?

REFERENCE LIST

Adam, SK: Lack of effect on mental efficiency of extra vitamin C. *Am J Clin Nutr* 34(9):1712, 1981.

Ajayi, OA; James, OA: Effect of riboflavin supplementation on riboflavin nutriture of a secondary school population in Nigeria. *Am J Clin Nutr* 39(5):787, 1984.

Appel, JA; Briggs, GM: Choline. In *Modern Nutrition in Health and Disease*, 6th ed. Edited by RB Goodhart; ME Shils. Philadelphia, Lea & Febiger, 1980, p. 282.

Balcke, P; Schmidt, P; Zazgornik, J; et al: Pyridoxine therapy in patients with renal calcium oxalate calculi. *Proc Eur Dial Transplant Assoc* 20:417, 1983.

Bamji, MS; Laxmi, AV: Interrelationship between riboflavin and pyridoxine and biochemical aetiology of lesions of the mouth. *Indian J Nutr Diet* 16(July):295, 1979.

Berger, A; Schaumburg, HH: More on neuropathy from pyridoxine abuse. *N Engl J Med* 311(15):987, 1984.

Bray, DL; Briggs, M: Carnitine. In *Modern Nutrition in Health and Disease*, 6th ed. Edited by RB Goodhart; ME Shils. Philadelphia, Lea & Febiger, 1980, p 291.

Campbell, CH: Lactic acidosis of thiamin deficiency. *Lancet* 2(August 25):446, 1984.

Committee on Diet, Nutrition and Cancer (CDNC): *Diet, Nutrition, and Cancer*. Washington, DC, National Academy Press, 1982.

Crawford, D: Excessive use of pyridoxine. *Can Med Assoc J* 130(4):343, 1984.

Creagan, ET; Moertel, C: Vitamin C therapy of advanced cancer. *N Engl J Med* 301(25):1399, 1979.

Crowell, GF; Roach, ES: Pyridoxine-dependent seizures. *Am Fam Physician* 27(3):183, 1983.

Dietary fiber and vitamin B_{12} balance. *Nutr Rev* 37(4):116, 1979.

Dubick, MA; Rucker, RB: Dietary supplements and health aids—critical evaluation. Part 1, Vitamins and minerals. *J Nutr Ed* 15(2):47, 1983.

Ejderhamn, J; Hamfelt, A: Pyridoxal phosphate concentration in blood in newborn infants and their mothers compared with the amount of extra pyridoxal taken during pregnancy and breast feeding. *Acta Paediatr* 69(3):327, 1980.

Enloe, C Jr; Hartley, GL: To dose or megadose. *Nutr Today* 13(2):6, 1978.

Farkas, CP: Potential for and implications of thiamine deficiency in northern Canadian Indian populations affected by mercury contamination. *Ecol Food Nutr* 8(1):11, 1979.

Herbert, V: Co-ingestion of ascorbic acid and vitamin B_{12}. *JAMA* 242(21):2285, 1979.

Herbert, V; Cohen, A; Schwartz, E: Vitamin C and iron overload. *N Engl J Med* 304(18):1108, 1981.

Herbert, V; Colman, N; Jacob, E: Folic acid and vitamin B_{12}. In *Modern Nutrition in Health and Disease*, 6th ed. Edited by RB Goodhart; ME Shils. Philadelphia, Lea & Febiger, 1980, p. 229.

Herbert, V; Jacob, E: Destruction of vitamin B_{12} by ascorbic acid. *JAMA* 230:244, 1974.

Hodges, RE: Ascorbic acid. In *Modern Nutrition in Health and Disease*, 6th ed. Edited by RB Goodhart; ME Shils. Philadelphia, Lea & Febiger, 1980, p 259.

Hoyt, CJ: Diarrhea from vitamin C. *JAMA* 244(15):1674, 1980.

Ink, SL; Henderson, LM: Vitamin B_6 metabolism. *Ann Rev Nutr* 4:445, 1984.

Irwin, MI; Hutchins, BK: A conspectus of research on vitamin C requirements of man. *J Nutrition* 106:823, 1976.

Jukes, T: Down the primrose path with "organic" foods. *Sch Foodserv J* 28(10):52, 1974.

Kalimer, AB; Hartman, D; Hornig, DH: On the requirements of ascorbic acid in man: Steady-state turnover and body pool in smokers. *Am J Clin Nutr* 34(7):1347, 1981.

Kirksey, A; Roepke, JLB; Styslinger, LM: The vitamin B_6 content in human milk. In *Methods in Vitamin B_6 Nutrition, Analysis and Status Assessment*. Edited by JE Leklem; RD Reynolds. New York, Plenum, 1980, p 269.

Lemoine, A; Devehat, CL: Codaccioni, JL; et al: Vitamin B_1, B_2, B_6 and C status in hospital inpatients. *Am J Clin Nutr* 33(12):2595, 1980.

Mandel, H; Berant, M; Hazani, A; et al: Thiamine-dependent beriberi in the "thiamine-responsive anemia syndrome." *N Engl J Med* 311(13):836, 1984.

Massey, LK; Davison, MA: Effects of oral contraceptives on nutritional status. *Am Fam Physician* 19(1):119, 1979.

McCollum, EV: *History of Nutrition*. Boston, Houghton Mifflin, 1957.

McLaren, DS: The luxus vitamins A and B_{12}. *Am J Clin Nutr* 34(8):1611, 1981.

Megavitamins and the hyperactive child. *Nutr Reviews*, 43(4):105, 1985.

Miller, BF; Keane, CB: *Encyclopedia and Dictionary of Medicine, Nursing, and Allied Health*, 4th ed. Philadelphia, W. B. Saunders Co, 1987.

Mitwalli, A; Blair, G; Oreopoulos, DG: Safety of intermediate doses of pyridoxine. *Can Med Assoc J* 131(1):14, 1984.

Park, GL; Avery, SM; Byers, JL; et al: Identification of bioflavonoids from citrus. *Food Tech* 37(12):98, 1983.

Pauling, L: *Vitamin C and the Common Cold*. San Francisco, W. H. Freeman and Co, 1970.

Pitt, HA; Costrini, AM: Vitamin C prophylaxis in Marine recruits. *JAMA* 241(9):908, 1979.

Ramirez, J; Flowers, NC: Leucocyte ascorbic acid and its relationship to coronary artery disease in man. *Am J Clin Nutr* 33(10):2079, 1980.

Reuler, JB; Broudy, VC; Cooney, TG: Adult scurvy. *JAMA* 253(6):805, 1985.

Rivlin, RS: Hormones, drugs and riboflavin. *Nutr Reviews* 37(August):241, 1979.

Rodriguez, MS: A conspectus of research on folacin requirements of man. *J Nutr*, 108(12):19, 1978.

Roepke, JLB; Kirksey, A: Vitamin B_6 nutriture during pregnancy and lactation. *Am J Clin Nutr* 32(11):2257, 1979.

Rosenberg, IH; Bowman, BB; Cooper, BA; et al: Folate nutrition in the elderly. *Am J Clin Nutr* 36(5 suppl):1060, 1982.

Sauberlich, HE; Canham, JE: Vitamin B_6. In *Modern Nutrition in Health and Disease*, 6th ed. Edited by RB Goodhart; ME Shils. Philadelphia, Lea & Febiger, 1980, p 216.

Schaumburg, H; Kaplan, J; Windebank, A; et al: Sensory neuropathy from pyridoxine abuse: A new megavitamin syndrome. *N Engl J Med* 309(8):445, 1983.

Szent-Györgyi, A; Stone, P; Harley, HL; et al: How vitamin C really works . . . or does it? *Nutr Today* 14(5):6, 1979.

Tanaka, K (ed): New light on biotin deficiency. *N Engl J Med* 304(14):839, 1981.

Tarr, JB; Tamura, T; Stokstad, ER: Availability of vitamin B_6 and pantothenate in an average American diet in man. *Am J Clin Nutr* 34(7):1328, 1981.

Walsh, JH; Wyse, BW; Hansen, RG: Pantothenic acid content of 75 processed and cooked foods. *J Am Diet Assoc* 78(2):140, 1981.

Weininger, J; Briggs, GM: Bioflavonoids. In *Modern Nutrition in Health and Disease*, 6th ed. Edited by RB Goodhart; ME Shils. Philadelphia, Lea & Febiger, 1980. p 279.

Further Study

Bailey, LB; Mahan, CS; Dimperio, D: Folacin and iron status in low-income pregnant adolescents and mature women. *Am J Clin Nutr* 33(9):1997, 1980.

Bates, CJ; Black, AE; Phillips, DR; et al: The discrepancy between normal folate intakes and the folate RDA. *Hum Nutr App Nutr* 36A(6):42, 1982.

Belko, AZ; Obarzanek, E; Roach, R; et al: Effects of aerobic exercise and weight loss on riboflavin requirements of moderately obese, marginally deficient young women. *Am J Clin Nutr* 40(3):553, 1984.

Benowicz, RJ: The age of vitamins. *Family Health* 12(Sept):28, 1980.

Bootman, JL; Wertheimer, AI: Patterns of vitamin usage in a sample of university students. *J Am Diet Assoc* 77(1):58, 1980.

Carpenter, KJ; Lewin, WJ: A reexamination of the composition of diets associated with pellagra. *J Nutr* 115(5):543, 1985.

Cerrato, PL: Vitamin C. Who needs it? And when? *RN* 48(8):59, 1985.

Hall, CA: Vitamin B_{12} deficiency and early rise in mean corpuscular volume. *JAMA* 245(11):1144, 1981.

Hecht, A: Vitamins over the counter: Take only when needed. *FDA Consumer* 13(4):17, 1979.

Innis, SM; Allardyce, DB: Possible biotin deficiency in adults receiving long-term total parenteral nutrition. *Am J Clin Nutr* 37(2):185, 1983.

Johnson, GE; Obenshain, SS: Nonresponsiveness of serum high-density lipoprotein cholesterol to high-dose ascorbic acid administration in normal men. *Am J Clin Nutr* 34(10):2088, 1981.

Jones, DY; Kumanyika, SK: Premenstrual syndrome: A review of possible dietary influences. *J Can Diet Assoc* 44:194, 1983.

Koehley, HH; Hard, MM: Vitamin contents of pre-prepared foods sampled from a hospital food service line. *J Am Diet Assoc* 82(6):622, 1983.

Rao, RH: Glucose tolerance in subclinical pyridoxine deficiency in man. *Am J Clin Nutr* 38(9):440, 1983.

Roth, KS: Biotin in clinical medicine. *Am J Clin Nutr* 34(9):1967, 1981.

Willett, W; Sampson, L; Bain, C; et al: Vitamin supplements used among registered nurses. *Am J Clin Nutr* 34(6):1121, 1981.

The Unique Minerals

12

THE STUDENT WILL BE ABLE TO:

- **List the macrominerals found in the body with their main physiological roles.**
- **List five trace elements found in the body that are probably better considered as contaminants than useful elements.**
- **Discuss the pros and cons of fluoridation of the water supply.**
- **List the advantages and disadvantages of mineral supplementation.**

Bioavailability
Calcium-to-phosphorus
  ratio
Fluorosis
Hemosiderosis
Hypogeusia
Iodine deficiency disorder
  (IDD)
Idiopathic hypercalcemia
Keshan disease
Macromineral
Metalloenzyme
Micromineral
Tetany
Total iron-binding capacity
  (TIBC)
Trabeculae of bone

When we gaze at the steep cut through a mountain to make a road and realize that the trace elements so vital to our lives come from that huge slice of rock, we are amazed. Eons are required to transform the minerals in rock into biologically available compounds: rock to soil to plants and animals and then to humans. Not only where the elements come from but the infinitesimal amounts needed by the body are difficult to fathom (Fig. 12–1).

A peculiar feature of nutritional deficiency may be due to geography—the possibility of living in a region where the soil is depleted of a vital trace element, such as iodine, or the good fortune to live where the soil is rich and bountiful. This is another reason to select a variety of foods from different regions.

Figure 12–1. *This graphic symbol is a generic illustration for all trace elements (TE).*

anatomical systems: (1) skeleton and teeth (calcium, phosphorus, and magnesium), (2) vitamin B$_{12}$ (cobalt), (3) hemoglobin (iron), (4) thyroid hormone (iodine), and (5) enzyme systems (most of the trace elements). Another role of minerals is to act as regulators to control body functions in:

1. Transmitting nerve impulses (sodium and potassium).
2. Maintaining acid-base balance.
3. Regulating osmotic pressure and water balance between intracellular and extracellular fluid.
4. Maintaining the permeability of cell membranes (calcium).

PUBLIC CONSUMPTION

Even in the United States where food is abundant, many individuals consume a diet inadequate in minerals. Eleven essential minerals are assessed in an annual study by the Food and Drug Administration (FDA). Such reports have revealed low levels of calcium, magnesium, iron, zinc, copper, and manganese (i.e., less than 80 percent of the RDAs or below the Estimated Safe and Adequate Daily Dietary Intake range) for some or all age-sex groups. Young children, teenage girls, adult women, and older women were most at risk of low intakes. Potassium, phosphorus, and selenium intakes were adequate for all groups (Pennington et al, 1986).

On the other hand, sodium intake exceeded the Estimated Safe and Adequate Daily Dietary Intake range for teenage boys and two-year-old children. This is of concern because of its relationship to hypertension. Even though iodine was above the RDA for all age-sex groups, no harmful effects are known. This high level is obtained by the excessive use of iodized salt (Pennington et al, 1986).

Classification of Minerals

All the metallic mineral elements in the body account for only about four percent of the total body weight, or 6 lbs. for a 150 lb. person. Minerals are divided into two groups: nonmetallic (or organic) elements and metallic (or inorganic) elements. The organic elements include carbon, hydrogen, oxygen, and nitrogen. They are responsible for the other 96 percent body weight. Minerals are also subdivided into those required in larger amounts, i.e., macronutrients such as calcium, and those required in smaller amounts, i.e., micronutrients such as zinc (Table 12–1).

Calcium

Calcium, a macronutrient, is a prevalent element in nature, as well as being vital for health.

PHYSIOLOGICAL ROLES

At least 99 percent of the total amount of calcium is found in the skeleton and teeth. The calcium deposited in teeth remains permanently. However, calcium (as well as phosphorus) in the bone actually is reserved for special body needs.

Physiological Functions of Minerals

Minerals have many functions. As structural components, minerals are part of the following

Table 12–1. Metallic Mineral Elements in the Body

Essential Macronutrients (100 mg or more/day)	Essential Micronutrients (Trace Elements: no higher than a few mg/day)	Possibly Essential Micronutrients (Trace Elements)	Trace Elements Found in the Body (Unknown Function or Contaminants)
1. Calcium (Ca)	1. Iron (Fe)	1. Nickel (Ni)	1. Aluminum (Al)
2. Phosphorus (P)	2. Copper (Cu)	2. Tin (Sn)	2. Cadmium (Cd)
3. Sodium (Na)	3. Cobalt (Co)	3. Silicon (Si)	3. Lead (Pb)
4. Potassium (K)	4. Zinc (Zn)	4. Vanadium (V)	4. Arsenic (As)
5. Magnesium (Mg)	5. Manganese (Mn)		5. Barium (Ba)
6. Chlorine (Cl)	6. Iodine (I)		6. Strontium (St)
7. Sulfur (S)	7. Molybdenum (Mo)		7. Mercury (Hg)
	8. Fluorine (Fl)		8. Silver (Ag)
	9. Selenium (Se)		9. Gold (Au)
	10. Chromium (Cr)		10. Antimony (Sb) and others

Bone is constantly changing as the osteoblasts deposit fresh calcium salts where new stresses have developed, and where osteoclasts are removing calcium deposits. In fact, one of the main purposes of the trabeculae of bone is to provide calcium for the blood. Despite this turnover, the calcium equilibrium is quite stable.

Even though only one percent of the calcium is found in blood, its functions are vital. Calcium is involved with the transmission of nerve impulses, muscle contraction and relaxation, blood clotting, structure and function of cell membranes, and absorption of vitamin B_{12}.

CALCIUM BALANCE

Calcium balance, i.e., an intake that equals excretion, is not just dependent on total calcium intake and utilization. Absorption is affected by many factors, including vitamin D, parathyroid hormone, protein intake, lactose, calcitonin, and steroid hormones (especially estrogen).

While several plant foods contain high amounts of calcium, absorption is poor. Oxalates in vegetables bind the calcium to reduce absorption, but they apparently do not interfere with calcium content from other sources (Allen, 1984). Phytates also have been considered to interfere with calcium absorption, as does excessive fiber. Other interference with absorption results from high-protein and/or high-alcohol intake (Allen, 1984). Since calcium from plant foods is not absorbed as well, the total amount in these foods cannot be considered available.

Weight-bearing exercise has more effect upon normal calcium deposits in bone than upon any other nutrient. Immobilization from a fracture, for example, immediately starts depletion. In the young person, recovery of calcium deposits is usually rapid, but the geriatric patient may never regain bone density. Calcium absorption from the gastrointestinal tract decreases with age.

When dietary intake is 800 mg of calcium (the RDA for children one to ten years of age and adults over 19), calcium balance is only slightly positive. An intake of 1200 mg of calcium more often results in optimal absorption, particularly in women (Spencer, 1986). Calcium intake for postmenopausal women should be increased to 1500 mg/day (NIADDKD, 1984).

CALCIUM-TO-PHOSPHORUS RATIO

Normally, the range of calcium in the blood is 9 to 11 mg/dl and phosphorus, 3 to 4.5 mg/dl. If the calcium level goes up, the phosphorus may go down or vice versa. This reciprocal relationship acts as a protective mechanism for preventing their combined concentrations from becoming so high in the extracellular fluid that calcium and phosphorus would react together with a subsequent calcification of soft tissue and stone formation.

When the calcium level multiplied by the phosphorus level is greater than 75, calcification and stone formation may result (Table 12–2). However, sufficient phosphorus intake is neces-

Table 12–2. Normal and Abnormal Calcium-to-Phosphorus Ratio*

Normal Blood Levels	Abnormal Blood Levels (renal disease)
Calcium = 10 mg/dl (average) Phosphorus = 4 mg/dl (average)	Example: Calcium = 8 mg/dl Phosphorus = 18 mg/dl
Ca × P = product 10 × 4 = 40 (Calcium and phosphorus are soluble in blood)	Ca × P = product 8 × 18 = 144 (Calcium and phosphorus precipitate causing calcification of soft tissue)

*From Lewis, CM: *Nutrition and Diet Therapy: Vitamins and Minerals.* Philadelphia, F. A. Davis Co., 1976, by permission.

Table 12–3. Calcium Equivalents

The following foods contain approximately the same amount of calcium as an 8 oz. cup of milk (approximately 300 mg):

Low-fat milk	1 cup
Buttermilk	1 cup
Cheddar cheese	1 ½ oz.
Cottage cheese	2 cups
Yogurt	1 cup
Processed cheese	1 ½ slices
Ice cream	1 ½ cups
Ice milk	1 ½ cups
Tofu*	8 oz.
Broccoli*	2 cups
Collard, turnip greens*	1 cup
Kale, mustard greens*	1 ½ cups
Oysters	1 ½ cups
Salmon	4 oz.
Sardines	2 ½ oz.

*Calcium from vegetable sources is not as easily absorbed by the intestine and is not as effective in fulfilling calcium requirements.

sary to decrease the loss of calcium with all intake levels of calcium. Recent studies show that absorption of calcium does not decrease during a high phosphorus intake up to 2000 mg/day. This finding indicates that the dietary calcium-to-phosphorus ratio probably does not play as important a role in the utilization of calcium under normal conditions as previously believed (Spencer, 1984; Spencer, 1986). However, under abnormal conditions or in certain diseases the calcium-to-phosphorus ratio can become an important assessment that may require adjusted intakes (see Chapter 33).

SOURCES

Milk and other dairy products supply most of the available calcium in our diet. Not only are they excellent sources because of the high calcium content, but lactose enhances the absorption. Table 12–3 lists the equivalent amounts of calcium in some foods. Appendix D-4 contains a more extensive list of foods with their calcium content.

The amount spent on calcium supplements is estimated to increase from $17 million in 1980 to $200 million by 1988. In addition to all the pharmaceutical products available, food producers are fortifying products such as all-purpose flour, soft drinks, and breakfast cereals. While it is not known whether all sources are equally utilized, it is assumed that most sources are absorbed with similar efficiency. A wise guideline would be to consume calcium with some form of sugar—lactose or sucrose—which enhances its absorption (Kelly et al, 1984).

DEFICIENCIES

A dietary deficiency of calcium is frequently observed. This could be due to (1) uninformed choices or just not selecting adequate amounts, (2) the mistaken belief that "milk is only for babies," or (3) economic hardships plus a lack of knowledge regarding inexpensive sources of calcium-rich foods.

Previously, calcium has been associated mainly with bone growth for children and osteoporosis in postmenopausal women. Current research proves that calcium intake is vitally important throughout life for both men and women. Other potential problems associated with a prolonged inadequate calcium intake include accelerated bone loss resulting in alveolar bone loss and accompanying oral health problems, and a rise in blood pressure (NDC, 1984).

Osteoporosis. One third of all postmenopausal Caucasian women suffer from osteoporosis (Allen, 1984). This "silent" disease is difficult to detect since 25 to 40 percent of bone is lost before it is detected (NDC, 1984). Loss of calcium in the jawbone, which may loosen teeth, and gum disease may be the initial signs (Allen, 1984). However, it usually goes unnoticed until pain or spontaneous fracture occurs. Further discussion on osteoporosis and osteomalacia is in Chapter 31.

Hypertension. High blood pressure is more

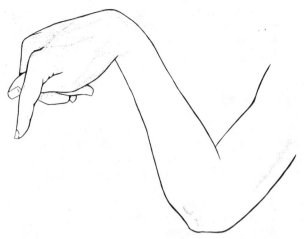

Figure 12–2. Trousseau's sign (carpopedal spasm) with hypocalcemia. (From Menzel LK: Clinical problems of electrolyte balance. Nursing Clinics of North America 15:559, September 1980.)

prevalent in people with a low-calcium intake (McCarron, 1983). An increased incidence of toxemia of pregnancy, a condition involving high blood pressure and other symptoms, has been linked to insufficient calcium intake (240 to 370 mg/day) (NDC, 1984).

Growth. Stunting of growth and rickets as well as vitamin D deficiency occur with calcium deficiency (see Chapter 10). Teeth and bones are porous and less dense.

Tetany. A neuromuscular disorder of uncontrollable muscular cramps and tremors involving the muscles of the face, hands, feet, and eventually the heart can result from hypocalcemia. Death may ensue. Trousseau's sign is a symptom of hypocalcemia (Fig. 12–2).

HYPER- OR HYPOCALCEMIA

Calcium exists in the blood in two forms: ionized and bound to protein (mainly albumin). For this reason, a protein determination should accompany each calcium level so the calcium value can be properly interpreted. A depressed concentration of total calcium can be due to hypoproteinemia (a low protein concentration), but it is the concentration of ionized calcium with which clinicians are concerned.

Hypoparathyroidism, some bone diseases, certain kidney diseases, and low serum protein levels are accompanied by depressed serum calcium levels (hypocalcemia). Adults may develop hypercalcemia, but the condition is observed more frequently in infants between five and eight months of age. It is caused by overdoses of cholecalciferol or excessive amounts of vitamin D preparations. Treatment involves providing a low-calcium diet with no vitamin D. Certain commercial products are designed to meet these requirements.

Adult Hypercalcemia. Hyperparathyroidism, certain types of bone disease, vitamin D poisoning, sarcoidosis, or prolonged excessive intake of milk may cause adult hypercalcemia. Milk-alkali syndrome (see Chapter 27) may result in this condition also.

Clinical Implications:

- No benefits have been observed for fracture healing when increased calcium or hormones are taken.
- Fatty acids form insoluble soaps with calcium, so patients unable to absorb fats have low calcium absorption.
- Drinking water can provide as much as 22 percent of the RDAs for calcium in hard-water areas. However, this is in the form of calcium bicarbonate (a salt), which can combine with zinc to render the calcium unavailable. Hard water can have a positive effect upon the utilization of zinc (Gibson et al, 1983).
- Persons predisposed to developing kidney stones (or those with a family history of this disorder) should consult their physicians before increasing calcium intake (Calcium, 1984).

Phosphorus

PHYSIOLOGICAL ROLES

Phosphorus is found mostly in bone along with calcium, but phosphorus is so abundant in plants and animals that deficiencies have not been observed. Phosphorus and calcium are the most abundant minerals in the body. However, phosphorus goes into every body cell and functions in almost every aspect of metabolism, including: (1) the structure of bones and teeth; (2) the transfer and release of energy stored as ATP; (3) a component of DNA and RNA; (4) cell permeability as phospholipids; and (5) metabolism of fats, carbohydrates, and proteins.

SOURCES

A diet adequate in calcium and protein already has enough phosphorus since it is present in the same foods (see Appendix D-4).

DEFICIENCIES

Hypophosphatemia may be seen with long-term ingestion of aluminum hydroxide antacids (Spencer, 1986) or in certain stress conditions where the calcium-to-phosphorus balance is disturbed. Even relatively small phosphorus depletions can cause increased calcium excretion resulting in negative calcium balance and bone loss (Spencer et al, 1982). Intestinal conditions, such as sprue and celiac disease, can result in phosphorus malabsorption deficiencies.

HYPERPHOSPHATEMIA

Excessive phosphorus may occur in cases of hypoparathyroidism or renal insufficiency (see Chapters 30 and 33).

Sodium

PHYSIOLOGICAL ROLES

Sodium is the principal cation in extracellular fluid. Its functions are the maintenance of osmotic equilibrium and body fluid, tissue formation, nerve transmission, and muscle contraction.

SOURCES

Sodium is found naturally in many foods (see Appendix D–3), thereby making extra intake un-

necessary to reach the recommended maximum intake of 6 to 8 gm/day. The addition of sodium in processed foods often becomes a problem for consumers.

DEFICIENCIES

Prolonged vomiting, renal disease, adrenal insufficiency, diarrhea, use of diuretics, or profuse sweating may result in deficiencies. If sodium and water are both lost, the volume of blood will be decreased, muscle cramps will occur and blood pressure may be low. (For sodium as an electrolyte, see Chapter 5; for sodium's role in hypertension, see Chapter 32.)

Potassium

PHYSIOLOGICAL ROLES

Potassium is the major intracellular electrolyte; it functions in conjunction with sodium to maintain the balance of body fluids. Its levels are also closely related to those of magnesium.

SOURCES

Some of the richest sources are meats, including veal and salmon, and fruits and vegetables (see Appendix D–3). It is so widely distributed among foods that a dietary deficiency is rare.

DEFICIENCIES

The most common causes of potassium deficiency are diuretics, fasting, starvation, infectious diarrhea, and vomiting.

Clinical Implications:

• Hypokalemia has been confirmed in zealous dieters who are overly concerned about not appearing obese or edematous. A high urine potassium level along with a low serum potassium level suggests the use of diuretics. Any urine with a potassium level of more than 30 mEq/L should be tested for diuretics (Rodman & Reidenberg, 1981).

- Hypokalemia results in cardiac arrhythmias, generalized muscle weakness, inability of the kidneys to retain sodium or produce acid urine, and inefficient use of protein and carbohydrates.
- Oral supplementation of potassium is safer than intravenous feedings.
- Potassium is more effective when given with meals to avoid gastrointestinal disturbances.

Magnesium

PHYSIOLOGICAL ROLES

Magnesium is vitally important in controlling normal cardiovascular function. Besides calcium and phosphorus, bones contain most of the body's 25 gm of magnesium. Magnesium has many functions, including an enzyme action fundamental to the production of energy (ATP), calcium and phosphorus metabolism in bone, and maintenance of the function and structural integrity of heart muscle as well as other muscles and nerves.

The RDA for magnesium is 300 mg/day for women and 400 mg/day for men. Increased intakes do not improve magnesium status in well nourished individuals, but high magnesium intake can lead to increased phosphorus excretion and a negative phosphorus balance (Spencer, 1986).

SOURCES

Whole-grain products, nuts, beans, and green leafy vegetables are some of the best sources of magnesium. Since it is part of the chlorophyll molecule chlorophyll-rich foods are good sources for magnesium.

DEFICIENCIES

In certain diseases or under stressful conditions, deficiencies may occur. While calcium has reserves in bone available for mobilization, magnesium in bone is not available to replace serum magnesium deficits. A deficiency may result from renal therapy, protein-energy malnutrition in infants (especially newborns) and children, postsurgical stress, diabetes, hyperthyroidism, acute alcoholism, burns, severe infections, gastrointestinal disorders, and diseases of the parathyroid. Chronic alcoholics may require magnesium therapy after an acute attack of delirium tremens caused by their low levels of serum magnesium because of high losses in the urine. Symptoms of a magnesium deficiency are neuromuscular dysfunction, personality changes, muscle spasms, convulsions (especially in infants), hyperexcitability, tremors, anorexia, nausea, apathy, decreased tendon reflexes and cardiac arrhythmias.

Clinical Implications:
- Decreased food intake and/or impaired absorption, use of certain diuretics and digitalis toxicity may be contributing factors to hypomagnesemia predisposing of cardiac arrhythmias and aggravating digitalis toxicity. Administration of magnesium may be useful (Shils, 1980).
- Hypomagnesia has been found in about one third of infants of diabetic mothers. This was related to the severity of maternal diabetes and premature birth (Shils, 1980).

Chlorine

Chlorine is the primary anion connected with sodium. These two minerals function in the maintenance of extracellular fluid, osmotic equilibrium, and electrolyte balance. Hydrochloric acid in the gastric juice is formed from chloride. Deficiencies are unlikely.

Sulfur

The main functions of sulfur include its role in blood clotting, bone formation, and muscle metabolism. It is also a structural component of two amino acids (methionine and cysteine), vitamins (thiamin and biotin) and cytoplasm of every cell. One of the most important functions of sulfur is its ability to neutralize toxins by combining with them to form harmless compounds that can then be released from the body.

Iron

If one trace mineral were to be selected as the most difficult to obtain in adequate amounts, it would be iron.

PHYSIOLOGICAL ROLES

Iron is needed by the bone marrow to form hemoglobin and for cellular oxidation. It transports oxygen from the lungs to the tissues, catalyzes many oxidative reactions within cells, and participates in the final steps of energy metabolism.

The body has about 4 gm of iron, which can be found in hemoglobin, myoglobin, and cytochromes as well as bound to protein. Total iron-binding capacity (TIBC) measures the iron bound to transferrin, which transports iron in the blood. A higher TIBC indicates lower stores of iron since it represents iron-carrying capacity.

REQUIREMENTS

The demand for iron replenishment is constant since the life of a red corpuscle is only about 120 days. As the body removes old or damaged cells, iron is liberated. The body conserves iron well, but menstruation, pregnancy, and birth deplete stores in women (see Chapter 15). During the reproduction phase of a woman's life, iron loss is at least double that of a man or of a post-menopausal woman.

SOURCES

While liver is the best source of iron, meats, egg yolk, dark green vegetables, enriched breads and cereals all contribute significant amounts (Table 12–4).

Iron intake can also be enhanced by cooking in an iron container (Table 12–5). Acidity, moisture content, cooking time, and the amount of stirring increase the iron content of the meal. The most acidic foods produce the highest increase in iron content (Brittin and Nossaman, 1986). Of course, if the iron pan has a Teflon coating, then iron cannot be released (Beutler, 1980). Because of the continual problem of sufficient iron intake among the general public, particularly women and children, encouraging individuals to use iron utensils is often recommended.

BIOAVAILABILITY

Most of the iron in food is in the oxidized form of ferric iron (Fe^{+++}), although some ferrous iron (Fe^{++}) has been found. Ferrous iron is absorbed better than ferric iron. The reduction of ferric to ferrous iron requires an acid medium, such as that found in the stomach or ascorbic acid from the diet (Cook et al, 1984). Iron is frequently taken as a supplement; the bioavailability for various sources is given in Table 12–6.

Absorption Factors. Another important factor for iron absorption is the physiological need. Efficiency of the absorption process parallels the need for this element. In a healthy individual, as little as 10 percent may be absorbed, compared with an anemic individual who utilizes as much as 50 percent. Absorption of copper, zinc, and manganese are related to that of iron; excesses of any one in the diet causes interference with the absorption and utilization of the others (NNC, 1978). Interfering substances, such as phytates from vegetables and cereals, decrease iron availability.

In addition, combinations of food can enhance iron absorption. A meal of roast beef (rich in iron) with potatoes (rich in vitamin C) and a tossed green salad (rich in folic acid) will increase iron availability. If iron supplements are taken, a source of vitamin C plus other foods will offer the greatest absorption with the least stomach disturbance.

Heme Iron. There are two categories of iron in foods—heme and nonheme compounds. Green leafy vegetables contain nonheme iron, but this is not absorbed as well as the heme iron from meat. Generally, heme iron in animal tissues amounts to an average of 40 percent of the total iron in all animal tissues (meat, liver, poultry, and fish). Nonheme iron represents the remaining 60 percent of iron in animal tissues and all the iron of vegetable products (CDA et al, 1981). If meat and vegetables are eaten at the same time, the absorption of iron from vegetables doubles. The ascorbic acid and heme content of foods determines the classification of nonheme iron as low, medium, or high availability. Monsen and colleagues (1978) describe this method in detail. Simply estimated, 10 percent of the total iron intake is absorbed.

Table 12–4. Iron Content of Foods in Milligrams per Serving*

0.3–0.7 mg/serving	0.7–1.4 mg/serving	1.5–2 mg/serving
Fruits, e.g., apples, bananas, cherries, melons, citrus, pineapple ....avg. size	Rice, cooked (brown or white enriched) ....1 cup	Barley ....½ cup
Corn grits ....1 cup	Tortilla (6 in. diam.) 1	Buckwheat ....½ cup
Popcorn (popped) ....1 cup	Cream of Wheat ....1 cup	Oatmeal ....1 cup
Bread (all varieties) ....1 slice	Wheatena ....⅔ cup	Chicken (all cuts) ....3–4 oz.
Enriched macaroni, spaghetti or noodles ....½ cup	Wheat germ ....1 Tbsp.	Bologna ....3–4 oz.
Peanut butter ....2 Tbsp.	Dry bulgur wheat ....2 Tbsp.	Ham ....2 oz.
Mushrooms ....⅓ cup	Pumpkin seeds ....1–2 Tbsp.	Dried apricot halves ....6 large
Eggplant ....½ cup	Berries (all) ....1 cup	Green beans ....1 cup
Tomato ....1 small	Broccoli ....1 cup	Brewer's yeast ....1 Tbsp.
	Carrots ....1 cup	
	Collards ....1 cup	
	Potato ....1 med.	

2–4 mg/serving	4–5 mg/serving
Amaranth ....3½ oz.	Beef (lean only), all cuts ......3 oz.
Figs, dried ....3 med.	Lamb (lean only), all cuts ....4 oz.
Cooked peas & beans ....½ cup	Calf's liver ....1 oz.
Black strap molasses ....1 Tbsp.	Raisins ....½ cup
Tofu (soybean curd)	

*From Winick, M: Nutritional anemias. *Nutrition & Health* 6(2), 1984, with permission.

DEFICIENCIES

Even though the iron requirement could be met by most diets, iron deficiency continues to be a worldwide problem, especially among children and women of childbearing age because of its erratic absorption as well as inadequate intake (Mertz, 1983). Deficiencies of iron result in a reduced capacity and lowered resistance to infections and eventually anemia (see Chapter 34).

HEMOSIDEROSIS

Excessive iron in blood (hemosiderosis) occurs when excessive iron is present in the body, which may occur with (1) excessive iron intake, (2) multiple blood transfusions, and (3) a failure to regulate absorption.

The increased absorption of iron when taken with an alcohol-containing carrier, such as beer or wine, has long been recognized as a therapy for anemia. Inexpensive red wines, also rich in iron, contain wide variation in content (10 to 350 mg/L). Hemosiderosis is common among chronic alcoholics who may drink over a liter of inexpensive wine daily (Davidson et al, 1975).

Clinical Implications:

- Since iron-deficiency anemia is so well emphasized and iron supplements are readily available, it is not surprising that many individuals may receive excessive amounts of iron that may cause serious problems. About 2000 cases of iron poisoning occur each year in the United States; this danger has not been given enough attention.
- Approximately 6.2 percent of all acute poisonings in children are due to consumption of ferrous sulfate medications. Few individuals realize the potential danger from these brightly-colored, sugar-coated iron preparations. While it may require several hundred pills to cause acute poisoning in an adult, as few as 6 to 12 tablets have caused the death of a child (NNC, 1978).

Copper

Copper, zinc, and iron are closely interrelated, and increases or decreases of one may affect the others.

PHYSIOLOGICAL ROLES

Copper is essential for the formation of red blood cells and many enzymes and the utilization of iron. Copper appears in the plasma in the form of ceruloplasmin.

SOURCES

Copper is widely distributed in our food supply. The richest sources include shellfish, oysters, crabs, calf's liver, hickory and Brazil nuts, sesame and sunflower seeds, legumes (such as soybeans and kidney, navy, and lima beans), and molasses. Milk is extremely low in copper.

DEFICIENCIES

An intake of 2 to 3 mg/day of copper is suggested by the National Research Council. The incidence of marginal copper nutriture may be greater than suspected (Sandstead, 1982; Mertz, 1983). Recent analysis of American diets has shown that many contain less than 1 mg/day of copper. Prolonged copper deficiency has resulted in a form of anemia not corrected by copper supplements. Most copper deficiencies have been detected under unusual conditions, such as total parenteral nutrition.

Some signs of copper deficiencies have been noted in cases of children recovering from protein-energy malnutrition on a diet mainly composed of milk. Failure to grow, anemia, and disturbances in bone development are the clinical manifestations; copper supplementation will reverse the symptoms (Mertz, 1983).

TOXICITY

Wilson's disease represents a special case of copper toxicosis in which an inborn error of metabolism permits large amounts of copper to accumulate in the liver, kidney, brain, and cornea. The concentration of copper in the cornea leads to a characteristic brown or green ring called the Kayser-Fleischer ring. Except for patients with Wilson's disease, copper toxicosis is seldom encountered.

Clinical Implications:

- Copper, iron, and zinc are lost through sweat; however, more supplementary copper is required for chemical equilibrium than either zinc or iron (Jacob, et al, 1981).
- Persons who consume diets high in zinc and low in protein are at risk of copper deficiency; high dietary fiber intakes increase the dietary requirement for copper (Sandstead, 1982).

Zinc

PHYSIOLOGICAL ROLES

For over half a century, zinc has been known as an essential dietary element. A multitude of research observations have confirmed its importance for growth, reproduction, and even for life itself. There are now over 70 metalloenzymes (an enzyme plus a metal or mineral) known to require zinc for their functions.

ABSORPTION

Zinc absorption is variable and highly dependent upon several factors, i.e., body size, the level of zinc in the diet, and the presence of other potentially interfering substances, such as calcium, phytates, fiber, and the chelating agents. However, phytates are not likely to interfere with zinc's bioavailability in people consuming a typical well-balanced diet (Forbes et al, 1984).

Table 12–5. *Iron Content of Foods Through Cooking Utensils**

| Food | Cooking Time | Iron Content | | |
		Glass Dish	Iron Skillet	Increase Factor
	min.	←——	mg/100gm	——→
Apple butter	120	0.47	52.5	112
Spaghetti sauce	180	3.0	87.5	29
Gravy	20	0.43	5.9	14
Potatoes, fried	30	0.45	3.8	8
Rice casserole	45	1.4	5.2	4
Beef hash	45	1.52	5.2	3
Scrambled eggs	3	1.7	4.1	2

*From Beutler, E: Iron. In *Modern Nutrition in Health and Disease*, 6th ed. Edited by RS Goodhart; ME Shils. Philadelphia, Lea & Febiger, 1980, with permission.

Table 12–6. Bioavailability of Iron from Various Iron Sources*

Source	%
Ferrous sulfate	100
Ferrous ammonium sulfate	99
Ferrous gluconate	97
Ferric citrate	73
Ferric pyrophosphate	45
Reduced iron	37
Ferric oxide	4
Ferrous carbonate	2

*National Academy of Sciences, Washington, D.C., 1975.

Zinc and vitamin A are apparently interrelated. A marginal zinc status may affect the vitamin A status, and when both of these nutrients are deficient, there is a synergistic effect on fetal malformations (Baly et al, 1984). Zinc and copper are also closely interrelated; high levels of copper potentiate the teratogenicity of zinc deficiency. When this occurs during pregnancy in experimental animals, malformations increase as the copper intake increases with zinc deficiency (Reinstein et al, 1984).

SOURCES

Foods with a high zinc content are also high in copper (Table 12–7). Normal daily intake for zinc is 12 to 15 mg in a well-balanced American diet containing adequate animal protein. The RDA for zinc is 15 mg/day. Zinc is more available from animal sources than plants, which means that vegetarians are more likely to be deficient.

DEFICIENCIES

Zinc deficiencies may be caused by a number of problems other than dietary intake, as shown in Table 12–8. Those at particular risk of zinc deficiency include people whose zinc requirements are relatively high (such as during periods of rapid growth) and persons subsisting on a poor diet consisting primarily of cereal proteins. Some of the most rewarding results from scientific investigations with zinc deficiency have been discovered by Prasad (1966) in the Middle East.

Growth. Prasad suggested that dwarfed, hypogonadal, clay-eating boys who were being studied in Iran might be deficient in zinc. The boys had marked growth retardation and were sexually underdeveloped with no facial, pubic, or body hair. Their livers and spleens were enlarged; their skin was rough and dry; they appeared lethargic. The nutritional history was interesting in that they ate only bread made of wheat flour. They also consumed nearly one pound of clay daily in order to satisfy hunger pangs. The habit of geophagia (clay-eating) is common in their locale. Supplemental zinc with adequate animal protein intake reversed the clinical manifestations of zinc deficiency.

Other Conditions. Such conditions as liver diseases, malabsorption syndrome, thermal burns, chronic uremia, alcoholism, malnutrition, and drug intake of penicillamine or parenteral histidine may cause zinc deficiency (Prasad, 1985).

Clinical manifestations of zinc deficiency are listed in Table 12–9. Severe zinc deficiency may even result in death (Prasad, 1985). When zinc deficiency is diagnosed, zinc supplementation is vital. Supplementation in zinc-depleted individuals

Table 12–7. Zinc Content of Foods in Milligrams per Serving*

0.2 to 0.5 mg/serving	0.5 to 1 mg/serving	1 to 1.5 mg/serving
Egg....................1 med.	Puffed wheat.............1 oz.	Clams ....3 oz.
Gefilte fish....................3½ oz.	Cheddar cheese ....1 oz.	Brown rice...................1 cup
Mango....................½ med.	Tuna....................3 oz.	Whole wheat bread.............2 slices
Applesauce....................1 cup	White rice....................1 cup	Popcorn ....2 cups
Pineapple juice....................8 oz.	White bread....................2 slices	Wheat germ ....1 Tbsp.
Tomato....................1 med.	Cranberry-apple drink ....8 oz.	Bran (cooked, dried)..............¾ cup
Potato cooked ....1 med.	Chicken breast....................3 oz.	
	Milk (whole or skim)..............8 oz.	

4 to 5 mg/serving	Other	
Beef (lean only)....................3½ oz.	9.4 mg Pacific oysters (raw)..3½ oz.	
Pork (lean only)....................3½ oz.	74.7 mg Atlantic oysters (raw)..3½ oz.	
Lamb (lean only)....................3½ oz.		
Liver (beef and calf) ....3 oz.		

*From Winick, M: Nutritional anemias. *Nutrition & Health* 6(2), 1984, with permission.

Table 12–8. Causes of Zinc Deficiency*

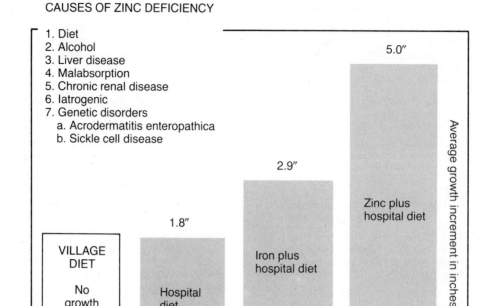

CAUSES OF ZINC DEFICIENCY

1. Diet
2. Alcohol
3. Liver disease
4. Malabsorption
5. Chronic renal disease
6. Iatrogenic
7. Genetic disorders
   a. Acrodermatitis enteropathica
   b. Sickle cell disease

Growth Response of
Zinc-Deficient Patients to Treatment

*From Prasad, AS: Nutritional zinc today. *Nutrition Today* 16(2):4, 1981. Reproduced with permission of *Nutrition Today* Magazine, P.O. Box 1829, Annapolis, MD.

is beneficial for wound healing but unnecessary for normal subjects (Prasad, 1985).

TOXICITY

Accidental consumption of high levels of zinc by humans normally causes vomiting and diarrhea but can result in renal damage, pancreatitis and even death. Thus, high zinc intake can be extremely toxic to man. Supplementation is recommended only under medical supervision.

Clinical Implications:

- Many patients with sickle-cell disease develop chronic leg ulcers that do not heal; zinc supplementation is beneficial (Prasad, 1981).
- Some patients with celiac disease who fail to respond to diet, steroids, and nutritional supplements, will make a remarkable recovery with administration of zinc (Prasad, 1981).

- Excessive zinc supplementation (10- to 20-fold excess of the RDA) could have deleterious effects by reducing immunological responses and reducing high-density lipoproteins while increasing low-density lipoproteins, thus affecting cardiovascular function (Chandra, 1984).
- High intakes of coffee, cocoa, and tea (because of their phytate content) may lower zinc levels if the zinc status is marginal (Harland & Oberless, 1985).
- Folic acid supplementation increases zinc excretion; zinc status must be satisfactory for maintenance with such supplementation (Milne et al, 1984).
- A considerable amount of zinc may be lost by excessive sweating during strenuous exercise (McDonald & Margen, 1980).
- Alcohol intake results in increased zinc excretion (McDonald & Margen, 1980).
- Some patients on total parenteral nutrition (TPN) have developed clinical manifestations of severe zinc deficiency, which can be fatal.
- An abnormality in zinc metabolism often occurs in patients with chronic renal failure, and

Table 12–9. *Manifestations of Zinc Deficiency**

Mild	Moderate	Severe
Oligospermia	Growth retardation	Bullous-pustular
Weight loss	Hypogonadism in	dermatitis
Hyperammonemia	males	Alopecia
	Skin changes	Diarrhea
	Poor appetite	Emotional disorder
	Mental lethargy	Weight loss
	Delayed wound	Intercurrent infections
	healing	Hypogonadism in
	Taste abnormalities	males
	Abnormal dark	Death
	adaptation	

*From Prasad, AS: Nutritional zinc today. *Nutr Today* 16(2):4, 1981. Reproduced with permission of *Nutrition Today* Magazine, P.O. Box 1829, Annapolis, MD.

it develops prior to the initiation of dialysis treatment (Prasad, 1981).
- Zinc supplements should be carefully monitored because of the risk of overdose.
- Large doses of zinc decrease the absorption of calcium when calcium intake is low but do not affect it if intakes are normal or higher (Spencer et al, 1985).
- Persons with abnormalities of taste due to zinc deficiency may respond to supplementation, but additional zinc is not effective in restoring normal taste acuity for other conditions.

Cobalt

Cobalt is a part of vitamin B_{12} and contributes to the formation of red blood cells. Cobalt deficiency is unknown in man since it is widely distributed in food.

Manganese

Manganese is essential in several enzyme systems, one of which is important for bone development and another for insulin production of the pancreas. Foods high in manganese are red meats, whole-grain cereals, legumes, green leafy vegetables, and tea. The manganese in green vegetables and cereals is not readily absorbed.

Usually, diets range from 2 to 5 mg/day; fre-
quently, intake is less than 2 mg/day (Kies, 1986). Vegetarian diets that contain very little absorbable manganese have resulted in poor bone healing and may put individuals at risk for osteoporosis (Saltman, 1985). The absorption of iron and manganese are inversely proportional, so a large amount of one causes a reduction in the other.

Besides being an essential trace mineral, manganese can be an environmental hazard. Inhaling manganese dusts can be toxic (Mertz, 1983). Miners in Chile, for example, have developed "manganese madness" (severe psychotic symptoms) and paralysis (Davidson et al, 1975).

Iodine

PHYSIOLOGICAL ROLES

Iodine is a part of thyroxine, the hormone secreted by the thyroid gland. It combines with the amino acid tyrosine to form thyroxine, which regulates the basal metabolic rate.

SOURCES

The only rich source of iodine is seafood. When eaten once or twice per week, the average intake is about 150 mcg/day. The best safeguard for an adequate intake is the use of iodized salt. Fortification of salt with iodine is not mandatory, so the plain unfortified salt is also available. Some health food promoters advocate sea salt, but this does not contain sufficient amounts of iodine.

Iodine supplementation of salt in the United States has been one of the most successful programs. Some areas of the world have used iodized poppyseed or walnut oil for injections or by mouth to help reduce goiter incidence. Others are contemplating iodinating water (Ziporyn, 1985).

DEFICIENCIES

More than 400 million people in Asia alone are iodine-deficient (Ziporyn, 1985). Since iodine is the essential element in thyroxine, a deficiency may cause profound metabolic and emotional influences ranging from a mild deceleration of catabolic functions, with sensitivity to cold, dry skin, mildly elevated blood lipids, and mild depression of mental functions (Mertz, 1983).

Goiters result from an iodine deficiency because the thyroid gland works harder to compensate for the deficiency. They are more prevalent in women than men. Long ago, many of the famous painters' models were women with large throats implying the prevalence of goiter. Endemic goiter occurs where the soil and/or water is low in iodine content. No particular pattern is evident for the distribution of iodine among the earth's surfaces. In childhood, the deficiency is more dramatic and results in cretinism (see Chapter 30).

Previously, goiter was considered the main disorder from low-iodine intake. However, current references to iodine deficiency disorders (IDD) include:

1. Stillbirths, abortions, and congenital anomalies.
2. Endemic cretinism usually characterized by mental deficiency, deaf mutism, and spastic diplegia and lesser degrees of neurological defect related to fetal iodine deficiency.
3. Impaired mental function of children and adults with goiter associated with subnormal concentrations of circulating thyroxine.

Iodine deficiency disorders rather than goiter is the more applicable terminology (Hetzel, 1983).

Molybdenum

The amount of molybdenum present in plants depends upon the soil content. It is more likely to be found in neutral or alkaline soils with high organic matter than in acid, sandy soil. Molybdenum has a role in iron metabolism. A very high incidence of gout in some areas of Russia has been attributed to extremely high intakes of molybdenum from local plants growing on the molybdenum-rich soil (Davidson et al, 1975).

Fluoride

PHYSIOLOGICAL ROLES

Notoriety for fluoride has come through its protection of teeth. Fluoride has been called a "bone seeker" because most of it is in the bone and dental enamel. There are some indications that an increase in fluoride intake above that normally available has a beneficial influence on skeletal tissue metabolism (see Chapter 31).

SOURCES

All foods contain some fluoride, but the amounts are insignificant (less than 1 ppm, except seafood, which may have 5 to 10 ppm). Food is not a major source of fluoride for adults, but infant foods are often fortified with fluoride.

Fluoridation of community water contributes to the intake of persons of all ages and is shown to be a practical, cost-effective means of achieving significant decreases in the prevalence of dental caries (Rao, 1984). Still, there is some discussion about the advantages of fluoridation of water when only about 1 percent is actually used for drinking. Yet, this is a universal method of reaching all socioeconomic groups and their children who are the main target population.

TOXICITY

Fluorine has the narrowest range of safe and adequate intakes of all elements. Mottling of tooth enamel results from slight overexposure, approximately three to four times the amount necessary to prevent caries (Figure 12–3). Further increases may result in toxicity (fluorosis) and bone deformities. Current fluoridation of drinking water at the level of 1 mg/L is safe (Mertz, 1983).

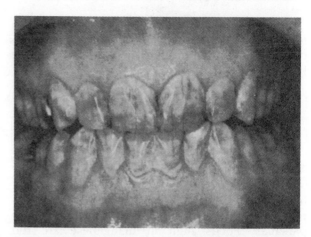

Figure 12–3. Mottled tooth enamel caused by fluorosis. (From Nizel, AE: Nutrition in Preventive Dentistry Science and Practice, 2nd ed. Philadelphia, W. B. Saunders Co, 1981, with permission.)

The ingestion of large amounts of fluoride can also result in adverse effects on skeletal tissue. These changes can increase in severity and eventually result in a general increase in bone density and considerable calcification of ligaments in the neck and vertebral column. It is difficult to determine exactly how much fluoride is required to produce these changes. A 5- to 10-fold margin of safety probably exists between the amount of fluoride needed to provide optimal protection against caries and that required for osteosclerotic changes. There is a 15- to 20-fold margin of safety against crippling fluorosis (NCC, 1978).

Clinical Implication:

- Aluminum in antacids decreases the absorption of fluoride (Spencer & Kramer, 1985).

Selenium

SOURCES

Both toxicity and deficiency have been seen in animals from irregular distribution of selenium (Se) in soil, but these are rarely seen in people. Cattle may develop chronic selenosis when they graze on soil high in selenium. Persons consuming products from such areas may first show vague symptoms of ill health such as fatigue, dizziness, or dermatitis (Rosenfield & Beath, 1964). Urinary selenium may be checked as an indicator of current dietary selenium (Sutherland et al, 1980).

Selenium concentration and biological availability of selenium in the soil determine the amount in feed and food plants. Areas with soil concentrations of less than 0.10 ppm of selenium will result in selenium deficiency disease (Combs & Combs, 1984).

A minimum of 0.05 mg and a maximum intake of 0.2 mg/day of selenium is considered safe and adequate for individuals over seven years of age. Indications suggest that adults may often exceed 0.2 mg/day without harmful effects. Selenium intake correlates closely with caloric and protein intake. Selenium in dairy products and eggs is more readily absorbed than that in other food groups (Palmer et al, 1983).

DEFICIENCIES

In the People's Republic of China, there is an endemic cardiomyopathy associated with severe selenium deficiency called Keshan disease. This disease is named for Keshan county in northeastern China where it was first described. It affects infants who have been weaned, children, and women of child-bearing age among the rural population. It has a fatality rate as high as 80 percent in the target age groups. Incidence of the disease varies with different seasons and years. These patients have the lowest blood selenium levels of any people worldwide (Combs & Combs, 1984). Oral selenium prophylaxis is extremely effective in reducing, but not completely eliminating, Keshan disease.

Chromium

PHYSIOLOGICAL ROLES

Chromium is involved in carbohydrate and lipid metabolism, especially in the utilization of glucose. Chromium is a cofactor for insulin, so a deficiency causes insulin resistance. A mild elevation of circulating insulin levels may be followed by disturbed glucose tolerance and elevated blood lipid levels. It may even develop into a syndrome closely resembling diabetes mellitus (Mertz, 1983).

SOURCES

Chromium is poorly absorbed, but it is found in meats, whole-grain cereals, brewer's yeast, and other foods. Although the minimum daily requirement of a healthy adult can be estimated with some confidence as between 0.05 and 0.02 mg/day, there is presently no way of translating this requirement into dietary recommendations.

DEFICIENCIES

Clearly identified deficiency states have not been observed, but tissues show a decrease in their amount with aging and repeated pregnancies.

Clinical Implications:

- Excessive industrial exposure to chromate dust results in increased incidence of cancer and ulcerations and irritations of the respiratory system (NNC, 1978).
- Chromium excretion is strongly dependent on the efficiency of carbohydrate metabolism; even a mild impairment of glucose tolerance has been shown to increase the chromium excretion (Mertz et al, 1977). It is not known whether increased intestinal absorption can compensate for the increased demand under these conditions.

Other Trace Minerals

Other trace minerals found in the body include aluminum, lead, cadmium, mercury, boron, tin, vanadium, silicon, and nickel. However, their physiological roles have not been identified, and it is not known whether they are essential to health. More attention has been given to them as contaminants in the environment and foods. Some are considered to have no harmful effects and are used therapeutically, such as aluminum in antacids.

• FALLACIES and FACTS

FALLACY: All women should take iron supplements throughout life.
- **FACT:** No supplementation should be taken unless laboratory tests show a deficiency and a physician prescribes the type and amount.

FALLACY: Bone meal or dolomite should be taken as calcium supplements.
- **FACT:** The search for a natural supplement of calcium, magnesium, phosphorus, and other minerals from a living source led to the recommendation of bone meal. Since this may come from the bones of old animals that have accumulated lead over their lifetime, prolonged use of bone meal can result in lead poisoning. An individual must always question whether such supplements have appropriate sanitation and quality control.

FALLACY: Sea salt is superior to regular salt.
- **FACT:** Sea salt contains chiefly sodium chloride along with small amounts of magnesium chloride, magnesium sulfate, and calcium sulfate. In the amounts usually ingested, the quantity of these other minerals is nutritionally insignificant. It is important to note that sea salt loses iodine in the drying process; therefore it is not considered a source of iodine. Iodized salt is the best choice. No evidence suggests that sea salt is more nutritious than ordinary table salt (Dubick & Rucker, 1983).

FALLACY: A selenium dietary supplement cures cancer, heart disease, sexual dysfunction, arthritis, various infectious diseases, heavy-metal poisoning, poor eyesight, skin and hair problems, and aging.
- **FACT:** A cause-and-effect relationship between selenium and disease in humans has yet to be established. In general, no evidence exists for selenium deficiency in the United States. It is estimated that a well-balanced diet furnishes about 0.15 mg/day, and an adequate and safe intake range for adults is 0.5 to 0.2 mg/day. There is no justification for recommending selenium supplementation for the general population.

FALLACY: Large doses of zinc increase virility and improve the sex drive.
- **FACT:** No evidence exists that zinc supplementation offers these benefits.

FALLACY: Athletes who are performing at maximum levels need supplements of magnesium, copper, and zinc.
- **FACT:** Physical training produces no deficiencies of these minerals; they are not needed as extra supplements (Lukaski et al, 1983).

FALLACY: Marinating less expensive cuts of meat tenderizes the meat.
- **FACT:** Marination improves tenderness only slightly. At the same time, substantial amounts of valuable minerals (zinc, magnesium, and iron) are lost with marination, and sodium content is increased (Howat et al, 1983). Cooking meat slowly with moisture for longer periods of time can enhance tenderness. Acids, such as those from tomatoes or wine, also help tenderize tough meat.

FALLACY: Senior citizens should drink hot coffee or tea with their meals.
- **FACT:** A warm beverage or soup or a glass of wine before meals will start the diges-

tive juices flowing and improve diges-tion, but there are other matters to con-sider. Coffee and tea both decrease the absorption of iron. The stronger the coffee or tea, the more iron is lost. No decrease in iron absorption occurs when coffee is drunk one hour before a meal, but the same degree of inhibition as with simultaneous ingestion is seen when coffee is taken one hour after the meal (Morch et al, 1983).

Summary

Mineral elements differ from other nutrients because they are available from sources other than food intake. Air pollution, direct contact of the skin or sources such as drinking water complicate assessment. Diets consisting of only a few foods may be not only missing needed trace elements but also polluted by the environment to give additional hazards.

Distribution of trace elements is uneven and constantly changing. It may not be possible to establish one ideal intake or requirement for an individual trace element. A definitive range over which homeostasis is effective is more logical. Supplements in excess of the safe and adequate intake ranges are dangerous. Large intakes of one trace element may be toxic and interfere with the absorption and/or metabolism of other trace elements.

Marginal deficiencies produce mild indications that something may be wrong, such as mild changes in glucose tolerance or blood lipids or slight impairment of taste acuity or wound healing. Growth rates may be slightly or dramatically altered, or immunity may be weakened against bacterial, viral, or chemical agents.

Since diagnostic procedures have not been developed to detect marginal toxicity adequately, trace elements should be obtained from a well-balanced diet, not from supplements.

Review Questions

1. A patient claims that she cannot drink milk. How would you advise her?
2. What are the main physiological roles of iron, fluoride, selenium and zinc?
3. How do trace elements differ from vitamins?
4. Why are iodine and fluoride supplemented for the general intake of the population but iron is not?
5. How would you respond to the remark that milk is only for babies?
6. Name other minerals or vitamins that either are required for metabolism of the mineral or function in such similar ways that they are called "sparers" for each other.
   - A. Calcium: _____ and _____
   - B. Selenium: _____
   - C. Sodium: _____
   - D. Zinc: _____ and _____
7. How can the iron content of foods be increased?
8. Name some trace elements that may be useful as well as poisonous to humans.
9. A patient who is slightly overweight and anemic is advised by a cook that red meats contain more calories than chicken and fish. Therefore, she decided to delete red meats from her diet. What advice would you offer her?

Case Study: Mrs. J.M. has been admitted to the unit for chronic alcoholism. On admission, she is noted to have hyperactive deep tendon reflexes and tremors. Laboratory data on admission reveal decreased serum magnesium.

1. What signs would you expect to see on physical examination?
2. What is the effect of increased calcium intake on serum magnesium?
3. Hypomagnesemia is clinically similar to what other electrolyte imbalance?
4. What other conditions may lead to decreased serum magnesium levels?
5. What effect would increased vitamin D have on serum magnesium?

REFERENCE LIST

Allen, LH: Calcium absorption and requirements during the life span. *Nutr News* 47(1):1, 1984.
Baly, DL; Golub, MS; Gershwin, ME; et al: Studies of marginal zinc deprivation on rhesus monkeys. III. Effects on vitamin A metabolism. *Am J Clin Nutr* 40(2):199, 1984.
Beutler, E: Iron. In *Modern Nutrition in Health and Disease*, 6th ed. Edited by RS Goodhart; ME Shils. Philadelphia, Lea & Febiger, 1980, p. 324.
Brittin, HC; and Nossaman, CE: Iron content of food cooked in iron utensils. *J Amer Diet Assoc* 86(7):897, 1986.
Calcium the forgotten nutrient. *Nutr Health News* 1(4):1, 1984.
Chandra, RK: Excessive intake of zinc impairs immune responses. *JAMA* 252(11):1443, 1984.
Chicago Dietetic Association (CDA) and South Suburban Dietetic Association of Cook and Will Counties: *Manual of*

Clinical Dietetics, 2nd ed. Philadelphia, W. B. Saunders Co., 1981.

Cook, JD; Watson, SS; Simpson, KM; et al: The effect of high ascorbic acid supplementation on body iron stores. *Blood* 64(3):721, 1984.

Combs, GF Jr; Combs, SB: The nutritional biochemistry of selenium. *Ann Rev Nutr* 4:257, 1984.

Davidson, Sir S; Passmore, R; Brock, JF; et al: *Human Nutrition and Dietetics*, 6th ed. New York, Churchill Livingstone, 1975.

Dubick, MA; Rucker, RB: Dietary supplements and health aids—a critical evaluation. Part 1. Vitamins and minerals. *J Nutr Ed* 15(2):47, 1983.

Forbes, RM; Parker, HM; Erdman, JW, Jr: Effects of dietary phytate, calcium, and magnesium levels on zinc bioavailability to rats. *J Nutr* 114(8):1421, 1984.

Gibson, RS; Anderson, BM; Scythes, CA: Regional differences in hair concentrations: A possible effect of water hardness. *Am J Clin Nutr* 37(1):37, 1983.

Harland, BF; Oberleas, D: Phytate and zinc contents of coffees, cocoas, and teas. *J Food Science* 50(3):832, 1985.

Hetzel, BS: Iodine deficiency disorders (IDD) and their eradication. *Lancet* 2(November 12):1126, 1983.

Howat, PM; Sievert, LM; Myers, PJ; et al: Effect of marination upon mineral content and tenderness of beef. *J Food Sci* 48(2):662, 1983.

Jacob, RA; Sandstead, HH; Munoz, JM; et al: Whole body surface loss of trace metals in normal males. *Am J Clin Nutr* 34(7):1379, 1981.

Kelly, SE; Shawla-Singh, K; Sellin; et al: Effect of meal composition on calcium absorption: Enhancing effect of carbohydrate polymers. *Gastroenterology* 87(3):596, 1984.

Kies, C: Bioavailability of manganese. Presented at *American Chemical Society Symposium: Bioavailability of Manganese*, September 8, 1986.

Lewis, CM: *Nutrition and Diet Therapy: Vitamins and Minerals.* Philadelphia, F. A. Davis Co., 1976.

Lukaski, HC; Bolonchuk, WW; Kelevay, LM; et al: Maximal oxygen consumption as related to magnesium, copper, and zinc nutriture. *Am J Clin Nutr* 37(3):407, 1983.

McCarron, DA: Calcium and magnesium nutrition in human hypertension. *Ann Intern Med* 98(5 Part 2):800, 1983.

McDonald, JT; Margen, S: Wine versus alcohol in human nutrition. IV. Zinc balance. *Am J Clin Nutr* 33(5):1096, 1980.

Mertz, W: Our most unique nutrients. *Nutr Today* 18(2):6, 1983.

Mertz, W; Wolf, WR; Roginski, EE: Relation of chromium excretion to glucose metabolism in human subjects. *Fed Proc* 36:1152, 1977.

Milne, DB; Canfield, WK; Mahalko, JR; et al: Effect of oral folic acid supplements on zinc, copper, and iron absorption and excretion. *Am J Clin Nutr* 39(4):535, 1984.

Morch, TA; Lynch, SR; Cook, JD: Inhibition of food iron absorption by coffee. *Am J Clin Nutr* 37(3):416, 1983.

National Dairy Council (NDC): The role of calcium in health. *Dairy Council Digest* 55(1), 1984.

National Institutes of Arthritis, Diabetes, and Digestive and Kidney Diseases (NIADDKD): Consensus Conference: Osteoporosis. *JAMA* 252:799, 1984.

National Nutrition Consortium, Inc (NNC): *Vitamin-mineral Safety, Toxicity and Misuse.* Chicago, American Dietetic Assoc., 1978.

Palmer, S; Olson, DE; Ketterling, LM; et al: Selenium intake and urinary excretion in persons living near a high selenium area. *J Am Diet Assoc* 82(5):511, 1983.

Pennington, JAT; Young, BE; Johnson, RD; et al: Mineral content of foods and total diets: The selected minerals in foods survey, 1982 to 1984. *J Amer Diet Assoc* 86(7):876, 1986.

Prasad, AS: Clinical manifestations of zinc deficiency. *Ann Rev Nutr* 5:341, 1985.

Prasad, AS: Nutritional zinc today. *Nutr Today* 16(2):4, 1981.

Prasad, AS: *Zinc Metabolism.* Springfield, IL, Charles C Thomas Co., 1966.

Rao, GS: Dietary intake and bioavailability of fluoride. *Ann Rev Nutr* 4:115, 1984.

Reinstein, NK; Lonnerdal, B; Keen, CL; et al: Zinc-copper interactions in the pregnant rat: Fetal outcome and maternal and fetal zinc, copper and iron. *J Nutr* 114(6):1266, 1984.

Rodman, JS; Reidenberg, MM: Symptomatic hypokalemia resulting from surreptitious diuretic ingestion. *JAMA* 246(15):1687, 1981.

Rosenfeld, I; Beath, DA: *Selenium, Geobotany, Biochemistry, Toxicity and Nutrition.* New York, Academic Press, 1964.

Saltman, P: Trace minerals in health and disease. In *Frontiers in Longevity Research.* Edited by RJ Morin. Springfield, IL, Charles C Thomas, 1985, p 162.

Sandstead, HH: Copper bioavailability and requirements. *Am J Clin Nutr* 35(4):809, 1982.

Sandstrom, B; Davidsson, L; Cederblad, A; et al: Oral iron, dietary ligands, and zinc absorption. *J Nutr* 115(3):411, 1985.

Shils, ME: Magnesium. In *Modern Nutrition in Health and Disease*, 6th ed. Edited by RS Goodhart; ME Shils. Philadelphia, Lea & Febiger, 1980, p. 310.

Spencer, H: Minerals and mineral interactions in human beings. *J Amer Diet Assoc* 86(7):864, 1986.

Spencer, H; Kramer, L; Norris, C; et al: Effect of small doses of aluminum-containing antacids on calcium and phosphorus metabolism. *Am J Clin Nutr* 36:32, 1982.

Spencer, H; Kramer, L; Osis, D: Effect of calcium on phosphorus metabolism in man. *Am J Clin Nutr* 40(8):219, 1984.

Spencer, H; Kramer, L: Osteoporosis: Calcium, fluoride, and aluminum interactions. *J Am Coll Nutr* 4:121, 1985.

Spencer, H; Kramer, L; Derler, J; et al: Studies of zinc metabolism during nutritional repletion. *Fed Proc* 44:1278, 1985.

Spencer, H; Kramer, L; Norris, C; et al: Inhibitory effect of zinc on the intestinal absorption of calcium. *Clin Res* 33:872, 1985.

Sutherland, B; Levander, DA; King, JC: Biochemical and physiological changes with selenium depletion and repletion in young men: Possible parameters for selenium status assessment. *Fed Proc* 39(3):435, 1980.

Ziporyn, T: For many, endemic goiter remains a baffling problem. *JAMA* 253:1846, 1985.

Further Study

Asseth, J; Thomassen, Y; Norheim, G: Decreased serum selenium in alcoholic cirrhosis. *N Engl J Med* 303(16):944, 1980.

Deluca, HF; Anast, CS (eds): *Pediatric Diseases Related to Calcium.* New York, Elsevier Science Publishing Co, 1980.

Dutta, SK; Miller, PA; Greenberg, LB; et al: Selenium and acute alcoholism. *Am J Clin Nutr* 30(11):713, 1983.

Felver, L: Understanding the electrolyte maze. *Am J Nurs* 80(9):1591, 1980.

Freeland-Graves, JH; Ebangit, ML; Bodzy, PW: Zinc and copper content of foods used in vegetarian diets. *J Am Diet Assoc* 77(6):648, 1980.

Gillies, ME; Paulin, HV: Estimations of daily mineral intakes from drinking water. *Hum Nutr Appl Nutr* 36A(4):287, 1982.

Greger, JL; Krystofiak, M: Phosphorus intake of Americans. *Food Tech* 35(12):78, 1981.

Hallberg, L: Iron absorption and iron deficiency. *Hum Nutr Clin Nutr* 36C(4):259, 1982.

Institute of Food Technologists. Dietary Salt. *Food Tech* 34(1):85, 1980.

Kaehny, WD; Hegg, AP; Alfrey, AC: Gastrointestinal absorption of aluminum from aluminum-containing antacids. *N Engl J Med* 296(24):1389, 1977.

Lawler, MR; Klevay, LM: Copper and zinc in selected foods. *J Am Diet Assoc* 84(9):1028, 1984.

Lindner, PG: Caution: All potassium supplements are not the same! *Obesity & Bariatric Med* 10(4):87, 1981.

McFadden, EA; Zaloga, GP; Chernow, B: Hypocalcemia: A medical emergency. *Am J Nurs* 83(2):227, 1983.

Monsen, ER; Hallberg, L; Layrisse, H; et al: Estimation of available dietary iron. *Am J Clin Nutr* 31(1):134, 1978.

Swanson, CA; King, JC: Human zinc nutrition. *J Nutr Ed* 11(4):181, 1979.

Tsongas, TA; Meglen, RR; Walravens, PA; et al: Molybdenum in diet: An estimate of average daily intake in the United States. *Am J Clin Nutr* 33(5):1103, 1980.

Wheater, RH: Aluminum and Alzheimer's disease. *JAMA* 253(15):2288, 1985.

Zoller, JM; Wolinsky, I; Paden, CA; et al: Fortification of non-staple food items with iron. *Food Tech* 34(1):38, 1980.

Food Sanitation
and Safety

13

THE STUDENT WILL BE ABLE TO:

- **Discuss toxicity versus the hazards of various food substances.**
- **List the four microorganisms responsible for most food-related illnesses.**
- **Discuss ways that nurses can help prevent foodborne illnesses.**
- **State four reasons to include additives in foods.**

OBJECTIVES

Aflatoxin
Bactericidal
Bacteriostatic
Botulism
Half-life
Hazard
Immunosuppression
Immunoincompetence
Mycotoxin
Pathogenesis
Salmonellosis
Staphylococcus
Tolerance
Toxicity
Trichinosis

TERMS TO KNOW

Foods contain thousands of chemicals; only a few are necessary for health. In addition to the essential nutrients supplied by food, the diet contains toxic and non-nutritive substances that may interact with nutrients or have no effect. These substances are either present naturally in foods or have been purposely added during processing (Fig. 13–1). Microorganisms are also found in foods; some are pathogenic while others are beneficial. Americans expect hygienically safe, nutritious foods as a basic component of life. Few understand chemicals; in a recent survey, 19% of the respondents felt chemicals are *never* good for us (McNutt et al, 1986).

Not only is the nutritional value of foods important, but also the possibility of harmful substances in the food must be considered. These harmful substances may be (1) natural, (2) inten-

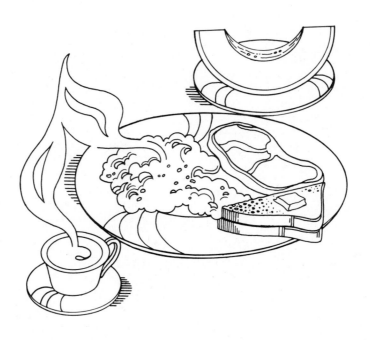

Coffee:

Caffeine
Methanol
Ethanol
Butanol
Methylbutanol
Acetaldehyde
Methyl formate
Dimethyl sulfide
Propionaldehyde
Pyridine
Acetic Acid
Furfural
Furfuryl alcohol
Acetone
Methyl acetate
Furan
Methylfuran
Diacetyl
Isoprene
Guaiacol
Hydrogen sulfide

Scrambled Eggs:

Biotin
Pantothenic acid
Riboflavin
  (vitamin B$_2$)
Thiamin
  (vitamin B$_1$)
Niacin
Pyridoxine
  (vitamin B$_6$)
Folic acid
  (folacin)
Cyanocobalamin
  (vitamin B$_{12}$)
Sodium chloride
Iron
Calcium
Phosphorus

Ovalbumin
Conalbumin
Ovomucoid
Mucin
Globulins
Amino acids
Lipovitellin
Livetin
Cholesterol
Lecithin
Choline
Lipids
  (fats)
Fatty acids
Lutein
Zeaxanthin
Vitamin A

Chilled cantaloupe:

Starches
Cellulose
Pectin
Fructose
Sucrose
Glucose
Malic acid
Citric acid
Succinic acid
Anisyl propionate
Amyl acetate
Ascorbic acid
  (vitamin C)
Beta-carotene
  (vitamin A)
Riboflavin
  (vitamin B$_2$)
Thiamin
  (vitamin B$_1$)
Niacin
Phosphorus
Potassium

Figure 13–1. *Naturally occurring chemicals in foods (listings are not necessarily complete). (Adapted from* Good Morning! Your Breakfast Chemicals. *Chemical Manufacturers Association, 2501 M Street, NW, Washington, DC, 20037, by permission.)*

tionally added, (3) unintentionally added from the environment or during processing, or (4) contaminated with microorganisms.

The possible problems of chronic exposure to toxic chemicals in processed and unprocessed food products are receiving considerable attention. Cancer, the second major cause of death in the United States, is possibly a cumulative disease caused by certain chemicals present in the environment and foods (Eys, 1984). While these factors are being investigated and are closely monitored, problems can even result from excessive ingestion of some dietary constituents that are essential in lesser quantities. For example, small amounts of vitamins A and D are essential, but large amounts have a toxic effect. Likewise, problems also arise from improper food handling, by both the consumer and producer.

The increased sensitivity of some individuals to normally nontoxic levels of particular foodborne substances or additives evokes allergic responses (see Chapter 35). This chapter addresses the potential hazards of ingesting known toxicants, contaminants, additives, and microorganisms and the problems caused by improper food handling.

Naturally-Occurring Food Toxicants

Toxicity is the capacity of a chemical substance to harm living organisms; a hazard has the capacity to produce injury under normal conditions of use (Strong, 1976). All substances are potentially toxic at some level; they are hazardous if large enough quantities are consumed. In general, only those substances capable of being harmful in small amounts are considered poisonous. Only a few chemicals naturally present in foods have been evaluated for toxicity. The risks involved vary with different toxicants and levels. In some instances, the risks must be weighed against the benefits. Specific regulations governing the use of chemical toxins in the U.S. food supply have established allowable tolerance levels, i.e., the amount of a contaminant that permits a food item to be considered unadulterated. Allowable levels must consider how the body metabolizes the chemical as well as toxicological data of similar substances.

In addition to the potential dangers of certain chemicals in foods, many microorganisms are commonly found. Problems occur from these organisms as a result of faulty processing, storage, or preparation.

INTRINSIC TISSUE COMPONENTS

Our diet consists of foods that are readily available; these foods seem to have agreed with our forefathers—in other words, they did not cause any immediate discomfort or death. Toxic chemicals present in most foods are too low to be harmful in amounts ordinarily consumed. In most instances, the body has metabolic ways of degrading, detoxifying, eliminating, or dealing effectively with most chemicals found in foods, provided excessive amounts of any one chemical are not consumed at any one time. If a person were to eat a year's normal intake of fish at one sitting, s/he might die from the natural content of arsenic. Certain species of mushrooms and the puffer fish contain poisons that are deadly even in small amounts.

Additionally, the hazards produced by these toxicants in a varied diet are relatively low for several reasons. The concentrations are so low that a grossly exaggerated consumption of food is required, usually over an extended period of time, to present a hazard. The toxicities of many chemicals in our diet are not cumulative. Many antagonistic interactions occur so that the toxicity of one element is offset by an adequate amount of another.

Foodborne toxicants can cause a decrease in nutrient availability or utilization, or they may damage the gastrointestinal tract and thereby adversely affect absorption (Taylor, 1982). Table 13–1 shows the many substances found in foods that affect nutritional status. Other chemicals in foods have other health-related effects; e.g., myristicin found in carrots is a hallucinogen.

Foodborne intoxications are usually associated with unusual dietary habits such as consumption of strange foods, foods prepared by abnormal methods, or excessive amounts of certain foods. Most of the nutrient-toxicant interactions are insignificant in terms of creating a health hazard.

Clinical Implication:

- Individuals who voluntarily adopt an unusual dietary pattern may consume excessive amounts of particular foods; they run the risk of encountering problems.

Table 13–1. Foodborne Toxicants

Food Factors	Nutrients Affected/Mechanism	Food Sources
Dietary fiber	Decreases absorption of minerals, vitamins, protein.	Plants.
Phytates	Decreased availability of zinc.	Oilseeds, grains.
Oxalates	Decreased absorption of calcium; implicated in kidney stones.	Spinach, rhubarb, tea, cocoa, beet greens, poke.
Gossypol	Decreased availability of iron, other minerals, protein.	Cottonseed.
Tannins	Decreased availability of protein, vitamin B_{12}, glucose, iron.	Many plants, tea.
Avidin (destroyed by cooking)	Binds with biotin.	Raw eggs.
Thiaminase	Decreases availability of thiamin.	Shellfish, carp, blackberries, red beets, Brussels sprouts, red cabbage, currants.
Pressor amines	Increases blood pressure.	Cheese, avocados, bananas, lemons.
Trypsin inhibitors (destroyed by cooking)	Inhibits protein digestion.	Raw soybeans, legumes.
Ovoinhibitor	Inhibits protein digestion.	Eggs.
Ovomucoid	Inhibits protein digestion.	Eggs.
Amylase inhibitors	Inhibits carbohydrate digestion	Legumes.
Dicumarol	Interferes with vitamin B and thrombin production.	Sweet clover, herbal teas.
Goitrogens	Inhibits iodine uptake by thyroid.	Cabbage, cauliflower, Brussels sprouts, broccoli, kale, kohlrabi, turnips, rutabagas, horseradish.
Phlorizin	Inhibits glucose absorption.	Apple bark and seeds.
Solanine	Anticholinesterase (transmission of nerve impulses).	Greenness under potato skins.
Saponins	Complexes with cholesterol reducing plasma cholesterol levels; causes hemolysis, diarrhea, and vomting when taken in large amounts.	Alfalfa, soybeans.

PATHOGENIC ORGANISMS

Many foods are an excellent culture medium in which organisms thrive. Microorganisms require (1) certain nutrients, (2) moisture, and (3) a neutral or slightly acidic pH environment. Foods naturally supply all these elements, and the microorganisms will thrive if they are also given (4) warmth and (5) time in which to multiply. Many organisms are naturally present in foods, while others are added unintentionally during food preparation and handling.

While illness from microbial contamination is rarely fatal, food contamination is of concern for several reasons. It can result in death, especially in immunosuppressed patients who cannot form antibodies to antigens present. Besides the discomfort of the illness, long-term factors may be associated with food contamination; the immune function is compromised and predisposes the individual to other infections. Economic factors may have far-reaching effects—from days absent from work to potential law suits. There is no excuse for serving contaminated food to people.

The "infamous four" microorganisms—*Staphylococcus aureus, Clostridium perfringens, Salmonella,* and *Clostridium botulinum*—account for 94 percent of all food-related illnesses. Although foodborne diseases do not have to be reported to public health authorities, between 1,400,000 and 3,400,000 cases are estimated to occur yearly (Foster, 1982). Characteristics of the illnesses, prevention, and therapeutic measures for those four microorganisms are shown in Table 13–2.

Foodborne infections are caused when specific bacteria are present in the food. *Salmonella* and *C. perfringens* bacteria grow and reproduce in the intestines to cause illness. When specific bacteria grow in the food and produce a toxin or poison, which causes the illness, food intoxication occurs. *Staphylococcus* and botulism organisms produce harmful toxins.

Botulism. *Clostridium botulinum* produces a toxin that affects the human nervous system and is often fatal. The organism is widely distributed in nature and occurs in cultivated and forest soils and water. The spores produced are anaerobic and remarkably resistant to heat, chemicals, and radiation. The neurotoxin enters the circulatory system via the small intestine when contaminated food is eaten. Foods involved in botulism vary according to food preservation and eating habits; al-

Table 13–2. Summary of Common Foodborne Organisms

Illness or Organism	Incubation Period	Duration	Symptoms	Foods Implicated	Prevention	Treatment
Salmonella	6–36 hours (usually 12 hours)	1–3 days	Diarrhea, nausea, abdominal cramps, prostration, chills, fever, and vomiting. Severe cases resemble typhoid.	Raw meat and poultry; cracked eggs and egg products; salads; milk and milk products; gravies, sauces, and warmed-over food.	Wash hands; adequately cook foods; immediate and adequate refrigeration of foods; clean work surfaces.	Rehydration.
Clostridium perfringens	8–24 hours	12–24 hours	Abdominal cramps, intestinal gas, and diarrhea; rarely, fever or vomiting.	Meats inadequately cooked and allowed to cook slowly or stand at room temperature.	Serve meats directly after cooking or refrigerate rapidly between cooking and serving.	Self-limited disease.
Clostridium botulinum	8–72 hours	Weeks; death may occur in 4–8 days	Early signs include fatigue, weakness, vertigo, and dry mouth followed by blurred vision and progressive difficulty in speaking and swallowing; bilateral sixth nerve dysfunction with or without ptosis or pupillary abnormalities.	Home-canned vegetables improperly processed—especially string beans, asparagus, spinach, and smoked fish.	Pressure cooking of home canned foods, especially vegetables.	Maintain adequate ventilation; trivalent antitoxin.
Staphylococcus	2–4 hours	Less than 24 hours	Abrupt and violent onset of nausea, vomiting, explosive diarrhea, prostration. No fever.	Cooked ham or other meats, cream-filled or custard pastries, and other dairy products; chicken, fish, meat, or potato salads; gravies, sauces, and dressings.	Handle food as little as possible with bare hands. Thoroughly cook foods; refrigerate foods immediately after cooking; frequent hand washing. Persons with infected lesions or nasal discharges should not be permitted to handle food.	Rehydration; antiemetics.
Trichinosis	24–72 hours (acute)	Year or more	Vomiting, cramps, and diarrhea for 2–3 days; followed by muscle pain and tenderness, fever, periorbital edema which subsides about one month after onset.	Inadequately cooked pork and pork products; whale, bear, walrus, and seal meats.	Adequate cooking of pork and pork products.	ACTH or corticosteroids.

most any type of nonacidic food will support growth and toxin formation, but botulism is typically found in foods kept in hermetically-sealed containers. All bulging cans should be discarded without being opened. Both the bacteria and toxin are destroyed by cooking or boiling for 10 minutes.

Salmonella. Foods can contain several species of *Salmonella*, which grow in the gastrointestinal tract and release an endotoxin. The microbe, which causes salmonellosis, is an inhabitant of the intestinal tract of all animals. Mishandling of poultry, meat, and dairy products is the most frequent cause of outbreaks. After an incubation period, sudden onsets of crampy, abdominal pain and diarrhea, occasionally containing mucus or blood, accompanies nausea and a low-grade fever. *Salmonella* is of increasing concern to public health officials because the number and severity of outbreaks are increasing yearly (Gast, 1985). According to the National Center for Disease Control (CDC), *Salmonella* infections were estimated at 3 to 4 million cases in 1984, with the disease probably contributing to several hundred deaths (Parmley, 1986).

Clostridium perfringens. While *C. perfringens* is widely distributed in the soil as well as the gastrointestinal tract, extensive growth of this microbe in food is necessary to cause illness. *C. perfringens* contamination can be classified as foodborne infection and intoxication. The organism inside the gastrointestinal tract grows and produces spores. A toxin is released from the spores that causes the symptoms. The microorganism is anaerobic with rather fastidious nutritional requirements—several preformed amino acids and vitamins. Meat, poultry, soups, and gravies are the foods generally implicated. Unlike other foodborne illnesses, nausea and vomiting are rare; the typical symptoms are abdominal cramps and pronounced diarrhea.

Staphylococcus aureus. Cases of true food poisoning are caused by *S. aureus*. These bacteria are usually present in the noses of 50 percent of healthy people and on the hands of 20 percent (Madlin et al, 1982). The microbes grow, producing an enterotoxin, which causes inflammation and irritation of the lining of the stomach and intestinal tract. The food poisoning can occur without demonstrating the presence of viable microorganisms in the food; only the toxin is needed. This is the most common type of foodborne illness occurring in the United States and is popularly called ptomaine poisoning. Foods contaminated with *Staphylococcus* do not have any obnoxious odors or flavor changes.

Mycotoxins. Fungal toxins (mycotoxins) naturally infect foodstuffs and often in spite of people's efforts. As certain food molds grow, mycotoxins are produced. Aflatoxin B_1, which is a fungal metabolite, is the most potent hepatic carcinogen known. Aflatoxins grow on grain and nut products such as peanuts, corn, cottonseed, soybeans, and other grains. Aflatoxins can grow very rapidly and contaminate the grain in the fields or stored under humid conditions.

The presence of aflatoxins cannot be determined by visual inspection. However, minute amounts of aflatoxin can be detected by available instruments, and the FDA enforces an upper limit on the aflatoxin content of foods. (Until 1960, only parts per million could be measured; now parts per trillion are routinely measured.)

Neither the taste nor the nutritive value of the food is affected by the presence of these organisms. It is not known how susceptible humans are to the toxic effect of aflatoxins. While aflatoxins are not immediately lethal, their effects are cumulative, being stored in fatty tissues.

The presence of visible mold does not mean aflatoxin is present, but excessively moldy foods should be discarded or returned to the store. Products such as peanuts that are processed into peanut butter in a local store may be a possible source of aflatoxin, because of the lack of controls or testing on the raw product used. Peanuts and other nuts in the shell should be examined before consumption; moldly, badly damaged, or shriveled nuts should be discarded.

Escherichia coli. A pathogenic toxin is produced by *E. coli*, which is a major cause of childhood diarrhea in developing nations and is the leading cause of travelers' diarrhea (see Chapter 28). Caused by endogenous bacteria in the gut, it was previously believed to be transmitted from person to person or through water contaminated with fecal material. Worldwide, several foods have been implicated in diarrheal outbreaks: meats, dairy products, vegetables, baked products, and coffee substitutes (Kronacki & Martyh, 1982; Taylor et al, 1982).

OTHER FOODBORNE ORGANISMS

Because food is a good culture medium, other infectious agents may be present including those that cause shigellosis or bacillary dysentery, streptococcal infections (such as strep throat or scarlet fever), brucellosis or undulant fever (especially from the raw milk of infected animals), tularemia or rabbit fever and infectious hepatitis. Eating raw shellfish may result in either bacterial gastroenteritis or hepatitis A infections. While the FDA has established strict requirements for harvesting and handling raw shellfish, frequent cases are reported in the United States, Europe, and Australia (Morse et al, 1986; Dupont, 1986). Trichinae, tapeworms, and other parasites may also be present in foods.

Trichinosis. Trichinae are tiny microscopic worms that live in the muscles; trichinosis is prevalent in hogs fed uncooked garbage. The parasites are killed by cooking the meat to 77°C (Kotula et al, 1982) or by freezing it for 20 days after purchasing it. Humans become hosts to the trichinae when they eat infected pork that is not fully cooked. Treatment is usually with ACTH or corticosteroids.

Amebic Dysentery. The parasitic protozoa *Entamoeba histolytica* causes amebic dysentery. It is transmitted through feces from a carrier who has not washed his/her hands, or by water contaminated with feces. The cyst from the ameba grows in the intestine and then burrows into the lining. Ulcers in the gastrointestinal tract and erosion of the mucosa cause profuse and bloody diarrhea.

PREVENTION OF FOODBORNE ILLNESSES

Preventing foodborne disease is usually a matter of sanitary food production and handling techniques. Foods are normally processed to destroy pathogenic organisms (bactericidal methods) and/or to prevent their growth (bacteriostatic methods). Food preservation also attempts to maintain optimum qualities of color, flavor, texture, and nutritive value.

Heat. Cooking kills most microorganisms, depending on the length of time and temperatures used.

Foods are frequently kept at cold temperatures to inhibit the growth of bacteria. Refrigerator temperatures (35–50°F) will retard spoilage by inhibiting the growth rate or pathogenic microorganisms; freezer temperatures (below 32°F) inhibit the growth of all microorganisms (Fig. 13–2). Neither refrigeration nor freezing methods are bacteriocidal but rather bacteriostatic.

Drying. Dehydration of foods prevents growth of microorganisms because they cannot grow without water. Freeze-drying is a process for removing water while the food is frozen.

Chemical Preservatives. The growth of microorganisms can be deterred by the use of chemical preservatives, which are discussed later in the chapter.

Fermentation. Fermentation is a method of utilizing microorganisms to preserve foods from pathogenic organisms. This oldest form of preservation is used in making cheese, bread, and wine. The end products of bacterial growth are inhibitory to the growth of pathogenic microorganisms. The addition of microorganisms to foods is considered a food additive (Smith & Palumbo, 1981).

Irradiation. Food irradiation is another food preservation technique to prevent food spoilage. Short-wavelength gamma rays, similar to x-rays, are used on foods to kill insects, bacteria, yeast, and molds that often contaminate foods and cause illness. The organisms are killed by very low dosages, so the food itself does not become radioactive. Changes in the food are similar to those of cooking the product, only slightly affecting color, taste, and texture.

In the United States, irradiation is permitted to sterilize spices, to inhibit potatoes from sprouting, to control organisms in stored wheat, wheat flour and fresh pork, and for foods used in the space program. Irradiation of fresh pork affects possible trichina worms that may be present so they cannot reproduce in the human body; the approved dosage is too low to kill other potential food poisons. The shelf life of pork is not extended by the process. Irradiation could be extended to kill insects on fruits and vegetables, thus eliminating the use of some pesticides, such as ethylene dibromide (EDB).

Safe Food-Handling Procedures. In health care, safe food-handling procedures are of paramount importance. Cleanliness and proper hygienic procedures cannot be overemphasized. Most foodborne illnesses are caused by consumers and food-service enterprises not following rules for safe food handling. Because of the debilitated conditions of patients as a result of illness or various medical therapies, many are extremely susceptible to problems caused by microorganisms. The following rules are not an extensive list for food handlers working directly with food, but are precautions for health care workers involved in delivering food to patients or maintaining a small on-the-floor kitchen for between-meal feedings.

1. Hot foods should be kept above 140°F until served; cold foods should be kept below 40°F until served. (The bacteria count can double every 15 to 30 minutes in cooked foods that are allowed to cool to between 45°F and 140°F.) Don't let food ready to serve stand longer than one hour at room temperature.
2. Always wash hands before and after working with food (even passing trays).
3. Handle foods as little as possible. Never touch utensils in areas that will come into contact with the mouth.
4. Be especially careful if you have touched any infections, especially a boil, which is probably full of staph.

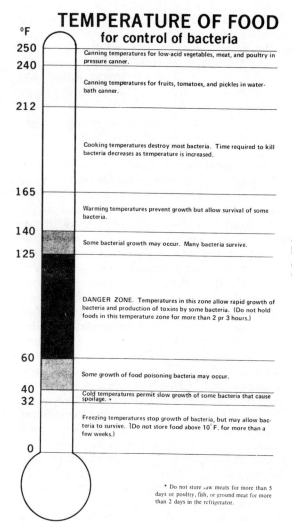

Figure 13–2. *Temperature of food for control of bacteria. (From Keeping Food Safe to Eat: A Guide for Homemakers.* U.S. Department of Agriculture, Home and Garden Bulletin No. 162. U.S. Government Printing Office, 1969.)

5. Do not allow a cut or infection on your hands to touch any food.
6. If you are ill, don't handle food.
7. Be sure to cover your mouth and nose for a cough or sneeze when working with food; then wash hands.
8. To prevent foods from becoming contaminated, keep them covered until in the patient's room.
9. Refrigerate perishable foods immediately when they are sent from the kitchen.
10. If a food doesn't look or smell right, throw it out.
11. Stock the floor's refrigerator with sufficient food for a 24-hour period. Date all foods when they are received; discard perishable items after 48 hours.

The general availability of efficient refrigeration and air conditioning makes it possible to provide carefully-controlled storage temperatures to prevent deterioration of food products and growth of organisms. Various terms that apply to storage of foods (including supplemental feedings) and drugs, as approved by the National Formulary Board, are clarified in Table 13–3.

Clinical Implications:

- Most people recover from foodborne illnesses in two to four days; however, children under four years of age, the elderly, and individuals already debilitated from certain diseases or therapies may become seriously ill.

- Call the kitchen to delay a tray if a patient is unable to eat at the regular time. The kitchen is better-equipped to keep the food at the appropriate temperature. Ideally, hot foods are prepared just before serving, and depending on the time element involved, the kitchen might be able to cook the food fresh.

- Because of the prevalence of staph bacteria in hospitals, and its rapid growth in eggs and milk, milkshakes and eggnog made with raw egg are not advisable. High-protein powders are frequently used to increase the nutrient content.

- Food brought from outside the facility to patients by relatives and friends should be monitored. If it is not eaten immediately, roaches, ants, and rodents are attracted to it. Left unrefrigerated, bacteria may grow rapidly.

- Family and friends who eat from patients' trays may endanger themselves, especially if the patient has a contagious condition, such as hepatitis.

- Cancer-causing chemicals in foods can cause immunoincompetence.

- Some cancer patients who are immunocompromised consume such bizarre "health" items as raw liver or rattlesnake pills. Many of these products contain contaminants, bacterial as well as chemical, further deteriorating their ability to fight invasion.

- *Clostridium botulinum* is present in raw honey. Infantile botulism occurs when children under two years of age are given raw honey.

- People should avoid raw or questionably cooked shellfish in areas where hepatitis A infection, cholera, or other forms of gastroenteritis are prevalent. Individuals with health problems (e.g., cancer, diabetes, or chronic gastrointestinal diseases) should avoid all uncooked shellfish (DuPont, 1986).

Table 13–3. *Storage Temperatures*

Terminology	Temperatures
Cold place	Not exceeding 8°C (46°F)
Refrigerator	Between 2 and 8°C (36 to 46°F)
Cool place	Between 8 and 15°C (46 to 59°F)
Room temperature	Between 15 and 30°C (59 to 86°F)
Excessive heat	About 40°C (104°F)

*This terminology designates storage temperatures approved by the National Formulary Board.

Environmental Contamination

Indirectly, some substances are added to our foods by environmental and industrial contamination and by the use of chemical fertilizers and pesticides. Nevertheless, foodborne illness due to environmental contaminants rarely occurs.

ENVIRONMENTAL AND INDUSTRIAL CONTAMINANTS

The presence of lead, mercury, cadmium, aluminum, and chlorine in our food supply has caused great concern. To date, there is little evidence of chronic disease associated with their presence in foods. Several of the metals are believed to be carcinogenic in man and lower animals; however, the valence of the metal and the type of compound associated with it are important considerations of its carcinogenic potential. As mentioned before, many of these compounds are found naturally in plants or animals.

Food has been a major source of lead because of the use of lead-containing vessels, lead pottery glazes, industrial air pollution, lead pipes, lead-based paint, and pesticides. These sources have been decreasing. Shellfish from contaminated waters may also contain high concentrations of lead (Newberne, 1980). Lead poisoning may cause anemia, peripheral neuropathy, or encephalopathy.

Mercury occurs naturally in foods but is also an environmental pollutant. Since mercury is toxic, the FDA has established allowable maximal levels for mercury in foods. From tests conducted, practically all foods contain levels of mercury concentration within the norms. Only fishery products, specifically tuna and swordfish, show concentrations greater than normal (IFT, 1973). Research has shown that some fish, including tuna, have a built-in mechanism for blocking and reducing the toxicity of mercury. Currently, industrial discharge of mercury and its use in agriculture are regulated to prevent any further problems.

Aluminum has recently been indicated as a possible cause of Alzheimer's disease. It has no known essential function in humans (Shore & Wyatt, 1983) and is poorly absorbed. Aluminum was previously believed to be harmless and is widely used in water purification.

It is also present in almost all foods. While many cooking utensils are aluminum, foods cooked in these dishes are only slightly higher in aluminum content, unless the food is acidic (Greger et al, 1985; Bjorksten, 1982). The amount of aluminum in foods is small compared to amounts present in medications such as antacids and buffered analgesics. Currently, there are no restrictions for aluminum in foods or drugs (Greger, 1985).

Cadmium has no known function at present. Although there is none in the body at birth, by 50 years of age, there may be 20 to 30 mg of cadmium. Excessive levels damage the kidneys. Cadmium is a recognized industrial hazard. Superphosphate used as a fertilizer may contain 15 to 21 mg/kg. Some municipal drinking water contains cadmium, and soft waters are likely to contain more after standing in galvanized pipes.

Some trace elements, even though they are essential to humans, have been recognized because of their excess or unbalanced concentration in food and water. Zinc, copper, manganese, and selenium all have relatively narrow margins of safety—they are necessary, but too much can have a toxic effect.

The role of other trace elements remains to be identified in the body. Arsenic appears to be a contaminant without an essential role, but a small amount is found in humans. Lithium is present in drinking water and some plants. It is used in the treatment of coronary heart disease and mental conditions.

In many instances, the risks involved must be weighed against the benefits. Chlorine can react with organic compounds in water to yield carcinogenic products. Yet, chlorine in the drinking water kills bacteria that cause illness.

CONTAMINATION FROM PESTICIDES AND FERTILIZERS

Substances that are needed or widely used but also considered hazardous are called economic poisons, e.g., insecticides, fungicides, and herbicides. An adequate food supply for the world's population could not be produced without the use of pesticides. Legal tolerances have been established by the Environmental Protection Agency (EPA), which limits the amount of residue that may remain on edible products.

Some of the pesticides originally permitted for use were considered to leave no residue. With the development of more sensitive analytic procedures, minute traces were detected in some, forcing their withdrawal. A problem of enforcing national regulations that control allowable levels (be it pesticide residue, additives, or other substances) is that FDA regulations are applicable only to products in interstate commerce.

Some pesticides have been implicated in carcinogenesis in animals. Because of these reports, some pesticides must be considered a potential problem, and their use has been banned or restricted. Drastic curtailment of DDT on crops has resulted in a decline of DDT-related pesticides. Poor-quality protein potentiates metabolic response to DDT and lindane; therefore, a diet high in good-quality proteins is protective (Newberne, 1980).

RESIDUE FROM DRUGS

Drugs given to animals that are to be eaten have received considerable attention because of the possibility of residues remaining in the food—meat, milk, or eggs. Medications are used for animal diseases, to increase the production of meat or to improve its texture and tenderness. Drugs that leave a residue in edible portions must be proven safe prior to their use. Regulations for the use of drugs in animals permit a certain amount of residues or their metabolites in the food supply. Where applicable, withdrawal intervals are required before milk or eggs are collected or the animal is slaughtered (Newberne, 1980).

One drug that has received widespread attention is diethystilbestrol (DES). Its use in food-producing animals has been banned because of the residue.

Recent evidence indicates subtherapeutic antimicrobials given to cattle can produce a species of *Salmonella* resistant to antimicrobials. Shortly after beginning antimicrobial medications, patients develop gastrointestinal problems, suggesting that they had an asymptomatic infection, which grew rapidly when the medication was started (Holmberg et al, 1984).

RADIOACTIVITY

Nuclear testing emits radioactive elements that fall back to earth. This contaminates many plants and animals that are eaten, and concern has been raised over the effects of radioactive compounds in the body.

Nuclear explosions have increased the amount of strontium-90 and iodine-131 in the soil. Strontium can be deposited in the bones and teeth, which is especially detrimental to the bone- and blood-forming cells in the marrow. When both strontium and calcium are in the gut competing for absorption, calcium is preferentially absorbed. Fortunately, most strontium is ingested through milk, which contains a large amount of calcium. Iodine-131 has been shown to increase the possibility of thyroid cancer. Fresh foods and milk are principal sources.

Most radioactive substances in foods are potassium-40 and carbon-14, which occur naturally. These have a very long half-life (i.e., the length of time before half of the element disintegrates). However, very little carbon-14 is absorbed; the potassium remains in the body for only a few months.

Excessive concentrations of radioactive elements may be carcinogenic. The Atomic Energy Commission and the U.S. Public Health Service regularly analyze the radioactive content of foods. At the present time, the current levels are well below any danger levels.

Clinical Implications:

- Residues from antibiotics frequently used for illnesses in animals are potential hazards to individuals allergic to them.
- One should insist that all foods are purchased from safe sources. Fish and shellfish from polluted waters, homemade canned foods, mushrooms gathered noncommercially, raw milk, and cracked eggs are no bargain if they cause illness.
- Poisonous materials, such as insecticides, should never be stored in the kitchen.
- Acidic beverages should not be stored in a galvanized container.
- Kitchens should be kept clean and free from rats, mice, and insects.
- All foods should be stored securely in sealed containers.

Food Additives

By definition, an incidental food additive is a substance other than the basic foodstuff that is present as a result of production, processing, storage, or packaging. *Intentional* additives are purposely added to perform specific functions; the amounts added are controlled and usually very small.

Many people believe the use of additives is the curse of modern civilization. Actually, the technique of using additives is not new; salt and vinegar were two additives used by early American settlers to preserve their food until the next crop. Today, approximately 2800 additives are used (Lehmann, 1982). This large number is misleading because most additives are used in trace amounts, although large quantities of a few are used. The three additives used in the largest amounts are sugar, corn syrup, and salt. When these are subtracted from the total consumption of additives, varying amounts of about 30 different additives are used, approximately 7.4 lb/year. Over half of these function as leavening agents or to adjust the acidity of foods. The remaining 20 percent (1.8 lbs.) includes more than 1900 additives, or slightly less than 0.008 oz. per capita per year of each additive (Hall, 1973).

PURPOSE OF ADDITIVES

The use of food additives makes many foods available that would otherwise be unobtainable. In many instances, additives can make food safer, cheaper, and more convenient. Table 13–4 shows some of the names of the additives, their purposes in food, and some foods in which they are most frequently used. One reason for people's apprehension about additives is the list of chemical names on the label. The unfamiliar terminology, even the names of vitamins added to foods, may sound frightening, e.g., thiamin mononitrate. There are four major reasons for adding substances to foods (Lehmann, 1982).

1. *Improve nutritional value.* Iodine was the first nutrient to be added to a seasoning (salt) in order to alleviate a nutritional deficiency due to the unavailability of iodine in the diet in certain regions (causing goiter and cretinism). Enrichment and fortification, discussed in Chapter 3, are used to increase the nutrient values in foods. Nutritive additives have helped to eradicate other deficiency diseases, such as rickets, scurvy, and pellagra. Because of the inherent dangers of excessive amounts of some nutrients, the FDA has guidelines for nutrient enrichment.

Table 13–4. A Guide to Food Additives*

Functions in Foods	Some Commonly Used Additives	Some Foods in Which Used
Preservatives		
Antioxidants are used to prvent oxidation resulting in rancidity of fats or browning of fruits	Butylated hydroxyanisole (BHA), tocopherols (vitamin E), citric acid, ascorbic acid.	Vegetable shortenings and oils, potato chips, pudding and pie filling mixes, whipped topping mix, canned and frozen fruits.
Other preservatives are used to control the growth of mold, bacteria, and yeast	Sodium benzoate, propionic acid, calcium propionate.	Table syrup, bread, cookies, cheese, fruit juices, pie fillings.
For Consistency and Texture		
Emulsifiers make it possible to uniformly disperse tiny particles of globules of one liquid in another liquid	Mono- and dyglycerides, lecithin, polysorbate 60, propylene glycol, monostearate.	Salad dressing mixes, margarine, cake mixes, whipped topping mix, pudding and pie filling mix, chocolate, bread.
Stabilizers and thickeners aid in maintaining smooth and uniform texture and consistency; provide desired thickness or gel.	Algin derivative, carrageenan, cellulose gum, guar gum, gum arabic, pectin, gelatin.	Instant pudding mixes, ice creams, cream cheese, frozen desserts, chocolate milk, baked goods, salad dressing mixes, frozen whipped toppings, jams and jellies, candies, sauces.
Acids/Bases		
Control the acidity and alkalinity of many foods, may act as buffers or neutralizing agents.	Citric acid, adipic acid, sodium bicarbonate, lactic acid, potassium acid tartrate.	Gelatin desserts, baking powder, baked goods, process cheese, instant soft drink mixes.
Nutrient Supplements		
Mainly vitamins and minerals—are added to improve the nutritive value of foods.	Potassium iodide (iodine), vitamin D, thiamine mononitrate (vitamin B_1), riboflavin (vitamin B_2), ascorbic acid (vitamin C), niacin (a B vitamin), vitamin A, palmitate, ferrous sulfate (iron).	Iodized salt, milk, margarine, enriched or fortified breakfast cereals, enriched macaroni, enriched rice, enriched flour, instant breakfast drink.
Flavors and Flavoring Agents		
Both natural and synthetic types are added to foods to give a wide variety of flavorful products without restrictions of season or geographic locale.	Natural lemon and orange flavors, dried garlic, herbs, spices, hydrolyzed vegetable protein, vanillin and other artificial flavors (mainly fruit flavors).	Pudding and pie filling and gelatin dessert mixes, cake mixes, salad dressing mixes, candies, soft drinks, ice cream, barbecue sauce.
Colorings		
Both natural and synthetic types are used to enhance the appearance of foods. Most colors used today are approved synthetic colors since there are not enough natural colors available.	Carotene, carmel color, beet powder, artificial colors.	Margarine, cheese, soft drink mixes, candies, jams and jellies, fruit-flavored gelatins, pudding and pie filling mixes.
Miscellaneous Additives		
Include anti-caking agents; anti-foaming agents; flavor enhancers; humectants; curing agents; sequestrants; and firming, bleaching, and maturing agents; nonnutritive sweeteners.	Sodium silicoaluminate, monosodium glutamate (MSG), glycerine, saccharin.	Dessert mixes, soft drink mixes, seasoned coating mixes, salad dressing mixes, flaked coconut, special diet products.

*From *Today's Food and Additives,* 1976. General Foods Corporation, 250 North Street, White Plains, NY 10425.

2. *Prevent oxidation and spoilage.* Antioxidants are a type of preservative that prevents the oxidation of fats and oils, fruits and vegetables. Oxidation of fruits and vegetables causes them to turn dark when exposed to air. Preservatives are also used to protect foods from bacterial growth. For instance, sodium nitrates and nitrites are used to prevent contamination of cured meats, fish, and poultry by the bacterial toxin from *C. botulinum.* In other words, these additives help to retard spoilage and to preserve natural color and flavor.

3. *Aid in processing or preparation.* A wide variety of substances used to maintain stability and consistency in products include emulsifiers, stabilizers, and thickeners. Emulsifiers enable

particles to mix and stay dispersed in a substance. One example is peanut butter, which separates into an oil layer at the top and a dry layer at the bottom unless emulsifiers are used. Stabilizers contribute to the smooth uniform texture of many foods and food products. Thickeners help provide body to certain foods and are used to make jams and jellies from fruits that do not naturally contain sufficient amounts of pectin. Leavening agents, such as yeast and baking powder, are used to make foods light in texture and baked goods rise; humectants retain moisture within a product; anticaking agents keep salts and powders free-flowing.

4. *Enhance flavor and appearance.* These substances are the most widely used and controversial additives. Included in this category are coloring agents, natural and synthetic flavors, spices, flavor enhancers, and sweeteners. In home cooking, spices are used, such as pepper, ginger, and sage, to make foods taste better. Likewise, if used in commercial food preparation, these substances are considered additives. Some flavoring agents, such as monosodium glutamate, are flavor enhancers and do not have a specific taste but rather bring out the natural flavor of the foods with which they are combined. Sweeteners are included in this group because they may be added to improve taste. Without spices and flavorings, foods would be less appealing. While many complex factors are involved in food choices, the overall appearance of food and its container influences selections and, hence, controls nutrient intake (Bender, 1981).

NECESSITY OF FOOD ADDITIVES

Since most foods are perishable or semiperishable, food processing helps to keep foods safe, and additives extend their availability by preventing spoilage. Year-round availability of foods adds variety to our diets. Because of judicious use of additives, our food is less expensive than in most other countries.

Additives are also beneficial to the hurried housewife by making foods more convenient to prepare. Convenience foods are partially prepared or cooked. They must remain stable for usually lengthy transportation and storage periods until consumers are ready to prepare them. Some additives are needed for each step of processing (Fig. 13–3). While it might be nice to renounce many additives, few people are willing to eliminate the conveniences of using at least some processed or convenience foods.

Health Applications: The Safety of Additives

The use of additives is regulated by law. Before a newly proposed additive can be used, it must undergo strict testing to establish its safety for the intended use. As with pesticides, safety levels of additives have been established limiting both the quantity and how the additive can be used. Currently, additives are specific, well-known substances that meet specifications for purity and have been shown as convincingly as possible by animal experimentation and human experience to be free from harmful effects in the amounts used.

Additives can be used in definite amounts for the specific reasons stated above. The FDA has established some criteria: They cannot be used to disguise inferior manufacturing processes and practices; to camouflage damaged, spoiled, or inferior goods; to deceive customers; or to lower nutritional quality. They must also not be used in amounts above the minimum required to achieve the intended effects (Packard, 1976).

During the 1950s, the Delaney committee, appointed by the U.S. House of Representatives, investigated the use of additives. Additives deemed to be harmless were labeled "generally recognized as safe" (GRAS). These substances met certain specifications of safety—in other words, they had been used for years without any known occurrence of health problems. The Delaney clause, which was added to the Food Additives Amendment of the Food, Drug, and Cosmetic Act, prohibits the use of any food additive if it is found to induce cancer in man or animals. At that time, there was scientific uncertainty about the potential carcinogenicity of most chemical substances. It is the general feeling of most persons in the scientific community, including the AMA (1980), that the Delaney clause should be amended to permit special additives, despite their potential hazard, provided the risk of using the substance is less than the risk of not using the substance.

In the 1970s, the FDA requested the Federation

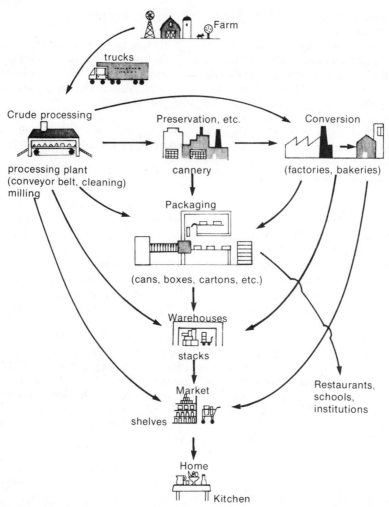

Figure 13–3. *Food channels from farm to consumer. (From* Nutrition and Physical Fitness, *11th ed, by George M. Briggs and Doris Howes Calloway. Copyright © 1984 by CBS College Publishing. Reprinted by permission of CBS College Publishing.)*

of American Societies for Experimental Biology (FASEB) to re-evaluate certain items on the GRAS list. The results of examining available scientific information regarding these substances are shown in Table 13–5.

Most food additives are derived from natural sources or are synthetically produced to be identical to the natural chemical substance. In many instances, the effects of chemicals naturally present in a food are observed, and this chemical is then added to other foods to achieve the same effect. For instance, calcium propionate in Swiss cheese was observed to retard mold. It was then added to bread to inhibit

mold growth. Less than one percent of the additives are not from natural food products.

Additives and Carcinogenesis. Additives have become a public issue because of several episodes regarding safety, especially their role in carcinogenesis. After nearly a century of being used, several studies linked the use of saccharin to tumor formation in rats. In 1972, saccharin was removed from the GRAS list, and in 1977 the FDA recommended that it be banned altogether. Since saccharin was the only artificial sweetener on the U.S. market at the time, Congress passed a moratorium preventing the FDA ban. Further studies confirm that the present level of saccha-

Table 13–5. Status of Additives on the GRAS* List

Status	Ingredients Involved	Glossary
Class I Considered safe for use at current levels and future anticipated levels under conditions of good manufacturing practices.	*Class I* 305 ingredients including vegetable oils, casein, tartrates, aluminum compounds, benzoates, protein hydrolyzates.	1. Alginates—derivatives of seaweeds used as emulsifiers and stabilizers in many food products including beverages, ice cream, and baked goods. 2. Aluminum compounds—compounds used as emulsifying, firming, and leavening agents in food products including baked goods, cheese, and relishes.
Class II Safe for use at current levels but more research is needed to determine whether a significant increase in consumption would constitute a dietary hazard.	*Class II* 68 substances including some zinc salts, alginates, iron and some iron salts, tannic acid, sucrose, vitamins A and D.	3. Benzoates—used as preservatives in many food products including baked goods, beverages, jellies, jams, and margarine. 4. BHA (butylated hydroxyanisole) and BHT (butylated hydroxytoluene)—man-made antioxidants (preservatives) used in many food products including oils and shortenings, chewing gum, dry breakfast cereals, nut products, and beverages.
Class III Additional studies recommended because of unresolved questions in research data.	*Class III* 19 substances including caffeine, BHA, and BHT.	5. Carnauba wax—derivative of palm tree leaves used to glaze candy. 6. Casein—the principal protein in cow's milk used predominantly as sodium caseinate as a texturized and nutrient source in food products, primarily dairy products and imitation dairy products.
Class IV FDA urged to establish safer conditions or prohibit addition of the ingredient to foods.	*Class IV* 5 substances: Salt and four modified starches—distarch glycerol and hydroxypropyl, acetylated and succinyl distarch glycerol.	7. Iron salts—used as a nutritional supplement in food products, particularly in bread. 8. Protein hydrolyzates—used as flavor enhancers, particularly in meat products. 9. Sucrose—used as a sweetener, flavor enhancer, moisture retainer, and preservative in many food products.
Class V Insufficient data on which to make a recommendation.	*Class V* 18 substances, some including glycerides, and certain iron salts and carnauba wax.	10. Tannic acid—occurs in tea and fruits, and is used to clarify beer and wine and as a component of caramel, brandy, and other flavors. 11. Tartrates—used as flavoring agent and buffers in foods including beverages, baked goods, candies, gelatins, jellies, jam, and preserves.

*GRAS = Generally recognized as safe.

From *Yesterday's Additives—Generally Safe*. FDA Consumer, HHS Publication No. (FDA) 81-2147. Washington, DC, Government Printing Office, 1981.

rin use presents an insignificant cancer risk (AMA, 1985; Scientific Review Group, 1985).

Nitrates and nitrites have also been implicated in cancer. These are added to foods, such as bacon and luncheon meats, to control bacterial growth (specifically botulism). More than 40 percent of the nitrates consumed are from the intake of lettuce, cabbage, spinach, and beets. Nitrates are reduced to nitrites by bacteria in the saliva. The nitrites react with secondary amines from protein to form nitrosamines, a reaction that also occurs in cooking nitrate-containing foods. Experiments have shown that nitrosamines are carcinogens in animals. So far, a suitable substitute to prevent microbial growth in meat products has not been found; however, food manufacturers have reduced the amounts of nitrates and nitrites to minimal levels in these products.

Fortunately, a varied diet contains chemicals (vitamins) that can detoxify chemical carcinogens. Vitamin C blocks the conversion of nitrite to nitrosamine; and vitamin E can inhibit cancer formation in animals exposed to various carcinogens (Slaga, 1981).

Other Safety Concerns. As with many natural substances, individuals are sometimes allergic to additives. One of the most frequently implicated is the yellow food coloring, called tartrazine or FD & C Yellow No. 5. Many aspirin-intolerant individuals are sensitive to this additive. Another additive that caused allergic reactions prior to any FDA ban is sulfite; this additive was used to maintain freshness after fresh fruits and vegetables are cut. Proper ingredient labeling of foods, beverages, and drugs enables individuals to abstain from these additives.

Some additives have been implicated by the late Dr. Ben Feingold to cause hyperkinesis and learning difficulties (see Chapter 16).

Currently, additives are as safe as science can make them. They are designed not to be toxic, and most of them would have to be ingested in very large single doses to produce acute symptoms. While the actual risk of cancer from any of these substances is unknown and the significance of environmental carcinogenesis cannot be defined yet, evidence is increasing that foods could be a major pathway for carcinogens. Research is being conducted in order to learn more about the effects of these substances.

Health care personnel need to be concerned and aware of progress and changes that may have beneficial health effects for consumers. Local, state, and federal legislation is necessary to assure a healthy food supply. Civic organizations are frequently organized and effective in enacting laws or other necessary actions.

· FALLACIES and FACTS

FALLACY: *Herbal teas have medicinal benefits and are better because they contain no caffeine.*

· **FACT:** *Some of these caffeine-free alternatives have been time-tested and have no adverse effects. Herbal teas are frequently inadequately labeled and are not standardized in their content. However, some problems have been discovered about various herb teas, and summarized in Table 13–6.*

FALLACY: *Raw milk contains more nutrients and is healthier.*

· **FACT:** *Milk is an excellent culture medium, and organisms can multiply rapidly in it. Most of the bacteria are nonpathogenic, but raw milk has been known to transmit tuberculosis and brucellosis. Consumption of raw milk from a dairy in Minnesota was associated with chronic diarrhea that lasted at least one year for 75 percent of the cases (Osterholm et al, 1986). Pasteurization destroys about 98 percent of all bacteria. It also inactivates about half of the vitamin C and about 15 percent of the thiamin. Since milk is not considered a major source of either of these nutrients, this presents no problem. Some enzymes are*

also inactivated; however these are not dietary essentials (Potter et al, 1984).

FALLACY: *Natural foods from health food stores have no pesticide residues or additives.*

· **FACT:** *Whether foods are labeled as health foods or not, they may contain traces of environmental contaminants. Traces of pesticides were higher in 55 products tested from health food stores than in similar products that were grown conventionally (Barrett & Knight, 1973). In another study, no pesticides were detected in either health or traditional foods, but seven samples of health food and three of traditional foods contained polychlorinated biphenyls (PCBs). While residues can often be found in both types of products, they are well below established tolerance levels; the major difference is the greater cost of health foods (Appledorf et al, 1973).*

FALLACY: *Biological control of insects and weeds with insect predators can eliminate the need for pesticides.*

· **FACT:** *Dr. Tschirley (1973) states: "In the United States there are about 10,000 species of insects, 1500 species of weeds, 500 species of nematodes, 8000 species of fungi, 250 viruses, and 160 bacteria that are considered pests. Thus, we must deal with about 20,000*

Table 13—6. Dangers of Herbal Teas*

Type of Herbal Tea	Possible Deleterious Effects
Chamomile tea or teas made from goldenrod, marigold, and yarrow flowers.	Anaphylactic reactions in individuals allergic to ragweed, asters, or chrysanthemums.
Teas made with burdock, catnip, juniper, hydrangea, and jimsonweed.	Anticholinergic effects.
Teas made with senna, aloe, buckthorn, and dock.	Severe diarrhea.
Licorice tea.	Sodium retention and potassium loss, severe diarrhea, elevated blood pressure.
Dandelion and quack grass tea.	Mild (probably harmless) diuretic action.
Teas made from juniper berries.	Gastrointestinal irritation.
Teas from shave grass or horsetail plants.	Acute neurotoxicity.
Sassafras tea.	Mild stimulant, contains a potent carcinogen, safrole.
Kavabava tea made from the kava plant.	Confusion, ataxia, impaired breathing, dimmed vision, dulled hearing, and hallucinations.
Nutmeg tea.	Nausea, dryness of mouth and throat, drowsiness, rapid pulse, flushed skin, disturbed vision, incoherent speech, vertigo, and hallucinations.

*Data from Herbal teas; sassafras and comfrey teas. *Nutrition and the MD* 8(5):3, 1982.

species of pests." *Biological control of insects and weeds is a good method when applicable, but this alone will not suffice. To suppress pests by nonchemical methods, several techniques are being investigated and can be used conjunctively with biological control. These include host resistance and chemical growth modifiers that alter growth, development, or behavior.*

FALLACY: *Modified food starch is an unnatural additive used in foods.*

• **FACT:** *Modified food starches are produced from tapioca, potatoes, and several cereals including wheat, rice, and corn. Each starch can be altered by use of chemical treatment to yield starches with the specific useful property needed (e.g., clarity, tolerance of acid, gel-forming ability, or blandness of flavor). In this process, the starch mole-* cule is partially split or restructured. This does not change its energy value or digestibility. However, modified food starches used in baby foods have been of concern when some infants' gastrointestinal tracts were unable to absorb the starch, resulting in diarrhea.

FALLACY: *Butylated hydroxytoluene (BHT), an antioxidant food preservative, is an effective treatment for herpes simplex virus type 2.*

• **FACT:** *BHT is associated with potentially serious side effects in animals, increasing the incidence of tumors in the lungs, liver, and bladder. Gastric irritation and even perforation is a potential hazard in humans when the drug is taken on an empty stomach (Smolinske, 1985). BHT has not been approved by the FDA as a treatment for herpes; well-controlled clinical studies have not been conducted (Shlian & Goldstone, 1986).*

Summary

All foods are made of chemicals: Some are necessary, some have no effect, and some are harmful. These chemicals may be a natural constituent of the foodstuff, or they may be added intentionally or unintentionally. Absolute safety does not exist; no food is totally harmless. Scientific research enables us to make wise decisions regarding acceptable versus hazardous food components.

While many potentially harmful substances occur naturally in foods and may be used as food additives, they do not present significant hazards to the consumer. Actually, more is known about the substances added to foods than is known about the naturally-occurring substances. The best protection from ingesting too much of a harmful substance is to practice moderation in eating habits. A variety of foods is important not only to supply nutrients but also in avoiding toxicological hazards.

The biggest controllable hazard in foods involves microorganisms that naturally thrive in foods. Proper handling is essential to prevent foodborne illnesses.

Review Questions

1. Choose three products that have been fortified and list the nutrients added.
2. What would you do if you opened a carton of milk for a patient that had an "off-odor," but the expiration date was still several days away?
3. List the "infamous four" microorganisms responsible for food poisoning.
4. What is meant by botulism? Trichinosis? What foods are generally suspect for causing each of these?
5. How are nursing personnel responsible for preventing food poisoning in patients?
6. A mother tells you her three-year-old refuses to eat anything but hot dogs. Why should she be concerned?
7. What are the four purposes of food additives? Using the ingredient label, list the additives in the following products and state their purpose: bread, processed cheese, bacon, salt, canned soup, crackers, and frozen pizza.
8. Frequently, family and friends want to bring foods into the hospital or nursing home for patients. Discuss the pros and cons of allowing this, provided the foods are allowed on the diet.

REFERENCE LIST

American Medical Association Council on Scientific Affairs (AMA): Saccharin. *JAMA* 254(18):2622, 1985.

American Medical Association Council on Scientific Affairs (AMA): Food safety and the Food, Drug, and Cosmetic Act (Delaney Clause). *Conn Med* 44(3):167, 1980.

Appledorf, H; Wheeler, WB; Koburger, JA: Health foods verus traditional foods: A comparison. *J Milk Food Technol* 36(4):242, 1973.

Barrett, S; Knight, G: Rodale presses on. *Nutr Notes* 9:6, 1973.

Bender, AE: The appearance and the nutritional value of food products. *J Human Nutr* 35(3):215, 1981.

Bjorksten, JA: Aluminum as a cause of senile dementia. *Compr Ther* 8(5):73, 1982.

DuPont, HL: Consumption of raw shellfish—Is the risk now unacceptable? *N Engl J Med* 314(11):707, 1986.

Eys, JV: Nutrition and neoplasia. In *Nutrition Review's Present Knowledge in Nutrition*, 5th ed, Washington DC, The Nutrition Foundation, 1984.

Foster, EM: Is there a food safety crisis? *Food Tech* 36(8):82, 1982.

Gast, LL: A response to today's food safety concerns. *Nutr News* 48(3):9 1985.

Greger, JL: Aluminum content of the American diet. *Food Tech* 39(5):73, 1985.

Greger, JL; Goetz, W; Sullivan, D: Aluminum levels in foods cooked and stored in aluminum pans, trays, and foil. *J Food Prot* 48(9):772, 1985.

Hall, RL: Food additives. *Nutr Today* 8(4):20, 1973.

Holmberg, SD; Osterholm, MT; Senger, KA; et al: Drug-resistant *Salmonella* from animals fed antimicrobials. *N Engl J Med* 311(10):617, 1984.

Institute of Food Technologists Expert Panel on Food Safety and Nutrition and the Committee on Public Information (IFT): Mercury in food. *J Food Sci* 38(4):729, 1973.

Kotula, AW; Murrell, KD; Acosta-Stein, L; et al: Influence of rapid cooking methods on the survival of *Trichinella spiralis* in pork chops from experimentally infected pigs. *J Food Sci* 47(3):1006, 1982.

Kronacki, JL; Marth, EH: Foodborne illness caused by *Escherichia coli*: A review. *J Food Prot* 45(11):1051, 1982.

Lehmann, P: *More Than You Ever Thought You Would Know About Food Additives*. FDA Consumer HHS Publication No. (FDA) 82-2160, Revised February 1982.

McNutt, KW; Powers, ME; Sloan, AE: Food colors, flavors, and safety. *Food Tech* 40(1):72, 1986.

Madlin, N: Life in the kitchen. *Food Management* 17(7):34, 1982.

Morse, DL; Guzewich, JJ; Hanrahan, JP; et al: Widespread outbreaks of clam and oyster-associated gastroenteritis: Roles of Norwalk virus. *N Engl J Med* 314(11):678, 1986.

Newberne, PM: Naturally occurring food-borne toxicants. In *Modern Nutrition in Health and Disease*, 6th ed. Edited by RS Goodhart; ME Shils. Philadelphia, Lea & Febiger, 1980, p. 463.

Osterholm, MT; MacDonald, KL; White, KE; et al: An outbreak of a newly recognized chronic diarrhea syndrome associated with raw milk consumption. *JAMA* 256(4):484, 1986.

Packard, VS: *Processed Foods and the Consumer: Additives Labeling, Standards, and Nutrition*. Minneapolis, University of Minnesota Press, 1976.

Parmley, MA: Salmonella—A closer look. *Food News for Consumers* 3(1):10, 1986.

Potter, ME; Kaufmann, AF; Black, PA; et al: Unpasteurized milk: The hazards of a health fetish. *JAMA* 252(15):2048, 1984.

Scientific Review Group: Saccharin—current status. *Food Chem Toxicology* 23(4/5):543, 1985.

Shlian, DM; Goldstone, J: Toxicity of butylated hydroxytoluene. *N Engl J Med* 314(10):648, 1986.

Shore, D; Wyatt, RJ: Aluminum and Alzheimer's disease. *J Nerv Ment Dis* 171(9):553, 1983.

Slaga, TJ: Food additives and contaminants as modifying factors in cancer inductions. In *Nutrition and Cancer: Etiology and Treatment*. Edited by GR Newell; NM Ellison. New York, Raven Press, 1981, p. 279.

Smith, JL; Palumbo, SA: Microorganisms as food additives. *J Food Prot* 44(12):936, 1981.

Smolinske, S: Butylated hydroxytoluene. In *Poisindex Information System* Vol 46. Edited by BH Rumach. Denver, Micromedex, Inc, 1985.

Strong, FM: Toxicants occurring naturally in foods. In *Nutrition Review's Present Knowledge in Nutrition*, 4th ed. New York, The Nutrition Foundation, 1976, p 516.

Taylor, SL: An overview of interactions between foodborne toxicants and nutrients. *Food Tech* 36(10):91, 1982.

Taylor, WR; Schill, WL; Wells, JG; et al: A foodborne outbreak of enterotoxigenic *Escherichia coli* diarrhea. *N Engl J Med* 306(18):1093, 1982.

Tschirley, FH: Pesticides-relations to environmental quality. *JAMA* 224(8):1157, 1973.

Further Study

Bain, RJI: Accidental digitalis poisoning due to drinking herbal tea. *Br Med J* 390(June 1):1624, 1985.

Brown, JL: Sulfite sensitivity. *JAMA* 254(6):825, 1985.

Cohen, SM: Saccharin: Past, present, and future. *J Am Diet Assoc* 86(7):929, 1986.

Frank-Stromborg, M; Krafka, B; Gale, D; et al: Carcinogens: Are some risks acceptable? *Am J Nurs* 86(7):814, 1986.

Glick, N: Bringing home the (nitrite-less) bacon. *FDA Consumer* 13(5):25, 1979.

Goldfrank, L; Weisman, R: Bacterial food poisoning: What to do if prevention fails. *Postgrad Med* 72(3):171, 1982.

Graham, T; Lee, W: The nurse's role in the prevention of food poisoning. I. Eat, drink, and be healthy. *Nurs Mirror* 152(13):37, 1981.

Graham, T; Lee, W: The nurse's role in the prevention of food poisoning. II. Now wash your hands please. *Nurs Mirror* 152(14):31, 1981.

Hatheway, CL; Whaley, DN; Dowell, VR: Epidemiological aspects of *Clostridium perfringens* foodborne illness. *Good Tech* 34(4)77, 1980.

Kuhn, PJ: What kind of food poisoning is it? *RN* 48(6):39, 1985.

Lecos, C: Of microbes and milk: Probing America's worst salmonella outbreak. *FDA Consumer* 20(1):22, 1986.

Lecos, C: The public health threat of food-borne diarrheal disease. *FDA Consumer* 19(9):19, 1985.

Lecos, C: Irradiation proposed to treat food. *FDA Consumer* 18(4):10, 1984.

Lehmann, P: More than you ever thought you would know about food additives. *FDA Consumer* 13(3):10; (4):18; (5):12, 1979.

Levine, AS; Labuza, TP; Morley, JE: Food technology: A primer for physicians. *N Engl J Med* 312(10):268, 1985.

Manufacturing Chemists Association: *Food Additives: Who Needs Them?* (1825 Connecticut Ave., N.W., Washington, D.C., 20009).

Morrison, RM: Food irradiation: An update. *Nat Food Review* 26:11, 1985.

Sheena, AZ; Stiles, ME: Efficacy of germicidal handwash agents on hygienic hand disinfection. *J Food Prot* 45(8):713, 1982.

Truswell, AS; Brand, JC: Processing food. *Br Med J* 291(October 26):1186, 1985.

Tse, CST: Food products containing tartrazine. *N Engl J Med* 306(11):681, 1982.

Optimal Nutrition for Health and Well-Being

14

OBJECTIVES

THE STUDENT WILL BE ABLE TO:

- *State the U.S. dietary guidelines and their purpose.*
- *Identify dietary selections in each food group that significantly affect intake of calories, fats, salt, and sugar.*
- *Cite some economical buys in each food group.*
- *Discuss food preparation and storage techniques that retain nutrient values.*
- *Refer clients to sources for economic resources or food and nutrition information.*

TERMS TO KNOW

Basic/complex/
convenience foods

235

The Surgeon General's report on healthy people (DHEW, 1979) stated that the people in the United States have never been healthier. Age-corrected mortality rates have been falling during this century; life expectancy is continuing to rise; the mortality rate for coronary heart disease has declined 20 percent during the last 20 years; death rates from cancers not associated with excessive cigarette smoking have not been rising. In spite of this positive report, only the tip of the iceberg has been touched as far as practicing preventive medicine.

Since a perfect food, required by each human being, does not exist, nutrition involves individual choices. Modern technology has permitted many foods to be readily available year round; this increase in the number of foods available complicates the decision-making process. Even in an affluent society, health problems and diseases related to poor nutrition exist—obesity, coronary heart disease, diabetes, tooth decay, osteoporosis, and anemia. Many of these nutrition-related health problems are associated with an overabundance of foods and an increasingly sedentary lifestyle. The remainder is frequently the result of poor food choices.

The U.S. food supply provides adequate quantities of nutrients to protect healthy Americans from deficiency diseases (FNB, 1980). How-

ever, selections are not always the wisest. Because of economic, educational, and cultural factors, equitable distribution of nutrients is not always accomplished. Inappropriate selections may result in over- or underconsumption of various nutrients, and nutritional status may be affected.

Affluence has not helped us to practice moderation in our eating habits. Unrestrained habits, especially overeating, have contributed to the development of many of these degenerative diseases. Obesity, a major problem in the United States, is a form of malnutrition, at least partly due to the abundance of appetizing food.

While nutritional status may be contingent on food choices, selections are rarely based on health considerations. Some of the current disease problems are sensitive to nutrition; others are not (Fig. 14–1). Most problems that are truly nutrition-dependent, such as scurvy and pellagra, have virtually been eliminated. Because so many factors are involved, a specific food plan to fit the needs of everyone is impossible; however, general guidelines contain information required to make informed individual decisions.

Dietary Goals

The Senate Select Committee on Nutrition and Human Needs published the 1977 Dietary Goals for the United States. This report emphasized the importance of cardiovascular disease, hypertension, certain forms of cancer, diabetes, obesity, and cirrhosis as causes of morbidity in the United States.

These goals have been widely debated within the medical community for several reasons. There is no guarantee that by following the recommendations, chronic degenerative diseases will be averted. Sound nutrition is not a panacea. As Clydesdale (1979) observes, people continue to seek magic in foods, "when all that food can give them is a fulfillment of their genetic potential." No single dietary recommendation will be appropriate for everyone.

Based on recommendations made from these goals, the United States Department of Agriculture (USDA) and the Department of Health, Education, and Welfare (USDHEW) arrived at some dietary guidelines for Americans (USDA & USDHEW, 1985), as shown in Figure 14–2. The guidelines are intended for healthy Americans who

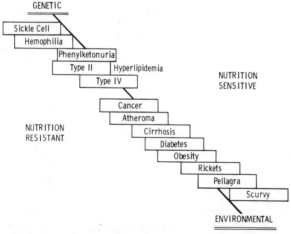

Figure 14–1. Diseases affected by environmental and genetic factors and their relationship to nutrition. Reciprocal genetic and environmental determinants of 13 diseases as shown on a linear scale. Extent to which nutritional intervention can modify the disease is indicated by the degree of displacement of each bar to the right of the line. (From Olson RE: Are professionals jumping the gun in the fight against chronic diseases? Copyright © 1979, The American Dietetic Association. Reprinted by permission from Journal of the American Dietetic Association 74:543, 1979.)

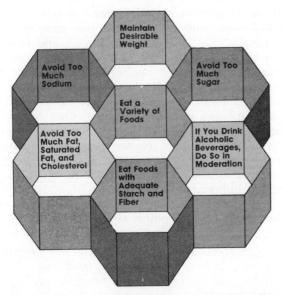

Figure 14–2. *Getting the right balance. Good nutrition is a balancing act: Choosing foods with enough protein, vitamins, minerals, and fiber, but not too much fat, sodium, sugar, and alcohol. Also, energy (calorie) intake must be balanced with energy expended. These seven dietary guidelines, used together, can help you select a healthful diet. (From U.S. Department of Agriculture, U.S. Department of Health and Human Services:* Dietary Guidelines for Americans, *2nd ed. Home and Garden Bulletin No. 232, 1985.)*

want to avoid nutritional deficiencies and reduce risks of some chronic health problems. They do not apply to those requiring special diets or having conditions that interfere with normal nutrition. They can be used by individuals who are at risk of developing chronic diseases, for instance, a family history of obesity, high blood pressure, or high cholesterol levels.

Eat a variety of foods. The merits of a varied diet cannot be overemphasized. A variety of foods is more likely to furnish adequate quantities of all the essential nutrients and lessen the chances of excessive intake of any one noxious compound. Actually no healthy person with a broad range of likes and who regularly eats a wide variety of fruits, vegetables, milk, cereals, and a small amount of animal protein at each meal will be in any danger of developing nutritional deficiencies. This goal can be met by emphasizing variety from each of the basic food groups.

Clinical Implication:

• Megadoses or large doses of supplements of any nutrient should be avoided.

Maintain desirable weight. Obesity involves persons of all ages and economic groups. Approximately 30 percent of middle-aged women and 15 percent of middle-aged men weigh more than 120 percent of their ideal body weight, according to the Health and Nutrition Examination Survey (USDHEW, 1977). Obesity increases the probability of developing hypertension, coronary heart disease, gallbladder disease, diabetes, and problems associated with osteoarthritis.

Obesity is an indicator that caloric intake has exceeded caloric output. Energy balance is most difficult to achieve with today's lifestyles and jobs, which are sedentary and low in energy expenditure. Weight reduction is covered in Chapter 24.

Moderation of calorie intake is the key to maintaining one's ideal weight; many consider it to be the most important dietary practice for Americans (Commentary, 1979). Moderation does not necessarily exclude any food category, but includes all the food groups for their essential nutrients. When the energy requirement is low, consumption of foods from the accessory food group (i.e., alcohol, sugar, and fats) should be especially reduced because these foods provide calories but few other nutrients.

Avoid too much fat, saturated fat, and cholesterol. The biggest change in dietary habits is reflected by the fact that, in the early 1900s, consumption of fat from animal and plant sources was 83 and 17 percent, respectively; in 1982, it was 57 and 43 percent. Consumption of vegetable sources of fats has increased the total dietary fat level, but animal sources still contribute the largest proportion (Marston & Welsh, 1984). Plant products do not contain cholesterol; however, some plant oils (coconut, cocoa butter, and palm oils) are rich in saturated fats.

Higher cholesterol levels are more prevalent in affluent countries than in developing ones (Harper, 1981). High blood cholesterol levels, whether in a population or an individual, denote an increased risk of coronary heart disease. In some people, excessive caloric intake can also increase blood cholesterol.

Additionally, plasma lipid concentrations should be analyzed especially for persons with genetic predisposition to cardiovascular diseases. Persons falling into high-risk categories on the basis of their plasma lipid profiles should be given a therapeutic diet based on the type of hyperlipidemia diagnosed (see Chapter 32) and encouraged to achieve or maintain desirable weight. Serum low-density lipoprotein–cholesterol levels can be lowered by a diet high in polyunsaturated fats and low in saturated fats and cholesterol.

While cholesterol and saturated fats are not essential nutrients, other essential nutrients are affected when beef, liver, and egg consumption is decreased. Each of these foods is a good source of iron, which is a difficult nutrient to obtain in adequate amounts from our food supply. In addition, liver and eggs are very economical for individuals on a low budget.

By decreasing the total amount of fat ingested and continuing to use more polyunsaturated fats (as is the trend), this goal can be met and practiced by the general public with no adverse effects by following these guidelines:

- Choose lean meat, fish, poultry, dry beans, and peas as protein sources. (USDA choice grades of grain-fed animals contain the largest amount of saturated fat and are therefore less desirable.)
- Men and postmenopausal women should use eggs and organ meats (such as liver) in moderation—about four eggs per week and one to two servings of liver per month).
- Use less butter, cream, hydrogenated margarine, shortenings and coconut oil, and foods containing such products.
- Trim excess fat off meats; remove skin from poultry.
- Broil, bake, or boil rather than fry.
- Read labels carefully to determine both the amount and types of fat contained in foods. Avoid products listing saturated or hydrogenated fats near the top of the ingredient list.
- Low-fat or skim milk can be substituted for whole milk in cooking and drinking for everyone except young children less than two years of age.
- Prepare soups and gravies ahead of time, chill, and remove hardened fat.
- Shellfish, although relatively high in cholesterol, are low in fat and acceptable occasionally.

Eat foods with adequate starch and fiber. A beneficial dietary change is the slight increased intake of fruit and vegetables in the United States since about 1925 (Prescott, 1981). Further increases in the consumption of fruits and vegetables are recommended to include more foods rich in vitamins A and C. These may help lower the risk of several types of cancer. Cruciferous vegetables (e.g., cabbage, broccoli, cauliflower, and Brussels sprouts) may also help prevent certain cancers (CDNC, 1982).

The intake of grains during this same period has decreased dramatically (Marston & Peterkin,

1980). Unrefined complex starches contain significant amounts of fiber and also vitamins and minerals, especially zinc, vitamin B_6, and folacin. An increase in the intake of complex starches would naturally have healthful benefits.

The accomplishment of this goal requires educational efforts to change food habits with different emphases in menu planning. One complication in implementing this goal is that foods containing complex carbohydrates are usually eaten with added fats or sugars. For example, sugar is usually added to cereal, and margarine is added to bread or potatoes.

To increase complex carbohydrates in the diet, the following points are important:

- Substitute starches for fats and sugars.
- Select foods that are good sources of fiber and starch, such as dried beans and peas, nuts, fruits and vegetables, and whole-grain breads and cereals.
- Eat more fruits and vegetables high in vitamins A and C.

Avoid too much sugar. Refined sugar contains calories and no other nutrients. This goal was not meant to decrease the intake of natural sugars found in fruits, vegetables, and milk.

Sugar is known to play a role in tooth decay; however, many other factors are involved in the formation of caries. Contrary to popular opinion, sugar does not cause diabetes mellitus or obesity, even though these patients may have to decrease their sugar intake in order to decrease the caloric intake.

Actually, the total amount of sugar ingested has remained relatively constant since 1935. More than two thirds of the refined sugar in the diet is now found in processed foods and beverages, whereas in the past, homemakers added it while cooking (Marston & Peterkin, 1980).

Many other sweeteners are now on the market as substitutes for sucrose. Several, including fructose, sorbitol, mannitol, and xylitol, contain the same number of calories as sucrose. "Dietetic" products containing these sweeteners can mislead one to believe they contain no calories. The long-term metabolic effects of large amounts of fructose-containing sweeteners are unknown (Lecos, 1980). While fructose is ordinarily thought of as a naturally-occurring fruit sugar, it has been implicated in increasing serum triglycerides (Simko, 1980; Hayford et al, 1979).

The newest high-intensity sweetener on the market, aspartame, is an excellent sugar substitute for diabetics but cannot be used by anyone with phenylketonuria. It may also be a problem for the more than four million undiagnosed Americans who are heterozygous for phenylketonuria (Wurtman, 1983).

Focus on Low-Calorie Sweeteners summarizes information about noncaloric sweeteners that are being added to foods as sugar substitutes. While consumption of these artificial sweeteners has increased considerably, total sweetener consumption has not decreased.

Guidelines for avoiding excessive amounts of sugars include:
- Use less of all sugars, including white, brown, or raw sugars; honey; and syrups.
- Consume less foods containing sugars, i.e., candy, soft drinks, ice creams, cakes, pies, and cookies.
- Select fresh fruits or those canned without sugar or in light, rather than heavy, syrup.
- Read food labels for information on sugar content. The following are all sugars: sucrose, glucose, maltose, dextrose, lactose, fructose, or syrups. If these appear at the beginning of a list of the ingredients, the product contains a large amount of sugar.

Avoid too much sodium. While no RDA for sodium or even a minimal requirement has been established, moderation in total salt intake is desirable. Wide ranges of salt consumption are tolerated well by most individuals. The average amount of salt intake in the United States is about 10 gm daily, which is approximately 20 times the amount thought to be necessary. More than one fourth of this is added by the individual.

About 20 percent of the population may be at risk of developing hypertension. Studies have shown that dietary salt restriction does not have a clinically significant effect on blood pressure in the majority of the population, but it is effective for a small subgroup of salt-sensitive individuals (Holden et al, 1983; Laragh & Pecker, 1983).

Individuals with a family history of hypertension or who are salt-sensitive should be identified. A low-salt intake begun at an early age may possibly protect against development of hypertension (De Swiet, 1982). In 1977, the practice of adding salt to infant foods was discontinued. The preferred amount of salt is dependent on the level of salt consumption; this preference can be lowered after reducing sodium intake for a while (Beauchamp et al, 1983; Bertino et al, 1982). This reinforces the importance of establishing good food habits early in life.

Voluntary labeling of the sodium content of foods (especially processed foods) is being encouraged, so consumers can make informed choices (AMA, 1983). The sodium content of many fast foods is significant (a cheeseburger and french fries may contain more than 1300 mg). Additionally, the FDA has suggested the amount of sodium added by food manufacturers be decreased.

Most sodium intake is from foods in the meat, grain, and milk food groups; these foods contribute to other essential nutrients currently being consumed in marginal amounts (e.g., calcium, iron, magnesium, and vitamin B_6). Reducing sodium intake by indiscriminately avoiding foods high in sodium may be eliminating essential nutrients (Engstrom & Tobelmann, 1983).

Another problem with general advice is that reduced sodium consumption may decrease the blood pressure in some individuals with low blood pressure. These individuals should also be identified and advised to continue on a moderate salt intake. Also, persons who are involved in activities in which perspiration is significant (outdoor work or athletic activities in the heat) should not severely restrict sodium intake. A high-salt intake is not necessary.

As the AMA recommendations (1979) state, "Prudence suggests that moderation in salt intake is desirable for the entire population." A few guidelines to avoid excessive sodium are:
- Learn to enjoy other seasonings or the natural flavors of foods; try other seasonings such as lemon, garlic, or ginger.
- Cook with only small amounts of added salt.
- Use little or no salt at the table.
- Limit the intake of salty foods, such as potato chips, pretzels, salted nuts and popcorn, condiments (e.g., soy sauce, steak sauce, or garlic salt), cheese, pickled foods, and cured meats.
- With better food labeling specifying the sodium content of processed foods and snack items and increased educational support from physicians, dietitians, and nurses, consumers will be able to expand their food choices to suit individual preferences as well as physiological needs.
- Emphasis should be on eliminating discretionary or added salt while selecting a balanced diet from the basic food groups.

If you drink alcoholic beverages, do so in moderation. Because of the increased incidence of alcoholism and the high-caloric, low-nutrient density of alcohol, this goal has been well-supported by the medical community. One or two drinks daily do

FOCUS ON Low-Calorie Sweeteners*

Saccharin

Description: Noncaloric sweetener discovered in 1879; used commercially to sweeten foods and beverages since early 1900s. Usage increased greatly during both world wars because of sugar shortages.

Relative Sweetness: 300 times sweeter than sucrose.

Metabolism: Slowly absorbed; not metabolized; rapidly excreted unchanged by the kidneys.

Assets: Stable shelf life; combines well with other sweeteners; synergistic effect when combined with aspartame and/or cyclamate; appropriate for widest range of applications.

Limitations: Slight aftertaste.

Applications: Primarily in soft drinks, tabletop sweeteners, and a wide range of other beverages and foods.

Aspartame

Description: Nutritive sweetener made from two amino acids (L-phenylalanine and L-aspartic acid). Because of its intense sweetness, the small amounts ingested are considered virtually noncaloric.

Relative Sweetness: 200 times sweeter than sucrose.

Metabolism: Digested as a protein; the resulting amino acids are metabolized normally.

Assets: Sugar-like taste; enhances some flavors; synergistic effect when combined with saccharin and/or cyclamate; appropriate for many applications.

Limitations: Unstable at prolonged high heat; not suitable for cooking or products that undergo heat sterilization. Breaks down gradually depending on temperature and acidity. Contraindicated with phenylketonuria (PKU).

Applications: Tabletop sweeteners, soft drinks, cold breakfast cereals, chewing gum, dry beverage mixes, instant coffee and tea, gelatins, puddings, fillings, toppings, refrigerated or frozen beverages, gelatin desserts, breath mints, and multi-vitamin supplements. Stability may pose problems.

Cyclamate

Description: Noncaloric sweetener discovered in 1937; used widely during the 1960s in low-calorie foods and beverages.

Relative Sweetness: 30 times sweeter than sucrose.

Metabolism: Partially absorbed; metabolized in the gut, not by the liver, excreted by kidneys unchanged.

Assets: Stable shelf life and appropriate for use in liquids; sugar-like taste; synergistic effect with saccharin and/or aspartame.

Limitations: Least "sweetening power" of the commercially acceptable noncaloric sweeteners.

Applications: Prior to 1970, widely used as tabletop sweetener, in sugar-free beverages and other low-calorie foods, particularly with saccharin.

Acesulfame K

Description: Noncaloric sweetener discovered in Germany and being developed by the American Hoechst Corp. Like saccharin and cyclamate, acesulfame K is an intensely sweet organic salt.

Relative Sweetness: 200 times sweeter than sucrose.

Metabolism: Not metabolized by the body.

Assets: Sweet taste is rapidly perceptible; good shelf life; relatively stable across temperature and pH ranges normally associated with food processing.

Limitations: Some aftertaste noted at levels required to achieve adequate sweetness when used alone.

Applications: Potentially useful for almost all applications—hot and cold beverages, baked goods, milk products, gums and candies, tabletop sweeteners, toothpaste, and pharmaceuticals.

FOCUS ON Low-Calorie Sweeteners*

Saccharin

Safety: Nearly a century of safe human use. Several studies found bladder tumors in rats exposed to high doses of saccharin—equivalent to a person drinking hundreds of cans of diet soda daily from birth. In other animal studies, saccharin has not been found to pose a carcinogenic risk. Human studies found no association between saccharin and bladder cancer. Recent data (1982) of a study has confirmed the National Cancer Institute's conclusion that there was "no evidence of increased risk with the long-term use of artificial sweeteners in any form or with use that began decades ago."

Status: A 1977 proposed ban on saccharin in the United States was stayed by Congress pending further research. Congressional moratorium on saccharin ban recently has been extended several times.

Aspartame

Safety: Extensive animal and human studies provide strong evidence that aspartame is no more hazardous than normal dietary protein consumption. The 1981 FDA approval included these conditions: a label cautioning "contains phenylalanine" for persons with PKU; directions not to use it in cooking; and monitoring the quantities of consumption. This is the first time FDA has required continued monitoring of an additive. Aspartame has been associated with potential toxicological effects, but the FDA concluded that "enormously large amounts of aspartame would have to be consumed by a normal individual before reaching even a cautiously estimated toxic threshold." In 1984, the FDA reaffirmed that aspartame is safe.

Status: Approved for use in more than 30 countries. Approved in the U.S. for use in specific products.

Cyclamate

Safety: Banned in the United States in 1970. Current petition for reapproval in the United States, includes data from 75 new studies supporting the safety of cyclamate.

Status: Petition for U.S. reapproval pending. Approved for use in more than 40 countries worldwide.

Acesulfame K

Safety: A multitude of safety studies has been conducted; no ill effects were reported.

Status: Petitions for the use of acesulfame K in foods have been filed in several countries, including the United States. Acesulfame K was recently approved for use in foods and beverages in the United Kingdom.

---

*Adapted from The multiple sweetener concept, June, 1983. *Calorie Control Commentary.* Calorie Control Council, 5775 Peachtree-Dunwoody Road, Suite 500-D, Atlanta, GA 30342.

Table 14—1. *Guidelines for Choosing Foods for Optimum Nutrition*

	Bread/Cereal Group	Fruit/Vegetable Group	Milk Group	Meat Group	Accessory Foods
High in cholesterol			Butter and cream.	Egg yolks, shrimp, organ meats, bacon, salt pork, and animal products.	Sauces and desserts prepared with cream and butter.
High in salt	Pretzels, salted crackers, highly seasoned rice, and pasta mixtures.	Pickled vegetables (pickles and sauerkraut), regular canned vegetables, vegetable juices with added salt.	Buttermilk.	Canned fish and meats, chipped beef, and textured vegetable protein analogs.	Canned and dehydrated soups and bouillon and instant seasoned sauces and mixes.
High in salt and fat	Salted snacks and chips.	Potato chips, frozen vegetables in sauce, and olives.	Natural cheeses, especially blue, Camembert, processed cheese, and cheese foods.	Canned, dried, salted, cured meats or fish such as bacon, salt pork, ham, corned beef, sausage, frankfurters, luncheon meat, and corned beef.	
High in fat		French fries, fried vegetables, and avocados.	Cream cheese, sour cream, whole milk, butter, and cream.	Duck, goose, nuts, brisket, oily fish (mackeral), and fish packed in oil.	Chocolate, coconut, solid shortening, and most nondairy creamers.*
High in sugar and fat	Commercial granola, doughnuts, and pastries.		Sweetened condensed milk, ice cream, malts and shakes, chocolate milk, whole-milk, fruit-flavored yogurt.		Sweetened coconut.*
High in sugar	Presweetened breakfast cereals.	Fruits canned or frozen in heavy syrup, juices with added sugar, and maraschino cherries.	Ice milk.		Sugars, jams, jellies, preserves, honey, syrups, most candies, and beverages sweetened with sugar.
Reduced in fiber; low in salt, fat, and sugar	Refined grains, especially white rice, degerminated cormeal or flour, and white flour.	Fruit juices and peeled fruits and vegetables.			
Wise food choices for optimum nutrition†	Use *whole grain* breads and cereals, predominantly rye bread, whole-wheat bread, brown rice, shredded wheat, oatmeal, and graham crackers.	Fresh fruits and vegetables, especially raw unsweetened frozen and canned fruits, frozen vegetables (plain), and dried fruits.	Fortified skim or low-fat milk (fresh, dry, or evaporated), low-fat cheeses (farmer, sapsago, mozzarella, Monterey Jack, cottage cheese), low-fat yogurt, and skimmed uncultured buttermilk.	Predominantly: fish, chicken and turkey (no skin), veal, and egg whites. Less frequently: lean meats (beef, pork, or lamb). Frequently: dried peas, beans, and lentils.	

*These products, like animal fats, are high in saturated fats.

†A food not listed as wise food choice is not necessarily bad. Most of these foods also contain vitally needed nutrients and do not need to be totally eliminated from the diet. Rather, they should be used in moderation.

not appear to be harmful to adults. Alcohol has been used medicinally to stimulate the appetite.

Nutritional complications can occur from drinking too much alcohol; it also can cause birth defects when ingested by pregnant women.

Summation of the Dietary Goals. These goals can be used as an adjunct to the basic food groups, to help clarify some points lacking in the food groups relating to optimal health, as shown in Table 14–1. Skim or low-fat milk is to be encouraged; foods from the fruit and vegetable group are to be emphasized as well as whole grains from the bread and cereal group. In the meat group, generally more chicken and fish as well as dried beans, peas, and nuts are desirable. To maintain one's ideal weight, less fat, sugar, and alcohol may be needed. Salt intake should be moderate.

It helps if you enjoy a variety of foods. As Davies (1972) states, "Eat a little of everything and not too much of any one thing."

Optimal Nutrition Using Economical Food Purchasing

While Americans are increasingly concerned about proper nutrition, they are also anxious about food prices and try to conserve their food dollars. Most Americans spend only about one fifth of their income on food. Even Americans on welfare are affluent in the eyes of most of the world's population who earn less than $600 a year (Padberg, 1981). Selecting the most nutritious products within one's available money is a common problem.

FOOD BUDGET

Many factors enter into food-budgeting decisions: (1) the number and ages of family members, (2) the number of meals eaten out, (3) kitchen equipment, (4) time allocated to food purchasing and preparation, (5) skill and educational level of the homemaker, (6) food preferences and priorities, (7) family income, and (8) special dietary needs. Health professionals who have a general knowledge of food costs can aid individuals in stretching their food dollar. High-priced foods are not necessarily the most nutritious; it is

possible to provide palatable, nutritious foods on a low budget. Sample meal plans containing the recommended amounts of nutrients and moderate levels of fat, cholesterol, sweeteners, and sodium were planned by the USDA and compared to actual household food expenditures (Peterkin, 1983). As shown in Figure 14–3, more of the food budget should be allocated for fruits and vegetables, grain products, milk, and dry beans, and less expenditures for meats and items in the accessory food group.

The USDA has established several food plans for different income levels: thrifty, low-cost, moderate-cost, and liberal. Persons on thrifty and low-cost food plans need more skill in buying, storing, and utilizing every penny to its fullest, but adequate nutrition can be provided. On these two food plans, it is necessary to (1) purchase the least expensive items in each basic food group, (2) rely on the minimal servings of meats, (3) utilize meat substitutes frequently (e.g., legumes and peanut butter), (4) serve larger quantities of grains, cereals, and pasta products, (5) prepare most foods from scratch rather than buying convenience foods, and (6) eliminate most highly processed foods that are expensive or have poor nutrient content (e.g., carbonated beverages and potato chips).

If the amount of calories is not of concern, foods supplying the most nutrients per dollar include beef liver, fresh potatoes, brown rice, wheat germ, milk, eggs, and peanut butter. On the basis of nutrient density (nutrient contribution per kilocalorie), the best buys are spinach, beef liver, tomatoes, canned tuna, nonfat and low-fat milk, tofu, dry-roasted peanuts, eggs, and fresh carrots (Schaus & Briggs, 1983).

MENU PLANNING AND ECONOMICAL SHOPPING

The best nutritional buys in the four basic food groups are listed in Table 14–2. A few basic suggestions can help consumers cut food costs and get more for their money:
1. Menus should be planned a week at a time, using the basic food groups.
2. Plan menus around seasonal foods or weekly specials advertised in newspapers.
3. Use meat alternatives, such as legumes, nuts, and cheese several times weekly. Protein sources are generally the most expensive budget items; however, it is not necessary to buy

How it was spent by
survey households:

How it might be spent for
better nutritional balance:

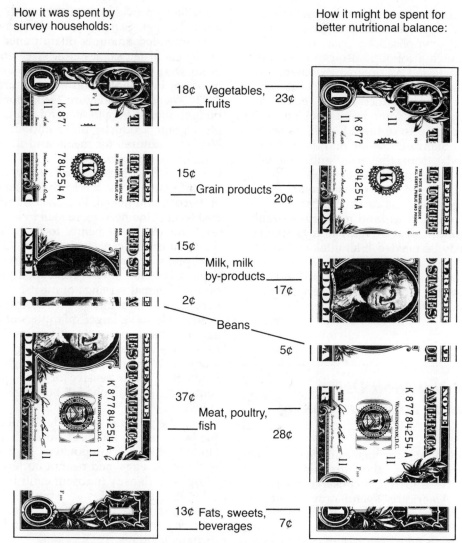

18¢ Vegetables,
fruits   23¢

15¢
Grain products   20¢

15¢
Milk, milk
by-products   17¢

2¢
Beans   5¢

37¢
Meat, poultry,
fish   28¢

13¢ Fats, sweets,
beverages   7¢

Figure 14–3. The food dollar. (From Peterkin BB: Making food dollars count. Family Economics Review 4:23, 1983.)

choice quality grades for good nutrition. Table 14–3 shows the relative cost of 20 grams of protein from various foods.

4. Store brands and generic products are almost always a good buy for the money.
5. Prepare a shopping list and stick to it. Avoid impulse buying but be prepared to make substitutions if a similar item is a better buy.
6. Plan menus around foods the family will eat.
7. Read labels to determine if similar products are comparable in nutritive value.
8. Unit pricing helps in comparing the costs of different products. Generally, the price per ounce is stated, which makes it easier to compare various sizes.
9. Larger sizes may be cheaper; they are only bargains if the food will be eaten before it spoils.
10. Shop at large supermarkets rather than small operations or convenience stores.
11. Snack foods and many sugar-coated breakfast cereals are not wise food purchases because of their low nutrient values. The price per ounce is astonishing.

CONVENIENCE FOODS AND ECONOMY

Convenience foods have been fully or partially prepared by food manufacturers and usually cost more because of extra handling and packaging. Convenience foods also require more preservatives.

Understanding the different types of convenience foods can be helpful in making wise food purchases (Odland & Axelson, 1982). *Basic* convenience foods have been subjected to basic processing techniques such as canning, freezing, or drying. Examples include peanut butter, pasteurized process cheese, instant coffee, and frozen orange juice. *Complex* convenience foods include those that have many ingredients and are timesavers for the cook who may have varying levels of experience in making items such as bread, luncheon meats, canned soups, or jellies and jams. *Manufactured* convenience foods cannot be prepared in the home and include items such as ready-to-eat cereals and carbonated beverages.

Convenience foods save time in meal preparation, planning, purchasing, buying, and cleanup. They also can expand the variety of foods served.

Some convenience foods are more expensive, while some cost about the same or even less than their counterparts prepared in the home. In general, basic convenience foods, especially vegetables, cost less than fresh ones cooked at home, although this varies with seasonal availability (Table 14–4). Complex convenience products generally cost more than foods made in the home (Table 14–5). Many manufactured convenience foods, such as carbonated beverages, offer many calories but few nutrients and are considered to be expensive accessory foods. When items, such as pizza, can be purchased in more than one form, those with more convenience usually cost more (Odland & Axelson, 1982), as shown in Tables 14–6 and 14–7.

Optimal Nutrition from Food Preparation

Even though food is carefully chosen for its nutritional value, its nourishment is affected by how food is handled and prepared before its consumption. As mentioned in Chapter 13, edibles must be handled with care to prevent contamination with foodborne organisms, and sometimes must be properly cooked to kill any organisms naturally present. Food is not nourishing if it causes illness.

FRAGILITY/STABILITY OF NUTRIENTS

Food and many of the nutrients it contains are very delicate and must be handled with care to conserve its nutrients. Many of the vitamins are especially susceptible to leaching, heat degradation, light, and oxidation (Table 14–8).

Since most food consumed in the United States is processed, it is important to consider the effect of processing, cooking, and storage on the nutrient content. In general, most minerals, carbohydrates, lipids, and proteins as well as vitamin K and niacin are stable (more than 85 percent retention) during processing and storage. Vitamins A, D, E, B_6, and B_{12}, riboflavin, pantothenic acid, and folacin are slightly less stable. Thiamin and ascorbic acid are the most likely to be seriously depleted by processing, storage, and home preparation of foods (Borenstein, 1980). The nutritional value of home-cooked foods is frequently about the same as processed foods (IFT, 1974). On the other hand, *highly processed* fruits and vegetables, such as potato chips, are not as nutritional as the fresh form, such as a baked potato.

PROCESSED FOODS

Because of lifestyles in the United States and the increasing number of women working full-time, more processed and convenience foods are being used. While we have more control over what happens to the food when it is homegrown and know what is added to it, this is an impossible task for most Americans. Many individuals feel that foods processed outside the home are not nutritious. As Clydesdale (1979) states:

> The public often feels that the manufacturer of a processed food takes the vitamins out of the food, puts them in his pocket, goes home and gives them to his kids, and leaves the consumer a processed food with nothing of value in it.

Not everything done to foods by industrial processing has been good; neither can it be said that the old-fashioned, "Virginia-cured," home-processed hams with their large amounts of salt and sugar were necessarily good either.

The milling process produces grain that is more stable to deterioration and, thereby, increases its shelf-life. Nutritionally, this is the most detrimental food processing technique; the bran coat of grains, which contains lipids that are rapidly oxidized, is mechanically removed, reducing the fiber content of the grain. Additionally, approximately 70 to 80 percent of the thiamin, ribo-

Table 14–2. Nutritional Bargains from the Basic Four*

Food Group	More Economical	More Expensive
Milk	Skim and 2% milk	Whole milk
	Nonfat dry milk	Whole milk
	Evaporated milk	
Cheese	Cheese in bulk	Grated, sliced, or individually-wrapped slices
	Cheese food	Cheese spreads
Ice cream	Ice milk or imitation ice cream	Ice cream or sherbet
Meat	Home-prepared meat	Luncheon meat, hot dogs, canned meat
	Regular hot dogs	All beef or all-meat hot dogs
	Less tender cuts	More tender cuts
	U.S. Good and Standard grades	U.S. Prime and Choice grades
	Bulk sausage	Sausage patties or links
	Pork or beef liver	Calves liver
	Heart, kidney, tongue,	
	Bologna	Specialty luncheon meats
Poultry	Large turkeys	Small turkeys
	Whole chickens	Cut-up chickens or individual parts
Eggs	Grade A eggs	Grade AA eggs
	Grade B eggs for cooking	
Fish	Fresh fish	Shellfish
	Chunk, flaked, or grated tuna	Fancy- or solid-pack tuna
	Coho, pink, or chum salmon (lighter in color)	Chinook, king, and sockeye salmon (deeper red in color)
Fruits and Vegetables	Locally grown fruits and vegetables in season	Out-of-season fruits and vegetables or those in short supply and exotic vegetables and fruits
	Grades B or C	Grade A or Fancy
	Cut up, pieces, or sliced	Whole
	Diced or short cut	Fancy-cut
	Mixed sizes	All the same size
	Fresh or canned	Frozen
	Plain vegetables	Mixed vegetables or vegetables in sauces
Fresh fruits	Apples	Cantaloupe
	Bananas	Grapes
	Oranges	Honeydew melon
	Tangerines	Peaches
		Plums
Fresh vegetables	Cabbage	Asparagus
	Carrots	Brussels sprouts
	Celery	Cauliflower
	Collard greens	Corn on the cob
	Kale	Mustard greens
	Lettuce	Spinach
	Onions	
	Potatoes	
	Sweet potatoes	

*From Green, ML; Harry, J: *Nutrition in Contemporary Nursing Practice.* Copyright © 1981, John Wiley & Sons, Inc. Reprinted by permission of John Wiley & Sons, Inc.

flavin, niacin, and vitamin B_6 is lost. Enrichment replenishes some of the nutrients lost in processing, but not all of them (Table 3–2).

Some food processing is designed for optimal retention of nutrients. Fresh fruits and vegetables have a higher nutritive value and better taste immediately after harvest but rapidly deteriorate if transported long distances or improperly stored.

By rapidly cooling fresh produce immediately after harvesting and by constant control of the temperature, nutrient quality is enhanced (Krochta & Feinberg, 1975).

Freezing and canning of fruits and vegetables are frequently done on site to harvest the fruits and vegetables at their peak ripeness. This means the taste is superior and nutrients are at their opti-

Table 14—2. Nutritional Bargains from the Basic Four* Continued

Food Group	More Economical	More Expensive
Canned fruits	Applesauce Peaches Citrus juices Other juices	Berries Cherries
Canned vegetables	Beans Beets Carrots Collard greens Corn Kale Mixed vegetables Peas Potatoes Pumpkin Sauerkraut Spinach Tomatoes Turnip greens	Asparagus Mushrooms
Frozen fruit	Concentrated citrus juices Other juices	Cherries Citrus sections Strawberries Other berries
Frozen vegetables	Beans Carrots Collard greens Corn Kale Mixed vegetables Peas Peas and carrots Potatoes Spinach Turnip greens	Asparagus Corn on the cob Vegetables, in pouch Vegetables, in cheese and other sauces
Dried fruits and vegetables	Potatoes	Apricots Dates Peaches
Breads and cereals	Day-old bread White enriched bread Cooked cereal Regular cooking oatmeal Plain rice Long-cooking rice Graham or soda crackers	Fresh bread Rolls, buns Whole grain Ready to eat cereals Quick cooking or instant oatmeal Seasoned rice Parboiled or instant rice Specialty crackers

mum level. Unless these foods are blanched to inactivate enzymes, vitamin losses may be significant (Hein & Hutchings, 1974). Frozen foods that are packed immediately after harvesting may be higher in nutritive value than their fresh counterparts available in the supermarket.

Foods subjected to drying and fermentation processes retain most of their vitamins if the finished foods are protected from oxygen by packaging or antioxidants (IFT, 1974). As discussed in Chapter 13, many additives are added in processing to protect the nutrient values of foods.

FOOD STORAGE

All foods can deteriorate and spoil over time. To maintain optimal nutritional value, taste, and appearance of foods, storage times and temperatures are important. Perishable items, including

Table 14–3. Meats and Meat Alternates
Cost of 20 grams of protein from specified meats and meat alternates

Food	Amount, Ready-to-Eat to Give 20 Grams of Protein[3]	Market Unit	Part of Market Unit to Give 20 Grams of Protein	Price per Market Unit[3]	Cost of 20 Grams of Protein
					(Dollars)
Dry beans	1½ cups	pound	.24	.57	.14
Bread, white enriched[4]	8 slices	22 oz	.37	.44	.16
Eggs, large	3⅓	dozen	.28	.80	.22
Beef liver	2⅔ oz	pound	.24	.96	.23
Turkey, ready-to-cook	2⅓ oz	pound	.33	.72	.24
Chicken, ready-to-cook	2⅓ oz	pound	.42	.62	.26
Peanut butter	4½ tbsp	12 oz	.23	1.19	.27
Milk, whole, fluid[5]	2½ cups	½ gal	.31	.98	.30
Bean soup, canned	2½ cups	11¼ oz	.82	.40	.33
Tuna canned	2½ oz. drained	6½ oz	.44	.87	.38
Cured ham, bone in	3⅓ oz	pound	.30	1.25	.38
Chicken breast halves	2½ oz	pound	.27	1.45	.39
Ground beef, lean	3 oz	pound	.25	1.89	.47
Processed American cheese	3¼ oz	8 oz	.40	1.23	.49
Frankfurters	4	pound	.39	1.39	.54
Chuck roast of beef, bone in	3¼ oz	pound	.35	1.63	.57
Ocean perch filet, frozen	3½ oz	pound	.31	1.94	.60
Rump roast of beef, boned	3 oz	pound	.26	2.40	.62
Round beefsteak, bone in	2½ oz	pound	.23	2.99	.69
Bacon, sliced	10½ slices	pound	.52	1.45	.75
Bologna	6 oz	8 oz	.75	1.04	.78
Pork chops, center	2¾ oz	pound	.35	2.66	.93
Porterhouse beefsteak	3⅔ oz	pound	.34	4.39	1.49

[1]From Junker, CC: Cost comparison tools to stretch your food dollar. In *Food from Farm to Table, USDA Yearbook of Agriculture.* Washington, DC, Government Printing Office, 1982.

[2]About one-third of the daily amount recommended for a man.

[3]Average prices from several Washington, DC area supermarkets. Prices for processed items are for the least costly brand in the market unit specified.

[4]Bread and other gram products, such as pasta and rice, are frequently used with a small amount of meat, poultry, fish, or cheese as main dishes in economy meats. In this way, the high-quality protein in meat and cheese enhances the lower quality of protein in cereal products.

[5]Although milk is not used to replace meats, it is an economical source of good quality protein.

produce, dairy products, fresh meats, and eggs are refrigerated at temperatures between 33 and 40°F. Frozen foods should be maintained at temperatures of 0°F or lower to minimize losses. Products that can be stored at room temperature should be kept in cool, dry areas in airtight containers.

PREPARATION TECHNIQUES

Many nutrient losses occur during preparation or cooking. In general, the less handling and pre-preparation of the food, the more nutrients are retained. A few guidelines can help preserve nutrients during food preparation:

1. Fresh produce should be prepared as near to serving time as possible.

2. Water-soluble vitamins are leached out in water; do not soak cut fruits and vegetables.

3. Utilize the outer portions of produce as much as possible by scrubbing fruits and vegetables instead of paring them. When necessary, pare as thinly as possible.

4. Utilize parings and portions of vegetables generally not consumable to make soup stock; these are a very rich source of potassium and water-soluble vitamins.

5. Leave produce whole or in large pieces so less surface area is available for oxidation of nutrients.

6. Store any fruits or vegetables that have been cut or otherwise processed, such as fruit juice, in air-tight containers. The container size should be appropriate for the amount to be stored to prevent excessive oxidation from the air inside the container.

Table 14–4. Cost Comparisons—Basic Convenience Foods*

	Relative cost
	(Percent)
Fresh green beans	100
Canned green beans	62
Frozen green beans	90
Home-prepared french-fried potatoes	100
Frozen french-fried potatoes	83
Juice squeezed from fresh oranges	100
Ready-to-drink orange juice reconstituted from frozen concentrate	65
Pasteurized orange juice	86
Canned orange juice	63
Frozen orange juice concentrate	46
Fluid skim milk	100
Instant nonfat dry milk	65

*From Odland, D; Axelson, J: Convenience foods—what they cost you. In *Food from Farm to Table, USDA Yearbook of Agriculture.* Washington, DC, Government Printing Office, 1982.

Table 14–5. Cost Comparisons—Complex-Convenience Foods*

		Relative Cost
		(Percent)
Main Dishes	Homemade fried chicken with mashed potatoes and carrots.	100
	Frozen, ready-to-heat fried chicken plate dinner.	144
	Homemade lasagna.	100
	Frozen lasagna.	144
Vegetables	Fresh broccoli with butter sauce.	100
	Frozen broccoli with butter sauce (boil-in-the-bag).	180
Baked Products	Homemade white bread.	100
	Ready-to-eat white bread (firm-crumb type).	227
	Ready-to-eat white bread (soft-crumb type).	82
	Homemade waffles.	100
	Frozen waffles.	268
	Homemade apple pie.	100
	Ready-to-eat apple pie.	185

*From Odland, D; Axelson, J: Convenience foods—what they cost you. In *Food from Farm to Table, USDA Yearbook of Agriculture.* Washington, DC, Government Printing Office, 1982.

COOKING METHODS

Many foods are cooked to enhance their palatability, to make them more easily digested, and to eliminate bacteria. Cooking affects acceptability as well as nutritional value.

Sufficiently high temperatures are necessary to destroy microorganisms, especially in pork. Cooked foods should be maintained at temperatures above 140°F to eliminate bacterial growth, or they should be promptly chilled.

Iron cookware used to be very common but has virtually been phased out. However, iron cookware can contribute to dietary iron (see Chapter 12). Well-seasoned iron skillets also help cook foods without adding large amounts of fats.

Cooking increases the digestibility of protein in meats. The cellulose in fresh produce is generally softened, decreasing the bulk so that a greater quantity is eaten. The addition of large amounts of fats in the cooking process, such as frying food, is to be discouraged.

A new method of cooking for most Americans is stir-frying, which is an old Oriental technique. This method is highly recommended and has the added benefit of being quick. Foods are cut in small pieces and cooked very briefly over high heat with or without a small amount of vegetable oil. The vegetables retain their nutrient value, color, and crispness.

The use of the microwave is another time-saver. Because of the shorter cooking time, and the smaller quantity of water added, this method is believed to conserve nutrients. However, vegetables cooked by a home microwave contain about the same vitamin levels as those boiled in small amounts of water (Hagen & Schweigert, 1983).

1. Cook foods just until tender or for the shortest time possible. A covered pan minimizes cooking time because steam increases the temperature inside.

Table 14–6. Cost Comparisons—Convenience Items Made From a Mix*

	Relative cost
	(Percent)
Homemade chili-macaroni	100
Chili-macaroni from a mix	116
Homemade macaroni and cheese	100
Macaroni and cheese from a mix	33
Homemade pancakes	100
Pancakes from a mix (just add water)	102
Homemade chocolate cake	100
Chocolate cake from a mix	53

*From Odland, D; Axelson, J: Convenience foods—what they cost you. In *Food from Farm to Table, USDA Yearbook of Agriculture.* Washington, DC, Government Printing Office, 1982.

Table 14–7. Pizza Cost Comparisons*

	Relative Cost
	(Percent)
Homemade pizza	100
Pizza from a mix	144
Frozen pizza	179

*From Odland, D; Axelson, J: Convenience foods—what they cost you. In *Food from Farm to Table, USDA Yearbook of Agriculture.* Washington, DC, Government Printing Office, 1982.

2. Use the least amount of liquid possible in cooking. Cover the pan to minimize the amount of water necessary. Use the leftover liquid, which contains water-soluble vitamins, in gravies and soups.
3. Serve vegetables as soon as they are cooked.
4. Do not add baking soda while cooking vegetables.

The Role of Fast Food in Optimal Nutrition

Fast food is served quickly and conveniently at a relatively low cost (Sheridan & McPherrin, 1981). Fast-food sales have increased dramatically over the last 10 years becoming an integral part of our fast-paced lifestyle.

While some believe that fast food is junk food, this is not necesarily true. Nutrient analysis by fast-food chains and independent studies reveal that their menu items contain rich sources of protein (30 to 50 percent of the RDAs). There are also items available that, if selected, provide 20 to 30 percent of the RDAs for thiamin, riboflavin, ascorbic acid, and calcium (Shannon & Parks, 1980). When a hamburger or roast beef sandwich is selected, substantial amounts of iron are furnished from the beef.

Most menus lack a rich source of vitamin A. In many cases, salads have been an added selection because of consumer demand (Fig. 14–4). This provides a source of vitamins A and C and also dietary fiber. Shortages of other nutrients, specifically biotin, folacin, pantothenic acid, iron, and copper are also reported (How nutritious, 1975).

Several other problems with fast foods have been of concern (Young et al, 1981):
1. *The calorie content* of a meal is generally between 900 to 1800 kcal—33 to 66 percent of the RDA for young men or 45 to 90 percent for young women.
2. *The sodium content* is very high, ranging from 1000 to 2515 mg.
3. *The fat content* of some fast-food meals can be as high as 51 percent of the calories consumed. The ratio of saturated to unsaturated fats in

Table 14–8. Stability of Nutrients*

Nutrient	Effect of pH			Air or Oxygen	Light	Heat	Max. Cooking Losses
	Neutral pH7	Acid < pH7	Alkaline > pH7				
Vitamins							%
Vitamin A	S	U	S	U	U	U	40
Ascorbic acid	U	S	U	U	U	U	100
Carotene	S	U	S	U	U	U	30
Cobalamin	S	S	S	U	U	S	10
Vitamin D	S		U	U	U	U	40
Folic acid	U	U	S	U	U	U	100
Vitamin K	S	U	U	S	U	S	5
Niacin	S	S	S	S	S	S	75
Pantothenic acid	S	U	U	S	S	U	50
Pyridoxine	S	S	S	S	U	U	40
Riboflavin	S	S	U	S	U	U	75
Thiamin	U	S	U	U	S	U	80
Tocopherol	S	S	S	U	U	U	55

S = stable (no important destruction).
U = unstable (significant destruction).
*Adapted from Harris, RS; Karmas, E: *Nutritional Evaluation of Food Processing,* 2nd ed. Copyright 1975 by AVI Publishing Company, Westport, CT.

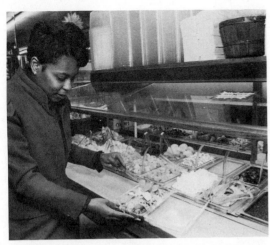

Figure 14–4. Variety and convenience have made salad bars a big hit with consumers, but is there an added price tag? A 1985 survey of three Washington, DC, supermarkets showed that the salad bar was two to seven times more expensive than what the individual ingredients cost in the same store. (Courtesy of USDA, Food News for Consumers Magazine 3(2):12, 1986.)

fast foods is not available. Tallow and lard (both animal fats that are predominantly saturated) used to be frequently used for deep-frying until public awareness and demand motivated most fast-food chains to change to vegetable fats. The method of preparation (deep-frying or grilling) as well as the temperature at which foods are fried, and whether the cooking fat is reused, affects the fat content.

The impact of fast foods on nutritional status depends on how frequently the individual consumes them, the composition of each item selected, and what other foods are eaten during the day. As Shannon and Parks (1980) state, "Occasional visits to fast food restaurants will obviously have little impact on the nutritive value of a week's diet." Wise choices are possible when consumers know their own nutritional needs and the content of menu items. Nutritional analysis of many items offered by the fast food chains is shown in the Appendix.

Optimal Nutrition Through Federal and Community Programs

While the health of all classes of people benefits from foods providing proper nutrition, fre-

quently people who are economically deprived or uneducated need special assistance. Widespread hunger is not prevalent in the United States, but it is a real problem in low-income areas, as evidenced by the increased numbers of children failing to thrive because of malnutrition and anemia (Shahoda, 1984). Zee and colleagues (1985) compared the nutritional status of children living in urban poverty in 1983 with a similar survey in 1977. Improvements were observed in median serum levels of vitamins A and C, hemoglobin, and red blood cell volume. Nevertheless, 9 to 19 percent of the children had low or deficient levels of vitamins A, B_1, B_2, and C as well as hemoglobin, serum iron, and transferrin saturation. This improvement was attributed to the fact that families in the 1983 group participated in a commodity supplementary food program. Malnourishment is also common among the growing number of elderly persons (Shahoda, 1984).

A variety of nutrition resources are available in the community to help financially, to assist with food budgeting, or to teach basic nutrition and meal planning (Table 14–9). It is important for health care professionals to identify individuals or families with nutritional needs and help them participate in various community and government programs. One of the best sources to check for community availability of special food programs is the city or county health department.

FEDERAL PROGRAMS

The federal government administers several nutrition programs through the Department of Agriculture (USDA) and the Department of Health and Human Services (DHHS). Several major federal programs provide supplemental food and nutrition education for the general public with special emphasis on high-risk groups—pregnant and lactating women, infants, children, and the elderly.

The food stamp program provides coupons to low-income households who meet certain requirements. The coupons are free to persons who qualify, which enables them to improve their diets by increasing food purchasing power. Local welfare offices administer the program and are widely distributed throughout the country.

Special Supplemental Food Program for Women, Infants, and Children (WIC) is available to pregnant and lactating women, infants, and children up to five years of age who are considered to be at nutritional risk. Criteria for nutritional risk are evi-

Table 14—9. Referral Chart for Community Nutrition Resources*

Population Group	Risk Factor	Referral Source	Contact
Pregnant and lactating women	Low income.	Food stamps.	Welfare office.
	Anemia, inadequate weight gain, age-related risk factor, inadequate diet,	WIC Program.	City, county, or state health department.
	adolescent pregnancy, inadequate health care, or lack of food and nutrition information.	Maternity and Infant Care Project. EFNEP. Prenatal education.	State health department. Land-grant universities. Prenatal clinic or private health care team.
Infants	Low birth weight, failure to thrive, or poor growth patterns.	WIC Program.	City, county, or state health department.
	Inadequate health care.	Children and Youth Project.	State health department.
Children	Poor growth patterns, inadequate diet, or anemia.	WIC Program (up to five years of age).	City, county, or state health department.
	Low income.	Children and Youth Project (up to 18 years of age).	State health department.
		Headstart (preschool).	Local community action project.
		School Lunch.	Board of education.
		School Breakfast.	Local community action project.
General Adult	Obesity	Weight Watchers International, Thin Within, Dieters workshop, TOPS, and other weight reduction groups.	Local chapters.
	Hyperlipidemia, cardiovascular disease, or hypertension.	American Heart Association.	Local chapter.
	Diabetes.	American Diabetes Association.	Local chapter.
	Low income.	Food stamps.	Welfare office.
	Lack of food and nutrition information.	EFNEP.	Land-grant universities.
	General consumer information for all populations.†	Community nutrition groups and community cooperatives.	Local groups
		American Dietetic Association.	Chicago, IL 60611.
		Center for Science in the Public Interest.	
		Nutrition Foundation.	Washington, DC 20009.
		Society for Nutrition Education.	Washington, DC 20006
		U.S. Government Printing Office.	Berkeley, CA 94704. Washington, DC 20402.
Elderly	Low income.	Food stamps.	Welfare office.
		Congregate meal sites.	Social service agency.
	Homebound.	Meals on Wheels.	Social service agency.
	Diabetes.	American Diabetes Association.	Local chapter.
	Obesity.	Weight reduction groups.	(See adult section.)
	Cardiovascular disease.	American Heart Association.	Local chapter.

*From Finkelhor, S: Nutrition resources. *Medical Clinics of North America* 63(5):1117, 1979.
†This is only a partial listing. Programs may vary in different parts of the country.

dence of iron deficiency, inadequate weight gain during pregnancy, teenage pregnancy, failure to thrive, poor growth patterns, and inadequate dietary patterns based on a scoring system of a 24-hour dietary recall. The WIC program is usually available through county and city health departments. Supplemental foods include iron-fortified formula, milk, cheeses, iron-enriched cereals, eggs, peanut butter, legumes, and fruit juices.

Breast-feeding is promoted. In addition to the supplemental foods, health care and nutritional education are provided.

The school breakfast and lunch programs provide nutritious meals for children at school. Nutritional standards mandated by law require that lunch must furnish at least one third of the RDAs for children.

The Nutrition Program for the Elderly provides

both group meals and home-delivered ones. Besides providing one hot meal to the elderly (containing one third of the RDAs, a variety of social services are also available.

The Expanded Food and Nutrition Education Program (EFNEP) is available through county extension services of land-grant universities. Nutrition aides, who are low-income homemakers, are trained to go into homes of other low-income individuals and to assist them with meal planning, budgeting, cooking, and other food and nutrition-related problems.

Headstart is a preschool educational program for low-income families. Meals are furnished for the children, and nutrition education is available for the parents.

Since these programs are all dependent on federal funding, any cutbacks, such as those anticipated by the Gramm-Rudman-Hollings (1985) deficit-reduction act, jeopardize their budgets. Although the food stamp program was automatically exempt from this reduction in monies, others are being affected to some degree. This may result in some changes in eligibility (home-delivered meals to the elderly), increased quotas per unit (EFNEP), and more prioritizing of clients to serve those who have the greatest need (WIC).

Some programs receive additional funding from state governments, but these budgets may have to be cut, too. The fact that most of these programs are popular, preventive forms of health care (which is cheaper than health care for the ill) is in their favor when budget cuts are made.

STATE AND COUNTY PROGRAMS

State and local health departments usually have various programs to provide nutrition services, such as Well Baby Clinics and Family Health Centers. The health department and county hospitals are excellent resources for information about the various programs available.

THE PRIVATE SECTOR

Many resources are available for food and nutrition information. Several are listed in Table 14-9 and Appendices E-1 and E-2. Local chapters of many of these organizations furnish free or inexpensive literature, audiovisual materials, and health-oriented programs on various topics. They can be located in the telephone book. Frequently, local churches will provide free meals or other help.

ROLE OF THE HEALTH PROFESSIONAL

Legislation regarding federal, state, and county programs is frequently updated. All programs must prove themselves cost-effective for continued funding. By being involved in civic organizations and communicating with legislative representatives, health professionals can become knowledgable regarding pending legislation and have a voice about possible changes affecting the health and well-being of Americans. Involvement with volunteer organizations, such as the American Heart Association, will help further their health-related programs for the community.

• FACTS and FALLACIES

FALLACY: *By following the U.S. dietary guidelines, all health-related problems can be prevented.*

• **FACT:** *The U.S. dietary guidelines are an advisable way to eat; however, they do not guarantee that all health-related problems, such as cancer, diabetes, and heart disease can be avoided. Other factors are important, such as heredity, smoking, environmental hazards, and exercise. Nutrition is only one part of good health.*

FALLACY: *According to the U.S. dietary guidelines, an infant should be given low-fat or skim milk when s/he is weaned from the breast or bottle.*

• **FACT:** *This is an incorrect assumption; children below two years of age (not on breast or formula milk) should be given whole milk, which provides more energy for their growing needs.*

FALLACY: *All persons would be healthier if they strictly adhered to the U.S. dietary guidelines.*

• **FACT:** *No one guideline is appropriate for all individuals. For instance, a laborer who works hard in the hot sun every day should not restrict his/her salt intake. Each person's health, age, heredity, activities, and other factors should be considered prior to making dietary changes.*

Summary

In promoting an optimal diet for better nutrition, many factors must be considered. Two rules of thumb are applicable (Goodhart, 1980): (1) regularly eat a variety of foods and (2) eat and drink in moderation. In other words, "experience foods widely: indulge appetite temperately" (Davies, 1972). The dietary goals can be used to help interpret the basic food groups about items that are of concern to consumers and to encourage moderation in food consumption.

An important aspect that cannot be overlooked is that food should be enjoyed. Meals should be more than edible; they should be palatable. No food has any nutritional value unless it is consumed. Eating has always been one of the pleasures of life, and it must fulfill both psychological and physiological needs.

Many food chocies are made for economic reasons. Even on a limited budget, nutritious foods are available. Individuals responsible for meals on limited funds must plan more carefully and need to have more information about economical foods high in nutrients. Many government and private organizations have information available to help with money management.

Care must also be taken in the preparation of the foods, or many of the nutrients may be lost. Optimal nutrition is not achieved by setting a plate in front of someone. A nutritious meal must have been chosen wisely with the individual's physiological needs and preferences in mind, prepared to conserve the nutrients, and, finally, enjoyed.

Review Questions

1. List the Dietary Goals for the United States. List your favorite food items from each category and the frequency of consumption. Are these moderate amounts? If not, what are some foods that you can substitute for them?
2. How would you counsel a family to feed their children if the overweight mother is hypertensive, the overweight father is diabetic, but the children are currently healthy and of normal weight for size and age?
3. Plan an inexpensive menu for a week, using low-cost foods.
4. Where could the following persons be referred for financial aid, food and nutrition information, or menu planning and budgeting:
   a. A family of six whose father has recently lost his job?
   b. A pregnant teenager?
   c. A low-income family with school-age children in which both parents work?
   d. A senior citizen living alone who is not inspired to prepare meals for himself?
   e. A pregnant mother of five children, ages 1, 3, 5, 6, and 8, whose husband has abandoned them?
   f. An elderly person living on social security who is on a bland, low-salt diet?

REFERENCE LIST

American Medical Association Council on Scientific Affairs (AMA): Sodium in processed foods. *JAMA* 249(6):784, 1983.

American Medical Association Council on Scientific Affairs (AMA): American Medical Association Concepts of Nutrition and Health, *JAMA* 242(21):2335, 1979.

Beauchamp, GK; Bertino, M; Engelman, K: Modification of salt taste. *Ann Intern Med* 98(5 pt 2):763, 1983.

Bertino, M; Beauchamp, GK; Engelman, K: Long-term reduction in dietary sodium alters the taste of salt. *Am J Clin Nutr* 36(6):1134, 1982.

Borenstein, B: Effect of processing on the nutritional values of foods. In *Modern Nutrition in Health and Disease*, 6th ed. Edited by RS Goodhart; ME Shils. Philadelphia, Lea & Febiger, 1980, p 497.

Clydesdale, FM: Toward nutritional adequacy. *Ross Timesaver Dietetic Currents* 6(1), 1979.

Commentary: Dietary Goals for the United States, 2nd ed. *J Am Diet Assoc* 74(5):529, 1979.

Committee on Diet, Nutrition, and Cancer (CDNC): *Diet, Nutrition and Cancer*. National Academy Press, 1982.

Davies, L: *Easy Cooking for One and Two*. Harmondsworth, England, Penguin Press, 1972.

Department of Health, Education and Welfare (DHEW): *Healthy People: The Surgeon General's Report on Health Promotion and Disease Prevention*. DHEW (PHS) Publication No. 79-55071, Washington, DC, 1979.

De Swiet, M: Blood pressure, sodium, and take-away food. *Arch Dis Child* 57(9):645, 1982.

Engstrom, AM; Tobelmann, RC: Nutritional consequences of reducing sodium intake. *Ann Intern Med* 98(5 Pt 2):870, 1983.

Food and Nutrition Board, National Research Council (FNB): *Toward Healthful Diets*. Washington, DC, National Academy of Sciences, 1980.

Goodhart, RS: Criteria of an adequate diet. In *Modern Nutrition in Health and Disease*, 6th ed. Edited by RS Goodhart; ME Shils. Philadelphia, Lea & Febiger, 1980, p 445.

Hagen, RE; Schweigert, BS: Nutrient contents of table-ready foods: Cooked, processed, and stored. *Contemporary Nutr* 8(2):1983.

Harper, AE: Dietary guidelines for Americans. *Am J Clin Nutr* 34(1):121, 1981.

Harris, RS: Losses of nutrients during large scale preparation for direct feeding. B. Effects of large scale preparation on nutrients of foods of plant origin. In *Nutritional Evaluation of Food Processing*. Edited by RS Harris; H Von Loesecks. New York, J. Wiley & Sons, 1960.

Hayford, JT; Donney, MM; Wiebe, D; et al: Triglyceride integrated concentration: Effect of variation of source and amount of dietary carbohydrate. *Am J Clin Nutr* 32(8):1670, 1979.

Hein, RE; Hutchings, IJ: Influence of processing on vitamin-mineral content and biological availability in foods. In *Nutrients in Processed Foods: Vitamins, Minerals*. Edited by PL White. Chicago, American Medical Association, 1974, p 59.

Holden, RA; Ostfeld, AM; Freeman, DH, Jr; et al: Dietary salt and blood pressure. *JAMA* 250(3):365, 1983.

How nutritious are fast food meals? *Consumer Reports* 40(5):278, 1975.

Institute of Food Technology, Expert Panel on Food Safety and Nutrition (IFT): The effects of food processing on nutritional values. *Food Tech* 28(10):77, 1974.

Krochta, JM; Feinberg, B: Effects of harvesting and handling on the composition of foods. Part 1. Effect of harvesting and handling on fruits and vegetables. In *Nutritional Evaluation of Food Processing*. Edited by RS Harris; E Karmas. Westport, CT, AVI Publishing Co, 1975, p 98.

Laragh, JH; Pecker, MS: Dietary sodium and essential hypertension: Some myths, hopes, and truths. *Ann Intern Med* 98(5 Pt 2):735, 1983.

Lecos, C: Fructose: Questionable diet aid. *FDA Consumer* 14(2):20, 1980.

Marston, RM; Peterkin, BB: Nutrient content of the national food supply. *Nat Food Review* 9(winter):21, 1980.

Marston, RM; Welsh, SO: Nutrient content of the United States food supply, 1982. *Nat Food Review* 25(winter):7, 1984.

Odland, D; Axelson, J: Convenience foods—what they cost you. In *Food from Farm to Table, 1982 Yearbook of Agriculture*. Washington, DC, Government Printing Office, 1982, p 343.

Padberg, DI: Pickin' and choosin' in the supermarket. In *Will There Be Enough Food? 1981 Yearbook of Agriculture*. Washington, DC, Government Printing Office, 1981, p 179.

Peterkin, BB: Making food dollars count. *Family Econ Rev* 4:23, 1983.

Prescott, R: Per capita food consumption highlights. *Nat Food Review* 16(fall):7, 1981.

Schaus, EE; Briggs, GM: Nutritionally economic foods. *J Nutr Ed* 15(4):130, 1983.

Select Committee on Nutrition and Human Needs. United States Senate. *Dietary Goals for the United States*, 2nd ed. Washington, DC, Government Printing Office, 1977.

Shahoda, T: Hunger problem is real: Medical experts. *Hospitals* 58(8):61, 1984.

Shannon, BM; Parks, SC: Fast foods: A perspective on their nutritional impact. *J Am Diet Assoc* 76(3):242, 1980.

Sheridan, MJ; McPherrin, EG: *Fast Food and the American Diet*. American Council on Science and Health (47 Maple Street, Summit, NJ 07901), November 1981.

Simko, V: Increase in serum lipids on feeding sucrose: The role of fructose and glucose. *Am J Clin Nutr* 33(10):2217, 1980.

U.S. Department of Agriculture and U.S. Health, Education, and Welfare (USDA & USHEW): *Nutrition and Your Health: Dietary Guidelines for Americans*, 2nd ed. Home and Garden Bulletin No. 232, 1985.

U.S. Department of Health, Education, and Welfare (USDHEW): *Dietary intake findings, United States, 1971–1974*. DHEW Publication No. 77–1647, 1977.

Wurtman, RJ: Neurochemical changes following high-dose aspartame with dietary carbohydrates (letter). *N Engl J Med* 309(7):429, 1983.

Young, EA; Brennan, EH; Irving, GL: Update: Nutritional analysis of fast foods. *Ross Timesaver Dietetic Currents* 8(2), 1981.

Zee, P; DeLeon, M; Roberson, P; et al: Nutritional improvement of poor urban preschool children: A 1983–1977 comparison. *JAMA* 253(22):3269, 1985.

Further Study

Ahrens, EH: The diet heart question in 1985: Has it really been settled? *Lancet* 1(May 11):1085, 1985.

Ahrens, EH, Jr; Connor, WE; Bierman, EL; et al: Symposium. The evidence relating six dietary factors to the nations' health. *Am J Clin Nutr* 32(suppl);2627, 1979.

Arlin, M: Controversies in nutrition, a brief review. *Nurs Clin North Am* 14(2):199, 1980.

Bowen, E; Mondschein, N: Help yourself! Give your patients a portion of good nutrition education. *J Pract Nurs* 30(November–December):23, 1980.

Brown, JG: Eat right in spite of yourself. *Health* 14(1):25, 1982.

Clark, RA; Blackburn, GL: The role of nutrition in disease prevention and health promotion. *Compr Ther* 9(4):12, 1983.

Cleveland, LE: Buying food for the nutrients it provides. In *Food from Farm to Table. 1982 Yearbook of Agriculture*. Washington, DC, Government Printing Office, 1982, p 285.

Council on Scientific Affairs: Aspartame: Review of safety issues. *JAMA* 254(3):400, 1985.

Farris, RP; Frank, GC; Webber, LS; et al: A nutrition curriculum for families with high blood pressure. *J Sch Health* 55(3):110, 1985.

Finkelhor, S: Nutrition resources. *Med Clin North Am* 63(5):1117, 1979.

Jones, J: *Jet Fuel*. New York, Random House, 1984.

Junker, CC: Cost comparison tools to stretch your food dollar. In *Food from Farm to Table. 1982 Yearbook of Agriculture*. Washington, DC, Government Printing Office, 1982, p 326.

Lecos, C: Dietary guidelines for Americans: No nonsense advice for healthy eating. *FDA Consumer* 19(9):10, 1985.

Lecos, C: What about nutrients in fast foods? *FDA Consumer* HHS Publication No. (FDA) 83–2172, May 1983.

Lecos, C: The sweet and sour history of saccharin, cyclamate, aspartame. *FDA Consumer* 15(7):8, 1981.

Levine, AS; Labuza, TP; Morley, JE: Food technology. A primer for physicians. *N Engl J Med* 312(10):628, 1985.

May, M: Nutrition: Eat, drink, and be healthy. *Nurs Mirror* 151(5):28, 1980.

Miller, RW: *How to Ignore Salt and Still Please the Palate*. FDA Consumer HHS Publication No. (FDA) 82–2165, April 1982.

Oliver, MF: Consensus or nonsensus conferences on coronary heart disease. *Lancet* 1(May 11):1087, 1985.

Wolf, ID; Peterkin, BB: Dietary guidelines: The USDA perspective. *Food Tech* 38(7):80, 1984.

Yes, reducing cholesterol does lower CHD incidence. *Am J Nurs* 84(3):297, 1984.

NUTRITION INTERVENTION THROUGHOUT THE LIFE CYCLE

Dietary Management for the Adult Woman: Pregnancy, Lactation, and Premenstrual Syndrome

15

THE STUDENT WILL BE ABLE TO:

- **Define the dietary measures applicable to toxemia.**
- **List nutrients (with the amounts) that are usually supplemented during pregnancy.**
- **Describe fetal alcohol syndrome.**
- **Plan the food intake for pregnancy.**
- **List high-risk factors for pregnancy.**
- **Evaluate the symptoms of a PMS sufferer and counsel her regarding dietary changes that may be beneficial.**

Acetonuria
Alveoli
Antepartum
Bifidus factor
Colostrum
Dystocia
Eclampsia
Fetal alcohol syndrome (FAS)
Full term (FT)
Gravida
Induced nonpuerperal lactation
Intrauterine growth rate (IUGR)
Low birth weight (LBW)
Mastitis
Neonatal
Oxytocin
Perinatal
Pregnancy-induced hypertension (PIH)
Pregravid weight
Premenstrual syndrome (PMS)
Prolactin
Relactation
Small for gestational age (SGA)
Terotogenesis
Toxemia
Very low birth weight (VLBW)

MALNUTRITION

Extensive literature is available on relationships of the pregnant woman, fetal development, newborn infant, and even anomalies occurring later in life for the newborn—all due to malnutrition and different nutrient deficiencies (Table 15–1). The vulnerable part of the body is dependent upon its stage of development and the extent of nutrient deprivation (Fig. 15–1). Briefly, poor nutrition during pregnancy for the mother results in higher incidence of hemorrhages, preeclampsia and eclampsia, and complications in labor and delivery (Luke, 1979). For the infant, poor eating habits of the mother result in a higher incidence of: (1) fetal distress, (2) asphyxia neonatorum, (3) congenital anomalies (30-fold increase in major anomalies with severe malnutrition), (4) prematurity and perinatal death, (5) neonatal mortality, and (6) congenital heart disease (a 16-fold increase with severe malnutrition).

Low birth weight and premature infants have more abnormalities as well as increased mortality. There is substantial evidence of an association between the level of intellectual functioning and low birth weight (i.e., 2000 to 2500 gm), which is even more marked in very low birth weight (VLBW) infants (i.e., 1500 gm) (Ricciuti, 1981).

AGE OF THE GRAVIDA

Pregravid Status. In addition to nutritional status, pregravid age and weight are also factors in the outcome of the pregnancy. According to Luke (1979), four major categories of nutritional risks exist: (1) juvenile gravidas—under 18 years old, (2) older gravidas—35 years of age or older, (3) low pregravid weight—10 percent or more under ideal weight, and (4) pregravid obesity—20 percent or more over ideal weight.

Adolescent Pregnancy. In the United States, a million teenagers become pregnant every year; 400,000 are under 18 years of age and 30,000 are less than 15 years old. About 60 percent of these adolescents continue pregnancy to delivery, and one fourth of them become pregnant again within a year (Beal, 1981).

Most females have not completed linear growth and achieved gynecological maturity until the age of 17. Not only are many of these young girls still growing and storing nutrients in their own bodies, but the majority have inadequate dietary intakes of calcium, iron, vitamin A, niacin, and calories for growth and energy. The socioeconomic disadvantages of these young mothers may

Table 15–1. Nutritional Risk Factors During Pregnancy*

The pregnant woman is very likely to be at nutritional risk if, at the onset of pregnancy, she

a. is an adolescent (15 years of age or less).
b. has had three or more pregnancies during the past 2 years.
c. has a history of poor obstetric or fetal performance.
d. is economically deprived.
e. is a food faddist ingesting a bizarre or nutritionally restrictive diet.
f. is a heavy smoker, drug addict, or alcoholic.
g. has a therapeutic diet for chronic systemic disease.
h. had a prepartum weight at her first prenatal visit of <85% or >120% of standard weight.

The pregnant woman is very likely to be at nutritional risk, if during prenatal care she

a. has a low or deficient hemoglobin/hematocrit.
b. has inadequate weight gain or any weight loss.
c. has excessive weight gain (more than 2 pounds per week).
d. is planning to breast feed her baby.

*Adapted from: Task Force on Nutrition: Assessment of Maternal Nutrition. American College of Obstetricians and Gynecologists, 1978.

affect their diet by the amount of food available and by their uninformed selections; thus the requirements of the fetus may not be met (McCormick et al, 1983). In addition to the nutritional risk for the gravida and infant, maternal and neonatal mortality rates are higher for younger gravidas (Miller & Field, 1984; McCormick et al, 1983).

In order for a teenager to gain adequate weight to support a successful pregnancy, more nutrient-dense foods should be eaten instead of merely increasing food intake (Table 15–2). Dietary intake should be based upon the RDAs for their age in addition to those for pregnant women. The average teenager will need an additional 300 kcal daily for the first trimester and an extra 600 to 650 kcal/day during the second and third trimester, rather than the routine RDA increase of 300 kcal (Miller & Field, 1984). Even with nutritional adjustments, the infants of adolescents are smaller and thinner than those of older women (Frisancho et al, 1983).

Older Pregnancies. Many couples today are choosing to postpone parenthood. Pregnancy after the age of 35 is influenced by the individual's overall health. In addition to finding that it is not as easy to become pregnant as expected, there are several maternal risks involving preexisting medical conditions, such as diabetes, kidney disease, hypertension, cardiovascular problems, and leiomyoma uteri. These conditions should be closely supervised to lessen their impact upon the fetus.

The older female needs to be particularly

CRITICAL PERIODS OF DEVELOPMENT

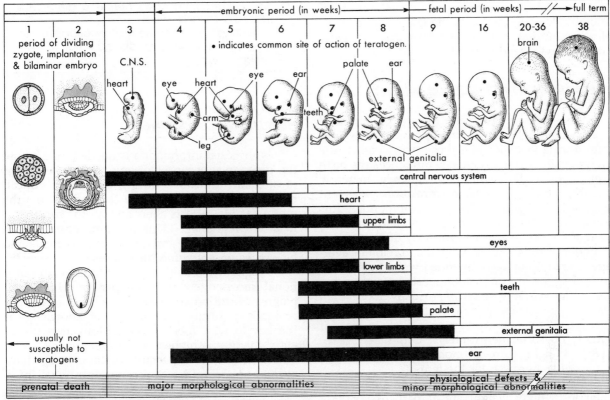

Figure 15–1. Periods of maximum fetal teratogenic vulnerability and critical periods of development. Black bar denotes highly sensitive periods. (From Moore KL: The Developing Human, 2nd ed. Philadelphia, W. B. Saunders Co, 1977, by permission.)

aware of maintaining her nutritional health if a later pregnancy is anticipated. As the mother's age increases, her baby is more likely to be premature and smaller than average (DeVore, 1983).

In all cases, primary factors for success are the previous nutritional status, adequate weight gain, and providing the essential nutrients during pregnancy. Caloric needs may be at least 4 per-

Table 15–2. Weight Gain Recommendation for a 15-year-old Gravida*

Basic data	
Age	15 years
Age of menarche	12.5 years
Body weight at conception	48 kg (105.6 lb.)
Body height at conception	62 cm (64 in.)
Adequate weight for height	55 kg (121 lb.)
Recommendation	
Estimated weight deficit	7 kg (15.4 lb.)
Estimated growth increments (9 months)	1.13 kg (2.48 lb.)
Average pregnancy gain	12.5 kg (27.5 lb.)
Total weight to be gained	20.6 kg (45.3 lb.)

*From Rosso, P; Lederman, SA: Nutrition in the pregnant adolescent. In *Adolescent Nutrition*. Edited by M. Winick. New York, John Wiley & Sons, 1982, with permission.

cent less than for a younger pregnant woman, owing to a lowered resting basal metabolism rate and less activity. Therefore, with this somewhat limited caloric restriction in the face of an increase of other nutrients, foods of high-nutrient density are required (Weigley, 1983).

PREGRAVID AND GESTATIONAL WEIGHT

Successful pregnancies depend upon ideal preconception weight plus appropriate weight gain during gestation. Of these two weights, the weight gain during pregnancy influences the birth weight more than the prepregnancy maternal weight, which is second in correlation. A weight gain of 1 to 2 kg (2 to 4 lbs.) is recommended during the first trimester of pregnancy, with a weight gain of 0.45 kg (about 1 lb.) weekly during the remainder of the pregnancy for the gravida of average weight. Total recommended weight gain is 10 to 12.3 kg, or 22 to 27 lbs. Suggested weight gains for underweight women are usually more than the average recommended weight gain—about 20 lbs. for overweight women and 15 to 16 lbs. for grossly obese women (Suter & Ott, 1984; Rosso, 1985). Weight gain is monitored regularly to achieve ideal growth for the fetus.

Gravidas who are 50 percent or more above their ideal body weight are at particular risk of gaining too little weight, resulting in a smaller than average or a low birth weight (LBW) infant (George et al, 1984).

If the expectant mother's weight is 10 percent below ideal, or 20 percent or more above the norm for her height and age group, both the gravida and infant are at nutritional risk. Twice as many LBW infants are born to underweight women as to women of normal weight.

Clinical Implications:

- Excessive weight gain during pregnancy does not cause the development of preeclampsia (CNMPC, 1981).
- Pregnancy is not an appropriate time for weight reduction because it may be accompanied by ketonuria, which may result in fetal neurological damage (Naeye & Chez, 1981). Ideally, weight adjustments (both losses and gains) are made before conception.
- Rapid weight gains during pregnancy usually are due to the accumulation of fluid rather than fat deposits.
- At one time, obstetricians recommended restricting weight. However, that was based upon easing delivery of the infant. This is not advisable today.

- After surgical bypass for obesity (for more normal weight of the newborn), a period of two years is recommended before a pregnancy (Gibbs & Seitchik, 1980).
- Unfortunately, the present preoccupation with slimness may result in attempts not to gain weight during pregnancy.

NUTRITION COUNSELING

Nutritional information is needed long before the pregnancy occurs. Not only are the selections of adequate nutrients during pregnancy critical, but food intake from the beginning of the mother's life affects her ability to support a healthy pregnancy. Plans for conception should encourage potential gravidas to choose foods and beverages wisely before pregnancy.

Pregnant women may have little or no nutritional knowledge despite aggressive school campaigns. Nutrition counseling is often unavailable or ignored during pregnancy, yet knowledge is the key to wise food choices. Motivation for dietary changes is highest during pregnancy.

Low-income expectant mothers may have several opportunities to receive nutritional information, but the private sector in many cases has no specific program. There are many benefits of a nutritional educational component incorporated into the obstetrician's treatment during the first trimester of pregnancy. In one such program, a registered dietitian meets with the expectant parents in an informal relaxed atmosphere to present nutrition information applicable to their needs. This helps the pregnant woman to understand her energy and nutrient needs; to cope with gastrointestinal problems, heartburn, morning sickness, and constipation; and to recognize risk factors. Not only are the gravida and fetus better fed, but the father and other members of the family become more conscious of the role of nutrition for better health (Allard, 1986).

Active listening to the pregnant woman is the only way to gain her confidence and learn about her particular eating habits. Open questions with no suggestion of an expected answer facilitate these conversations, such as: Is there any food or beverage that you do not eat? Is there anything that you crave and eat often? Do you know of any special foods to be eaten or avoided during pregnancy?

Some women have special cravings while they are pregnant. Inquiring about any unusual eating habits, such as eating clay (pica), ice, or starch is important (see Chapter 18). A discussion of the results and causes of these habits is more effective than telling them to stop eating those items.

Most importantly, it is helpful to determine whether the gravida understands what foods she should be eating. This can be tested by allowing her to plan some daily menus that meet the RDA guidelines for pregnancy. *Focus on a Sample Menu for Pregnancy* shows an adequate menu pattern. Counseling is successful if the gravida can plan nutritionally adequate menus that incorporate her favorite foods. Attempts should be made to consume foods in spite of morning sickness (which may occur at any time during the day).

CLINICAL LABORATORY ASSESSMENT

Physical evidence of poor nutrition tends to appear late and may be subtle and nonspecific, making clinical laboratory assessment imperative. Because of the many biochemical and physiological changes occurring during pregnancy, normal female values are not valid. Table 15–3 lists laboratory tests for assessing nutritional status during pregnancy.

Minimum laboratory tests include:
1. Urine: glucose and protein (albumin) for diabetes, preeclampsia, or renal disease.
2. Serum hemoglobin and hematocrit, vitamin B_{12}, iron and ferritin, and red cell folate.

NUTRITIONAL FACTORS

The RDAs for pregnancy (see inside cover) should be included daily for optimum health of mother and fetus; however, the 10-State Nutrition

---

FOCUS ON	A SAMPLE MENU FOR PREGNANCY

BEFORE RISING: Crackers (if desired).
BREAKFAST: Orange juice (4 oz.)
    Bran flakes (½ cup) with skim milk (4 oz.) and sugar (1 tsp.)
    Raisin toast (1 slice) with margarine (1 pat)
    Skim milk (8 oz.)
MIDMORNING: Low-fat strawberry yogurt (8 oz.)
    Graham crackers
LUNCH: Turkey (2 oz.) sandwich on cracked whole-wheat bread with margarine (1 pat) plus low-fat mayonnaise (1 Tbsp.)
    Tossed green salad with Italian dressing (1 to 2 Tbsp.) (vinegar plus safflower or corn oil plus seasonings)
    Skim milk (8 oz.)
MIDAFTERNOON: Tomato juice (8 oz.)
    Hard-cooked egg
DINNER: Roast beef (3 oz.)
    Baked potato with margarine (1 pat)
    Celery and carrot sticks
    Nectarine with low-fat cottage cheese
BEDTIME: Oatmeal cookies (2)
    Skim milk (8 oz.)

Note: Water throughout day with/or between snacks and meals. Adjustments in kilocalories and specific nutrients as required for various ages and physical conditions.

Survey (USDA, 1972) revealed that pregnant women have diets below standard for energy, iron, calcium, vitamin A, and protein. Zinc, folacin, and magnesium are poorly supplied by foods

---

Table 15–3. Nutritional Assessment in Pregnancy: Laboratory Tests

Laboratory Tests	Normal Range	
	Nonpregnant	*Pregnant*
Serum protein, total	6.5 to 8.5 gm per 100 ml	6 to 8 ·
Serum albumen	3.5 to 5 gm per 100 ml	3 to 4.5
Blood urea nitrogen	10 to 25 mg per 100 ml	5 to 15
FBS	70 to 110 mg per 100 ml	65 to 100
2-hr postprandial blood sugar	<110 mg per 100 ml	<120
Folic acid, serum	5 to 21 ng per ml	3 to 15
Vitamin B_{12} serum	330 to 1025 pg per ml	Decreased
Hgb/Hct	>12/36	11/33
Serum Fe/Fe binding capacity	>50/250 to 400 mcg per 100 ml	>40/300 to 450

consumed normally and may be low during pregnancy (Suter & Ott, 1984). Table 15-4 helps to translate RDAs for a pregnant woman into servings from the basic food groups.

Energy. During pregnancy, the amount of calories is increased to ensure nutrient and energy needs. The RDAs state that an additional 300 kcal or 36 kcal/kg of body weight per day is needed. Additional energy is needed (1) to build the new tissues (including those of the fetus, placenta, and amniotic fluid and increases in extracellular fluid, uterus, breasts, and blood volume), (2) to support the increased metabolic expenditure, and (3) to

move the additional weight. Energy requirements will reflect changes in normal physical activities. While the pregnant woman may gradually slow her pace, obstetricians usually advise to continue exercising as much as possible; moderation is always the key. Appropriate weight gain reflects the adequacy of energy intake.

Protein. Since protein is the basic nutrient for growth, an additional 30 gm of protein daily of the RDA for the gravida's age group is recommended. This is usually accomplished by an increase of two cups of milk (16 gm of protein) and two additional ounces of meat or meat substitute

Table 15-4. Examples of Daily Food Pattern Guidelines for Optimal Nutrition During Pregnancy

Food	Servings	Measure	Kcal	Protein (gm)	Calcium (mg)	Major Nutrients
Milk products (Vitamin D–fortified)	4					Calcium, protein
Milk, skim, or		8 oz.	88	8.8	296	
Yogurt (low-fat "LF")		8 oz.	113	7.7	271	
Cottage Cheese (LF)		4 oz.	96	19.2	104	
Cheese, American		1 slice	100	6.3	188	
Ice Cream		1 cup	257	6.0	194	
Egg	1	whole	72	5.7	24	
Meat (lean), Legumes, Nuts	2		(at least 4 oz. total)			Protein, iron
Beef, Chicken, Fish, or Pork		3 oz.		20.0		
Liver once/week						Exceptionally nutritious
Legumes, Dried Beans (Great Northern)		½ cup	101	14.0	90	
Nuts						
Peanut Butter		1 Tbsp.	94	4.0	9	
Fruit and Vegetables	4 +					
Citrus Fruits or equivalents	2					Vitamin C
Orange Juice		4 oz.				
Tomato Juice		8 oz.				
Grapefruit		½				
Green, yellow, orange Vegetable	1					Carotene (vitamin A)
Other Fruits and Vegetables	1 +					
Raw Fruit/Vegetable	1					Folic acid
Bread and Cereal (Whole-grain or enriched)	4					B Vitamins
Bread		1 slice				
Cereal		½ cup				
Vegetable oil or margarine (corn or safflower)	3	1 Tbsp.				Linoleic acid
Water (fluoridated)	*					Fluid, fluoride
Iodized Salt in moderation						Iodine
Supplements						Optional
Iron			30 to 60 mg or more as needed			
Folic Acid			400 mcg			
Zinc			10 to 12 mg + 8 to 10 mg/foods†			
Copper			2.0 mg + 1.00 mg/foods†			
Pyridoxine (B₆)			4.0 mg			

Note: General modifications above the RDAs include an additional 300 kcal for pregnancy, 500 kcal for lactation, 30 grams protein, double the folic acid and calcium.

*Water: 1 gm water/kcal (Stumbo et al, 1985). (8 oz. = 240 gm, so about 10 to 11 (8 oz.) glasses, or the equivalent from foods, per 2500 kcal. See Chapter 5.)

†Taper, LJ; Oliva, JT; Ritchey, SJ: Zinc and copper retention during pregnancy: The adequacy of prenatal diets with and without dietary supplementation. *American Journal of Clinical Nutrition* 41:1184, 1985.

(14 gm of protein). Additionally, kilocalories must be adequate to prevent protein from being used for energy.

B Vitamins. Several of the B vitamin requirements are based on energy intake; usually, their intake increases automatically with increased calories. Adequate intake of several B vitamins is difficult to achieve without careful selection of foods or supplementation. Most women from late pregnancy through six months postpartum are substantially below the Estimated Safe and Adequate Daily Dietary Intake of 4 to 7 mg/day of pantothenic acid without supplements. Studies with experimental animals have shown a variety of complications and defects in offspring due to pantothenic acid deficiency (Song et al, 1985).

Vitamin B₆. The current RDA for vitamin B_6 is 2 to 6 mg daily. However, some studies of pregnant women suggest that an advisable level is between 5.5 and 7.6 mg/day (diet plus supplement as pyridoxine equivalents) to maintain plasma pyridoxal levels (Schuster et al, 1984). Prescriptions may be given to pregnant women for a multivitamin supplement containing 4.0 mg vitamin B_6 daily. This, in addition to the amounts supplied by foods, supplies a total intake of about 5.1 to 5.4 mg of vitamin B_6 (Reynolds et al, 1984).

Vitamin B_6 is critical to normal development of infants. Convulsive seizures and hyperirritability occur in infants with very low intakes from formula or breast milk (Reynolds et al, 1984). These findings concerning placental transfer plus the increased requirement for this vitamin with greater protein intake add credibility to a modest supplementation during gestation (Pitkin, 1981). However, as discussed in Chapter 10, too much vitamin B_6 can cause nerve damage.

Folic Acid. The RDA for folic acid during pregnancy is double the nonpregnant allowance (from 400 to 800 mcg). Since folic acid is a cofactor in DNA synthesis, pregnancy increases its demand. A marked depletion of this vitamin can cause megaloblastic anemia in the mother, but even a mild deficiency has been associated with low birth weight of infants and some obstetrical complications (Thenen, 1982).

Plasma folate levels fall as pregnancy advances so that at term they are about half the nonpregnant values. Red cell folate is a more useful index, even though the turnover of red blood cells is slow and there will be a delay before a deficiency causes significant reductions in the folate concentrations of the red cells. There is evidence that patients who have low red cell folate levels at the beginning of pregnancy develop megaloblastic anemia in the third trimester (Letsky, 1982).

The requirement for folic acid is difficult to meet by food intake alone without conscientious daily selections of raw fruits and vegetables, especially green leafy vegetables. Folacin-fortified breakfast cereals, milk, and orange juice may supply significant amounts (Thenen, 1982). Other good sources are listed in Chapter 11.

There is considerable debate over the time to start supplementation of folic acid. Supplementation of an additional 400 mcg/day is usually recommended during the last half of pregnancy because of increased metabolism and urinary excretion (Suter & Ott, 1984). However, Truswell (1985) claims that since a good intake of folate is important in preventing neural tube defects in a minority of women, supplementation of folic acid should be periconceptional because this vitamin is needed around 28 days after ovulation.

Clinical Implication:

- Excretion of formiminoglutamic acid (FIGLU) increases when there is a folate deficiency, but this test is no longer recommended since increased FIGLU excretion occurs normally in early pregnancy (Letsky, 1982).

Iron. It has been estimated that as many as 25 percent of low-income pregnant women have deficient hemoglobin levels (Gibbs & Seitchik, 1980). Hemoglobin and hematocrit are tested at least once or twice during pregnancy; in some facilities, they are tested monthly.

The gestational requirement of iron averages 800 mg (500 mg for maternal erythropoiesis and 300 mg for the fetus and placenta) or approximately 4 mg/day over the last three-quarters of gestation (Table 15–5). An average of 30 mg of iron stored in the reticuloendothelial cells of the bone marrow is marginally adequate. With this

Table 15–5. *Iron "Costs" of Normal Pregnancy**

Iron contributed to fetus	200–370 mg
In placenta and cord	30–170
In blood loss at delivery	90–310
In milk, lactation 6 months	100–180
	420–1030 mg
Average per day (pregnancy 9 mo, lactation 6 mo)	1–2.5

*From Beutler, E: Iron. In *Modern Nutrition in Health and Disease*, 6th ed. Edited by RS Goodhart; ME Shils, Philadelphia, Lea & Febiger, 1980, with permission.

storage amount plus 1 to 1.5 mg/day from food sources, the gravida can meet this need (Pitkin, 1981).

Even though absorption of iron is enhanced during the last two-thirds of the pregnancy, supplemental iron is ordinarily prescribed. Prevention of iron deficiency is accomplished by oral supplementation of 30 to 60 mg of iron/day as a simple ferrous salt (150 to 300 mg of USP ferrous sulfate) for women with iron stores. Women without iron stores may require 120 to 240 mg iron/day or 600 to 1200 mg USP ferrous sulfate (Letsky, 1982).

Some women may experience adverse symptoms, i.e., nausea or constipation, from iron supplementation, which may account for poor compliance (Orr & Simmons, 1979). Yet when iron supplementation is taken with meals, adverse symptoms are rare. Also, iron absorption is enhanced by the presence of vitamin C and protein, so these nutrients should be included in the meals.

An intramuscular injection of iron (1000 mg) can be given to women who cannot be given iron by the oral route either because of noncompliance or because of unacceptable side effects. This one injection assures iron sufficiency for that pregnancy. However, the injections are painful and can stain the skin, but there is no extra risk of incurring malignancy at the injection site as once reported (Letsky, 1982).

Calcium. The RDA of 1200 mg/day of calcium is easily met by four servings of milk or milk products. Low-fat or skim milk may be used to control weight as well as saturated fat intake. Milk may be incorporated into cooking or used in different forms such as cheese, ice cream, or yogurt for variety. The vitamin D requirement should be from a fortified calcium source.

Iodine. During the second half of pregnancy, the basal metabolic rate may increase up to 23 percent because of increased activity of the thyroid gland. Goiter is likely to develop during pregnancy unless the needed iodine is supplied. A deficiency may cause cretinism in infants. Iodized salt can supply the additional 25 mg iodine requirement through larger amounts of seasoned foods.

Sodium. In pregnancy sodium retention is a normal physiological adjustment. Because of the increased amounts of food consumed in the latter stages of pregnancy, edema is more likely to develop as more sodium is ingested. Resting with the feet elevated may be recommended. If excessive salting of foods is practiced, these amounts may be reduced. Sodium restriction is an obsolete concept and no longer advisable; diuretics are not recommended during pregnancy either (Suter & Ott, 1984).

Zinc. The recommendations for zinc as well as suggested copper intake are rarely met by dietary measures without supplementation (Taper et al, 1985). Higher-than-normal incidences of delivery complications (including postmaturity and difficult deliveries) can be anticipated in women consuming inadequate dietary zinc (Golub et al, 1984). If supplementation is desired, 15 to 25 mg of elemental zinc is prescribed. If the supplementation of iron exceeds 60 mg, an adjustment should be made to increase zinc since excessive iron reduces the serum zinc levels (Breskin et al, 1983).

Fluids. The gravida should be reminded to drink more than six glasses of fluids (mainly water) per day. Total fluid intake should be 1 gm water/kcal (Stumbo et al, 1985). Since 8 oz. equals 240 gm, about 10 to 11 (8 oz.) glasses, or the equivalent from foods, would be recommended. Of course a large part of this fluid intake can come from fruits and vegetables.

Not only is fluoridated water preferable, but fluoride supplementation has been suggested by some studies. Primary dentition begins at 10 to 12 weeks of pregnancy (Worthington-Roberts et al, 1981). Fewer caries were seen in infants whose mothers were given 1 mg fluoride daily, as well as fluoridated water (Glenn et al, 1982).

Clinical Implications:

- Vitamin B_{12} supplements are advisable for vegetarians (who exclude all animal products) to prevent megaloblastic anemia during pregnancy (Farthington, 1981).
- Inadequate dietary habits cannot be corrected simply by vitamin and mineral supplementation. With a well-balanced diet, only iron and folacin supplementation may be suggested.
- Nutritional reserves may be depleted with multiparous interconceptional periods of less than a year. A previous history of aborted, stillborn, premature, or low birth weight infants indicates inadequate nutritional status.
- The least expensive iron tablets should be tried first; they are usually quite acceptable by the individual with few, if any, side effects and may even be absorbed better than more expensive brands (Letsky, 1982).
- If the hemoglobin values of an iron-deficient patient do not increase 1 gm/dl per week, a transfusion may be indicated (Letsky, 1982).

- Sodium restriction during pregnancy should be prescribed only if some specific complication such as cardiac failure occurs (Weigley, 1983).

Other Influential Factors

Medications. Drugs and medications can affect the fetus and nursing infant (Table 15–6). These include such common items as aspirin, antihistamines, vitamin preparations, caffeine, and alcohol. A previous recent history of oral contraceptives indicates an increased need for vitamins C, B_6, and B_{12} and folacin. Each of these influences on the gravida's nutritional status should be discussed with her early in the pregnancy.

Smoking. Both smoking and psychological stress are directly related to low birth weight because of decreased utilization of kilocalories. Despite increased energy intakes, smoking results in low birth weight with greater risk of perinatal mortality. Infants of smoking mothers are significantly lighter, shorter, and have smaller head and arm circumferences (Harrison et al, 1983).

Caffeine. Pregnant women should avoid, or use sparingly, foods, beverages, and drugs containing caffeine. Studies in Finland (the country with the highest per capita coffee consumption) have linked the amount of coffee consumed during pregnancy to malformed children (Kurppa et al, 1983). Pregnant women who consume large quantities of coffee apparently have an increased incidence of spontaneous abortions, premature labor, and small for gestational age infants.

Not only is caffeine found in coffee, tea, chocolate, cocoa, and some soft drinks, but it may be

Table 15–6. Drugs Excreted in Human Milk*

Drug	Implication for Mother	Implication for Nursing Infant
Antibiotics (broad- and medium-spectrum)	Mother should not take certain ones.	Sensitization of baby may occur, especially with penicillin Anemia, shock, death Hepatotoxic
Anticoagulants	Mother should not take.	Infant can develop serious hemorrhage
Anticonvulsants	No problem except with primidone (Mysoline).	Drowsiness in infant
Antimigraine agents, e.g., ergotamine (Cafergot)	Mother should not take.	May cause vomiting, diarrhea, shock, and hypertension
Antitumor drugs	Mother should not take.	May harm infant's developing cells
Antispasmodics and anticholinergics, e.g., trihexyphenidyl (Artane) and nylidrin (Arlidin)	Mother should not take.	Diminish lactation and may cause heart irregularities in baby
Aspirin, phenacetin, and combinations	Mother should not take.	May cause bleeding in infant May cause a macular rash
Hypotensives in combination with diuretics	Mother should not take; may cause galactorrhea.	Hazardous to infant because may cause increased respiratory tract secretions, cyanosis, and anorexia
Isoniazid	Mother should not take.	Causes mental retardation in infant
Laxatives	Present in milk.	Can cause diarrhea in baby
Propranolol	Mother should not take.	May cause bronchospasm, bradycardia, hypotension, congestive heart failure, and hypoglycemia in baby
Psychotropic drugs	Mother should not take.	Drowsiness, other unknown effects in infant
Radioactive iodine	Mother should not be given.	Suppresses infant's thyroid
Steroids	Mother should not take; decrease lactation.	Decrease lactation and thus infant growth Cause gynecomastia in baby
Thiazide diuretics	Present in milk.	May cause dehydration in infant
Urinary anti-infectives	Present in milk; mother should not take sulfonamides.	May be noxious to infant if taken by mother continuously Sulfonamides noxious to infants less than 2 months old
Vaginal medications (Flagyl vaginal inserts, AVC cream, other sulfonamides)	Mother should not use.	Cause jaundice of newborn

*From Rothermel, PC; Faber, MM: Drugs in breast-milk—a consumer's guide. *Birth Family Journal* 2:76, 1975.

in over-the-counter drugs for headache, colds, allergy, and menstrual and pain-killing compounds as well as stay-awake pills and many prescription drugs. The caffeine content of various foods and beverages is listed in Appendix D–4. The FDA advises the avoidance of caffeine until further studies clarify the exact limits (Lecos, 1982).

Alcohol. As little as 2 oz./day of alcohol can cause fetal alcohol syndrome (FAS), a condition characterized by irreversible brain damage and mental retardation. The first trimester is the most vulnerable time for the fetus, yet the woman may not even be aware of the pregnancy, especially during the first crucial month. Four to five drinks a day, or at least 45 drinks per month, can produce the full FAS syndrome with its obvious characteristics (Table 15–7).

The FAS child has specific physiological deformities, as shown in Figure 15–2. The mental and physical abnormalities cannot be reversed (Iber, 1981).

Even with adequate nutrition, normal development of fetal organs is jeopardized. Other proclivities that usually accompany alcohol consumption (e.g., smoking, excessive amounts of coffee the morning after, poor eating habits with little attention to needed nutrients, and perhaps tranquilizers) may also adversely affect the unborn child.

Because the brain has a special affinity for alcohol, it is one of the first organs affected. Even at birth, the circumference of the head is small (microcephaly), indicating abnormal brain capacity (i.e., 140 gm in a FAS infant compared to a normal brain weighing 400 gm) (Iber, 1981). Fewer brain cells exist. Additionally, some of the cells may be damaged preventing normal functioning; fewer neurons result in disorganized thought. The thinking ability of the brain is permanently disturbed.

Additionally, there are fewer total body cells, which mean abnormal weight gain. LBW babies are born as though all the body cells have been affected by alcohol, which depletes fluids and affects normal cell development and growth. The tragedy of FAS is that many gravidas simply do not know about this condition before and during pregnancy.

COMMON CONDITIONS DURING PREGNANCY

Nausea and Vomiting. Morning sickness may occur only in the morning or may last throughout the day during the first trimester. A diet high in protein and low in carbohydrate may predispose the gravida to periods of nausea and vomiting. An increase in carbohydrate intake will be useful. If the demand during the first trimester for glucose is not readily met from the diet and/or when the liver glycogen-glucose turnover is inadequate, sickness may occur more often (Pickard, 1982). Other relevant tips for morning sickness include:

1. Eat dry toast, crackers, or some dry cereal about half an hour before getting out of bed. Jelly may be used, but no fat, such as butter or margarine.
2. In the morning, get up slowly and avoid sudden movements.
3. Eat small, frequent meals without going very long with no food. An empty stomach causes nausea. Several small snacks (even as many as eight) may be better tolerated than a few large meals.
4. Rest after a meal.
5. Avoid fatty foods, spicy foods such as pizza, caffeine, and rich foods such as pastries.

---

*Table 15–7. Fetal Alcohol Syndrome**

1. Irreversible mental retardation.
2. Head too small (microcephaly).
3. Irritability in infancy and hyperactivity in childhood.
4. Less growth in height and weight with more discrepancy in height prenatally and throughout life.
5. Eyes
   a. Too close together.
   b. Mongolian look; a fold of skin starting at the root of the nose goes to the point where the eyebrow starts and may cover the inner corner of the eye (epicanthus).
   c. Drooping of upper eye lid (ptosis).
   d. Uncontrollable squinting (strabismus).
   e. Nearsightedness (myopia).
6. Nose
   a. Undefined, short, and upturned; remains too short for life.
   b. No bridge from the forehead to the nose.
   c. Normal pair of ridges with an indentation between them from the bottom of the nose to the upper lip is not seen.
7. Ears are poorly formed and incorrectly placed.
8. Mouth
   a. Prominent ridges in palate.
   b. Cleft lip.
   c. Cleft palate.
   d. Small teeth with faulty enamel.
   e. Small jaws.
9. Poor coordination.
10. Weak skeletal muscles seen as weakness and floppiness in babies with less ability and strength later in life (hypotonia).
11. Bones and joints underdeveloped.
12. Heart—atrial and ventricular membrane wall defects.

---

*Iber, FL: The fetal alcohol syndrome. *Nutrition Today* 15(5):4, 1980, with permission.

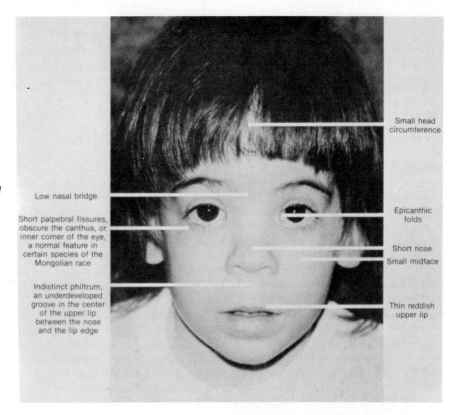

Small head circumference

Low nasal bridge

Epicanthic folds

Short palpebral fissures, obscure the canthus, or inner corner of the eye, a normal feature in certain species of the Mongolian race

Short nose
Small midface

Indistinct philtrum, an underdeveloped groove in the center of the upper lip between the nose and the lip edge

Thin reddish upper lip

Figure 15–2. Child with fetal alcohol syndrome. (Courtesy of Nutrition Today 15(5):5, 1980, by permission.)

6. Fruits, cold foods, and complex carbohydrates (e.g, rice, potatoes, and noodles) are tolerated better.
7. Keep the kitchen well ventilated to avoid odors during food preparation.
8. Liquids such as weak tea or apple juice may be drunk between meals, but should be avoided during meals.
9. Relax and stay calm.

Vitamin B$_6$ deficiency has also been linked to morning sickness (Pickard, 1982). Some reports claim that a higher carbohydrate intake with foods containing all of the B vitamins is sufficient. On the other hand, supplementation of 5 to 10 mg/day of pyridoxine hydrochloride is reported to relieve morning sickness and the mental depression often experienced (Wheatley, 1977). Individuals who have been using oral contraceptives for a long time may require higher supplementation of 15 mg or more (Roepke & Kirksey, 1981).

Lactose Intolerance. If gastrointestinal disorders occur frequently, the person may be lactose intolerant, which is very common in some minority groups (see Chapter 7). The importance of calcium intake from tolerated foods needs to be emphasized. Calcium supplementation may be useful.

Leg Cramps. Frequently, pregnant women have painful leg cramps at night. Although not clearly defined, neuromuscular irritability is thought to be caused by low serum calcium and high serum phosphate. Milk intake is eliminated, or at least reduced for a time because it is high in both phosphorus and calcium. Supplementary calcium (calcium lactate or carbonate) may be used until the cramps stop.

Constipation. Later in pregnancy, hemorrhoids or constipation may be caused by the pressure of the fetus. The usual remedies of more fiber, water, dried prunes, and exercise are recommended. The patient may need to be reminded to allow enough time for this routine and to try to relax.

Heartburn. Indigestion, delayed gastric emptying, or gas may be due to the pressure from the fetus. Heartburn occurs so frequently during pregnancy that a discussion of this subject is in order during the first prenatal conference. Suggestions for coping with heartburn are detailed in Chapter 27.

Clinical Implications:

- Hyperemesis (excessive vomiting) should be assessed by the physician. Hospitalization may be required to treat dehydration.
- Self-medication with laxatives is not advised; the physician should be consulted.

DISORDERS OF PREGNANCY

Pregnancy-Induced Hypertension. Toxemia, or pregnancy-induced hypertension (PIH), refers to elevated blood pressure commonly seen in pregnancy. When PIH is accompanied with convulsions, it is called eclampsia. Preeclampsia is a more accurate term for toxemia. Perinatal and maternal morbidity and mortality are increased in cases of hypertensive complications of pregnancy. Toxemia of pregnancy is a misnomer because no toxins have been found to cause this disorder.

Preeclampsia usually occurs after the 20th week of conception and disappears after the pregnancy. The three symptoms are (1) edema with sudden weight gain, (2) proteinuria, which may be very low even in serious cases, and (3) hypertension. Preeclampsia is more common among primiparae, adolescents (especially those under 15 years of age), underweight women, pregnancies with multiple fetuses, and low-income populations (because of poor nutritional intake). Preeclampsia also tends to occur in underweight women when they fail to gain weight normally.

Clear-cut answers are not available for the cause or prevention of this serious condition that threatens both the mother and fetus. Malnutrition is generally common among these individuals. Apparently, a causal relationship exists between preeclampsia and malnutrition, particularly a deficiency of protein, iron, calcium, and thiamin. A well-balanced diet designed to compensate for the deficiencies is recommended.

Anemia. Three different causes of anemia may appear during pregnancy. First, iron deficiency anemia is common as a result of the extra demands for iron. For this reason, supplementation is usually provided.

Abnormal complications due to ruptured tubal pregnancy or abortion may precede hemorrhaging and necessitate transfusions. Even then, iron supplementation is required to reestablish normal blood values.

Folic acid may be reduced, causing megaloblastic anemia. As a precaution, supplementation is ordinarily included at least during the later stages of pregnancy.

Diabetes Mellitus. See Chapter 29 for information related to pregnancy in women with diabetes mellitus.

LACTATION

Since the decision to feed the newborn by bottle or breast is generally made during pregnancy, an informative discussion with the gravida is appropriate to help her make the best decision for herself and her infant. However, she should not feel pressured in her decision. If breast-feeding is chosen, there are some exercises and suggestions that the mother should begin prior to the infant's birth to ensure success.

At least 95 percent of mothers can and do successfully breast-feed in communities where breast-feeding is the rule rather than the exception (Khan, 1980). Even though breast-feeding is physiologically natural, nearly all mothers need to be taught and guided with their first newborn. In ancient Greece, a "doula" (a woman slave) stayed with the primigravida to guide her through each step of mothering and nursing (Raphael, 1973). In the United States, the primigravida is usually surrounded by other mothers using bottle-feeding and may not have any extended family member with previous breast-feeding experience, and no doula. Some proposed advantages of breast-feeding for the mother are the following:

- Human milk, designed for human infants is nutritionally superior to alternatives.
- Human milk is sanitary and free from harmful bacteria.
- Breast-fed infants have fewer allergies (Kreiger, 1982).
- Breast-fed babies are less likely to be overfed (though it is controversial as to whether this relates to future weight).
- Mother-infant bonding is enhanced.
- Breast-feeding is more convenient because it is always available at the proper temperature and needs no preparation.
- Breast-feeding results in less gastrointestinal disturbances (diarrhea or constipation).

It is commonly accepted that breast milk has certain anti-infectious properties. However, some clinical studies in industrialized countries have disagreed with this assumption. Bauchner and colleagues (1986) scrutinized 20 studies with methodological standards to evaluate their scientific validity. Because of research flaws, they concluded that breast-feeding has only a minimal protective effect against infections.

Disadvantages of breast-feeding include:

- Some of the medications that might be necessary for the gravida's health could be contraindicated in breast-feeding (see Table 15–6).
- Unless expressed milk is given, the mother is the only one who can feed the infant.
- If the mother returns to work, she may not want to express milk on a regular basis.
- Breast-feeding is contraindicated if the nipples are cracked or fissured (temporarily) or if the mother has mastitis or an acute illness.
- Breast milk is not appropriate for infants with such inborn errors of metabolism as galactosemia or phenylketonuria.
- If the mother's stores of thiamin or vitamin B_{12} are depleted, breast-fed infants may become deficient in these vitamins.

Breast-fed babies are most vulnerable to hemorrhagic disease of the newborn since breast milk contains less vitamin K than infant formulas. However, a prophylactic dose of vitamin K is routinely given to newborns at birth to prevent this problem.

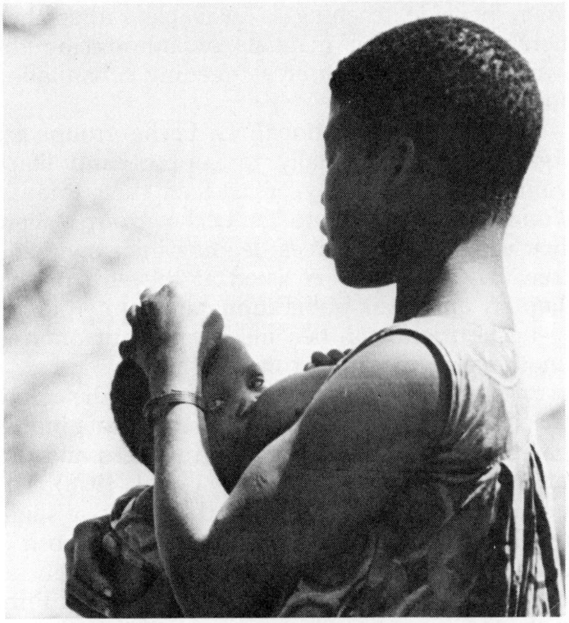

Figure 15–3. "Health for all by the year 2000." Promotion of healthy mothers who breast-feed their infants is an important part of mother and child care programs. (Photo courtesy of WHO/J Mohr.)

Breast-Feeding

Even though more mothers are now breast-feeding their infants when discharged from the hospital, about one-third of these women stop breast-feeding within six weeks—before lactation is fully established (MacLean, 1982) (Fig. 15–3). Only 25 percent are still breast-feeding at five to six months postpartum (Axelson et al, 1986). More primiparae than multiparae and more highly educated women are breast-feeding (Foman et al, 1985).

There are two main steps to successful breast-feeding: believing that one can breast-feed and allowing the infant to suck enough for release of the milk. Confidence is not as easy to obtain for the new mother as might be expected. Without support and valid information, she can easily become discouraged with rumors, superstitions, and questions about her ability to produce adequate milk.

Health Care Professionals. For mothers who decide to breast-feed, health care professionals must assume a supportive role—one of sharing information and providing the primigravida with contacts, rather than being an ever-present nursemaid. Health care professionals must be thoroughly knowledgeable, and preferably those who have breast-fed their own children will be assigned to work with and support the primigravida.

Stories of actual breast-feeding experiences can be most encouraging to the new mother. Also, realizing that her fears and anxieties are typical and common among women can be a great relief. Relaying positive statements to reinforce the primigravida can be most beneficial (Helsing & King, 1982).

Discussing the environment of the new mother with her and the members of her family can be useful in obtaining a peaceful, undisturbed setting with plenty of rest for the gravida. Most women need a period of seclusion, rest, and adaptation without extra responsibilities other than the new infant and herself (Helsing & King, 1982).

A potential breast-feeder must not only be eager to breast-feed, but must be aware of the factors involved. Prenatal classes promote confidence and supply pertinent information. However, the medical facility must support the mother who chooses to breast-feed. Rooming-in without the rigid restrictions of routine feedings is helpful. Breast-feeding is more often successful when bedside teaching is available rather than merely distributing manuals or announcing the availability of a call-in breast-feeding consultation (Johnson et al, 1984).

La Leche International. La Leche groups are organized internationally to support and teach women to successfully breast-feed their infants. Women who belong to La Leche groups share their experiences of breast-feeding their own children. Their address is listed at the end of this chapter, and their publications are numerous. A La Leche friend can become a confidant offering emotional support and comradeship.

Techniques of Breast-feeding. Studies indicate that putting the newborn to the breast immediately after birth increases both success and duration of breast-feeding (Salariya et al, 1978). The mother should be reassured that only a slight amount of milk is released when the newborn is allowed to suck for a few minutes immediately after and even for a few days following birth. Prior to the delivery of milk, colostrum, a thin yellow fluid, is secreted. It is thought to be a source of various antibodies that protects the newborn against infections and diseases (Foman, 1974).

The newborn should be given to the mother and put to the breast as soon as the mother feels ready. Early sucking helps the milk to "come in" and the newborn to start sucking and to prepare his/her digestive tract by removing meconium, which is the first bowel movement. No bottle feedings are offered because the difference in sucking can be confusing to the newborn (Fig. 15–4). Once the newborn becomes adjusted to taking a bottle, it becomes much harder to get him/her to take the breast, but not vice versa. If the breast is taken well first, then the competition from the bottle is insignificant (Helsing & King, 1982).

Milk production and infant sucking both require some time to adjust to one another. Occasionally, too much milk is produced immediately after birth. Blood and fluid in the supporting tissue cause enlargement of the breasts and some pain at this time.

It is unnecessary to clean the nipples before a feeding, since human milk is bacteriostatic. When bathing, only water is used; nothing should be put on the nipples that will require washing off before nursing, such as soap, lotions, or medication. The skin should be thoroughly dry before anything is put on it, or the moisture will make the skin softer and weaker. Edible oils, A & D Ointment, vitamin E ointment, Vasoline, lanolin, or some of the breast milk may be applied. Alcohol or alcohol-containing lotions are too drying.

In breast-feeding, the nipple plus the areola must be offered instead of only the nipple. Figure 15–4 shows the difference in sucking in breast-feeding compared to a bottle. Most infants take 80 to 90 percent of the milk from each breast in the first four minutes (Lucas et al, 1979). If a newborn sucks longer than 10 minutes, check the position. Some infants do take longer, but it is important to observe that s/he is sucking correctly. Feedings of one to two minutes are too brief and leave the breasts engorged.

Physiological Reflexes. Basically, breast-feeding depends on three automatic body reactions in the mother and three reflexes in the infant. For the mother, they are: (1) the nipple-erection reflex, (2) the prolactin reflex, which produces milk, and (3) the oxytocin reflex, which ejects the milk. The infant's responses include: (1) the rooting reflex, which causes him/her to turn the mouth toward the breast when s/he is touched on the cheek, (2) the sucking reflex, and (3) the swallowing reflex.

Both sets of reflexes are dependent upon each other; therefore, the amount of milk needed by an individual infant is produced by the mother upon the initiation of sucking. When the quantity of milk appears to be inadequate (hypogalactia), the infant should be put to the breast more often to allow more sucking. Hypogalactia is more common during the growth spurts that usually occur at about three weeks, six weeks, and three months of life. The more often a baby nurses, the more milk is produced.

The Mother's Reflexes. As the newborn sucks, the sensory nerve endings in the nipple are stimulated sending impulses to the hypothalamus in the brain (Fig. 15–5). The hypothalamus stimulates the anterior pituitary to release prolactin into the blood. As it reaches the breast, it causes milk-secreting cells to release milk. The more the infant sucks, the more milk is released.

Another hormone, oxytocin, is released upon sucking. This hormone causes the myoepithelial cells around the alveoli and ducts to contract, which squeezes milk from the alveoli, ducts, and sinuses towards the nipple. Milk is ejected, or thrown out, to the infant as the sucking starts. Sometimes the milk may come so fast that it can choke the infant. If this is anticipated, the mother may express her breast slightly before offering it to the infant. This reflex of the milk being ejected is called the let-down reflex. Often a woman may feel a tense or prickling sensation beneath her nipples as this starts. Ways to establish the let-down reflex include taking a warm shower or drinking warm milk or tea before nursing and nursing in a darkened, quiet room in a comfortable chair.

When the let-down reflex does not function, the milk-producing cells produce fewer fatty globules and the caloric content of the milk is decreased. The resulting milk has only five to ten kcal/oz. instead of the normal 20 kcal or more. That is why babies getting such milk are so hungry. The mother thinks that she has a lot of milk, but its quality is greatly decreased (Applebaum, 1976). This cycle often ends with engorgement or a breast infection in the mother and loss of weight in the baby.

The milk-ejection reflex may cause sexual sensations during nursing, or vice versa (sexual activities may cause milk flow). To prevent women from feeling guilty about these sensa-

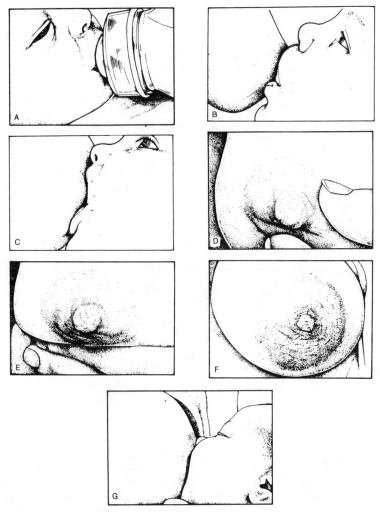

Figure 15—4. Position of infant's mouth: A) Both the sucking action and the position of the baby's lips are different with bottle-feeding. B) The baby is sucking the nipple as if it were a bottle and is pulling the nipple out, which can cause soreness. C) The baby is sucking in a good position, with most of the areola in its mouth; notice that its head is very close to the breast, and it is not pulling the nipple out unnecessarily. D) The mother is holding the nipple out for her baby as if it were a teat on a bottle; she is only offering the nipple itself. E) Here the mother is offering her whole breast to the baby, so it can take the nipple and areola into its mouth. F) Sometimes the areola of a breast is very big, and then the baby cannot get the whole areola into its mouth. G) The baby sucking from a breast with a very large areola. The baby cannot possibly get the whole areola into its mouth, but you can see that its head is in a good position (Fisher 1981). (Drawings by Ivanson Kayaii from photographs by Margaret Bristol, ARPS, of the Oxford University Department of Medical Illustration. From Helsing E, King FS: Breast-Feeding in Practice. Oxford, Oxford University Press, 1982, by permission.)

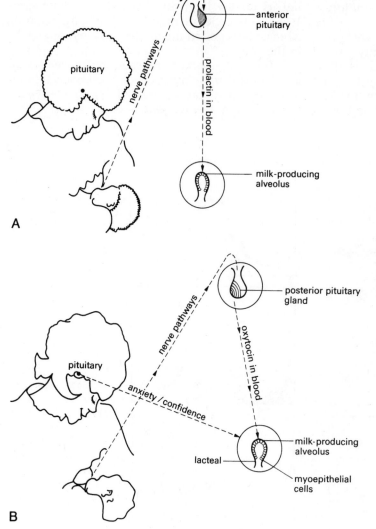

Figure 15–5. Milk production: A) The prolactin, or milk-producing, reflex simplified. B) The oxytocin, or milk-ejection, reflex simplified. (From Helsing E, King FS: Breast-Feeding in Practice. Oxford, Oxford University Press, 1982, by permission.)

tions, they should know that this is nature's way of making nursing enjoyable for the survival of the species. It is normal and quite acceptable (Helsing & King, 1982).

Additionally, this interaction between the uterus and lactation causes the uterus muscle to contract, helping the delivery of the placenta, controlling hemorrhage, and helping the uterus regain its normal size. Just after birth, these contractions may cause pains, but the woman who understands that they are beneficial will be more tolerant.

Because the milk-ejection is easily inhibited, the nursing mother needs empathy and sympathy with guidance to prevent anxiety and fears and to give her confidence. "Drying-up" may occur easily with embarrassment, anger, fear, or getting chilled.

Clinical Implication:

- Pharmacological doses of vitamin B6 given to lactating women may inhibit plasma prolactin. Lower doses (0.5 to 4.0 mg/day) will increase

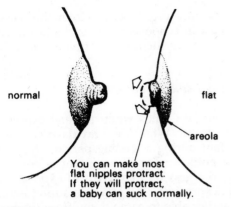

Figure 15–6. *Normal and flat nipples. (From Helsing E, King FS: Breast-Feeding in Practice. Oxford, Oxford University Press, 1982, by permission.)*

plasma concentrations of pyridoxal phosphate and vitamin B$_6$ in breast milk without impairing lactation (Andon et al, 1985).

SUCCESSFUL BREAST-FEEDING

Normal infant weight gain is the criterion for successful breast-feeding. Most women can produce enough milk for three to nine months, with others going 12 months or longer (Ahn & MacLean, 1980). It may be appropriate to assess maternal nursing behavior when breast-fed infants are experiencing unacceptable growth deceleration. Apparent lactation failure may only reflect infrequent nursings. Ordinarily, weight increases with more frequent nursing periods (Matheny & Picciano, 1986)

NIPPLE CONDITIONING

Successful breast-feeding partially depends on prenatal preparation and correct information to prevent possible difficulties. Examination of the nipple early in pregnancy is important. Nipples may be normal and protractile, which enhance sucking, or inverted, flat, short, or nonprotractile. Figure 15–6 shows a normal and flat nipple.

Several methods can be used to condition the nipple, which is especially helpful for some women with inverted nipples. The woman should gently roll the nipple between the thumb and index finger repeatedly for five minutes twice a day during the last trimester. Wearing a glass or rubber nipple shield inside a well-fitting brassiere may also be helpful (Figs. 15–7 & 15–8). Some women find that the nipple areas become less sensitive if given a brisk rubbing with a terry towel after bathing.

LACTATION PROBLEMS

Frequently encountered problems with lactation include flat or inverted nipples, soreness, engorgement, and breast infections. Management approaches to these problems is presented in Table 15–8.

Sore nipples can be extremely painful. Initially, soreness can occur at the beginning of breast-feeding and may be caused by faulty sucking technique, engorged breasts, flat nipples, or a thrush infection in the infant. Short, frequent nursings promote speedy healing.

Early breast engorgement may occur when the milk is first produced (Fig. 15–9), but this can

Figure 15–7. *A) Glass nipple shell showing two parts; B) nipple shell, put together; C) flat nipple; D) same nipple with glass shell in use. Notice how nipple sticks out beneath the dome. (From Helsing E, King FS: Breast-Feeding in Practice. Oxford, Oxford University Press, 1982, by permission.)*

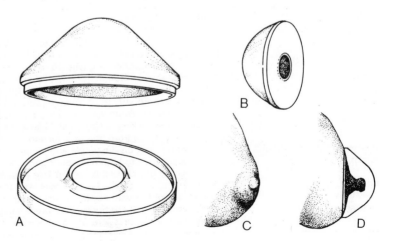

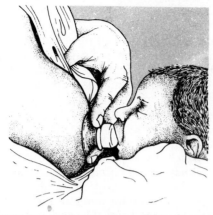

Figure 15–8. *A baby breast-feeding with the help of a nipple shield. This shield has a glass base and a rubber teat. Some women like glass shields because you can see the milk flowing through them. The National Childbirth Trust recommends an all-rubber shield, which some women find easier and simpler to use. (From Helsing E, King FS: Breast-Feeding in Practice. Oxford, Oxford University Press, 1982, by permission.)*

be avoided by frequent feedings from birth. Not only is milk production stimulated, but excess milk is also removed, which otherwise becomes trapped. In engorgement, milk-producing cells are compressed and traumatized from the back pressure of the milk, so the mother produces less. Additionally, the cells that contract to cause letdown may be injured.

When the breasts become infected, weaning is contraindicated because it will produce engorgement, stasis, cracked nipples, and more infection. Antibiotics are seldom needed if hot packs and frequent nursing are initiated early. If antibiotics are prescribed, neither the bacteria of the breast infection nor the antibiotics have been shown to harm the infant (Applebaum, 1976).

MANUAL EXPRESSION OF MILK

There are times when manual expression of milk is useful. When the gravida wishes to leave her infant during a feeding period, she may prepare a bottle earlier. If an infant is born prematurely, the gravida may wish to express milk for her newborn until the infant is strong enough to suck and/or able to come home from the hospital.

With both hands around the breast against the chest wall, place the thumbs above and the fingers below Moving the hands (not just the fingers), massage the whole surface of the breast toward the edges of the areola (Figure 15–10). Gently press the edges of the areola between fingers and thumb of the hand from the opposite side of the body, with the other hand supporting the breast (Helsing & King, 1982). There are also several types of breast pumps available.

MISTAKEN IDEAS ABOUT BREAST-FEEDING

Many statements are offered as reasons to discontinue breast-feeding. However, the reasons may not be valid but rather excuses to allow the mother to stop. The primigravida should not be pressured to breast-feed if she does not want to. However, she deserves to thoroughly understand the benefits of breast-feeding.

Table 15–8. *Lactation Problems and Their Management*

Problem	Prevention or Therapy
Flat nipples	Manipulate the nipple before offering it to the infant to make it more erect and easy to grasp. Wearing a nipple shield before birth may be helpful (Fig. 15–7). The nipple shield with a rubber tip may be used when breastfeeding (Fig. 15–8).
Inverted nipples	Wear a nipple shield inside the brassiere during the last trimester. The rolling exercise, as described in the section on nipple conditioning, may be helpful.
Sore nipple	Offer the breasts properly to encourage proper sucking (Fig. 15–4). Hold the baby in different positions to decrease continuous pressure on the same breast. Initially offer the breast that is least sore when the sucking is strongest. Expose the breast to the air. Wear breast shields to keep the nipple dry and free from brassiere friction.
Cracked or fissured nipples	Put some of the milk on the nipple and areola and allow to dry. Expose to the air.
Breast engorgement	Frequent feedings from birth are best. Manual expression of milk when the infant is not eating well (e.g., because of sickness) is helpful. Use a breast pump to prevent entrapment of the milk.
Infection	Place hot washcloths on the breast, cover with thin plastic wrap and lie down. Maintain heat with a heating pad or hot-water bottle. Nurse frequently. Take analgesics if necessary.
Leakage	Cross the arms against the breasts and press firmly. Breast pads with an outside plastic coating may be worn inside the brassiere. These should be changed frequently.

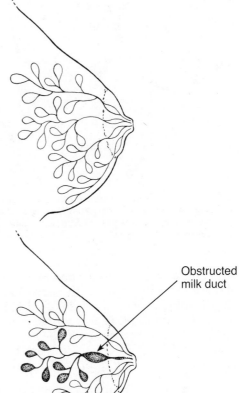

Figure 15–9. *Breast engorgement due to poor drainage from obstructed milk duct.*

Obstructed milk duct

Clinical Implications:

- Infants nursed by vegetarians frequently are malnourished and have lower growth rates. Many older vegetarian children are both lighter and shorter than their nonvegetarian counterparts. Vegetarian lactating women and their children must understand the importance of a balanced diet with appropriate weaning foods in sufficient quantities (Finley et al, 1985).
- An infant who is upset should be calmed before being offered the breast.
- Rest is essential for the mother and the infant.
- Since ovulation occurs two weeks before menstruation begins, the cessation of menses during breast-feeding is not a reliable way to manage future pregnancies.
- Some infants reject the breast for a day or so when menstruation begins, but then return to normal.
- Manual expression of the breast during pregnancy is not advocated. Colostrum for the infant is lost, and it may cause premature labor (Lawrence, 1985).

PREMENSTRUAL SYNDROME

Premenstrual syndrome (PMS) may affect some females from the time their menses begin until menopause, or it may not begin until later. Estimates of the prevalence of PMS among men-

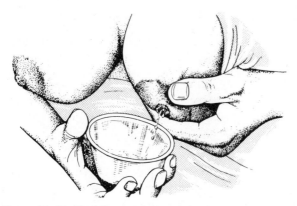

Figure 15—10. *Mother in a special care baby unit in rural Africa manually expressing her milk. (From Helsing E, King FS:* Breast-Feeding in Practice. *Oxford, Oxford University Press, 1982. Drawing by Ivanson Kayaii.)*

struating women in the United States range from about 60 to 90 percent, with approximately 10 to 15 percent experiencing severe or disabling symptoms (Rossignol, 1985). Supportive therapy, stress reduction, and exercise should be basic treatments (Table 15–9). While the underlying cause is unknown, some dietary recommendations may offer relief.

Dr. Katherine Dalton in England and Dr. Guy Abraham in California *claim* fantastic results with many of their patients. However, much of their work is not supported by conclusive scientific studies; when some of their theories are subjected to double blind studies, the placebo has as much effect as the drug or nutrient being tested. Therefore, their work is highly criticized by the conservative medical profession.

There is a wide range of symptoms for PMS with individuals being affected differently. The

Table 15—9. *Guidelines for Premenstrual Syndrome*

1. Eat a varied well-balanced diet that utilizes all the basic food groups.
2. Rigid caloric restrictions should not be imposed during the week before menses.
3. Increase consumption of complex carbohydrates, especially whole-grain products, to 60 percent of total caloric intake.
4. Avoid excessive amounts of caffeine when mastalgia (breast tenderness) is a problem.
5. Use salt in moderation if premenstrual water retention is a major problem, especially during that time of the cycle.
6. Limit dairy products to two servings per day.
7. Include at least one or two tablespoons of a food source high in linoleic acid and vitamin E (e.g., salad dressings or margarines high in corn or safflower oil).
8. If a supplement is needed, take moderate amounts of vitamins and minerals and avoid megadoses.

one common factor is that the symptoms are cyclic, appearing three to seven days before menses, and dramatically disappearing after menstruation. One of the most common symptoms of PMS is nervous tension, exhibited by irritability, anxiety, crying, loneliness, restlessness, mood swings, and depression. Headaches, backaches, fatigue, less motor control (accident prone), poor judgement, and nausea may also be present. These emotions influence levels of activity as well as personal relationships. It is believed that these women have high estrogen-to-progesterone ratios. Since vitamin B_6 is involved in the regulation of neurotransmitters in the brain, it has been used for PMS patients with mood changes. A few small double-blind studies using B_6 have inconsistent results. Vitamin B_6 may be beneficial for some patients, but large doses are harmful, and intake should remain well below 500 mg/day. Doses as low as 50 mg/day are less likely to be harmful, and some studies indicate they may be helpful for some women (Meister, 1985).

Other PMS sufferers are affected by excessive water and salt retention, abdominal bloating, painful breasts, skin disorders, and weight gain. In some cases, spironolactone, a mild diuretic that counters the effects of the hormone aldosterone, is prescribed based on the hypothesis that this hormone is elevated during the premenstrual phase of the menstrual cycle (Meister, 1985). Others have suggested a decreased sodium intake (3 gm/day) at this time or no salt added to foods.

Vitamin E, at doses of 150 to 300 mg/day, has been used effectively for treating several PMS symptoms (London et al, 1984). Since it has been used to reduce symptoms in benign breast disease, it is not surprising that it is effective in relieving sore breasts. So, while vitamin E may be used to treat PMS, a deficiency of vitamin E is not the cause for PMS.

Another group of PMS patients crave sweets, have an increased appetite and low serum magnesium levels. Their symptoms are characterized by fatigue, fainting spells, headache, palpitation, and even trembling (Abraham, 1983). Whether a relative deficiency of this mineral is responsible for the symptoms is not known. Magnesium supplementation appears to be safe in small doses for healthy individuals. High intakes of milk products interfere with magnesium levels since calcium blocks magnesium absorption. Since the long-term effects of calcium-poor diets increase the risk of osteoporosis, calcium should not be omitted from the diet.

The craving for sweets has been treated with

a low-sugar, high-protein diet. Since the symptoms of PMS are not relieved by eating, it seems unlikely that hypoglycemia is responsible (Sharma, 1982). However, these individuals may benefit from eating more frequently and increasing the amount of complex carbohydrates, e.g., pasta and legumes. This also reduces the appetite by avoiding glycemic fluctuations.

Evening primrose oil has become popular as another nutritional treatment. This substance contains unsaturated fatty acids and vitamin E. There is no scientific evidence to support the use of evening primrose oil for PMS (Meister, 1985).

Clinical Implications:

- Nonprescription PMS supplements are available, but they may or may not offer the desired nutrients. For example, magnesium may be a component (desirable), or calcium may be a component (usually undesirable for this condition).
- Many of the PMS supplements are megadoses of vitamins; they should be taken cautiously under a physician's care.

• FACTS and FALLACIES

FALLACY: *If the pregnant woman craves raspberry ice cream at midnight or pizza at 2:00 AM, all efforts should be made to get them. The pregnant woman has a natural instinct that causes a craving of nutrients needed.*

- **FACT:** *This cannot be considered accurate. Nutrient needs must be met by deliberate preplanning and knowledgeable food choices. Abnormal appetites do occur, but nutrient information is essential for correct assessment.*

FALLACY: *It does not matter what the gravida eats; her fetus will obtain whatever s/he needs from her body if the nutrients are not available from food sources.*

- **FACT:** *The gravida cannot be considered a source of all essential nutrients for her fetus unless she consumes an adequate diet during gestation and also has optimum stores before conception (Tufts Univ., 1985).*

FALLACY: *When a pregnant woman has gas or indigestion caused by the pressure of the fetus, she should take antacids.*

- **FACT:** *Small frequent meals are more advisable. Antacids or baking soda can cause alkalemia, or even anemia as the result of the antacid combining with iron.*

FALLACY: *A pregnant woman should not consume non-nutritive sweeteners.*

- **FACT:** *Cyclamates cannot be used in the United States because of reported carcinogenicity. Reports on saccharin vary; aspartame seems to be widely accepted. Since aspartame contains the amino acids phenylalanine and aspartic acid, the question arises to its safety for mothers with heterozygous phenylketonuria (PKU) and its possible effects upon a PKU fetus. No specific data is available at this time. Plasma phenylalanine levels increase after consumption but return to baseline within four hours. Presently, aspartame appears safe as a sweetening agent for use by children two years of age or older (Horwitz & Bauer-Nehrling, 1983).*

FALLACY: *A pregnant woman should eat twice as much food when she is pregnant as she is eating for two.*

- **FACT:** *A pregnant woman only needs about 15 percent more calories (about 150 extra kcal/day) during the first three months and an additional 350 kcal/day for the remainder of the pregnancy. However, the requirement for iron nearly triples; for folic acid, it doubles, and for calcium, it increases by 50 percent (Tufts Univ., 1985).*

FALLACY: *Pregnant women should not exercise.*

- **FACT:** *A normal pregnant woman who does not have medical problems should continue exercises such as walking, swimming, stationary cycling, and modified forms of dancing, and calisthenics as long as her pulse rate does not exceed 140 beats a minute and strenuous activity is not engaged in for more than 15 minutes. Specific exercise programs should be discussed with her physician (Tufts Univ., 1985).*

FALLACY: *If twins are expected, food intake should be doubled.*

- **FACT:** *Specific research on nutrient needs of women expecting multiple births is sparse. Some research indicates that the healthiest babies were born to mothers who gained about 41 lbs. during the typical twin pregnancy time of*

36 weeks. Tall or thin women who are expecting twins should gain somewhat more than that. Increases in folic acid and protein should be included (Tufts Univ., 1985).

FALLACY: By taking calcium supplements instead of drinking milk, the pregnant woman can avoid gaining excessive weight.

• **FACT:** Milk provides an excellent source of high-quality protein as well as other nutrients. The calcium is better absorbed from milk than from supplements; also the intake of calcium and iron supplements is contraindicated at the same time (Tufts Univ., 1985). Other adjustments are preferred to control weight.

FALLACY: Small breasts cannot produce enough milk.

• **FACT:** The size does not indicate anything about the success or failure of breast-feeding.

FALLACY: The milk is too thin.

• **FACT:** Breast milk is normally thin. Despite its consistency and slightly bluish color, it is ideal as a source of food and water for the infant.

FALLACY: The baby does not gain as much weight as an infant on formula.

• **FACT:** Infants fed formula are usually heavier than those who are breast-fed, but that does not mean healthier. Each infant must be evaluated individually.

FALLACY: Breast-feeding distorts the shape of breasts.

• **FACT:** Expressing milk when the breasts become too full can relieve the pressure and protect their shape. Both breasts should be offered to the infant at each feeding. Wearing a brassiere that is properly fitted and comfortable during both pregnancy and lactation will support breast tissue. Breasts are larger just after delivery, but they will reduce to their former size (or possibly remain slightly smaller or larger). If these measures are followed, there should not be any difference other than the changes that might occur from being pregnant without nursing.

FALLACY: If one doesn't have enough milk for the infant, one feeding should be skipped to have more milk available later.

• **FACT:** The milk supply diminishes with reduced sucking. Putting the infant to breast more often (not less often) will increase the milk supply. Since milk cannot be stored within the breast, it should be expressed and refrigerated or frozen for later use.

SUMMARY

The most important factor in a successful pregnancy is an average weight gain of 22 to 27.3 lbs. The ideal age for becoming pregnant is the early twenties when the body has reached full growth stature and has built up a nutrient reserve. Women who are younger or older and heavier or lighter than their ideal weight are at greater risk.

The most successful pregnancies producing a healthy newborn require optimum nutrient intake for the gravida from the beginning of her own life until the birth of her infant.

The quality of the diet is as critical as the total weight gain. An abundant supply of high biological value protein, four daily servings of milk fortified with 400 IU of vitamin D, optimum intakes of vitamins, and possibly supplementation of iron, folic acid, and zinc may be recommended. Iodized salt should be used in a normal manner; if edema occurs, it should be treated with bedrest. Restriction of salt and use of diuretics are not useful and may be harmful.

Adequate complex carbohydrates (50 to 60 percent of the diet) will provide energy and help prevent nausea and vomiting. Carbohydrates are needed to provide sufficient glucose and glycogen stores for the fetus. Linoleic acid should be supplied from the fat intake.

Weight reduction is not desirable because the nutrient content often becomes deficient. Also, no periods of starvation are desirable, including skipping breakfast. No alcohol should be consumed; caffeine intake is not recommended.

A thorough discussion of breast-feeding should occur as early in pregnancy as possible. This provides the gravida an opportunity to investigate valid information and decide what is most desirable for herself. Then she will have adequate time to prepare her breasts if she decides to breast-feed.

Review Questions

1. What is toxemia of pregnancy? Why is this term a misnomer?

2. Plan the food intake for one day for a pregnant woman and discuss your decisions.
3. What are the high-risk factors for pregnancy?
4. Discuss fetal alcohol syndrome and explain how alcohol affects the fetus.
5. What supplemental nutrients are usually prescribed during pregnancy?
6. Why would a high-potency vitamin pill not protect the expectant mother?
7. Discuss advantages and disadvantages of breast-feeding.

Case Study: Mrs. M.A. is a 30-year-old primigravida. She is now in the first trimester. Prior to her pregnancy, she weighed 55 kg; she is 166 cm tall. She has always been weight-conscious and carefully guards against weight gain. Mr. and Mrs. A drink two to three cocktails each week and occasionally have wine with dinner. While she is very excited about her pregnancy, she expresses concern to the nutritionist about gaining weight. Her hemoglobin, hematocrit, and serum albumin are within normal limits.

1. How much weight should she gain in the first trimester? The second trimester? The third trimester?
2. Mrs. M.A. does not care for milk. How much milk should she drink each day? What would you suggest to her to increase her calcium intake?
3. How would you counsel her about the alcohol usually consumed?
4. Mrs. M.A. asks if she should reduce her salt intake. What would you tell her?
5. What are some helpful hints for dealing with morning sickness?
6. Her physician has prescribed vitamin and mineral supplements. Why are these frequently recommended?

REFERENCE LIST

Abraham, GE: Nutritional factors in the etiology of the premenstrual syndrome. *J Reproductive Med* 28(7):446, 1983.

Ahn, CH; MacLean, WC, Jr: Growth of the exclusively breastfed infant. *Am J Clin Nutr* 33(2):183, 1980.

Allard, JP: Maternal nutrition for clients in the private sector. *J Am Diet Assoc* 86(8):1069, 1986.

Andon, MB; Howard, MP; Moser, PB; et al: Nutritionally relevant supplementation of vitamin B_6 on lactating women: Effect on plasma prolactin. *Pediatrics* 76(5):769, 1985.

Applebaum, RM: Management of lactation problems. In *Symposium on Human Lactation*. Edited by LR Waletzky. Rockville, MD, U.S. Dept Health, Education, and Welfare, 1976, p 69.

Bauchner, H; Leventhal, JM; Shapiro, ED: Studies of breastfeeding and infection: How good is the evidence? *JAMA* 256(7):887, 1986.

Beal, VA: Assessment of nutritional status in pregnancy—II. *Am J Clin Nutr* 34(4):691, 1981.

Breskin, MW; Worthington-Roberts, BS; Knopp, RH; et al: First trimester serum zinc concentrations in human pregnancy. *Am J Clin Nutr* 38(6):943, 1983.

Committee on Nutrition of the Mother and the Preschool Child (CNMPC), Food and Nutrition Board: *Nutrition Services in Perinatal Care*. Washington, DC, National Academy Press, 1981.

Department of Continuing Education of Harvard Medical School (DCEHMS): Pregnancy: Age and outcome. *The Harvard Medical School Health Letter* X(12):1, 1985.

DeVore, NE: Parenthood postponed. *Am J Nurs* 83(8):1160, 1983.

Farthington, MA: Prenatal nutritional guidance for the vegetarian mother. In *Nutrition and Vegetarianism*. Edited by JB Anderson. Chapel Hill, School of Public Health, University of North Carolina, May 1981.

Finley, DA; Lonnerdal, B; Dewey, KG; et al: Breast milk composition: Fat content and fatty acid composition in vegetarians and nonvegetarians. *Am J Clin Nutr* 41(4):787, 1985.

Foman, SJ: *Infant Nutrition*, 2nd ed. Philadelphia, W. B. Saunders Co, 1974.

Foman, SJ: Breast-feeding and evolution. *J Am Diet Assoc* 86(3):317, 1986.

Foman, MR; Fetterly, K; Barry, BS; et al: Exclusive breast-feeding of newborns among married women in the United States: The National Natality Surveys of 1969 and 1980. *Am J Clin Nutr* 42(11):864, 1985.

Frisancho, AR; Matos, J; Flegel, P: Maternal nutritional status and adolescent pregnancy outcome. *Am J Clin Nutr* 38(5):739, 1983.

George, NN; Kim, SK; Duhring, JL: Prepregnancy weights and weight gains related to birth weights of infants born to overweight women. *J Am Diet Assoc* 84(4):450, 1984.

Gibbs, CE; Seitchik, J: Nutrition in Pregnancy. In *Modern Nutrition in Health and Disease*, 6th ed. Edited by RS Goodhart; ME Shils. Philadelphia, Lea & Febiger, 1980.

Golub, MS; Gershwin, ME; Hurley, LS; et al: Studies of marginal zinc deprivation in rhesus monkeys: II. Pregnancy outcome. *Am J Clin Nutr* 39(6):879, 1984.

Glenn, FB; Glenn, WD; Duncan, RC: Fluoride tablet supplementation during pregnancy for caries immunity: A study of the offspring produced. *Am J Obstet Gynecol* 143(5):560, 1982.

Harrison, GG; Branson, RS; Vaucher, YE: Association of maternal smoking with body composition of the newborn. *Am J Clin Nutr* 38(5):757, 1983.

Helsing, E; King, FS: *Breast-feeding in Practice*. Oxford, Oxford University Press, 1982.

Horwitz, DL; Bauer-Nehrling, JK: Can aspartame meet our expectations? *J Am Diet Assoc* 83(2):142, 1983.

Iber, FL: The fetal alcohol syndrome. *Nutrition Today* 15(5):4, 1980.

Johnson, CA; Garza, C; Nichols, B: A teaching intervention to improve breastfeeding success. *J Nutr Ed* 16(1):19, 1984.

Khan, M: Infant feeding practices in rural Meheran, Comilla, Bangladesh. *Am J Clin Nutr* 33(11):2356, 1980.

Klaus, MH; Kennell, JH: *Maternal-Infant Bonding. The Impact of Early Separation or Loss on Family Development*. St. Louis, C. V. Mosby Co, 1976.

Krieger, I: *Pediatric Disorders of Feeding, Nutrition and Metabolism*. New York, John Wiley & Sons, 1982.

Kurppa, K; Holmberg, PC; Kuosma, E; et al: Coffee consumption during pregnancy and selected congenital malformations: A nationwide case-control study. *Am J Public Health* 73(12):1397, 1983.

Lawrence, RA: *Breast-feeding: A Guide for the Medical Profession*, 2nd ed, St. Louis, C. V. Mosby Co, 1985.

Lecos, C: Pregnant women need advice. *FDA Consumer* 16(2):16, 1982.

Letsky, EA: Nutrition and blood. 2. The need for haematinics in pregnancy. *Hum Nutr Appl Nutr* 36A(4):245, 1982.

London, RS; Sundaram, G; Manimekalai, S; et al: The effect of alpha-tocopherol on premenstrual symptomatology: A double-blind study. II. Endocrine correlates. *J Am College Nutr* 3:351, 1984.

Loris, P; Dewey, KG; Poirier-Brode, K: Weight gain and dietary intake of pregnant teenagers. *J Am Diet Assoc* 85(10):296, 1985.

Lozoff, B; Brittenham, GM; Trause, MA; et al: The mother-newborn relationship: Limits of adaptability. *J Pediatr* 91(1):1, 1977.

Lucas, A; Lucas, PJ; Baum, JD: Pattern of milk flow in breast-fed infants. *Lancet* 2(July 14):57, 1979.

Luke, B: *Maternal Nutrition*. Boston, Little, Brown & Co, 1979.

Luke, B; Jonaitis, MA; Petrie, RH: A consideration of height as a function of prepregnancy nutritional background and its potential influence on birth weight. *J Am Diet Assoc* 84(2):176, 1984.

McCormick, MC; Shapiro, S; Starfield, B: High-risk young mothers: Infant mortality and morbidity in four areas in the United States, 1973–1978. *Am J Public Health* 73(12):18, 1983.

MacLean, H: The breastfeeding experience. *J Canadian Diet Assoc* 43(10):300, 1982.

Matheny, R; Picciano, MF: Feeding and growth characteristics of human milk-fed infants. *J Am Diet Assoc* 86(3):327, 1986.

Meister, KA: *Premenstrual Syndrome*. Summit, NJ, American Council on Science and Health, 1985.

Miller, KA; Field, CS: Adolescent pregnancy: A combined obstetric and pediatric management approach. *Mayo Clinic Proc* 59(5):311, 1984.

Naeye, RL; Chez, RA: Effects of maternal acetonuria and low pregnancy weight gain on children's psychomotor development. *Am J Obstet Gynecol* 139(2):189, 1981.

Niswander, KR; Gordon, M: *The Women and Their Pregnancies*. DHEW Publication No. (NIG) 73, 1972.

Orr, RD; Simmons, JJ: Nutritional care in pregnancy: The patient's view. *J Am Diet Assoc* 75(2):136, 1979.

Pickard, BM: Some preliminary observations on the relationship between preconceptional diet and nausea and vomiting in early pregnancy. *Proc Nutr Soc* 41(3):94A, 1982.

Pitkin, RM: Assessment of nutritional status of mother, fetus, and newborn. *Am J Clin Nutr* 34(4):658, 1981.

Raphael, D: *The Tender Gift: Breastfeeding*. Englewood Cliffs, NJ, Prentice-Hall, 1973.

Reames, ES: Opinions of physicians and hospitals of current breast-feeding recommendations. *J Am Diet Assoc* 85(1):79, 1985.

Reynolds, RD; Polansky, M; Moser, PB: Analyzed vitamin B_6 intakes of pregnant and postpartum lactating and nonlactating women. *J Am Diet Assoc* 84(11):1339, 1984.

Ricciuti, HN: Adverse environmental and nutritional influences on mental development: A perspective. *J Am Diet Assoc* 79(2):115, 1981.

Roepke, JLB; Kirksey, A: Effects of vitamin B_6 supplementation during pregnancy on the vitamin B_6 nutriture of previous long-term oral contraceptive users and nonusers. *Fed Proc* 40(3):863, 1981.

Rossignol, AM: Caffeine-containing beverages and premenstrual syndrome in young women. *Am J Pub Health* 75(10):1335, 1985.

Rosso, P: A new chart to monitor weight gain during pregnancy. *Am J Clin Nutr* 41(3):664, 1985.

Salariya, EM; Easton, PM; Cater, JI: Duration of breast-feeding after early initiation and frequent feeding. *Lancet* 2(November 25):1141, 1978.

Schuster, K; Bailey, LB; Mahan, CS: Effect of maternal pyridoxine-HCl supplementation on the vitamin B_6 status of mother and infant and on pregnancy outcome. *J Nutr* 114(5):977, 1984.

Sharma, V: Premenstrual syndrome. *Practitioner* 226:1091, 1982.

Song, WO; Wyse, BW; Hansen, RG: Pantothenic acid status of pregnant and lactating women. *J Am Diet Assoc* 85(2):192, 1985.

Stumbo, PJ; Booth, BM; Eichenberger, JM; et al: Water intakes of lactating women. *Am J Clin Nutr* 42(11):870, 1985.

Suter, CB; Ott, DB: Maternal and infant nutrition recommendations: A review. *J Am Diet Assoc* 84(5):572, 1984.

Taper, LJ; Oliva, JT; Ritchey, SJ: Zinc and copper retention during pregnancy: The adequacy of prenatal diets with and without dietary supplementation. *Am J Clin Nutr* 41(6):1184, 1985.

Thenen, SW: Folacin content of supplemental foods for pregnancy. *J Am Diet Assoc* 80(3):237, 1982.

Truswell, AS: Nutrition for pregnancy. *British Med J* 291(27):203, 1985.

Tufts University: Facts and fallacies about eating and pregnancy. *Diet and Nutrition Letter* 3(10):3, 1985.

U.S. Department of Agriculture (USDA): *Ten State Nutrition Survey (1960–1970). IV. Biochemical*. DHEW Publ. No. (HMS) 72-8132, 1972.

Waletzky, LR; Herman, EC: Relactation. *Am Fam Physician* 14(2):69, 1976.

Weigley, ES: Nutrition and the older primigravida. *J Am Diet Assoc* 82(5):529, 1983.

Wheatley, D: Treatment of pregnancy sickness. *Br J Obstet Gynecol* 84:444, 1977.

Worthington-Roberts, BS; Vermeersch, J; Williams, SR: *Nutrition in Pregnancy and Lactation*, 2nd ed. St. Louis, C. V. Mosby Co, 1981.

Further Study

Axelson, ML; Kurinij, N; Sahlroot, JT; et al: Primiparas' beliefs about breast feeding. *J Am Diet Assoc* 85(1):77, 1985.

Brown, JE; Toma, RB: Taste changes during pregnancy. *Am J Clin Nutr* 43(3):414, 1986.

Cerrato, PL: When your patient is eating for two. *RN* 49(6):67, 1986.

Finley, DA; Dewey, KG; Lonnerdal, B; et al: Food choices of vegetarians and nonvegetarians during pregnancy and lactation. *Am J Diet Assoc* 85(6):678, 1985.

Frank, EP: What are nurses doing to help PMS patients? *Am J Nurs* 86(2):137, 1986.

Jewell, ME: Breast feeding. *Am Family Physician* 30(7):167, 1984.

Palmer, JL; Jennings, GE; Massey, L: Development of an assessment form: Attitude toward weight gain during pregnancy. *J Am Diet Assoc* 85(8):946, 1985.

American Academy of Pediatrics Committee on Nutrition. Statement on teenage pregnancy. *Pediatrics* 63(5):795, 1979.

Daniels, P; Weingarten, K: A new look at the medical risks in late childbearing. *Women Health* 4(spring):5, 1979.

Gueri, M; Jutsum, P; Sorhaindo, B: Anthropometric assessment of nutritional status in pregnant women: A reference table of weight-for-height by week of pregnancy. *Am J Clin Nutr* 35(3):609, 1982.

Johnson, EM; Schwartz, NE: Physicians' opinions and counseling practices in maternal and infant nutrition. *J Am Diet Assoc* 73(3):246, 1978.

Leonard, LG: Pregnancy and the underweight. *Am J Maternal Child Nurs* 9(5):331, 1984.

Luke, B: Megavitamins and pregnancy: A dangerous combination. *Am J Maternal Child Nurs* 10(1):18, 1985.

Barsivala, V; Virkar, K: The effects of oral contraceptives on concentrations of various components of human milk. *Contraception* 7(4):307, 1973.

Blinick, G; Wallach, RC; Jerez, E: Drug addiction in pregnancy and the neonate. *Am J Obstet Gynecol* 125(2):135, 1976.

Avery, JL: *Induced Lactation: A Guide for Counseling and Management.* Denver, CO, Resources in Human Nurturing, 1979.

Brown, RE: Relactation: An overview. *Pediatrics* 60(1):116, 1977.

Hormann, E: *A Study of Induced Lactation.* Franklin Park, IL, La Leche League International, 1976.

Garza, C; Goldman, AS: Effect of maternal nutritional status on lactation performance and infant nutrition. *Perinat Neonat* 9(2):11, 1985.

Jones, D: Breastfeeding Problems. *Nurs Times* 80(33):53,1984.

Psiaki, D; Olson, D; Kaplowitz, D: *Current Knowledge on Breastfeeding.* Ithaca, NY, Cornell University, 1980.

Resources

International Childbirth Education Association
2763 N W 70th Street
Seattle, WA 98167

La Leche League International, Inc.
9616 Minneapolis Avenue
Franklin Park, IL 60131

Breast Pumps:
Egnel, Inc.
412 Park Avenue
Cary, IL 60013

Other breast pumps available from medical supply houses and pharmacies.

Dietary Management of Infancy, Childhood, and Adolescence

THE STUDENT WILL BE ABLE TO:

- *Outline the procedure for additional foods for the infant after the initial stage of feeding by bottle or breast.*
- *Plan daily meals with adequate nutrients for a six-year-old and 12-year-old child as well as a 17-year-old male adolescent according to the RDAs.*
- *Suggest ways to handle these typical problems: diarrhea, colic, and food jags.*

OBJECTIVES

TERMS TO KNOW

Attention deficit disorder
  (ADD)
Beikost
Failure to thrive (FTT)
Defined diet
Hyperactivity
Hypogalactia
Renal solute load
Small for gestational age
  (SGA)
Suckling versus sucking

Not only the present health, but the future lifelong health for the newborn depends upon the loving care and feeding from the mother or caretaker (Fig. 16–1).

National nutrition objectives were established by the Public Health Service (1980) to reduce dietary risks that face Americans and to aid in planning programs targeted at nutrition and health problems. Some objectives that should be implemented by 1990 are to:

1. Eliminate growth retardation of infants caused by inadequate diet.
2. Increase the percentage of breast-fed infants to 75 percent at hospital discharge and 35 percent at six months of age.
3. Decrease the mean serum cholesterol level in children ages one to 14 to 150 mg/dl or below. (Mean serum cholesterol level was 176 mg/dl for children ages one to 17 from 1971 to 1974.)

Hopefully, our nation can achieve these nutritional goals for the optimal health of infants and children in the near future.

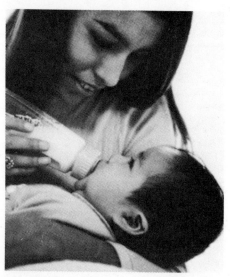

Figure 16–1. Mother feeding her infant with a bottle. (Courtesy of Gerber Products Company.)

Nutrient Intake for the Infant

Nutrient intake is intricately woven throughout life with the physical, mental, and emotional status of the human being. The period most critical to growth of the brain begins nine months before birth and continues into the second year. During this time, the actual number of cells and the size of the head (cell mass) depend upon optimum nutrients. Head circumference achieves two thirds of its postnatal growth by 24 months of age (Pipes, 1986). Therefore, food intake during infancy is most important for mental performance later in life.

The obstetrician should suggest a prenatal conference with the pediatrician to discuss whether the newborn will be breast-fed or bottle-fed. Certainly, the mother should not be pressured into making her decision. However, the medical profession as a group has been so hesitant to recommend either method to the mother that conferences or discussions are rare. Both the father and mother have the right to understand the advantages and disadvantages of both methods to be able to make the best selection for the infant and themselves. In general, mothers who bottle-feed are influenced by their mothers and friends; they usually do not attend childbirth classes. In contrast, breast-feeding mothers are less influenced by their peers; most attend childbirth classes (Lawrence, 1980).

BREAST-FEEDING

Human milk is a natural substance that offers optimum nutrients specifically designed for the newborn. It is believed that each mother's milk is uniquely suited to her infant. For example, the protein content is higher if the infant is premature (Krieger, 1982). Formulas are designed to simulate breast milk with remarkable success. Table 16–1 lists the nutrients in human milk, cow's milk, and formula.

For the optimal health of the breast-fed infant, the following nutrient supplements are recommended (Fomon, 1986):

1. An initial injection of vitamin K immediately after birth will prevent the possibility of vitamin K deficiency, which might cause intracranial bleeding.
2. Fluoride supplementation (0.25 mg/day) is without hazard to the infant and may possibly be of some benefit in protecting against dental caries.
3. A daily supplement of 400 IU of vitamin D should be given unless the infant is light-skinned and the head, forearms, and hands are exposed for about one hour per week to sunlight.
4. Daily iron supplementation of 0.5 to 1.0 mg is suggested.

Table 16–1. Daily Dietary Allowance for Infants and Nutrient Content of Human Milk, Cow's Milk, and Infant Formula*

Nutrient	Daily Allowances		Human Milk	Cow's Milk	Typical Formula
	0 to 6 month	6 to 12 month	(per liter)		
Kilocalories	117/kg	108/kg	750	670	680
Protein (gm)	2.2/kg	2.0/kg	11	36	16
Casein (gm)	–	–	4.4	29.5	13.1
Lactalbumin (gm)	–	–	6.7	6.5	2.9
Lactose (gm)	–	–	68	49	72
Fat (gm)	–	–	45	36	36
Polyunsaturated (gm)	–	–	7	1.4	8
Monounsaturated (gm)	–	–	21	11	5
Saturated (gm)	–	–	17	21	21
Cholesterol (mg)	–	–	200	113	160
Vitamin A (IU)	1400	2000	1898	1447	2500
Vitamin D (IU)	400	400	22[a]	400	400
Vitamin E (IU)	4	5	2.7	1.5	15
Vitamin C (mg)	35	35	43	10	55
Folacin (mcg)	50	50	52	55	50
Niacin (mg equiv)	5	8	1.5	9.5	7.0
Riboflavin (mg)	0.4	0.6	0.36	1.8	1.0
Thiamin (mg)	0.3	0.5	0.16	0.3	0.6
Vitamin B_6 (mg)	0.3	0.4	0.1	0.5	0.4
Vitamin B_{12} (mcg)	0.3	0.3	0.3	5.3	1.5
Vitamin K (mcg)	15[b]	15[b]	15	60	65
Calcium (mg)	360	540	340	1220	510
Phosphorus (mg)	240	400	140	960	390
Iodine (mcg)	35	45	30	47	68
Iron (mg)	10	15	0.2[c]	0.5	1.5[d]
Magnesium (mg)	60	70	40	120	41
Zinc (mg)	3	5	1.6[c]	4	5
Copper (mcg)	60/kg[e]	60/kg[e]	240[c]	300	400
Sodium (mEq)[g]	8[f]	6[f]	7	22	10
Potassium (mEq)	7[f]	6[f]	13	38	18
Chloride (mEq)	7[f]	6[f]	11	28	15
Renal solute load (mOsm/L)[h]			79	232	105

*From Krause, MV; Mahan, LK: *Food, Nutrition and Diet Therapy,* 7th ed. Philadelphia, W.B. Saunders Co, 1984, with permission.
[a]May be higher if vitamin D sulfate is included (360 IU). Lakdawala and Widdowson. *Lancet* 1:167, 1977. Not known if vitamin D sulfate form is biologically active in neonate.
[b]Advisable intake.
[c]Picciano and Guthrie. *Am J Clin Nutr* 29:242, 1976.
[d]Also available with 12.6 mg/L.
[e]Estimated requirement.
[f]Advisable intakes.
[g]Milliequivalents.
[h]Milliosmoles/L.

BOTTLE-FEEDING

In spite of the rise in breast-feeding plus the recommendation by the American Academy of Pediatrics (AAP, 1976) that infants be breast-fed during their first year, 48 percent of all newborns in 1981 were formula-fed. One of the main reasons for formula-feeding is the number of women who return to work immediately after birth. It is possible for these women to breast-feed if they desire, but it may be difficult to manage all the demands without stress. Another problem is the lack of support and encouragement for breast-feeding. In the United States, formula-feeding is a safe and acceptable choice.

One main advantage of bottle-feeding is that the infant can be fed by other people. Bottle-feeding is better if the mother is taking contraindicated medicines or if she wishes to return to oral contraceptives immediately.

Table 16–2. Nutrient Levels of Infant Formulas[a]

| Nutrient | Requirements of the Infant Formula Act of 1980 | |
	Minimum (per 100 kcal)	Maximum (per 100 kcal)
Protein (gm)	1.8[b]	4.5
Fat		
(gm)	3.3	6.0
(% cal)	30.0	54.0
Essential fatty acids (linoleate)		
(% cal)	2.7	
(mg)	300.0	
Vitamins		
A (IU)	250.0 (75 mcg)[c]	750.0 (225 mcg)[c]
D (IU)	40.0	100.0
K (μg)	4.0	
E (IU)	0.7 (with 0.7 IU/gm linoleic acid)	
C (ascorbic acid) (mg)	8.0	
B_1 (thiamine) (mca)	40.0	
B_2 (riboflavin) (mcg)	60.0	
B_6 (pyridoxine (mcg)	35.0 (with 15 μg/gm of protein in formula)	
B_{12} (mcg)	0.15	
Niacin (mcg)	250.0	
Folic acid (mcg)	4.0	
Pantothenic acid (mcg)	300.0	
Biotin (mcg)	1.5[d]	
Choline (mg)	7.0[d]	
Inositol (mg)	4.0[d]	
Minerals		
Calcium (mg)	50.0[e]	
Phosphorus (mg)	25.0[e]	
Magnesium (mg)	6.0	
Iron (mg)	0.15	
Iodine (mcg)	5.0	
Zinc (mg)	0.5	
Copper (mcg)	60.0	
Manganese (mcg)	5.0	
Sodium (mg)	20.0	60.0
Potassium (mg)	80.0	200.0
Chloride (mg)	55.0	150.0

[a]From Anderson, SA; Chinn, HI; Fisher, KD: History and current status of infant formulas. *American Journal of Clinical Nutrition* 35:381–397, 1982, reprinted with permission.

[b]The source of protein shall be at least nutritionally equivalent to casein.

[c]Retinol equivalents.

[d]Required to be included in this amount only in formulas that are not milk-based.

[e]Calcium-to-phosphorus ratio must be no less than 1.1 or more than 2.0.

Commerical Formulas. In 1980, the Infant Formula Act (Table 16–2) was enacted to provide recommendations of nutrients in the standard 20 cal/oz. for full-term infants (Wink, 1985). While nutrients differ slightly for various brands, all comply with these standards set by the Infant Formula Act. Table 16–3 lists these commercial formulas with their nutrient content; Table 16–4 shows the carbohydrate, protein, and fat sources of the formulas as well as indications for their use.

In formula selection, several factors need to be considered. The renal system in infants is im-

mature and may be unable to concentrate urine. Protein in a formula produces urea, which along with the electrolytes sodium, potassium, and chloride, contributes to the renal solute load. If the renal solute is too high or fluids are restricted, hypertonic dehydration may result. Because of its high renal solute load, fresh cow's milk is not suitable for newborn infants.

The osmolality of a formula influences the gastrointestinal tolerance of a formula. The osmolality is determined by the number of particles in the solution. Hydrolyzed proteins, monosaccha-

Table 16–3. Nutritional Values of Infant Formulas (per 1000 ml)*

	Vit A (IU)	Vit D (IU)	Vit E (IU)	Vit K (mg)	Vit C (mg)	Folic Acid (mg)	Thiamine (mg)	Riboflavin (mg)	B₆ (mg)	B₁₂ (mcg)	Niacin (mg)	Choline (mg)	Biotin (mg)	Pantothenic Acid (mg)	Sodium (mEq)	Potassium (mEq)	Chloride (mEq)	Calcium (gm)	Phosphorus (gm)	Magnesium (mg)	Iodine (mcg)	Manganese (mg)	Copper (mg)	Zinc (mg)	Iron (mg)
Enfamil	1690	422	12.7	96	55	.1	.5	.6	.4	2.1	8.4	47.5	.016	3.17	10.1	17.3	13.3	.528	.444	47.5	69	1.0	.6	4.2	1.48
Enfamil with Iron	1690	422	12.7	96	55	.1	.5	.6	.4	2.1	8.4	47.5	.016	3.17	10.1	17.3	13.3	.528	.444	47.5	69	1.0	.6	4.2	12.7
Similac 20 Kcal/oz.	2500	400	17	30	55		.65	1.0	.4	1.5	7.0	102	.01	3.0	10.9	20	14.9	.51	.39	41	100	.03	.6	5.0	1.5
Similac with Iron	2500	400	17	30	55		.65	1.0	.4	1.5	7.0	102	.01	3.0	10.9	20	14.9	.51	.39	41	100	.03	.6	5	12
Similac 24 LBW	3000	480	18	NA	100	.1	1.0	1.2	.5	2.0	8.4	NA	.015	3.6	16.1	30.8	24.8	.73	.56	80	120	.04	.8	8	3.0
Advance	2400	400	12	20	50	.1	.75	.9	.6	2.5	10	NA	.008	4.0	13	22	14	.51	.39	64	60	.027	.9	6.0	12
Enfamil Premature (20 cal/oz.)	2080	416	13	62	56	.2	.5	.6	.4	2.0	8.3	47.5	.016	3.0	11.3	18.9	15.8	.78	.39	70	53	.17	.6	6.7	1.0
Enfamil Premature (24 cal/oz.)	2496	499	16	75	68	.24	.6	.7	.5	2.5	10	57	.019	3.7	13.6	22.7	26.4	.94	.47	83	63	.2	.7	8	1.3
PM 60/40	2500	400	15	30	55	.05	.65	1.0	.3	1.4	7.3	128	.01	3.0	6.9	14.9	7.0	.4	.2	42	40	.03	.4	4.0	2.6
Special Care (20 kcal/oz.)	4580	1000	25	83	250	.25	1.7	4.2	1.7	3.7	20	67	.025	12.5	12.6	21.3	15.2	1.2	.6	83	125	.17	1.7	10	2.5
Special Care (24 kcal/oz.)	5500	1200	30	100	300	.3	2.0	5	2	4.5	24	80	.03	15	15.2	25.6	18.3	1.4	.72	100	150	.2	2.0	12	3
SMA	2647	423	9.5	58	58	.05	.7	1.0	.4	1.0	10.2	88	.015	2.1	6.5	14.4	10.5	.45	.33	53	69	.16	.5	3.7	13
"Preemie" SMA	3200	510	15	70	70	.1	.8	1.3	.8	2	6.3	165	.018	3.6	14	19	15	.75	.4	70	83	.2	.7	5	3
Prosobee	2112	422	10.6	106	55	.11	.53	.63	.42	2.1	8.4	52.7	.05	3.2	12.6	21	15.5	.63	.50	74	69	.2	.6	5.3	12.7
Isomil	2500	400	17	150	55	.1	.4	.6	.4	3.0	9.0	NA	.03	5.0	13	18.2	15	.7	.5	50	150	.2	.5	5.0	12
Isomil SF20	2500	400	17	150	55	.1	.4	.6	.5	3.0	9.0	NA	.03	5.0	13	18	15	.7	.5	50	150	.2	.5	5.0	12
Isomil SF Concentrate	2500	400	17	150	55	.1	.4	.6	.4	3.0	9.0	NA	.03	5.0	13	18	15	.7	.5	50	150	.2	.5	5.0	12
RCF—Module	2500	400	17	150	55	.1	.4	.6	.4	3.0	9.0	NA	.03	5.0	17	18	15	.7	.5	50	100	.2	.5	1.5	1.5
Lofenolac	1690	422	10.6	106	55	.1	.5	.6	.4	2.1	8.4	90	.05	3.17	14	18	13.3	.63	.47	74	48	1.06	.63	4.2	12.7
Nutramagin	1690	422	10.6	106	55	.1	.5	.6	.4	2.1	8.4	90	.05	3.17	14	18	13.3	.63	.47	74	48	1.06	.63	4.2	12.7
Progestimil	2090	419	15	107	54	.1	.5	.6	.4	2.0	8.4	90	.05	6.6	14	14.8	17	.60	.42	74	47	.2	.6	4.0	13
Meat Base Formula	1778	467	6	NA	60	.03	.6	1.0	.87	8.7	7.3	NA	NA	2.0	7.9	9.8	NA	1.0	.67	40	33	NA	.4	2.8	14

*From Rombeau, JL; Caldwell, MD: Enteral and Tube Feeding. Philadelphia, W. B. Saunders Co, 1984, with permission.

Table 16–4. Nutritional Values of Infant Formulas (per 1000 ml)*

Manufacturer	Product	Carbohydrate Sources	Protein Sources	Fat Sources	Kcal/Ml	mOsm/L	CHO GMS	PRO GMS	Fat GMS	Comments
I. Milk-Based Indications: Normal GI tract; for infants greater than 36 weeks gestation.										
1. Mead Johnson	Enfamil	Lactose	Nonfat milk	Soy oil Coconut oil	.68	290	70	15	37	
2. Mead Johnson	Enfamil with iron	Lactose	Nonfat milk	Soy oil Coconut oil	.68	290	70	15	37	
3. Ross	Similac	Lactose	Nonfat milk	Coconut oil Soy oil Coconut oil	.68	262	72.3	15.5	36.1	Also available at 13 cal/oz., 24 cal/oz. and 27 cal/oz. dilutions
4. Ross	Similac with iron	Lactose	Nonfat milk	Soy oil Coconut oil	.68	262	72.3	15.5	36.1	
5. Ross	Similac 24 LBW	Corn syrup solids Lactose	Nonfat milk	Soy oil Corn oil MCT oil	.81	300	84.9	22	44.9	For feeding LBW infants (<2500 gm)
6. Ross	Advance	Corn syrup solids Lactose	Nonfat milk Soy isolate	Soy oil Corn oil	.54	210	55	20	27	For older infants
II. Whey Adjusted Diets Indications: Normal or immature GI tract; for infants less than 36 weeks gestation.										
7. Mead Johnson	Enfamil Premature (20 cal/oz.)	Corn syrup solids (60%) Lactose (40%)	Whey (lactalbumin) (60%) Casein (40%)	Coconut oil (20%) Corn oil (40%) MCT oil (40%)	68	244	74	20	34	
8. Mead Johnson	Enfamil Premature (24 cal/oz.)	Corn syrup solids (60%) Lactose (40%)	Whey (lactalbumin) (60%) Casein (40%)	Coconut oil (20%) Corn oil (40%) MCT oil (40%)	.81	300	89	24	41	
9. Ross	PM 60/40	Lactose	Whey (lactalbumin) (60%) Casein (40%)	Coconut oil Corn oil	.68	260	68.8	15.8	37.6	
10. Ross	Special Care (20 cal/oz.)	Corn syrup solids (50%) Lactose (50%)	Whey lactalbumin (60%) Casein (40%)	Coconut oil (30%) Corn oil (20%) MCT oil (50%)	.68	300	71.7	18.3	36.7	
11. Ross	Special Care (24 cal/oz.)	Corn syrup solids (50%) Lactose (50%)	Whey (lactalbumin) (60%) Casein (40%)	Coconut oil (30%) Corn oil (20%) MCT oil (50%)	.81	300	86	22	44	

	Product	Carbohydrate	Protein	Fat						Comments
12. Wyeth	SMA	Lactose	Whey (lactalbumin) (60%) Casein (40%)	Coconut oil Safflower oil Soy oil	.68	296	71.8	14.9	35.9	
13. Wyeth	"Preemie" SMA	Lactose (50%) Dextrose polymers (50%)	Whey (lactalbumin) (60%) Casein (40%)	Soy Safflower oil Soy oil MCT oil	.81	268	86	20	44	

III. Soy Isolate
Indications: Cow's milk intolerance; otherwise normal GI tract.

	Product	Carbohydrate	Protein	Fat						Comments
14. Mead Johnson	Prosobee	Corn syrup solids	Soy isolate	Soy oil (80%) Coconut oil (20%)	.68	200	69	20	36	Lactose-free
15. Ross	Isomil	Corn syrup solids Sucrose	Soy isolate	Soy oil Coconut oil	.68	250	68	20	36	Lactose-free
16. Ross	Isomil SF20 Ready to Feed	Corn syrup solids	Soy isolate	Soy oil Coconut oil	.68	250	68	20	36	Lactose-free
17. Ross	Isomil SF Concentrated Liquid	Corn syrup solids	Soy isolate	Soy oil Coconut oil	.68	250	68	20	36	Lactose-free
18. Ross	RCF	—	Soy isolate	Soy oil Coconut oil	.68	N/A	—	20	36	Module carbohydrate-free

IV. Casein Hydrolysate
Indications: Protein sensitivity; malabsorption; short bowel syndrome; galactosemia.

	Product	Carbohydrate	Protein	Fat						Comments
19. Mead Johnson	Lofenolac	Corn syrup solids Tapioca starch	Casein hydrolysate	Corn oil	.68	NA	87.6	21.9	27	Lactose-free, low phenylalanine, for use in infants and children with PKU
20. Mead Johnson	Nutramagin	Sucrose Modified tapioca starch	Casein hydrolysate	Corn oil	.68	NA	87.6	22	26	Lactose-free
21. Mead Johnson	Pregestimil	Corn syrup solids (85%) Modified tapioca starch (15%)	Casein hydrolysate	Corn oil (60%) MCT oil (40%)	.68	338	91	19	27	Lactose-free

V. Meat-Based Diets
Indications: Cow's milk intolerance; galactosemia.

	Product	Carbohydrate	Protein	Fat						Comments
22. Gerber	Meat Base Formula	Cane sugar Modified tapioca starch	Beef hearts	Sesame oil	.68	NA	63.3	28.7	33.3	Lactose-free

*From Rombeau, JL; Caldwell, MD: *Enteral and Tube Feeding.* Philadelphia, W. B. Saunders Co, 1984, with permission.

rides, and disaccharides increase the osmolality. This can result in abdominal distention, diarrhea, and vomiting.

Breast milk is about 300 milliosmoles (mOsm)/kg. Formulas are limited to no greater than 400 mOsm/kg with a caloric density of 20 kcal/oz. (AAP, 1976). The incidence of necrotizing enterocolitis is thought to be higher among infants who are fed hyperosmolar solutions (Wink, 1985).

Nonfat cow's milk is the basis for most infant formulas with modifications to resemble human milk. These formulas, whether predominantly whey or casein, provide similar growth rates to those of breast-fed infants. Since the amino acid taurine is in breast milk, it is added even though the precise need in undefined (Wink, 1985).

Because skim milk is not satisfactory for normal infant growth, fat must be added to these formulas. Linoleic acid is the essential fatty acid required, but too much linoleic acid can cause hemolytic anemia and raise vitamin E requirements, especially in the preterm infant (Martinez & Dodd, 1983). The saturated fats of cow's milk are poorly digested and absorbed, so combinations of unsaturated vegetable and/or medium-chain triglyceride (MCT) oils are added (Wink, 1985).

Breast milk, the ideal infant food, contains more cholesterol than cow's milk or commercial formulas. During the growth period, an adequate intake of cholesterol may be necessary for myelination of the nervous system and for the production of bile acids and hormones. Therefore, the American Academy of Pediatrics (AAP) Committee on Nutrition questions the wisdom of limiting fat and cholesterol intake in newborns (AAP, 1986).

Soy protein formulas are used most often when milk protein is not appropriate. Even with the addition of the amino acid methionine, the growth rate is not maintained as well as with breast milk or milk-based commercial formulas. Soy protein formulas are not recommended for the preterm infant except for a limited time. They are appropriate for infants who have a temporary lactase deficiency secondary to diarrhea and for those with congenital lactase deficiency or galactosemia. They may also be the preferred formula for infants whose parents are vegetarians. If an allergy to cow's milk is present or potentially a factor, soy formula may be used. Many other specialized formulas are available for specific medical conditions, e.g., Lofenolac (Mead Johnson) for phenylketonuria or Meat Base Formula (Gerber) for cow's milk intolerance.

Diluted formulas containing less than 20 kcal/oz. are used only briefly when appropriate. On the other hand, infants may require a higher caloric intake or a more concentrated formula. When protein and mineral levels are increased, the osmolality is increased and the infant must be carefully observed for gastric distress (Wink, 1985).

Standards for the premature infant are not clearly defined. However, special formulas are available such as "Preemie" SMA (Wyeth), Enfamil Premature Formula (Mead Johnson), and Special Care (Ross). When the infant weighs 2 kg, a standard formula may be initiated (AAP, 1977).

Vitamins and minerals are added to formulas. Formulas for preterm infants contain generous amounts of vitamin E because excessive iron as well as linoleic acid increases the vitamin E requirements by interfering with its absorption and utilization (AAP, 1977).

For the first four months of life, 26 to 32 oz./day of formula will satisfy infants. Fluid requirements are usually met by breast milk, but they may or may not be met via formula.

Amount of Formula. To determine the plan for a formula: (1) Estimate the kilocalories required for the weight of the baby by multiplying 100 kcal by the body weight in kilograms; (2) decide how much formula is needed (using the kilocalories required); (3) divide this by the number of feedings desired. Contrary to rigid feeding schedules enforced in the past, infants today are generally fed on demand, i.e., when they are hungry. A pattern usually develops by the infant feeding on demand to eat six times per day at four-hour intervals (2 AM, 6 AM, 10 AM, 2 PM, 6 PM, and 10 PM). By two to three months of age, the 2 AM feeding will be dropped, and by six months of age, only four feedings are demanded (6 AM, 11 AM, 4 PM, and 10 PM).

PREPARATION OF FORMULA

Most commercial formulas are available as ready-to-feed liquids or concentrated preparations (liquid or powder) to be diluted with water. In many homes in the United States today, the preparation of formula consists of mixing one feeding at a time without all the former sterilization procedures. This is possible because of new products, the higher degree of sanitation by automatic dishwashers, and the higher temperatures of hot water tanks. For sanitation reasons, one feeding at a time is usually recommended when terminal sterilization is not used. There are large popula-

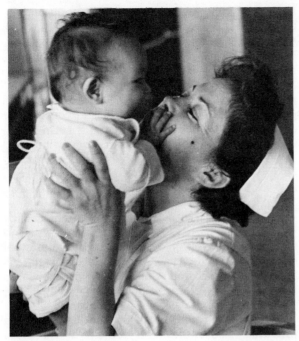

Figure 16–2. Tender loving care—the hallmark of good nursing—is as essential for growth as food. (Courtesy of World Health Organization. Photo by E. Schwab.)

tions still in the United States as well as worldwide that must practice more complicated sterilization methods. An even larger population worldwide must depend upon breast-feeding to protect the newborn from fatal infections.

Techniques for Bottle-Feeding. The position for bottle-feeding should be as much like breast-feeding as possible. Touching helps to strengthen feelings of love, security, and trust and is as important as the nutrients in the formula (Fig. 16–2). The bottle is held at an angle so that the nipple is kept full of milk, and the baby is held with the head at breast level. The hole in the nipple should be large enough to permit the milk to drip out of the bottle without shaking. Smaller holes will make the baby suck in too much air, which may lead to vomiting. The bottle should never be forced on the baby to be finished. On the other hand, if s/he cries after finishing the bottle, more formula may be needed. A constant weight gain according to growth charts is a wise guide to follow. After feeding, the baby should be placed over the shoulder and patted gently on the back to expel air.

Clinical Implications:

- Errors in dilution are serious and can be hazardous for the infant. Undiluted concentrated formula can lead to hypernatremia and tetany from solute loads that are too heavy for the kidneys to excrete. Cases of cerebral damage and gangrene of the extremities have been reported to be the result of hypernatremic dehydration and metabolic acidosis (Pipes, 1986).
- Heating infant formulas or food particularly in a microwave oven can result in severe burns to the infant's mouth and throat due to the build-up of heat after removal from the microwave. Shaking formula and stirring food immediately after removal from the microwave can help dissipate heat; however, the temperature must be checked immediately before feeding and several times following to prevent extreme temperatures.
- Equipment cannot be satisfactorily sanitized in a microwave oven.

Infant Size and Growth

THE PREMATURE INFANT

Normal birth weight is 6½ lbs. (3500 gm) or more. A newborn that weighs less than 5½ lbs. (2500 gm) or has a gestational age of less than 37 weeks is considered premature. Usually, a poor nutritional status of the mother before or during pregnancy with a less-than-ideal weight gain during pregnancy or premature delivery results in a low birth weight (LBW) infant. The small for gestational age (SGA) infant is usually full term, but the birth weight is less than 2500 gm.

Premature infants are at high risk for many complications. They are slow to catch up to normal growth rates. Their bodies contain more water and less protein and fat, their bones are poorly calcified, normal sucking reflexes are poorly developed, and the gastrointestinal tract and renal functions are not fully developed. Additionally, the liver is immature in its enzyme system and iron stores. For these reasons, feeding for the premature infant is specially tailored to the infant's problems.

The neuromuscular abilities of the SGA infant may be sufficient enough to suck and digest food, so tube feedings are not necessary; however, increased levels of nutrients are needed to grow to larger size. The SGA baby who weighs more than 1750 gm (almost 4 lbs.) can usually be fed as a term infant.

Premature babies, especially LBW infants, may require tube feedings because of the poorly developed sucking reflex. Feedings are cautiously administered to avoid overloading the tiny immature digestive tract (Helsing & King, 1982).

If the weight is less than 1800 gm, 0.1 gm of folic acid per week is recommended (Helsing & King, 1982). To prevent rickets, 600 IU/day of vitamin D may be started at one month of age. At one month, 25 mg/day of vitamin C may be given. Energy needs are increased from 100 kcal/kg/day for a normal infant to 140 kcal/kg/day for the LBW infant (MacKeith & Wood, 1977).

GROWTH RATES

Growth is the definitive test of wellness (Fig. 16–3). The birth weight doubles in four months (from 7½ to 14 lbs.), and another 7½ lbs. is added in the next eight months. Usually, the growth spurt slows down, and the infant gains only another 4 to 6 lbs. until two years old. Appendices C–6a and C–6b show the average growth of girls and boys for the first 36 months of life.

FAILURE TO THRIVE

When the weight of children is less than 80 percent of the median for age, the term "failure to thrive" (FTT) is used. This complex condition may be caused by organic and/or psychosocial factors; a multidisciplinary team approach is essential. Tender human contact is a requirement just as much as nutrients from food.

Nonorganic failure to thrive may be characterized by vomiting, diarrhea, rumination, and persistent feeding disorders (poor appetite, poor ability to suck, easily fatigued, crying during feedings, refusing to change from liquids to solid food). Organic failure to thrive may be characterized by sleep disturbances, elimination problems, self-stimulation, and aggression (Peterson et al, 1984).

Catch-up growth for the FTT infant can be phenomenal. Early recovery rates for height and weight can be as high as 15 times those of normal children the same age. As FTT children approach the growth of normal children, the rate slows to three times that of normal children (Peterson et al, 1984).

However, catch-up growth is dependent on providing kilocalories and protein in excess of normal needs. General energy needs may be 50 percent above normal. The protein-to-kilocalorie ratio is inflated during catch-up growth, increasing from 0.05 to 0.08 kg/kcal (Peterson et al, 1984).

Fortification may be used to increase the caloric density of foods, i.e., concentration of formula and addition of carbohydrate, protein, and fat sources to beverages. The feeding environment must be pleasant and without distractions. Emotional support is equally critical.

Clinical Implications:

- A newborn infant will lose weight for the first few days, but should not lose more than 10 percent of its birth weight or take longer than 10 to 14 days to regain it.
- Breast-fed babies grow at a slower rate than formula-fed infants. Whether this has an effect on weight later in life is controversial.

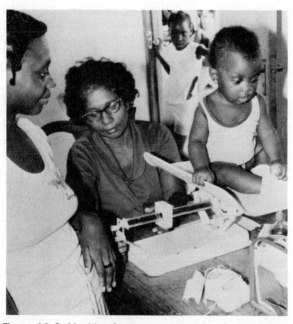

Figure 16–3. *Nutritional status monitored by physical growth. In many places—Jamaica, for example—mothers gather to monitor their children's growth. This is a guarantee of future good health. (Courtesy of World Health Organization. Photo by D. Anand.)*

Progression of Infant Feeding (to 12 Months of Age)

Consideration of the developmental stage of the infant is necessary for a successful feeding regimen. For the infant, nutrition is related to the neuromuscular maturation (Table 16–5).

Table 16–5. Developmental Stages of Eating: Progression in Feeding Behaviors During the First Two Years of Life*

Age	Developmental Landmarks	Appropriate Foods
Birth to 3 months (normal weight, 6½ lbs. or more)	Rooting reflex. Suckling. Tongue pushes food forward and out of mouth when jaw drops. Puts hand or thumb in mouth.	Human milk or formula.
3 to 4 months	Sucking.	
4 to 5 months	Tongue moves back and forth.	Beikost. Iron-fortified rice cereal.
5 to 6 months (birth weight doubled)	Beginning of chewing movements (jaw moves up and down). Drools. Drinks from cup.	Strained vegetables then strained meats and strained fruits. Semisolid and pureed foods. Tuna fish, mashed potatoes, well-cooked mashed vegetables, ground meats in gravy and sauces, soft diced fruit (bananas, peaches, pears), flavored yogurt, and egg yolk.
6 to 9 months	Sits with support. Self-feeds by securing large pieces with a palmar grasp.	Chopped foods. Add finger foods, such as arrowroot biscuits, oven-dried toast, and zwieback. Food should be soluble in mouth to prevent choking. Variety of textures mandatory for acceptance of new foods later in life.
9 to 12 months (birth weight tripled by first year)	Sits alone. Holds bottle. Refined digital grasp. Rotary chewing pattern. Uses fingers to grasp small pieces of food and utensils. Pushes food.	Increase the use of small-sized finger foods as the pincher grasp develops. Cheese sticks, dry cereal, peas, small pieces of meat. Add well-cooked mashed or chopped table foods, prepared without added salt or sugar. Canned fruit, not mashed, spaghetti, macaroni.
12 to 15 months	Tries to use spoon and cup but spills from them.	Foods that will adhere to spoon when scooped, e.g., mashed potatoes, applesauce, cooked cereal, and cottage cheese.
15 to 24 months	Walks alone. May seek and get food independently. Uses spoon to self-feed. Holds glass with both hands. Ulnar deviation of wrist develops. More skilled at cup and spoon feeding. Names food, expresses preferences; prefers unmixed foods. Experiences food jags. Appetite appears to decrease.	Chopped fibrous meats, e.g., a roast or steak. Solid foods. Introduce raw vegetables and fruits gradually. Food of high nutrient value should be available. Balanced food intake should be offered, but the child should be permitted to develop transitory food preferences.

*Adapted from Pipes, P: Nutrition in Infancy and Childhood. St. Louis, C. V. Mosby Co, 1981, with permission.

Note: At birth, the stomach holds 2 Tbsp.; at one year, it holds one cup. The stomach of an adult can hold two quarts.

NEUROMUSCULAR MATURATION

This orderly fashion of development begins with the rooting reflex. The caretaker should be careful not to touch the baby's cheek during feeding, as this distraction will cause the infant to turn his/her head away from the breast or bottle. This reflex depends upon being hungry; when the infant is full, it is not as strong.

Suckling is the manner in which the infant obtains milk during the first three to four months. Its vigorous up-and-down movement seems more like biting and can be painful. *Sucking* is developed later when the orofacial muscles are used with the mouth more pursed, and the tongue moving back and forth. This backward movement of the tongue makes the smacking noises that occur (Krieger, 1982). Breast-fed infants ordinarily do not require separate feedings of water, but bottle-fed infants are usually offered water (Table 16–6).

A forward motion of the tongue on dropping the lower jaw is typical during the first three months. If semisolid foods are offered at this time, the tongue will force the food out, which might be interpreted as dislike. No discriminating taste is occurring though, just reflex action.

The sucking motion becomes developed enough to eat and handle semisolid foods from a spoon around four to six months of age. From six to eight months, motility increases and the infant can receive food and pass it between the gums in a chewing motion.

At seven months, the baby can chew, so pureed foods are not required; some variety of texture is mandatory if the infant is going to accept unfamiliar foods later in life (Endres & Rockwell, 1980). Similar changes in foods offered must be made as the baby continues to grow. Buying separate baby foods is not necessary. Selected foods

Table 16–6. *Fluid Requirements of Infants and Children**

Age	Amount of water (ml/kg/day)
1 week	80 to 100
2 weeks	125 to 150
3 months	140 to 160
6 months	130 to 155
9 months	125 to 145
1 year	120 to 135
2 years	115 to 125

*Adapted from Vaughan, VC; McKay RJ (eds): *Nelson Textbook of Pediatrics*, 10th ed. Philadelphia. W. B. Saunders Co, 1975, with permission.

from the family menu can be pureed for use. The following guidelines are useful when preparing baby food at home:

1. Fruits, vegetables, and meats should be fresh and of high quality.
2. High sanitation standards must be maintained; utensils and hands should be thoroughly clean.
3. Follow the standards in Chapter 14 to maintain the nutrient content of the food. (Do not overcook; use minimal amounts of water.)
4. Seasonings and spices are not necessary. Do not use salt, and use minimal amounts of sugar.
5. Avoid using processed foods with a high salt content, such as ham, bacon, and hot dogs.
6. Honey should *not* be added to foods prepared for infants under one year of age.*
7. Use a blender, food mill, or baby food grinder to puree the food; sufficient water must be added for a smooth consistency.
8. Divide the pureed food into individual-sized portions and store them in the freezer.
9. Thaw only the amount for single feeding prior to serving.
10. Leftover portions should be thrown away. Reheating will result in the loss of some nutrients, and the food may become contaminated with bacteria.

Beikost. This German word means "food other than milk." Some foods are added between four and six months so that the amount of formula stays near 32 oz., with these foods supplementing the kilocalories and nutrient intake.

Three disadvantages in starting beikost too early (before four months) are: (1) unnecessary costs, (2) high probability of overfeeding, and (3) more supplementation resulting in less hunger and less sucking by the infant, which means less milk intake. By four to five months of age, the ability to swallow foods is more developed as well as the infant's digestive system. There is also less possibility of development of food allergies.

Iron. Supplementation of iron is recommended for formula-fed infants after four months of age, breast-fed infants four to six months of age, and preterm infants after two months of age. Iron given to a LBW infant at an earlier age can increase the infant's liability to certain infections; additionally, the infant is less able to use the iron earlier (Helsing & King, 1982). Iron supplementation (usually ferrous sulfate or ferric ammonium

*Honey frequently contains botulism spores; the immune systems of young infants do not have the capacity to resist botulism.

Table 16–7. *Fluoride Supplementation for Infants and Children (mg/day)**

Age	Concentration of Fluoride in Drinking Water (ppm)		
	< .3	0.3 to 0.7	> 0.7
2 weeks to 2 years	0.25	0	0
2 to 3 years	0.50	0.25	0
3 to 16 years	1.00	0.50	0

*2.2 mg of sodium fluoride contains 1 mg of fluoride.

From Committee on Nutrition: Fluoride supplementation: revised dosage schedule. *Pediatrics 63*:150, 1979, with permission.

citrate) is ordinarily given as liquid drops or fortified cereals.

Other Foods. Semisolids are offered before milk at feeding time, yet the amounts are limited in order to reserve some appetite for milk. All foods should be served alone rather than mixed together to observe acceptance and tolerance of the food.

No sugar or salt is added to baby food. Infant foods should not be salted until at least after the first year of life (Yeung, 1984). Salt intake in adulthood seems to be associated with salt intake in early childhood, leading to hypertension in those who are salt-sensitive. Salt is an acquired habit and not related to enjoyment of food unless one is accustomed to it.

Initially, 1 tsp. of iron-fortified dry cereal is mixed with 1 to 2 Tbsp. of formula or breast milk daily. After this is well accepted for two to three weeks, up to 3 Tbsp. of another food may be introduced. Rice cereal is initiated first because it is less allergenic than other cereal products. Fluoride supplementation is recommended for infants and children to increase the strength of teeth (Table 16–7). If the water is not fluoridated, vitamin supplements containing fluoride may be given.

The introduction of vegetables, meats, and fruits varies among pediatricians. Some prefer the introduction of vegetables after cereals, then meats followed by fruits. Because sweet flavors are well accepted, the other foods are offered first. Fruits that are added to cereals usually have sugar in them, so they should not be chosen.

Basal caloric requirements for infants and children may be estimated according to Table 16–8. From the beginning of beikost, the direction of feeding should be to include the food groups as soon as possible to assure a well-balanced diet (Table 16–9). When the infant is consuming at least one third of the energy intake from supplemental foods, homogenized milk fortified with vitamin D may be used. This may occur during the

Table 16–8. *Calculation of Basal Caloric Requirements for Infants and Children**

For a child less than 5 years of age, the basal caloric requirement for 24 hours is computed by multiplying the standard weight for the measured height by the basal requirement for calories per pound per 24 hours for the appropriate age (see table of "Basal Requirement for Calories per Pound per 24 Hours" below). The height is that of the child measured without shoes. The weight to be used is an estimate of a desirable weight based on evaluation of the child's muscular development and body fat.... The age to be used is that of the child to the nearest year or half year. Depending on activity, actual calorie expenditure of a child is generally 50 to 80% greater than basal expenditure.

Basal Requirement for Calories per Pound per 24 Hours

	Calories	
Age	Boys	Girls
6 months	25.0	25.0
1 year	25.5	25.5
2 years	25.0	24.5
3 years	23.5	23.5
4 years	23.0	22.0

*Pemberton, CM; Gastineau, CF (eds): *Mayo Clinic Diet Manual.* Philadelphia: W. B. Saunders Co, 1981, with permission.

second six months of life. Pasteurized milk that has a reduced fat content is inappropriate during the first year of life (AAP, 1986).

Clinical Implication:

• As the infant begins cutting teeth through the next few years, great care should be given to not offering the infant foods conducive to choking. Texture is important from six months to one year, but the food must be easily dissolved, e.g., crackers or zwieback. When chewing has fully developed, soft raw vegetables such as peeled zucchini may be offered. Raw carrots, celery, popcorn, nuts, and hard candies should be postponed for a few more years for safety.

Infant Problems Related to Nutrition

DIARRHEA

When diarrhea is accompanied by a fever over 101°F, by vomiting that lasts more than 24 hours, or by severe diarrhea with stools more

Table 16–9. *Recommended Food Intake for Good Nutrition According to Food Groups and the Average Size of Servings at Different Age Levels**

Food Group	Servings Per Day	Average Size of Servings					
		1 Year	2 to 3 Years	4 to 5 Years	6 to 9 Years	10 to 12 Years	13 to 18 Years
Milk and Cheese (1.5 oz. cheese = 1 cup milk	4	1/2 cup	1/2 to 3/4 cup	3/4 cup	3/4 to 1 cup	1 cup	1 cup
Meat Group (protein foods)	3 or more						
Egg		1	1	1	1	1	1 or more
Lean meat, fish, poultry		2 Tbsp.	2 Tbsp.	2 oz.	2 to 3 oz.	3 to 4 oz.	4 oz. or more
Peanut butter		1 Tbsp.	1 Tbsp.	2 Tbsp.	2 to 3 Tbsp.	3 Tbsp.	3 Tbsp.
Fruits and Vegetables	At least 4						
Vitamin C source	1 or more	1/3 cup or equivalent	1/2 cup or equivalent	1/2 cup or equivalent	1/2 cup or equivalent	1/2 cup or equivalent	1/2 cup or equivalent
Vitamin A source	1	2 Tbsp.	3 Tbsp.	1/4 cup	1/4 cup	1/3 cup	1/2 cup
Other vegetables (e.g., potato and legumes) or	2	2 Tbsp.	3 Tbsp.	1/4 cup	1/3 cup	1/2 cup	3/4 cup
Other fruits (e.g., apples)		1/4 cup	1/3 cup	1/2 cup	1 medium	1 medium	1 medium
Breads and Cereals (whole grain or enriched)	At least 4						
Bread		1/2 slice	1 slice	1 to 1/2 slices	1 to 2 slices	2 slices	2 slices
Ready-to-eat cereal		1/2 oz.	3/4 oz.	1 oz.	1 oz.	1 oz.	1 oz.
Cooked cereal (e.g., macaroni, spaghetti, and rice)		1/4 cup	1/3 cup	1/2 cup	1/2 cup	3/4 cup	1 cup
Fats and Carbohydrates							
Butter, margarine, oils, mayonnaise, and so forth (1 tsp. = 45 calories)		Number of servings and portion sizes to meet caloric needs					
Desserts and sweets (e.g., 100 calories = 1/3 cup pudding or ice cream; 2 cookies; 1 oz. cake; 2 Tbsp. jelly, and jam)		Number of servings and portion sizes to meet caloric needs					

*Chicago Dietetic Association: *Manual of Clinical Dietetics.* Philadelphia, W. B. Saunders Co, 1981, with permission.

than 10 times/day with a large volume of water lost, immediate attention must be given to correct the condition (Endres & Rockwell, 1980). Diarrhea refers to unformed, watery stools that are unlike the usual ones. Acute diarrhea of one to four days requires replacement of fluid, sodium, and potassium.

The physician should be contacted to ensure that nutrients and electrolytes are replaced. For mild diarrhea, foods are normally withheld for the first 24 to 48 hours with fluids given to replace fluid and electrolyte losses. A general outline of dietary management of mild diarrhea is given in Table 16–10. Commercially available solutions, such as Lytren (Mead Johnson) and Pedialyte (Ross), contain a safe concentration of replace-

ment electrolytes. They can be used full strength or diluted to decrease the osmolar load. Additionally, calories should be provided to decrease catabolism.

With fluid intake of 120 ml/kg/day plus an amount of fluid equal to that lost in feces, water balance will be maintained unless insensible water losses are excessive because of fever or elevated environmental temperature. If fluid intake is less than 120 ml/kg during the first 24 hours of therapy, the infant should be clinically evaluated to determine the osmolality of the urine. Urine concentration greater than 400 mOSm/L generally indicates the desirability of initiating parenteral fluid therapy. If fever is present or the environmental temperature high, intakes of 150 ml/kg/day

Table 16–10. *General Outline of Dietary Management of Mild Diarrhea**

Time	Diet
First 8 to 12 hours	Small amounts (15 to 30 ml every 1/2 to 1 hour) of sweetened dilute tea, dilute cola, ginger ale, sugar water, or dilute Jell-O water.
12 to 24 hours (if number of stools has lessened or not increased in frequency)	Increase clear fluids to 60 to 90 ml every 2 hours.
24 hours (if definite improvement)	Plain solids such as Jell-O, bananas, applesauce, or salt crackers.
36 to 48 hours	Gradual return to regular diet (dry toast, baked potato without butter, infant cereals mixed with water, fruits).
3 to 5 days	Gradual addition of milk and milk products, begin with half-strength skim, then full-strength skim, half-strength whole milk, and finally undiluted whole milk.

*From Rombeau, JL; Caldwell, MD: *Enteral and Tube Feeding.* Philadelphia, W. B. Saunders Co, 1984.

for maintenance are desirable. While refeeding should be resumed as soon as possible, acute infections may cause transient lactose deficiency. Lactose-free formulas (made from soy protein or casein hydrolysate) may be introduced after the first 12 to 24 hours (or after good oral hydration is maintained). Either regular formula or soy-based formula is initially ¼ to ½ strength, gradually increased to full strength in 24 to 36 hours if the patient continues to do well clinically.

Clinical Implications:

- If vomiting does not accompany diarrhea, more liberal amounts of fluids can be given.
- When carbohydrates are fed during the course of severe diarrhea, two or three stools (immediately after intake) should be examined daily to determine carbohydrate intolerance. The Clinitest tablets may be used with 0.25 percent or more indicating carbohydrate intolerance, or a pH less than 6. Tests should be repeated several times for verification before changing to a lactose-free diet. If necessary, a soy-isolate of casein hydrolysate may be used for several weeks or months until recovery is well advanced (Fomon, 1974).
- Room temperature fluids are better tolerated.
- Artificial sweeteners are a known cause of diarrhea in infants and children (Lipin, 1984).

- Apple juice has been identified as a cause of diarrhea in infants as a result of carbohydrate malabsorption (Hyams & Leichtner, 1985).
- The diarrhea regimen described in Table 16–9 is deficient in protein, fat, and energy. Prolonged use has precipitated nutritional problems (Self, 1986).

REGURGITATION

During the first six months, regurgitation (spitting up) is common but gradually diminishes. The baby is burped by holding him/her over the shoulder or in a sitting position and patting on the back. Handling the baby gently and placing him/her on the right side or abdomen with the head slightly elevated during naps is also helpful. Most people burp a baby during and immediately after feedings, but some babies may need to be held in a sitting position from a few minutes to an hour and then burped again. Vomiting is a more serious situation than spitting up, and the physician should be consulted.

CONSTIPATION

A hard, dry stool passed with straining indicates constipation. The frequency of the stools or the number of stools will vary with each individual. Daily elimination of one or more stools is not necessary. Breast-fed infants rarely are constipated or have diarrhea. If the bottle-fed infant is receiving an appropriate diet, s/he should not have either condition.

Solid foods may cause some constipation, and if so, more fruit, cereal, or water may help this condition. A ½ oz. of prune juice with a ½ oz. of water will help soften stools. Dark corn syrup, ½ to 1 tsp. per feeding, is usually effective (Gellis & Kagan, 1982). If constipation continues, the diet should be reviewed along with total fluid intake.

HICCUPS

Swallowed air bubbles can cause the hiccups. One should offer the infant water and resume the regular feeding method.

MILK ANEMIA

Infants frequently develop anemia when given milk, usually because they do not eat sufficient amounts of iron-rich foods. The baby should be given iron-rich food (such as cereals) before being offered milk.

NURSING BOTTLE SYNDROME

When the baby is put in bed with a baby bottle, s/he may fall asleep with milk in the mouth, which results in "nursing bottle syndrome." Baby teeth are destroyed when exposed to milk for long periods of time; this condition is accelerated if other beverages with high sugar content are given, e.g., fruit juice (Fig. 16–4).

COLIC

Unhappy, fussy babies who continue to cry for hours, often until completely exhausted, are described as having "colic." The firstborn is a more likely candidate for this condition, which usually starts late in the afternoon. The term "colic" derives from the impression that the pain is due to spasms of the colon, since relief sometimes follows the passage of feces or flatus. The stomach is tense with the legs drawn up toward the body. A thorough physical of the infant is in order to be sure nothing is wrong that can be treated. If an infant is allowed an empty bottle or if the nipple holes are too small (requires more sucking) or too large (forces the infant to gulp to keep up with the flow of milk), the infant swallows too much air. Air may go into the intestines, where distension can cause spasms.

In the breast-fed infant, gas can be produced

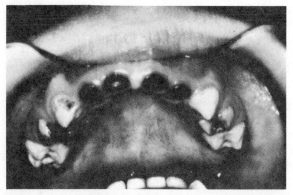

Figure 16–4. *Nursing bottle syndrome: Rampant caries due to use of nursing bottle with sugar-sweetened beverages as a pacifier. (From Nizel AE: Nutrition in Preventive Dentistry: Science and Practice, 2nd ed. Philadelphia, W. B. Saunders Co, 1980, by permission.)*

by foods that the mother eats, causing colic in the baby. Such foods include garlic, onion, broccoli, cabbage, sauerkraut, and pickles. Too much chocolate, or any other food, may cause indigestion. Nuts, berries, and citrus fruits also present problems. Of course, the simplest cause may be the baby's nursing position, which allows too much air to be swallowed (Applebaum, 1976).

Allergies may also cause colic. For example, excess intestinal air results from carbohydrate fermentation due to lactose intolerance. Cow's milk and eggs are both frequent offenders (see Chapter 35). If milk allergy is expected, a trial on soybean milk may be used (Gellis & Kagan, 1982).

Relaxation of the infant and mother may be a useful goal to reduce colic. An overtired baby cries a lot. While some claim that the following practices are not effective, others have found them useful: rhythmic rocking, being walked, humming noises, a pacifier, and wrapping a baby snugly in a blanket and holding firmly. If a mother has been breast-feeding, she may eliminate strong-flavored foods, such as cabbage or onions, for a trial.

With a physician's recommendation, medication may be used to interrupt the cycle. Sometimes elixir of phenobarbital (20 mg/5 cc), in a dosage of ½ tsp. four times a day, may be given for a short period (Gellis & Kagan, 1982). As suddenly as the colic period starts, it stops at about three to four months of age (Krieger, 1982).

ASPHYXIATION BY FOOD

One death occurs approximately every five days from food-related asphyxiations in infants and children up to nine years of age (Harris et al, 1984). Three phases of food asphyxiation are penetration, occlusion, and expulsion. A common cause is choking on bones, seeds, or regurgitated formula or juice.

Several characteristics influence the chance of food penetrating the defenses of the mouth and pharynx. Food that is small, thin, smooth, or slick when wet may inadvertently slip through and enter the pharynx. Hard or tough foods resist mastication and may enter the pharynx prematurely without being properly chewed and mixed with saliva. Then the cough or gag reflex may be triggered after a deep inhalation that causes food to lodge in the airway. Highly viscous foods, such as peanut butter, mold to the airway. Round or cylindrical and pliable or compressible foods can easily plug the airway.

Round foods are hazardous, and hot dog products cause the most deaths. Other foods most often listed as causing asphyxia include apples, cookies, beans, carrots, bread, nuts, peanut butter, chewing gum, hard candy, and grapes. Hot dogs, apple pieces, and cookies or biscuits cause half the deaths in infants under one year old. Peanuts and grapes are the most dangerous items among two-year-olds. Hot dogs remain very risky even for three-year-olds (Harris et al, 1984).

Distractions during eating or poor caretaker supervision can play a role not only by failing to prevent asphyxiation initially but also by averting proper rescue attempts. Information regarding choking risks in children should be disseminated not only to parents and caretakers but also to the food industry and health professionals.

Feeding the Toddler (One to Three Years of Age)

MEAL SUGGESTIONS

Children like regularity, so eating at the same time is preferable and helps control appetite. Regular meals also help to avoid fatigue, which can interfere with emotions as well as appetite.

More food is eaten by the child when the parents eat at the same time, rather than just offering food for the child to eat alone (Hertzler, 1983). Children like to be asked what they want to eat (when it is appropriate) without the parents assuming they know (Birch, 1979).

TYPES OF FOOD

One tart, one mild, and one crisp food is a good rule. Strong-flavored vegetables are more popular if eaten raw, e.g., turnips. Color is especially appealing to children. A tiny sprig of parsley, a carrot stick, or a slice of tomato is appreciated. Bright colors such as green, yellow, red, and orange are all liked.

Two to three year olds may find meat hard to chew; thrice-ground meat is easier. Cooked dried beans are suitable for part of the protein intake, but their poor digestibility is a limiting factor for older children as well as for infants and small children (Graham et al, 1979).

Preschool Children (Four to Six Years Old)

The preschool child's rate of growth is slower than the infant's; however, the activity level is usually high because they play hard and are constantly active. Consequently, nutrient needs are relatively high. Poor nutritional status (as measured by growth rate and biochemical indices) is generally more prevalent in lower socioeconomic groups where the amounts and variety of foods may be limited. Approximately 10 percent of all children, regardless of socioeconomic background, may be iron-deficient. Vitamins A and C are also frequently deficient in the diet.

FEEDING CONCERNS

Preschoolers are relatively independent at the table as far as feeding themselves. Certain factors need to be considered to make the mealtime pleasant rather than an ordeal. While sturdy child-size tables and chairs may be used, booster chairs allow the family to eat together. Family mealtime is important for socialization. Children will imitate others at the table in both manners and food habits.

Nonbreakable dishes should be heavy enough to resist spilling. Beverages should be in small squatty containers that are about ½ to ¾ full.

Small amounts of food are offered several times a day. Serving sizes should be based on appetite, but initially about 1 Tbsp. can be offered for each year of age. Snacks can contribute significantly to the nutrient intake. Some wholesome snacks enjoyed by this age group include cheese cubes, fresh fruit, raw vegetable sticks, milk, and fruit juices.

Children who are tired will not eat well. A short rest period should be allowed prior to the meal if they have been very active.

Parental attitudes and eating habits are the most influential factors on the child's food preferences. This may occur for several reasons. Foods that are disliked by one or both parents will not be served very often or may not be served at all. Additionally, children will mimic their parents and tend to enjoy foods the parents like.

When planning menus, the child's food preferences must be considered; however, offering

Table 16–11. Food Pattern for Preschool Child[a]

Food	Portion size	Number of portions advised ages (yr) 2 to 4	4 to 6
Milk and dairy products			
Milk[b]	4 oz.	3 to 6	3 to 4
Cheese	1/2 to 3/4 oz.	May be substituted for one portion of liquid milk	
Yogurt	1/4 to 1/2 cup	May be substituted for one portion of liquid milk	
Powdered skim milk	2 Tbsp.	May be substituted for one portion of liquid milk	
Meat and meat equivalents			
Meat,[c] fish,[d] poultry	1 to 2 oz.	2	2
Egg	1	1	1
Peanut butter	1 to 2 Tbsp.		
Legumes—dried peas and beans	1/4 to 1/3 cup cooked		
Vegetables and fruits			
Vegetables		4 to 5 to include 1 green leafy or yellow[e]	4 to 5 to include 1 green leafy or yellow
Cooked	2 to 4 Tbsp.		
Raw	Few pieces		
Fruit		1 citrus fruit or other vegetable or fruit rich in vitamin C	1 citrus fruit or other vegetable or fruit rich in vitamin C
Canned	4 to 8 Tbsp.		
Raw	1/2 to 1 small		
Fruit juice	3 to 4 oz.		
Bread and cereal grains			
Whole grain or enriched white bread	1/2 to 1 slice	3	3
Cooked cereal	1/4 to 1/2 cup	May be substituted for one serving of bread	
Ready-to-serve dry cereals	1/2 to 1 cup		
Spaghetti, macaroni, noodles, rice	1/4 to 1/2 cup		
Crackers	2 to 3		
Fat			
Bacon	1 slice	Not to be substituted for meat	
Butter or vitamin A–fortified margarine	1 tsp.	3	3 to 4
Desserts	1/4 to 1/2 cup	As demanded by calorie needs	
Sugars	1/2 to 1 tsp.	2	2

From Pipes, PL: *Nutrition in Infancy and Childhood.* St. Louis, The C. V. Mosby Co, 1977, with permission.
[a]Diets should be monitored for adequacy of iron and vitamin D intake.
[b]Approximately 2/3 cup can easily be incorporated in a child's food during cooking.
[c]Liver once a week can be used as liver sausage or cooked liver.
[d]Should be served once or twice per week to substitute for meat.
[e]If child's preferences are limited, use double portions of preferred vegetables until appetite for other vegetables develops.

foods that are disliked may eventually result in their acceptance. Strong-flavored vegetables (overcooked cabbage and onions) are generally disliked. Crisp, raw vegetables are well accepted. Tough stringy fibers, such as those in celery or string beans, should be removed. Since these children still enjoy eating with their fingers, cutting fruits and vegetables into small pieces will increase their acceptance. They generally prefer their foods separate; casseroles and stews are not well liked. Foods that can be easily chewed are more readily accepted.

Food jags are common among this age group; they may refuse to eat anything except one food at each meal. This may be a way for the child to assert his/her new independence. This typical developmental stage is temporary. While a child cannot be forced to eat, the parent should maintain control by determining what foods are offered. A variety of foods should be available. Refusing to eat is a way to attract attention. The food obsession may cause parental concern, but overreaction may prolong rather than correct such behaviors. Food should not be used as a bribe or reward.

At times during this period, growth is slow and appetite decreases. Parents can be assured that this is normal and should not force the child to eat when s/he is not hungry.

Children should not be made to clean their plates. If sufficient amounts are not eaten, the parent may limit snacking or should be certain that the snacks are nutrient-dense. This is a critical period during which lifelong food habits are forming; good habits established at this time will affect to some extent the individual's health throughout life. Table 16–11 offers a food pattern for preschool children.

School-Age Children (7 to 12 Years Old)

During the school years, growth is slow and steady; food intake gradually increases while the energy needs per unit of body weight decline. These middle childhood years are the result of early growth and development; reserves are laid down for upcoming rapid adolescent growth. New activities and new friends begin to influence choices and broaden one's horizons. S/He will be exposed to different foods and food patterns. These new ideas may have an effect on food choices at home.

While food preferences are established early, children begin to accept more foods. Almost all foods are liked; vegetables are the least favorite of the food groups. Planning menus around the food groups is important to include all the necessary nutrients. While accessory foods containing mostly sugars or fats are not eliminated, they should not replace essential items of the diet.

The appetite is usually good; but food habits and intake may suffer because the children do not like to take time for meals. It may be wise to require that the child spend a specific amount of time at the table (15 to 20 minutes) to prevent the child from forming the habit of gulping down food. Additionally, the appetite may be adversely affected by stresses, such as schoolwork and emotional difficulties.

Good manners can and should be learned at this age; however, punishment or continuous correction at the table is not appropriate. Good manners are learned by the child imitating adults. While manners should not be overemphasized, family mealtime is when children will learn from the parents.

Students are ravenous after school. Although bakery products, soft drinks, candy, and chips are favorites, nutritious food should be available at home.

At this stage of life, it is also important for children to form good exercise habits. Many children are driven to school and may watch television for several hours in the afternoon and evening with no physical exercise other than that obtained in the physical education course. Sports interests should be cultivated while the child is young. Although team sports are important, activities that rely more on individual participation such as swimming can be maintained throughout life. Even at this early age, weight control is a balance between physical activity and food intake. Good habits need to be cultivated early in life.

Adolescents

It is not surprising that nutritional deficiencies are more prevalent among adolescents than any other age group; rapid growth rates and maturation changes cause them to be particularly susceptible (Bailey et al, 1984). Adolescent boys have greater nutritional needs than adolescent girls because of the rates of growth and changes in body composition (Mahan & Rees, 1984). A 15-year-old boy requires 3000 kcal, as compared to 2100 kcal for a 15-year-old girl. Research shows that teenagers have poor diets that are likely to be deficient in calcium and vitamin C. Six out of ten girls eat only two thirds of the nutrients required. Girls tend to have diets also deficient in the recommended amounts of iron, and boys are more likely to lack thiamin as well.

PEAK GROWTH

A girl's peak growth usually occurs between 10¼ and 13½ years of age; for boys, growth spurts occur between 11¾ and 14½ years of age. Energy needs of boys 11 to 14 years old will exceed those of girls by 500 kcal, although height and weight are similar and the growth rates even higher in girls. Sufficient zinc intake is critical to growth and sexual development of adolescent boys; adolescent girls apparently can develop normally with lower levels as their dietary intakes are frequently below the recommended level (Thompson et al, 1986). Energy needs are highest (2100 to 3900 kcal) in boys 15 to 18 years old when growth in muscle mass is greatest. Appendices C–6c and C–6d show physical growth of girls and boys from 2 to 18 years of age.

INFLUENTIAL FACTORS ON EATING HABITS OF ADOLESCENTS

Several mental, psychological, psychosocial, and physiological changes add strain to the adolescent's growth period.

Peer Pressure. Probably the strongest influential factor among teenagers is peer pressure. Not only are food choices affected, but the times available to eat may be determined by group activities.

Stress may be defined as physical, mental, or emotional strain or tension. Most adolescents have stress in their lives because of continual changes. Sexuality, body image, scholastic and athletic pressures, relationships with friends and relatives, finances, career plans, and ideological beliefs may cause conflicts as the adolescent tries to understand his/her identity.

Lack of sleep can push the limits of the teenager emotionally and physically. The presence of stress can decrease the utilization of several nutrients, particularly vitamin C and calcium.

Reduction Diets. Adolescents are eager to try fad diets, and girls are often obsessed about being thin. This is unfortunate because the nutrients during this period are necessary to build the basic strength of their bodies to last a lifetime.

Obesity, anorexia nervosa, and bulimia are serious health concerns amenable to early treatment. Guidelines for preventing these problems are discussed in Chapter 24. Prevention may be the only successful treatment in some cases.

Snacks and Fast Foods. Adolescents frequently have excessive intakes of sodium, sugar, and fat. For the teenage boy, these high-calorie foods may be useful, but for the teenage girl, a typical fast-food meal of 900 to 1300 kcal may be too much for her day's allowance. These snacks do, however, offer significant nutrients and can be improved with the substitution of a shake for a cola, or by adding orange juice. The nutrient value of fast foods may be seen in Appendix A–3.

Teenagers frequently substitute soft drinks for milk at meals as well as for snacks. This may contribute to their low intakes of certain nutrients that are already below the RDA, e.g., calcium and riboflavin (Guenther, 1986).

Education. Probably the best tactic for nutrition education among adolescents is to appeal to their physical image or their muscular development for sports. The earlier information is presented, the more likely it is to be accepted and used later by teenagers.

Parental Guidance

Parents play a role in influencing the eating behavior of children of all ages. When parents are authoritarian and rigid, refusal of food may be used to express rebellion. Ill feelings between the parents and children may be reflected by poor food intake. However this does not mean that a laissez-faire approach is appropriate. Parents can stock the kitchen with nutritious snack foods, e.g., cooked meats, raw vegetables, milk, cheese, fruit, nuts, peanut butter, raisins, and popcorn, to encourage good eating habits. Additionally, parents can support nutrition education curriculum in the school.

Parents cannot effectively tell their children to eat a certain way or a particular food when they are not practicing their own advice. They may not place enough importance upon having the whole family eat together. When they do eat together, the television may be on most of the time, blocking interpersonal relationships and preventing a relaxed, friendly atmosphere.

Breakfast

The meal most likely to be skipped by all school-age children is breakfast. Usually, the main reason is lack of time. However, waking children earlier and preparing or providing breakfast can improve the chances of their eating it. The morning meal may help to improve attitude, increase work output, and result in a better attention span. Children omitting breakfast are more likely to be careless and listless in the late morning hours. Breakfasts are offered by some schools.

The federal school breakfast program requires three food components to provide children with a good start toward meeting their daily nutritional needs. Each breakfast must contain at a *minimum*:
1. *Milk*—½ pint pasteurized fluid, whole, skim, low-fat milk or cultured buttermilk served as a beverage or on cereal.
2. *Vegetables and fruits*—½ cup of fruit or vegetables or ½ cup of full-strength fruit or vegetable juice.
3. *Bread or cereal*—a serving of bread or ¾ cup (or 1 oz.) of cereal, or an equivalent combination. (The variation in serving size for cereal allows for a smaller serving of the high-density granola-type cereals.)

To help children meet nutritional needs, breakfast should also contain as often as possible a meat or meat alternate—1 oz. (edible portion as served) of meat, poultry, or fish; or 1 oz. of cheese, or 1 egg, or 2 Tbsp. of peanut butter; or an equivalent amount of any combination of these foods.

Breakfast should furnish at least a quarter to a third of the nutrients for the day. In general, fruits and vegetables are most often the factors limiting optimal dietary intake of children, with many having no sources of vitamin A or C during the day (Caliendo et al, 1977). Since a fruit source high in vitamin C at breakfast is the easiest, surest protection of this nutrient, eating breakfast is especially significant.

As children reach adolescence, meal skipping becomes more frequent for all meals, with girls skipping meals more often than boys. Girls who scored high on personal adjustment, emotional stability, family relations, and conformity missed fewer meals and had better diets than other girls (Mahan & Rees, 1984).

School Lunch

The child's lunch may be provided by the school or brought from home. The federal government requires its school lunch program to provide approximately one third of the RDAs for children. New, different, and disliked foods are introduced to the child in a setting where the child is anxious to conform. Free or reduced-price meals are available for low-income families.

Many changes have been implemented in the school lunch program in recent years. Popular items, such as pizza or burritos, may appear on the menu; skim or low-fat milk or cultured buttermilk must be offered; whole milk may be offered; fresh fruits are provided rather than desserts such as cake (Table 16–12).

"Offer versus serve" was designed to reduce plate waste and food costs in the lunch program without sacrificing the nutritional integrity of the meals. It allows students to refuse one or two items that they do not intend to consume. In other words, of the five items on the menu, the student must take only three or four.

The school lunch program is usually more nutritious, not because it is a hot meal, but because box lunches generally contain less variety. Normally, only favorite foods are carried. They are also limited to foods that travel well and do not need heating or refrigeration.

A Healthy Diet

What constitutes a healthy and protective diet for all infants and children is of concern; however, there is considerable controversy surrounding this subject. The American Heart Association (Weidman et al, 1983), American Health Foundation (Berenson & Epstein, 1983), and National Institutes of Health (Consensus Development Panel, 1985) have recommended dietary changes that are in line with the dietary goals for the United States for all persons over the age of two. (The major thrust is to limit dietary fats to 30 percent of total calories, rather than the current 40 percent). These groups feel that atherosclerosis begins in childhood and that a reduction of fats and cholesterol in the diet will decrease the risk of this disease.

The American Academy of Pediatrics' Committee on Nutrition states that these dietary restrictions have not proved "effective in lowering serum cholesterol levels during the first two decades of life" and that they will not "adequately support growth and development, especially during the adolescent growth spurt" (AAP, 1986). Therefore, this committee recommends a more moderate amount of fat—30 to 40 percent of total energy intake. Diets restricted in fat and cholesterol usually reduce the intake of red meat and milk, both of which are major sources of protein, iron, calcium, and other minerals necessary for growth. The best assurance of nutritional adequacy is a varied diet that includes all of the food groups. The committee also cautions against parents who go to extremes in adopting a dietary restriction, endangering the health of the child. Children under two years of age who are at risk because of family history should be screened by at least two serum cholesterol measurements. Diet and/or medication should be initiated if appropriate.

The AAP Committee on Nutrition has endorsed a prudent lifestyle that includes other factors that affect blood lipids. Early detection of obesity and hypertension is advocated; counseling for the maintenance of ideal body weight and regular physical exercise should be a routine part of all health check-ups. Smoking should be avoided.

Table 16–12. School Lunch Patterns for Various Age/Grade Group

COMPONENTS	Preschool ages 1-2 (Group I)	Preschool ages 3-4 (Group II)	Grades K-3 ages 5-8 (Group III)	Grades 4-12 age 9 & over (Group IV)	RECOMMENDED QUANTITIES[2] Grades 7-12 age 12 & over (Group V)	SPECIFIC REQUIREMENTS
MEAT OR MEAT ALTERNATE — A serving of one of the following or a combination to give an equivalent quantity:						• Must be served in the main dish or the main dish and one other menu item. • **Vegetable protein products, cheese alternate** products, and enriched macaroni with fortified protein may be used to meet part of the meat/meat alternate requirement. Fact sheets on each of these alternate foods give detailed instructions for use.
Lean meat, poultry, or fish (edible portion as served)	1 oz	1½ oz	1½ oz	2 oz	3 oz	
Cheese	1 oz	1½ oz	1½ oz	2 oz	3 oz	
Large egg(s)	½	¾	¾	1	1½	
Cooked dry beans or peas	¼ cup	3/8 cup	3/8 cup	½ cup	¾ cup	
Peanut butter	2 Tbsp	3 Tbsp	3 Tbsp	4 Tbsp	6 Tbsp	
VEGETABLE AND/OR FRUIT — Two or more servings of vegetable or fruit or both to total	½ cup	½ cup	½ cup	¾ cup	¾ cup	• No more than one-half of the total requirement may be met with full-strength fruit or vegetable juice. • Cooked dry beans or peas may be used as a meat alternate or as a vegetable but not as both in the same meal.
BREAD OR BREAD ALTERNATE — Servings of bread or bread alternate A serving is: • 1 slice of whole-grain or enriched bread • A whole-grain or enriched biscuit, roll, muffin, etc. • ½ cup of cooked whole-grain or enriched rice, macaroni, noodles, whole-grain or enriched pasta products, or other cereal grains such as bulgur or corn grits • A combination of any of the above	5 per week	8 per week	8 per week	8 per week	10 per week	• At least ½ serving of bread or an equivalent quantity of bread alternate for Group I, and 1 serving for Groups II-V, must be served daily. • Enriched macaroni with fortified protein may be used as a meat alternate or as a bread alternate but not as both in the same meal. NOTE: *Food Buying Guide for Child Nutrition Programs*, PA-1331 (1983) provides the information for the minimum weight of a serving.
MILK — A serving of fluid milk	¾ cup (6 fl oz)	¾ cup (6 fl oz)	½ pint (8 fl oz)	½ pint (8 fl oz)	½ pint (8 fl oz)	At least one of the following forms of milk must be offered: • Unflavored lowfat milk • Unflavored skim milk • Unflavored buttermilk NOTE: This requirement does not prohibit offering other milks, such as whole milk or flavored milk, along with one or more of the above.

U.S. Department of Agriculture, National School Lunch Program

USDA recommends, but does not require, that you adjust portions by age/grade group to better meet the food and nutritional needs of children according to their ages. If you adjust portions, Groups I-IV are minimum requirements for the ages/grade groups specified. If you do not adjust portions, the Group IV portions are the portions to serve all children.

[1] Group IV is highlighted because it is the one meal pattern which will satisfy all requirements if no portion size adjustments are made.

[2] Group V specifies recommended, not required, quantities for students 12 years and older. These students may request smaller portions, but not smaller than those specified in Group IV.

Dental Caries

Since tooth formations begin before birth and are not completed until about 12 years of age, the actual structure of the tooth is affected by food intake. Poorly developed teeth are more susceptible to decay later in life. A clear relationship has been shown in several studies between nutritional deficiency during tooth development and tooth size, tooth formation, time of tooth eruption, and susceptibility to caries. Calcium with vitamin D must be present to form normal teeth. Both are essential for proper calcification of the dentin and normal enamel. Vitamin D is critical to tooth development; later deficiency can promote tooth decay.

Teeth are more dense and hard when one part fluoride per million parts of drinking water is added during their formation. Excessive fluoride in water can cause permanent mottling of teeth. A 60 percent reduction of caries is gained by using fluoridated water during earlier growth periods. The topical administration of fluoride to teeth can result in about 20 percent reduction in tooth decay.

Sealants are a new method that act as a barrier protecting the decay-prone areas of the teeth from plaque and acid. It is a clear or shaded plastic material that is applied to the biting or chewing surfaces of permanent teeth.

Food selection and patterns of consumption influence dental health. Use of a toothbrush with dental floss, fluoride toothpaste, and sealants cannot completely control caries formation. Not only do foods influence tooth development, but they influence cariogenicity by the sucrose content, physical properties, and the frequency of consumption (see Chapter 7).

Hyperactivity

Attention deficit disorder (ADD) is the latest term for hyperkinetic behavior syndrome (HBS), hyperactivity, learning disabilities, or minimal brain dysfunction. This condition refers to an elevated activity level with deviations from the normal behavior patterns in children. These children are usually inattentive, impulsive, hasty, emotionally bland, and defensive with social ineptness.

The late Dr. Benjamin Feingold, a pediatrician and allergist at Kaiser Medical Center in San Francisco, suggested a diet for ADD that is still used by an estimated 200,000 American children under the guidance of 100 self-help groups, even though it is unsubstantiated and the very concept of hyperactivity, or hyperkinesis, remains poorly defined (Hadley, 1984).

The Feingold Diet eliminates two groups of foods: Group 1 consists of almonds, cucumbers, tomatoes, berries, apples, oranges, and several other fruits having high levels of naturally occurring salicylates. Group 2 includes foods that contain artificial colors and flavors (most are perceived by the public as processed). This category includes additives and is largely selected on the basis of ingredient labeling and standards of food identity. With the exception of butylated hydroxytoluene (BHT), foods containing preservatives are not excluded from the original Feingold diet. Commercially prepared desserts and other foods that have high amounts of sucrose are usually not allowed because they contain artificial colors or flavors, even though no restrictions are placed on homemade sweets (Consensus Development Conference, 1982).

Since the diet excludes many fruits, nutritional intake may be compromised, especially for vitamin C. Several studies that tested the effectiveness of the diet have concluded that it may reduce hyperactive behavior in approximately 10 percent of the children (Swanson & Kinsbourne, 1980; Weiss et al, 1980).

The National Advisory Committee on Hyperkinesis and Food Additives (1980) reviewed a number of carefully controlled double-blind studies and reported no consistent dramatic change in behavior of hyperactive children. The children followed a diet that eliminated artificial food colorings and then underwent challenge testing with them.

However, many children have been treated with highly favorable results. A major influential factor is probably the mandatory rule for the entire family to assume the same diet. Changing the child's status in a family by letting him/her become the dominant family member who determines what everyone else eats is an extremely influential factor (Lipton & Mayo, 1983). More attention is focused on the child when the diet is used. Additionally, all family members have high expectations, which may influence the results.

Clinical Implications:

- The main responsibility for the dietitian, physician, and other paraprofessionals involved

with the patient is to be sure that a well-bal-anced diet is eaten to meet the RDAs even though it may be an additive-free diet.
- Treatment on the basis of a placebo effect can be harmful if it prevents a child from re-ceiving appropriate medical or psychiatric treatment.

Lead Toxicity

Children are more susceptible to lead than adults. The goal set for 1990 is a lead toxicity of less than 500 cases per 100,000 children up to five years old (Neggers & Stitt, 1986).

To decrease lead toxicity, several preventive measures should be implemented. Canned milk products are a major source of lead in the diets of infants and children; changing from cans to jars has reduced the lead contamination from fruits and juices. Lead is also ingested from toddlers' normal hand-to-mouth activities; in older children, playing with dirt or lead-contaminated objects may result in lead ingestion (Neggers & Stitt, 1986).

Screening for lead toxicity can prevent irreversible physiological damage and fatality. A careful dietary analysis that includes an assessment of pica habits and living environments can also be used to detect lead poisoning. Early symptoms of lead ingestion are nonspecific: vomiting, irritability, weight loss, general malaise, headache, and insomnia. As a result, the correct diagnosis of lead poisoning is easily overlooked.

As the lead levels increase, general cognitive, verbal, and perceptual abilities decrease learning aptitudes. Although good nutrition is not a cure for lead poisoning, deficiencies in calcium, iron, zinc, protein, and fat enhance lead toxicity (Neggers & Stitt, 1986). Calcium competes with lead absorption; a diet high in calcium is recommended. Zinc and iron also decrease lead absorption (Mahaffey, 1981).

Illness

Children who are ill at home or in the hospital require special treatment to meet their nutri-tional needs while their appetite is poor. A temporary decrease in food intake during short periods of illness does not pose any major problem. Parents need not try to force food during this time. Children with chronic or very severe illnesses or injuries must be watched more closely.

Dehydration can occur very rapidly in young children and babies when body fluids are lost and not adequately replaced (fever, vomiting, and diarrhea). In order to insure against dehydration, offer the child small amounts of favorite beverages at least hourly, expecting him/her to take some. Water or carbonated beverages may be given. Beverages sweetened with sugar, rather than artificially, are preferred because they offer some calories as well as fluid. Foods that have a high water content, e.g., congealed gelatin, Popsicles, sherbet, should be offered frequently.

A hospitalized child who understands some of the conditions and problems may be more co-operative; understanding the environment will ease the fears and frustrations and make it seem more familiar. Most of all, the presence of a parent is of utmost importance to help allay fears. While food intake is to be encouraged, too much coaxing and attention will cause the child to rebel and become manipulative.

Plain foods low in fat and delicately seasoned are better tolerated and have more appeal to the sick child. Frequent small meals, rather than three larger ones, will also increase intake.

The environment is important to encourage the sick child to eat. Colorful and cleverly designed straws, napkins, and plates can induce children to eat. Food intake can also be increased by socialization during the meal. Children who are hospitalized should be allowed to eat together. If not, someone should sit and talk with the child during mealtime. Including the parents in planning the care and having them readily available to encourage the child help provide security and support.

Clinical Implications:
- Involve the child (if old enough) in charting his/her fluid intake.
- To promote food intake during a hospital stay, determine foods the child likes and dislikes and his/her normal habits so that favorite foods can be served. A bit of pampering is appreciated by the child, and favorite foods can help spur the desire to eat.

• FALLACIES and FACTS

FALLACY: *Infant foods should be tasted by the adult to see if they are flavorful.*
• **FACT:** *Adults prefer more seasoning in their foods, but infants do not appreciate them. Most health professionals feel that seasonings, especially salt, should be omitted from infant foods until after the first year of life (Yeung et al, 1982). The amount of salt intake in adulthood seems to be associated with salt intake in early childhood.*

FALLACY: *Orange juice is the first fruit juice to offer an infant.*
• **FACT:** *On the contrary, orange juice is one of the last fruit juices offered. It is not recommended because of its high frequency of allergies. The main advantage is its vitamin C content. Mother's milk and commercial formulas contain sufficient ascorbic acid to prevent scurvy.*

FALLACY: *Goat's milk should be given to babies who are allergic.*
• **FACT:** *Goat's milk has been promoted by health food advocates; however, its alleged nutritional and medical superiority has not been scientifically documented. The solute load of goat's milk is high as well as the content of sodium, potassium, and protein. It is deficient in iron; vitamins C, D, and B_{12}; and folic acid; it should be avoided (Taitz & Armitage, 1984; Sawaya et al, 1984). Hypoallergenic formulas are more appropriate for the allergic infant.*

FALLACY: *Food should be withheld from an infant with diarrhea to allow the digestive tract to rest.*
• **FACT:** *This is an old-fashioned idea. Diarrhea may quickly result in serious electrolyte imbalances, so fluids are critical to the infant. Intestinal damage is compounded by a caloric deficiency, leading to a decline in protein stores as catabolism begins (Self, 1986). A recent study concluded that a soy-based, lactose-free formula for infants with acute diarrheal illness is safe and effective and results in more reduction of stool volume and a shorter duration of the illness as compared to "gut rest" (San-*

tosham et al, 1985). Nutrients must be continued as soon as tolerated.

FALLACY: *Cereal should be introduced at six weeks of age.*
• **FACT:** *The digestion of cereal will not be complete because the ability to fully absorb starch is usually undeveloped until four months of age. If iron supplementation is the goal, drops can be given (Kreiger, 1982).*

FALLACY: *Cereal before bedtime will help an infant sleep through the night.*
• **FACT:** *Cereals do not satisfy the infant any more than formula or breast milk. Actually, the caloric content of cereal is less than that of formula. Feeding as late as possible will be useful.*

FALLACY: *Vitamin E should not be used for premature infants to prevent potential blindness because several deaths have occurred from the use of an intravenous form of this vitamin.*
• **FACT:** *The retinopathy of prematurity (ROP), or the blindness common to premature babies, can be delayed to allow time for preventive treatment or can be avoided completely when the correct amounts of vitamin E are given; the vitamin E form that resulted in deaths was one that had not been approved by the FDA. When this particular form was used, the amount was incorrectly estimated to be similar to the other.*

Summary

From infancy to adolescence, adequate nutrition is essential to support the rapid growth and development during the different stages of life. The nutritional needs of infants are best met by breast milk; however, formula feedings simulate breast milk and are suitable alternatives. They offer different advantages to the mother. For the first four to six months of life, no other foods are necessary. After that time, pureed foods are introduced one at a time. As the infant's neuromuscular system matures and teeth erupt, foods that require chewing are given. Eventually, children are able to feed themselves and to choose what they want to eat.

Growth by height and weight are key techniques to evaluate the health status of children. Nutrient intake influences the physical, emotional, and mental abilities of each individual.

Nutrient needs for all stages of growth can be met by providing a well-balanced diet based on all the food groups. Different amounts of foods are required for each stage. Habits are formed early and are likely to affect eating patterns throughout life. These habits are principally determined by parental influences. Adolescents require a high food intake for skeletal and muscular maturation; failure to meet these requirements will affect future health.

Regardless of the growth rate or state of health, the critical need for nutritional education is constantly present. All health care professionals can help teach good practices for optimal nutrition.

Review Questions

1. Plan meals for a family for one day with a two-year-old toddler, a 10-year-old boy, and a 15-year-old girl who is trying to reduce.
2. What is the treatment for an infant with diarrhea?
3. What are the differences between low birth weight and small for gestational age infants, and how do these differences affect their food intake?
4. Discuss feeding a newborn infant from birth to age one.
5. What is beikost?
6. What is considered normal weight for a newborn infant? How much should it be expected to gain during the first year of life?

Case Study: Shanna P. is a 13-year-old who was brought to the physician's office for a yearly physical examination. Her weight at this time is 90.7 kg and height is 174.8 cm.

Questions by the nurse indicate that Shanna has always been overweight but has gained approximately 25 lbs. since starting junior high school. She is a finicky eater and refuses many meat and vegetable dishes. She does not exercise except in physical education class and spends most of her time at home watching television. All lab work was normal, but elevated blood pressure (130/88) was noted.

Exogenous obesity with hypertension is diagnosed, and the patient and her family are referred for dietary counseling.
1. Why are the early adolescent years so important for weight?
2. At what other times in the life cycle is excess weight a particular problem?

3. What factors have prompted the development of this child's obesity?
4. What should she weigh?
5. What tentative nursing diagnoses could you develop?
6. List goals for this patient.
7. In your nursing care plan, develop a diet plan for Shanna.

Case Study: Jennifer C. is brought to the physician's office for a six-month checkup. She weighed 3.2 kg at birth and now weighs 6.9 kg. She was bottle-fed from birth. At three months, she was started on cereals but has resisted all attempts to increase her solid food intake. She is allowed to go to sleep with a bottle and is often propped up in her crib with a bottle at the day-care center.

1. What additional assessment data would you need?
2. Is Jennifer's weight gain within the expected range?
3. How much should she gain in the next six months?
4. What tentative nursing diagnosis could you derive?
5. The nurse encourages Jennifer's mother to discontinue the habit of allowing her to go to sleep with a bottle and to request that the day-care center do the same. Why?
6. The physician recommends that solid foods be introduced gradually to Jennifer. What foods should be introduced first?
7. Should Jennifer's mother decide to prepare the food at home, what procedures should she use?
8. When will Jennifer be old enough for finger foods?
9. Why should egg whites be withheld until one year of age?
10. Explain nursing bottle syndrome.

REFERENCE LIST

American Academy of Pediatrics (AAP) Committee on Nutrition: Prudent life-style for children: Dietary fat and cholesterol. *Pediatrics* 78(3):521, 1986.

American Academy of Pediatrics (AAP) Committee on Nutrition: Nutritional needs of low-birth-weight infants. *Pediatrics* 60(10):519, 1977.

American Academy of Pediatrics (AAP) Committee on Nutrition: Commentary on breastfeeding and infant formulas. *Pediatrics* 57(2):278, 1976.

Applebaum, RM: Management of lactation problems. In *Symposium on Human Lactation*. Edited by LR Waletzky. Rockville, MD, U.S. Dept. of Health, Education and Welfare, 1976.

Bailey, LB; Wagner, PA; Davis, CG; et al: Food frequency related to folacin status in adolescents. *J Am Diet Assoc* 84(7):801, 1984.

Berenson, GS; Epstein, FH; et al: Summary and recommendations of the conference on blood lipids in children: Optimal levels for early prevention of coronary artery disease. *Prev Med* 12(6):738, 1983.

Birch, LL: Preschool children's food preferences and consumption patterns. *J Nutr Ed* 11(4):189, 1979.

Brown, JE: Nutrition services for pregnant women, infants, children and adolescents. *Clinical Nutr* 3(3):100, 1984.

Caliendo, MA; Sanjur, D; Wright, J; et al: Nutritional status of preschool children. *J Am Diet Assoc* 71(1):20, 1977.

Consensus Development Conference: Defined diets and child-hood hyperactivity. *JAMA* 248(3):290, 1982.

Consensus Development Panel: Lowering blood cholesterol to prevent heart disease. *JAMA* 253(14):2080, 1985.

Endres, JB; Rockwell, RE: *Food, Nutrition, and the Young Child.* St. Louis, C. V. Mosby Co, 1980.

Foman, SJ: Breast-feeding and evolution. *J Am Diet Assoc* 86(3):317, 1986.

Foman, SJ: *Infant Nutrition,* 2nd ed. Philadelphia, W. B. Saunders Co, 1974.

Gellis, SS; Kagan, BM: *Current Pediatric Therapy 10.* Philadelphia, W. B. Saunders Co, 1982.

Graham, GG; Morales, E; Placko, RP; et al: Nutritive value of brown and black beans for infants and small children. *Am J Clin Nutr* 32(11):2362, 1979.

Guenther, PM: Beverages in the diets of American teenagers. *J Am Diet Assoc* 86(4):493, 1986.

Hadley, J: Facts about childhood hyperactivity. *Children Today* 13(January-February):8, 1984.

Harris, CS; Baker, SP; Smith, GA; Harris, RM: Childhood asphyxiation by food. *JAMA* 251(17):2231, 1984.

Helsing, E; King, FS: *Breast-Feeding in Practice.* Oxford, Oxford University Press, 1982.

Hertzler, AA: Children's food patterns. A Review: I. Food preferences and feeding problems. *J Am Diet Assoc* 83(5):551, 1983.

Hyams, JS; Leichtner, AM: Apple juice an unappreciated cause of chronic diarrhea. *Am J Dis Child* 139(5):503, 1985.

Kreiger, I: *Pediatric Disorders of Feeding, Nutrition and Metabolism.* New York, John Wiley & Sons, 1982.

Lawrence, RA: *Breast-Feeding, A Guide for the Medical Profession.* St. Louis, C. V. Mosby Co, 1980.

Lipin, R: Outbreak of diarrhea linked to dietetic candies—New Hampshire. *JAMA* 252(13):1672, 1984.

Lipton, MA; Mayo, JP: Diet and hyperkinesis—an update. *J Am Diet Assoc* 83(8):132, 1983.

MacKeith, R; Wood, CBS: *Infant Feeding and Feeding Difficulties.* London, Churchill Livingstone, 1977.

Mahaffey, KR: Nutritional factors in lead poisoning. *Nutr Rev* 39(10):353, 1981.

Mahan, LK; Rees, JM: *Nutrition in Adolescence.* St. Louis, C. V. Mosby Co, 1984.

Martinez, GA; Dodd, DA: Milk feeding patterns in the U.S. during the first 12 months of life. *Pediatrics* 71(2):166, 1983.

Matsukubo, T: Cariogenic potential index and classification of foodstuffs using in vitro assessment. *J Dent Res Program and Abstracts* 61(1079):298, 1982.

National Advisory Committee on Hyperkinesis and Food Additives: *Final Report to the Nutrition Foundation.* New York, Nutrition Foundation, 1980.

Neggers, YH; Stitt, KR: Effects of high lead intake in children. *J Am Diet Assoc* 86(7):938, 1986.

Pemberton, CM; Gastineau, CF (eds): *Mayo Clinic Diet Manual,* 5th ed. Philadelphia, W. B Saunders Co, 1981.

Peterson, KE; Washington, J; Rathbun, JM: Team management of failure to thrive. *J Am Diet Assoc* 84(7):810, 1984.

Pipes, PL: *Nutrition in Infancy and Childhood.* St Louis: The C. V. Mosby Co, 1986.

Public Health Service: *Promoting Health, Preventing Disease: Objectives for the Nation.* Washington, DC, U.S. Dept. of Health and Human Services, 1980.

Santosham, M; Foster, J; Reed, R; et al: Role of soy-based lactose-free formula during treatment of acute diarrhea. *Pediatrics* 76(2):292, 1985.

Sawaya, WN; Khalil, JK; Al-Shalhat, AF: Mineral and vitamin content of goat's milk. *J Am Diet Assoc* 84(4):433, 1984.

Self, TW: Pitfalls of the "BRAT" diet. *Nutr and the MD* 12(4):1, 1986.

Swanson, JM; Kinsbourne, M: Food dyes impair performance of hyperactive children in a laboratory learning test. *Science* 207 (March 28):1485, 1980.

Sweeten, MK: *Fact Sheet: Nutrition and the Teen Scene.* College Station, TX, Texas Agricultural Extension Services, Texas A & M University System, 1978.

Taitz, LS; Armitage, BL: Goat's milk for infants and children. *Br Med J* 288(Jan 28):428, 1984.

Thompson, P; Roseborough, R; Russek, E; et al: Zinc status and sexual development in adolescent girls. *J Am Diet Assoc* 86(7):892, 1986.

Weidman, W; Kwiterovich, P; Jesse, MJ: Diet in the healthy child. *Circulation* 67(6):1411A, 1983.

Weiss, B; Williams, JH; Margen, S; et al: Behavioral responses to artificial food colors. *Science* 207(March 28):1487, 1980.

White-Graves, MV; Schiller, MR: History of foods in the caries process. *J Am Diet Assoc* 86(2):241, 1986.

Wink, D: Getting through the maze of infant formulas. *Am J Nurs* 85(4):388, 1985.

Wolraich, ML; Stumbo, PJ; Milch, R; et al: Dietary characteristics of hyperactive and control boys. *J Am Diet Assoc* 86(4):500, 1986.

Yeung, DL: Infant nutrition update. *J Can Diet Assoc* 45(1):20, 1984.

Yeung, DL; Hall, J; Leung, M; et al: Sodium intakes of infants from 1 to 18 months of age. *J Am Diet Assoc* 80(3):242, 1982.

Further Study

Ashbrook, S; Doyle, M: Infants' acceptance of strong- and mild-flavored vegetables. *J Nutr Ed* 17(2):1985.

Brown, JE: Nutrition services for pregnant women, infants, children and adolescents. *Clin Nutr* 3(3):100, 1984.

Canadian Pediatric Society Nutrition Committee: Infant feeding. *J Can Diet Assoc* 41(June):46, 1980.

Cheung, S: Issues in nutrition for the school-age athlete. *J School Health* 55(1):35, 1985.

George, DE: Chronic diarrhea in infants and children. *Am Fam Physician* 29(5):280, 1984.

Hadley, J: Facts about childhood hyperactivity. *Children Today* 13(July-August):8, 1984.

Ideas for counseling children on diet. *Diab Ed* 7(2):42, 1981.

Johnson, GH; Purvis, GA; Wallace, RD: What nutrients do our infants really get? *Nutr Today* 16(4):4, 1981.

Jones, DY; Nesheim, MC; Habicht, J-P: Influences in child growth associated with poverty in the 1970's: An examination of HANES I and HANES II, cross-sectional US national surveys. *Am J Clin Nutr* 42(4):714, 1985.

Morgan, BLG: Nutritional needs of the female adolescent. *Women Health* 9(2/3):15, 1984.

National Institute of Allergy and Infectious Diseases: *Defined Diets Bibliography.* Available from National Institutes of Health, Medical Applications of Research, Bldg. 1, Room 216, Bethesda, MD 20205.

Truswell, AS: Children and adolescents. *Br Med J* 291(Aug 10):397, 1985.

Van Swearingen, JM: Nutrition and the growing athlete. *J Orthop Sports Phys Ther* 6(3):173, 1984.

Maturity in the Life Span

17

THE STUDENT WILL BE ABLE TO:

- *List and describe factors that influence the food intake of the older person.*
- *Explain procedures for maintaining the individual's ego and self-integrity as dietary care is required.*
- *Discuss dietary changes that could be made to provide optimum nutrient intake.*
- *List potential dietary deficiencies that have symptoms similar to senility.*

Atrophy
Degeneration
Geriatric
Gerontology
Senescence
Senile
Senile purpura

OBJECTIVES

TERMS TO KNOW

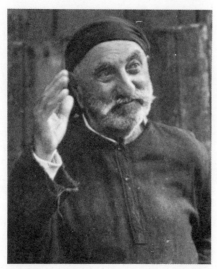

Figure 17–1. *The centenarians. (From* Nutrition Today *13(3): 8, 1978, by permission.)*

3. Their food intake is high in vegetables and milk products; sour milk and low-fat cheese are the main source for protein. Tea and small amounts of homemade wines are the principal beverages.
4. And, last of all, they exaggerate their age. These elderly people have discovered that more respect is accorded them if they start overstating their age after about their seventieth birthday (Enloe, 1978).

Another paradise lost? No, even though these people are not supercentenarians, a second look clearly shows an active mental and physical population seldom seen in the United States (Fig. 17–1). Their program of work, rest, friends, and diet could be used as a suitable model.

What are the problems of aging and what can be done to improve this period of life? Aging is not merely the passing of years, but also the accumulation of mental, physical, spiritual, and social changes.

Remarkably old people have been reported living in Pakistan, Russia, and Ecuador high in the mountains. Their extraordinary health, high spirits, and wonderfully full and productive lives have been envied. After several visits with these people, Leaf (1975) noted some similarities:
1. Throughout their lives, these people are constantly busy with heavy work such as farming or household chores as well as walking the steep mountain slopes.
2. These older people have a pattern of resting more than usual—10 hours per night plus afternoon naps. Pleasant relaxation before bedtime involves their friends and families.

LIFE SPAN

Can nutrition add longevity to life? Certainly, it can reduce the severity of signs and symptoms of a variety of conditions that cause metabolic problems. In this way, it may enhance the quality of life and increase longevity within the individual's biologically determined life span.

Senescence is the process of growing old; senile refers to the characteristics of being old. Whether the individual is a tottering oldster at 60, or a "youth" at 80, depends in large measure on past and present food intake. A sexagenarian may be frail, feeble, unsteady, easily fatigued, slow-

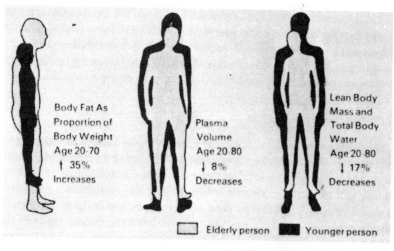

Figure 17–2. *Changes in the body with aging. (From Vestal RE:* Drugs and the Elderly *(1979). NIH Publication No. 79-1449, U.S. Department of Health, Education and Welfare, Washington, DC.)*

moving, short of breath, and dulled in sensibilities. All of these traits could be the result of poor nutrition and/or pathophysiological conditions. Their similarities and intermingling of borderline states make medical evaluations more complex. On the other hand, an octogenarian may display a surprising amount of stamina, stability, endurance, and alertness.

New terminology is based on the technical life span of man (TLS), which is 115 years (Watkin, 1982). The following terms are based on the proportion of the TLS survived:

> aged: 86 years and older
> elderly: 77 to 85 years old
> aging: 69 to 76 years old
> mature: 55 to 68 years old

Preventive nutrition for aging should begin, of course, before birth and continue throughout life. Good nutrition plays its most significant role during youth and middle age in the prevention of those diseases that ultimately manifest themselves as serious disabilities among the aged. Gerontology, the study of aging and problems of the aged, is distinct from geriatrics, the treatment of diseases in the aged. Today, a few clues exist for altering the process of aging by nutritional means.

Physiological Factors

A number of physiological changes (Fig. 17–2) may significantly influence nutritional requirements of the elderly person. Maximum efficiency for many organ systems occurs between 20 and 30 years of age with a gradual decline at different rates for various individuals (Harper, 1982).

BODY WEIGHT

Too much or too little food intake reduces longevity. People with a weight-to-height ratio in the highest or lowest 10 percent of the population have substantially more illness and less longevity than those in the middle 80 percent (Palmore, 1980). Obesity is an underlying cause of many pathological conditions.

COGNITIVE ABILITY

Past studies have shown that nursing home patients with severe nutritional deficiencies suffer a moderate-to-severe impairment in thinking and memory; nutritional supplements improve cogni-

tion. Protein, vitamin C, folic acid, niacin, pyridoxine, riboflavin, thiamin, and vitamin B_{12} are of particular importance for the ability to think and remember (Treichel, 1983).

GASTROINTESTINAL FUNCTION

Secretions of hydrochloric acid and digestive enzymes decrease with age. Hypochlorhydria may interfere with iron and vitamin B_{12} absorption, possibly resulting in anemia (Albanese, 1980). Still, only a small part of nutritional deficiency in the elderly can be attributed to the decline of their digestive functions (unless there are complications from illness, disease, or drugs), primarily because the digestive system is very adaptive (Rosenberg & Bowman, 1983). Chronic problems, such as constipation, hiatus hernia, or ulcer, may be aggravated by medications.

Motility of the intestinal tract and secretions of intestinal mucosa also decrease, causing problems with bowel movements. Practically all elderly individuals suffer from constipation and may have a long history of cathartic abuse or laxative use. Many institutions habitually offer laxatives rather than trying to correct the problem through dietary intake of fresh fruits and vegetables, prune juice, and fiber. Constipation is usually safely remedied by an increase in dietary fiber, such as brown rice, whole-wheat breads, and cereals. Wheat bran, if used, should be added gradually to the diet and fluid should be increased by at least six ounces per teaspoon of bran (Rozovski, 1983).

Persistent constipation may also be relieved by doubling the amount of fluid consumed (Rozovski, 1983). Encouraging exercise and increasing fluid intake, especially warm beverages upon waking in the morning, can help avoid constipation. When constipation, diarrhea, or urinary or fecal incontinence is a problem, the elderly person frequently becomes apprehensive about eating or drinking.

RENAL SYSTEM

Kidney function is reduced; renal plasma flow is decreased, sometimes by as much as 50 percent (Albanese, 1980). Fever, which in the healthy individual can lead to mild dehydration, can result in severe dehydration in individuals with impaired renal function from reduced reabsorption of water. A large intake of water can aid impaired renal functions by reducing the osmotic concentration of fluids being filtered by the kidney (Watkin, 1980).

BREATHING CAPACITY AND NEUROMUSCULAR ABILITIES

Maximal breathing capacity may be 40 percent and vital capacity 60 percent of normal values in the elderly (Tobin, 1975). Motor function (handgrip strength) also declines. Responses to environmental stimuli are slower with age (Masoro, 1976). Such normal physical changes may lead an older person to mistakingly believe s/he is "anemic" because of less endurance and strength.

SENSORY ORGANS

The visual, auditory, and olfactory sensory organs are impaired with age. In addition to the dulled senses of taste and smell, other factors, e.g., antihypertensive drugs, hypoglycemic agents, anti-Parkinson compounds, and other drugs, can alter taste perception (Schiffman, 1983). This explains why adults prefer their food more highly seasoned than younger persons. Renal failure also leads to deterioration of taste sensitivity (Kamath, 1982). When sugar and salt restrictions are necessary, alternative seasonings will enhance natural sweetness (allspice, cinnamon, cloves, ginger, and nutmeg). Other food flavors can provide added taste sensations (see Chapter 32 for alternatives to salt).

However, taste acuity is not solely responsible for food intake. Poor vision makes food preparation not only difficult but hazardous. Poor hearing increases isolation and decreases socialization. Other psychosocial, psychological, and physiological factors also cause food to be less well received.

MASTICATORY ABILITY

Generally, individuals who wear dentures have reduced masticatory efficiency, and those with seriously compromised natural dentition or ill-fitting dentures tend to alter their food choices to reduce chewing. Figure 17–3 compares improperly fitted dentures with correctly fitting ones in the same patient.

The logical sequence of eating food is biting,

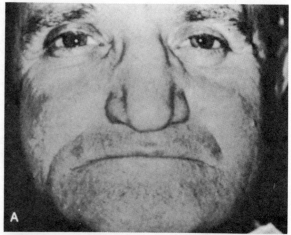

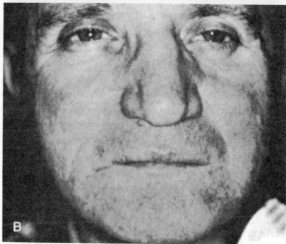

Figure 17–3. A) Geriatric patient wearing dentures with incorrect occlusal vertical dimension; note overclosure. B) Same patient with correct occlusal vertical dimension; note improvement in facial appearance. (From Nizel AE: Nutrition in Preventive Dentistry: Science and Practice, 2nd ed, Philadelphia, W. B. Saunders Co, 1980, by permission.)

chewing, and swallowing. New denture wearers should be encouraged to reverse this order—namely, they should learn to swallow a liquid diet with the dentures first, then chew soft foods, and last, bite regular foods (Nizel, 1981). Concentrating on one act at a time is easier and protects the mouth from becoming sore throughout.

Abnormalities in lip posture, masticatory muscle, tongue functions, and swallowing increase with age (Age, 1983). Masticatory efficiency changes food choices. Consumption of some meat and fresh fruits and vegetables usually decreases, which results in reduced energy, iron, and vitamin C intakes. Other problems may include increased gastrointestinal irritation and increased mortality from choking.

BASAL METABOLISM

The basal metabolic rate starts to diminish early in adulthood and continues to decline throughout life. Energy needs decline with age at about two percent per decade, due to decreases in the basal metabolic rate as well as physical activity. In older persons, the rate may be as much as 10 to 12 percent below the level of 20-year-olds (See Chapter 9). While a 55-year-old man may require 2400 kcal for his total energy needs, only 2050 kcal may be needed at age 76; a woman may need 1800 kcal at age 55 and only 1600 at age 76.

Nutrients

RDAs

Current RDAs provide guidelines for the nutrient requirements of two groups of adults, those 23 to 50 years old and those over 51. The RDAs for the over-51 group are largely based on extrapolation because most data regarding nutrient requirements have been based on young adults. Obviously, many differences (both physiologically and in health status) exist among people between the ages of 51 and 90. Dynamic changes (previously mentioned) during this period affect nutrient absorption, metabolism, and utilization. Additionally, many degenerative diseases and heavy drug use affect the availability of nutrients and requirements.

The RDAs are intended for healthy persons, not taking into consideration the frequent diseases and disorders that occur within this age group. Sugar and/or salt restrictions are not uncommon.

As the percentage of elderly in the population increases, the need for more nutrition information based on scientific data pertinent to this age group will become more valuable. While many nutrients are altered for the elderly, vitamin and mineral supplements are taken on the basis of irrational knowledge; some may be inappropriate to real needs.

ENERGY

Only energy requirements decrease with age; other nutrients are required in the same amounts throughout adulthood, and some may even be increased. Deliberate food choices must be carefully preplanned, or the nutrient needs are not met and unwanted weight is gained. More nutrient-dense foods are required to maintain optimum health. Energy and nutrient requirements for adults are listed on the endsheets.

PROTEIN

An intake of 12 percent or more of the energy needs should come from protein foods, or a minimum of 54 gm in an 1800 kcal diet (Matthews, 1983). The RDA is 0.8 gm/kg/day. There is some controversy over protein for older adults; some feel it should be increased to avoid negative nitrogen balance, and others believe it should be reduced (Lee, 1984; Gersovitz et al, 1982). With this in mind, the individual should be assessed and recommendations prescribed. Added stress from injury, gastrointestinal disease, or high drug usage increases catabolism, thereby increasing the level of dietary protein required to maintain nitrogen balance.

Chronic inadequate protein intake can result in hypoproteinemia, characterized by edema and muscular weakness and wasting. The overlapping of symptoms caused by aging, dietary deficiencies, and disease obviously complicates treatment of the elderly. Checking food intake becomes a basic priority and one that can alleviate unnecessary suffering.

One unusual finding is that elderly men require more than twice the amount of methionine and lysine needed for nitrogen equilibrium or retention than young adults (Watkin, 1980). Cereal grains (low in the essential amino acid lysine but adequate in methionine) are complemented by legumes having adequate lysine but little methionine.

The main reason the elderly consume less protein is lack of money to buy the best sources, i.e., red meat, fish, poultry, eggs, and milk. Protein from plant and animal sources should be combined to balance the amino acid content. Protein from leguminous plants (e.g., dry beans, dry peas, lentils, nuts, peanut butter, and soybean products) is of good quality, economical, and contains valuable nutrients; these may replace some animal source proteins but should be combined with complementary proteins, as discussed in Chapter 6.

Clinical Implications:

- For persons who have had strokes or have difficulty in swallowing, adequate protein intake requires specific planning and attention.
- Since the aged have impaired renal function, excessive protein intake should be avoided. Blood urea nitrogen levels normally regulated by renal filtration may increase dramatically if the rate of renal filtration is reduced, resulting in azotemia.
- Appropriate nutrition counseling can provide information on complete and incomplete sources of proteins to help people live within a limited budget.

CARBOHYDRATE

Carbohydrate foods are readily available and economical, need little preparation, and require less time and effort to eat in comparison to proteins and fats. Complex carbohydrates are needed for fiber and bulk and some are economical sources of incomplete protein. Fifty to 60 percent of a person's total kilocalories should be from carbohydrates.

FAT

An increase of carbohydrate intake is balanced by a decrease in fat intake for elderly individuals. About 20 to 30 percent of the energy requirement should come from fat. The benefits of fat, which are satiety and flavor, may be even more important with increases in age and possible restrictions such as sodium.

Dietary fat restriction is necessary if fat malabsorption occurs. Decreased fat absorption in the elderly has been related to reduced digestive capacity occurring with age and may also be a consequence of drug therapy, gastrointestinal surgery, or disease. In these cases, calories from readily absorbable fats can be provided by medium-chain triglycerides (MCT) that need no bile acid emulsification and minimal enzymes for digestion and absorption.

ELECTROLYTES

For the elderly, dietary mineral intake may need to be adjusted either up or down, based on evaluation of the patient's nutritional status. Excess or even normal dietary levels can have deleterious consequences in certain diseases, particularly chronic illness. For example, since sodium is the primary determinant of the extracellular fluid volume, in conditions of excessive retention of extracellular fluid (congestive heart failure and hypertension), restriction of dietary sodium is essential to reduce extracellular fluid volume (see Chapter 31). On the other hand, rigid and severe restriction of sodium may seriously affect food acceptance; the use of diuretics may be preferred.

Restriction of dietary phosphorus may be necessary since hyperphosphatemia is a common companion of azotemia in renal disease. In such cases, a diet low in phosphorus as well as protein is prescribed (Watkin, 1980).

Calcium. Elderly people (especially women) usually have a negative calcium balance and are losing bone mass. Inadequate calcium intake is believed to be one of the main reasons for these conditions. Decreased physical activity and chronic acid-base imbalance contribute to calcium loss over the years. The combined use of alcohol, antacids, and drugs also disturbs calcium reserves (Spencer et al, 1982). This decrease in skeletal mass may lead to spontaneous fractures. In the United States, about 190,000 hip fractures and 100,000 broken wrists occur yearly (Weinstein, 1983).

Not only are older people not eating as much calcium as the RDA suggests, but many nutrition experts insist that the calcium level of 800 mg is too low. Daily intake should be at least 1200 to 1500 mg except in individuals with special problems of sarcoidosis, active tuberculosis, or other absorptive hypercalciuric syndromes (Heaney et al, 1982).

Magnesium. While magnesium deficiency is rare in humans, certain disorders of the elderly, such as chronic renal disease and drug-induced diuresis, make them prime candidates. Signs of this deficiency are personality changes, nausea, apathy, and muscle tremor.

Potassium. Dietary potassium requirements may be increased as a result of disease or trauma where accelerated protein breakdown occurs. Increased potassium losses have been noted following surgical operations, malnutrition, drugs, and fever. The chief features of potassium deficiency are muscular weakness and mental confusion.

Iron. No differences have been found between young adults and active older persons in their ability to absorb iron in the form of ferrous sulfate, but disease conditions are major contributors to iron deficiency, either directly or indirectly (Nordstrom, 1982).

Some elderly persons take large amounts of aspirin for osteoarthritis, which causes gastritis and bleeding and may result in iron deficiency anemia (Hardison, 1983). Many gastrointestinal diseases can significantly reduce dietary iron absorption, and GI bleeding leads to increased iron losses. Therapeutic drug use can markedly alter dietary iron utilization.

Lack of iron leads to anemia, which, if severe, gives rise to symptoms such as fatigue, lack of energy, and shortness of breath upon exertion. A combination of nutritional anemias may coexist in the elderly person, which most often includes folic acid, vitamin B_{12}, and iron deficiency anemia (see Chapter 34). The mean iron intake of older healthy Americans is generally adequate until the age of 75. Then meat consumption (the most utilizable source of iron) is decreased with a rise in breakfast cereal intake (Sandstead et al, 1982).

Zinc. Older adults seem to consume only marginal amounts of zinc (less than 45 percent of the RDA) because of lower protein consumption with advancing years (Betts & Vivian, 1984; Nordstrom, 1982). In addition, intestinal absorption is decreased in those over 65 years of age (Sandstead et al, 1982). Dietary zinc appears to be related closely to energy intake and can be adequate with careful food selection on a modest calorie intake (Rosenberg et al, 1982). Marginal zinc deficiency may manifest such clinical symptoms as decreased taste acuity, mental lethargy, slow wound healing, and immune dysfunction.

Clinical Implication:

- Even though zinc supplementation is popular, self-medication with amounts of zinc above the RDA (15 mg) may be harmful; a physician's diagnosis and recommendation should be obtained. Supplementation is more important for those with low caloric intake (Rosenberg et al, 1982).

WATER-SOLUBLE VITAMINS

Since water-soluble vitamins are not stored in the body for long periods, adequate daily food intakes are needed to maintain these vitamins. If foods are limited in variety or in quantity, deficiencies result.

Ascorbic Acid. Many elderly individuals have low ascorbic acid intakes. Stress, such as that from burns, surgery, or aging, can increase vitamin C excretion and decrease vitamin C tissue levels. In addition, corticosteroids increase urinary excretion of vitamin C. Anti-inflammatory drugs such as aspirin, indomethacin, and phenylbutazone inhibit ascorbic acid metabolism. The superior ascorbic acid status of people living at home compared to those residing in institutional settings perhaps indicates the destruction of ascorbic acid during prolonged cooking or holding periods of foods.

Because vitamin C is active in so many different reactions in the body, an analysis of intake is imperative. Plasma and tissue levels of vitamin C tend to decrease with age. Ideally, a generous food source of vitamin C would be included in most meals. Recommended plasma concentrations of vitamin C in elderly subjects may be maintained with an intake of 60 mg/day (Newton et al, 1985).

Thiamin. The lowest intake of thiamin is among black elderly males with incomes below the poverty level (Blumberg, 1986). Thiamin may be deficient because of impaired digestive functions, defective utilization in the tissues, or alcoholic polyneuritis. Since evidence suggests that elderly individuals may use thiamin less efficiently and that it is required in larger amounts to saturate tissues, an intake of 1 mg/day is recommended even if less than 2000 kcal/day are consumed (Albanese, 1980).

Niacin. Since tryptophan is a precursor of niacin and a main source of tryptophan is milk, niacin is frequently deficient in the elderly. Early signs of niacin deficiency are lassitude, anorexia, mild digestive disturbances (especially heartburn, glossitis, and diarrhea), and psychic and emotional changes (such as anxiety, irritability, and depression). The tongue is sore, red, and often swollen. A diagnosis of mild niacin deficiency is not easy in the absence of characteristic dermatitis. The presence of glossitis, diarrhea, and mild mental changes in a person whose diet has been low in niacin and protein is highly suggestive of deficiency.

Folacin. Erythrocyte-folate concentrations reflect total folate stores while recent folic acid intake is reflected by serum-folate concentrations. The absorption of folacin is not affected by age. Folacin inadequacy in healthy older people may be related to insufficient dietary intake (Bailey et al, 1984). Factors such as chronic drug use (cimetidine, phenytoin, sulfasalazine, and antacids), alcohol consumption, and prior gastrointestinal surgery have a negative influence on folacin status. Conditions such as gastric atrophy and hypochlorhydria, which occur more frequently in the elderly, will result in decreased intestinal folate absorption (Russell et al, 1980). Low serum folate levels have been correlated with mental disorders.

Pyridoxine (Vitamin B₆). With increasing age, serum pyridoxal phosphate decreases. Clinical evidence (such as an increased prevalence of carpal tunnel syndrome) and biochemical indices suggest an altered vitamin B_6 metabolism that could result in a higher requirement of the vitamin (Guilland et al, 1984).

Vitamin B₁₂. Cobalamin is less available in the elderly person because of decreased gastric juice and less meat consumption. Men have consistently lower levels than women (Watkin, 1980). More common deficiency signs are neurological manifestations as well as the expected pernicious anemia.

In one study of elderly individuals who complained of fatigue, symptoms disappeared in 89 percent of those given a supplement of vitamin B_{12} (Schlenker, 1973). Confusion and disorientation in the elderly population have also been attributed to a deficiency of vitamin B_{12}. Some patients with neurological symptoms (without anemia) responded positively to vitamin B_{12} treatment. A deficiency can be diagnosed by measuring serum B_{12} levels.

Clinical Implications:

- The elderly patient may have reactivation of dormant infections, such as tuberculosis. Isoniazid, a drug frequently used to treat tuberculosis, may result in drug-induced vitamin B_6 deficiency and, in turn, peripheral neuropathy. Prophylactic administration of pyridoxine at a level of 25 to 30 mg/day can avoid this side effect (Roe, 1985).
- The possibility of folate deficiency anemia should be included in the examinations of elderly hospitalized patients on certain drugs (anticonvulsants and sulfasalazine) and in alcoholics (Iber et al, 1982).

FAT-SOLUBLE VITAMINS

Fat-soluble vitamins are stored longer in the body, so the deficiency states do not appear as rapidly. However, one must be careful to provide each fat-soluble vitamin in optimal amounts.

Vitamin A. Absorption of vitamin A by the intestine is increased with age (Watkin, 1980), but less consumption of fruits and vegetables results in intakes below the RDAs. Also fat-soluble vitamins are not absorbed when mineral oil is taken, which may be a frequent practice among those with constipation. However, the popularity of vitamin supplements among the elderly may cause more of a problem with hypervitaminiosis A than with vitamin A deficiency.

Vitamin D. A deficiency of vitamin D may be the result of several causes: dietary insufficiency, malabsorption, kidney disease, and inadequate exposure to sunlight. Vitamin D stores decline with age for most people, particularly those confined to institutions or homes. Because of the effect of sunlight on individuals who are not housebound, a definite seasonal difference exists in the amount of vitamin D because of available sunlight. The vitamin D requirement increases with age to 15 to 20 mcg/day (600 to 800 IU) from all sources (Lynch et al, 1982).

Impaired bone mineralization in the absence of vitamin D in the aged is referred to as senile osteomalacia—the adult counterpart of rickets. Progressive decalcification of the bone results in symptomatic pain in sites such as the ribs, lower lumbar vertebrae, pelvis, and legs. Osteomalacia and osteoporosis are similar in some of their pathological problems, e.g., hip fractures. Table 17–1 compares these two conditions. Osteoporosis, however, occurs more often than osteomalacia in the elderly person.

Subclinical osteomalacia in the elderly may be corrected by relatively low doses of alfacalcidol (0.5 mcg/day) or vitamin D_2 (25 mcg/day) given for three months. The treatment is safe and not accompanied by a serious risk of hypercalcemia or renal impairment (Hoskins et al, 1984).

Both calcium and vitamin D, which are important in maintaining bone mineralization, are abundant in fortified milk. The liquid nature of milk also makes it readily consumable by the elderly in whom problems of dentition or other physical handicaps often limit ingestion of nutritious solid foods. However, regular consumption of milk by the elderly is unpopular because of its expense and the frequent trips needed to purchase it. The use of dry milk is also unpopular.

Clinical Implication:

- Excess intake of vitamin D may result in hypercalcemia and extraosseous calcification, particularly in the kidney, leading to chronic renal failure. Individual reaction varies in accordance with different doses of vitamin D; therefore, monitoring is essential for satisfactory results.

Table 17–1. Skeletal Calcium Imbalance*

Imbalance	Causes	Effects

Rickets and osteomalacia:	Diminished bone mineralization due to:
	1. dietary deficiency of calcium and/or vitamin D.
	2. calcium and/or vitamin D deficiency secondary to:
	   a. fat malabsorption or
	   b. chronic renal disease.
		Low mineral content in bone resulting in:
		1. soft, flexible bones and skeletal deformities;
		2. bone pain and generalized weakness;
		3. spontaneous fractures in adults.

Osteoporosis (most common problem):	1. Excessive bone resorption due to:
	   a. immobilization;
	   b. hyperparathyroidism.
	2. Diminished hormonal secretion with aging.
	3. Long-term inadequate dietary calcium intake.
		Diminished total bone mass resulting in:
		1. shortened stature and stooped posture;
		2. fractures;
		3. low back pain.

*Lewis, CM: *Nutrition Vitamins and Minerals: Sodium and Potassium.* Philadelphia, F. A. Davis Co, 1976, with permission.

Vitamin E. This vitamin is unusual because small amounts are present in the body during infancy. Peak values are reached during adolescence then slowly decrease with age until the concentrations are as low as during infancy. The exact requirement is still unknown. There is no support for the theory of this vitamin being more essential to prolong life than others.

Vitamin K. Senile purpura may occur from impaired absorption or inadequate utilization of vitamin K. Purpura refers to the spontaneous hemorrhagic disorders of petechiae (small red spots) and ecchymoses (bruises) that can easily be seen through the epidermis. No supplementation is recommended, however.

WATER

Fluid intake and water content of diets is of particular concern because of chronic illnesses that lead to impairment of the various homeostatic mechanisms controlling water balance. A progressive decrease in homeostatic capability continues with aging. Older men require more time to correct their water deficits, and they are less thirsty than younger men. Seemingly mild stresses—such as the imposed fluid restriction in preparation for some laboratory procedures; the presence of fever, infection, or diarrhea; or the use of diuretics—can upset the normal physiological state. In the hospital setting, such minor disturbances are cumulative, often occurring too frequently to permit the sluggish corrective responses of the elderly until profound and even potentially fatal derangements have occurred (Leaf, 1984).

Since secretion of saliva and gastric juices decrease, water can be a useful aid in washing down partially masticated food that might otherwise prove too difficult to swallow. Problems of elimination can also be improved by increased intake of fluids.

Plain water, however, is not highly favored by the elderly. Rarely do they drink optimum quantities of water but are more receptive to soups, juices, milk products, soft drinks, tea, and coffee. Care should be taken to maintain a good appetite and not let beverages prevent adequate food intake. Six to eight glasses per day are recommended.

Clinical Implications:

- Patients confined to bed or paralyzed by an accident or disease often need water intakes as high as 3 to 4 L/day to prevent kidney stone formation.
- Great care must be given to the water requirements of tube-fed patients, especially to those who are comatose and unable to respond to the sensation of thirst. If hypernatremia occurs, the appropriate treatment is the administration of water, enough to add 4 percent of the body weight in kilograms for each 10 mEq/L increase in serum sodium above normal (Watkin, 1980).
- Constipation, a chronic problem in the elderly, frequently occurs in persons with low fluid intake. A rectal examination by the physician should be considered a mandatory part of the evaluation of a patient who has distension or is vomiting, because fecal impaction can be a cause of vomiting (Daly, 1977).

- An elderly person may intentionally restrict fluids because of nocturia or incontinence. Careful attention should be given to the fluid needs of the elderly to avoid the many causes of dehydration, especially in hot weather.

ALCOHOL

Pleasure from "vices" can be tolerated in old age and, better still, planned to offer diversion and joy. Total abstinence for an individual who is accustomed to small amounts of alcohol may do more harm than good. The hypertensive patient, chronic nephritic, and diabetic can safely take their daily nip in moderation. Even the elderly gout patient may be allowed a modest portion of whiskey, but not wine or malt drinks (Cecil, 1981).

While too much alcohol can be harmful (see Chapter 28), several studies have proved the remarkable value of a brief cocktail period or happy hour in nursing homes and residential institutions for the elderly. (Alcoholics were given a substitute beverage.) Complaints dwindled. Beds were not as uncomfortable, food criticisms ceased, and personnel got better marks. Whether the sociability or the physiological reaction to the little nip improved appetite and digestion is not known, but the results were most successful (Kastenbaum, 1985).

Research on the effects of wine for geriatric patients demonstrates that its moderate use is beneficial; more zest for life, improved morale, more social interaction, more restful sleep at night, and reduction in use of psychotropic drugs are benefits that have been noted. Increased self-esteem of patients, a feeling of maturity and conviviality, feeling once again grown-up and part of a social group are psychosocial benefits (Kastenbaum, 1985).

Poor sleep may be attributable to a deficit of gama-aminobutyric acid (GABA), a substance found in the body as it prepares for sleep that is also found in wine. Attention should be given to educate not only the elderly person but the health care staff (Kastenbaum, 1985).

On the other hand, the possibility of alcohol abuse should always be considered in a malnourished elderly patient. Alcoholism has been diagnosed in 18 to 56 percent of the elderly patients admitted to various general hospitals, and in 23 percent of psychiatric admissions (Korsten & Leiber, 1983). Guidelines for safe levels of alcohol are given in Chapter 28.

Pharmaceuticals

Although drug-nutrient interactions can compromise anyone's nutritional status, these problems are accentuated in the elderly because of physiologic and pathophysiologic changes. Because older citizens are less likely to be healthy or free from disease, they have more problems with nutrient absorption and utilization. Since the elderly take half of all pharmaceuticals consumed, they are the major prescription and over-the-counter (OTC) drug users. Those living independently may take three or more drugs; the residents in long-term care facilities may take more than 10 drugs (Roe, 1985). Excessive use of OTC drugs is common. It is most difficult to know precisely what senior citizens are taking when they are on their own and even more difficult to predict how effective the drug will be. They may share drugs with friends and start or stop medications whenever they choose.

The most common reason for discontinuing a drug, other than cure, is that the drug is ineffective. Of course, it may be ineffective for any number of reasons or simply because the patient is not taking it. With all these interfering factors, the physician cannot predict the absorption of an oral dose in his patients. S/He must work with the patient to find the right amount and the correct drug. The elderly patient may not even report back to the physician, much less follow directions for a successful program (Roe, 1985). The discussion on food-drug interaction in Chapter 22 is especially relevant to this group of patients.

However, some nutrient-drug interactions more common to this group are vitamin B_6 deficiency in cancer victims; decreases in magnesium, phosphate, calcium, and potassium caused by diuretics; and decreased folate and iron levels caused by chronic aspirin intake (Sempos et al, 1982).

Eating Patterns

DEFICIENCIES

Such surveys as the 10-State Nutrition Survey, the Health and Nutrition Examination Survey (HANES), and USDA food consumption studies have clearly shown that persons 50 years of age and older consume far less food than younger adults. Dairy products, fruits, and vegetables were omitted from the diets of one third to one half of all participants (men and women) in one study (Betts & Vivian, 1984).

Senior citizens typically consume low amounts of vitamin A, ascorbic acid, calcium, thiamin, and iron. Men consume more protein, fat, and riboflavin than women. As age increases, intakes of fat, protein, iron, thiamin, and niacin decrease (LeClerc & Thornbury, 1983). Deficiencies of calcium, iron, zinc, thiamin, and folate may be related to specific diseases or disorders frequently observed in older persons (Heaney et al, 1982).

Nutrient intakes of men are consistently higher than those of the women in all environments. Both men and women who live at home have the highest intake of most nutrients (Murphy, 1982). In several studies, the sterotype of elderly men and women eating bread and jam because they are unwilling or unable to cook for themselves was definitely not supported.

A survey of Wisconsin nursing homes found that residents had low levels of energy, magnesium, zinc, vitamin B_6, and folic acid (Sempos et al, 1982). Vitamin and mineral supplements are advisable for most of the elderly population. Frequent monitoring of the individual's status is essential; periodic monitoring of menus and food supply is also mandatory to determine the adequacy of food intake. Nutrient-dense foods should be used primarily to protect those persons who should have a low-calorie intake.

Elderly individuals who are most likely to be at nutritional risk are women, persons with the least education, and persons who have recently experienced a drastic change in lifestyle, e.g., moving from their home to an apartment or institution (O'Hanlon et al, 1983). Chronic disease and financial burdens imposed by limited income are among the most important factors influencing nutritional status. About 80 percent of the elderly individuals, as compared with 40 percent of those under 65 years of age, have one or more chronic diseases (Weimer, 1983).

SNACKS

Snacks continue to be popular, averaging two per day, usually in the afternoon and evening. These may provide important additional energy,

but they are often high only in carbohydrate, particularly sucrose (Singleton et al, 1983).

SUPPLEMENTS

A milk-based food supplement, i.e., an instant breakfast mix with dry milk, may be given rather than a commercial liquid supplement to help economize while preventing nutrient deficiencies. The supplement increases the protein, ascorbic acid, folic acid, vitamin D, and thiamin concentration of the diet (Katakity et al, 1983).

Clinical Implications:

- Nursing and nutrition professionals must take time to document cost savings along with improved patient outcome, e.g., the cost of laxatives and stool softeners versus the cost of whole-wheat bread and adding bran to appropriate foods. A pureed diet costs less than half as much as a blended formula (Matthews, 1983).
- Loneliness and depression are often associated with poor appetite, e.g., after the loss of a spouse.
- Constant surveillance of weight can prevent serious nutrient depletions. Aggressive nutritional support is more successful than recovery of lost status.
- An older person usually requires more time to eat, and rapid satiety is reached by some. Rather than three meals a day, frequent feedings of smaller amounts as well as liquid supplements are beneficial.
- Even though the individual has dentures, s/he may not wear them or be able to use them to chew or because the gums may be sore. Observe food intake carefully to be sure that adequate food is consumed.

ADAPTIVE EQUIPMENT

One of the most basic and rewarding of all self-care skills is that of feeding oneself. While disabled people have used adaptive equipment to feed themselves, little attention has been given to the elderly who survive illnesses that leave them with limited mobility. Once an individual is fed by others, continued dependency frequently develops, rather than attempting to regain his/her own independent abilities (see Figs. 31–1 to 31–4).

Independence in eating results in several other rewards. Obviously, there is increased personal pride, self-respect, and dignity. Morale improves in some cases when individuals are able to join others in the dining room and leave the facility to visit relatives and friends in their homes. Another benefit is an increased appetite. Adaptive equipment offers elderly patients with limited mobility as much potential as any other disabled group.

Community Services

ELDERLY POPULATION

By the year 2000, more than 28 million persons will be over 65 years of age. In 1980, one of every eight persons (more than 25.5 million) was in this age group (LeClerc & Thornbury, 1983). Projections are that a 68-year-old man has an expectancy of about nine years of independent living. This is followed by about four years of progressively decreasing capacity necessitating assistance from others. Women have an expectancy of about 11 years of independent living followed by about nine years of progressive disability requiring assistance from others (Sandstead, 1985).

The average resident in a skilled nursing facility is 81 years old and will remain in the facility for two years and eight months. Most suffer from at least one chronic disease in addition to general debilitation. Diabetes, strokes, organic brain syndrome, cardiac insufficiency, Alzheimer's and Parkinson's disease are among the frequent admitting diagnoses (Matthews, 1982). However, one of the main goals for senior citizens is to maintain their independence and health as long as possible. The government has taken a giant step forward with a nutrition program for this purpose.

PROGRAMS

In 1972, Congress created a comprehensive nutrition program for elderly individuals designed to relieve social as well as nutritional problems by providing meals predominantly in congregate settings. The Nutrition Program for the Elderly, mandated by the Title VII amendment to the Older Americans Act, has become a significant program in promoting better health among senior citizens by providing food and nutritional education through federal funding to the states. Future plans emphasize increasing self-sufficiency

---

Table 17–2. Nation's Goals and Specific Objectives of Healthy Older Adults*

Goal: To improve the health and quality of life for older adults and, by 1990, to reduce the average annual number of days of restricted activity due to acute and chronic conditions by 20 percent, to fewer than 30 days per year for older people ages 65 and older.

Improved Health Status
   a. By 1990, at least 60 percent of the estimated population having definite high blood pressure (160/95) should have attained successful long-term blood pressure control, i.e., a blood pressure at or below 140/90 for two or more years. [High blood pressure control rates vary among communities and states, with the range generally being from 25 to 60 percent based on current data.]
   b. By 1990, the cirrhosis mortality rate should be reduced to 12 per 100,000 per year. [In 1978, the rate was 13.8 per 100,000 per year.]

Reduced Risk Factors
   a. By 1990, the prevalence of significant overweight (120 percent of "desired" weight) among the U.S. adult population should be decreased to 10 percent of men and 17 percent of women, without nutritional impairment. [In 1971–74, 14 percent of adult men and 24 percent of women were more than 120 percent of "desired" weight.]
   b. By 1990, the average daily sodium ingestion (as measured by excretion) by adults should be reduced at least to the 3 to 6 gm range. [In 1979, estimates ranged between averages of 4 and 10 gm sodium. NOTE: One gram of salt provides approximately 0.4 gm sodium.]
   c. By 1990, the mean serum cholesterol level in the adult population aged 18 to 74 should be at or below 200 mg/dl. [In 1971–74, for male and female adults ages 18 to 74, the mean serum cholesterol level was 223 mg/dl. For a smaller population sample in 1972–75, mean blood plasma cholesterol levels were about 211 mg/dl for males ages 40 to 59 and about 210 mg/dl for females ages 40 to 59.]
   d. By 1990, the proportion of adults 18 to 65 participating regularly in vigorous physical exercise should be greater than 60 percent. [In 1978, the proportion who regularly exercised was estimated at over 35 percent.]
   e. By 1990, 50 percent of adults 65 years and older should be engaging in appropriate physical activity, e.g., regular walking, swimming, or other aerobic activity. [In 1975, about 36 percent took regular walks.]
   f. By 1990, the proportion of adults who smoke should be reduced to below 25 percent. [In 1979, the proportion of the U.S. population that smoked was 33 percent.]

---

*From Lee, SL: Nutrition services for adults and the elderly. *Clinical Nutrition* 3(3):109, 1984, with permission.

through improved health for the later years to delay the less desirable and more costly nursing home care.

These programs provide food that will meet a significant amount of the RDAs for one day at minimal or no cost. This alleviates some of the problems for those with fixed income, no transportation, and little incentive to cook for themselves. The nutrition program helps reduce the isolation of older persons by offering them the opportunity to participate in leisure time and recreational activities and to combine food with friendship.

The primary thrust of the nutrition program for the elderly is to provide meals in a group setting. Meals may also be delivered to those participants who are homebound because of illness, incapacitating disability, or extreme transportation problems. The spouse of the homebound participant may also receive a home-delivered meal, regardless of age or condition. In such cases, food is often delivered by senior volunteers who visit with the shut-ins while they eat.

Since many elderly individuals are reluctant to participate in nutrition programs if the meals are labeled "free," participants are given an opportunity to contribute to all or part of the meal cost, but no one may be turned away from a meal for inability to pay. Only the participant will determine if and how much s/he will pay. In most cases, participants pay something for their meals, even those who are employed by the project or who assist as volunteers. Contributions are handled in strict confidence. These funds are used to increase the number of meals served.

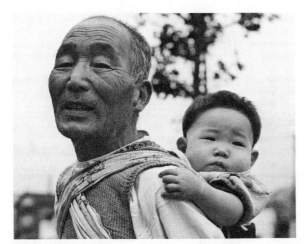

Figure 17–4. Grandfather is pleased and proud to "mind the baby" while parents are at work; a task which underlines an elderly person's sense of belonging to the family. (Courtesy of World Health Organization.)

Food stamps are another useful nutrition support system. However, many elderly people are hesitant to ask for any financial help. Transportation may also be a problem.

These programs are estimated to reach only 20 percent of the elderly who need them (Schuster, 1983). Collective imagination by national and local governments as well as the private sector is crucial to maintain these programs now and in the future. Many of the poor elderly survive by whatever free shelters and food may be found. Hopefully, the nation's goals and objectives for healthy older adults shown in Table 17–2 will be met by more people in the future. Attention to appropriate nutrient intake from birth can result in healthier, happier, and more productive older Americans (Fig. 17–4).

• FALLACIES and FACTS

FALLACY: Ground nutmeat of apricot kernels (laetrile) can slow down the process of aging and cure cancer.

• **FACT:** Whether the oil from apricot kernels in some parts of the world is beneficial has not been chemically investigated. Lethal amounts of cyanide are found in oils extracted from the kernels of American apricots or peaches.

FALLACY: Mineral oil is a good inexpensive laxative.

• **FACT:** Deficiencies in fat-soluble vitamins among adults in the United States are usually secondary to consumption of low-fat diets, habitual ingestion of mineral oil as a laxative, or diseases characterized by steatorrhea. Because mineral oil interferes with absorption of fat-soluble vitamins, it should not be used.

FALLACY: All fruits are "acid."

• **FACT:** Most fruits would appear to be acidic, but in the digestive process, they are actually alkaline. Only a few fruits for example, cranberries and plums, are acid-producing.

FALLACY: Elderly people don't need much to eat because they are not growing.

• **FACT:** The body has certain cells that are constantly being repaired and replaced, which is quite similar to earlier growth periods. Metabolism for the function of the body requires all the same nutrients. In fact, nutrients may need to be increased because of stress and disease.

FALLACY: *Antioxidants increase the life span.*
- **FACT:** *Aging has been theorized as free-radical reactions produced during normal metabolism that leads to cellular damage. Fortunately, people possess efficient free-radical "scavengers," two of which are vitamins C and E. Superoxide dismutase (SOD) tablets, which are marketed to prolong life, have not been shown to have a consistent effect on aging. In fact, this enzyme is hydrolyzed in the gastrointestinal tract so that blood serum shows no increase over normal amounts after its ingestion (Schneider & Reed, 1985).*

Summary

Little has changed since the days of Ponce de León. Everyone would like to know the secrets of longevity. Although the following suggestions may sound simple, the implications of present-day nutritional knowledge suggest that longevity is affected by (1) choosing a variety of foods from the basic food groups, (2) planning menus to provide the desirable nutrients, and (3) avoiding overindulgence and overweight. Moderate exercise and frequent medical and dental check-ups are also important.

One of the most outstanding revelations from studying the nutritional needs of the elderly is that so many nutrient deficiencies cause behavioral changes that mimic psychiatric problems. Serious attention must be given to the physical examination with proper laboratory tests to identify nutrient status, the disease symptoms, and last of all, possible age-related symptoms.

Age affects the older person's nutritional requirements in many ways. Physiological changes in body organs, rates of absorption, medications, illnesses or abnormal physical conditions, availability of food, and attitude toward life all play intricate parts in this complex nutritional regimen. In fact, good nutrition throughout life may make the difference between older people who are active and productive and those who need frequent medical care, hospital admission, and even institutionalization for physical or emotional disabilities.

Review Questions

1. Plan a day's menus for a geriatric patient without dentures.
2. What are some of the nutrients that might be harmful because of excessive intake?
3. What are some vitamins and minerals that might influence mental attitudes because of their deficiencies?
4. Discuss the reasons elderly persons might not eat adequately.
5. Visit a group meal program. Review the menu and discuss the beneficial effects of the program's various activities.

REFERENCE LIST

Age, masticatory ability and swallowing. *Nutr Rev* 41(11):344, 1983.

Albanese, AA: *Nutrition for the Elderly.* New York, Alan R. Liss, Inc, 1980.

Bailey, LB; Cerda, JJ; Bloch, BS; et al: Effect of age on poly- and mono-glutamyl folacin absorption in human subjects. *J Nutr* 114(9):1770, 1984.

Betts, NM; Vivian, VM: The dietary intake of noninstitutionalized elderly. *J. Nutr Elderly* 3(4):3, 1984.

Blumberg, JB: Nutrient requirements for the healthy elderly. *Cont Nutr* XI(6), 1986.

Bowman, BB; Rosenberg, IH: Digestive function and aging. *Hum Nutr Clin Nutr* 37C(2):75, 1983.

Cecil, RL: Old age and the vices. *J Am Geriatr Soc* 29(12):550, 1981.

Daly, JM, editor: Nutritional problems of the elderly. *Dialogues in Nutrition* 2(3), 1977.

Enloe, CF: Paradise lost. *Nutr Today* 13(3):6, 1978.

Gersovitz, M; Motil, I; Munro, HN; et al: Human protein requirements: Assessment of the adequacy of the current recommended dietary allowances for dietary protein. *Am J Clin Nutr* 35(1):6, 1982.

Guilland, JC; Berguig, B; Leqacu, B, et al: Evaluation of pyridoxine intake and pyridoxine status among aged institutionalized people. *Int J Vit Nutr Res* 54(2–3):185, 1984.

Hardison, JE: An ice crusher for Aunt Linna. *JAMA* 249(20):2769, 1983.

Harper, AE: Nutrition, aging and longevity. *Am J Clin Nutr* 36(4 suppl):737, 1982.

Heaney, RP; Gallagher, JC; Johnston, CC; et al: Calcium nutrition and bone health in the elderly. *Am J Clin Nutr* 36(5 suppl):986, 1982.

Hoskins, DJ; Campbell, GA; Kemm, JR; et al: Safety of treatment for subclinical osteomalacia in the elderly. *Br Med J* 289(Sept 29):785, 1984.

Iber, FL; Blass, JP; Brin, M; et al: Thiamin in the elderly—relation to alcoholism and to neurological degenerative disease. *Am J Clin Nutr* 36 (5 suppl):1067, 1982.

Kamath, SK: Taste acuity and aging. *Am J Clin Nutr* 36(4 suppl):766, 1982.

Kastenbaum, R: Wine and the elderly person. *J Nutr Elderly* 4(3):15, 1985.

Katakity, M; Webb, JF; Dickerson, JWT: Some effects of food supplement in elderly hospital patients: A longitudinal study. *Hum Nutr Appl Nutr* 37A(2):85, 1983.

Korsten, MA; Leiber, CS: The elderly alcoholic. In *Nutrition in Middle and Later Years.* Edited by E Feldman. Boston, John Wright PSG, Inc, 1983.

Leaf, A: *Youth in Old Age.* New York, McGraw-Hill, 1975.

Leaf, A: Dehydration in the elderly. *New Engl J Med* 311(12):791, 1984.

LeClerc, HL; Thornbury, ME: Dietary intakes of Title III meal program recipients and nonrecipients. *J Am Diet Assoc* 83(5):573, 1983.

Lee, SL: Nutrition services for adults and the elderly, *Clin Nutr* 3(3):109, 1984.

Lynch, SR; Finch, CA; Monsen, ER; et al: Iron status of elderly Americans. *Am J Clin Nutr* 36(5 suppl):1032, 1982.

Masoro, EJ: Physiologic changes with aging. In *Nutrition and Aging*. Edited by M Winick. New York, John Wiley & Sons, 1976.

Matthews, LE: Protein requirements in the elderly. *J Nutr Elderly* 2(2):35, 1983.

Murphy, C: Diets of the elderly. *J New Zealand Diet Assoc* 36(October):10, 1982.

Newton, HMV; Schorah, CJ; Habibzadeh, N; et al: The cause and correction of the low blood vitamin C concentrations in the elderly. *Am J Clin Nutr* 42(4):656, 1985.

Nizel, AE: *Nutrition in Preventive Dentistry Science and Practice*, 2nd ed. Philadelphia: W. B. Saunders Co, 1981.

Nordstrom, JW: Trace mineral nutrition in the elderly. *Am J Clin Nutr* 36(4 suppl):788, 1982.

O'Hanlon, P; Kohrs, MB; Hilderbrand, E; et al: Socioeconomic factors and dietary intakes of elderly Missourians. *J Am Diet Assoc* 82(6):676, 1983.

Palmore, E: Predictors of longevity. In *Epidemiology of Aging*. Edited by SG Haynes; M Feinleib. Bethesda, MD, National Institute of Aging, 1980.

Roe, DA: *Drugs and Nutrition in the Geriatric Patient*. New York, Churchill Livingstone, 1984.

Rosenberg, IH; Bowman, BB; Cooper, BA; et al: Folate nutrition in the elderly. *Am J Clin Nutr* 36(5 suppl):1060, 1982.

Rozovski, JF: Nutrition for older American. *Nutr Health* 5(3):1, 1983.

Russell, RM; Krosinski, SD; Somloff, IM: Correction of impaired folic acid absorption by orally administered HCl in subjects with gastric atrophy. *Am J Clin Nutr* 39(4):656, 1984.

Sandstead, HH: Some relations between nutrition and aging. *J Am Diet Assoc* 85(2):171, 1985.

Sandstead, HH; Henriksen, LK; Greger, JL; et al: Zinc nutriture in the elderly in relation to taste acuity, immune response, and wound healing. *Am J Clin Nutr* 36(11):1046, 1982.

Schiffman, SS: Taste and smell in disease. *N Engl J Med* 308(21):1275, 1983.

Schneider, EL; Reed, JD, Jr.: Life extension. *New Engl J Med* 312(18):1159, 1985.

Schlenker, ED: Nutrition and health of older people. *Am J Clin Nutr* 26(10):1111, 1973.

Schuster, K: The politics of feeding the elderly. *Food Management* 18(2):46, 1983.

Sempos, CT; Johnson, NE; Elmer, PJ; et al: A dietary survey of 14 Wisconsin nursing homes. *J Am Diet Assoc* 81(1):35, 1982.

Singleton, N; Kirby, AL; Overstreet, MH: Snacking patterns of elderly females. *J Nutr Elderly* 2(2):3, 1983.

Spencer, H; Kramer, L; Osis, D: Factors contributing to calcium loss in aging. *Am J Clin Nutr* 36(4 suppl):776, 1982.

Tobin, JD: Normal aging—the inevitability syndrome. In *The Quality of Life, The Later Years*. Edited by LE Brown. Acton, MA, Publishing Sciences Group, 1975.

Treichel, JA: Food for thought in the elderly. *Science News* 123(23):358, 1983.

Watkin, DM: The physiology of aging. *Am J Clin Nutr* 36(5 suppl):750, 1982.

Watkin, DM: Nutrition for the aging and the aged. In *Modern Nutrition in Health and Disease*, 6th ed. Edited by RS Goodhart; ME Shils. Philadelphia, Lea & Febiger, 1980, p 781.

Weinstein, RS: The histological heterogeneity of osteopenia in the middle-aged and elderly patient. In *Nutrition in Middle and Later Years*. Edited by E Feldman. Boston, John Wright, PSG, Inc, 1983.

Further Study

Bidlack, WR; Kirsch, A; Meskin, MS: Nutrition requirements of the elderly. *Food Tech* 40(2):61, 1986.

Cerrato, PL: Hidden malnutrition in geriatric patients. *RN* 48(7):60, 1985.

Cerrato, PL: Helping elderly patients resist infection. *RN* 49(5):69, 1986.

Creative dining program makes eating fun. *Hospitals* 57(2):46, 1983.

Danovitch, SH: Gastrointestinal function after forty. *Am Fam Physician* 29(2):205, 1984.

Endres, JM; Theobald, L; Galligos, CR; et al: Energy and nutrient content of menus, foods served, and foods consumed by institutionalized elderly. *J Nutr Elderly* 2(1):3, 1982.

Epstein, M: Aging and the kidney: Clinical implications. *Am Fam Physician* 31(4):123, 1985.

Fuller, ES: What's a sound diet for the elderly? *Patient Care* 20(11):90, 1986.

Goodwin, JS; Goodwin, JM; Garry, PJ: Association between nutritional status and cognitive functioning in a healthy elderly population. *JAMA* 249(21):2917, 1983.

Hickler, RB; Wayne, KS: Nutrition and the elderly. *Am Fam Physician* 29(3):137, 1984.

Hogstel, M (ed): *Nursing Care of the Older Adult in the Hospital, Nursing Home and Community*. New York: John Wiley & Sons, 1981.

Hyams, DE: Drug usage by the elderly, in *Drugs and Nutrition in the Geriatric Patient*. Edited by DA Roe. New York, Churchill Livingstone, 1984.

Kohrs, MB: A rational diet for the elderly. *Am J Clin Nutr* 36(4 suppl):796, 1982.

Lecos, CW: Diet and the elderly. *FDA Consumer* 18(10):7, 1984–85.

Nagami, PH; Yosikawa, TT: Tuberculosis in the geriatric patient. *J Am Geriatr Soc* 32(6):356, 1983.

National Agricultural Library: *Nutrition and the Elderly: A Selected Annotated Bibliography for Nutrition and Health Professionals*. Washington, DC, Government Printing Office, 1985.

Newman, JM: Cultural, religious, and regional food practices of the elderly. *J Nutr Elderly* 5(1):15, 1985.

Newton-Rice, L: Dietary guidelines for the institutionalized elderly. *Community Nutritionist* 2(May-June):23, 1983.

Parfitt, AM; Gallagher, JC; Heaney, RP; et al: Vitamin D and bone health in the elderly. *Am J Clin Nutr* 36(5 suppl):1014, 1982.

Roe, DA: Therapeutic effects of drug-nutrient interactions in the elderly. *J Am Diet Assoc* 85(2):174, 1985.

Russell, RM; Whinston-Perry, R: Geriatric nutrition: Considerations essential to an accurate assessment. *Consultant* 24(8):67, 1984.

Wayler, AH; Muench, ME; Kapur, KK; et al: Masticatory performance and food acceptability in persons with removable partial dentures, full dentures, and intact natural dentition. *J Gerontol* 39(3):284, 1984.

Ethnic and Religious Influences

18

- *State reasons people have food patterns.*
- *Recognize that each culture has some unique but beneficial food traditions.*
- *Relate individual feeding problems within an institution to cultural influences.*
- *Suggest ways to adapt a menu to suit particular cultural patterns.*
- *Suggest ways to adapt a hospital menu to comply with strict Jewish dietary laws.*

Food pattern
Geophagia
Hot-cold theory
Pica
Yin and yang

OBJECTIVES

TERMS TO KNOW

Food Patterns

HABITS OR PATTERNS

In terms of food choices, people are creatures of habit (Zifferblatt et al, 1980). Patterns throughout societies are quite evident; however, the term "habit" connotes inflexibility. Individuals do change their habits for numerous reasons, hence the term "food patterns" is more descriptive of food choices. Many factors are associated with the formation of food patterns and preferences. Food patterns are generally developed during childhood and reflect the family's lifestyle as well as its ethnic or cultural, social, religious, geographic, economic, and psychological components. All of these influence an individual's attitudes, feelings, and beliefs about food. However, the factors that seem to predominate food choices are cultural and economic.

CULTURAL FACTORS

One of the most interesting and visible ways cultural differences are expressed is through the foods an individual eats or does not eat. Although milk is the *only* food used by everybody worldwide, many cultures consider it appropriate only for infants and children.

Children of different cultures, exposed to what adults eat, do not question whether this is what they should be eating. Cultural food patterns establish the foundation for a child's lifelong eating customs regarding time and number of meals per day, foods acceptable for specific meals, preparation methods, likes and dislikes, foods suitable for specific members of a group, table manners, the social role of foods and eating, and attitudes toward eating and health. Patterns and attitudes that develop throughout childhood are very complex and promote a sense of stability and security when the individual is older (Fig. 18–1).

Not only do many ethnic groups coexist in this country, but literally thousands of localized patterns have developed because of food availability. As Schwerin and colleagues (1982) have discovered ". . . distinct and discrete patterns of consuming foods in different combinations exist; and these patterns have remained quite consistent over the past decade." For example, few people in the northern United States would routinely choose grits, and many Southerners would not recognize lentils. While American diets are diversified, they have become more homogeneous because of transportation, advertising, mobility, new methods of production, changes in income

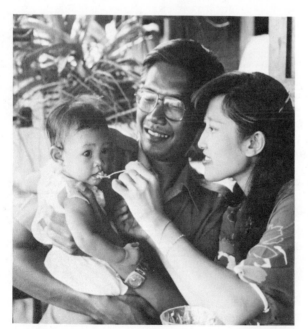

Figure 18–1. *Eating habits are established at a very young age. (WHO photo by T. Kelly.)*

distribution, and appreciation of one another's heritage (Riggs, 1980).

No culture has ever been known to make food choices solely on the basis of nutritional and health values of food. For example, broccoli is one of the most nutritious vegetables (based on nutrient density) available in the United States, but ranks 21st in the amount consumed; whereas, the tomato, the most commonly eaten vegetable, rates sixteenth as a source of vitamins and minerals (Farb & Armelagos, 1980).

Individual preferences do not ordinarily influence the nutritional adequacy of the diet. Insufficient quantities of basic food items (milk, bread, cereals, and eggs) have the greatest effect on nutritional adequacy rather than specific aversions, such as to turnips or rye bread.

ECONOMIC FACTORS

When persons relocate, established food habits are carried to the new location; however, these habits are retained only if the foods are available at an affordable price. Therefore, problems arising within various cultural groups are economic rather than the fault of traditional food patterns. Foods from the "old country," which were cheapest at "home," are very expensive or possibly not even available in their new location. Gradually, the diet conforms to the food resources of the new location. Evidence of malnutrition increases as income level decreases.

STATUS AND SYMBOLIC INFLUENCES

A food in various cultures will have a different prestige or status within the society. For example, beef is regarded as a high status food among most people in the United States, but Hindus from India consider cows sacred and do not eat beef. Foods may obtain their status rating from religious beliefs, availability, cost, cultural values, and traditions or because a highly respected individual has endorsed it.

Even today in many cultures, males are more highly valued than females. Thus, male members of the household may be fed first with the females and children being allowed to eat only after the males are filled. Consequently, females and children may receive insufficient quantities and less variety of foods.

Because of symbolic meanings of food, which have nothing to do with nutriture, eating becomes associated with sentiments and assumptions about oneself and the world (Farb & Armelagos, 1980). Foods sometimes become symbolic to people not only because of religious connotations but because foods are often used as rewards. After a child has fallen, a mother may give the child candy to help him/her forget the pain and to stop crying. How many times has a mother been overheard to say, "Just be good while I'm doing this, and I'll buy you an ice cream cone"? Sometimes, food is withheld for bad behavior.

Working with People with Different Food Patterns

RESPECT FOR OTHER EATING PATTERNS

Health care professionals must be prepared to meet the unexpected. Recognizing that eating habits and patterns vary with individuals and that characteristic cultural patterns are usually observed among different nationalities and religious groups is important. Of course, individuals are partial to their own food pattern; however, too many individuals, including health care professionals, are convinced that their own beliefs, attitudes, and practices are the best way and assume that everyone should follow them. It is important when working with persons who have strong cultural ties to be sensitive to their preferences and to avoid being judgmental. Only by avoiding cultural biases will people open up to reveal crucial information that will allow the professional to help them.

Even when the facts are known, an analysis of the situation may be clouded because of uniquely individual habits. Information should be obtained regarding food habits by open-ended questions rather than questions that put words into a person's mouth. For example, "Did you have anything to eat this morning?" might elicit a different response than, "What did you have for breakfast this morning?"

Individuals sometimes refuse to eat a particular food or to comply with a diet regimen because of cultural or religious beliefs. Generally, if preferred foods are known, an adequate diet can be

Table 18–1. *Cultural and Regional Foods*

Name of Food	Culture/Region	Type of Food	Description
Adobo	Filipino	Meat	Meat with soy sauce
Ajinomoto	Japanese	Grain	Wheat germ
Anadama	New England	Grain	Cornmeal-molasses yeast bread
Arroz blanco	Puerto Rican	Grain	Enriched white rice
Bacalao	Puerto Rican	Meat	Salted codfish
Bagels	Jewish	Grain	Bread dough, doughnut-shaped, boiled in water and baked
Baklava	Greek	Dessert	Layered pastry made with honey
Bok choy	Oriental	Vegetable	Green leafy, stalk-like vegetable
Brioche	French	Grain	Egg-rich cake bread, used as sweet roll or shell for entrees
Bulgur	Middle Eastern	Grain	Granular wheat product with nut-like flavor
Burrito	Mexican	Combination	Sandwich; tortilla filled with beef-bean mixture and fried or baked
Café con leche	Latin American	Beverage	Coffee with milk
Cape Cod turkey	New England	Meat	Codfish balls
Challah	Jewish	Grain	Sabbath or holiday twisted eggbread
Chayote	Mexican	Vegetable	Squash-like vegetable
Chitterlings	Southern U.S.	Meat	Intestine of young pigs, soaked, boiled, and fried
Chorizo	Mexican	Meat	Sausage
Cilantro	Mexican	Seasoning	Coriander, similar to parsley
Crackling	Southern U.S.	Snack	Crispy pieces of fried pork fat
Croissants	French	Grain	Buttery, flaky, crescent-shaped rolls
Crumpets	English	Grain	Muffin-like product cooked on griddle then toasted
Cush	Montana	Grain	Cornbread mixed with butter and water and fried
Dandelion greens	Southern U.S.	Vegetable	Leaves from dandelion plant
Dolmathes	Greek	Combination	Grape leaves stuffed with beef
Enchiladas	Mexican	Combination	Tortilla filled with meat and cheese
Escargots	French	Meat	Snails
Falafel	Jewish	Meat	Mashed chick peas mixed with spices and fried
Fatback	Southern U.S.	Fat	Fat from loin of pig
Feijoada	Brazilian	Meat	Black beans with meat
Feta	Greek	Milk	Soft, salty white cheese from sheep's or goat's milk
Finnan haddie	Scottish	Milk	Salted, smoked haddock
Frijoles fritos	Mexican	Meat	Refried pinto beans
Gazpacho	Spanish	Soup	Cold soup with chopped tomatoes, green peppers, and cucumbers
Gefilte fish	Jewish	Meat	Seasoned fish ground and shaped into balls
Goulash	Hungarian	Meat	Stew seasoned with paprika
Grits	Southern U.S.	Grain	Hulled and coarsely ground corn
Guava	Cuban	Fruit	Small, yellow or red sweet tropical fruit
Gumbo	Creole	Combination	Well-seasoned okra stew with meat or seafood
Hangtown fry	California	Meat	Fried oysters and eggs
Hoe cake	Southeast U.S.	Grain	Thin corn cake
Hog maw	Southern U.S.	Meat	Stomach of pig
Hoppin' John	Southern U.S.	Combination	Blackeyed peas and rice
Hushpuppies	Southern U.S.	Grain	Fried cornbread
Jalapeños	Latin American	Vegetable	Hot peppers
Jambalaya	Creole	Combination	Well-seasoned combination of seafoods, tomatoes, and rice
Kale	Southern U.S.	Vegetable	Dark green leafy vegetable, similar to spinach
Kasha	Jewish	Grain	Coarsely ground buckwheat, toasted before cooking in liquid
Kelp	Oriental	Vegetable	Seaweed
Kibbeh	Middle East	Meat	Fresh raw lamb, ground and seasoned, similar to meat loaf
Kielbasa	Polish	Meat	Sausage
Kimchi	Korean	Vegetable	Peppery fermented combination of pickled cabbage, turnips, radishes, and other vegetables
Kuchen	German	Dessert	Yeast cake
Latkas	Jewish	Grain	Pancakes, sometimes from potatoes
Lard	—	Fat	Shortening-like product from pork
Limpa	Swedish	Grain	Rye bread
Lox	Jewish	Meat	Smoked salmon
Matsoh	Jewish	Grain	Unleavened bread
Menudo	Mexican	Meat	Stew made with tripe (cow's stomach)
Minestrone	Italian	Soup	Vegetable soup
Miso	Oriental	Meat	Fermented soybean paste
Moussaka	Greek	Combination	Meat and eggplant casserole

Table 18–1. Cultural and Regional Foods Continued

Name of Food	Culture/Region	Type of Food	Description
Mush	Southwest U.S.	Grain	Cooked cereal, usually cornmeal
Pan Dowdy	New England	Dessert	Dumplings and fruit
Papaya	—	Fruit	Large, yellow melon-like tropical fruit
Pasta	Italian	Grain	Macaroni, spaghetti, and noodles in various shapes made from wheat
Pepperoni	Italian	Meat	Hot sausage
Phyllo	Greek	Grain	Paper-thin pastry for making meat, vegetables, cheese and egg dishes, and sweet pastries
Pilaf	Middle Eastern	Grain	Rice enriched with fat and sometimes vegetables, bits of meat, and spices
Poi	Polynesian	Vegetable	Root vegetable, especially taro, cooked and pounded, mixed with water, and sometimes fermented
Polenta	Italian	Grain	Cornmeal or cornmeal mush
Polk	Southern U.S.	Vegetable	Dark green leafy vegetable
Potato knishes	Jewish	Vegetable	Potato pancakes
Pot liquor (likker)	Southern U.S.	Vegetable	Liquid from cooking green vegetables or bones
Proscuitto	Italian	Meat	Ready-to-eat, cured, smoked ham
Prickly pear	Native American	Fruit	Fruit of cactus
Pumpernickel	—	Grain	Yeast bread with wheat, corn, rye, and potatoes
Ratatouille	French	Vegetable	Well-seasoned casserole of eggplant, zucchini, tomato, and green pepper
Red-eye gravy	Southern U.S.	Gravy	Fried ham gravy
Sake	Oriental	Beverage	Rice wine
Salt pork	Southern U.S.	Fat	Salted pork fat from the belly
Sancocho	Puerto Rican	Combination	Soup with meat and viandas
Sashimi	Japanese	Meat	Raw fish
Sauerbraten	German	Meat	Pot roast in spicy, aromatic, sweet-and-sour marinade
Scones	English	Grain	Round, flat, unleavened sweetened bread
Scrapple	Pennsylvania Dutch	Combination	Solid mush from cornmeal and the by-products of hog butchering
Shoofly pie	Pennsylvania Dutch	Dessert	Molasses pie
Shoyu	Japanese	Seasoning	Soy sauce
Sofrito	Puerto Rican	Seasoning	Specially seasoned tomato sauce
Sopapillos	Mexican	Grain	Rich fried bread
Spatzle	German	Grain	Small dumplings
Spoonbread	Virginia	Grain	Baked dish with cornmeal
Spumoni	Italian	Dessert	Fruited ice cream
Stollen	German	Dessert	Christmas fruitcake
Strickle sheets	Pennsylvania Dutch	Dessert	Coffee cake
Strudel	German	Dessert	Light pastry, filled with fruit or cheese
Tacos	Mexican	Combination	Fried tortillas, filled with meat, vegetables, and hot sauce
Tamales	Mexican	Grain	Pancake-like leathery bread
Tempura	Japanese	Combination	Deep-fried seafood or vegetables
Teriyaki sauce	Hawaiian	Accessory	Sweetened soy sauce
Tofu	Oriental	Meat	Soybean curd
Trotters	Southern U.S.	Meat	Pig's feet
Viandas	Puerto Rican	Vegetable	Starchy tropical vegetables, including plantain, green bananas, and sweet potatoes

planned around them, and the individual is more receptive to minor changes in the diet pattern.

EFFECTING CHANGE

In addition to knowing about usual food practices, the level of nutrition knowledge enables one to make nutritional suggestions that can be understood and are culturally appropriate (Dewey et al, 1984). Several basic facts will help in ap-proaching persons from various ethnic groups in order to promote sound nutritional practices (Suitor & Crowley, 1984):

1. One can find faults and advantages in each cultural food pattern. These patterns have contributed to the survival of the group in a particular environment. People have a remarkable ability to obtain a nutritious diet out of available foodstuffs. Some eating patterns that appear strange may actually be adaptive by enhancing or preserving nutritional value.

2. Other food patterns are nutritionally superior or at least comparable to "ordinary" American traditions.

3. Each food, food behavior, and tradition can be categorized as useful, neutral, or potentially harmful. A food that is beneficial promotes health by contributing necessary nutrients, such as the tofu in Oriental cooking, which increases the protein and calcium content of the diet. Neutral foods are not especially beneficial but are not harmful to health. Some customs may be harmful, and efforts should be made to alter these practices. For example, since many water-soluble vitamins are destroyed by heat, the practice of cooking foods (especially vegetables) for long periods of time is to be discouraged unless the liquids are consumed and/or iron cookware is used.

4. Food patterns are generally deeply ingrained, contribute to psychological stability, and are hard to change. If it is necessary to change the diet for health or medical reasons, suggest minimal alterations to traditional foods of the client and present the information with options to the whole family. Additionally, compliance is improved when the individual has some control over food choices, understands the meal plan, and feels responsible for following the suggestions (Maras & Adolphi, 1985).

5. Cultural patterns tend to be used more consistently by older family members.

The unique characteristics of several of the more prevalent ethnic and religious groups are presented in this chapter to provide some understanding of a few food practices that might affect the patient's acceptance of food and his/her ability to adjust to a special diet. It is not possible to cover the dietary practices of all cultures and religions. Furthermore, individuals from any culture have different tastes and preferences; therefore, it is important not to stereotype cultural groups. It is also important for the health care professional to become especially familiar with patterns common in his/her local area. Table 18–1 categorizes foods of different cultures and regions with a brief description to help introduce some unique and interesting foods.

Black American

Food of black Americans is not significantly different from other people living in the same area. Distinct differences exist between those living and raised in the North compared with those in the South. As a cultural group, many blacks are in lower socioeconomic groups, which of itself may precipitate nutritional problems. Nutrients that are often inadequate include iron, calcium, riboflavin, and vitamin A. As mentioned earlier, the frequency of deficiency for all nutrients is associated with economic factors.

Black Americans tend to have medical problems somewhat different from white Americans. Hypertension, twice as great among blacks than whites, is the major killer. Obesity, especially in women, and dental caries are other problems.

Soul foods have generally been cooked for long periods of time and are well-seasoned. Southern blacks economize in their cooking by preparing such foods as chicken wings, ribs, and chitterlings. Poke salad, collards, and many other greens and vegetables are combined with fatback and cooked for long periods.

Pica, or consumption of non-food items, was originally a cultural pattern among pregnant black women resulting from nutritional needs.

Geophagia, or the eating of earthy substances such as dirt or clay, is most common among children under three years of age and pregnant women and to some extent among males. It is found mainly in lower socioeconomic groups.

In many African societies, the biological need for calcium, iron, and other minerals by pregnant and lactating women is partially met by eating clays from nutrient-rich sources. Analysis of some clay "eggs" reveals comparable amounts of calcium, magnesium, potassium, copper, zinc, and iron as in supplements prescribed for pregnant women in modern societies (Farb & Armelagos, 1980). After arrival in the United States, they continued to eat clay, which is still sold in some areas of the South and shipped to relatives in the North. Geophagia leads to iron deficiency because the clay inhibits the absorption of iron and perhaps also potassium and zinc (Halsted, 1968). It is therefore believed that geophagia is both a cause and consequence of anemia.

When clay is not available, laundry starch is sometimes substituted, which can irritate the stomach and is almost entirely lacking in valuable minerals.

Clinical Implications:

• Blacks normally have lower hemoglobin levels and hematocrits (Garn et al, 1980; Dallman et al, 1978). While this may be partially caused by genetics, some studies suggest that nutritional factors may be responsible (Jackson et al, 1983).

- Many black people are lactose intolerant but can tolerate buttermilk, yogurt, and fermented cheese or sometimes small quantities of milk.
- Intake of iron, calcium, and vitamin A should be especially noted in a diet history since these nutrients are known to be low in the black American diet.
- Because of the high incidence of hypertension, sometimes necessitating a low-sodium diet, special attention should be given to the importance of seasoning foods to make them acceptable while limiting the use of salt.

Mexican

FOCUS ON *A TYPICAL MEXICAN MENU*

Breakfast
Fried eggs
Bacon
Tortillas
Café con leche

Lunch
Soup with noodles
Rice
Refried beans
Jalapeño peppers
Soda

Dinner
Beef stew with vegetables
Refried beans
Tortillas
Lettuce and tomato salad
Soda

Throughout Latin America, foods and illnesses are believed to possess varying degrees of "hot" and "cold." The classification is not rigidly defined, and foods placed in these two categories vary from person to person. The hot-cold theory is not based on the temperature of food. The degree of a food's hotness comes from the sun and refers to the energy contained by the plant or animal while it was alive. Cold foods include most fresh vegetables, staples, corn, beans and squash, most tropical fruits, and low-prestige meats (goat, fish, and chicken). Hot foods include chili peppers, onion, garlic, milk, cereal grains, beef, and most oils. Coldness can also come from contact with water; boiling hot soups are "cold" foods because of their water content. Hot foods are believed to be more easily digested than cold foods. A balanced intake of the contrasting "hot-cold" foods is supposed to maintain health. Contrasting foods eaten simultaneously blend in the stomach, tempering each other.

Mexican food is a fascinating combination of both Spanish and Indian influences, utilizing many foods native to America: beans, corn, tomatoes, avocados, and pumpkins (see *Focus on a Typical Mexican Menu*). Rice, olives, and almonds are also used extensively. Many flavors and seasonings are creatively combined. For example, they may combine nutmeg, chocolate, cinnamon, red pepper, and onions plus other seasonings in one recipe. Nothing that is typical of most cuisines is ordinarily done. There seems to be no limitations as to what seasonings can be combined.

The most typical dishes are the native Mexican ones, made with masa (corn kernels soaked in lime water then ground to a meal). These include tortillas (the bread of the Mexican culture), tamales, tacos, enchiladas, tostadas, and many others. Tortillas prepared from corn treated with lime water increases the calcium content about 15 times over that in the original corn, and possibly increases the availability of certain amino acids (Katz et al, 1974). Tortillas are now being prepared from wheat flour, so this excellent source of calcium is lost. However, flour tortillas are comparable nutritionally to white bread when enriched flour is used (Saldana & Brown, 1984). Yeast breads are increasingly replacing the tortilla.

Milk is usually limited in the diet, but some cheeses, especially Monterey Jack, are used in meal preparation. Meats, such as chicken, pork chops, wieners, cold cuts, and hamburger, are used several times a week. Dried beans, either pinto or calico, are staples of the Mexican diet, eaten at every meal. They are usually cooked, mashed, and refried and provide a good source of protein, iron, and calcium. Eggs are used frequently.

Basic vegetables include potatoes, fresh tomatoes, onions, carrots, and chilies from green and red peppers. Chili peppers, used as a seasoning, are a valuable source of vitamin A, supply some vitamin C, and even small amounts of the B vitamins. Where the intake of vitamins is marginal, they can make important nutritional contributions, even though they cannot be eaten in large amounts. Chili peppers contain capsaicin, which will lower the body temperature by causing sweating. Hot peppers have other attributes: (1) they facilitate the digestion of starches, (2) increase gastric secretions (Rosin, 1978), (3) stimulate the appetite by adding variety and increasing fluid intake and (4) inhibit the growth of some bacteria—namely, *Staphylococcus* and *Salmonella* (Pangborn, 1975). Chili pepper, onion, and garlic are the seasonings most frequently used. Lard, salt pork, and bacon fat are used for frying.

Most vegetables in the Mexican home are cooked so long that much of the original nutritive value is lost. Bananas and melons are popular fruits.

The most popular breakfast cereal used to be oatmeal, but it is being replaced by ready-to-eat cereals.

While the native Mexicans eat three large meals a day, families in the United States usually serve one main meal with leftovers or easily prepared snacks for the other meals. Candy and soft drinks are common snacks.

Clinical Implications

- Flour, cereal, and pasta products should be enriched.
- Intake of milk or cheese is normally low and might need to be increased.
- More dark green and deep yellow vegetables and foods rich in vitamin C could be incorporated into the diet.
- The use of fried foods probably should be decreased.
- Tortillas made with lime-treated cornmeal should be encouraged.

Puerto Rican

Similar to other Latin American cultural beliefs, many Puerto Ricans subscribe to the hot-cold theory of health and disease. However, they classify diseases as hot and cold, and food and medications as hot, cold, and cool.

As in other Latin American countries, both Indian and Spanish influences are reflected in the popular Puerto Rican national dishes. Rice (cooked grainy) and dry red or white beans stewed with bacon or olive oil, garlic, and onions

and often peppers are daily foods of the people. *Safrito* is a tasty mixture of tomatoes, green peppers, sweet chili peppers, onions, garlic, oregano, and fresh coriander cooked together in lard or vegetable oil and used as a relish to season foods.

A variety of fruits and vegetables—*viandas* (starchy vegetables including plantains, sweet potatoes, green bananas, cassava, and breadfruit), acerola, mango, avocado, corn, okra, chayotes, tubers, and citrus fruits—are eaten regularly in Puerto Rico. The acerola (also called the West Indian or Barbados cherry) is the highest known natural source of vitamin C (1000 mg/100 gm portion). However, many of these items are very expensive in the United States because they have to be imported. Fruits are usually eaten as snacks. Very few dark green leafy vegetables are used.

Chicken, pork, and beef are normally fried but are usually limited in the diet because they are expensive. Salted dried codfish (*bacalao*) is a popular dish. Eggs are frequently used as the main dish in the form of an omelet.

Even though milk is very well liked, it is seldom drunk as a beverage. Intake may be low because of its cost. *Café con leche* (coffee with milk) contains 2 to 5 oz. of milk and constitutes the largest part of milk intake. Native white cheese is popular but expensive.

Most foods are cooked a very long time or fried. Lard and salt pork are used to flavor many dishes. Malt beer has an exaggerated reputation for being very nutritious and may be given to children and lactating women.

A typical breakfast might consist of *café con leche* with or without bread; if income permits, butter, eggs, oatmeal, and fruit may be added. Lunch and dinner generally include rice and beans and/or *viandas,* sometimes with codfish and oil. As income permits, meats and a greater variety of foods are included. Dessert is not an essential part of the meal.

Clinical Implications:

- Pregnant Puerto Ricans have a high incidence of megaloblastic anemia and should possibly increase their intake of foods high in folic acid (Parker & Bowering, 1976).
- The diet of Puerto Ricans living in mainland cities may lack variety because of the inability to afford island foods they are accustomed to.
- For patients needing to control carbohydrate intake, *viandas* are counted as bread exchanges.

Cuban

Cubans enjoy many cut-up vegetables, fine stews, and casseroles flavored with sage, parsley, bay leaves, thyme, cinnamon, curry powder, capers, onions, cloves, garlic, and saffron. Saffron is such an integral part of Cuban foods that some dishes are considered anemic-looking and unpalatable unless they have a deep golden saffron hue.

Cubans serve soup at least once a day. Chicken, fish, or a meat soup is served before each major meal. A bowl of salad is always brought to the table, whether it is eaten or not. Fried foods, especially fish, poultry, and eggs, are popular.

Everyone eats rice and beans of many kinds. Fruits and vegetables are plentiful; however, Cuban refugees state that fruits and vegetables are not consumed regularly (Gordon, 1982). Cubans use a lot of plantains. A sample main meal, generally served at noon, is shown in *Focus on a Typical Cuban Dinner*.

Normally, breakfast is coffee and bread. Adults drink a lot of strong coffee and rum; milk and carbonated beverages are given to children.

Clinical Implications:

- Calcium intake is normally low; one should incorporate some cheese and milk into the diet.
- Teaching other methods of food preparation to replace frying and long cooking periods is beneficial.

Native American

Food scarcity and a lack of variety is still a problem for Native Americans living on reservations. Fresh fruits, vegetables, and meats are very expensive, if available at all. Traditional foods vary among tribes, but the basic Native American diet consists of corn, beans, and squashes. Corn is a status food for most tribes. Chili peppers add spice to the diet and are a good source of vitamin C.

Diets on some reservations are considered to be poor, supplying less than two thirds of the RDAs for one or more nutrients (Miller, 1981). Generally, diets tend to be inadequate in calories,

---

> **FOCUS ON** A TYPICAL CUBAN DINNER
>
> **Dinner**
> Rum
> Bean soup
> Bacalao
> (Salted dried codfish)
> Rice or Black Beans
> Boiled sweet potatoes
> Guava paste and cheese
> Coffee

---

calcium, iron, iodine, riboflavin, and vitamins A and C (Owen et al, 1981; Bass & Wakefield, 1974).

Several leading causes of death among Indians, especially tuberculosis, and high maternal and infant death rates are attributable to poverty and isolated living conditions. Poor nutrition is directly related to several leading causes of death. Heart diseases and cirrhosis of the liver are common; diabetes is three times more common in some tribes than the national average (Miller, 1981). Indians have the highest reported prevalance of noninsulin-dependent (Type II) diabetes mellitus. Hyperinsulinemia in the Pima tribe reflects a resistance to insulin action (Nagulesparan et al, 1982). Low hemoglobin values have been well documented, and mild thyroid deficiency is also frequent (ICND & DIPH, 1964).

Clinical Implications:

- Diets of most tribes tend to be inadequate in protein, calcium, and vitamins C and A, which should be noted. However, the biggest problem may be availability and economics.
- Lactase deficiency is prevalent among Indians; calcium and riboflavin sources other than milk should be encouraged.
- The request for dietary change must be accompanied by an understanding of the patient's lifestyle in order for the health care professional to help the individual implement the program (Glasbrenner, 1985).

Chinese

The Chinese feel that eating is truly one of the joys of life. Nourishment of the body for a happier and longer life is considered most important, thereby leading to the development of hygienic food and the belief in a harmonious mixture of foods.

The yin-yang concept reflects these beliefs. Foods and diseases are categorized as yin or yang, relating to the reaction a food has within the body and not its temperature or seasoning. Yin is a passive feminine force that complements the active, masculine yang. Yin foods are generally bland, such as grains and vegetables. Yang foods are very spicy, take a long time to prepare, contain a lot of fat, and are necessary for health and strength. Most meats, alcoholic beverages, and deep-fried dishes are considered yang.

Nutritionally, the yin-yang system has been beneficial, creating variety in the diet and balancing the amounts of animal protein, grains, and vegetables. The Chinese favor moderation in diet and would reject extreme diets (such as one allowing only raw fruits and vegetables). If a proposed diet is not balanced in terms of yin and yang foods, it may not be followed.

China is a very large country, and regional differences in eating habits exist, reflecting food availability and styles of cooking. In the northern areas (especially around Peking), wheat flour made into noodles, steamed bread, and dumplings are the staples. Foods are generally light and delicately seasoned, frequently with wine stock, garlic, and scallions.

Throughout the southern regions of China, rice is not only a staple but symbolizes life and fertility. Cuisine in southern regions (especially around Canton) offers the most varied menu. Cantonese cooking is subtle and the least greasy of all the regional styles, and excels at stir-frying. Szechwan cooking (southwestern China) is highly seasoned with fagara pepper, which is very strong and hot. Cooks from the coastal region in southeast China use more soy sauce and sugar and specialize in salty and gravy-laden dishes.

In general, the preparation of Chinese food takes longer than the actual cooking. The cutting technique is of prime importance. A properly planned dinner has small portions of several dishes. Although it may not have a main course, the meal will present a variety of colors, textures, and flavors.

Pork is the primary meat, eaten almost daily. Variety of flavor is also important, and small portions of chicken, duck, and lamb are bought by the ounce to garnish rice or to add to vegetable dishes.

Soybean products are abundant and cheap; hence, they are used in many ways in Oriental cuisine. Soybeans yield tofu (soybean curd), soy sauce, oil, and bean sprouts. Tofu is a good source of protein and iron, easily digested, and popular. It can also be a good source of calcium if calcium salts are used to precipitate the curd. Sweet-and-sour spareribs are frequently craved by expectant Chinese mothers. The preparation is nutritively adaptive since the use of vinegar leaches calcium from the rib bones into the meat, making it available to the body (Farb & Armelagos, 1980).

The Chinese use many different vegetables in cooking—bean sprouts, bamboo shoots, water chestnuts, gourds, and others. These are normally stir-fried or briefly cooked in hot water. A Chinese broth may cook for hours, but vegetables are not added until a short time before the soup is served. However, raw vegetables are rarely served. Popular seasonings are ginger, soy sauce, and garlic. While soybean oil, peanut oil, and lard are the most frequently used fats, the diet is low in fat.

Clinical Implications:

- The typical Chinese diet may be low in protein, calcium, and vitamin D; however, Christakis and colleagues (1968) reported that Chinese children in the United States had better diets than other ethnic groups examined.
- Because of the prevalence of lactose intolerance, milk and milk products are not normally used. However, tofu may be substituted, and milk in the form of cheese, custard, or ice cream may be accepted.
- Brown or enriched rice furnishes more vitamins, and its use should be encouraged.
- Raw vegetables may be refused because, in China, uncooked vegetables are often contaminated from organic fertilizer and may cause illness (Chang, 1974).
- Patients may refuse iced water because it is believed to shock the system and is harmful (Chang, 1974).
- Soy sauce becomes a problem in a sodium-restricted diet. Greater success has been attained by having patients measure and severely limit the use of soy sauce (Chang, 1974).

Japanese

Many Japanese dishes are ideally suited to American life, most being very economical and nutritious. The Japanese take great pride in the visual effects of foods they use. The arrangement of food, color contrast, and even shape are as important as cooking and seasoning. The rules for picking up chopsticks, holding bowls and teacups, and eating soups are well established.

Much of the food is cooked on a hibachi (a small grill) by broiling, steaming, boiling, and stir-frying. Stir-fry cooking preserves vitamins because the food is cooked only briefly.

Because meat is expensive in Japan, it is stretched with vegetables. Fish is used in many fascinating ways. Soybean products are an important source of protein. Tofu (soybean curd) is used extensively.

Many vegetables, usually steamed and served with soy sauce, are included. Seaweed, bamboo shoots, and bean sprouts are common vegetables. Few salads are served. Rice or noodles are staples and take the place of bread.

Fruit is the usual dessert, especially melons, berries, and tangerines. Other Japanese sweets are made of bean paste.

The use of extraordinary flavors is typical of Japanese cuisine; their wheat germ powder, called *ajinomoto*, enhances flavors. Soy sauce is also an important seasoning.

Unsweetened green tea is the national beverage, but beer and sake are popular and served with the meal. Milk is included in the children's diet, but rarely used by adults (see *Focus on a Typical Japanese Menu*).

Clinical Implications:

- Lactose intolerance is common among the Japanese, so other sources of calcium, such as tofu, are needed.
- One should encourage the use of enriched rice and discourage washing the grains before cooking to preserve nutrient value.
- For patients needing a sodium restricted diet, seasonings such as soy sauce and the many types of pickles ordinarily eaten should be noted.
- The intake of raw fish has been implicated in stomach cancer (Qureshi, 1981), carries a risk of infestation with fish tapeworms (Goldman, 1985), and has been associated with outbreaks of gastroenteritis (Morse et al, 1986).

FOCUS ON A TYPICAL JAPANESE MENU

Breakfast
Rice
Miso shiru
(Bean Paste Soup)
Egg (usually raw)
Tsukudami
(Fish cooked in shoyu)
Umeboski
(Salted plum)
Green tea

Lunch
Rice or noodles
(Saba, udon, or somen)
Boiled vegetables
Broiled fish
Green tea

Dinner
Rice
Suimono
(Clear soup)
Sashimi
(Raw fish)
Teriyaki fish
(Deep fried)
Chawani mushi
(Steamed custard)
Tsukemono
(Pickles)
Tempura
Green tea

Vietnamese

A blending of Chinese and French cuisines has resulted in the light and subtle tastes of Vietnamese cuisine. White rice and other foods are served separately rather than mixing them together; vegetables are stir-fried. As in other Oriental cultures, rice is a staple and may be eaten at all three meals. Because of the use of chopsticks, all items are cut in bite-size pieces before cooking.

Nuoc mam is a salty condiment added to almost every cooked dish. It is the liquid drained from wooden casks in which alternating layers of fresh fish and salt have been tightly packed and allowed to ferment. Other condiments may be added to *nuoc mam*, such as chili, garlic, and sugar, to vary the taste for blending with different foods.

One of the most popular dishes is a delicate beef-and-noodle soup called *pho*. Beef, beef bones, onions, ginger, and cinnamon are simmered all day long with water being added when necessary. Just before serving, freshly cut scallions, onions, more thinly sliced beef, bean sprouts, and thin white rice noodles are added and cooked briefly. *Nuoc mam*, may be added for flavor. Chicken soups, quite different from the Western type, are equally popular.

A wide variety of vegetables, such as bamboo shoots, bok choy, broccoli, carrots, cauliflower, cabbage, sweet potatoes, squash, watercress, and spinach are generally stir-fried or steamed. Many fruits are eaten raw. Sugar cane is plentiful.

Vietnamese from southern areas prefer spicier food than the people in the north; they also use a lot of coconut.

Very little fresh milk is available but may be given to the children. Sweetened condensed milk is available for coffee. Lactose intolerance is common.

Vietnamese prefer their foods as fat-free as possible and use vegetable oil for frying. Tea is the most popular beverage.

Clinical Implications:

- The amount of *nuoc mam* sauce used would be of concern for anyone on a sodium-restricted diet.
- Various ways of increasing the calcium content of the diet should be encouraged.

Korean

The main staple of the Korean diet is rice mixed with other grains, since a diet consisting only of white rice causes health problems. White rice is often mixed with barley, millet, and red beans.

The Koreans eat three hearty daily meals, all about the same proportion (see *Focus on a Typical Korean Menu*). The use of chopsticks makes it important to serve food cut into small pieces. Many foodstuffs are grilled. Soups, containing seaweed, meat, or fish are always served.

One of the most respected products in Korea is ginseng, whose root is said to resemble the hu-

---

FOCUS ON *A TYPICAL DAILY KOREAN MENU*

Breakfast
Cream of corn soup
Rice
Kimchi
Barley tea

Lunch
Soup
Hot turnip slices
Kimchi (two or more types)
Toasted seaweed
Rice
Barley tea

Dinner
Spinach salad
seasoned with sugar,
vinegar, and sesame oil
Kimchi (two or more types)
Dried fish
Rice
Barley tea

---

man fetus. It is said to be a panacea for curing illnesses regardless of age or sex and is considered an aphrodisiac.

Since Korea is surrounded on three sides by water, fish products abound and account for 85 percent of the nation's animal protein intake. Every conceivable kind of fish is served, either raw, freshly steamed, or salted and dried. Eggs are scarce and, therefore, expensive. Beef is the preferred meat. Meat marinades contain a lot of sugar and provide a crispy coating.

Kimchi is one of the most nutritious preservation processes available not requiring refrigeration. Chopped vegetables are highly seasoned, salted, and fermented underground or in special earthenware containers. *Kimchi* can be made from naturally grown vegetables, such as cabbage, turnips, cucumbers, and other seasonable vegetables. These vegetables are soaked in salted water overnight and seasoned the following day with garlic, scallions, ginger, and hot pepper. *Kimchi* must ferment without being disturbed for at least a month and is best after two or three months. At least one variety is served at each meal.

Many vegetables grow in Korea, and both fresh and *à la kimchi* ones are preferred staples. Vegetables are never overcooked. Vegetable dishes are seasoned with red and black pepper, garlic, sesame seed oil, and soy sauce. Many types of seaweed are available and are highly prized for their nutritive value; seaweed soup is a must for expectant mothers. Noodles, made from rice flour, are popular.

Many fresh fruits are available—apples, peaches, strawberries, pears, watermelon, blackberries, pomegranates, currants, cherries, and pears. Fruit is served morning and afternoon and with each meal. Although cakes and pastries are not usually served with meals, many small shops specialize in such goodies.

A number of products essential to the Korean diet are made from soybeans: soy sauce, soybean pastes, bean sprouts, bean curd, and soy milk. Bean curd and soy milk are the "dairy products" of Korea.

Since there is no room for a dairy industry in this densely populated country, only children are given milk, which may be purchased daily in very small (about 90 ml) containers. Because of the scarcity of milk, babies are often weaned as late as two years of age.

The basic seasonings of Korean cooking consist of soy sauce, bean paste, and red pepper paste. Other important ingredients that make the taste distinct are sesame seed, sesame oil, garlic, green onion, red pepper, vinegar, sugar, rice wine, mustard, and red pepper. Vegetable fats, such as sesame oil and bean oil (made from brown beans), are used for cooking.

Korea has never been a tea-drinking nation. Ginseng is made into a very popular drink. The beverage that usually accompanies a Korean meal is barley water, served cold in summer and warm in winter. Instead of wasting any grains stuck to the pan after the rice for the meal has been removed, a cup or two of water is added. This rice water simmers slowly while the meal is being eaten and is then served after the meal.

Clinical Implications:
- The medicinal properties of ginseng are poorly researched (Barna, 1985).
- Long-term abuse of ginseng may be associated with hypertension. Other adverse reactions (less frequently seen) can include nervousness, sleeplessness, skin eruptions, morning diarrhea, edema (Siegel, 1979), and irregularities in blood sugar level (Ginseng, 1980).
- Since rice in the United States is not mixed with other grains (as practiced in Korea) to in-

crease its nutritive value, the use of whole-grain or enriched rice should be encouraged.
- Stronger-tasting greens (turnip greens, kale, and mustard greens) might be substituted for the popular, but expensive, seaweed.
- Tofu and other sources of calcium for lactose-intolerant people is important.
- When sugar intake must be limited (as in diabetes), a sugar substitute can be dissolved in hot water and poured over the meat, which is broiled until the crispy texture is achieved (Maras & Adolphi, 1985).
- *Kimchi* provides a zesty accompaniment to plain boiled foods, but because it is not readily available in the United States, a Mexican salsa may be an acceptable substitute (Maras & Adolphi, 1985).

Italian

Italians have preserved their cultural heritage partly because of the importance they place on sharing food with families and friends. Mealtime is leisurely and associated with warmth and fellowship. Normally, breakfast is light and the largest meal is at noon with a smaller evening meal (see *Focus on a Typical Italian Lunch and Dinner*).

The Italians, with their fertile imagination, have developed two simple ingredients, flour and water, into numerous pastas, food that is deli-

FOCUS ON A TYPICAL ITALIAN LUNCH AND DINNER

Lunch
Risotto alla Milanese
(Rice, Milan style)
Zucchini e pepperoni fritti
(Summer squash with green peppers)
Fruit
Wine

Dinner
Olives and Insalata
Minestrone
Paticcio di Polenta
(Cornmeal dish with mushroom filling)
Wine

ciously filling, and a "budget stretcher" of expensive meats. Parmesan cheese is used as an accompaniment for flavoring many dishes. The native cheese is freshly grated into a wooden bowl before each meal and added to spaghetti, soup, or whatever the main course may be.

A healthy Italian habit is the eating of many greens. Salads are served whenever possible, at lunches and dinners. Popular vegetables are broccoli, escarole, asparagus, cauliflower, and mushrooms.

Veal, fish (fresh, dried, and pickled), highly seasoned cold cuts (salami, coppa, and prosciutto), and chicken are frequently used meats. Bread is essential to every meal. Heavy desserts are not desired, so the meal may be finished off with fresh fruit and cheese. Garlic, wine, olive oil, tomato puree, and a mixture of herbs (thyme, basil, oregano) are used to season foods.

Wine and black coffee are the beverages most frequently chosen. Milk is generally avoided because of milk-borne epidemics common in Italy in the past. Italians generally believe wine is good for adults to drink with a meal and even a small amount for children is good.

Clinical Implications:

- Since milk is seldom used as a beverage, one should determine if enough calcium is provided by the diet (especially for children).
- Italian breads may not be enriched and may not contain milk; the use of whole-grain or enriched breads should be encouraged.
- Domestic oils, such as soybean, cottonseed, and corn, are less expensive for cooking and seasoning foods than olive oil.

Middle Eastern

Nine separate countries around the eastern Mediterranean Sea (Greece, Turkey, Lebanon, Syria, Iraq, Iran, Israel, Jordan, and Egypt) are bound together by foods and certain attitudes toward food.

Lamb and goat are staple meats of the Middle East. Beef is not favored, where neither pasturage nor climate is suitable for cattle. A very popular meat dish is *dolma*, made of ground meat mixed with rice, herbs, and spices, and wrapped in leaves or stuffed into vegetables. The eastern Mediterranean countries enjoy all varieties of saltwater and fresh-water fish, shellfish, and roe. Many Moslems avoid pork and wild birds. Vegetables and legumes are frequently the main dish.

Bread is the staple of life: Each mouthful of food is eaten with a bite of bread (Valassi, 1962). A meal without bread is unthinkable, and the bread is usually homemade, fresh, and warm. The more compact dark bread is preferred to refined white bread.

Pilaf is a festive dish for the entire Near East. Beans and lentils rank just behind bread and rice in popularity. Boiled beans are served cold at breakfast with a dressing of olive oil and lemon juice—and perhaps a bit of garlic for extra taste.

A variety of vegetables, both cooked and raw, are served. The most frequent seasonings used in their preparation are onions, fresh tomatoes or tomato paste, olive oil, and parsley. In the Middle East, there are more than 120 ways of preparing eggplant.

The best-known sweet is baklava. However, sweets are served mostly on holidays or social calls, seldom as dessert. A bowl of fresh fruit is the usual dessert. This may consist of cucumbers, guavas, mangos, citrus fruits, dates, figs, pomegranates, or bananas.

Cooking fats used in Middle Eastern cooking include olive and sesame oil, butter, and *ghee* (clarified butter from goat, sheep, or camel milk). Animal fat is used when the dish is to be eaten hot; oil, when it is likely to be eaten cold. A meal is not regarded as tasteful and well prepared unless a large quantity of fat has been added. Mint, oregano, and cinnamon are popular spices; the most popular herb is garlic (except in Iran where it is considered vulgar). Olives in dozens of shapes and colors are popular.

Milk is not normally consumed as a beverage by adults; however, it is given to children. Many Middle Easterners feel yogurt is the supreme health food, curing many ills, conferring long life and good looks, prolonging youth and fortifying the soul. Yogurt is used in many ways: mixed with diced cucumber as an appetizer; as a topping on rice, fried vegetables, and desserts; or eaten plain. Thin yogurt (diluted with water) is safer and less perishable than milk and very thirst-quenching. A Greek specialty cheese is feta, a white cheese from sheep's or goat's milk.

The Moslem faith forbids wine, and many people in the Near East do not drink alcoholic beverages. Christians and Jews, of course, follow a different tradition. No meal is ended without coffee or tea, but coffee takes precedence most of the time. In Iran, the favorite drink is tea, hot and sweet.

Clinical Implications:

- The protein and calcium content of the diet can be increased by encouraging intake of yogurt and white cheese.
- In planning carbohydrate-limited diets, one of the difficulties is to decrease bread consumption.
- The amount of fat in the diet could pose problems for low-kilocalorie, diabetic, or low-fat diets.
- The traditional feta cheese and olives, two favorite foods, are high in sodium and would have to be eliminated from a sodium-restricted diet.

Religious Food Restrictions

Religious beliefs affect eating patterns, attaching symbolic meanings to food and drink. Some examples of this are the bread and wine served during the Christian communion service and the Hindu reverence for the cow. These patterns do not usually result in any nutritional problems but could affect patients' food intake during a hospital stay or make them uncooperative about a dietary prescription.

JEWISH

The Jewish dietary laws are adhered to in varying degrees owing to the differences in interpre-

1. Only meat from the forequarter of cloven-hoofed quadrupeds that chew cud (cattle, sheep, goat, or deer) is allowed. The animals must have been killed observing rigid rules that result in minimal pain to the animal and maximal blood drainage. Preparations of koshered meats may be by one of two methods.
   A. The meat is soaked in cold water for half an hour; salted with coarse salt; and drained to let blood run off. It is then thoroughly washed under cold running water and drained again before cooking.
   B. The meat is first prepared by quick searing, which permits liver to be eaten since it cannot be prepared by the above method.
2. Meat and dairy products cannot be served at the same meal, nor can they be cooked or served in the same set of dishes. Milk or milk products may be consumed just before a meal, but not until six hours after eating a meal with meat products. Fish or eggs can be eaten with dairy products or meat meals. Eggs that have a blood spot are not allowed.
3. Only fish with fins and scales are allowed; no shellfish or scavenger fish may be eaten.

tation and importance placed by the three basic groups: (1) Orthodox—strict observance, (2) Conservative—nominal observance, and (3) Reform—less ceremonial emphasis and minimum observance of the general dietary laws.

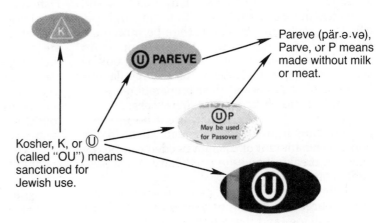

Figure 18–2: Kosher food labeling: All designations mean kosher; the Ⓤ signifies the endorsement of the Union of Orthodox Rabbis, which honors the strictest Jewish laws. Other designations, such as "K," are usually local sanctions.

Pareve (pär·ə·və), Parve, or P means made without milk or meat.

Kosher, K, or Ⓤ (called "OU") means sanctioned for Jewish use.

Table 18–2. *Food Restrictions of Various Religions*

Religious Group and Food Restrictions	Clinical Implications with Institutional Situations or with Modified Diets
Catholic Abstinence from meat, meat soups, or gravy on Ash Wednesday and Fridays during Lent.	Fish or other meat substitutes are generally offered on these days.
Mormons No alcoholic beverages. No stimulants.	Substitutes should be given to patients for regular coffee, tea, and most carbonated beverages, especially if the patient is on a liquid diet.
Moslems No pork or pork products. No animal shortenings. Only kosher meats allowed. Regular gelatin, marshmallow, and other confections containing gelatin are not allowed. No alcoholic products or beverages (including extracts such as vanilla or lemon). Fasting is common (mandatory for one month each year). Recommended foods: honey, milk, dates, meat, seafood, and vegetable and olive oil (Sakr, 1971).	Hospitalized patients may need assistance in selecting from hospital menus to see that the vegetables are not cooked with any animal shortenings or pork seasonings. While institutional meats are not normally kosher, they may be purchased. One should assist the patient in selecting from the hospital menu to be certain s/he receives adequate food considering these restrictions. Fasting can be precarious with some medical problems, especially diabetes and hypoglycemia. Some of these foods may be contraindicated on a special diet (honey on a diabetic diet) and should be noted.
Seventh-Day Adventists Optional vegetarianism: (1) strict vegetarianism, (2) lactoovovegetarianism, (3) no pork or pork products, shellfish, or blood.	If sodium is restricted, the use of soy-based meat analogs should be noted because they are high in sodium. Strict vegetarians need assistance to select a well-balanced menu from the regular hospital diet. Assist patients in choosing from hospital menu to receive foods not seasoned with pork.
No alcoholic beverages. No beverages containing caffeine. Snacking between meals is discouraged (mealtimes are at intervals of five to six hours).	Substitutes should be made for the regular coffee, tea, and some carbonated beverages ordinarily given, especially if the patient is on a liquid diet. Some diabetic, hypoglycemic, and ulcer-type diets require more frequent feedings.

Regulations about the types of food that may or may not be eaten are derived from biblical laws. Jewish people observe many holidays and holy days that are associated with fasting and specific food traditions. Foods that are permitted are called kosher, which means fitting or proper. An example of labels identifying kosher foods is shown in Figure 18–2. Some of the regulations with regard to foods and their preparation are described in *Focus on Jewish Food Restrictions*.

The Jewish dietary laws present no problem in providing nutritionally adequate diets in the home. (The amount of calcium needed can be obtained at breakfast and the one "dairy" meal ordinarily consumed.)

Other than food restrictions, Jewish cookery is influenced by the country or locale in which they are living, and the country from which they migrated (e.g., France or Germany). The diet is rich in pastries, cakes, preserves, and relishes. Fish and dairy products are used abundantly.

Because of a high incidence of diabetes, obesity, and coronary heart disease, therapeutic diets are often necessary. To insure compliance with a diet, it is important to take a careful dietary history. Diabetic and weight reduction diets can be planned to provide variety within compliance of the restrictions and to include some favorite foods, such as bagels or matzoh.

Clinical Implications:

Kosher meats are not generally purchased for the hospital but are available from wholesale distributors.

- Foods can be cooked in foiled-lined pans and served on disposable plates.
- Frequently, some foods that are not kosher are overlooked, including crackers, margarine, bread, gelatin, and broth-type soups.
- Special attention should be given to the insulin-requiring diabetic for special holiday traditions, especially those requiring fasting and serving wine in religious celebrations.
- Sodium-restricted diets also present problems because kosher meat may contain twice as much sodium as conventionally-processed meat. However, soaking beef or veal in a large amount of water removes all the added salt (Burns & Neubort, 1984; Kisch, 1953). Many favorite Jewish foods are highly salted and must be noted.

OTHER RELIGIONS

Table 18–2 lists food restrictions and practices of several religious groups. These restrictions need consideration only in institutional settings and sometimes when the individual is on a modified diet.

Summary

Once again, we are reminded of the basic concept of nutrition whereby the body needs nutrients, not specific foods. Nutritionally, individuals have traits reflecting their culture and heritage, their religion, and their social or economic status. Various cultural food patterns have resulted in the survival of that culture; problems resulting from these patterns are generally due to extenuating circumstances, such as economic problems. When nutritional problems are manifest, it is our responsibility to assist individuals to make compromises or subtle changes, not by trying to change their whole diet. A knowledge of the nutrients in many foods will help them to supplement the dietary intake in deficient areas.

Review Questions

1. What ethnic groups are most prevalent in your area?
   a. List dietary problems and some suggestions for altering the diet.
   b. Plan a two-day menu that would fulfill the RDAs and utilize many of their favorite foods or habits.
   c. Would an individual have any problem being able to follow that menu, such as economic hardship or the local availability of special foods?
2. What are the two main determinants for food choices?
3. In working with individuals whose food patterns are different, what five facts should be remembered?
4. Other than good foods to eat, what other life-long eating customs are learned as a child?
5. State some reasons why all Caucasians in the United States do not have the same eating patterns.
6. You notice on the chart that a new patient is Jewish. Discuss the consequences of each of the following actions:
   a. Calling in the regular diet order written by the physician, ignoring the fact the patient is Jewish.
   b. Calling the dietitian to come talk to the patient immediately.
   c. Checking with the patient to see if s/he has food preferences that would necessitate special foods.
7. Why is it important to be especially sensitive to an individual's eating habits when they are ill?
8. Define geophagia and pica. Are these practices helpful or harmful and why?
9. Name the cultures associated with the following terms:
   a. Soul food
   b. Hot-cold foods
   c. Pasta
   d. Yin and Yang

Case Study: A community health nurse is assigned to an area of the city that has a concentration of Southeast Asians. In assessing the nutritional status of an individual, she makes the following observations:
- Many of the new immigrants are at nutritional risk because they may have lived in areas with decreased availability of food or have been in prison camps for up to five years.
- Pregnant women often restrict their food intake during the last trimester to ensure small babies and easier deliveries. Little emphasis is placed on the pregnant woman's diet.
- Fruits and vegetables are often restricted in the first month postpartum.
- There is minimal intake of dairy products.
- Babies are usually bottle-fed, which may lead to problems with sanitation and proper preparation of the formula.

- Bottles filled with milk or sweetened liquids are used as pacifiers.

What nutritional problems can you identify from this data? How can the community health team work together to eliminate these problems?

REFERENCE LIST

Barna, P: Food or drug? The case of ginseng. *Lancet* 2(September 7):548, 1985.

Bass, MA; Wakefield, LM: Nutrient intake and food patterns of Indians on Standing Rock reservation. *J Am Diet Assoc* 64(1):36, 1974.

Burns, ER; Neubort, S: Sodium content of koshered meat (letter). *JAMA* 252(21):2960, 1984.

Chang, B: Some dietary beliefs in Chinese folk culture. *J Am Diet Assoc* 65(4):436, 1974.

Christakis, G; Miridjianian, A; Nath, L; et al: A nutritional epidemiologic investigation of 642 New York City children. *Am J Clin Nutr* 21(1):107, 1968.

Dallman, PR; Barr, GD; Allen, CM; et al: Hemoglobin concentration in white, black and oriental children: Is there a need for separate criteria in screening for anemia? *Am J Clin Nutr* 31(3):377, 1978.

Dewey, KG; Metallinos, ES; Strode, MA; et al: Combining nutrition research and nutrition education—dietary change among Mexican-American families. *J Nutr Ed* 16(1):5, 1984.

Farb, P; Armelagos, G: *Consuming Passions: The Anthropology of Eating.* Boston, Houghton Mifflin Co, 1980.

Garn, SM; Ryan, AS; Abraham, S: The black-white difference in hemoglobin levels after age, sex and income matching. *Ecol Food Nutr* 10(2):69, 1980.

Glasbrenner, K: Seeking Indian-acceptable ways to fight hypertension. *JAMA* 254(14):1877, 1985.

Ginseng. *Med Lett Drugs Ther* 22(17):72, 1980.

Goldman, DR: Hold the sushi (letter). *JAMA* 253(17):2495, 1985.

Gordon, AM, Jr: Nutritional status of Cuban refugees: A field study on the health and nutriture of refugees processed at Opa Locka, Florida. *Am J Clin Nutr* 35(3):582, 1982.

Halsted, JA: Geophagia in man: Its nature and nutritional effects. *Am J Clin Nutr* 21(12):1384, 1968.

Interdepartmental Commission of National Defense and Division of Indian Public Health (ICND & DIPH): *Fort Belknap Indian Reservation: Nutrition Survey.* Washington, DC: U.S. Public Health Service, 1964.

Jackson, RT; Sauberlich, HE; Skala, JH; et al: Comparison of hemoglobin values in black and white male U.S. military personnel. *J Nutr* 113(1):165, 1983.

Katz, SH; Hediger, ML; Valleroy, LA: Traditional maize processing techniques in the New World. *Science* 184(May 17):765, 1974.

Kisch, B: Salt poor diet and Jewish dietary laws. *JAMA* 153(16):1472, 1953.

Maras, ML; Adolphi, CL: Ethnic tailoring improves dietary compliance. *Diab Ed* 11(4):47, 1985.

Miller, MB: Supplementing and adding variety to the diets of Indians on a reservation in Minnesota. *J Am Diet Assoc* 78(6):626, 1981.

Morse, DL; Guzewich, JJ; Hanrahan, JP: Widespread outbreaks of clam- and oyster-associated gastroenteritis. *N Engl J Med* 314(11):678, 1986.

Nagulesparan, M; Savage, PJ; Knowler, WC; et al: Increased in vivo insulin resistance in nondiabetic Pima Indians compared with Caucasians. *Diabetes* 31(11):952, 1982.

Owen, GM: Garry, PJ; Seymore, RD; et al: Nutrition studies with White Mountain Apache pre-school children in 1976 and 1969. *Am J Clin Nutr* 34(2):266, 1981.

Pangborn, RM: Cross-cultural aspects of flavor preferences. *Food Tech* 29(6):34, 1975.

Parker, SL; Bowering, J: Folacin in diets of Puerto Rican and black women in relation to food practices. *J Nutr Ed* 8(2):73, 1976.

Qureshi, BA: Nutrition and multi-ethnic groups. *Royal Soc Health J* 101(5):187, 1981.

Riggs, S: Tastes of America: Regionality. *Institutions* 87(12):76, 1980.

Rosin, P: The use of characteristic flavorings in human culinary practice. In *Flavor: Its Chemical, Behavioral and Commercial Aspects.* Edited by CM Apt. Boulder, CO, Westview Press, 1978, p 101.

Sakr, A: Dietary regulations and food habits of Muslims. *J Am Diet Assoc* 58(2):126, 1971.

Saldana, G; Brown, HE: Nutritional composition of corn and flour tortillas. *J Food Sci* 49(4):202, 1984.

Schwerin, HS; Stanton, JL; Smith, JL; et al: Food, eating habits, and health: A further examination of the relationship between food eating patterns and nutritional health. *Am J Clin Nutr* 35(5 Suppl):1319, 1982.

Siegel, RK: Ginseng abuse syndrome. Problems with the panacea. *JAMA* 241(15):1614, 1979.

Suitor, CW; Crowley, MF: *Nutrition: Principles and Applications in Health Promotion,* 2nd ed. Philadelphia, J. B. Lippincott Co, 1984.

Valassi, KV: Food habits of Greek Americans. *Am J Clin Nutr* 11(3):240, 1962.

Zifferblatt, SM; Wilbur, CS; Pinsky, JL: Understanding food habits. *J Am Diet Assoc* 76(1):9, 1980.

Further Study

Cantoni, M: Adapting therapeutic diets to the eating patterns of Italian Americans. *Am J Clin Nutr* 6(5):548, 1958.

Cultural Food Patterns in the U.S.A. Chicago, American Dietetic Association, 1976.

Cusor, D; Wagner, MG: The changing role of the service professional within the ghetto. *J Am Diet Assoc* 60(1):21, 1972.

DeGracia, R: Cultural influences on Filipino patients. *Am J Nurs* 79(8):1412, 1979.

Fathauer, G: Food habits—an anthropologist's view. *J Am Diet Assoc* 37(4):335, 1960.

Gordon, JH; Kilgore, V: Planning ethnic menus. *Hospitals* 45(November 1):87, 1971.

Guinn, B: Emotions and obesity among Mexican American children. *J School Health* 55(3):113, 1985.

Hallman, P: A view of the Chinese family. *J Home Ec* 77(summer):28, 1985.

Hongladarom, H; Russell, M: An ethnic difference—lactose intolerance. *Nurs Outlook* 24(12):764, 1976.

James, S: When your patient is black West Indian. *Am J Nurs* 78(11):1908, 1978.

Koh, ET; Chi, MS: Clinical signs found in association with nutritional deficiencies as related to race, sex, and age for adults. *Am J Clin Nutr* 34(8):1562, 1981.

Ludman, EK; Newman, JM: Yin and yang in the health-related food practices of three Chinese groups. *J Nutr Ed* 16(1):3, 1984.

Nutrition Education and the Spanish-Speaking American: An Annotated Bibliography, 1961–72. *J Nutr Ed* 5(suppl 1), 1973.

Pasqualis, EA: The impact of acculturation on the eating habits of elderly immigrants: A Cuban example. *J Nutr Elderly* 5(1):27, 1985.

Peterson, DB; Datlani, JT; Baylis, JM; et al: Dietary practices of Asian diabetics. *Br Med J* 292(January 18):170, 1986.

Primeaux, M: Caring for the American Indian patient. *Am J Nurs* 77(1):91, 1977.

Roberts, LJ: A basic food pattern for Puerto Rico. *J Am Diet Assoc* 30(5):1097, 1954.

Spillman, DM: Some practical considerations of the Jewish dietary laws. *J Nutr Elderly* 5(1):47, 1985.

Wilson, CS: Food-Custom and Nurture. *J Nutr Ed* 11(suppl 1), 1979 (contains an annotated bibliography on sociocultural and biocultural aspects of nutrition).

DIET THERAPY

Basic Dietary Management of Patients

19

THE STUDENT WILL BE ABLE TO:

- *State the purposes of diet modifications.*
- *Explain the effect of illness on appetite and nutritional status.*
- *Define the basic modified diets.*
- *List nutritional information that should be recorded on the patient chart.*
- *Properly prepare the patient for feeding.*
- *Discuss the role of nursing in implementing and evaluating the nutrition care plan.*
- *Demonstrate proper procedures for serving trays.*
- *Determine when patients' dietary orders should be changed.*

Diet therapy
Diets—clear-liquid, full-liquid, pureed, mechanical-soft, light, dental-liquid, and as tolerated

OBJECTIVES

TERMS TO KNOW

Section I discussed the basic principles for good nutrition; Section II discussed how nutritional requirements and status are affected during various stages of life and cultural influences on eating habits; Section III involves nutrition for illnesses or disease states. A diet modification involves deviation from the normal diet to meet the physiological needs for specific disease requirements. Conditions or diseases alter the body's physiological needs or utilization of different nutrients; in spite of this, the individual's requirement for other nutrients must be maintained. This sometimes can become complicated because, as you have seen from studying basic nutrition principles, each food contributes an assortment of nutrients. For example, milk provides not only calcium but also protein, lactose, and riboflavin and may also be a source of saturated fats. Knowledge of nutrient content of foods, physiological requirements, and nutrient utilization is necessary to be able to participate in nutritional care.

Many of the vitamin-deficiency diseases, such as scurvy, pellagra, and rickets, have virtually been eliminated because of nutritional knowledge, enrichment and fortification, and a better food supply. Nevertheless, many conditions exist in which diet modification can lengthen the life span and improve the quality of life.

Diet Therapy

DEFINITION

A therapeutic or modified diet may be regarded as a modification of the normal diet to treat the disease or illness. Recommended nutrient allowances for healthy individuals are a first consideration, then necessary adaptations of specific conditions in relation to the disease state are made. Usually, the diet is an adjunct to medical or surgical care; in instances such as phenylketonuria, it may be the principal treatment. Sodium restriction or weight reduction can reduce or eliminate medication for hypertension or diabetes. On the other hand, such a close correlation may not be evident, but diet is always essential in cell maintenance, growth, and repair.

Physical problems may require different feeding patterns, such as tube feedings due to surgery or restrictions in the digestive tract. Nutrients may not be utilized because of conditions such as sprue. Whatever the past or present status, the goal for diet therapy is optimal nutriture for the patient. If the gastrointestinal tract is functional, the oral method of feeding is preferred to other feeding modalities. The advantages of gastrointestinal feedings (as opposed to intravenous feedings) are discussed in Chapter 21.

PURPOSES

A modified diet may change one or more dietary factors, as shown in Table 19–1. Modified diets may be prescribed as a preventive measure for individuals who are genetically predisposed to heart disease or hypertension (see Chapter 14). A combination of diet modifications may also be used. An example of this is a 1500 kcal, 1 gm sodium diet that might be necessary for a diabetic with hypertension.

Nutritionally inadequate diets are sometimes temporarily required to correct a serious problem. While a low-residue diet is inadequate in nutrients, it may be necessary to rest the gastrointestinal tract during acute digestive disorders. Inadequate diets are usually labeled as such in the diet manual, and supplementation with missing nutrients is possible.

Goals for diet therapy can be any one or a combination of the following:
1. To maintain normal or optimal nutritional status even though illnesses may increase requirements, e.g., a high-protein diet for persons in traction.
2. To correct nutritional deficiencies that may occur, e.g., anemia.
3. To correct body weight in over- or underweight patients.
4. To provide rest for the body or for certain organs, e.g., a low-protein diet for kidney disease.

Table 19–1. *Modification of Dietary Factors*

Modification	Example
Consistency	Liquid
Texture	Low residue
Seasoning or flavor	Bland
Energy value	Caloric modification
Nutrient levels (such as for fat, carbohydrate protein, or sodium)	1 gm sodium, 40 gm protein

5. To adjust nutrient intake to a level the body can properly metabolize, e.g., the diabetic diet.

Diet Manual

The American Dietetic Association (ADA) has prepared the *Handbook of Clinical Dietetics* (1981), which documents the scientific basis for dietary modification in treatment of specific disorders and includes food lists and sample menus for various modified diets. Even though these guidelines are established for all therapeutic diets, each facility decides on its own manual.

Under Medicare's *Conditions of Participation for Hospitals,* the hospital is required to have an up-to-date manual that has been jointly approved by the medical and dietary staffs. A committee may combine efforts to write a manual for a specific area. A copy of the adopted manual is usually available in the main office, or at the head nurse's desk for the convenience of physicians and nurses, at all nursing stations, and of course, in the dietary department.

A good diet manual states the exact regimen to be followed with clearly-defined restrictions to avoid decisions being made by those who are not sufficiently trained. Slight variations in diet manuals occur, but the overall principles will be consistent. Local eating habits are generally reflected in them in order to clarify whether favorite items are allowed on the various regimens. These manuals are written to provide:

- Guidance for food preparation.
- Information about available dietary regimens for particular conditions and their nutritional adequacy.
- A specific list of foods allowed and avoided.
- Standards for monitoring the patient by all professional staff members.

DIET NOMENCLATURE

Titles of diets, ideally, should specifically describe the diet. Naming the disease, such as "ulcer diet," is not as accurate as "bland diet." People do not like being labeled by their conditions, nor does it increase morale. The more precise terminology allows the diet to be used for patients with an ulcer or several other conditions requiring chemically and mechanically nonirritating foods. (The "diabetic diet" is the exception to this rule, since it is still called by the name of the condition.)

High- or low-calorie or other nutrient diets are not precise enough; the diet should specify the number of kilocalories or grams of nutrients to be controlled. A "low-sodium" request can be more accurately filled when the order reads "500 mg sodium."

In the past, several diet plans become known by the author's name—Sippy's, Muelengracht's, and Kempner's diets; these have become obsolete as a result of new knowledge and changing philosophies, which led to the development of more appropriate diets.

THE DIET PRESCRIPTION

In most instances, the physician orders an appropriate diet for every patient admitted, whether it is a regular (or normal) or modified diet. This should be a reflection of the patient's symptoms, laboratory tests, and nutritional needs.

The patient's diet prescription, reflecting the disease condition, should vary as little as possible from the patient's normal diet. The diet should take into consideration various personal factors that could interfere with an individual's ability to follow the diet: food habits and preferences, economic status, religious beliefs, who prepares the meals, and where the meals are eaten. For instance, a traveling salesman frequently has problems following a bland or sodium-restricted diet.

The medical prescription is vital to the client, as is the prescribed diet. The two are closely interrelated. The diet prescription, like one for drugs, should specify the type of nutrients, amount (kilocalories or dosage), frequency or time of administration, route of food ingestion or drug administration when applicable, and the necessity of nutrient supplementation compromised by the modifications. The patient should be involved in the decision-making process to determine the expected outcome or goals.

Depending on the patient's condition, the order may vary from nothing by mouth (NPO) to any of the specific therapeutic diets or the regular diet. Records of this order are sent by the nurse's station to the dietary department. As the patient's condition is monitored, the diet order changes appropriately.

Basic Diet Modifications

In spite of numerous diet modifications available for various abnormal conditions, most hospital diets are based on a regular diet with variations in texture and consistency. As shown in Tables 19–2 and 19–3, hospital diets are designed to follow a sequence. Normally, the patient is NPO for a few hours before surgery. After surgery, clear-liquid diets help the patient return to normal absorption and digestion patterns. The full-liquid diet is then instituted, followed by the soft, and then the regular diet. The main concern is to provide continuous dietary support to the fullest degree possible for the prevailing circumstances.

CLEAR-LIQUID DIET

Only clear liquids or clear substances that liquefy at room temperature (e.g., gelatin) are allowed.

Indications. The clear-liquid diet provides clear fluids to relieve thirst, prevent dehydration, maintain electrolyte balance, yield minimal bowel residue, and test the ability to tolerate oral feedings. Broth provides some sodium; carbonated beverages, sugar; and fruit juices, a small amount of carbohydrate and potassium. Clear liquids are indicated for short-term use, usually no longer than 24 to 48 hours, following periods of acute vomiting or diarrhea or surgery.

A new progressive trend is to increase the nutrient intake during this period. A few institutions have even phased out the clear-liquid diet because of its nutritional inadequacies in favor of specific items that promote optimum nutrition and decrease the length of stay in the hospital. Several supplements of high-nutrient content are appropriate. High-protein broth mixes (such as Delmark's) provide high-quality protein and more calories yet contain half as much sodium as a standard broth. Citrotein beverages (Doyle) and Surgical Liquid Diet (Ross SLD) are nutritionally balanced, have specified osmolarities and are suggested for use until the patient can tolerate normal foods of higher nutrient content (Murray et al, 1985).

Characteristics. The amount of fluid in a given feeding on the clear-liquid diet is usually restricted to 30 to 60 ml/hr at first, gradually increasing the amount as tolerance improves. Some facilities allow only apple juice on the very strict clear-liquid diet; others may allow all juices except prune and tomato. (Some juices, e.g., orange, may not be well-tolerated, causing stomach distention.) The most preferred items on this diet are tea, ginger ale, and apple juice.

Some facilities require decaffeinated coffee while others do not. Such policies should be verified in the diet manual.

them to be of practical value to replace electrolytes lost in vomitus and diarrheal fluid. Commercial supplements provide more nutrients.

FULL-LIQUID DIET

Foods that are liquid or liquefy at room temperature, including all items on the clear-liquid diet plus milk and some milk-containing products, make up the full-liquid diet (Turner, 1970).

Indications. The full-liquid diet frequently is indicated for individuals who (1) are unable to chew, swallow, or tolerate solid foods; (2) have acute infections and fever of short duration; or (3) lack appetite. Nourishment in the form of full liquids may be necessary following oral surgery or plastic surgery of the face and neck, for example,

Table 19–2. Foods Allowed in Progressive Hospital Diets

Food Group	General	Mechanical-Soft	Soft or Light	Full-Liquid	Clear-Liquid
Milk and calcium equivalents	All	Milk and milk beverages, eggnog, yogurt, ice cream, pudding, cream soups, cottage cheese, cheese, and custards.	Same as mechanical-soft plus mild cheese.	Milk and milk beverages, eggnog, yogurt, ice cream, pudding, and custard.	None
Meat and protein equivalents	All	Eggs, tender meats or meats processed by grinding or chopping, peanut butter, creamed meats, and casseroles.	Tender or ground chicken, fish, beef, lamb, liver, veal; eggs; and simple casseroles.	Pureed meats added to cream soups.	None
Fruits and vegetables	All	All juices, all pureed fruits and vegetables, applesauce, ripe banana, cooked or canned tender fruits and vegetables, and mashed potatoes.	Cooked low-fiber vegetables; boiled, mashed, creamed, scalloped, or baked potatoes; fruit juices; cooked and canned fruits (without seeds, coarse skins, or fiber); and bananas.	Strained fruit juices, whipped potatoes, vegetable juices, and vegetable puree in soup.	Grape, cranberry, apple juice, other strained fruit juices, and vegetable water.
Grain	All	Cooked cereals, dry cereals served with milk, cooked noodles, rice, enriched and whole-wheat bread, refined crackers, simple cakes, and plain cookies served with a beverage.	Refined or finely ground cooked cereals, noodles, rice, spaghetti and macaroni (not highly seasoned), fine whole grain, rye without seeds, enriched white breads, toast, crackers, melba toast, zwieback, graham crackers, plain cookies, and cake.	Cooked refined cereals, strained or blended gruels.	None
Other beverages	All	All	All	All	Carbonated beverages, tea, coffee, clear broth, clear fruit-flavored drinks.
Fat	All	Butter, margarine, cream sauces, and gravies.	Broth, strained cream soups, butter, margarine, gravy, and plain sauces.	Margarine, butter, gravy, and cream.	None
Sweets	All	Puddings, pies, sherbet, and gelatin desserts.	Gelatin and sherbet.	Clear candies, honey, sugar, Popsicles, plain sugar-sweetened gelatin, syrup, and sherbet.	Syrup, clear candies, honey, sugar, Popsicles, sugar sweetened gelatin, and ices.
Miscellaneous	All	Soups, seasonings.	Mild seasonings.		

Table 19–3. *Meal Plans for Progressive Diets*

	General	Mechanical-Soft	Soft	Full-Liquid	Clear-Liquid
Breakfast	Orange juice, scrambled eggs, bacon, buttered toast, apricot preserves, and coffee or tea.	Orange juice, scrambled eggs, buttered toast, grape jelly, and coffee or tea.	Orange juice, scrambled eggs, buttered toast, grape jelly, and coffee or tea.	Apple juice, Cream of Wheat with butter or margarine and sugar, orange gelatin, and coffee with cream and sugar. Vanilla ice cream.	Apple juice, chicken broth, high-calorie orange gelatin, and coffee or tea with sugar.
Morning nourishment					Carbonated beverage.
Lunch	Roast beef with gravy, rice, green beans, bran muffin with margarine, apple pie, and iced tea or milk.	Chopped roast beef, rice, chopped green beans, roll with margarine, chopped apple cobbler, and iced tea or milk.	Roast beef, rice, green beans, rolls with margarine, apple sauce, and iced tea or milk.	Tomato juice, beef broth with strained roast beef; vanilla pudding; milk; and tea with sugar, lemon, or cream. Eggnog (commercial preparation).	Grape juice, beef broth, high-calorie strawberry gelatin, and coffee or tea with sugar.
Afternoon nourishment					Tea and Popsicle.
Supper	Baked chicken, baked potato, buttered carrots, tossed salad, rolls with margarine, pineapple sherbet, and cookies.	Chopped baked chicken, baked potato, chopped carrots, pear half (canned), roll with margarine, pineapple sherbet, and milk.	Baked chicken, baked potato, buttered carrots, pear half (canned), rolls with margarine, pineapple sherbet, and milk.	Orange juice, cream of potato soup, strawberry gelatin, pineapple sherbet, and tea with sugar, lemon, or cream.	Cranberry juice, chicken broth, carbonated beverage, Popsicle, and tea with sugar.
Evening nourishment				Hot chocolate.	High-calorie gelatin.

and in patients with esophageal strictures or mandibular fractures. The full-liquid diet has traditionally been used as a step in the progression from clear liquids to solid foods, but often this is unnecessary (see Table 19–2).

Characteristics. The main criterion for foods on the full-liquid diet is that they "pour." The diet should be smooth, easy to swallow, require no chewing, have minimal amounts of fiber, and become liquid at room or body temperature. Protein and kilocalories are easily increased to higher energy levels if desired. The goal is for maximum nutrients per serving, so each serving is usually fortified with other foods as much as possible.

A variety of foods may be used, including milk, plain frozen desserts, pasteurized eggs, fruit juices, vegetable juices, cereal gruels, broth, and milk and egg substitutes. The diet can be supplemented with commercial products such as Ensure (Ross) or Carnation Instant Breakfast to provide adequate nutrients (see Chapter 21). Six feedings or more per day are served.

A dental-liquid diet may be necessary for long periods of time for those who have wired jaws. Blended foods all taste the same and rapidly become monotonous. Meat tastes chalky and gritty. No original flavor remains, so most patients find such diets especially undesirable. Freeze-dehydration in combination with blenderizing has produced items that are identifiable, including beef burgundy, beef stroganoff, beef with gravy, beef with spaghetti, chili, and chicken and pork concoctions. Other items will be available in the future (Bannar, 1980).

Supplementation. A vitamin-mineral supplement plus high-energy, high-protein supplements are recommended if the full-liquid diet is to be used for more than a few days. Most individuals are able to tolerate the addition of finely homogenized, strained meat (used for infant feeding) added to bouillon or tomato juice. The protein level of the full-fluid diet may be supplemented by including nonfat dry milk in allowable foods or commercial polymeric formulas (see Chapter 21).

For additional kilocalories, butter or fortified margarine may be added to hot liquids, and powdered glucose or glucose polymers may be dissolved in fruit juices. The use of a glucose polymer, which is not as sweet as sucrose, permits larger amounts to be added.

If a low-sodium diet is indicated, low-sodium soups, eggnogs, and custard can be offered.

Clinical Implications:

- Postsurgical patients who experience nausea, vomiting, distension, or diarrhea when given a full-liquid diet may temporarily be lactose intolerant. Lactose-hydrolyzed milk or lactose-free supplements may be substituted.
- Because of its high concentration of simple carbohydrates, the full-liquid diet may be contraindicated following gastric surgery.
- Special attention should be given to planning full-liquid diets for patients with diabetes mellitus or functional hypoglycemia in order to provide proper amounts of carbohydrates.
- Since this diet tends to be high in cholesterol, modifications can be effected if it is to be used on a long-term basis in patients with hypercholesterolemia. Skim milk can be substituted for whole milk, and polyunsaturated fats and oils can be utilized (ADA, 1981).
- Following tonsillectomy or throat surgery, a cold semiliquid diet may be used because it is chemically, mechanically, and thermally nonirritating to the throat (see Chapter 27).

PUREED DIET

Easily swallowed foods requiring no mastication are classified as purees. The pureed diet is very similar to the full-liquid diet except foods are semiliquid instead of more free-flowing. Persons with neurological disorders who may need retraining in swallowing without aspiration may require this diet; those with wired or fractured jaws would also be candidates. Cancer patients with head and neck abnormalities and stroke patients may also require such a diet.

Clinical Implications:

- Special attention may be required for optimal food intake, since these patients particularly may be under more stressful conditions than others, which in turn, means less absorption of available nutrients.
- Consistency may be varied according to the individual's preference and ability. The nurse and dietitian should evaluate this with the client.

MECHANICAL-SOFT (DENTAL-SOFT) DIET

Nonchewy foods are provided for the person who has no teeth or who has difficulty in chewing or swallowing owing to the absence of several teeth, loose dentures or sore gums, cancer of the head or neck region, esophageal repair, or certain neurological disorders. This diet may be used indefinitely. The sole criterion is that foods can be eaten without chewing. Pureed foods are not as well received as chopped or ground foods. Foods that should be avoided include tough meats; fruits or vegetables with membranes, tough skins, or tough fibers; hard rolls; bacon; nuts; and caramels.

SOFT DIET

Liquid foods and solid foods that contain a restricted amount of indigestible carbohydrate and no tough connective tissue are allowed. The soft diet may also be called a "low-fiber diet."

Indications. A soft diet is used postoperatively after the full-liquid and before a general diet and for acute infections or gastrointestinal disturbances. Distension caused by bulky food and bowel movements may elicit pain. This is typical in acute gastrointestinal disturbances or following surgery. The diet is indicated whenever inflammatory changes have progressed to stenosis of the intestinal or esophageal lumen or in some instances of esophageal varices (ADA, 1981).

Characteristics. Foods are cooked simply. Tender meats or those tenderized in the cooking process are used to decrease the amount of connective tissue. These are low in residue and readily digested. Fried foods and rich pastries are omitted. Other fat-rich foods, such as pork (except bacon), salad dressing, nuts, and coconut, as well as strong seasonings are avoided.

Vegetables must be cooked, not raw. Strongly flavored vegetables, such as onions, leeks, radishes, dried beans, and vegetables of the cabbage family (Brussels sprouts, cauliflower, broccoli, and turnips), have commonly been omitted. Strongly flavored or "gas-forming" vegetables may cause discomfort when cooked improperly. To minimize these effects, such vegetables should be cooked quickly; the cooking utensil is kept uncovered to prevent the water from becoming acid, and one should drain and serve promptly (Turner, 1970). Rather than prohibit all strongly flavored vegetables, options by the staff and clients should be exercised.

Some fruits such as bananas, grapefruit, or orange sections without membrane are permitted. All others are avoided as well as brans, coarse grains, and alcoholic beverages.

Clinical Implications:

- Some facilities define a light or convalescent diet separately from a soft diet. Others use these terms interchangeably. The diet manual can be consulted to distinguish each policy.
- Fiber-deficient diets are associated with prolonged intestinal transit and small infrequent stools. Continued use of a low-fiber diet may be associated with diverticular colon disease. A low-fiber diet may actually aggravate symptoms and is contraindicated in irritable bowel syndrome or in diverticulosis.

REGULAR OR GENERAL DIET

Self-selected diets offered by the facility allow the patient some options. The regular diet normally meets the basic nutrient requirements to maintain healthy body tissues plus additional demands necessary for new growth and repair.

Indications. This diet is ordered for the client without restrictions or modifications.

Characteristics. Individual preferences, tolerances, and aversions vary considerably among patients. Some believe that they cannot eat a certain food, whether that is true or not. There is no reason to push such foods when substitutes can be found.

Clinical Implications:

- When individuals are under stressful conditions, even though the diet is designed to meet the RDAs, these may not be adequate because of increased requirements.
- While all diets need a variety of foods for optimal health, the restrictions for different therapeutic diets may make this harder to achieve. Without a wide variety, the RDAs may not be met.
- Attention to actual intake is important. Check the returned tray for food consumption.
- Discover (and share with the dietary staff) distinctive qualities of the client's background, such as religious, cultural, ethnic, and financial factors, that might influence acceptance or rejection of the menus.

DIET AS TOLERATED

On admission or postoperatively, the order may read "diet as tolerated." Postoperatively, the clear-liquid to regular-diet progression is the standard routine. However, the diet-as-tolerated order permits a patient's preferences to be considered at the discretion of the nurse and dietitian. For instance, a patient who refuses to eat congealed gelatin and apple juice but who feels "in the mood" for chicken soup and crackers should be allowed to select them. On the other hand, if the request postoperatively is pizza, judicious nurses would advise against such foods, which are hard to digest and could cause problems.

On admission, the diet-as-tolerated order also requires consultation with the patient. Digestive problems or strong preferences can influence the ingestion of many foods; this warrants consideration of the foods given for nourishment. This order is an excellent opportunity for interaction between the nurse, dietitian, and patient to plan a diet that is eaten, well tolerated, and therefore nourishing.

The Hospitalized Patient

In addition to the nutritional needs of the patient, physiological, cultural, economic, emotional, and spiritual needs are important in the healing process. Hospitalization naturally elicits psychological stress, which also occurs with most illnesses or health problems. The patient in a hospital or any other type of institution is in a formidable environment. S/He is unfamiliar with the surroundings and routines, apprehensive or frightened about what is going to happen, and dependent on others for his/her care, meals, and all other needs. These factors can contribute to anorexia (Johnston, 1981).

Each patient is individually coping with this stress. S/He may become defensive, self-centered, angry, depressed, withdrawn, or irritable. Acceptance of the hospital routine is more difficult for some persons. In general, illnesses do not bring out the best in anyone. Many become finicky and frequently make special demands. They may prefer their cultural patterns from childhood. Stress seems to strengthen a neophobia for foods and may result in the rejection of anything but familiar ones. It is beyond the scope of this book to cover the different problems and their interpretation; the article by Luckmann and Sorensen (1975) is highly recommended for an understanding of the subject.

Frequently, food comes under attack because this is something the patient knows about—how to feed himself/herself. Institutional mealtimes are not a social experience as they ordinarily are in the home. The food pattern, preparation, and times are different from the individual's regular customs. Eating in bed from a tray can be an awkward task.

Opinions about food are very strong; a certain food that is intensely disliked may provoke a patient to refuse everything. A brief dietary history on admission can help avoid some of these conflicts. Criticisms of the food may be a way to draw attention. They should be acknowledged and appropriate changes made if possible. Generally, patients have different impressions of food and are better satisfied if they are able to choose from a selective menu.

Health care professionals must encourage good food habits for better nutrition. Trying to help people for their own good can sometimes be a frustrating task, especially if the individual stubbornly opposes the efforts. Many individuals resist change because they don't feel it's safe to trust outsiders.

ILLNESS AND APPETITE

Decreased appetite is prevalent during illnesses because of apathy, anorexia, drugs, inactivity, or many other reasons. A modified diet is for the comfort and treatment of the patient, but it may cause distress rather than provide immediate comfort if the patient is not given some explanation for the diet. The nurse plays a vital role in explaining to the patient the expectations of the dietary regimen toward his/her overall care.

ILLNESS AND NUTRITION

Stress can be both the cause and the consequence of malnutrition. While stress cannot directly be measured, intense stress or anxiety can reduce the absorption of a variety of nutrients, particularly protein and vitamin C. While increased intake of nutrients is not a remedy for stress, nutrient losses can be replaced. Deficiency

of any of the essential nutrients diminishes the body's resistance, which can initiate or aggravate other diseases. Hence, the provision of a well-balanced diet during periods of stress is essential to promote faster recovery. Supplying excessive amounts of nutrients is rarely of value, unless a deficiency exists.

As you will learn in the upcoming chapters, different physiological conditions increase losses of various electrolytes and nitrogen; others increase metabolic rate, thereby increasing vitamin requirements. While disease states usually increase nutrient requirements of the body, lack of appetite, vomiting, and pain often interfere with intake of sufficient quantities of nutrients. Drug therapy profoundly affects intake, absorption, and utilization of nutrients (see Chapter 22). To compound the problem of increased requirements during illness, a dietary restriction frequently alters the taste of food and thereby negatively affects appetite. However, for many patients, dietary modification is not required. Nutritional care for these patients is supplied by a normal diet that provides the patients' optimal nutritional requirements and meets their psychological and aesthetic needs for appetite appeal.

Meal Frequency

Especially in therapeutic diets, frequent meals that are smaller in size may be better tolerated than the usual three meals daily. For example, four to six daily meals (i.e., small meals every two hours) are often advisable. Three meals a day is a simplistic conception most often adopted for convenience of work schedules than for optimal health care. When a person is ill, meals served more often may be better accepted for several reasons:

- Food intolerances caused by acute illness or surgery (anorexia nervosa, vomiting, diarrhea, or stress).
- Reduced capacity as a result of partial or total gastrectomy.
- Lack of appetite.
- Increased need for kilocalories and nutrients.
- For specific disease conditions (one should increase fluids for urinary tract infections but restrict fluids in cases of renal failure, congestive heart failure, or increased intracranial pressure).

• Satiety and comfort (i.e., full- or clear-liquid diets have limitations to the amount that can be consumed at one time but have a low-satiety value).

Including the basic food groups in each meal (or even in snacks as far as possible) will help the body to obtain optimal nutritive value from each food eaten.

Federal regulations require the time lapse between the last meal of one day and the first meal of the next to be not more than 14 hours. Meals should be 1½ to three hours apart, or not more than five hours apart between 7:00 AM and 10:00 PM. The kilocalories should be divided among these meals with 10 percent or more from protein. Items such as juice or ice cream may be counted as snacks but do not consitute a meal.

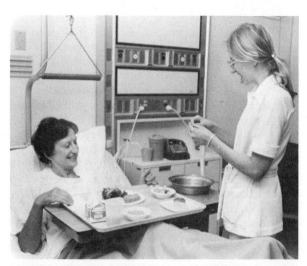

Figure 19–1. The nurse has an important role in the patient's food intake. (Courtesy of University of Arkansas Medical Sciences, Department of Nursing and Campus Media Services, Little Rock, AR.)

Nutritional Teamwork

All members of the health care team work towards obtaining optimal health for the client. Successful nutritional management requires complementary teamwork between the client, physician, nurse, and dietitian or dietetic technician. Sometimes, the cooperative efforts of this team are less obvious than others; but the shared responsibility for the patient only varies in intensity, not in overall support. Observation, documentation, and communication are the critical operating factors between these team members for a successful outcome (see Chapter 20).

Providing nutritious, appetizing food is usually a function of the dietary department. The dietitian plans the diet and may assess the nutritional status of the patient. Nursing service has an important role in seeing that the patient eats the food, progresses toward improved health, and is satisfied with his/her dietary plan (Fig. 19–1).

Input from the family can provide additional information about the patient's food habits or problems that may arise in implementing a diet at home. When all factors are considered, the diet will be more acceptable and is more likely to be followed.

While the patient needs to know what the diet does not permit, emphasis should be placed on foods that are allowed as well as enjoyed. This emphasis can also help to motivate the patient. Motivation is best ensured by the patient's understanding and knowledge. An awareness of the role of the diet in his/her health and recovery process or in minimizing the discomforts of the disease will more likely elicit cooperation from the patient.

Because of close contact with the patient and his/her family, the nurse can frequently motivate the patient to eat or to follow a diet at home. Through informal but "planned" conversations during meals, the patient can learn more about his/her diet and nutritional needs. Patience, tact, kindness, ingenuity, and firmness bolster patient morale. Continual education throughout the hospital stay by input from both nursing and dietary staffs is much more effective than one formal diet instruction period just prior to discharge. While formal diet instruction may be provided by dietary staff, nursing service can have a great impact on patient cooperation.

With current knowledge about the importance of nutrition, nurses can no longer turn their backs on the nutritional status, optimistic that patients will regain strength when they get well. An adequate supply of nutrients is necessary for recovery. Admission weight and height should be recorded when the condition permits. Nurses can remind physicians of how many meals have been missed because of testing or how long the patient has been on intravenous or nutritionally inadequate diets (either the diet or the intake may be inadequate).

Food on the tray does not meet its goal of providing nourishment if left uneaten. Assessment of intake can be requested from the dietary department when problems with intake are observed. Since the nurse is usually with the patient at mealtimes, his/her attitude and understanding of nutritional concepts can influence whether the patient eats. Observing, listening, and reporting are vital responsibilities. Observations can be made regarding how well the patient eats, what kinds and amounts of food are refused, and the patient's attitude toward the food. Observations made during mealtime are essential to any care plan. When a patient states s/he will eat something, yet it lies untouched on the tray, more adjustments must be made. By listening, one can learn which foods are preferred and why. Without communication between the nursing staff and the dietary department about the patient's needs and preferences, success in providing nutritional support will be minimal.

Promoting Food Intake

Adequate nutrition may mean the difference between a speedy recovery and a prolonged hospital stay. Inadequate amounts of nutrients to meet the requirements cause changes in body functions that may affect the outcome of disease and cause therapeutic measures to be unsuccessful. Promoting adequate nutrition includes providing a pleasant eating environment, helping the patient obtain nutritious, palatable food by assisting with the meal service, and helping the patient eat. The subject of feeding sick and hospitalized children is covered in Chapter 16.

ASSISTING WITH MENU SELECTION

In some institutions, patients can select from a menu, whether on a therapeutic or regular diet. While it is thought that this gives the individual an opportunity to order the foods that appeal to him/her, some problems arise with this system. Assistance is needed for those who have visual problems or difficulty in reading or writing. Some are apathetic; these selections become a chore. Institutional food terminology, while fairly standard, is unfamiliar to some; patients are hesitant to select items that are unfamiliar to them (Schutz et al, 1972).

When menus are filled out after completion of a meal, the patient is not hungry and does not know how s/he will feel the next day. Thus, s/he may fail to select enough food. Occasionally, every item on the menu will be checked; this would result in too many calories. Finicky eaters may not find anything on the menu that whets their appetite. Many individuals need guidance in selecting their foods to assure that they receive an appropriate amount.

An excellent learning opportunity occurs when patients on modified diets are allowed to select from a menu. Explanations can be given why certain foods are not on the diet or why only limited amounts are allowed.

PLEASANT ENVIRONMENT

Nursing service is generally responsible for helping the patient obtain and enjoy the foods by creating a pleasant environment for eating. If possible, an ambulatory patient should be taken to a dining room, where the social experience during mealtime is more conducive to eating. Some facilities have cafeterias for ambulatory patients; others provide a dining room. These areas should be bright, cheerful, and seasonally decorated.

Some patients who are clumsy or have difficulty chewing or swallowing may be embarrassed and prefer to eat alone. The perceptive nurse will be aware of and respect these feelings.

PREPARING THE PATIENT

In many circumstances, tray service is necessary. If proper preparations are completed before tray service, food can be delivered faster, reaching the patient at its proper temperature. Individuals in pleasant surroundings, ready to eat when the tray arrives, are more likely to eat. Remember, the objective with hospitalized patients is usually to entice them to eat even though their appetite is poor.

Clinical Implications:

- Make the patient as comfortable as possible—raise the bed if permitted. Sitting in an armchair is the preferred position for eating.
- Offer bedpans and urinals ahead of time, and remove them prior to mealtime.

- Try to ensure that the room is clean and free of odors.
- Wash the patient's face and hands; provide necessary oral hygiene; insert dentures.
- Clear the bedtray and place it in front of the patient.
- Some visitors are a hindrance to the patient's eating and should be asked to leave; others will encourage the patient to eat or even feed him/her.

SERVING THE TRAYS

Preparation of the trays is usually the responsibility of the dietary department, but interdepartmental cooperation will assure better care of the patient. An attractive tray served in a warm, cheerful manner will help ensure its being eaten. This gives the nurse an opportunity to learn more about the patient, discuss the diet, and see how well the food is tolerated. Certain procedures will ensure that the proper tray is served in the right manner so it can be eaten by the patient:

1. Check the patient's name with the name on the tray.
2. Always check the food on the tray to be sure the correct diet is being served.
3. Check the tray to be certain everything needed is on the tray. (In some instances, if the patient has not circled sugar, salt, pepper, or margarine, these items will be omitted from the tray.)
4. Serve trays promptly so the food is at its best.
5. Serve trays first to the patients who require less assistance.
6. Position everything on the tray so it is within easy reach.
7. Remove covers from foods. Open food containers, butter bread, pour beverages, cut meat, and otherwise assist, *as needed*. This is especially necessary when one arm cannot be used.
8. Encourage the patient to eat, but do not rush him/her.
9. A hand towel to protect the gown or pajamas may be suggested for those with coordination problems or who are slightly reclining on the bed.
10. Remove the tray promptly when the patient has finished eating.
11. After the patient is finished eating, provide an opportunity for proper mouth care and washing his/her hands.

12. If the tray cannot be eaten immediately because of tests or treatment, make arrangements to keep the food at the proper temperature or to receive the tray at a later time.

Foods brought in by family and friends should be judged for their suitability for the patient's diet and condition. If these items interfere with the intake of nutritious foods, they should be discouraged.

FEEDING THE PATIENT

Most individuals prefer to feed themselves, but acutely ill or handicapped patients, for example, warrant being fed. To encourage their self-esteem, patients should be allowed to do as much as they are capable of. Providing unnecessary assistance can be offensive to a person or nudge him/her into a dependent role. Occasionally, individuals will not eat rather than request assistance. In determining how much assistance is necessary, consider both the individual's nutritional needs and the physical capacity.

The types of food served may affect one's ability to self-feed. Gelatin, baked custard, and peas are very difficult to spoon if only one hand can be used. Sometimes finger foods are easier for patients to handle and allows them to maintain an independent role. Encourage foods that are nutritious and preferred by the patient, even though they may be messy.

Clinical Implications:

- Sit down while feeding the patient and appear at ease and unhurried.
- For blind patients, attractively describe the food. Caution them about foods that seem to be very hot, and identify each food before placing it in their mouth. Many blind persons can feed themselves if they know where the food is located on the tray. The items can be described in relation to the numbers on a clock.
- Offer small amounts of food at a time, encouraging the patient to chew the food well.
- Find out how the patient prefers to eat the items: Some eat all of one food; others alternate one food with another. Switching from one food to another during a meal generally increases intake (Rolls et al, 1982).
- Flexible straws are helpful for those who cannot use a cup.
- Allow ample time for the patient to chew and swallow or rest between mouthfuls.

- Try to be neat and not spill foods; wipe the patient's mouth with a napkin as needed during the meal.
- Pleasant and supportive conversation can make the patient feel more at ease.

Anytime the patient does not eat well, whether s/he is feeding himself or being fed, try to determine the cause and a remedy. Recording is the best way to communicate this information with other team members. Make judgments about the quantity of food by determining whether the patient is satisfied afterward. If it is not adequate, snacks may be permitted. Large quantities of food can be upsetting to some—they become discouraged just looking at it or become concerned that they are wasting food. Small frequent meals are sometimes required. If foods are not eaten, offer substitutions. Discuss any unsolved dietary problems with the charge nurse or dietitian.

Fluid Intake

Fluids can indicate liquids taken orally or parenterally. As discussed in Chapter 5, the body's requirement for the nutrient water is indispensable. Tissue hydration is essential for normal physiological functions. Included in fluid intake are substances taken into the body that are liquids at body temperature, such as gelatin, ice cream, and other frozen liquids.

Normal fluid intake should be 1500 to 2000 ml, or approximately 2 qt. daily. Fever, infection, and increased losses from sweating or diarrhea increase fluid requirements. While thirst normally regulates a person's fluid intake to maintain proper fluid and electrolyte balance, patients are sometimes too weak to get themselves a drink. Bedridden patients may purposely curtail fluid intake to avoid bothering the nurse for a bedpan.

When oral fluid is not sufficient, parenteral infusions are necessary; these should not routinely replace oral intake. Several measures to increase fluid intake include:

1. Be familiar with a patient's beverage preferences and offer them frequently, if they are permitted on the diet.
2. Offer fluids frequently throughout the day.
3. Serve fluids in small glasses.
4. Offer fluid alternatives such as ice cream or gelatin.
5. A straw is more accommodating for beverage intake with bedfast patients.

Before an operation and for various testing procedures, fluid may be withheld for 8 to 10 hr. However, sufficient amounts of fluid should be offered before and after these periods.

During certain disease conditions, fluids may be limited. The total allotment should be divided proportionately over the 24-hour period. It is usually advisable to serve fluids between meals rather than at mealtimes. Denying a patient's request for fluids is hard to do; tips to alleviate problems associated with limited fluid intake are given in Chapter 5.

• FALLACIES and FACTS

FALLACY: *Add raw eggs to blender beverages for more nutrient value.*
  • **FACT:** *Even though many recipes call for whole raw eggs or egg whites, this is not a safe policy. Because of the danger of Salmonella infection when raw egg is used, a pasteurized, commercial eggnog preparation or other high-protein supplement is recommended. Raw egg also contains an enzyme, avidin, which binds the B vitamin biotin and renders it unavailable.*

FALLACY: *Milk should never be given to a patient with fever.*
  • **FACT:** *The patient's temperature has no bearing on the ability to take milk. Cool liquids help reduce elevated body temperature.*

FALLACY: *Many people believe that milk and cheese are constipating.*
  • **FACT:** *This is not true. Milk and cheese are easily digested and leave little residue. If the diet is lacking in the foods that provide bulk, constipation can result, regardless of whether milk and cheese are eaten.*

FALLACY: *Frozen orange juice is not as nutritious as fresh orange juice.*
  • **FACT:** *On the average, a six-ounce glass of any orange juice provides 100 percent or more of an adult's daily requirement of vitamin C (60 mg); however, the big difference is in the flavor, which is changed by the processing. Freshly*

squeezed juice may taste best to some individuals, but frozen juices are quite similar in taste and cost less than half the price of fresh juice. Chilled, bottled orange juice costs about the same, or possibly more than the frozen, but the flavor has seriously deteriorated (Orange juice, 1983).

Summary

The diet prescription is as vital to the patient's physical recovery as a drug prescription. Nutrition is an integral component of total patient care, affecting the recovery process as much as other therapies. Following a diet requires considerable self-discipline and is never an easy task. During illness, appetite is generally decreased while requirements are increased. The patient's food should be appetizing and enjoyable as well as suitable for his/her physical condition and served in an atmosphere conducive to eating. A conscientious nurse with a fundamental knowledge of diet therapy can elicit patient cooperation and diet adherence.

Insidious developments often caused by poor nutrition are frequently unnoticed until there is gross weight loss. With cooperative teamwork, this can be avoided. The nurse, who has constant and personal contact with the patient, must be aware that the food both is suitable and is being eaten. When this is questionable for any reason, the physician and the dietitian should be consulted.

For optimal nutritional planning, implementation, and evaluation, the nurse's input is invaluable. Information about the patient is obtained during discussions with the patient and family and during physical observations. A record of food intake and the patient's attitude to the food or diet are important as well as information regarding cultural, religious, and social background. Physical observations include a record of weight changes, poorly fitting dentures, arthritic problems, and other problems that may interfere with food intake. The nurse's role involves providing informal, correct dietary information about the implementation and reason for a diet, ensuring a pleasant environment for eating, assisting patients to obtain their food, and encouraging food intake.

Review Questions

1. Discuss how illness affects dietary intake and body requirements.
2. What is diet therapy? What are the purposes of diet therapy?
3. Write one day's menu plans for each of these diets with modifications based upon the general diet: general, mechanical-soft, soft, full-liquid, and clear-liquid.
4. Explain the rationale for each of the above modifications and describe foods allowed and avoided.
5. Review three other diet manuals besides the one in your facility. (Ask the dietitian where to get these.) How are they different? Why do these changes occur? Rank them in order of your preferences and state reasons for these decisions.
6. What are some available options for patients who constantly complain about the food?
7. How can the nursing and dietetic staffs work together for the utmost benefit to the client?
8. How can a nurse be influential in the patient's food intake?
9. What should the nurse do to assure adequate nutrition for a patient?

REFERENCE LIST

American Dietetic Association (ADA): *Handbook of Clinical Dietetics.* New Haven, Yale University Press, 1981.
Bannar, R: Liquified foods taste good. *Food Eng* 52(3):14, 1980.
Johnston, IDA: The relevance of nutritional care to the hospital patient. *Acta Chir Scand* 507(suppl):289, 1981.
Luckmann, J; Sorensen, KC: What patients' actions tell you about their feelings, fears, and needs. *Nursing* 5(2):54, 1975.
Murray, DP; Welsh, JD; Rankin, RA; et al: Survey: Use of clear and full liquid diets with or without commercially produced formulas. *JPEN* 9(6):732, 1985.
Orange juice: Frozen, refrigerated, canned. *Consumers' Reports 1983 Buying Guide*, p. 60.
Rolls, BJ; Rowe, EA; Rolls, ET: How flavour and appearance affect human feeding. *Proc Nutr Soc* 41(2):109, 1982.
Schutz, HG; Rucker, MH; Hunt, JD: Hospital patients' and employees' reactions to food-use combinations. *J Am Diet Assoc* 60(3):207, 1972.
Selye, H: On just being sick. *Nutr Today* 5(1):2, 1970.
Turner, D: *Handbook of Diet Therapy.* Chicago, University of Chicago Press, 1970.

Further Study

Boulden, L: Food! glorious food! . . . and dysnourishment. *Aust Nurs J* 12(1):28, 1982.
Cerrato, PL: Does your patient's food affect his mood? *RN* 86(3):62, 1986.
Chappelle, ML: The language of food. *Am J Nurs* 72(7):1294, 1972.

Cooper, LF: Florence Nightingale's contribution to dietetics. *J Am Diet Assoc* 30(2):121, 1954.

Cousins, N: Anatomy of an illness (as perceived by the patient). *N Engl J Med* 295(26):1458, 1976.

Davies, GJ; Evans, E; Stock, A; Yudkin, J: Special diets in hospitals: Discrepancies between what is prescribed and what is eaten. *Br Med J* 1(Jan 25):200, 1975.

Davis, J; Hodges, RE: A "new" approach to diet therapy. *Dietetic Currents* 1(5), 1974.

Donovan, L: Is the doctor starving your patient? *RN* 41(7):36, 1978.

Dornon, V: Diet in terms of illness. *Nurs Mirror* 160(8):38, 1985.

Greenburg, JL: Why your hospitalized patient won't eat. *Consultant* 19(9):119, 1979.

Hadley, A: Care about food: Campaign for real food . . . the separation of the nurse from the patient's dietary concerns. *Nurs Times* 81(12):43, 1985.

Holmes, S: Care about food: differing needs . . . Patient's nutritional needs vary. *Nurs Times* 81(13):35, 1985.

Jones, D: Patient's food: Careful diet. *Nurs Mirror* 151(4):30, 1980.

MacGregor, FC: Uncooperative patients: Some cultural interpretations. *Am J Nurs* 67(1):88, 1967.

Tobias, AL; Van Itallie, TB: Nutritional problems of hospitalized patients. *J Am Diet Assoc* 71(3):253, 1977.

Truswell, AS: Therapeutic diets. *Br Med J* 291(September 21):807, 1985.

Dietary Management of Malnutrition: Assessments

20

THE STUDENT WILL BE ABLE TO:

- *Identify physiological factors that have nutritional implications.*
- *Distinguish between kwashiorkor and marasmus, in terms of physiological symptoms and dietary causes.*
- *State the nurse's role in nutritional assessments.*
- *List four important facets of nutritional assessments.*

OBJECTIVES

Albumin
Anergy
Anthropometric
Assessment
Creatine-height index
Immunocompetency
Marasmic kwashiorkor
Nutrition screening
Protein-energy
*   malnutrition (PEM)*
Total lymphocyte count
Transferrin
Weight-height index

TERMS TO KNOW

With the alleviation of most vitamin deficiency diseases, malnutrition was virtually forgotten by many health professionals. Even in the United States, some cases of malnutrition remain. Those who most commonly develop nutritional deficiencies in the United States include the poorly educated, low-income families, the mentally or physically disabled, the elderly, alcoholics, drug addicts, food faddists, and the institutionalized (those in acute care hospitals, long-term care facilities, or prisons). In general, nutritional deficiencies in our country tend to be subclinical for individuals living outside hospitals (Roe, 1979). In addition to nutritional deficiencies, another form of malnutrition exists—obesity (see Chapter 24).

In 1974, Butterworth uncovered a "skeleton in the hospital closet"—iatrogenic, or physician-induced, malnutrition. The prevalence of this problem within a hospital depends on the type of people served, total patient care, nutritional screening techniques, and the availability of a nutrition support team (Roe, 1979). Malnutrition is especially common among patients hospitalized longer than two weeks; clinically significant protein-energy malnutrition affects more than 15 percent of the patients in acute care hospitals (Blackburn & Harvey, 1982).

Iatrogenic malnutrition does not mean that physicians have malicious intentions or a disregard for a patient's welfare. The condition is a result of emphasis on different types of treatments to cure a physiological problem while fundamental principles of nutrition are ignored. Conventional forms of medical and surgical therapy may not be sufficient: Antibiotics do not replace host defenses, sterile gauzes and sutures do not heal wounds. Many symptoms for this condition are more likely to be observed by nurses involved in routine patient care than by anyone else on the team.

Under the DRGs, malnutrition is classified as a "comorbidity" or "complicating condition" (CC). Comorbidity is an existing condition when the patient is admitted to the hospital; it results in at least one additional day of hospitalization in 75 percent of patients by virtue of associated complications (YUHSMG, 1981). A complication developing during hospitalization also results in an additional day of hospitalization.

Illness, stress, and trauma have catabolic effects increasing requirements while oral intake is minimal. Certain conditions—namely cancer, gastrointestinal disorders, chronic heart failure, alcoholism, and conditions with high metabolic needs—are more frequently associated with malnutrition. Additionally, a number of institutional

Table 20–1. *Undesirable Practices Affecting the Nutritional Health of Hospital Patients**

- Failure to record height and weight.
- Rotation of staff at frequent intervals.
- Diffusion of responsibility for patient care.
- Prolonged use of glucose and saline intravenous feedings.
- Failure to observe patients' food intake.
- Withholding meals because of diagnostic tests.
- Use of tube feedings in inadequate amounts, of uncertain composition, and under unsanitary conditions.
- Ignorance of the composition of vitamin mixtures and other nutritional products.
- Failure to recognize increased nutritional needs due to injury or illness.
- Performance of surgical procedures without first making certain that the patient is optimally nourished, and failure to give the body nutritional support after surgery.
- Failure to appreciate the role of nutrition in the prevention of and recovery from infection; unwarranted reliance on antibiotics.
- Lack of communication and interaction between physician and dietitian. As staff professionals, dietitians should be concerned with the nutritional health of *every* hospital patient.
- Delay of nutrition support until the patient is in an advanced state of depletion, which is sometimes irreversible.
- Limited availability of laboratory tests to assess nutritional status; failure to use those that are available.

*From Butterworth, CE: The skeleton in the hospital closet. *Nutrition Today* 9(2):4, 1974. Reproduced with permission of *Nutrition Today* Magazine, P.O. Box 1829, Annapolis, MD 21404.

practices are contrary to optimal nutrition care, as listed in Table 20–1.

Protein-energy deficiency, which is the most frequently observed consequence of malnutrition with serious implications, has been shown to (1) reduce synthesis of enzymes and plasma proteins, (2) increase susceptibility to infection, (3) impede wound healing, and (4) cause mental lassitude. In other words, it contributes to patient morbidity and mortality.

Nutritional Care

Nutritional care is the process of helping people choose foods that are nourishing to their bodies or of providing the body with nutrients in a utilizable form in the amounts required. Individual nutritional needs change throughout life for different conditions. For example, an infant requires different foods than a teenager; a diabetic must modify eating patterns.

The first step to prevent malnutrition or to reverse the process is a nutritional screening. This process identifies patients at high risk for nutritional problems. These problems are usually correctable; however, recognition of the problem (or screening) is imperative. The screening requires the cooperation of paraprofessionals and nursing staff to gather basic information.

A thorough nutritional assessment includes a compilation of information including dietary history, recent influential factors (e.g., surgery, medications, or illness), biochemical information, and sometimes immunological testing. This assessment process is similar to the assessment phase in the nursing process described in Chapter 1 and is followed by the other steps outlined—analysis, goals and objectives, implementation, and evaluation. The care plan becomes a management tool that ensures appropriate care. The patient is included in the process of developing the objectives, as appropriate. After implementation, reassessment determines the effectiveness of the plan (see Fig. 1–2). Nurses and dietitians must work together in developing and assessing care plans to provide adequate nutrition for the patient.

Each institution organizes the screening-assessment process to utilize the expertise of their personnel in the best manner. The ultimate goal is to make use of the limited time of all personnel and provide adequate care for patients.

Most hospitals employ registered dietitians and/or dietetic technicians, but they may be unable to assess the needs of all admissions. While they may routinely have contact with patients receiving modified diets, according to the screening standards of one acute care community hospital (Christensen & Gstundtner, 1985), 31 percent of the patients receiving routine diets (regular, soft, full-liquid, clear-liquid, or NPO) and 33 percent of patients placed on modified diets were malnourished on admission.

Malnutrition is underdiagnosed or frequently omitted from the discharge summary. Under the DRGs, hospitals can expect additional reimbursement simply by diagnosing all cases of malnutrition. Nutritional screening is used to determine patients at risk of developing malnutrition or those malnourished on admission in order to implement nutritional support. This lowers costs associated with treatment by avoiding complications. Not only does the hospital benefit, but patients may experience less suffering and are protected from potentially fatal consequences.

Early intervention for high-risk patients cannot be implemented unless nutritional screening is carried out on patients on admission or soon thereafter (Kamath et al, 1986).

In some institutions, the nutrition questionnaire is completed by the patient in the hospital admissions office, the patient's height and weight are measured by an admissions nurse, and the biochemical information is gathered by a registered dietitian who also makes recommendations for nutrition intervention, as shown in *Focus on the Screening Nutritional Profile*. Some hospitals utilize dietetic technicians to help gather the information, while many long-term care facilities utilize the food service director (Matthews, 1984).

In most instances, nursing staff members gather much of the data necessary for nutritional screening and assessment in their nursing assessment; this information must be coordinated for effective implementation of nutrition care without duplication of efforts. *By using information gathered in the clinical examination, the patient's history, and the laboratory data, the nurse can identify patients considered at high risk nutritionally.* They should then be referred to the dietitian, the physician, or the nutrition support team (as applicable for the institution).

For example, some information from a nursing history can indicate the individual's ability to obtain and prepare food: The social profile includes marital status, place where s/he lives, and who prepares the food. A knowledge of the person's occupation and daily activities can indicate general caloric needs. Financial problems frequently have significant nutritional impact.

Nutrient deficiency is not only attributed to inadequate intake; other possible causes must be evaluated: concurrent disease, drugs, or genetic effects modifying an individual's absorption, utilization, requirement, destruction, or excretion of nutrients. Most of these facts are also generated from the nursing history. This places another responsibility on the nurse, who has constant and personal contact with the patient: to know about nutrition and the individual patient (Swan & Rohrback, 1982).

In the hospitalized patient, nutritional care is very complex. Simply providing food is not sufficient. Careful monitoring will detect inadequate intake so that corrective actions can rectify the problem (counseling the patient, providing encouragement, or initiating nutritional support by supplemental feeding, tube feeding, or parenteral nutrition). Early recognition and referral of nutritional problems enhance the quality of patient care.

FOCUS ON THE SCREENING NUTRITIONAL PROFILE

Herman Hospital

Nutritional History Information

Patient's name _____

Age _____   Room number _____

Admission date _____

___ Yes ___ No 1. Have you lost more than 10 lbs. in the last six months without trying to lose weight? (Pediatrics, any weight loss)

___ Yes ___ No 2. Have you had a recent appetite loss causing you to miss meals for five days or more?

___ Yes ___ No 3. Do you have daily problems with vomiting or diarrhea?

4. Do you have any of the following medical conditions:

___ Yes ___ No   a. Crohn's disease or ulcerative colitis?

___ Yes ___ No   b. Chronic renal failure?

___ Yes ___ No   c. Chronic liver disease?

___ Yes ___ No   d. Cancer?

___ Yes ___ No   e. Diabetes?

___ Yes ___ No   f. Bedsores?

___ Yes ___ No 5. Have you had surgery in the last month, or a chronic illness lasting more than three weeks?

___ Yes ___ No 6. Have you had a temperature higher than 100.4° F. for more than three days?

7. Are you presently restricting any of the following items in your diet?

___ Yes ___ No   a. Salt?

___ Yes ___ No   b. Sugar?

Dietary History

A diet history supplies subjective information regarding eating habits, living conditions, and other factors that affect food choices.

I. Fluids
   A. Usual fluid intake amount
   B. Recent changes in amount (increased, decreased, or unchanged)
   C. Beverage preferences
   D. Frequency of intake
   E. Beverages not tolerated

II. Nutrition
   A. Teeth/mouth
      1. Condition of teeth
      2. Dentures
      3. Chewing difficulties
      4. Soreness in mouth
      5. Difficulty in swallowing
      6. Problems with choking
      7. Recent changes in taste
   B. Recent weight changes
   C. Appetite/food preferences
      1. Recent appetite changes (increased, decreased, or unchanged)
      2. Favorite foods
      3. Foods disliked
      4. Foods not tolerated and why
      5. Allergies
      6. Where meals are taken
      7. Who purchases and prepares the food
      8. Snacking habits
      9. Number of feedings per day
      10. Vitamin or mineral supplements
      11. Budgeting problems
      12. Alcohol intake (type and amount)
      13. Personal or religious restrictions (e.g., kosher or vegetarian)

___ Yes ___ No   c. Fat?
___ Yes ___ No   d. Protein?
___ Yes ___ No   e. Special (for example, food allergies)? Specify: _____

    8. Are you presently taking any of the following medications:

___ Yes ___ No   a. Steroids? (Prednisone or cortisone)
___ Yes ___ No   b. Antibiotics?
___ Yes ___ No   c. Vitamins?
___ Yes ___ No   d. Insulin?

Completed by: _____
Relation to patient: _____

Anthropometric Information

1. Height _____ inches   Completed by: _____
2. Weight _____ lbs.   Admissions Nurse
3. Head circumference _____ cm

Laboratory Information

Serum albumin _____ mg/dl

Summary _____
_____

Recommendation _____

Completed by: _____ R.D.

Courtesy of Herman Hospital, Houston, Texas. Reprinted by permission.

D. Diet
    1. Type of special diet
    2. Problems or concerns with diet
III. Gastrointestinal problems
    A. Excessive belching or heartburn
    B. Indigestion
    C. Nausea
    D. Vomiting
IV. Elimination
    A. Bowels
        1. Constipation or diarrhea
        2. Recent changes in bowel movements
        3. Frequency of bowel movements
        4. Use of laxatives or enemas, or other practices
    B. Difficulty of urination
        1. Recent changes (increased, decreased, or unchanged)
V. Current medications

Food habits are closely associated with cultural, religious, and socioeconomic background. Also, emotional factors should not be ignored in planning the patient's diet. In addition to revealing food preferences and quality and quantity of nutrients, a good diet history should disclose information regarding inadequate food and fluid intake, inadequate nutrient absorption, abnormal fluid losses, recent weight changes, decreased nutrient utilization, and increased losses and requirements. Thorough questioning may reveal physical or psychological handicaps to eating. A dietary history is also recommended so that the hospitalized patient will receive foods that s/he likes.

There are several techniques for determining actual and habitual dietary intake. Sometimes a nutrient intake record (such as a 24-hour recall, food diary, or food-frequency form) is used to provide a rough estimate of the amounts of nutrients eaten. The dietary recall or food diary is more precise than a diet history for determining intake for a short period, but the diet history is more accurate because the intake of nearly all foods and the interrelationships of diet, medications, lifestyle, and physiological conditions are considered. Totals of nutrients eaten are compared with the RDAs to determine the adequacy of the diet. Frequently, only key nutrients—calories, protein, fat, dietary fiber, and vitamins A and C—may be used as indices to assess overall nutrient intake (Byers et al, 1985). This minimizes time and expense involved in such studies.

A *food diary* is maintained by the patient for three to seven days, including one weekend day. Records of foods eaten, the amounts, method of preparation, where the food is eaten, and time of day are kept.

The *24-hour recall* is easier and quicker but less accurate than a food diary. In the 24-hour recall, the individual records all foods and amounts eaten for the previous day.

The *food-frequency form* ascertains the number of times per day, week, or month that specific foods or categories of foods are eaten. This information can be easily analyzed and translated to estimate nutritional adequacy of the diet.

Clinical Implications:

- In the hospital, all food consumption (including foods not on the tray) should be charted along with notations about adequacy of intake (Metheny & Snively, 1983). This is especially important if nutrient analysis of intake is necessary.
- Note all routes of fluid intake and output, and chart if appropriate.

Anthropometric Measurements

Anthropometric measurements (human body measurements) are an objective technique for assessments. Body measurements are compared with standards. Basic measurements include height, weight, ideal body weight, percent of weight loss, triceps skinfold, and arm-muscle circumference.

WEIGHT AND HEIGHT

These are important parameters that should be measured directly and accurately for all admis-

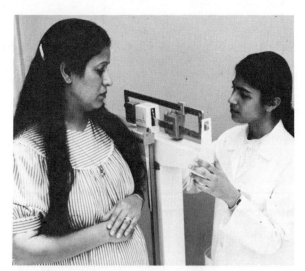

Figure 20–1. Body weight and weight changes are important indices of nutritional status. (WHO photo by T. Kelly.)

sions. Height and weight can be obtained from the patient or family if direct measurements are impossible.

Body weight is one of the most expedient and helpful indicators of nutritional status (Fig. 20–1). It is a nonspecific measure of all body components, including fat and protein.

In order to accurately determine ideal body weight, body frame size (small, medium, or large) must be known. The wrist is measured at its smallest circumference distal to the styloid process of the radius and ulna and then classified as shown in Appendix C–2.

Ideal weights can be determined from the Metropolitan Life Insurance Company charts (see Appendix C–1). This compares the weight of patient with normal values of other individuals of the same height and gender. By comparing the

Table 20–2. Possible Indications of Weight-Height Index Deviations

Weight-Height Index	Indication
> 90 percent*	Moderate depletion
> 80 percent*	Severe depletion
< 110 percent†	Moderately overweight
< 129 percent†	Grossly overweight

*Data from Blackburn, GL; Harvey, KB: Nutritional assessment as a routine in clinical medicine. *Postgraduate Medicine* 71(5):46, 1982.
†Data from Weinsier, RL; Butterworth, CE, Jr: *Handbook of Clinical Nutrition.* St. Louis, The C. V. Mosby Co, 1981.

actual weight (in kilograms) with the ideal weight for a patient's height (in centimeters), the weight-height index can be determined.

$$\frac{\text{actual body weight}}{\text{ideal body weight}} \times 100 = \text{weight-height index}$$

Deviations from the normal (100%) weight-height index indicate the degree of depletion or overweight, as shown in Table 20–2.

WEIGHT LOSS

If fluid loss is not significant, weight loss is a better indication of current nutritional status; it reflects the use of body stores for energy. This occurs rapidly when caloric intake is grossly inadequate. If a high-stress condition exists, and especially if intravenous dextrose solutions are being administered, protein stores are catabolized.

Weight status may be maintained, falsely indicating adequate nutrition, because water and collagen replace fat and muscle tissue being catabolized (Shils, 1981). This common finding in protein-energy malnutrition (PEM) occurs particularly in the obese patient.

The rate of weight loss is important (Table 20–3). More rapid weight loss indicates more severe nutritional consequences. For nutritional assessment, the short-term (within the past 6 to 12 months) involuntary weight loss is significant. Daily weight fluctuations reflect body fluid changes. Trends over a period of time are more helpful for indicating nutritional status. An involuntary weight loss of five percent in one month or 10 percent over six months is significant (Blackburn & Harvey, 1982).

Clinical Implications:

- Record height and weight for all admissions and at regular intervals throughout hospitalization.
- Rapid weight loss of six percent (even in an obese patient) may diminish a patient's ability to withstand stress from medical or surgical therapies (Roy et al, 1985).
- If edema is present, weight may be maintained, with a false indication of adequate nutritional status (Butterworth & Weinsier, 1980).
- The reliability of body weight as an indicator of nutritional status is particularly limited in obese or edematous patients (Blackburn & Harvey, 1982).
- During stress or trauma, the obese patient should not be calorically restricted (Butterworth & Weinsier, 1980).
- Patients with a weight-height index of less than 80 percent are at high risk of nutritional deficiency (Blackburn & Harvey, 1982).
- A weight loss of 10 percent or more over a period of one to three months is an excellent clue of impending PEM (Blackburn & Thornton, 1979).
- Weight losses of 10 percent or more over a period of two weeks (when infection is absent) reflect negative fluid balance rather than loss of protein or fat stores (Blackburn & Thornton, 1979).

SKINFOLD MEASUREMENTS

The amount of body fat, indirectly measured by skinfold measurements, is also an indirect indicator of previous caloric balance (intake versus requirement). Since 50 percent of fat stores are subcutaneous, the skinfold thickness indicates the amount of caloric reserves. Special skinfold calipers are required for this technique (Fig. 20–2). Triceps and subscapular skinfold measurements are most commonly used. Three consecutive measurements of the nondominant midarm-triceps skinfold are averaged. Percentiles for triceps skinfold are shown in Appendix C–3.

Clinical Implications:

- Skinfold measurements are more difficult and less accurate in the obese (Bistrian & Blackburn, 1983).
- Very low fat stores indicate a significant nutritional problem because the body's adaptive mechanism during starvation is unable to use endogenous fat for fuel (Blackburn & Harvey, 1982).

Table 20–3. *Evaluation of Weight Change**

Time	Significant Weight Loss	Severe Weight Loss
1 week	1 to 2 percent	> 2 percent
1 month	5 percent	> 5 percent
3 months	7.5 percent	> 7.5 percent
6 months	10 percent	> 10 percent

$$\text{Percent weight change} = \frac{(\text{Usual weight} - \text{Actual weight})}{\text{Usual weight}} \times 100$$

*From Blackburn, GL; Thornton, PA: Nutritional assessment of the hospitalized patient. *Medical Clinics of North America* 63(5):1103, 1979, by permission.

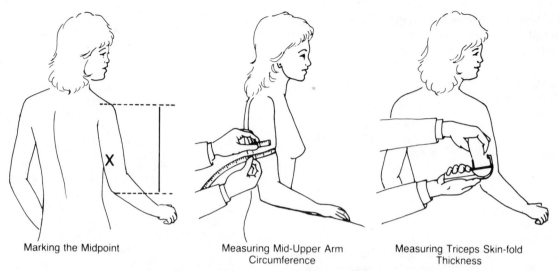

Marking the Midpoint

Measuring Mid-Upper Arm
Circumference

Measuring Triceps Skin-fold
Thickness

Figure 20–2. Measuring mid–upper arm circumference and triceps skinfold thickness. (From Poleman CM, Capra CL: Shackelton's Nutrition Essentials and Diet Therapy, 5th ed. Philadelphia, W. B. Saunders Co, 1984, by permission.)

MIDARM CIRCUMFERENCE

Body fat and protein or skeletal muscle mass are assessed by midarm circumference (MAC), which is an index of the arm's total area (see Fig. 20–2). This also reflects caloric adequacy. Using a mathematical equation, the amount of subcutaneous fat (measured by skinfold thickness) can be subtracted from the MAC to estimate the lean tissue in the arm, called the midarm muscle circumference (MAMC). This can also be determined by using the normogram in Appendix C–5a. MAMC is a measurement of protein stores or the amount of muscle. (Lean body mass can also be measured by laboratory determinations, discussed later in this chapter.) MAMC correlates well with other estimates of body protein status, such as serum albumin. Percentiles of upper arm circumference and arm muscle circumference are in Appendix C–4.

Disuse atrophy, common in hospitalized patients, produces changes similar to those seen when muscles are catabolized for energy and must be considered. Temporal muscles are less likely to be affected by atrophy (Weinsier & Butterworth, 1981).

Clinical Implications:

- Weight-height index underestimates protein-energy malnutrition in patients with edema from cardiac, renal, or hepatic disease. MAMC is more indicative of nutritional status (Blackburn & Harvey, 1982).
- Visual observations of muscles in the scapular, pelvic, and calf areas may indicate muscle wastage.

HEAD AND CHEST CIRCUMFERENCE

During infancy and childhood, these measurements are utilized to assess growth rate.

GROWTH CHARTS

In children, weight-height charts evaluate growth rate in relation to reference standards (see Appendix C–6). Measurements place the child in a certain percentile; measurements between the 25th and 75th percentiles are considered normal. Above normal deviations may be an indication of obesity; below normal may suggest failure to thrive or inadequate nutrition. These observations are good indicators of nutritional adequacy.

Clinical Assessment

A physical examination can reveal existing nutritional deficiencies. Losses of protein and fat stores are usually accompanied by vitamin and mineral depletion. Even well-nourished patients can develop clinical symptoms of malnutrition in a short time: Kwashiorkor may evolve within two weeks; water-soluble vitamin deficiencies may be seen in one to two months (Gerson, 1980). Mineral deficiencies (iron, calcium, magnesium, and zinc) accompany stress situations and anorexia. Even though this occurs rapidly, it is not the result of a person's not eating properly for one day; it is a reflection of improper long-term nutritional habits. Hypovitaminosis is prevalent in alcoholics and in patients with vascular disease and malabsorption syndromes. The most common chronic deficiency seen in the United States is iron-deficiency anemia (see Chapter 34).

Signs of malnutrition are often nonspecific; different problems may produce the same specific clinical finding. For this reason, clinical findings should be correlated with laboratory data or dietary intake. When attempting to identify the cause for clinical symptoms, many factors must be taken into consideration to establish or rule out primary nutritional deficiency, including (1) illness and its metabolic effects, (2) drugs being administered, (3) liver and kidney functions, (4) cardiac function, (5) gastrointestinal function, (6) different modalities of treatment (such as radia-

tion or chemotherapy), (7) presence of edema or dehydration, (8) possibility of an undiagnosed metabolic problem, and (9) environmental considerations (Table 20–4). Clinical variables also affect the method of nutritional repletion once a nutrient deficiency has been determined.

In human nutrition, deficiencies of several nutrients are more prevalent than an isolated nutrient deficiency (Solomons & Allen, 1983). Signs of malnutrition are most frequently evident in the skin, eyes, mouth, skeleton, and nervous system (Table 20–5). A close look at these areas is important for a thorough assessment. Important indices to observe include evidence of recent weight changes (muscle atrophy), fissures and scales around the mouth, inflamed tongue, pallor, multiple petechiae or hyperpigmentation, abnormal wound healing, rough skin, brittle or pitted nails, edema, or apathetic attitude. Clinical assessments and judgments are as important as any test (Hall et al, 1982) but should be used concurrently with dietary and biochemical assessments.

Clinical Implication:

- Never assume the physician has observed physical changes that may be obvious only during nursing care (Wood, 1982).

Table 20–4. Common Causes of Nutrient Deficiencies*

If Evidence for Deficiency of	Suspect History of
Vitamin A	Fat malabsorption; use of cholestyramine, mineral oil.
Carotene	Fat malabsorption; avoidance of fruit and vegetables; use of cholestyramine, mineral oil, neomycin.
Thiamine	Alcoholism; use of anatacids, cyclophosphamide.
Pyridoxine	Alcoholism; use of cycloserine, ethionamide, isoniazid, oral contraceptive agents, para-aminosalicylic acid (PAS), penicillamine, tetracycline.
Riboflavin	Alcoholism; use of tetracycline.
Niacin	Alcoholism; carcinoid syndrome.
Folic acid	Alcoholism, sprue; avoidance of fruit and vegetables; use of anticonvulsants, cycloserine, methotrexate, nitrofurantoin, oral contraceptive agents, PAS, trimethoprim.
Vitamin B_{12}	Pernicious anemia, resection of terminal ileum, total gastrectomy, intestinal bacterial overgrowth, sprue; avoidance of all animal and dairy foods; use of anticonvulsants, methotrexate, PAS, tetracycline.
Vitamin C	Avoidance of fruits and vegetables; cigarette smoking.
Vitamin D	Fat malabsorption, renal insufficiency; use of anticonvulsants, cholestyramine, mineral oil.
Vitamin E	Dietary deficiency unusual; fat malabsorption and premature infancy are predisposing factors.
Vitamin K	Fat malabsorption, sterilization of gut; use of anticonvulsants, cholestyramine, warfarin, mineral oil.
Calcium	Fat malabsorption, vitamin D deficiency (dietary deficiency of calcium per se is unlikely); use of actinomycin D, antacids, anticonvulsants, cholestyramine, mithramycin, neomycin.
Iron	Bleeding, gastrectomy, pregnancies; poor intake of meats, fruits, and vegetables; use of cholestyramine, chloramphenicol, neomycin.
Magnesium	Fat malabsorption, alcoholism; use of amphotericin.
Phosphorus	Alcoholism, chronic acidosis, hyperparathyroidism, vitamin D deficiency; use of antacids.
Zinc	Alcoholism, fat malabsorption, sickle cell disease, acute hepatitis, burns, diabetes mellitus, nephrotic syndrome, dialysis; use of diuretics, penicillamine.

*From Weinsier, RL; Butterworth, CE, Jr: Handbook of Clinical Nutrition. St. Louis, The C. V. Mosby Co, 1981, by permission.

Table 20–5. Clinical Nutrition Examination*

Clinical Findings	Consider Deficiency of	Consider Excess of
Hair, Nails		
Flag sign (transverse depigmentation of hair)	Protein, copper	
Hair easily pluckable	Protein	
Hair thin, sparse	Protein, biotin, zinc	Vitamin A
Nails spoon-shaped	Iron	
Nails lackluster, transverse ridging	Protein-calories	
Skin		
Dry, scaling	Vitamin A, zinc, essential fatty acids	Vitamin A
Erythematous eruption (sunburn-like)		Vitamin A
Flaky paint dermatosis	Protein	
Follicular hyperkeratosis	Vitamins A and C, essential fatty acids	
Nasolabial seborrhea	Niacin, pyridoxine, riboflavin	
Petechiae, purpura	Ascorbic acid, vitamin K	
Pigmentation, desquamation (sun-exposed area)	Niacin (pellagra)	
Subcutaneous fat loss	Calories	
Yellow pigmentation sparing sclerae (benign)		Carotene
Eyes		
Angular palpebritis	Riboflavin	
Band keratitis		Vitamin D
Corneal vascularization	Riboflavin	
Dull, dry conjunctiva	Vitamin A	
Fundal capillary microaneurysms	Ascorbic acid	
Papilledema		Vitamin A
Scleral icterus, mild	Pyridoxine	
Perioral		
Angular stomatitis	Riboflavin	
Cheilosis	Riboflavin	
Oral		
Atrophic lingual papillae	Niacin, iron, riboflavin, folate, vitamin B_{12}	
Glossitis (scarlet, raw)	Niacin, pyridoxine, riboflavin, vitamin B_{12}, folate	
Hypogeusesthesia (also hyposmia)	Zinc, vitamin A	
Magenta tongue	Riboflavin	
Swollen, bleeding gums (if teeth present)	Ascorbic acid	
Tongue fissuring, edema	Niacin	

*From Weinsier, RL; Butterworth, CE, Jr: *Handbook of Clinical Nutrition.* St. Louis, The C. V. Mosby Co, 1981, by permission.

Specific Diagnostic Procedures

BIOCHEMICAL INFORMATION

Laboratory data provide objective indicators for nutritional status and are frequently ordered when the diet history is questionable or unavailable. Laboratory findings are remarkably accurate, indicating existing and potential problems (Fig. 20–3). Marginal nutritional deficiencies can be detected before overt clinical signs appear. A thorough inspection of laboratory values sometimes reveals a direct relationship between a person's diet and his/her physical condition. In general, clinical and dietary assessments can be substantiated from laboratory data by confirming suspicions or indicating possible causes.

Biochemical indicators of nutritional status utilize blood and urine analyses. Urine is routinely checked for protein, glucose, pH, and acetone. As a general rule, urinary excretion levels fluctuate more than serum levels, reflecting recent rather than usual intake. Blood is usually tested for hemoglobin, hematocrit, total protein, serum albumin or prealbumin, and total lymphocyte count (TLC). Determinations of sodium and potassium, glucose, and cholesterol and triglyceride

Table 20–5. Clinical Nutrition Examintion Continued

Clinical Findings	Consider Deficiency of	Consider Excess of
Glands		
Parotid enlargement	Protein	
Sicca syndrome	Ascorbic acid	
Thyroid enlargement	Iodine	
Heart		
Enlargement, tachycardia, high output failure	Thiamine (wet beriberi)	
Small heart, decreased output	Calories	
Sudden failure, death	Ascorbic acid	
Abdomen		
Hepatomegaly	Protein	Vitamin A
Muscles, Extremities		
Calf tenderness	Thiamine, ascorbic acid (hemorrhage into muscle)	
Edema	Protein, thiamine	
Muscle wastage (especially temporal area, dorsum of hand, spine)	Calories	
Bones, Joints		
Beading of ribs (child)	Vitamins C and D	
Bone and joint tenderness (child)	Ascorbic acid (subperiosteal hemorrhage)	Vitamin A
Bone tenderness (adult)	Vitamin D, calcium, phosphorus (osteomalacia)	
Bulging fontanelle (child)		Vitamin A
Craniotabes, bossing (child)		Vitamin D
Neurological		
Confabulation, disorientation	Thiamine (Korsakoff's psychosis)	
Decreased position and vibratory senses, ataxia	Vitamin B$_{12}$, thiamine	
Decreased tendon reflexes, slowed relaxation phase	Thiamine	
Drowsiness, lethargy		Vitamins A and D
Ophthalmoplegia	Thiamine, phosphorus	
Weakness, paresthesias, decreased fine tactile sensation	Vitamin B$_{12}$, pyridoxine, thiamine	
Other		
Delayed healing and tissue repair (e.g., wound, infarct, abscess)	Ascorbic acid, zinc, protein	
Fever (low-grade)		Vitamin A

levels are indicative of electrolyte balance, carbohydrate metabolism, and lipid metabolism, respectively. Routine laboratory tests used for determining nutritional status are shown in Table 20–6.

VITAMIN LEVELS

Elaborate testing techniques are required for determining most vitamin levels. These tests are expensive and many hospitals are not equipped to provide them on a routine basis. To determine the nutritional status for vitamins, different techniques are implemented, as applicable for the vitamin being measured: vitamin levels in blood and urine, abnormal metabolic products in blood or urine, alterations in activities of certain blood enzymes, vitamin metabolites in urine, and saturation or load tests for certain vitamins (Laboratory indices, 1979). The more common (but infrequent) tests include those for urinary thiamin, riboflavin, and N'-methylnicotinamide and serum levels for carotene and vitamins A and C. By early detection of vitamin deficiency from laboratory tests, more serious complications can be prevented. Table 20–7 shows the various stages of vitamin deficiency. When nutrient intake is inadequate, the body's first adaptation is decreased urinary excretion of the nutrient or its metabolite. Secondly, biochemical changes indicate impaired function or cellular depletion. With further stages of depletion, clinical deficiencies are evident.

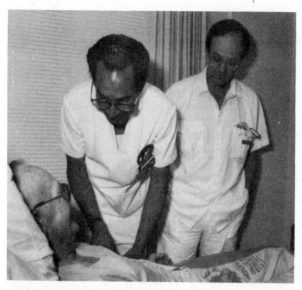

Figure 20–3. Nurses taking a blood sample as part of a nutrition investigation at the Dallas Veterans Administration Medical Association. (Courtesy of Eugene R. Davies, photographer.)

PROTEIN STATUS

Biochemical evaluation of protein status can be determined by several tests: creatinine-height index, 24-hour urine urea nitrogen excretion, and serum transferrin and albumin.

Creatinine-Height Index (CHI). Because all muscles produce a substance called creatinine, the amount of creatinine is directly proportional to skeletal muscle mass and is used to estimate lean body mass. Therefore, a person with smaller amounts of muscle or a malnourished person whose muscle mass has been used for energy produces less creatinine.

To determine the adequacy of muscle mass, 24-hour urinary creatinine content can be compared with standard values for a given height (Fig. 20–4). A creatinine-height index of less than 80 percent indicates a moderate deficit in lean body mass; a value less than 60 percent indicates a severe deficit. Creatinine measurements assume that there are no significant dietary sources of creatinine since it is rapidly excreted in the urine (Munro & Crim, 1980). Accurate results for this test require normal renal and liver function and state of hydration.

Blood Serum Proteins. Visceral protein stores are reflected in serum albumin, prealbumin, and transferrin levels. During malnutrition, protein synthesis is decreased, and albumin and transferrin may be catabolized for energy. Serum transferrin and albumin levels are closely correlated. However, transferrin, an iron-carrying protein, has a shorter half-life, and its measurement is more sensitive of current status. Albumin levels correlate better with changes in MAMC (Bistrian et al, 1974). Low serum levels indicate either depletion of body protein or decreased availability of amino acids for protein synthesis. Low levels of either indicate protein deficiency, which is accompanied by increased risks of anergy, sepsis, and mortality.

Thyroxine-binding prealbumin reflects recent changes in hepatic protein synthesis and is used as a marker for visceral protein stores (Tuten et al, 1985). Acute metabolic stress, accompanied by protein synthesis, causes a sharp, quick drop in prealbumin levels and reflects recent malnutrition.

Nitrogen Balance. A 24-hour urine urea nitrogen clearance test can be used to determine the extent of protein catabolism and nitrogen balance. Urea is the major waste product of protein catabolism. (Ammonia, a toxic substance, is transformed to urea in the liver and excreted in the urine.) In catabolic patients (negative nitrogen balance), protein breakdown is much higher than rates of synthesis; approximately three fourths of the ingested nitrogen is excreted (Steffee et al, 1981). The following formula is used to calculate the estimated nitrogen balance (ENB) (Mackenzie et al, 1974).

$$ENB = \frac{\text{protein input (gm)}}{6.25} - \text{24-hour urine urea N (gm)} + 4$$

By establishing a baseline in the unfed state, the protein and caloric adequacy of a nutrition support program can be monitored (Munro & Crim, 1980). A three-day average, utilizing the preceding formula, should be positive by more than 0.04 gm of nitrogen/kg/day to assure positive nitrogen balance (Weinsier & Butterworth, 1981).

IMMUNE SYSTEM

Malnutrition can also be determined by measuring immune response. Synthesis of antibodies and antibody response to stimulation are decreased in malnutrition. Two different types of laboratory tests are used—total lymphocyte count and skin antigen testing.

Table 20—6. Routine Laboratory Tests in Nutritional Assessment*

Laboratory Findings	Consider Deficiency of	Comment
↓ Albumin, serum	Protein	If no liver disease present
Albuminuria, mild	Protein and calories	If no renal disease present
Anemia		
Normocytic	Protein	
Microcytic	Iron, copper, pyridoxine	
Macrocytic	Folate (in months), vitamin B$_{12}$ (in years), ascorbic acid	
↓ Calcium, serum	Vitamin D, calcium	Consider fat malabsorption, ↓ serum magnesium
↓ Carotene, serum	Carotene (vegetable precursor of vitamin A)	Consider fat malabsorption
↓ Creatinine, serum	Calories	Reflects muscle wastage
Lymphopenia (< 1,200/cu mm)	Protein	Suggests impaired cell-mediated immunity
↓ Phosphorus, serum	Vitamin D, phosphorus	Consider phosphate-binding antacids, rapid glucose infusion, alcoholism
↑ Prothrombin time	Vitamin K	Consider fat malabsorption, biliary obstruction, sterile bowel if no liver disease
Skin tests (nonreactivity)	Protein	Suggests impaired cell-mediated immunity
↓ Transferrin or iron-binding capacity	Protein	Also decreased in chronic disease
↓ Urea, serum	Recent protein intake	If liver not severely impaired

*From Weinsier, RL; Butterworth, CE, Jr: *Handbook of Clinical Nutrition.* St. Louis, The C. V. Mosby Co, 1981, by permission.

Total Lymphocyte Count (TLC). The immune status is reflected in the TLC. A depressed TLC in malnourished patients predisposes them to infection. TLC can be calculated from the complete blood count and the percent of lymphocytes reported with the white blood count (WBC) by using the following formula:

$$TLC/ml = \frac{percent\ of\ Lymphocytes \times WBC}{100}$$

Moderate malnutrition is characterized by a TLC between 800 and 1200. Below 800, patients are considered to be severely malnourished (Blackburn & Thornton, 1979).

Skin Antigen Testing. Intradermal skin tests of recall antigens—mumps, *Candida albicans,* and streptokinase-streptodornase (SK-SD)—are administered to determine the cellular immune response. The tuberculin-skin test (PPD) may be used as a control. An immunocompetent patient will have a response within 24 hours; the malnourished patient may have a delayed or no response. Failure to respond positively (greater than 5 mm induration) may be an indicator of immunoincompetence. No response within 48 hours is termed *anergy.* Reestablishment of immunocompetence can be accomplished by two weeks of aggressive nutritional repletion (MacLean, 1979). While poor nutritional status is not the only causative factor to affect skin response, the dangers of the condition warrant an assessment to determine the cause.

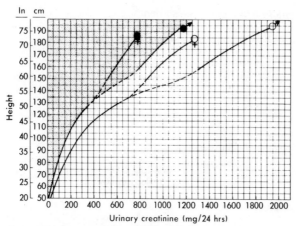

Figure 20–4. *Creatinine height index reference standard (all ages). Broken line represents extrapolated data. Stippled area represents severe muscle mass deficit (< 60% std). ♀ & ♂ = average (standard) values. ♀ & ♂ = 60% of standard. (From Weinsier RL, Butterworth CE Jr: Handbook of Clinical Nutrition. St. Louis, The C. V. Mosby Co, 1981, by permission.)*

Clinical Implications:

- A creatinine-height index less than 60 percent of standard indicates that the patient is at increased risk for anergy, sepsis, and death (Blackburn & Harvey, 1982).
- Profound deficiencies in visceral proteins develop before significant changes in anthropometric measurements in patients with stress secondary to surgery, trauma, or sepsis (Blackburn & Harvey, 1982).

Table 20–7. *Development of Vitamin Deficiency**

Sequence	Deficiency State	Demonstrable Symptoms and Comments
1	Preliminary	Inadequate availability of vitamin due to diet, malabsorption, and abnormal metabolism.
2	Biochemical	Enzyme-coenzyme activity depressed. Urinary vitamin reduced to negligible levels.
3	Physiological	Loss of body weight concurrent with appetite loss, general malaise, insomnia, and increased irritability.
4	Clinical	Increased malaise, loss of body weight with the appearance of deficiency syndromes.
5	Anatomical	Establishment of specific deficiency disease with specific tissue pathology. Unless reversed by repletion, death results.

*From Brin, M; Roe, D: Drug-diet interactions. *Journal of the Florida Medical Association* 66(4):424, 1979, by permission.

- A serum albumin level less than 3 gm/dl and/or serum transferrin levels less than 150 and 170 mg/dl represent significant depletion, and are usually accompanied by anergy and edema (Blackburn & Harvey, 1982).
- Transferrin and albumin are not as significantly affected when only energy deficiency is a problem (marasmus) as compared with protein deficiency (kwashiorkor) (Bistrian & Blackburn, 1983).
- Skin tests may be unreliable when steroid therapy is being administered (Metheny & Snively, 1983).
- Negative skin tests may be indicative of a low concentration of zinc or vitamin A rather than protein-energy malnutrition (Skin tests, 1979).

Referral Parameters

Because of the emphasis on cost containment, unnecessary tests and measurements or elaborate dietary histories are discouraged. However, all patients should be interviewed within 24 hours after admission with a simple, brief, but effective screening procedure to identify those who need more intensive nutritional evaluation. This also establishes a data base from which further changes in their condition can be assessed, reveals any inconspicuous symptoms, and quantifies elements that should be incorporated into a care plan. Identifying change is a significant factor in assessments. Table 20–8 lists commonly available information and routines that provide minimal nutritional screening.

Preliminary clues that are learned in a nursing assessment can be used as indicators of a poorly nourished state and thereby necessitate further nutritional evaluation. A patient should be referred to the dietitian or metabolic specialist for further evaluation of any of the following conditions:

1. A recent weight loss of more than six percent.
2. A low serum albumin and transferrin level.
3. Low lymphocyte or immune function.

The decision tree in Figure 20–5 provides a simple technique to determine nutritional status for predicting outcomes of other therapies or the need for nutritional support prior to those therapies. A synopsis of possible interrelationships among the four parameters used in nutritional assessment is given in Appendix C–9.

Table 20–8. Minimal Assessment of Nutritional Status

	Medical and Socioeconomic	Dietary	Anthropometric Measurements	Clinical Evaluation	Laboratory Evaluation
Infants	Birth weight Length of gestation	Bottle- or breast-fed Supplemental feedings (fluids, solids, method of preparation, weaning, self-feeding) Source of iron Vitamin supplements	Weight Length Overall rate of growth Head circumference	Skin color, turgor Malformations	Hematocrit Hemoglobin
Children	Birth weight Chronic/recent illness Physical activity	Food intake* Appetite Feeding jags, pica Snacking habits Vitamin/mineral supplements Arrangements for eating away from home	Weight Height Arm circumference Overall rate of growth	Skin color, turgor Muscle tone Subcutaneous fat Dental caries	Hematocrit Hemoglobin BUN
Adolescents	Medical history/allergies Socioeconomic data Physical activity Family history Medications	Food intake* (assess for excessive salt or sugar) Where and when foods are eaten Snacking habits Fad diets (especially females) Vitamin/mineral supplements Alcohol intake	Weight Height Recent weight changes	General appearance of hair, skin, eyes Muscle tone Subcutaneous fat Dental caries	Hemoglobin Urine protein Blood sugar
Adults	Medical history Age Number in family Socioeconomic data Physical activity Family history Medications	Food intake* (assess for saturated fat, cholesterol, sugar, salt; iron and calcium in females) Snacking habits Vitamin/mineral supplements Alcohol intake	Weight Height Recent weight changes	General appearance and maintenance of hair, skin, eyes, muscles Dental caries Blood pressure	Hemoglobin Urine protein Blood sugar Urinary pH
Elderly persons	Chronic illness or disability Use of tobacco, alcohol, drugs Source of income; amount for food Any physical changes (bleeding, bowel/ urinary patterns, fainting, headaches	Food intake* and patterns Supplements (protein, vitamins, minerals) Who purchases and prepares food Changes in food habits Taste changes Dietary restrictions	Weight Height Recent weight changes	Skin color, pallor Blood pressure Dentition	Hemoglobin Blood sugar Urinalysis Feces

*Question about the frequency of use of the basic food groups.

Malnutrition

BODY METABOLISM DURING STARVATION

When a patient's intake is inadequate to meet the physiological requirements over an extended period of time, the body is virtually starved, as endogenous energy stores are used for body functions. The degree of starvation and presence of stress determine the extent and type of malnutrition (Bistrian & Blackburn, 1983).

After the onset of starvation, glycogen stores are the first source of energy, rapidly depleted within 16 to 24 hours (Fig. 20–6). With continued

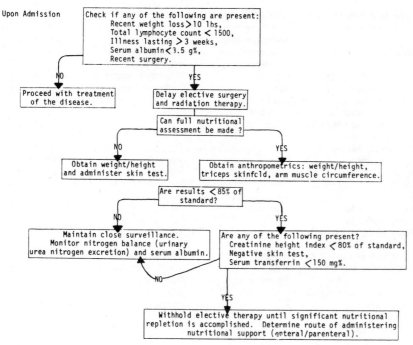

Figure 20–5. *Decision tree for nutritional support. (From Backburn GL, Harvey KB: Prognostic strength of nutritional assessment.* Progress in Clinical and Biological Research *77: 689, 1981, New York, Alan R. Liss, Inc, by permission.)*

starvation, skeletal muscle, visceral protein (body protein within the soft organs), and fat stores are catabolized for energy. Protein present in the visceral organs is necessary; mild protein losses from these areas can impair vital functions. Normal amounts of fat stores can provide more than 150,000 kcal and are the largest supply of energy. The body contains no reserve depots of protein that can be used when protein is not available. Protein deficits compounded with acute stress have a profound impact on many body functions.

The obligatory need for glucose requires a

Table 20–9. *Schematic Hormonal Adaptive Mechanisms in Malnutrition**

Hormone	Stimulus	Results	Hormonal Activities in	
			Calorie Deprivation	Protein-Calorie Deprivation
Insulin	↑ Glucose ↑ Amino acids	↑ Protein synthesis (muscle) ↑ Growth ↑ Lipogenesis	Decreased	Decreased
Growth hormone	↓ Glucose ↑ Amino acids	↑ Protein synthesis (body) ↑ Growth ↑ Lipolysis ↓ Urea synthesis	Variable, generally normal	Increased
Glucocorticoids	↓ Glucose ↓ Amino acids	↑ Protein catabolism (muscle) ↑ Protein turnover (viscera) ↑ Neoglucogenesis ↑ Lipolysis	Increased	Variable, generally normal
Thyroid hromones	↑ Energy metabolism	Energy homeostasis ↑ Protein turnover	Decreased	Decreased

*From Viteri, FE; Torun, B: Protein-calorie malnutrition. In Modern Nutrition in Health and Disease, *6th ed. Edited by RS Goodhart; ME Shils. Philadelphia, Lea & Febiger, 1980, by permission.*

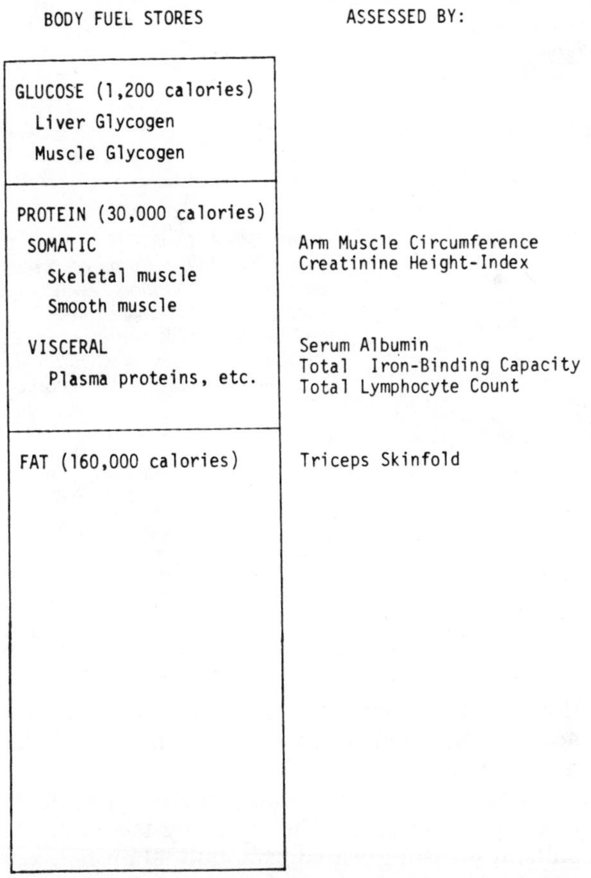

```
BODY FUEL STORES          ASSESSED BY:

┌──────────────────────────────────┐
│ GLUCOSE (1,200 calories)          │
│   Liver Glycogen                  │
│   Muscle Glycogen                 │
├──────────────────────────────────┤
│ PROTEIN (30,000 calories)         │
│   SOMATIC             Arm Muscle Circumference
│     Skeletal muscle   Creatinine Height-Index
│     Smooth muscle                 │
│                                   │
│   VISCERAL            Serum Albumin
│     Plasma proteins, etc.  Total  Iron-Binding Capacity
│                       Total Lymphocyte Count
├──────────────────────────────────┤
│ FAT (160,000 calories)   Triceps Skinfold
│                                   │
│                                   │
│                                   │
└──────────────────────────────────┘
```

Figure 20–6. Composition of body fuel stores and their nutritional assessment. (Adapted from Keithley JK: Infection and the malnourished patient. Heart and Lung 12(1):23, 1983, by permission.)

source. Because fatty acids cannot be converted to glucose, protein is the only source of gluconeogenesis after depletion of glycogen stores. Fortunately, with prolonged starvation, the body will adapt and use ketone bodies rather than glucose, thereby decreasing the rate of protein catabolism (Barrocas et al, 1982). In addition to these adaptive alterations during starvation, hormonal responses are modified, resulting in increased fat mobilization from adipose tissue, as shown in Table 20–9.

CLASSIFICATION

Protein-energy malnutrition (PEM) involves two distinct deficiency states: marasmus and kwashiorkor (Table 20–10). The combination of protein and calorie deficiency is called marasmic kwashiorkor.

Marasmus or Energy Deficiency. In the face of inadequate caloric intake, fat and muscle provide the necessary energy. Marasmus is based on the physical diagnosis of severe fat and muscle wastage. Weight loss is due to loss of muscle and fat; diminished skinfold thickness reflects the loss of fat stores; reduced midarm circumference reflects utilization of skeletal muscle. However, there is normal muscle mass, normal visceral protein (albumin and transferrin), and normal immune competence (Fig. 20–7).

Marasmus is a chronic illness. Nutritionally, it should be approached with the goal of gradually reversing the downward trend to allow for readaptation of metabolic and intestinal functions, rather than with aggressive treatment. Serum phosphate levels should be normal before intravenous dextrose feedings are initiated. Enteral feed-

Table 20–10. Comparison of Marasmus and Kwashiorkor*

	Marasmus	**Kwashiorkor**
Clinical setting	Calories	↓ Protein + stress
Time course to develop	Months, years	Weeks
Clinical features	Starved appearance Weight-height < 80 percent standard Triceps skinfold < 3 mm Midarm muscle circumference < 15 cm Creatinine-height index < 60 percent standard	Well-nourished appearance Hair easily pluckable Edema
Laboratory findings		Serum albumin < 2.8 gm/100 ml Serum transferrin <150 mg/100 ml Lymphocytes < 1200 cells/mm³ Nonreactive skin tests
Clinical course	Reasonably preserved responsiveness to short-term stress	↓ Wound healing ↓ Immuno-competence ↑ Infectious or other complications
Mortality	Low (unless related to underlying disease process)	High

*From Weinsier, RL; Butterworth, CE, Jr: Handbook of Clinical Nutrition. St. Louis, The C. V. Mosby Co, 1981, by permission.

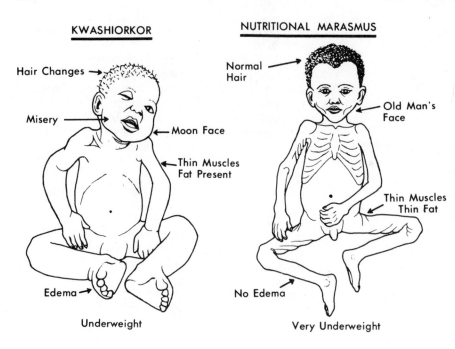

KWASHIORKOR

Hair Changes →

Misery →

Moon Face ←

Thin Muscles
Fat Present ←

Edema →

Underweight

NUTRITIONAL MARASMUS

Normal
Hair →

Old Man's
Face ←

Thin Muscles
Thin Fat ←

No Edema →

Very Underweight

Figure 20–7. *Clinical features of the two main severe forms of protein-calorie malnutrition—kwashiorkor contrasted with marasmus. (From Jelliffe DR: Child Nutrition in Developing Countries. Washington, DC, U.S. Department of State, 1969.)*

ings are the best method of treatment (see Chapter 21).

Marasmus is not particularly life-threatening, but should be corrected because it can readily develop into hypoalbuminemia (kwashiorkor) if stress or trauma is incurred (Fig. 20–8).

Kwashiorkor or Protein Deficiency. In the hospital, kwashiorkor occurs with insufficient dietary intake accompanied by the stress of major surgery, injury, or infection. Typical cases are adults under acute stress who have been on dextrose solutions for an extended period of time (two weeks or more). The continuous carbohy-

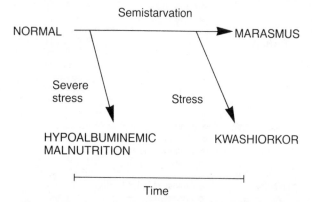

NORMAL → Semistarvation → MARASMUS

Severe
stress

Stress

HYPOALBUMINEMIC
MALNUTRITION

KWASHIORKOR

Time

Figure 20–8. *Factors leading to development of marasmus, hypoalbuminemic malnutrition, and kwashiorkor in adults. (From Blackburn GL, Harvey KB: Nutritional assessment as a routine in clinical medicine. Postgraduate Medicine 71(5):46, 1982, by permission.)*

drate supply interferes with the body's normal adaptive functions during starvation whereby fats are catabolized for energy.

Kwashiorkor, as summarized in Table 20–10, can be diagnosed principally using laboratory results. It is distinguished by a gradual protein loss, with severely depressed serum albumin and transferrin. Visceral organ functions are impaired, as exhibited by the presence of decreased immune competence and hypoalbuminemia. Body weight may remain stable. In some cases, the classic symptoms of kwashiorkor, i.e., skin changes, edema, and easily pluckable hair, are present (see Fig. 20–7).

Aggressive nutritional support is necessary for kwashiorkor. Without this, prognosis is very poor. Parenteral feedings (see Chapter 21) are often implicated to rapidly restore normal metabolic homeostasis (Weinsier & Butterworth, 1981).

Protein-Energy Malnutrition. The result of acute stress in addition to chronic starvation is PEM. Decreased body weight, muscle mass, skinfold thickness, and immune competence are evident. It is an extremely serious, life-threatening situation. Vigorous nutritional therapy is essential.

Vitamin and Mineral Deficiencies. Other deficiencies have been observed during hospitalization and can lead to specific problems. These can be diagnosed by clinical signs and various biochemical tests (see Appendix C–9). These conditions are compounded when they occur concurrently with protein or calorie deficiency. For instance, depressed vitamin C and protein levels result in poor wound healing.

Bollet and Owens (1973) found substantially fewer clinical cases of vitamin or mineral deficiencies than protein-energy malnutrition in hospitalized patients. Deficiency symptoms for vitamins and minerals are discussed in Chapters 10 to 12 under the specific vitamin or mineral. Since vitamins and minerals are required in small amounts, they can be supplemented orally or parenterally.

• FALLACIES and FACTS

FALLACY: *Analysis of hair is a good assessment tool for determining nutritional status.*
 • **FACT:** *Hair analysis has a number of potential pitfalls, including contamination by sweat, environmental pollutants, cosmetics (e.g., shampoos, bleaches, or dyes), and other factors. Several other factors alter the mineral content of hair—age, sex, hormonal levels, and disease. To date, it is not known what the various levels of trace elements mean in terms of health. Concentrations of copper and zinc are variable with increasing distance from the scalp (the farther from the scalp, the higher the values). Hair analysis appears to be of no value in assessing vitamin status. On the other hand, hair analysis for certain heavy metals, such as mercury, arsenic, and lead, can be very sensitive (Hambidge, 1982).*

 So many variables influence the results of hair analysis that little value is derived from a random examination of hair; under no circumstances should it be relied upon as the sole criterion of nutritional status for therapeutic recommendations (Rivlin, 1983).
FALLACY: *Ascorbic acid status can be determined by a lingual test in which a color indicator reacts with ascorbic acid in the saliva.*
 • **FACT:** *Scientific studies have found no significant correlation between either the lingual test and serum levels of ascorbic acid or the lingual test and the estimate of dietary ascorbic acid. Therefore, it is not a reliable diagnostic tool (Ascorbic acid, 1986).*

Summary

Successful nutrition care through the health care process is contingent on the professional's knowledge of nutrition, an awareness of various factors that have nutritional implications, and an ability to communicate observations to others. The nurse has the best opportunity to recognize high-risk patients and to help them before the onset of serious effects of malnutrition. Components of a nutritional support program include (1) observation and assessment of the patient's status, (2) determining requirements and ways to meet them (evaluating routes of access and formulas or types of diet), (3) setting goals for treatment, (4) initiating the plan of care, (5) monitoring biochemical and clinical status or general medical needs of the patient, and (6) evaluating the treatment and the patient's progress.

Early referral of potential problems enables the dietitian to provide more effective nutritional care. An initial screening on admission is important to determine a patient's nutritional state and to implement adequate techniques for either maintenance of good nutrition or rehabilitation.

The patient's diet, a medical history, plus some simple, inexpensive anthropometric measurements (at least weight and height), and routine basic laboratory findings usually suffice to alert the health care team to the possibility of malnutrition. A thorough nutritional assessment will utilize more sophisticated biochemical or laboratory studies of the blood and urine.

PEM can be described as a continuum between marasmus and kwashiorkor. Marasmus is simply an insufficient amount of calories, in which fat stores are used for energy. In the face of stress, when energy and protein requirements are high and not met, kwashiorkor develops. This situation is life-threatening because of delayed wound healing and the impaired resistance to infection. Certain vitamin and mineral deficiencies frequently accompany PEM and should be evaluated. The deficiencies seen most often involve vitamins A, C, and D as well as zinc, copper, and calcium.

Once malnutrition is identified, a plan for nutritional support must be implemented. The refeeding process may also precipitate shortages of potassium, phosphate, and magnesium, thereby necessitating continual reassessments. It is obvious that good nutritional care requires the combined attentive efforts of physician, nurse, and dietitian. With such a supportive team, recovery time can be shortened because there are fewer complications.

Review Questions

1. Discuss the role of nursing in nutritional assessments.
2. What parameters can nursing use to refer the patient for further nutritional assessment?
3. Compare marasmus and kwashiorkor in terms of dietary deficiencies and rehabilitation, clinical findings, and laboratory data.
4. List nutritional implications for each of the following assessment techniques: weight-height index, weight loss, clinical assessments, creatinine-height index, serum albumin and transferrin levels, and immune system evaluation.

Case Study: Mr. S.R., a 75-year-old retired farmer, has been living alone since his wife died 12 years ago. He has been progressively withdrawn over the past months and increasingly despondent over his failing health. His son found him unconscious on the kitchen floor. On admission, he is extremely thin (height, 70 inches; weight, 110 lbs.); there are multiple bruises present and several small open lesions on his arms and legs. He is admitted to the hospital for malnutrition.

1. What diagnostic studies would you anticipate for Mr. R?
2. Assuming a medium frame, determine Mr. R.'s ideal body weight.
3. Why is the total lymphocyte count an important aspect of nutritional assessment?
4. What is the significance of minimal or absent reactions to skin testing?
5. Why must scrupulous care be administered to any open wound or invasive procedure for this patient?

REFERENCE LIST

Ascorbic acid intake and salivary ascorbate levels. *Nutr Reviews* 44(10):328, 1986.

Barrocas, A; Webb, GL; Webb, WR; et al: Nutritional considerations in the critically ill. *South Med J* 75(7):848, 1982.

Bistrian, BR; Blackburn, GL: Assessment of protein-calorie malnutrition in the hospitalized patient. In *Nutritional Support of Medical Practice*, 2nd ed. Edited by HA Schneider; CE Anderson; DB Coursin. Philadelphia, J.B. Lippincott Co, 1983, p 128.

Bistrian, BR; Blackburn, GL; Hallowell, E; et al: Protein status of general surgical patients. *JAMA* 230(6):858, 1974.

Blackburn, GL; Harvey, KB: Nutritional assessment as a routine in clinical medicine. *Postgrad Med* 71(5):46, 1982.

Blackburn, GL; Thornton, PA: Nutritional assessment of the hospitalized patient. *Med Clin North Am* 63(5):1103, 1979.

Bollet, AJ; Owens, SD: Evaluation of nutritional status in selected hospitalized patients. *Am J Clin Nutr* 26(9):931, 1973.

Butterworth, CE, Jr: The skeleton in the hospital closet. *Nutr Today* 9(2):4, 1974.

Butterworth, CE, Jr; Weinsier, RL: Malnutrition in hospital patients: Assessments and treatment. In *Modern Nutrition in Health and Disease*, 6th ed. Edited by RS Goodhart; ME Shils. Philadelphia, Lea & Febiger, 1980, p 667.

Byers, T; Marshall, J; Fiedler, R; et al: Assessing nutrient intake with an abbreviated dietary interview. *Am J Epidemiol* 122(1):41, 1985.

Christensen, KS; Gstundtner, KM: Hospital-wide screening improves basis for nutrition intervention. *J Am Diet Assoc* 85(6):704, 1985.

Gerson, CD: Malnutrition: Do you always recognize it? *Consultant* 20(4):53, 1980.

Hall, CA; Baker, JP; Detsky, AS; et al: Nutritional assessment. *N Engl J Med* 307(12):754, 1982.

Hambidge, KM: Hair analyses: Worthless for vitamins, limited for minerals. *Am J Clin Nutr* 36(5):943, 1982.

Kamath, SK; Lawler, M; Smith, AE; et al: Hospital malnutrition: A 33-hospital screening study. *J Am Diet Assoc* 86(2):203, 1986.

Laboratory indices of nutritional status. *Nutrition and the MD* V(5):1, 1979.

Mackenzie, T; Blackburn, G; Flatt, JB: Clinical assessment of nutritional status using nitrogen balance. *Fed Proc* 33:683, 1974.

MacLean, LD: Host resistance in surgical patients. *J Trauma* 19(5):297, 1979.

Matthews, LE: Practical nutritional assessment: Maximizing limited resources. *J Nutr Elderly* 4(1):43, 1984.

Metheny, N; Snively, W: *Nurses' Handbook of Fluid Balance*, 4th ed. Philadelphia, J. B. Lippincott Co, 1983.

Munro, HN; Crim, MC: The proteins and amino acids. In *Modern Nutrition in Health and Disease*, 6th ed. Edited by RS Goodhart; ME Shils. Philadelphia, Lea & Febiger, 1980, p 51.

Rivlin, RS: Misuse of hair analysis for nutritional assessment. *Am J Med* 75(3):489, 1983.

Roe, D: *Clinical Nutrition for the Health Scientist*. Boca Ratan, FL, CRC Press, 1979.

Roy, LB; Edwards, PA; Barr, LH: The value of nutritional assessment in the surgical patient. *JPEN* 9(2):170, 1985.

Shils, ME: Indices of the nutritional status of the individual. *Prog Clin Biol Res* 67:71, 1981.

Skin tests as a measure of nutritional status. *Nutrition and the MD* V(5):3, 1979.

Solomons, NW; Allen, LH: The functional assessment of nutritional status: Principles, practice and potential. *Nutr Rev* 41(2):33, 1983.

Steffee, WP; Anderson, CF; Young, VR: An evaluation of diurnal rhythm of urea excretion in healthy young adults. *JPEN* 5(5):378, 1981.

Swan, E; Rohrback, C: Nutritional assessment—an investigative interview. *Nutr Support Services* 2(5):12, 1982.

Tuten, MP; Wogt S; Dasse, F; et al: Utilization of prealbumin as a nutritional parameter. *JPEN* 9(6):709, 1985.

Weinsier, RL; Butterworth, CE, Jr: *Handbook of Clinical Nutrition*. St. Louis, The C. V. Mosby Co, 1981.

Wood, SR: The nurse and nutritional support. In *Clinical Nutrition '81*. Edited by RIC Wesdorp; PB Soeters. New York, Churchill Livingstone Press, 1982, p 323.

Yale University Health Systems Management Group (YUH-SMG): *The New ICD-9-CM Diagnosis-Related Groups Classification Scheme, Volume I: User Manual*. U.S. Dept. of Commerce, National Technical Information Service (PB 83-155085), December 1981.

Further Study

Assessment Tips: Nurse's quick guide to nutritional disorders. *Nursing* 13(4):56, 1983.

Barrett, S: Commercial hair analysis: Science or scam? *JAMA* 254(8):1041, 1985.

Block, AS: Developing nutrition screening/assessments forms. *Am J IV Ther Clin Nutr* 7(6):17, 1980.

Butterworth, CE: Hospital malnutrition. *Nutr Today* 10(2):8, 1975.

Caly, JC: Helping people eat for health: Assessing adults' nutrition. *Am J Nurs* 77(10):1605, 1977.

Carpenito, LJ: Diagnosing nutritional problems. *Am J Nurs* 85(5):584, 1985.

Dansky, KH: Assessing children's nutrition. *Am J Nurs* 77(10):1610, 1977.

Fuller, E: Who is malnourished? *Patient Care* 20(11):143, 1986.

Henson, LR: Nutritional assessment and management of the hospitalized patient. *Crit Care Nurse* 5(2):53, 1985.

Keithley, JK: Proper nutrition assessment can prevent hospital malnutrition. *Nursing* 9(12):68, 1979.

MacBurney, M; Wilmore, D: Rational decision making in nutritional care. *Surg Clin North Am* 61(3):571, 1981.

Mallison, MB: Food for thought . . . malnourished patients. *Am J Nurs* 85(3):233, 1985.

Michel, L; Serrano, A; Malt, RA: Nutrition support of hospitalized patients. *N Engl J Med* 304(19):1147, 1981.

Monteith, M; Nakagawa, A: A flow chart approach to nutritional screening and assessment in long-term care facilities. *J Am Diet Assoc* 75(6): 684, 1979.

Moore, MC; Greene, HL: What you can learn from weighing a patient. *RN* 86(4):65, 1986.

Orr, JW; Shingleton, HM: Importance of nutritional assessment and support in surgical and cancer patients. *J Reprod Med* 29(9):635, 1984.

Salmond, SW: How to assess the nutritional status of the acutely ill patients. *Am J Nurs* 80(5):922, 1980.

Sauerblich, HE; Dowdy, RP; Skala, JH: *Laboratory Tests for the Assessment of Nutritional Status.* Cleveland, CRC Press, 1974.

Truswell, AS: Measuring nutrition. *Br Med J* 291(Nov 2):1258, 1985.

Wright, RA: Nutritional assessment. *JAMA* 244(6):539, 1980.

Enteral & Parenteral Nutrition

21

STUDENTS WILL BE ABLE TO:

- *Identify conditions that warrant supplemental feedings and/or tube feedings.*
- *List the different types of enteral feedings and characteristic features of each.*
- *State the advantages of enteral feedings over parenteral feedings.*
- *Identify the various routes and methods of delivery for tube feedings.*
- *List the precautions to check before and during a tube feeding.*
- *Cite sanitation techniques important in handling tube feedings.*
- *Describe techniques in administering tube feedings that affect the patient's comfort and adaptation.*
- *Explain the cause, prevention, and treatment of hyperglycemic hyperosmolar nonketotic dehydration.*
- *State why standard intravenous feedings cannot adequately nourish patients.*
- *State reasons for and limitations of peripheral and central parenteral nutrition.*
- *Explain tonicity and its importance in both enteral and parenteral feedings.*
- *Explain why fat emulsions are used in TPN.*
- *State the role of the floor nurse and nutritional support in TPN.*
- *List problems and complications commonly associated with TPN.*

Calorie-to-nitrogen ratio
Elemental
Enteral
Hyperalimentation
Hyperglycemic
  hyperosmolar
  nonketotic (HHNK)
  dehydration
Intravenous (IV)
Iso-, hypo-, and
  hypertonic
Monomeric
Osmolarity
Parenteral
Polymeric
Sepsis
Total parenteral nutrition
  (TPN)

OBJECTIVES

TERMS TO KNOW

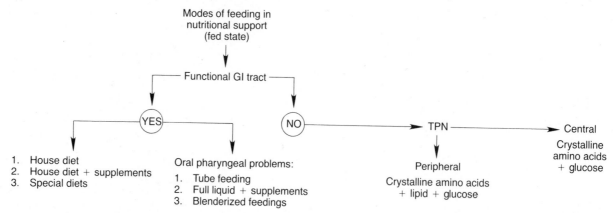

Figure 21–1. *Nutritional support systems. (Adapted from Hopkins BS, Bistrian BR, Blackburn GL: Protein-calorie management in the hospitalized patient, in Schneider HA, Anderson CE, Coursin DB (eds): Nutritional Support of Medical Practice, 2nd ed. Philadelphia, Harper & Row, 1983, p 145, by permission.)*

The catabolic stresses of illness, surgery, trauma, and some therapeutic measures demand aggressive nutrition support: Anywhere from 2500 to 4000 kcal/day or more are required for recovery. Thus, few patients can afford to remain NPO for extended periods. Standard dextrose intravenous (IV) feedings are not considered a form of nutritional support; a liter of D₅W provides only 170 kcal. These dextrose solutions are used to prevent or correct more imminent problems of fluid and electrolyte balance (see Chapter 5).

Unless preventive nutritional support is instituted early in the course of an illness before nutritional status deteriorates, physiologically stressed patients can develop nutritional disturbances rapidly. Without adequate nutrition, a state of "self-cannibalism" results, with the patient utilizing his/her own tissues to procure the necessary amino acids and energy for healing. Chronically ill patients who become malnourished are usually anorectic and hypermetabolic and have malabsorption problems. Consequently, they have impaired cell-mediated immunity, increased susceptibility to infection, poor wound healing, and weakness. Since oral intake is inadequate, other measures are necessary to assure that nutritional requirements are met.

An assessment of individuals whose intake is inadequate (either because they *cannot* or *do not* ingest adequate nutrients) will aid in precisely tailoring a plan to provide nutritional support for them. A variety of feeding modalities are available (Fig. 21–1). These may include modifications in consistency and flavor of foods, oral supplements, enteral feedings (using the gastrointestinal tract), and parenteral nutrition (intravenous feedings via peripheral or central veins).

Chernoff (1981) has established guidelines to determine the form of nutritional support for maintaining or renourishing a patient. The most appropriate method is to supply a normal diet. If intake is not adequate, oral supplements of nutritionally complete enteral feedings can be an adjunct to the normal diet. If nutritional status cannot be maintained from oral feedings, tube feedings may be an alternative. As a last resort, when the gastrointestinal tract is incapacitated or should be rested, parenteral (intravenous) feedings are in order.

Enteral Feedings

If the gastrointestinal tract is functional, it should be used, even if oral intake is not feasible. Tube feeding is a convenient, economical method of nutritional support when patients are unable to orally ingest adequate nutriment to meet their metabolic needs (Fig. 21–2). It can be used as the only feeding method or as a supplement to oral intake.

TYPES OF ENTERAL FEEDINGS

Several types of feedings are available utilizing the gastrointestinal tract to meet nutritional

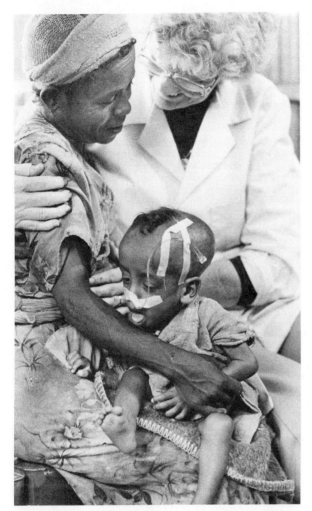

Figure 21-2. *A missionary volunteer nurse comforts a mother whose 12-pound, 22-month-old child came to the feeding—health care center in Rabel, Ethiopia, on the verge of death. The baby was fed with a nasogastric tube because his blood vessels were too small for normal intravenous feeding. (Photo by Don Rutledge, reprinted by permission, Foreign Mission Board, Southern Baptist Convention, Richmond, VA.)*

needs for different disease states, feeding modes, and digestive and absorptive functions (Table 21–1). With more than 50 enteral feeding products available, the formulations differ in osmolality (concentration of osmotically active particles in solution), digestibility, caloric density, lactose content, viscosity, and fat content (see Appendix A–2). Changes are constantly made (new formulas and composition of old formulas) in each of the classes of feedings as a result of new knowledge.

Blended Tube Feedings. Normal foods are blended to a liquid consistency for use as a tube feeding. Since the proportions of carbohydrate, protein, and fat are similar to the regular diet, the feeding is well tolerated by patients who have difficulty with swallowing or oral problems but an otherwise normally functioning gastrointestinal tract.

Sometimes regular foods are blenderized. Baby foods may be utilized with the addition of some liquid. Blended tube feedings of this type may be preferred, especially by some outpatients, because of better palatability, variety, and reduced cost. However, if the particle size is too large or the mixture too thick, the feeding tube may become clogged.

Commercially available blended products are Vitaneed (Biosearch), Formula 2 (Cutter), and Compleat-B (Doyle). They contain natural foodstuffs plus additional vitamins and minerals and moderate amounts of residue.

Polymeric Formulas. Tube feedings or oral supplements are commercially prepared products that can be used to increase nutrient intake or to provide complete enteral nutrition. Polymeric formulas provide intact nutrients in a complex form (whole proteins and long-chain triglycerides), which require a normally functioning gastrointestinal tract. Some polymeric formulas are flavored, increasing their acceptance as oral supplements.

Formulations are available as a powder to be mixed with milk or water and in ready-to-use liquid form. These have extended shelf life and are relatively palatable.

Because of the prevalence of lactose intolerance, many commercially prepared formulas are lactose-free. Most are made with caseinate and soy proteins as the source of protein, but some contain egg albumin. Various sweeteners are used; more complex carbohydrates, such as maltodextrin, help to decrease the osmolality of the formula. Fats are supplied from soy oil, medium-chain triglycerides (MCT), and corn oil.

Besides their convenience, commercially prepared formulas are microbiologically safe and are consistent in their nutrient content. Most contain 1 kcal/ml. When the patient is given 1000 to 2000 ml of formula, the RDAs for vitamins and minerals are met. (While the RDAs are used as a standard, these amounts may not be adequate for many patients.) They usually have a low osmolality and are relatively low in residue.

Monomeric Formulas. When the gastrointestinal tract is not wholly functional (as in short gut syndrome) or when fecal residue should be minimal (as before an operation), monomeric formulas

Table 21-1. *Classification of Tube Feedings*

Type	Commercial Preparations	Comments
Blenderized	Compleat B (Doyle) Formula 2 (Cutter) Vitaneed (Biosearch)	Blended natural foods; ready-to-use.
Polymeric milk-based	Meritene (Doyle) Instant Breakfast (Carnation) Sustacal Powder (Mead Johnson)	Pleasant-tasting oral supplements; provide intact nutrients.
Polymeric lactose-free	Enrich with fiber (Ross) Ensure (Ross) Isocal (Mead Johnson) Osmolite (Ross) Precision Isotonic (Doyle) Nutri 1000 (Cutter) Renu (Biosearch) Sustacal (Mead Johnson) Travasorb (Travenol)	Used as tube feeding, meal replacement, or oral supplement; made with intact protein isolates, oligosaccharides and starches, and fats; provide 1 kcal/cc (others available providing up to 2 kcal/cc); in adequate quantities meet RDAs for vitamins and minerals; ready to use (except Precision Isotonic); isotonic (except Ensure, Sustacal, and Travasorb).
Elemental or monomeric formulas	Criticare (Mead Johnson) Vipep (Cutter) Vital (Ross) Vivonex (Eaton) Travasorb Standard (Travenol)	Partially digested nutrients for feeding; hypertonic; require reconstitution.

are appropriate. (They are also called chemically defined or elemental diets.) Most are powders that are to be mixed with water to form hypertonic solutions. Monomeric diets require minimal digestion since the basic nutrients are ready-to-absorb and do not overly stimulate pancreatic, biliary, and intestinal secretions. The protein source is a balanced mixture of short-chain peptides or pure amino acids. The carbohydrate is glucose or dextrins. These diets contain very little fat. Electrolytes, minerals, and trace elements are also present.

Nutrients from monomeric diets are rapidly absorbed in the proximal small intestine and are adequately absorbed even in some cases of short-bowel syndrome. On the other hand, for individuals with a normally functioning gastrointestinal tract, there is no evidence that monomeric formulas are superior to polymeric formulas (Jones et al, 1983). The high osmolality of these formulas can cause an osmotic effect, drawing fluid into the gastrointestinal tract to dilute the concentration of the formula. The result is gastric distention, nausea, diarrhea, and dehydration. Adequate fluid intake is essential, and biochemical and nutritional monitoring is important.

Because of their amino acid and peptide content, chemically defined diets are not very palatable and are usually administered by tube. If patients are to take these solutions orally, smell and taste bud contact should be minimized. Only small amounts taken over a period of time can be tolerated. Incorporating even meager quantities of these formulas into clear liquids can significantly increase nutrient density of clear-liquid diets.

Modular Feeding Components. Individual nutrients can be used to increase the nutrient content of foods or commercial formulas or can be combined to tailor nutritional support for the specific requirements of the patient. Protein, carbohydrate, and fat components are produced commercially for this purpose. A nutritionally complete enteral formula can be made from the protein, carbohydrate, and fat entities with the addition of vitamins, trace elements, and electrolytes. These have been useful for renal diseases, hepatic diseases, and glucose tolerance tests. They are most frequently used to manipulate potassium, fluid, and glucose.

Carbohydrate supplements, Polycose (Ross) and Sumacal (Biosearch), are made from maltodextrin or cornstarch, contain 2 kcal/cc, and can be added to liquids without significantly affecting the flavor. Corn syrup could also be used.

Fat supplements (e.g., MCT oil by Mead Johnson) contain 7.7 kcal/cc and can be utilized in malabsorption syndromes (although essential fatty acids are not included). Microlipid (Biosearch) is a fat emulsion supplement containing essential fatty acids.

Protein formulations are also available: Casec (Mead Johnson), Pro Mix (Navaco), or Propac (Biosearch).

Specialty Feedings. Special formulations are

produced for patients with normally functioning gastrointestinal tracts but with metabolic problems. Amin-aid (McGaw) and Travasorb (Travenol) for renal diseases supply kilocalories and essential amino acids with the necessary low-electrolyte content (see Chapter 33). Hepatic-Aid (McGaw), for patients with advanced liver disease, contains a high percentage of branched-chain amino acids (leucine, isoleucine, or valine), low amounts of the aromatic amino acids (phenylalanine, tryrosine, or tryptophan), electrolytes, and kilocalories (see Chapter 28). These special formulations can be used as oral supplements or tube feedings. Vitamins and electrolytes are supplemented according to the metabolic status of the patient.

ADVANTAGES

The advantages of enteral feedings are obvious. They are physiologically more natural; nutrients are utilized more efficiently; metabolic upsets are less likely to occur; tonicity of the gastrointestinal tract is maintained; they are less expensive and more nutritionally complete than intravenous solutions. Demands on nursing personnel are less than with parenteral feedings. The elemental diet requires minimal digestive capabilities, decreases gastric and pancreatic enzyme secretions, and presents little residue in the colon.

Clinical Implications:

- When polymeric nutritional formulas are to be consumed between meals for additional nutrient support, the formula should be maintained in a chilled bedside container for easy patient accessibility.
- If the formula is to be taken orally, a variety of flavors helps to prevent "flavor fatigue" (Arnold, 1981).
- While elemental diets are available in several flavors, they are relatively unpalatable. They will be more acceptable if served as a fast-food beverage (on ice, covered, and with a straw) and sipped slowly. Leave a small amount in ice at the patient's bedside.

INDICATIONS FOR USE

The uses for tube feedings and oral supplements have expanded in recent years. Used both pre- and postoperatively, they provide more nutritional support to build up the patient and to prevent cachexia that can result from some treatments. Oral supplemental feedings may be used anytime it is felt that nutrient requirements exceed the amount of nutrients the patient is able to ingest. Tube feedings can be used for the following conditions:

1. Physical impairments that cause swallowing difficulties, dental disorders, dysphagia, stroke complications, comatose states (with caution), or esophageal obstruction.
2. Upper gastrointestinal problems such as esophageal fistula; partial obstructions in the esophagus or pylorus; and surgery or radiation therapy of the upper alimentary tract, neck, upper respiratory system, or oropharynx.
3. Mental disturbances such as anorexia or depression.
4. Hypermetabolic states that produce increased nutritional needs, such as burns, sepsis, multiple injuries, cancer, or hyperthyroidism.

In some instances, tube feedings may provide effective nutritional support for patients who have abnormal gastrointestinal tracts: inflammatory bowel disease (such as Crohn's disease), colitis, malabsorption syndromes, enterocutaneous fistulae, pancreatic insufficiency, short-bowel syndrome, and partial bowel obstruction. Conditions such as renal or hepatic failure and neurological dysfunctions may require the use of some of these specially developed products.

ROUTES FOR ADMINISTRATION

Tube feedings can be administered through a number of routes (Fig. 21–3). Recent development of soft, nonirritating tubes has proved to be an advantage over the stiff Levin tubes formerly used. The mercury- or tungsten-weighted tubes are radiopaque so the tip location can be checked by x-ray films. The smaller, soft-bore tubes made of polyurethane or silicon elastomers are available in several sizes and come with stylets to facilitate their placement. If the interior of the lumen has been lubricated, removal of the stylet is easier (Matarese, 1982).

The most common route is a nasogastric (NG) tube inserted into the stomach (intragastric route). This is satisfactory for short-term feeding, but the presence of the tube interferes with normal functioning of the lower esophageal sphincter (LES). Reflux esophagitis is a problem; regurgitation and aspiration are risks especially in the comatose pa-

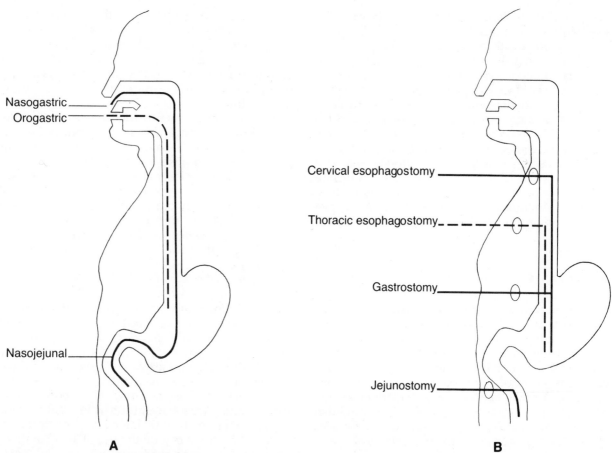

Figure 21–3. *Types of enteral tube feedings. A) Nasogastric tube: A weighted tube is passed through the nose into the stomach; prolonged use may irritate mucous membranes. Nasojejunal tube: Regurgitation and aspiration are minimized when tube is passed into the jejunum; adequate digestion of intact nutrients. Orogastric tube: Tube is passed through the mouth and removed after feedings. B) Esophagostomy: A temporary or permanent opening (stoma) is made through the neck or chest for patients with chewing or swallowing problems; entire GI tract is used; easy to care for, few complications, and appropriate for extended use. Gastrostomy: Temporary or permanent stoma feeds directly into the stomach; entire GI tract is used; appropriate for long-term use when the esophagus is impaired. Jejunostomy: Stoma bypasses the stomach; least acceptable method because of high incidence of dumping syndrome and diarrhea; large-gauge needle is sometimes used to place a small catheter into the jejunum; elemental formulas are used.*

tient. On the other hand, intragastric feeding permits full utilization of digestion and absorption functions and lessens the chances of a hyperosmolar solution causing gastric distention, nausea, vomiting, and sweating.

Longer, more flexible weighted tubes can also be passed to the duodenum (nasoduodenal) and the jejunum (nasojejunum). Intact nutrients can still be digested and the problem of regurgitation is lessened.

Gastrostomy, esophagostomy, or jejunostomy is more suitable for long-term use. The tube is surgically inserted at the appropriate location and sutured in place.

METHODS OF DELIVERY

Tube feedings can be administered intermittently (bolus feedings) or continuously. Bolus feedings, delivered only to the stomach, are normally given every three to four hours and resemble normal meal-feeding patterns. About 100 to 400 cc are administered at each feeding by either Asepto syringe or slow gravity drip.

Tube feeding by a syringe (called a bolus feeding) is an obsolete technique and should be discouraged. Feedings are infused within a few minutes (often too rapidly) and are poorly tolerated. Complications include gastric retention, pulmonary aspiration, nausea, diarrhea, distention, and cramps.

Disposable gravity-flow gastric feeding units control the flow rate and are therefore better tolerated. The prescribed volume of formula is infused over a 20- to 30-minute period.

Continuous feedings can be administered by gravity flow or a mechanical pump over a 16- to 24-hour period. A mechanical pump is more dependable than the gravity drip method, which is subject to an uneven flow rate. A small tube with a lumen smaller than No. 8 French requires a pump for continuous infusion (Campbell et al, 1984). The continuous feeding technique generally improves absorption, reduces diarrhea, and achieves nitrogen balance sooner. Pumps are now equipped with an alarm to indicate malfunction. Continuous pump infusions are recommended, especially for feedings into the distal duodenum or proximal jejunum, for monomeric formula, and for patients who have a limited absorptive area. Precise flow rates are important and should be checked every hour for accuracy.

ORDERING THE ENTERAL FEEDING

Tube feedings should be ordered to meet individual nutritional requirements and capabilities. A nutritional assessment (see Chapter 20) helps to determine the patient's requirements and tolerances and to select an appropriate formula. Unfortunately, patients with severe malnutrition and sepsis, requiring intensive nutritional support, are least able to tolerate a tube feeding. Patients with a serum albumin level of less than 3 gm/dl are probably not able to tolerate a full-strength formula (Cobb et al, 1981).

If tube feeding is the only feeding modality used, the total kilocaloric value must be adequate but not excessive. The amount and quality of protein in the formula is important. A high-protein formula (more than 16 percent) can cause dehydration, especially if the patient is unable to request fluids. Monomeric formulas must contain the essential amino acids to produce and maintain nitrogen balance. It the patient is intolerant of lactose, maltose, or sucrose, formulas are available that do not contain these carbohydrates.

Electrolyte imbalances or overload must be avoided. The amount of sodium in the formula should be of special consideration for patients with fluid retention.

Selecting the right formula can be a crucial element in the patient's recovery. Tube feedings that cause diarrhea or an oral supplement that is not consumed will not help the patient. Elemental formula diets are indicated only when malabsorption or maldigestion is present. They are sometimes given indiscriminately, even though the patient could benefit from the less expensive (and better-tasting) polymeric formulas (Hinsdale et al, 1985). Postoperative patients and those with moderate small-bowel impairment tolerate polymeric formulas better than the elemental feeding (Fairfull-Smith et al, 1980).

The dietary order should include: (1) the type of feeding (e.g., blended, polymeric, or monomeric), (2) the route of administration, (3) the volume to be administered daily, (4) the number of kilocalories per day, (5) the number of feedings per day, and (6) any other pertinent information such as the amount of protein or other nutrients desired.

Since these patients are in a high risk category for developing protein calorie malnutrition, the proper formula and amount must be prescribed and it must be delivered to the patient. Frequently inadequate amounts of tube feedings are given because of interruptions for diagnostic tests, physical and respiratory therapy, and a lack of an institutional protocol for compensatory rates of delivery.

PRINCIPLES AND PROCEDURES FOR TUBE FEEDINGS

Feedings administered directly into the intestinal tract should be easily digestible, almost isotonic (about 300 mOsm/L), and dispensed slowly. Tonicity refers to the relationship of the solution to the osmotic pressure of body fluids. Isotonic solutions have the same osmolality as the body fluids and do not cause rapid fluid shifts into or from the gastrointestinal tract.

If the individual has had food in the gastrointestinal tract in the previous 24 hours, a full-strength polymeric formula is appropriate. When the person has been without nourishment for a while, a formula low in calories, nutrients, and volume (50 to 100 cc per feeding) should be given.

While dilutions can be made by adding water, this procedure should be performed only by the department (usually dietary or pharmacy) responsible for preparing the formula. A diluted concentration of the formula with water means that, for a given volume of intake, the patient is receiving fewer kilocalories. If additional formula is needed (e.g., because of spillage), this should be obtained from the department responsible. One should not dilute the formula without checking with the responsible department.

Prior to beginning a tube feeding, the procedure should be explained to the patient to obtain his/her cooperation. Several precautions are imperative:

1. Allow 30 minutes after intubation before initiating feeding.
2. Do not feed anything into the tube unless the tip location is known.
3. Begin with formula that has been diluted 1/4 to 1/2 strength (by the responsible department) unless the formula is isotonic (300 mOsm/kg) or the patient has eaten within the last 24 hours.
4. Deliver slowly (start at a rate of 50 ml/hr).
5. Observe for glucosuria and diarrhea.
6. Increase the rate by 25 ml/hr at 8- to 12-hour intervals (until the desired rate is reached), provided glucosuria or diarrhea is not present.
7. Increase formula strength as tolerated *after* achieving the desired feeding rate.

By increasing the volume (rate) for administering an isotonic formula, fluid and electrolyte needs are achieved more quickly. Three to five days may be required for the patient's adaption to the formula. Increasing the concentration or amount of feeding too soon may have negative results and require starting the adaptive process over again. Even if the feeding falls behind schedule, one should not attempt to catch up.

During feeding, the patient's head should be elevated at least to a 30° angle during and for one hour after feeding to prevent aspiration. Gastric residuals for bolus feedings are checked before the feeding to determine gastric stasis.

Tube feedings require sanitary techniques to prevent bacterial contamination, especially when pouches are hung for extended periods of time. Unopened cans do not require refrigeration. Opened containers of formula should be dated, refrigerated, and discarded if not used within 24 to 48 hours.

The administration of cold formula causes cramping accompanied by diarrhea in some individuals (Kagawa-Busby et al, 1980). Before a tube feeding is administered, refrigerated formula should be placed in a container of hot water, and warmed to room temperature; feedings should be shaken to make sure particles are in suspension.

Adequate fluid intake is imperative. Additional water is usually necessary to maintain a satisfactory urinary output. Schulte (1978) advocates 0.5 ml of water for each milliliter of tube feeding to prevent osmotic dehydration. Patients who are able to take fluids by mouth are encouraged to do so. Additional water is especially necessary with a larger protein and electrolyte load and when the patient has fever, decreased renal concentrating

ability, or extensive tissue breakdown (Metheny & Snively, 1983). The amount of fluid necessary can be determined by fluid intake and output, clinical signs, and laboratory data, such as BUN and sodium levels.

Intermittent feedings should be preceded and followed by 20 to 50 ml of lukewarm water. This procedure moistens the tube to prevent the feeding mixture from adhering to it and flushes it out after the feeding.

Even though the patient is not taking food orally, routine oral hygiene is important.

COMPLICATIONS

Serious complications from enteral feedings may occur; however, most are preventable if the nurse is knowledgeable about nutritional requirements and physiological symptoms, and if s/he monitors the patient's responses. Most complications can be prevented by correct formula selection and proper administration techniques (Table 21–2). Some type of chart containing pertinent information on one page should be developed and used to prevent problems and complications (see *Focus on Enteral Feeding Chart*).

The most frequent complications of commercially prepared formula are dehydration, diarrhea, and nausea, which are related to diuresis caused by the hyperosmotic solution. Hyperglycemia is one of the first detectable signs (other than nausea and abdominal cramps) of this problem. Hyperglycemia occurs in 10 to 30 percent of tube-fed patients (Vanlandingham et al, 1981). The rate or concentration of the formula may be decreased or intermediate-acting insulin administered until the blood sugar is approximately 200 mg/dl (Bernard & Forlaw, 1984).

If this is left unchecked, hyperglycemic hyperosmolar nonketotic (HHNK) dehydration deteriorating into a coma may result. The syndrome of hyperglycemic hyperosmolar nonketosis develops when insulin reserves are adequate to prevent ketosis but inadequate to control serum glucose. The elevated blood sugar rises to cause osmotic diuresis and eventually dehydration. Because of careful monitoring of tube-fed patients, this complication is not observed frequently. Small doses of insulin and large amounts of fluids are given to correct the situation (Bernard & Forlaw, 1984).

Patients on steroid therapy and diabetics are more intolerant of large carbohydrate loads and must be monitored more closely. While urine could be tested for glucosuria, blood glucose monitoring using a visual blood glucose testing stick

Table 21–2. *Complications of Enteral Nutritional Support and Recommendations for Management**

Complication	Considerations	Management
A. Gastrointestinal 1. Diarrhea, bloating, hypermotility.	Hyperosmolar solution.	Use isotonic formula; dilute solution.
	Rapid administration of feeding.	Reduce infusion rate; gradually increase as tolerated.
	Lactose intolerance.	Use lactose-free formula.
	Bacterial contamination.	Use aseptic technique.
	Tube placement.	Reposition tube.
	Formula temperature.	Administer formula at room temperature.
	Treatment side effects.	Evaluate drug and radiation therapies. Antidiarrheal medications may be indicated.
2. Constipation.	Inadequate fluids, dehydration.	Increase fluid intake, monitor intake and output.
	Low residue content of formula.	Use fiber-containing formula.
	Medications.	Adjustment of medications.
3. Nausea, vomiting, abdominal cramping.	Hyperosmolar formula.	Use isotonic formula; dilute solution.
	Rapid administration of feeding.	Reduce infusion rate; gradually increase as tolerated.
	Lactose intolerance.	Use lactose-free formula.
	Bacterial contamination.	Use aseptic technique.
	Formula temperature.	Administer formula at room temperature.
	Delayed gastric emptying or gastric residual.	If ≥100 ml, hold feeding 2 to 8 hr. Resume at reduced/diluted flow rate.
	Gastric distention.	Ambulation may alleviate.
	Possible GI obstruction.	Discontinue feeding until problem is identified and corrected.
B. Mechanical 1. Aspiration.	Head of bed not elevated.	30 to 45° elevation of head of bed at all times.
	Incorrect tube placement.	Verify proper tube placement before/during feeding.
	Regurgitation in high-risk patients (weak, comatose, patients with neuromuscular disorders).	Consider gastrostomy or jejunostomy.
	Tube too large (commonly causes reflux at gastroesophageal sphincter).	Use smallest tube through which formula will flow.
	Delayed gastric emptying or gastric residual.	If ≥100 ml, hold feeding 2 to 8 hr. Resume at reduced/diluted flow rate. Maintain residual >100 ml.
2. Tube obstruction.	Inadequate flushing with water.	Flush tube with ≥25 ml of water after each intermittent feeding or every 2 to 9 hr during continuous feeding.
	Formula viscosity.	Adjust tube size; small-bore tubings (6 to 8 French) are not recommended for highly viscous formulas.
	Improper administration of medications through tube.	Use liquid medications when possible. Always flush tube with 25 ml of water before and after administration of medications through tube to prevent clogging.

*Courtesy of the Fort Worth Dietetic Association: *Enteral Nutrition Formula Handbook,* Fort Worth, TX, 1985.

Table continued on following page

Table 21—2. Complications of Enteral Nutritional Support and Recommendations for Management Continued

Complication	Considerations	Management
3. Nasoesophageal erosion.	Tube irritation, esophagitis.	Discontinue NG feeding. Adjust tube size and position. Consider gastrostomy or jejunostomy.
C. Metabolic 1. Dehydration.	Impaired glucose utilization.	Monitor serum and urine glucose.
Symptoms: Output > intake; rapid weight loss; thirst; dry skin; increased serum electrolytes; increased specific gravity of urine.	Inadequate fluid intake; excessive fluid losses.	Monitor intake and output; provide added fluids as needed.
2. Overhydration.	Renal, hepatic, cardiac failure; malnutrition; hypoalbuminemia.	Use calorie-dense formula; avoid rapid infusion of fluids, including IVs.
Symptoms: Intake > output; rapid weight gain; edema; decreased serum electrolytes; decreased specific gravity of urine.		Monitor intake and output and serum electrolytes.
3. Hyponatremia	Abnormal fluid retention.	Fluid restriction.
Symptoms: Serum Na$^+$ < 135 mEq/L; rapid weight loss; confusion; lethargy.	Abnormal sodium loss (vomiting, diarrhea, fistula). Excess fluid due to concurrent transfusion and IV administration.	Sodium supplementation if indicated. Decrease IV rate as tube feeding is increased.
4. Hypernatremia. *Symptoms:* Serum Na$^+$ > 150 mEq/L; dehydration.	Excessive solute load; inadequate fluid intake (diarrhea, profuse sweating, or osmotic diuresis).	Increase fluid intake; check formula osmolarity; monitor serum glucose.
5. Hypokalemia. *Symptoms:* Serum K$^+$ < 3.5 mEq/L; muscle cramps; weakness; confusion; apathy; cardiac arrhythmias.	Metabolic alkalosis; diarrhea; vomiting. Trauma recovery.	Control vomiting/diarrhea. Supplementary potassium. 4 mEq K$^+$/gm N recommended for tissue synthesis.
6. Hyperkalemia. *Symptoms:* Serum K$^+$ ≥ 6 mEq/L; diarrhea; nausea; irritability; weakness; cardiac arrhythmias.	Metabolic acidosis (shock, severe dehydration).	Provide fluids and potassium-wasting diuretics. Administer glucose and insulin to force K$^+$ into cells; adjust formula concentration.
7. Hyperglycemia.	Insufficiency of insulin.	Administer insulin; decrease infusion rate; try higher fat formula.
8. Hypoglycemia.	Secondary to hypoglycemic medications or sudden cessation of tube feeding.	Taper feedings slowly; monitor urine for sugar acetone every 4 hours.
9. Hyperphosphatemia.	Insulin administration; malnutrition.	Phosphate supplement in enteral or IV solution.
10. Hyperphosphatemia.	Renal insufficiency.	Change to formula with lower phosphorus content; phosphorus-binding antacid.

or glucose-monitoring instrument is more accurate.

The onset of hyperglycemia in a patient who has been adapted to the regimen with no complications can be a sign that an inadvertent amount of nutrient solution has been given. The flow rate should be checked, and, when flow has fallen behind, the rate should not be increased to attempt to catch up. Hyperglycemia in a patient whose glucose level was previously normal may be an indication of sepsis (Page & Clibon, 1982).

Mechanical complications can occur because

FOCUS ON *ENTERAL FEEDING FLOW SHEET**

Date					
Total calories (kcal)					
Total protein (gm)					
Total carbohydrate (gm)					
Total fat (gm)					
FOOD Carbohydrate (gm)					
Protein (gm)					
Fat (gm)					
Brand name					
FORMULA Carbohydrate (gm)					
Protein (gm)					
Fat (gm)					
Total calories: Nitrogen (gm)					
Caloric goal /% MET					
Protein goal /% MET					
Glucose 60 to 90 mg/dl					
Albumin 4.0 to 5.2 gm/dl					
BUN 7 to 26 mg/dl					
K					
Na					
Urine glucose					
UUN					
Total intake fluid (cc)					
IV					
PO					
Enteral tube					
Total output (cc)					
Urine					
Net fluid balance					
Other					
Weight (kg)					

*From Allen, TM: An enteral feeding protocol. Reprinted with permission from *Nutritional Support Services,* vol. 2, No. 3, March 1982.

of an incorrectly placed tube. This can be avoided by confirming the tip position roentgenographically.

Clinical Implications:

- When initiating a tube feeding, assure the patient that this is a temporary situation to facilitate his/her recovery.
- All tube feedings are perishable, readily support bacterial growth, and must be refrigerated after being reconstituted or opened. No more than a 24-hour supply should be prepared; it can be hung safely for up to 8 hours (Hostetler et al, 1982). One should pour only the amount required for a feeding and allow it to come to room temperature before administration (do not heat).
- A volume of 2000 cc usually furnishes 2000 kcal and the RDAs for vitamins and minerals. Malnourished patients may need this quantity or more, but others may gain weight on this amount (Arnold, 1981).
- Never increase the volume (rate) and concentration at the same time. By increasing the rate and then the concentration, complications such as abdominal cramping, diarrhea, or electrolyte imbalances are lessened.
- Be certain staff on all shifts know the formula being used and its dilution, even though they are not responsible for the dilution.
- The higher the osmolality, the greater the possibility that the formula will be poorly tolerated without gradual adaptations.
- When patients are on intermittent tube feedings, check gastric residual before each feeding. If 150 ml are aspirated, the usual rule is to withhold the feeding. Because of the useful gastric secretions and electrolytes, the residual should be reinstilled immediately.
- Optimal feeding rate for bolus tube feedings is 400 to 600 ml every 20 to 30 minutes (Page & Clibon, 1982).
- Additional fluids are mandatory, especially in infants and children, to prevent dehydration. Solute overload from protein and electrolytes is particularly hazardous.
- The duodenum and jejunum are more sensitive than the stomach to volume and tonicity. Therefore, feedings into these areas require more gradual advancement of caloric density of the diet, especially when hypertonic elemental feedings are used (Page & Clibon, 1982).
- Monomeric formulas are used for malabsorption or maldigestion (when the gastrointestinal tract is unable to properly digest or absorb nutrients); polymeric formulas are utilized whenever possible (Arnold, 1981).

- If an elemental diet furnishes less than two percent of the kilocalories as polyunsaturated fats, fatty acid deficiency may occur. Patients might require additional fat sources. Any vegetable oil (long-chain triglycerides) can be used.
- When a patient is unable to eat or drink, the tongue, mouth, and throat tend to become inflamed. Good oral hygiene is essential.
- Small tubes may become clogged when thick formulas and/or crushed medications are given. Several methods are used to open them:
  1. One teaspoon of meat tenderizer per 4 oz. of water is injected into the tube and clamped for one hour.
  2. Either cola beverages or cranberry juice (20 ml every two hours) can be injected into the tube.

Parenteral Nutrition

Parenteral nutrition is delivered via routes other than the alimentary tract (usually intravenously) when nutrient needs cannot be met solely by enteral intake. Standard intravenous (IV) therapy (D_5W with added electrolytes) through peripheral veins maintains fluid and electrolyte balance, contains no protein, and provides about 200 to 600 kcal (170 kcal/L) daily for energy needs until the patient is able to eat. Total parenteral nutrition (TPN) indicates that all necessary nutrients are being provided via veins; either peripheral veins or a central vein can be used. Peripheral vein TPN (sometimes referred to as PPN) is normally used for brief periods; TPN or CPN generally denotes central-vein parenteral nutrition.

Hyperalimentation means that nutrients are provided in excess of maintenance needs. TPN, especially when a central vein is used, is sometimes erroneously called hyperalimentation. Normally, TPN provides only the nutriment needed for tissue maintenance, in the range of 1800 to 3000 kcal/day. Under severe stress or tauma, patients may require "hyper" amounts of energy, which can be met with TPN therapy.

FLUID BALANCE

Fluid requirement in adults without abnormal losses is 2500 to 3000 ml/day (35 ml/kg). The total kilocaloric needs are supplied within and limited to approximately this quantity of water unless fluid requirements are increased because of increased fluid losses (e.g., vomiting, diarrhea, diaphoresis, or wound drainage) or hypermetabolic states (e.g., fever or hyperthyroidism). Fluid requirements may also be reduced because of inadequate kidney function or immediately after myocardial infarction.

Excess fluids can lead to overhydration, fluid overload, pulmonary edema, and water intoxication. Monitoring fluid balance is especially important in patients with cardiac, renal, and hepatic impairment.

Clinical Implications:

- Because of a higher percentage of body water in infants and children, fluid losses are more critical.
- The elderly have less fluid reserve and often poorly functioning kidneys (an inability to concentrate the urine) and should be closely monitored.

TONICITY

As with enteral feedings, solutions are classified as isotonic, hypotonic, or hypertonic. The tonicity of the parenteral solution determines its method of administration. A hypotonic or isotonic solution can be administered through peripheral veins; hypertonic solutions are administered via a central vein in order for the increased blood volume to dilute them.

Isotonic solutions are used to provide some energy, but their primary purpose is fluid replacement. A five percent dextrose solution is considered isotonic, requiring only 1 1/2 hours for assimilation in a 70 kg individual. Ten percent dextrose is hypertonic; however, moderately hypertonic solutions of dextrose can be administered peripherally. Isotonic solutions do not provide adequate fluids to meet physiological needs—renal excretion, insensible losses, and metabolic uses.

Protein is used in parenteral solutions in concentrations of 3 to 10 percent. The 3 1/2 percent protein solution is nearly isotonic and can safely be used peripherally, whereas a seven percent solution is hypertonic and is used in central venous feedings. Fat emulsions can significantly increase the caloric content without being hypertonic.

Hypertonic solutions have greater osmotic pressure than blood. Fluid is drawn into the bloodstream and can damage the blood vessels. Parenteral infusions of highly hypertonic solutions (more than 10 percent) can cause sclerosis, phlebitis, clotting, and swelling. Hypertonic solutions are sometimes used in patients with renal insufficiency (if edema is not present), but should be administered very slowly, and monitored closely.

Determining whether the solution will be hypertonic or isotonic depends on several factors including the energy requirement, amount of fluid the patient can safely tolerate, and whether or not fats are used. Glucose concentration of the three techniques for parenteral nutrition with the total amount of energy provided can be compared as shown in Table 21–3.

PARENTERAL NUTRIENTS

All the basic nutrients required by the body can be given intravenously: carbohydrates, proteins, fat emulsions, vitamins, water, and electrolytes. In addition, alcohol can be utilized as a source of energy.

Kilocalories. The amount of kilocalories is usually supplied by and calculated on the basis of carbohydrate content of the solution (unless fat or alcohol is used). Dextrose provides 3.4 kcal/gm. Protein infusions can contribute to the kilocalories (4.0 kcal/gm), but their objective is mainly for protein repletion. Thus, they are not usually counted for kilocalories or administered in high concentrations because of the increased urea production if used for energy. Energy nutrients can be determined by the equations shown in *Focus on Estimating Kilocalories in Parenteral Solutions*.

Table 21–3. *Energy Content and Tonicity of Parenteral Solutions**

Route of Administration	Glucose Concentration	Calorie Density
Central vein	25 to 35%	2550 to 3570 kcal/3 L
Peripheral vein (60% of the calories from lipids)	10%	1780 kcal/3 L
Peripheral vein (without lipids)	10%	1020 kcal/3 L

*From Weinsier, RL; Butterworth, CE, Jr: *Handbook of Clinical Nutrition.* St Louis, The C. V. Mosby Co, 1981.

FOCUS ON *ESTIMATING KILOCALORIES IN PARENTERAL SOLUTIONS*

Glucose or amino acid* solutions:

$$\text{Milliliters of solution} \times \begin{array}{c}\text{Concentration}\\\text{of nutrient}\\\text{in solution}\end{array} = \begin{array}{c}\text{Grams of glucose}\\\text{or amino acid infused}\end{array}$$

$$\text{Grams of nutrient} \times \begin{array}{c}\text{Physiological}\\\text{fuel factor}\end{array} = \text{Kilocalories}$$

Sample calculations:

To determine the number of kilocalories per gram in 3000 cc of D_5W:

$$3000 \text{ cc} \times \frac{5 \text{ mg of glucose}}{100 \text{ cc}} = 150 \text{ gm of glucose} \times \frac{3.4 \text{ kcal}}{\text{gm}} = 510 \text{ kcal}$$

To determine the number of kilocalories per gram in 3000 cc of 3.5 percent amino acid solution:

$$3000 \text{ cc} \times \frac{3.5 \text{ gm of amino acid}}{100 \text{ cc}} = 105 \text{ gm of amino acids (or protein)}$$

$$70 \text{ gm of amino acid} \times \frac{4 \text{ kcal}}{\text{gm}} = 280 \text{ kcal/gm}$$

To calculate the number of kilocalories for fat emulsions: 1 ml of 10 percent fat emulsion provides 1.1 kcal.

$$\text{Number of milliliters} \times 1.1 = \text{Number of kilocalories provided}$$

In simpler terms, the number of milliliters of fat emulsion roughly equals the number of kilocalories provided.

---

*While the amount of protein supplied is important to determine adequacy, the number of calories from protein is normally unimportant because protein is usually given in minimal amounts to support protein synthesis and anabolism.

Energy needs can be met by various combinations of dextrose and/or fat emulsions. An adult of normal weight requires approximately 30 kcal/kg body weight. Generally, 2400 to 3000 kcal/day supplies the energy needs for an underweight or slightly hypermetabolic patient (Butterworth & Weinsier, 1980). However, an assessment of the patient's condition (including nutritional status and amount of protein catabolism) and anthropometric parameters can be helpful in determining caloric requirements (see Chapter 20).

Kilocalories supplied parenterally are utilized less efficiently than those given enterally (Bivins & Rapp, 1980). Earlier, it was felt that an intravenous diet must provide two to three times the nutritional needs of the basal energy expenditure; however, recent studies have indicated that this may be excessive (Quebbeman et al, 1982). Excessive energy intake has been shown to produce undesirable metabolic complications, such as hepatomegaly, liver dysfunction, and respiratory insufficiency.

Carbohydrate. The monosaccharides (dextrose, fructose, and invert sugar) are used for intravenous feedings; all can be absorbed from the bloodstream. Table 21–4 shows the number of kilocalories provided by various dextrose solutions. Insulin may be administered to prevent hyperglycemia (and glucosuria) when hypertonic dextrose solutions are given.

Fructose may be less irritating to the vein, which is especially of concern in peripheral infu-

Table 21–4. Parenteral Carbohydrate Solutions*

Types of Solutions	Calories/Liter	Tonicity
Dextrose		
2½%	85	Hypotonic
5%	170	Isotonic
10%	340	Hypertonic
20%	680	Hypertonic
50%	1700	Hypertonic
Fructose		
10%	375	Hypertonic
Invert sugar		
5%	190	Isotonic
10%	375	Hypertonic

*From Metheny, N; Snively, W: *Nurses Handbook of Fluid Balance.* Philadelphia, J. B. Lippincott Co, 1983, by permission.

Table 21–5. Protein-Nitrogen Requirements

	Protein Requirements	Nitrogen Requirements
Healthy adults (70 kg)	0.5 to 1 gm/kg/day	5.6 to 11 gm
Adults with major wounds (70 kg)	1.0 to 1.5 gm/kg/day	11 to 16.8 gm
Infants	2.0 gm/kg/day	

sions. However, fructose has no significant advantage over glucose, except in postoperative and trauma patients who have increased insulin resistance and glucose intolerance (Twiggs & Nwangwu, 1982). Fructose can cause a rise in the serum level of lactic acid and is therefore contraindicated when metabolic acidosis is likely.

Dextrans are polymers of glucose, but are not used for energy. They are used in hemorrhaging patients as plasma volume expanders. They simulate albumin by binding with fluids; they last about 24 hours before being degraded and excreted (Metheny & Snively, 1983).

Protein. When parenteral fluids are required for more than three to four days, protein solutions are recommended (Goldberger, 1986). These crystalline compounds contain both essential and nonessential amino acids. They are well tolerated, enhance protein synthesis, and improve nitrogen balance when adequate amounts are used.

Amino acid concentrates are very expensive, so minimal amounts are used to provide the nitrogen requirement. Shizgal and Forse (1980) have determined that amino acids account for 81 percent of the cost of a TPN solution containing 2.5 percent amino acids. Increasing the concentrates to five percent increases the cost by 84 percent but does not increase the rate of anabolism.

Branched-chain amino acids (BCAA) have been used successfully in the severely stressed or septic patient and in those with impaired hepatic function (see Chapters 26 and 28, respectively).

For intravenous feedings, protein requirements are discussed in terms of nitrogen, since positive nitrogen balance is the ultimate goal. Considering that 1 gm of nitrogen is present in 6.25 gm of protein, nitrogen requirements are derived from protein demands (Table 21–5).

In severe stress or sepsis, greater quantities of nitrogen may be required; this can be determined by nitrogen balance studies. A liter of 5 percent amino acid solution contains 6.2 gm of nitrogen and 175 kcal.

Adequate amounts of nonprotein kilocalories must be given to achieve nitrogen balance and promote protein synthesis. This is generally referred to as the kilocalorie-to-nitrogen ratio. A ratio of 160 to 1 has been shown to promote optimal utilization of nitrogen in patients (Peters & Fischer, 1980). However, different disease states may require different levels.

Clinical Implications:

- Positive nitrogen balance and good visceral protein function are normally obtained in patients receiving TPN wtih 1.0 to 1.5 gm protein/kg/day and 30 to 40 kcal/kg/day (Blackburn & Harvey, 1982).
- Supplemental medications and other additives should not be added to protein solutions without first checking with the pharmacist.
- Protein solutions should be carefully examined before use and discarded if particulate matter is present or if cloudy.
- Crystalline amino acids, prepared as salts of hydrochloric acid, may lead to hyperchloremic acidosis.
- Protein should be initiated cautiously in patients with chronic protein-energy deprivation to avoid ammonia intoxication.
- Patients with hepatic or renal failure must be closely monitored when protein solutions are used; infusion rates should be slower. Special formulations are available and may be necessary.

Fat Emulsions. More than two times as much energy is provided from fat emulsions as from protein or carbohydrate emulsions. Fats are protein-sparing and are comparable to glucose in promoting positive nitrogen balance (Jeejeebhoy et al, 1976). These emulsions can be used in conjunction with carbohydrates and amino acids peripherally or in central venous alimentation. Fat emulsions significantly increase the kilocalorie infusion because of their high kilocaloric density and low tonicity. The development of three-liter bags has made the mixing of fat emulsions with dextrose and amino acids possible.

Two fat emulsions currently available in the United States are Intralipid from Cutter, a soybean oil emulsion, and Liposyn from Abbott, a safflower oil emulsion. Both are produced with a small amount of glycerol added to make the emulsion isotonic. A 10 percent solution provides 1.1 kcal/gm. A 20 percent solution of Intralipid provides 2 kcal/gm for individuals requiring more concentrated kilocalories.

Fat emulsions are necessary when TPN continues more than two to three weeks in order to prevent essential fatty acid (EFA) deficiency. The most common procedure is to use dextrose as the energy source in TPN, with fat emulsions used twice weekly to supply EFA for long-term TPN patients. However, the amount of fat utilized in the formulation for ventilator-dependent patients is high in order to increase the ratio of fat to carbohydrate kilocalories, which will decrease the respiratory quotient (see Chapter 26).

Fat infusions are initiated slowly, and the rate is increased as tolerated by the patient. Such adverse symptoms as palpitations, tachypnea, or an allergic reaction indicate that the rate of lipid administration should be decreased or discontinued.

Fat emulsions cause a rise in serum lipid levels and are contraindicated in patients with hyperlipemia, lipoid nephrosis, severe liver damage, and acute pancreatitis accompanied by hyperlipemia. Patients receiving fat emulsions should be observed for allergic reactions, hyperlipemia, hypercoagulability, nausea and vomiting, headache, flushing, dyspnea, fever, sweating, back or chest pain, and dizziness. The patient's liver function and ability to eliminate the infused fat from the circulation (the lipemia should clear between daily infusions) should be frequently monitored (Metheny & Snively, 1983).

Clinical Implications:

- Fat emulsions can be given in conjunction with amino acids or dextrose and administered via a Y-tube or three-way stopcock near the infusion site. Elevate more than the dextrose/amino acid preparation to prevent backflow and mixing of solutions.

- Nursing personnel should not mix fat emulsions with electrolyte or other nutrient solutions (dextrose or amino acids).
- Refrigerate Intralipid for storage; remove from refrigeration at least 30 minutes before use.
- *Do not shake fat emulsions.* Dispose of any bottle in which there appears to be any separation or if there is an inconsistency in texture or color.
- Heparin may be used to speed the clearance of lipids from the blood.
- Do not use filters with fat emulsions.
- Throw away bottles that have been opened; do not refrigerate.
- Eczematous skin lesions, bleeding tendencies, sparse hair growth, and decreased healing ability are signs of fatty acid deficiency.

Alcohol. Since alcohol has a greater kilocaloric value (7 kcal/gm) than carbohydrates or proteins, small amounts can be used. However, it is not practical as a major source of energy because of its inebriating effects. Combined with dextrose, alcohol is burned preferentially, permitting the glucose to be stored as glycogen. Alcohol provides readily utilizable kilocalories and has a sedating effect, which may be desirable for pain. (Sedation can be achieved without intoxication.) An improved sense of well-being or euphoria is another beneficial effect. Alcohol does not depend on the presence of insulin for metabolism.

When parenterally administered, it may have undesirable effects of dulled memory, decreased concentration, increased respiration and pulse, and vasodilation. Alcohol can be given at a rate of 1.5 gm/kg of body weight per 24 hours at a concentration not exceeding four percent. When the rate of administration of alcohol exceeds its metabolism, restlessness, inebriation, and coma may occur.

Vitamins. While multivitamin preparations are essential for use in long-term TPN, it is difficult to determine their required levels. Since vitamins are frequently catalysts used to metabolize carbohydrates, protein, and fat, when large amounts of the energy nutrients are given, it stands to reason that vitamin requirements would also be increased.

Greater requirements are also anticipated because larger amounts of vitamins are excreted in the urine of patients on intravenous fluids than on oral intake (Borgen, 1978). In 1975, the Nutrition Advisory Group of the American Medical Association recommended specific amounts of 12 vi-

Table 21–6. American Medical Association's Vitamin Recommendations for Parenteral Feedings*

Vitamin	Up to Age 11	Age 11 and Older
A	2,300 IU	3,300 IU
D	400 IU	200 IU
E	7 IU	10 IU
Ascorbic acid	80 mg	100 mg
Folacin	140 mcg	400 mcg
Niacin	17 mg	40 mg
Riboflavin	1.4 mg	3.6 mg
Thiamin	1.2 mg	3 mg
B_6 (pyridoxine)	1 mg	4 mg
B_{12} (cyanocobalamin)	1 mcg	5 mcg
Pantothenic acid	5 mg	15 mg
Biotin	20 mcg	60 mcg

*From AMA Department of Foods and Nutrition: *Guidelines for Multivitamin Preparations for Parenteral Use.* Chicago, American Medical Association, 1975.

Table 21–7. Electrolyte and Mineral Requirements During Parenteral Nutrition*

Electrolyte	Normal Range of Daily Requirements
Sodium	40 to 150 mEq as sodium chloride and sodium lactate.
Potassium	70 to 150 mEq as potassium chloride and potassium phosphate.
Chloride	Equal to sodium to prevent acid-base disturbances.
Calcium	0.2 to 0.3 mEq/kg/day added as calcium gluconate.
Magnesium	0.35 to 0.45 mEq/kg/day added as magnesium sulfate; give more if increased losses are present.
Phosphorus	7 to 10 mmol per 1000 kcal, extremely variable—adjust to keep serum concentrations normal.

*From Grant, JP: *Handbook of Total Parenteral Nutrition.* Philadelphia, W. B. Saunders Co, 1980.

tamins (AMA, 1979). The recommendations, shown in Table 21–6 are based largely on the oral RDAs and do not take into consideration the amount of kilocalories given to the patient or their solubility or excretion rate. The amounts recommended are minimal with close monitoring of clinical and laboratory values to indicate an increased need.

Water-soluble vitamins (B complex and C) and water-miscible forms of fat-soluble vitamins (A, D, and E) that adhere to published guidelines are available as intravenous multivitamin preparations. Intravenous multiple vitamin preparations do not contain folic acid, vitamin K, or vitamin B_{12}. Folic acid and vitamin K can be given weekly; vitamin B_{12} can be administered monthly. One should be certain that all vitamins have been ordered.

Electrolytes and Trace Elements. Serious complications have been reported when patients receiving TPN for extended periods did not have trace elements added to their formulas. Measures should be taken to ensure adequate amounts. Varying amounts of electrolytes are added to some commercial preparations. Sodium, potassium, chloride, phosphorus, magnesium, and calcium are essential and included in TPN therapy as indicated in Table 21–7. The amount of sodium added is dependent on the patient's condition, considering cardiovascular, renal, gastrointestinal, and endocrine status. Sodium may be as low as 15 mEq (350 mg).

Larger quantities of potassium are required for parenteral solutions than for the standard five percent dextrose solution because of increased anabolism. Tissue synthesis requires 3.5 mEq of potassium per gram of nitrogen. However, potassium should not be given if urine flow is inadequate. Hyperkalemia may cause cardiac arrest; potassium solutions should be carefully monitored and diluted 20 to 40 mEq/L for adults.

Chloride is usually given as the chloride salt; however, the ratio of sodium to chloride should be one to one in order to prevent acid-base disturbances.

Magnesium and phosphorus are important in energy synthesis and wound healing; the requirements may be increased if advanced malnutrition is a problem. Serum magnesium concentration depends on intake and elimination by the kidneys. If the magnesium level falls, there is a concomitant fall in calcium, causing neurological impairment and adverse gastrointestinal effects. The body needs 4 mEq of phosphate per gram of nitrogen for anabolism.

Calcium is an important element but must be administered slowly and in diluted solutions to deter cardiac arrest. Initiating calcium solutions slowly allows time to detect signs of hypersensitivity in patients.

While iron can be given intravenously or intramuscularly, the need for supplemental iron must be individually evaluated. Those receiving frequent transfusions will not need iron supplementation.

Deficiency symptoms for copper, chromium, molybdenum, iodine, selenium, and especially zinc (Fig. 21–4) have been observed in long-term

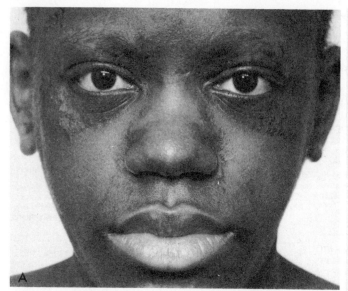
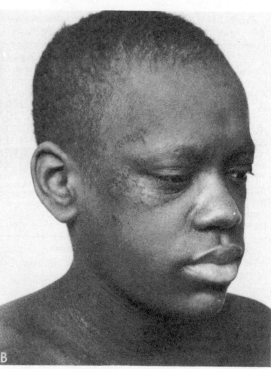

Figure 21–4. (A & B) Skin manifestations of acute zinc deficiency during parenteral nutrition. Nonpruritic dermatitis about mouth and eyes and over nose and chin is evident. (From Grant JP: Handbook of Total Parenteral Nutrition. Philadelphia, W. B. Saunders Co, 1980, by permission.)

TPN patients (Rudman & Williams, 1985; West, 1981). Standard TPN solutions contain small amounts of these elements as contaminants. Serum levels of these trace elements should be monitored and supplementation given during long-term TPN (Table 21–8). The needs vary with the patient's condition. Depleted, catabolic states and anabolism increase the amount of trace elements needed.

Clinical Implications:

- Magnesium infusions should be questioned in oliguric patients.

Table 21–8. Suggested Daily Intravenous Intake of Essential Trace Elements[a]

	Pediatric Patients, mcg/kg[b]	Stable Adult	Adult in Acute Catabolic State[c]	Stable Adult with Intestinal Losses[c]
Zinc	300[d] 100[e]	2.5 to 4.0 mg	Additional 2.0 mg	Add 12.2 mg/L small-bowel fluid lost; 17.1 mg/kg of stool or ileostomy output.[f]
Copper	20	0.5 to 1.5 mg		
Chromium	0.14 to 0.2	10 to 15 mcg		
Manganese	2 to 10	0.15 to 0.8 mg		20 mcg[g]

[a]From AMA Department of Foods and Nutrition: Guidelines for essential trace element preparations for parenteral use. *JAMA* 241(May 11):2051, 1979. Copyright 1979, by American Medical Association.
[b]Limited data are available for infants weighing less than 1500 gm. Their requirements may be more than the recommendations because of their low body reserves and increased requirements for growth.
[c]Frequent monitoring of blood levels in these patients is essential to provide proper dosage.
[d]Premature infants (weight less than 1500 gm) up to 3 kg of body weight. Thereafter, the recommendations for full-term infants apply.
[e]Full-term infants and children up to 5 years old. Thereafter, the recommendations for adults apply, up to a maximum dosage of 4 mg/day.
[f]Values derived by mathematical fitting of balance data from a 71-patient-week study in 24 patients.
[g]Mean from balance study.

- Calcium gluconate injected intravenously is used for emergency therapy of hypermagnesemia.
- Calcium salts should not be added to intravenous solutions containing sodium bicarbonate or phosphate. (Salts will form and precipitate.)
- Calcium is contraindicated in digitalized patients.
- Antibiotics degrade in a lowered pH. These additives should not be mixed with multiple vitamin complexes that contain ascorbic acid or in TPN solutions (Metheny & Snively, 1983).

PERIPHERAL INFUSIONS

For the quickest delivery of water, electrolytes, and glucose, peripheral infusions are utilized. They are generally used for short-term nutritional support. When enteral feeding is not possible, peripheral infusion is the safest route, if good peripheral veins are available. Isotonic solutions are less likely to damage the veins, but about 9 L of D_5W (five percent) glucose solution would be required to provide 1500 kcal. The large amount of fluid necessary for dilution to make the solution isotonic increases the risk of fluid overload. Thus, the limitations of energy and fluid volume restrict the amount of nutrients that can safely be infused through a peripheral vein.

In general, the objective of peripheral parenteral nutrition (PPN) is to prevent deterioration (achieve homeostasis) rather than to promote cell growth and repletion (Bivins & Rapp, 1980). It is applicable when patients require only supplementary or low-calorie support, and when low concentrations of glucose and amino acids and/or lipids are sufficient. If the patient is unable to tolerate enteral feedings within seven to ten days, another form of nutritional support should be instituted to prevent subcutaneous fat and muscle protein being used for energy (Chernoff, 1982).

More aggressive PPN would include fat emulsion in addition to carbohydrate and amino acids. Positive nitrogen balance and weight gain can be achieved, but this therapy is not routinely practiced.

Clinical Implications:

- Never break or interrupt the IV line to draw blood or administer medications.
- TPN solutions are an excellent medium for bacterial growth; they should not be allowed to hang for more than 12 hours.

- The Centers for Disease Control recommend a peripheral venipuncture device be changed at 48-hour intervals and not left in place longer than 72 hours (Metheny & Snively, 1983).

CENTRAL VEIN PARENTERAL NUTRITION

When nutrients are provided intravenously in sufficient quality and quantity for hypermetabolic patients who cannot be fed enterally, the central vein is normally used. This method has also been incorrectly labeled intravenous hyperalimentation because it is possible to provide more kilocalories than required. In the United States, central vein parenteral nutrition utilizes an indwelling catheter placed in either the internal jugular or the subclavian vein, terminating in the superior vena cava. When caloric requirements are high, central venous alimentation is usually the best form of nutritional support. Because the hypertonic solution is introduced in the superior vena cava, the large volume of blood flow dilutes it rapidly. Therefore, high-kilocalorie hypertonic glucose solutions in quantities of 2500 to 3000 ml can be given daily.

The purpose of central vein parenteral nutrition is to provide nutrients to maintain or increase lean body mass over an extended period; it can provide needed kilocalories, restore positive nitrogen balance, and replace essential vitamins, electrolytes, minerals, and trace elements.

Early recognition of problems that require TPN (e.g., patients who are going to be unable to eat for long periods or whose hypermetabolic status make it impossible for them to obtain sufficient amounts of nutrients) and initiation of the therapy are important (Shils, 1980). Weinsier and Butterworth (1981) advocate TPN in the following situations:

1. Incapacitated gastrointestinal tract.
2. Anticipation of a nonfunctioning gastrointestinal tract (to maintain anabolism).
3. To minimize intestinal activity.
4. As an alternative to enteral feeding in critical situations to avoid uncertainties of nutrient uptake or utilization.

Principles and Procedures. In general, the TPN solution is individualized to meet the specific requirements of each patient. Table 21–9 is indicative of a typical central-vein solution. Guild and Cerda (1979) have described five basic principles for the management of TPN:

1. Evaluate the patient. Nutritional assessment helps to determine the amount of energy and protein needed as well as to assess the risks and benefits of TPN for the patient. In addition to determining nutritional needs of the patient, an assessment forms a data base against which changes may be compared. A flow chart similar to that shown in _Focus on Adult TPN Monitor Flow Chart_ is a part of the permanent record assessing the patient's status.

2. A route for intravenous feeding should be established. If the final concentration of the dextrose solution is greater than 10 percent, the subclavian vein is catheterized by a physician under strict aseptic conditions.

3. Infusion of nutrients is administered slowly at first in order to allow the body to adjust. Generally, only 1 L of TPN formula is administered on the first day, 2 L on the second day, and 3 L on the third day if blood glucose levels are acceptable. Blood sugar and urine acetone levels are checked four times daily until they are consistently negative for 72 hours after the maintenance fluid rate has been reached.

4. Provide the patient with sufficient nonprotein kilocalories (carbohydrate and fat). This ensures that the amino acids are being used for protein synthe-

Table 21–10. _Physical and Laboratory Values That Require Regular Monitoring in Total Parenteral Nutrition (TPN) Solutions*_

Daily measurements:
  weight
  intake and output
  fractional urines (every 4 to 6 hr)
  temperature (4 times a day)
  blood pressure
  pulse
  respirations

Daily until a constant volume of TPN solution is ordered, then three times a week:
  hematocrit
  sodium
  potassium
  chloride
  carbon dioxide
  total protein
  creatinine
  blood sugar
  BUN

Weekly measurements:
  calcium
  phosphorus
  magnesium
  complete blood count
  prothrombin time
  liver function tests
  copper
  zinc

*From Swenson, JP; Edwards, D; Chamberlain, M; et al: A total parenteral nutrition protocol. _Drug Intelligence and Clinical Pharmacy_ 11(12):714, 1977.

sis, which can be monitored by comparing urinary nitrogen excretion with nitrogen intake (Table 21–10).

5. Establish a steady rate of delivery to minimize metabolic fluctuations. The flow rate of the infusion must be constant and uninterrupted. A pump is used for TPN administration to protect patients from air embolisms, erratic drip rates, and power failures. The rate must be monitored hourly. If the rate is too slow, hypoglycemia may result and there will be an insufficient amount of nutrients absorbed. Too rapid flow rate could lead to hyperglycemia and osmotic diuresis. Trying to catch up to the proper rate is not permitted.

Nutrition Support Team. Because of the many minute details involved in a successful TPN program, some hospitals maintain a nutritional support team, consisting of a physician, nurse, pharmacist, and dietitian, with other medical personnel incorporated as needed. Team members may be responsible for technical aspects of care and initiating the feeding and carefully monitoring the patient's condition, weight change, and

Table 21–9. _Solution for Parenteral Nutrition[a]_

Component	Amount/Liter	Amount/Day
Glucose (monohydrate)	250 gm	750 gm
Glucose calories[b]	850 kcal	2550 kcal
Amino acids[c]	35 gm	105 gm
Nitrogen	5.5 gm	15.5 gm
Protein equivalent	34.4 gm	103.2 gm
Na^+	35 mEq	105 mEq
K^+	40 mEq	120 mEq
Ca^{++}	4.5 mEq	13.5 mEq
Mg^{++}	10 mEq	30 mEq
Cl^-	48 mEq	144 mEq
Acetate⁻	70 mEq	210 mEq
P (inorganic phosphorus)	465 mg	1395 mg
$ZnSO_4$	5 mg	15.0 mg
Iron	1.0 mg	3.0 mg
Vitamins[d]	1.4 ml	4.2 ml

[a]From Meng, HC: Parenteral nutrition—principles, nutrient requirements, techniques, and clinical applications. In _Nutritional Support of Medical Practice_, 2nd ed. Edited by HA Schneider; CE Anderson; DB Coursin. Philadelphia, Harper & Row, 1983, p 203.

[b]Glucose monohydrate (USP) was used, and 3.4 kcal/L/gm of glucose was used for the calculation of calories/liter.

[c]Aminosyn 7 percent solution with electrolytes was used.

[d]Vitamins were given as aqueous multivitamin infusion solution (MVI) 5 ml ampule. Folate and B_{12} were added to the infusate separately. Iron was added as Imferon.

ADULT
TPN MONITOR
FLOW CHART

Unshaded area = recommended monitoring schedule

NAME _____

ROOM _____

HOSPITAL NUMBER _____

DATE				
SKIN TESTS	Baseline	Wk2	Wk4	Wk6
PPD 5 TU				
CANDIDA 1:100				
SK/SD				
MUMPS				

		PreTPN Baseline	DATE DAY 1	DAY 2	DAY 3	DAY 4	DAY 5	DAY 6	DAY 7	DAY 8	DAY 9	DAY 10	DAY 11	DAY 12	DAY 13	DAY 14
T P N S O L U T I O N	Calories															
	Glucose															
	Nitrogen															
	Na															
	K															
	Ca															
	Mg															
	Cl															
	PO4															
	MVI															
	Folic Acid															
	Insulin															
	Lipid															
	Total Volume															
I N T A K E	PO															
	IV															
	Total															
O U T P U T	Urine															
	Stool															
	Suction															
	Other															
	Total															
WGT.																
U R I N E	Glucose (Q6H)															
	Acetone (Q6H)															
	24 Nitrogen															
B L O O D	Na															
	K															
	Cl															
	Mg															
	Phos															
	Ca															
	BUN															
	Creat															
	Glucose															
	WBC															
	Lymphocytes															
	Hct															
	Hgb															
	SGOT															
	Albumin															
	Protime Pt/Con															
	PTT Pt/Con															
	Platelets															
	Triglycerides															
	Cholesterol															
	Zinc															

92632 (5-80)

*Courtesy of Oakwood Hospital, Dearborn, MI, with permission.

daily fluid intake and output. The nurse's role may encompass maintaining patient care, educating the nursing staff, assisting with CPN catheter placement and care, and educating the patient and family regarding this method of nutrition support (Hoying, 1983). A physical therapist may assist in maintaining the patient's dynamic state of tissue.

Staff nurses are still responsible for constant delivery of nutrient solution and supplemental additives (Fig. 21–5). They must also identify problems and initiate corrective action when needed. Emotional support is important for the patient in adjusting to this drastically different method of feeding. Institutions that have this teamwork report fewer complications of TPN therapy.

Preparation and Storage. In most institutions, the TPN solution is prepared by the pharmacist under a laminar flow hood. Because amino acids can be oxidized, the solution should be infused as soon as possible after mixing. The TPN solution can be safely stored at 4°C in the dark for up to 48 hours. The mixture should be removed from the refrigerator and allowed to come to room temperature before using. It should not be heated by any method.

Problems and Complications. A thorough investigation of other alternatives is warranted be-fore a final decision for TPN use is made. Another problem with TPN therapy is its cost—10 times more expensive than a normal hospital feeding (Chernoff, 1982).

Sepsis is one of the most frequent complications of TPN therapy. Strict control in mixing and storage of the infusion is essential to prevent bacterial contamination. Aseptic techniques are essential. One of the first signs of sepsis is glucose intolerance (provided it was not a previously existing condition).

Metabolic abnormalities related to the infusion of large amounts of glucose are common, including hyper- and hypoglycemia. If not corrected, a fatty liver may develop and, unless appropriate action is taken, may prove fatal (Ivey, 1979). The rate of glucose infusion should be decreased; exogenous insulin may be needed. Careful monitoring of clinical and laboratory data is important (see Table 21–10 and *Focus on Adult TPN Monitor Flow Chart*).

Other problems have been associated with excessive or deficient amounts of almost all the required nutrients: protein, fats, trace elements, electrolytes, and many of the vitamins (Table 21–11). Deficiency symptoms from many of the nutrients—copper, chromium, and biotin—were seldom or never observed before TPN therapy was developed. The article by Ivey (1979) is recom-

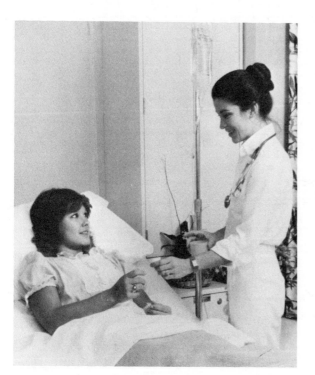

Figure 21–5. *Nursing service is responsible for a parenteral or intravenous feeding, which is the "nutrition" for the patient. (Courtesy of University of Arkansas Medical Sciences, Department of Nursing & Campus Media Services, Little Rock, AR.)*

Table 21–11. *Potential Metabolic Complications of Intravenous Hyperalimentation**

Problems	Possible Etiologies
I. Glucose metabolism	
A. Hyperglycemia, glycosuria, osmotic diuresis, hyperosmolar nonketotic dehydration and coma.	Excessive total dose or rate of infusion of glucose; inadequate endogenous insulin; glucocorticoids; sepsis.
B. Ketoacidosis in diabetes mellitus.	Inadequate endogenous insulin response; inadequate exogenous insulin therapy.
C. Postinfusion (rebound) hypoglycemia.	Persistence of endogenous insulin production secondary to prolonged stimulation of islet cells by high-carbohydrate infusion.
II. Amino acid metabolism	
A. Hyperchloremic metabolic acidosis.	Excessive chloride and monohydrochloride content of crystalline amino acid solutions.
B. Serum amino acid imbalance.	Unphysiologic amino acid profile of the nutrient solution; differential amino acid utilization with various disorders.
C. Hyperammonemia.	Excessive ammonia in protein hydrolysate solutions; arginine, ornithine, aspartic acid and/or glutamic acid deficiency in amino acid solutions; primary hepatic disorder.
D. Prerenal azotemia.	Excessive protein hydrolysate or amino acid infusion.
III. Calcium and phosphorus metabolism	
A. Hypophosphatemia: 1. Decreased erythrocyte 2,3-diphosphoglycerate. 2. Increased affinity of hemoglobin for oxygen. 3. Aberrations of erythrocyte intermediary metabolites.	Inadequate phosphorus administration, redistribution of serum phosphorus into cells and/or bone.
B. Hypocalcemia.	Inadequate calcium administration; reciprocal response to phosphorus repletion without simultaneous calcium infusion; hypoalbuminemia.
C. Hypercalcemia.	Excessive calcium administration with or without high doses of albumin; excessive vitamin D administration.
D. Vitamin D deficiency; hypervitaminosis D.	Inadequate or excessive vitamin D administration.
IV. Essential fatty acid metabolism	
Serum deficiences of phospholipid linoleic and/or arachidonic acids, serum elevation of Δ-5,8,11-eicosatrienoic acid.	Inadequate essential fatty acid administration; inadequate vitamin E administration.
V. Miscellaneous	
A. Hypokalemia.	Inadequate potassium intake relative to increased requirements for protein anabolism; diuresis.
B. Hyperkalemia.	Excessive potassium administration especially in metabolic acidosis; renal decompensation.
C. Hypomagnesemia.	Inadequate magnesium administration relative to increased requirements for protein anabolism and glucose metabolism.
D. Hypermagnesemia.	Excessive magnesium administration; renal decompensation.
E. Anemia.	iron deficiency; folic acid deficiency; vitamin B_{12} deficiency; copper deficiency; other deficiencies.
F. Bleeding.	Vitamin K deficiency.
G. Hypervitaminosis A.	Excessive vitamin A administration.
H. Elevations in SGOT, SGPT, and serum alkaline phosphatase.	Enzyme induction secondary to amino acid imbalance; excessive glycogen and/or fat deposition in the liver.
I. Cholestatic hepatitis.	Decreased water content of bile.

*From Duke, JH, Jr; Dudrick, JF: Parenteral feeding. In *Manual of Surgical Nutrition.* Edited by WF Ballinger; JA Collins; WR Drucker; et al. Philadelphia, W. B. Saunders Co, 1975, by permission.

mended for a discussion of these imbalances and deficiencies.

Clinical Implications:

- Dressings should be changed every other day using aseptic procedures; intravenous tubing and filters are changed daily.

- Total parenteral feedings are not advised for terminal or irreversible conditions.
- Hypertonic dextrose solutions administered too rapidly may cause hyperinsulinism, which may result in hypoglycemia unless the infusion is tapered off or followed by an isotonic solution.
- Hypertonic solutions are sometimes useful in causing osmotic diuresis, as utilized for cere-

bral edema. Hypertonic mannitol helps to eliminate fluids from the body.

Transitional Feedings

A change from one feeding mode to another is considered a transitional feeding or weaning period. This requires careful attention in order to maintain nutritional status while returning the patient to the most normal intake possible. The transition period, or tapering, is important to avoid "rebound" hypoglycemia (Colley & Wilson, 1979). Anytime the TPN solution must be discontinued abruptly, a solution of five percent dextrose in quarter-strength saline can be given for approximately 12 to 24 hours, until insulin secretion decreases (Metheny & Snively, 1983).

PARENTERAL TO ORAL FEEDING

The patient can be encouraged to take easily digested liquids. Clear liquids and polymeric formulas that are lactose-free with a low osmolarity are usually well-tolerated. Intravenous feeding may be gradually decreased as oral intake improves. Only with complete documentation of oral intake can the infusion be decreased appropriately. Intravenous feeding can be discontinued when kilocalorie intake consistently exceeds two thirds of the energy requirements.

PARENTERAL TO TUBE FEEDING

Enteral formulas should be initiated at half strength to prevent hyperosmotic diarrhea and bloating. As the enteral kilocalorie intake is increased, an equivalent amount is decreased in the intravenous feeding. Intravenous feedings are discontinued after the patient is stabilized on tube feeding.

TUBE TO ORAL FEEDING

This transition may be surprisingly difficult for many patients. Be sure that the swallowing function is consistent and regular. Begin with liquids, followed by soft or pureed foods. Because of the prevalence of lactose and fat malabsorption,

these should be initially excluded. When oral intake reaches 500 kcal or more, tube feedings can be proportionately and gradually decreased (the tube should be clamped for one hour before and after meals). When oral intake consistently exceeds two thirds of the patient's kilocalorie requirements, discontinue tube feedings (Transitional feedings, 1983).

Clinical Implication:

- Patients who have been on parenteral or continuous tube feedings for a long time may not feel hungry. A patient may need to be encouraged to begin eating again. A good start is to serve the patient's favorite foods (if at all possible) in an appetizing manner.

Home Enteral and Parenteral Nutrition

Amazingly, individuals can be sustained at home via enteral or parenteral feedings. If possible, enteral nutrition should be selected over parenteral nutrition (Chrysomilides & Kaminski, 1981). Flexibility and patient involvement are key components in developing a successful plan. For either therapy, it requires teaching specialized skills through an intensive training program to both the patient and a home health care agency and carefully following up in the home setting. Clear, concise materials and instructions prior to discharge contribute to the patient's confidence and ease in the transition. An interdisciplinary effort—by a physician, nurse, dietitian, psychiatrist, social worker, pharmacist, and discharge planner who are knowledgeable about the problems the patient is likely to face—can instruct qualifying patients and their caretakers in formula preparation, catheter care, feeding administration, and related techniques (Adams & Wirsching, 1984; Lees et al, 1981). Several centers have organized home parenteral training programs that teach multispecialty groups to manage these difficult patients (Fleming et al, 1980).

Feedings are given nocturnally to approximate daily requirements, while encouraging normal activities during the day. Although both systems are expensive, home care costs substantially less than hospital therapy, and the individual can return to a near-normal life. For those who require alternative nutritional modes but not acute or extended medical care, home feedings can be managed effectively, safely, and economically on an outpatient basis (Greene et al, 1981; Fleming et al, 1980).

Summary

When individuals have physical problems that interfere with the normal ability to ingest food orally, a plan for nutritional support is essential. Enteral and parenteral feedings are alternatives for individuals who are unable or unwilling to receive adequate nourishment from a normal diet. Once an implementation plan of nutritional support has been initiated, careful clinical and biochemical monitoring is essential to determine progress.

Enteral feedings utilize a functioning gastrointestinal tract and are the physiologically natural method of feeding because they permit more efficient use of the nutrients. Most tube feedings are commercial preparations made from intact nutrients (carbohydrate, protein, and fat). With sufficient energy intake, these provide 100 percent of the RDAs for vitamins and minerals. Monomeric enteral feedings contain basic nutrients ready for absorption for conditions requiring minimal digestion.

Parenteral alimentation is an accepted mode of intravenous delivery of essential nutrients to maintain a patient in nutritional equilibrium. It is indicated when enteral intake is impossible, potentially hazardous, or insufficient. Standard intravenous therapy does not provide sufficient kilocalories or protein. Peripheral infusions of dextrose, amino acids, and fat emulsions can provide about 1800 kcal, a sufficient amount to maintain a patient's ordinary needs. If large amounts of kilocalories (2000 to 5000 kcal) are needed, central vein intravenous feedings should be used.

Review Questions

1. List the alternative methods of feeding and list two conditions that warrant using them.
2. Discuss the advantages and disadvantages of a home-blended formula with commercially prepared formulas.
3. What is an elemental formula and for what conditions is it used?
4. What measures are taken to prevent glucosuria? Why is it important?
5. You notice that a patient in the nursing home is receiving 1800 kcal via intermittent feedings and has diarrhea. What are the possible causes and solutions for the problem?
6. The physician orders 1800 cc/1800 kcal for a bedridden patient who has been on IV feedings for three days. What should you do in initiating the formula to prevent complications?
7. A TPN formula contains the following components: 500 ml of a 10 percent fat emulsion, 500 ml of a five percent amino acid solution, and 1 L of $D_{10}W$. Calculate the amount of protein and energy provided.

Case Study: Ms B.D., a 23-year-old musician has been admitted to the hospital for exacerbation of Crohn's disease (regional enteritis). Since her nutritional status is poor, the physician decides to use parenteral feedings during the acute phase of bowel inflammation. A subclavian venous catheter is inserted and the TPN is begun.

1. Describe a regimen that might be used as the TPN therapy is begun.
2. Why must the blood glucose be monitored carefully?
3. What are the complications of TPN therapy?
4. Why is an infusion pump desirable for the administration of TPN?
5. What measures should the nurse take if the patient does not receive the prescribed amount of TPN fluid?

REFERENCE LIST

Adams, MM; Wirsching, RG: Guidelines for home enteral feedings. *J Am Diet Assoc* 84(1):68, 1984.

American Medical Association (AMA) Department of Food and Nutrition: Multivitamin preparations for parenteral use. A statement by the Nutrition Advisory Group. *JPEN* 3(4):258, 1979.

Arnold, C: Why that liquid formula diet may not work (and what to do about it). *RN* 44(11):34, 1981.

Bernard, M; Forlaw, L: Complications and their prevention. In *Enteral and Tube Feeding.* Edited by JL Rombeau; MD Caldwell. Philadelphia, W. B. Saunders Co, 1984.

Bivins, BA; Rapp, RP: Central versus peripheral nutrition: The controversy. *Am J IV Clin Nutr* 7(3):25, 1980.

Blackburn, GL; Harvey, KB: Nutritional assessment as a routine in clinical medicine. *Postgrad Med* 71(5):46, 1982.

Borgen, L: Total parenteral nutrition in adults. *Am J Nurs* 78(2):224, 1978.

Butterworth, CE, Jr; Weinsier, RL: Malnutrition in hospitalized patients: Assessment and treatment. In *Modern Nutrition in Health and Disease*, 6th ed. Edited by RS Goodhart; ME Shils. Philadelphia, Lea & Febiger, 1980, p 667.

Campbell, SM; Carpenter, JT; Dillon, SR; et al: Methods of nutritional support for hospitalized patients. *Am Fam Physician* 29(5):215, 1984.

Chernoff, R: Stress, surgery, burns and nutritional care. In *Nutrition in Clinical Care*, 2nd ed. Edited by RB Howard; NH Herbold. New York, McGraw-Hill Book Co, 1982, p 654.

Chernoff, R: Nutritional support: Formulas and delivery of enteral feeding. I. Enteral formulas. *J Am Diet Assoc* 79(4):426, 1981.

Chrysomilides, SA; Kaminski, MV, Jr: Home enteral and parenteral nutritional support: A comparison. *Am J Clin Nutr* 34(10):2271, 1981.

Cobb, LM; Cartmill, AM; Gilsdorf, RB: Early postoperative nutritional support using the serosal tunnel jejunostomy. *JPEN* 5(5):397, 1981.

Colley, R; Wilson, J: Managing the patient on hyperalimentation: Meeting patients' nutritional needs with hyperalimentation. *Nursing* 9(6):57, 1979.

Fairfull-Smith, R; Abunassar, R; Freeman, JB; et al: Rational use of elemental and non-elemental diets in hospitalized patients. *Ann Surg* 192(5):600, 1980.

Fleming, CR; Beart, RW, Jr; Berkner, S; et al: Home parenteral nutrition for management of the severely malnourished adult patient. *Gastroenterology* 79(1):11, 1980.

Goldberger, E: *A Primer of Water, Electrolytes, and Acid-Base Syndromes*, 7th ed. Philadelphia, Lea & Febiger, 1986.

Greene, HL; Helinek, GL; Folk, CC; et al: Nasogastric tube feeding at home: A method for adjunctive nutritional support of malnourished patients. *Am J Clin Nutr* 34(6):1131, 1981.

Guild, RT; Cerda, JJ: Total parenteral nutrition. *J Fla Med Assoc* 66(4):401, 1979.

Hinsdale, JG; Lipkowitz, GS; Pollock, TW; et al: Prolonged enteral nutrition in malnourished patients with nonelemental feeding. Reappraisal of surgical technique, safety, and costs. *Am J Surg* 149(3):334, 1985.

Hostetler, C; Lipman, TO; Geraghty, M; et al: Bacterial safety of reconstituted continuous drip tube feedings. *JPEN* 6(3):232, 1982.

Hoying, CL: Nutrition support—nurses' role in nursing management. *Nutr Support Serv* 3(6):28, 1983.

Ivey, MF: The status of parenteral nutrition. *Nurs Clin North Am* 14(2):285, 1979.

Jeejeebhoy, KN; Anderson, GH; Nakhooda, AF; et al: Metabolic studies in total parenteral nutrition with lipid in man. Comparison with glucose. *J Clin Invest* 57(1):125, 1976.

Jones, BJM; Lees, R; Andrews, J; et al: Comparison of an elemental and polymeric enteral diet in patients with normal gastrointestinal function. *Gut* 24(1):78, 1983.

Kagawa-Busby, KS; Heitkemper, MM; Hansen, BC; et al: Effects of diet temperature on tolerance of enteral feedings. *Nurs Res* 29(5):276, 1980.

Lees, CD; Steiger, E; Hooley, RA; et al: Home parenteral nutrition. *Surg Clin North Am* 61(3):621, 1981.

Matarese, LE: Enteral alimentation: Equipment. Part III. *Nutr Support Serv* 2(2):48, 1982.

Metheny, N; Snively, W: *Nurses' Handbook of Fluid Balance*, 4th ed. Philadelphia, J. B. Lippincott Co, 1983.

Page, CP; Clibon, U: A method of enterally feeding defined formula diet. *Am J IV Ther Clin Nutr* 9(1):9, 1982.

Peters, C; Fischer, JE: Studies on calorie-to-nitrogen ratio for total parenteral nutrition. *Surg Gynecol Obstet* 151(1):1, 1980.

Quebbeman, EJ; Ausman, RK; Schneider, TC: A re-evaluation of energy expenditure during parenteral nutrition. *Ann Surg* 195(3):282, 1982.

Rudman, D; Williams, PJ: Nutrient deficiencies during total parenteral nutrition. *Nutr Rev* 43(1):1, 1985.

Schulte, WJ: Surgical nutrition. In *Manual of Surgical Therapeutics*, 4th ed. Edited by R Condon; L Nyhus. Boston, Little, Brown & Co, 1978, p 246.

Shils, ME: Parenteral nutrition. In *Modern Nutrition in Health and Disease*, 6th ed. Edited by RS Goodhart; ME Shils. Philadelphia, Lea & Febiger, 1980, p 1125.

Shizgal, HM; Forse, RA: Protein and calorie requirements with total parenteral nutrition. *Ann Surg* 192(4):562, 1980.

Transitional feedings. *Nutrition and the MD* IX(6):4, 1983.

Twiggs, LC; Nwangwu, PU: Perspectives on the peripheral use of fructose containing hypertonic solutions in nutritional support. *Am J IV Ther Clin Nutr* 9(2):9, 1982.

Vanlandingham, S; Simpson, S, Daniel, P; et al: Metabolic abnormalities in patients supported with enteral tube feeding. *JPEN* 5(4):322, 1981.

West, KH: The importance of trace elements in total parenteral nutrition. *Am J IV Ther Clin Nutr* 8(9):11, 1981.

Weinsier, RL; Butterworth, CE: *Handbook of Clinical Nutrition*. St. Louis, C. V. Mosby Co, 1981.

Further Study

Anderson, BJ: Tube feeding: Is diarrhea inevitable? *Am J Nurs* 86(6):704, 1986.

Atkins, JM; Oakley, CW: A nurse's guide to TPN. *RN* 49(6):20, 1986.

Bayless, E: Taste tray increases acceptance of nutritional supplements. *J Am Diet Assoc* 73(5):542, 1978.

Bayer, LM; Scholl, DE; Ford, EG: Tube feeding at home. *Am J Nurs* 83(9):1321, 1983.

Campbell, SM; Carpenter, JT; Dillon, SR; et al: methods of nutritional support for hospitalized patients. *Am Fam Physician* 29(5):215, 1984.

Carr, P: When the patient needs TPN at home. *RN* 49(6):25, 1986.

Chernoff, R: Nutritional support: Formula and delivery of enteral feeding. II. Delivery systems. *J Am Diet Assoc* 79(4):431, 1981.

Chernoff, R: *Directory of PEN Products and Services*. Silver Spring, MD, American Society for Parenteral and Enteral Nutrition, 1985.

Colley, R; Wilson, J: How to begin hyperalimentation therapy. *Nursing* 9(5):76, 1979.

Colley, R; Wilson, J: Managing the patient on hyperalimentation. *Nursing* 9(6):57, 1979.

Colley, R; Wilson, J: Mabel, D: Providing hyperalimentation for infants and children. *Nursing* 9(7):50, 1979.

DeCristofaro, J: *A Selected Bibliography in Nutrition Support: Nutrition Assessment, Enteral and Parenteral Nutrition and Other Related Topics*. Chicago, Dietitians in Critical Care, The American Dietetic Association, 1983.

Giordano, C; Conly, D: Taking the worry out of hyperalimentation. Part I. *RN* 44(6):42, 1981.

Gordon, AM Jr: Enteral nutritional support: Guidelines for feeding product selection. *Postgrad Med* 72(1):72, 1983.

Griggs, BA; Hoppe, MC: Update: Nasogastric tube feeding. *Am J Nurs* 79(3):481, 1979.

Guhlow, LJ; Kolb, J: Pediatric IVs: Special measures you must take. *RN* 42(3):40, 1979.

Guiness, R: How to use the new small-bore feeding tubes. *Nursing* 16(4):51, 1986.

Heimburger, DC; Weinsier, RL: Guidelines for evaluating and categorizing enteral feeding formulas according to therapeutic equivalence. *JPEN* 3(1):61, 1985.

Hushen, SC: Questioning TPN as the answer. *Am J Nurs* 82(5):852, 1982.

Ivey, MF: The status of parenteral nutrition. *Nurs Clin North Am* 14(2):285, 1979.

Jacobson, NT: How to administer those tricky lipid emulsions. *RN* 42(6):63, 1979.

Journal of Nursing: Nursing Photo Book. *Managing IV Therapy.* Horsham, PA, Intermed Communications Inc, 1980.

Konstantinides, NN; Shron, E: Tube feeding: Managing the basics. *Am J Nurs* 83(9):1312, 1983.

Macfie, J: Towards cheaper intravenous nutrition. *Br Med J* 292(January 11):107, 1986.

Meguid, MM; Eldar, S; Wahba, A: The delivery of nutritional support: A potpourri of new devices and methods. *Cancer* 55(1 suppl):279, 1985.

Metheny, NM: 20 ways to prevent tube-feeding complications. *Nursing* 15(1):47, 1985.

Muller, RJ: The role of trace elements in intravenous nutrition. *Am J IV Ther Clin Nutr* 7(4):14, 1980.

Shea, M; McCreary, M: Early postoperative feeding. *Am J Nurs* 84(10):1230, 1984.

Skipper, A: Specialized formulas for enteral nutrition support. *J Am Diet Assoc* 86(5):654, 1986.

Walravens, PA: Keeping TPN on course with lab monitoring. *Diagn Med* 4(4):38, 1981.

Wilson, D: Make mouth care a must for your patients. *RN* 49(2):39, 1986.

Wilson, J; Colley, R: Teaching patients to administer hyperalimentation at home. *Nursing* 9(8):56, 1979.

Wilson, J; Colley, R: Administering peripheral and enteral feedings. *Nursing* 9(9):62, 1979.

Food-Drug Interactions

22

THE STUDENT WILL BE ABLE TO:

- *Identify drugs that can potentially affect nutritional status.*
- *List three ways drugs may affect appetite.*
- *State why the time of administration of a drug is important.*
- *Discuss how nutrients and non-nutritive substances can alter drug metabolism/absorption.*
- *Discuss how drugs can alter nutrient utilization.*

Amphetamines
Analgesic
Anorexiants
Antacids
Anticholinergic
Anti-infective
Antilipemics
Anticonvulsants
Antineoplastic
Cachexia
Caffeine
Chemotherapeutic
Cytotoxic
Diuretics
Lipophyilic
Monoamine oxidase inhibitor (MAOI)
Peristaltic stimulants
Saline cathartics
Tyramine
Xanthines

Drugs Versus Nutrients

Multiple techniques are employed to maintain or restore health and to alleviate disease symptoms, including diet and drug therapies. Drugs, like foods, are complex chemical substances. In contrast to foods needed for nourishment, drugs are used to diagnose, heal, or prevent an illness or disease or to produce chemical and biological effects in the body.

However, medications can frequently affect or be affected by nutrition. Additionally, foods may interact with drugs and thereby modify their absorption, metabolism, or excretion. While drug-drug interactions are more common than food-drug interactions, the latter have the potential to cause some of the erratic drug responses observed.

In contrast to medications, foods are made up of nutrients that are necessary for metabolic processes. In some cases, nutrients are used pharmacologically in very large amounts to produce chemical and biological effects, such as large doses of vitamin C (ascorbic acid) to acidify the urine during bladder infections. This chapter is concerned with how nutrients, functioning in their nutritional role, are affected by drugs and how drugs may be influenced by foods.

Nutritional Status

Chemicals in foods and drugs can affect each other to such an extent that some medications may not be able to perform their intended function or the body may not obtain adequate amounts of required nutrients. With the current concerns about iatrogenic malnutrition, food-drug interactions have received widespread attention. Although sometimes intentional, the interaction may be undesirable or even unexpected in other situations.

All nutrients, especially vitamins and minerals, can be affected by many drugs (see Appendix C–8). The nutrient intake, absorption, or metabolism are usually impaired. Drugs can affect nutritional status by: (1) stimulating appetite; (2) precipitating anorexia, nausea, or vomiting; (3) increasing excretion of nutrients in the stool or urine; and (4) competing with the nutrient at its site of action. These effects are more significant in patients with poor nutritional status or when long-term intake of drugs is necessary. By accentuating preexisting subclinical malnutrition, drug-nutrient effects may precipitate clinical symptoms of nutrient deficiency.

The extent of interaction between food and drugs is largely dependent on the individual's nutritional status, considering (1) the adequacy of nutrient intake, (2) the efficiency of nutrient absorption and excretion, and (3) the body's reserve stores of the nutrient.

A drug is less effective if (1) its bioavailability is decreased by food, (2) its metabolism is accelerated by a nutrient, or (3) the patient's nutritional status is poor. A person with adequate nutrient stores might have an increased tolerance for a drug and may be able to handle larger amounts (Roe, 1982). To maximize drug effectiveness, individuals should be monitored for their nutritional status while being treated with drugs. Dietary habits should be evaluated. The consumption of a well-balanced, nutritionally adequate diet can reduce the risk of nutritional disorders or altered drug efficacy. Other factors to consider are body weight, age, ethnic background, renal function, alcohol intake, smoking, and the time of administering the drug in relation to food intake (Zallen, 1979).

Hydration status can influence the therapeutic action of drugs and their retention in the body. The rate of urine elimination affects the rate of excretion of the drug; urine elimination may be decreased in dehydrated or edematous patients, causing increased drug levels in the body.

Health Care Teamwork

The patient, physician, pharmacist, nurse, and dietitian can coordinate efforts to reduce the number of ineffective drug therapies and the number of nutritionally depleted patients due to food-drug interactions. All drugs, prescription and nonprescription, should be taken into consideration in establishing health care plans (Roe,

1976). Although the nurse is in the pivotal position of knowing the medications and foods a patient is consuming, the pharmacist and dietitian can offer precautions about possible interactions that may affect therapeutic effectiveness of the drugs or diet.

Effect of Drugs on Food Intake

Drugs can reduce food intake by causing sedation, altering taste and smell, decreasing appetite, or causing an adverse response (nausea or vomiting) when foods are eaten (Table 22–1). Occasionally, drugs are used therapeutically to diminish or to stimulate appetite; more frequently though, these are undesirable side effects.

DECREASED FOOD INTAKE

Amphetamines and phenylpropanolamine are used for weight control; both depress the appetite by a direct effect on the central nervous system. While these are effective in weight reduction as long as they are taken, they are a crutch with a rebounding weight gain after the appetite suppressant is discontinued (Phenylpropanolamine, 1984; Stunkard, 1982, Freedman et al, 1982). Children given amphetamines to control hyperkinesis generally exhibit a slow growth rate during drug therapy but experience a growth rebound when the drugs are discontinued (Safer et al, 1972 and 1975).

Bulk-forming agents, such as those listed in Table 22–1, have been used in attempts to decrease food intake. They have not been shown to be consistently effective, although they do seem to stimulate gastric motility. The use of these agents in weight reduction programs is discussed in Chapter 24.

Decreased Appetite. Decreased food intake is a side effect of drugs that cause gastrointestinal distress (most frequently nausea or vomiting). The most notable of these are cancer chemotherapeutic agents. Patients who are already debilitated because of the cancer are likely to have a poor appetite; chemotherapy compounds the problem and hastens cachexia.

Abnormalities in Taste. Drug-induced loss of taste acuity (dysgeusia) will also result in anorexia. Drugs frequently implicated include griseofulvin (an antibiotic), penicillamine (an antiarthritic), lincomycin (an antibiotic), many of the antilipemics, phenytoin (an anticonvulsant), and methimazole (an antithyroid).

When medications have an unpleasant, difficult-to-mask taste, appetite may be depressed, especially if given with food. Potassium supplements, chloral hydrate (hypnotic), and vitamin B complex liquids are examples.

A metallic or a bitter taste accompanies some medications because they are excreted in the saliva. Streptomycin (even when given parenterally) and many antineoplastic drugs may alter taste acuity and cause an aversion to food. Frequently, decreased taste acuity may be caused by the drug chelating trace metals, which results in less nutrient availability. Zinc (Hambidge et al, 1972) and sometimes copper and nickel are usually involved (Use of copper, 1973; Cohen et al, 1973).

INCREASED APPETITE

Several tranquilizers and other psychoactive drugs stimulate appetite and may result in increased body weight. Weight gain is common in mental institutions, partially because of the side effects of drugs necessary to treat psychiatric problems.

Anabolic steroids may indirectly increase the appetite by creating a euphoric state, which sometimes offsets the anorectic effects of chemotherapy. Cyproheptadine, an appetite stimulator, has been successfully used in nutritional rehabilitation of malnourished individuals (Pawan, 1974; Stiel et al, 1970).

Clinical Implications:

- Some drugs, including digoxin and chemotherapeutic agents, can cause nausea and anorexia to such an extent that the patient's nutritional status deteriorates.
- Chemotherapy patients require appropriate nutritional support before, during, and between courses of drug therapy. Polymeric formulas can be used to increase nutrient and energy intake (see Chapter 25).
- For persons on phenothiazines and diazepam, weight should be carefully monitored. Encour-

Table 22–1. Drugs Affecting Food Intake

	Uses	Mechanism of Action	Examples
Decreases Appetite			
Amphetamines	Stimulant; used for weight control and hyperkinesis.	Depresses appetite via a central mechanism.	D-Amphetamine (Dexedrine), phenmetrazine (Preludin), and methylphenidate (Ritalin).
Cholinergic agents	Stimulates gut motility and alleviates urinary retention.	Nausea and anorexia; diarrhea.	Bethanechol chloride (Urecholine).
Narcotics	Analgesics; cough suppressants.	Nausea, anorexia, or sedation.	Morphine, codeine, and meperidine (Demerol).
Glyceryl guaiacolate	Expectorant.	Nausea and anorexia.	Robitussin.
High-fiber or bulk-forming medications	Stimulates gut motility.	Creates a feeling of fullness.	Methylcellulose, guar gum, and psyllium hydrophilic mucilloid (Metamucil, Konsyl).
Cytotoxic drugs	Cancer therapy.	Anorexia and inflammatory reaction in the upper gastrointestinal tract.	Methotrexate, procarbazine, Cytoxan, BiCNU, dactinomycin, 5-mercaptopyridoxal, and cisplatin.
Cardiac glycosides	Congestive heart failure.	Anorexia and nausea.	Digitalis (Crystodigin), digoxin (Lanoxin).
Griseofulvin	Antifungal.	Decreases taste acuity.	Fulvicin-U/F and Grifulvin V.
D-Penicillamine	Wilson's disease.	Induces zinc deficiency.	Cuprimine.
Lincomycin	Systemic infection.	Decreases taste acuity.	Lincocin.
Isoniazid	Tuberculosis.	Nausea, vomiting, and epigastric distress.	Isoniazid.
Antilipemics	Lowers blood lipids.	Decreases taste acuity; nausea.	Clofibrate (Atromid-S); cholestyramine (Questran).
Phenytoin	Anticonvulsant.	Decreases taste acuity.	Diphenylhydantoin (Dilantin).
Methimazole	Antithyroid.	Decreases taste acuity.	
Methythiouracil	Antithyroid.	Decreases taste acuity.	
Streptomycin	Antibiotic.	Metallic taste.	
Potassium iodide or potassium chloride	Potassium supplements.	Tastes bad and leaves a bad taste in the mouth.	Potassium chloride (K-Lyte; Kaochlor; Kayciel); potassium iodide (Mudrane).

age the intake of low-calorie foods. Evaluate the intake of various beverages used to relieve thirst.

- While phenothiazines usually increase the appetite, drowsiness and sedation are observed in the elderly; the patient's weight should be monitored regularly.
- Appetite-reducing drugs can contribute significantly to development of nutritional deficiencies, especially if the diet is marginal.
- In addition to deficiencies of zinc, copper, and nickel, nutritional deficiencies of niacin and vitamin A can also cause taste abnormalities (Hodges, 1972; Green, 1971).
- Zinc and niacin are prevalent in meats, and vitamin A precursors are found in vegetables; therefore, patients who have difficulty chewing are likely to develop decreased taste acuity.
- Consider specific taste alterations to make food more acceptable to patients. Suggest additional sugar, salt or spices, as applicable.

Effects of Absorption on Bioavailability of Nutrients and Drugs

Since both nutrients and drugs are blended in the gastrointestinal tract prior to absorption, many different things can happen to the nutrient, the drug, or the gastrointestinal tract that can affect absorption. Most food-drug interactions occur in the gastrointestinal tract, affecting the bioavailability of the ingested drug or nutrient. Drug absorption is somewhat different than nutrient absorption (Krondl, 1970). Whereas nutrients must usually be digested prior to absorption and require a specific pH as well as digestive enzymes, these factors are not necessary for the absorption of drugs.

Table 22–1. *Drugs Affecting Food Intake Continued*

	Uses	Mechanism of Action	Examples
Bromide-containing medications		Salty bitter taste in the mouth.	
Flagyl	Trichomoniasis.	Metallic taste.	
Chloral hydrate	Hypnotic.	Tastes bad.	Noctec.
Paraldehyde	Hypnotic.	Tastes bad.	
Vitamin B preparations		Tastes bad.	
Increases Appetite			
Phenothiazines	Tranquilizers and antipsychotics.	Central brain effects or improvement in mental condition.	Chlorpromazine (Thorazine), chlordiazepoxide (Librium), thioridazine (Mellaril), and trifluoperazine (Stelazine).
Benzodiazepines	Antianxiety.	Central brain effects and/or improvement in mental condition.	Diazepam (Valium).
Monoamine oxidase inhibitors (MAOIs)	Antidepressant.	Central brain effects and/or improvement in mental condition.	Eutonyl, Parnate, and Marplan.
Tricyclic antidepressants.	Antidepressant.	Crave sweets and carbohydrates.	Amitriptyline (Elavil) and imipramine (Tofranil).
Lithium carbonate	Antidepressant.	Central brain effects and/or improvement in mental condition.	
Oral contraceptives	Birth control.		Ortho-Novum, Enovid, and Ovral.
Anabolic steroids	Protein builder.		Testosterone.
Insulin	Hyperglycemia.	Increased appetite when hypoglycemia is present.	
Small amounts of alcohol/wine		Increases saliva and gastric secretions.	
Sulfonylureas	Oral hypoglycemia.		Orinase.
Cyproheptadine	Antihistamine (anticholinergic).		Periactin.

Drug absorption is dependent on lipid solubility, rate of dissociation, gastrointestinal pH, particle size, and physical form. Drugs are absorbed by passive diffusion. Weakly acidic drugs are absorbed in the stomach. Most drugs (especially neutral and basic ones) are absorbed in the small intestine (Roe, 1983).

DRUGS AND NUTRIENT ABSORPTION

Some of the more common drugs that affect absorption of specific nutrients are listed in Table 22–2. The fact that a drug reduces nutrient absorption does not mean that a deficiency will occur. Medications that are generally of concern include those used for chronic diseases over an extended period of time.

The types of drugs that most frequently cause malabsorption problems are laxatives, antacids, hypocholesterolemics, oral contraceptives, oral hypoglycemics, anticonvulsants, alcohol, and cytotoxic (i.e., tumor-inhibiting medications that are harmful to cells) drugs. Many antibiotics and colchicine (used to treat gout) are associated with malabsorption, but they are not generally prescribed for long-term therapy. The following conditions may result in drug-induced malabsorption of nutrients (Roe, 1976).

1. Decreased solubility of the nutrient. Absorption of nutrients may be affected by altered pH or by decreased solubility (the nutrient is bound to another agent that is not absorbed). An example of this involves malabsorption of fat-soluble vitamins with concomitant mineral oil ingestion. An acidic pH in the gastrointestinal tract is necessary for folic acid absorption and for intrinsic factor to combine with vitamin B_{12} for absorption. Long-

Table 22–2. *Malabsorption of Nutrients Due to Drug Intake*

Drug Classification	Nutrient(s) Detrimentally Affected
Antacids Aluminum or magnesium hydroxide.	Phosphate, folacin, and calcium.
Laxatives (when abused) Bisacodyl (Dulcolax). Phenolphthalein (in Ex-Lax). Mineral oil, milk of magnesia, and Haley's M-O.	 Potassium and calcium Potassium, calcium, and vitamin D. Fats and fat-soluble vitamins.
Antilipemics Clofibrate (Atromid S) and cholestyramine.	Fats; vitamins A, B_{12}, D, and K; folacin; and iron
Antineoplastics Cisplatin. Aminopterin, cytotoxic agents, and methotrexate.	 Magnesium and zinc. Calcium, folacin, lactose, and vitamin B_{12}.
Alcohol	Lactose, amino acids, electrolytes, long-chain fatty acids, thiamin, folacin, vitamin B_{12}, and magnesium.
Anticonvulsants Dilantin, phenytoin, and phenobarbital.	Folacin and calcium.
Oral contraceptives	Folacin and vitamin B_6.
Glucocorticoids and corticosteroids	Calcium and potassium.
Anti-infectives Neomycin. Sulfasalazine (Azulfidine).	 Fat, nitrogen, sodium, potassium, calcium, iron, lactose, sucrose, vitamins B_{12} and K. Folacin.

term antacid therapy and potassium chloride supplements neutralize the gastric hydrochloric acid, thereby preventing absorption of these vitamins. A high pH also interferes with conversion of ferric iron to the reduced, absorbent ferrous form.

2. *Adsorption of bile salts.* Antilipemics adsorb bile salts. Not only is cholesterol excreted, but fat-soluble vitamins are bound along with bile salts by the drug, resulting in their excretion. Deficiencies of vitamins A, D, and K may occur because of this nutrient-drug interaction (Heaton et al, 1972; Longenecker & Basu, 1965).

3. *Damage of the intestinal mucosa.* Drugs can decrease the amount of enzymes available and thereby interfere with the transport system of nutrient absorption. Methotrexate and 5-fluorouracil (both chemotherapeutic drugs) and colchicine inhibit rapid mitosis (i.e., cell division) of the epithelial cells throughout the gastrointestinal tract (Webb et al, 1968; Trier, 1962). Since colchicine is not used for long-term therapy, these effects are not considered serious. On the other hand, methotrexate causes malabsorption of several nutrients—vitamin B_{12}, folate, and calcium (Roe, 1984).

4. *Inactivation of intestinal enzymes.* While some carbohydrate-involving enzymes may be affected, the complex enzyme system required for absorption of vitamins B_6 and B_{12} is frequently rendered ineffective. Phenytoin (an anticonvulsant) and sulfasalazine (an anti-inflammatory) inhibit enzymes present in the intestinal epithelium thereby decreasing absorption of naturally-occurring folate. Anticonvulsants and the antitubercular drug para-aminosalicylic acid (PAS) also inhibit enzymatic mechanisms responsible for the absorption of vitamin B_{12} (Waxman et al, 1970; Reynolds et al, 1965).

5. *Decreased gastrointestinal transit time.* Laxatives decrease the amount of time for nutrient absorption in the intestinal tract. Peristaltic stimulants (containing bisacodyl or phenolphthalein) can interfere with the intestinal uptake of glucose, potassium, and calcium. Saline cathartics (milk of magnesia, magnesium sulfate, and sodium phosphate) are hypertonic, and water is osmotically attracted into the lumen. Although overuse may decrease nutrient availability, cathartics are not as hazardous nutritionally as peristaltic stimulants.

6. *Increased absorption.* Few drugs enhance nutrient absorption. However, increased absorption of cholesterol has been documented with long-term use of the laxative docusate sodium (Hartshorn, 1977) and the tranquilizer chlorpromazine (Clark et al, 1970).

Clinical Implications:

- When long-term therapy warrants drugs known to interfere with absorption, nutritional status should be routinely assessed and appropriate dietary changes or nutrient supplements implemented.
- Following colchicine treatment, temporary lactase deficiency may be observed (Smith & Bidlack, 1984).
- Vegetable bulk laxatives (e.g., Konsyl, Metamucil) are the least likely to cause nutrient malabsorption (ADA, 1981).
- Hypocholesterolemic agents may decrease the amount of long-chain triglycerides and fat-soluble vitamins absorbed. Medium-chain triglycerides (MCT) (ADA, 1981) and water-miscible forms of vitamins A, D, and K (Heaton et al, 1972) alleviate this problem.
- Antacids containing aluminum or magnesium hydroxide antacids (e.g., Amphojel, Basaljel, or Gelusil) complex with the phosphate ion, decreasing its absorption (Lindeman, 1979). For long-term use, serum phosphate levels should be monitored.
- The use of mineral oil as a laxative should be discouraged.
- Habitual use of milk of magnesia as an antacid can result in diarrhea.
- Encourage patients taking phenytoin and sulfasalazine to eat a varied and adequate diet rather than using folacin supplements (Smith & Bidlack, 1984).

FOODS AND DRUG ABSORPTION

Intake of food as well as the composition of food affects drug absorption. Physiological changes in the gastrointestinal tract or physical or chemical interactions among food components and drugs influence drug bioavailability. These factors can reduce, delay, or increase absorption of the drug or have no effect at all. Since a decrease in the percentage of drug absorbed is equivalent to a decrease in dosage, the time a drug is given in relation to food intake has clinical and economic implications. The established time of day for drug administration in health care institutions may conflict with the optimal bioavailability of the drug (Harper & Higgins, 1983).

Rate of Absorption. In most cases, the absorption of drugs is delayed by concomitant food intake; this may or may not decrease the amount of drug absorption. Thus, other considerations determine whether to give the drug with food. If a rapid effect is necessary (such as with analgesics, hypnotics, or anti-infectives for acute infections), the drug is taken on an empty stomach (Table 22–3). In general, a decreased rate of absorption is more significant when single doses of drugs are given. Aspirin is absorbed more rapidly when taken with 8 oz. of water on an empty stomach and, theoretically, is more quickly effective.

When a drug is given regularly to maintain a constant serum level rather than to provide a rapid peak, the rate of absorption is not the primary concern. Thus, the drug may be taken with food if total absorption is not significantly decreased. If absorbed too slowly, the drug may not reach an effective level in the blood, or the effects of the drug may be prolonged.

Amount of Absorption. Since types of foods eaten can affect the transit rate through the gastrointestinal tract, a drug is especially affected by diet and dietary changes if it (1) dissolves at an unusually slow rate, (2) is absorbed at a particular site, or (3) is in sustained-release form. In general, most drugs are water-soluble. If taken with fatty food, absorption is significantly delayed.

On the other hand, griseofulvin (used to treat fungal infection of the skin and nails) is lipophilic, and its absorption is markedly enhanced by fatty foods. Some drugs should be taken with food because their absorption is enhanced by prolonged time in the stomach, better solubility, presence of specific nutrients in foods, and increased blood flow to the gastrointestinal tract (Table 22–4).

Gastrointestinal distress is a common side effect of many drugs; therefore, trade-offs must sometimes be made. These drugs may need to be taken with food, even if absorption is decreased. By suggesting types of foods that can prevent stomach upsets, patient compliance can be increased.

While aspirin is absorbed more rapidly from an empty stomach, the use of 1 to 3 gm aspirin tablets causes a blood loss of 5 ml and an iron loss of 2 mg (Moore & Powers, 1982). Habitual users of aspirin may benefit by taking aspirin with food to minimize gastric irritation, which could contribute to iron deficiency anemia.

Many irritating drugs, such as nitrofurantoin (an antimicrobial), phenylbutazone (an analgesic), and para-aminosalicylic acid (an antitubercular) may be administered with, or immediately after, meals. Anticholinergic drugs, prescribed to re-

Table 22–3. Drugs to be Taken on an Empty Stomach*

Drugs and Classification	Rationale
Analgesics	
Acetaminophen (Datril, Phenaphen, Tylenol)	Food delays absorption.
Enteric-coated acetylsalicylic acid	Food delays absorption.
Antitubercular	
Para-aminosalicylic acid (PAS)	Food decreases absorption; however, the drug may be given with small amounts of food to minimize nausea and vomiting.
Antiarthritic	
Penicillamine (Cuprimine)	Food decreases absorption.
Anti-infective	
Amoxicillin (Amoxil, Larotid, Polymox, Robamox, Sumox)	Food decreases absorption; take with 8 oz. water.
Ampicillin (Amcill, Omnipen, Penbritin, Pensyn, Polycillin, others)	Food decreases absorption; take with 8 oz. water.
Cephalexin (Keflex)	Food delays absorption.
Cloxacillin (Tegopen)	Food decreases absorption; take with 8 oz. water.
Erythromycin/Erythromycin salts (Erythromycin Base, E.E.S., Pediamycin, others)	Food decreases absorption; *enteric-coated* erythromycin base and erythromycin ethylsuccinate may be given with food. Take with 8 oz. water.
Lincomycin (Lincocin)	Food decreases absorption.
Methacycline (Rondomycin)	Food decreases absorption.
Penicillin G Potassium (Pentids, others)	Food decreases absorption; take with 8 oz. water.
Penicillin V (V-Cillin K)	Food decreases absorption.
Sulfonamides (Gantrisin, others)	Food delays absorption.
Tetracyclines (Achromycin-V, Declomycin)	Food decreases absorption; will chelate with iron, magnesium, or calcium.
Cardiac drugs	
Digoxin (Lanoxin).	Food delays absorption; high-fiber meal decreases absorption. Maintain high potassium intake.
Pentaerythritol tetranitrate (Peritrate).	Take with 8 oz. of water.
Spasmolytic agents	
Theophylline (e.g., Slo-Phyllin).	Food delays absorption; take with 8 oz. water.
Anti-Parkinsonism agent	
Levodopa.	Food decreases absorption; take more than three hours after high-protein foods.
Laxative	
Bisacodyl.	Take with at least 250 ml water and at least one hour after a meal.
Mineral oil.	Interferes with absorption of food.

*These drugs should be taken on an empty stomach for efficient absorption, one hour before or three hours after a meal.

duce gastric acid secretion and gut motility, should be administered shortly before a meal for optimal effectiveness. These and other drugs, such as anorexiants, should be given a half hour before meals (Table 22–5). Antacids should be given 30 minutes to one hour after a meal; however, antacids are sometimes contraindicated by certain drugs (Table 22–6).

Tetracycline frequently causes gastrointestinal upsets. However, when given with food (milk and milk products) or supplements containing calcium, magnesium or aluminum (especially certain antacids), and iron and sodium bicarbonate, both the ion and tetracycline are malabsorbed. Methotrexate absorption is also decreased by milk intake (Pinkerton et al, 1980). Table 22–7 identifies drugs that should not be taken with milk or milk products.

The absorption, safety, and effectiveness of many drugs are enhanced by fluid intake, especially water (Table 22–8).

Acid-labile drugs are more effective if given one hour before or two hours after meals so that stomach acidity is reduced and the drug is in the

Table 22–4. Drugs to be Taken with Food*

Classification and Drugs	Rationale
Analgesics	
Aspirin (A.S.A., Ecotrin, Empirin); aspirin with codeine; ibuprofen (Motrin); indomethacin (Indocin); phenylbutazone (Butazolidin); mefenamic acid (Ponstel); and others.	Food delays and reduces absorption but prevents nausea, vomiting, and gastrointestinal irritation.
Propoxyphene (Darvon).	Food increases absorption.
Antineoplastic agents	
Busulfan (Myleran), cyclophosphamide (Cytoxan), hydroxyurea (Hydrea), melphalan (Alkeran), mercaptopurine (Purinethol), methotrexate, and thioguanine.	Generally given on a full stomach. Food may be withheld if the nausea and vomiting associated with these drugs occurs. Force fluids.
Sedatives and hypnotics	
Chloral hydrate (Noctec, SK-Chloral Hydrate, and others).	Food minimizes nausea and vomiting. Give with 8 oz. of liquid.
Tranquilizers	
Phenothiazines (Thorazine, Chlorpromazine, Mellaril, others).	Food minimizes gastrointestinal side effects.
Diazepam (Valium).	Food increases solubilization; increases absorption.
Lithium (Lithane, Eskalith).	Food increases absorption.
Antidiabetic agents	
Chlorpropamide (Diabinese).	Food delays absorption but minimizes gastrointestinal upsets.
Tolbutamide (Orinase).	
Steroids	
Cortisone (Cortone), methylprednisolone (Medrol), prednisone (Meticorten and Servisone), dexamethasone (Decadron), hydrocortisone (Cortef), and prednisolone (Delta).	Absorption is delayed by food, but more consistent blood levels are established when given with food.
Antilipemic agents	
Cholestyramine (Questran).	Take immediately before meals for clinical effect.
Clofibrate (Atromid-S).	Food decreases absorption, but minimizes gastrointestinal side effects.
Anticoagulants	
Dicumarol (Dufalone).	Food enhances absorption; limit foods with vitamin K.
Anticonvulsants	
Diphenylhydantoin, phenytoin (Dilantin), Carbamazepin (Tegretol).	Food enhances absorption and minimizes gastric irritation; food enhances absorption.
Anti-infective drugs	
Griseofulvin (Fulvicin).	High-fat meals enhance absorption.
Metronidazole (Flagyl).	Food delays absorption but minimizes gastric irritation.
Nitrofurantoin (Furadantin).	Food increases absorption.
Doxycycline (Vibramycin) and minocycline (Minocin).	Unlike other tetracyclines, better tolerated with food.
Isoniazide (INH)	Food decreases absorption but minimizes gastric irritation.
Para-aminosalicylic acid (PAS).	Food minimizes gastric irritation.
Hypotensive drugs	
Hydralazine (Apresoline).	Food enhances absorption.
Propranolol (Inderal).	Food enhances absorption.
Reserpine (Serpasil and Ser-Ap-Es).	Food minimizes gastric irritation.
Rauwolfia serpentina (Raudixin).	Food minimizes gastric irritation.
Diuretics	
Chlorthalidone (Hygroton), triamterene (Dyrenium), chlorothiazide (Diuril), and furosemide (Lasix).	Food minimizes stomach upset and delays absorption, but bioavailability is not affected.
Spironolactone (Aldactone) and hydrochlorothiazide (Dyazide).	Food increases absorption; prevents nausea and vomiting.
Antisecretory drugs	
Cimetidine (Tagamet).	Food delays absorption, but bioavailability is not affected.
Antiarthritic and antigout	
Allopurinol (Zyloprim), phenylbutazone (Butazolidin), trihexyphenidyl (Artane), and oxyphenbutazone (Tandearil).	Food delays absorption and prevents nausea and vomiting, but bioavailability is not significantly affected.
Replacement supplements	
Potassium products.	Food delays absorption, but minimizes gastrointestinal irritation.
Iron preparations.	Food minimizes gastrointestinal side effects.

*These drugs are too irritating to be taken on an empty stomach or their absorption is enhanced when taken immediately before, during, or after meals or with milk.

Table 22–5. Drugs to be Taken Prior to Meals*

Classification and Drug	Rationale
Anticholinergic agents Atropine sulfate (Antispasmodic), clidinium bromide (Librax), methscopolamine (Pamine), belladonna and its alkaloids (Donnatal and Donnagel), and propantheline (Pro-Banthine).	Anticholinergic drugs inhibit vagal effects on gastric glands and gastric secretion when the gastric acid is reaching a maximum. They are more effective against basal secretion when taken after gastric secretions are stimulated.
Antidepressants Monoamine oxidase inhibitors (Nardil, Parnate) and methylphenidate (Ritalin).	Give 30 minutes before meals to avoid interference with absorption.
Anorexiants Phentermine (Ionamin) and phenmetrazine (Preludin).	For maximum psychological and pharmacological effectiveness.

*These drugs should be given 30 minutes before meals.

stomach the least amount of time. Drugs that should not be given with acidic fruit or vegetable juices or carbonated beverages include: penicillin G (Pentids and SK-Penicillin G), cloxacillin (Tegopen), erythromycin base (E.E.S., E-Mycin E, and Pediamycin), erythromycin stearate (Bristamycin and Erythrocin), ampicillin, and levodopa.

Since the timing of drug administration is frequently the responsibility of the nursing staff, charts such as those given in this chapter should be readily available at each nursing station; if the drug is not listed, a pharmacist should be consulted.

Many patients, especially children and the elderly, have difficulty swallowing tablets or capsules. Different types of oral medication are formulated to be released over a long period of time or at predetermined intervals. These formulations include extended-release, enteric-coated, encapsulated beads, wax matrix, and sublingual products. Crushing, chewing, or breaking these products can dramatically affect their rate of absorption and increase the risk of adverse or toxic side effects.

Tablets that are hard to crush or appear to have a special hard coating or capsules that contain beads should alert the nurse to consult the pharmacist to determine if crushing is appropriate (Mitchell, 1984).

Clinical Implications:

- Drastic changes in dietary intake (such as a high-protein diet) can affect drug absorption, and patients should be advised to check with their physician before radical dietary changes (Roe, 1981).
- The absorption of acetaminophen is reduced by pectin present in foods such as jelly and apples.

Table 22–6. Drugs Not to be Taken with Antacids

Drugs	Rationale
Bisacodyl (Dulcolax).	Enteric coating dissolves in antacids, releasing the irritant drug in the stomach.
Iron preparations.	Complexed by antacids, which decreases absorption.
Tetracycline and its derivatives such as demeclocycline (Declomycin) and doxycycline (Vibramycin).	Complexes with antacids, which decreases absorption.

Table 22–7. Drugs Not to be Taken with Milk or Milk Products

Drugs	Rationale
Enteric-coated aspirin (Ecotrin).	Enteric coating dissolves in basic medium such as milk.
Bisacodyl (Dulcolax).	Enteric coating dissolves in basic medium such as milk.
Potassium chloride or iodide.	Complexed by the alkaline medium, decreasing absorption.
Methacycline (Rondomycin).	Complexed by the alkaline medium, decreasing absorption.
Tetracycline and its derivatives (Vibramycin, Sumycin, and Achromycin).	Complexes with the alkaline, very poorly absorbed.
Coated erythromycin (E-Mycin and Erythrocin).	Milk enhances dissolution of the protective coating, which protects the acid-labile drug from degradation in the stomach.
Methotrexate.	Complexes with the alkaline, decreasing absorption.

Table 22–8. Drugs Requiring Large Amounts of Fluid*

Drugs	Rationale
Aspirin, iron preparations, methotrexate, tetracycline.	Full glass of water (8 oz.) promotes dispersion and dissolution of the drug and reduces the risk of esophageal or peptic ulceration, or minimizes acid degradation in the stomach and enhances bioavailability.
Liquid potassium chloride (Kaochlor, Kaon, Kay Ciel, and K-Lyte).	Liquid potassium preparations must be diluted with water to avoid gastrointestinal injury. (Doses of 78 mg of potassium should be taken with at least 3 or 4 oz. of water, fruit juice, or a carbonated beverage).
Ampicillin (Ampicin and Penbritin); cloxacillin (Orbenin and Tegopen); erythromycin base (Erythromid and Robimycin); erythromycin stearate (Erythrocin); and penicillin G (Falapen, Hylenta, and Megacillin).	A full glass of water (8 oz.) enhances gastric emptying and dilutes the gastric contents of these acid-labile drugs.
Allopurinol (Zyloprim), probenecid (Benemid), and sulfonamides.	At least 8 oz. of water should be taken with these drugs; 8 to 10 glasses a day prevents crystalluria or the formation of urinary calculi.
Methylcellulose and psyllium hydrophilic mucilloid (Metamucil).	To be taken with at least 8 oz. of water; a generous quantity of fluid is necessary for the bulk-forming effect of these laxatives and to prevent obstruction.
Penicillamine (Cuprimine).	Patients with cysteinuria should drink about 1 pint of water at bedtime and again during the night, when the urine is more acid.
Cyclophosphamide (Procytox).	To ensure prompt excretion of toxic active metabolites, drug administration should be followed by 2000 to 3000 ml of fluid.

*These drugs should be administered with at least 8 oz. of fluid.

From Tuttle, CB: Harmony with drugs and food. Originally published in *Canadian Medical Association Journal,* volume 126, May 15, 1982.

- Patients should be told the best time to take medications in relation to meals for consistent and optimal absorption.
- Total abstention from milk and milk products during tetracycline therapy is discouraged. Foods or supplements containing calcium, iron, or magnesium can be given two to three hours before or after taking tetracycline.
- Optimal absorption of griseofulvin is associated with a high-fat meal; when it is prescribed for patients on a low-fat diet, its absorption can be increased by using a micronized formulation or by suspending the drug in a small amount of corn oil (Roe, 1981).
- Medications designed for gradual release, such as sustained-release tablets and capsule formulations, should not be broken or crushed.
- For individuals unable to swallow whole tablets or capsules, use a liquid or suspension form of medication.
- Enteric-coated drugs are designed to be released in the small intestine; foods in the stomach delay gastric-emptying time and interfere with the absorption of these drugs. These medications should not be crushed and should be taken one hour before or two hours after meals.

- Alcohol and hot beverages can cause premature erosion of pH-sensitive, enteric-coated tablets.
- Laxatives and high-fiber foods tend to reduce the bioavailability of poorly soluble drugs, such as digoxin (Rodman, 1980).
- Levodopa and methyldopa compete with absorption of amino acids. They should be taken with carbohydrate-rich snacks at least three hours before or after eating a high-protein meal.

Effect of Drug-Nutrient Interactions on Metabolism

Drugs and nutrients both affect metabolic processes in the body; they sometimes interfere with the metabolism of each other. In some instances, the therapeutic action of a drug directly interferes with the body's use of a particular nutrient; in others, non-nutritive substances in foods act as drugs to alter metabolism (e.g., caffeine).

DETRIMENTAL INTERACTIONS

Many drugs interfere with normal metabolism of pyridoxine (B_6). Isoniazid (INH), an antitubercular drug, and levadopa, used in the treatment of Parkinson's disease, complex with the nutrient making pyridoxine unavailable for normal metabolic purposes. A daily 50 mg supplement of pyridoxine protects against isoniazid-induced neuropathy (Visconti, 1977). Exogenous pyridoxine decreases the effect of levodopa (Mars, 1974; Van Woert, 1972). While the amount of pyridoxine supplied by a normal diet is acceptable, patients should not be given a supplement containing large amounts of vitamin B_6 (ADA, 1981).

Anticoagulating Medications. Coumarin derivatives interfere with the action of vitamin K and reduce the production of several clotting factors. If individuals on any of the coumarins or indanedione derivatives ingest large amounts of vitamin K in foods (e.g., liver or green leafy vegetables) or take vitamin K supplements, the effectiveness of the drugs are lessened.

Anticonvulsants. About one percent of the population, or 2.4 million Americans, suffer from active epilepsy (CCEC, 1977). Anticonvulsant drugs (primidone, phenobarbital, and phenytoin) increase vitamin D and K metabolism. The amount of vitamin D required to prevent bone demineralization caused by anticonvulsant therapy is estimated to be 600 to 1000 IU/day (Hahn et al, 1972). Folic acid deficiencies are also observed with prolonged usage. However, deficiency symptoms caused by anticonvulsant drugs are generally associated with a marginal diet containing low amounts of the vitamins. High doses of folic acid decrease effectiveness of these drugs (Baylis et al, 1971), but up to 5 mg/day can be used to improve serum folic acid levels (Moore & Ball, 1972).

Corticosteroids. The metabolism of carbohydrate, protein, and fat is affected by corticosteroids (Eisenstein, 1973). Glycogen is broken down to glucose, resulting in hyperglycemia; protein is catabolized, resulting in tissue-wasting; and fats are mobilized to certain areas of the body. Thus, the typical moon face and buffalo hump are found in patients on long-term steroid therapy.

Oral Contraceptives. Most nutrients are affected by oral contraceptives. While metabolic changes suggest an increased metabolic requirement for several nutrients, few clinical correlations have been identified. Patients on the pill for extended periods may become depleted of B vitamins, especially folic acid and vitamin B_6. However, vitamin deficiencies have been identified only in marginal diets. Particular attention should be given to the intake of foods containing folic acid and vitamin B_6. Supplements are not necessarily indicated, except for high-risk patients in whom other factors, such as deficient diet or disease, could increase the chances for a deficiency to develop (Sriwatanakul & Weintraub, 1983).

Antacids. Long-term use of antacids containing magnesium or aluminum hydroxide has a detrimental effect on mineral metabolism. Phosphate depletion is the first effect, followed by large calcium losses and vitamin D deficiencies (Spencer et al, 1975). Milk-alkali syndrome, caused by the overuse of antacids, is discussed in Chapter 27.

Antibiotics. Many antibiotics, particularly tetracyclines, can inhibit bacterial synthesis of vitamin K in the gastrointestinal tract (Wilson, 1974). Frequently, buttermilk or yogurt is advised to replace gastrointestinal microorganisms.

Monoamine Oxidase Inhibitors. The use of monoamine oxidase inhibitors (MAOIs) was prevalent for the treatment of depression in the 1960s and 1970s. MAOIs interfere with the natural enzyme monoamine oxidase. Because of the severity of the problems encountered with food-drug interactions, they are no longer widely used.

Norepinephrine, a hormone, acts as a neurotransmitter. The enzyme MAO (naturally present) maintains normal levels of norepinephrine by inactivating norepinephrine and preventing the absorption of tyramine (found in foods). Tyramine can cause the release of norepinephrine.

When MAOIs are given, norepinephrine builds up in the brain, improving moods. However, since the patient receiving MAOIs has no natural mechanism to inactivate norepinephrine and inhibit absorption of tyramine, foods containing tyramine should be eliminated from the diet. Tyramine is found in aged cheeses and derived from protein degradation; any protein-containing food that has undergone degradation can become dangerous to patients on MAOIs. They should eat only fresh protein (Folks, 1983). Table 22–9 indicates a hierarchy of foods that should definitely be avoided and those that are safe in moderate amounts. This diet may be called the low-tyramine or the MAOI diet.

When large amounts of norepinephrine accumulate, patients get nose bleeds, high blood pres-

Table 22–9. Restricted Tyramine Diet*

Food Group	Unrestricted Foods (< 5 mcg/g)	Foods Allowed in Moderation (5 to 20 mcg/g)	Foods to Avoid (> 20 mcg/g)
Cheese	Cottage cheese, ricotta, cream cheese	Processed American cheese, Gouda	Aged cheeses—brick, blue, cheddar, Camembert, Swiss, Romano, Roquefort, Stilton, mozzarella, Parmesan, provolone, Emmantaler, boursin, sour cream, brie
Beverages	Milk	Coffee, hot chocolate, cola drinks (1–3 cups per day)	Ale, beer, sherry, red and white wines,† yogurt, bouillon
Meats	Fresh or fresh frozen meat, poultry		Canned meats, chicken liver, beef liver, fermented (hard) sausage or salami, pepperoni, summer sausage, bologna, genoa salami
Fish	Fresh or fresh frozen fish or shellfish		Salt herring, dried fish, caviar
Vegetables	Most		Italian flat beans, Chinese pea pods, broad (fava) beans, mixed Chinese vegetables, eggplant
Fruit	Most		Figs, avocados
Miscellaneous			Chocolate, soy sauce, protein extracts, yeast concentrates or products made with them

*From Alpers, DH; Clouse, RE; Stenson, WF: *Manual of Nutritional Therapeutics.* Boston, Little, Brown & Company, © 1983.

†Fermentation of wine and beer does not ordinarily involve processes that result in the production of tyramine. Despite this, levels in beer are variable. The production of appreciable amounts of tyramine in red wines results from contamination with other than the usual fermenting organisms and from the inclusion of grape pulp and seeds in the process. These potential sources of amino acids are not used in making white wines. Because of the unpredictable variability in tyramine levels, all of the beverages listed are generally excluded (*Med. Lett. Drugs Ther.* 18(17):32, 1976).

sure, and hypertensive crisis. Other drugs associated with similar reactions include procarbazine (an antineoplastic) and isoniazid (an antitubercular).

Alcohol. Regardless of whether alcohol (ethanol) is considered a drug or a food, it does affect nutrient and drug metabolism. Large amounts of alcohol inhibit liver enzymes that metabolize drugs (Rubin et al, 1970), whereas chronically large amounts of alcohol speed up the metabolism of many drugs (Kater et al, 1969). Alcohol potentiates the effect of many types of drugs, including antidepressants, antihistamines, barbiturates, sedatives, hypnotics, narcotic analgesics, tranquilizers, diphenoxylate (Lomotil), disulfiram (Antabuse), MAOIs (Nardil and Parnate), meclizine (Antivert), methaqualone (Quaalude and Mequin), metronidazole (Flagyl), oral hypoglycemics (Diabinese, Dymelor, Orinase, Tolbutamide, and Tolinase); phentolamine (Regitine), and chloramphenicol (Chloromycetin). Consuming alcohol with some drugs increases the potential for gastric irritation and bleeding.

Ethanol metabolism is affected by disulfiram (Antabuse), a drug used in the treatment of alcoholism. When alcohol in any form is given to individuals taking disulfiram, blood acetaldehyde concentration rises, causing flushing, nausea, vomiting, and severe hypotension. This reaction also occurs when other drugs are given: metronidazole, furazolidone, chlorpropamide, griseofulvin, quinacrine, and procarbazine (Roe, 1984). Since alcohol reacts with so many medications, its avoidance is wise when any type of prescription or over-the-counter medication is used.

Caffeine. Although caffeine is a non-nutritive substance in food, it is probably the most widely used drug consumed in the United States and Europe (Pozniak, 1985). It is frequently ingested in large enough quantities to alter metabolism. Caffeine, theophylline, and theobromine are all chemically similar compounds called methylated xanthines. They are found naturally in coffee, tea, cocoa, and cola beverages (Table 22–10).

In general, caffeine has a greater metabolic effect than theophylline (theobromine has the least effect). These compounds affect body metabolism by:

- Stimulating the central nervous system (more rapid and clearer thinking, reduced drowsiness and fatigue, keener appreciation of sensory stimuli, and decreased reaction time).
- Stimulating the kidney and producing diuresis (especially theophylline).

Table 22–10. *Xanthine Content of Beverages**

Beverage	Caffeine	Theophylline	Theobromine
Coffee (1 cup)	85 mg	–	–
Tea (1 cup)	50 mg	1 mg	–
Cocoa (1 cup)	5 mg	–	250 mg
Cola (12 oz.)	50 mg	–	–

*Data from Rall, TW: Central nervous system stimulants. In *Goodman & Gilman's The Pharmacological Basis of Therapeutics*, 7th ed. Edited by AG Gilman; LS Goodman; TW Rall; et al. New York, Macmillan, 1985.

- Stimulating the cardiac muscle (especially theophylline). Excessively large doses can cause tachycardia and heart irregularities and lower venous pressure.
- Relaxing smooth muscles (especially the bronchoesophageal muscle).
- Increasing the basal metabolic rate.
- Increasing gastric secretions.

While caffeine intake has been linked to many types of cancer, no causal relationship has been established; few relationships can be correlated to dosage or duration of intake (Pozniak, 1985). However, because of its questionable safety, as shown in Table 13–5, caffeine was removed from the Class I GRAS list and placed in the class in which additional studies are needed.

There is no conclusive evidence that moderate amounts of caffeine are harmful to the average healthy adult (IFT, 1984); however, its use should be minimized during pregnancy, even though its link to birth defects is inconclusive (AMA, 1984). Caffeine may or may not be allowed for patients with hypertension, depending on the individual physician. Many drugs are affected by caffeine; it is definitely contraindicated when sedatives are given.

More than 1000 over-the-counter drugs contain caffeine; it is most frequently found in weight-control remedies (Dexatrim), alertness or stay-awake tablets (Vivarin), headache and pain-relief remedies (Excedrin), cold products (Triaminicin), and diuretics (Aqua-Ban). While the label does not state the quantity of caffeine, its presence is noted (Lecos, 1984).

The caffeine content of various beverages and foods is listed in Appendix D–5. While the AMA (1984) considered endorsement for labeling the caffeine content of foods and beverages, the major sources of caffeine—coffee and tea—contain variable amounts depending on the type of coffee bean or tea leaf, method of preparation, strength, and serving size. Therefore, it is difficult to determine accurately the caffeine in an "average" cup of coffee or tea and to put this on the label.

Licorice. Another natural food substance that can alter body metabolism is licorice. Natural licorice flavoring in excessive amounts can cause hypokalemia, salt and water retention, hypertension, and alkalosis. American-manufactured licorice contains synthetic flavoring, which does not have this effect. However, imported licorice is contraindicated especially in patients on non-potassium-sparing diuretics and low-salt diets.

RATE OF DRUG METABOLISM

Foods and the type of diet may also increase degradation and excretion of a drug by enhancing its metabolism owing to increased activity of drug-metabolizing enzymes (Bidlack & Smith, 1984; Rogers & Chir, 1982). In general, drugs are metabolized faster when the diet is high in protein and low in carbohydrates rather than the reverse (Anderson et al, 1982). The inclusion of cruciferous vegetables (e.g., cabbage and cauliflower) produces an increase in the rate of drug metabolism (Bidlack & Smith, 1984). Charcoal-broiled foods may increase the metabolism of drugs, especially phenacetin (present in Empirin and aspirin) (Kappas et al, 1978; Conney et al, 1976).

The metabolism of many drugs is reduced with marginal nutritional deficiencies of magnesium and vitamins A, E, and C (Bidlack & Smith, 1984). This could result in the drug's increased residence time in the body and may potentiate its action (Brin & Roe, 1979).

Clinical Implications:

- Patients consuming large amounts of caffeine while being treated with theophylline (a bronchial dilator) may be at risk of developing enhanced drug side effects, resulting from similar metabolic actions of the compounds.
- The nurse should be aware of patients who are habitual users of coffee, tea, and cola drinks. If the effectiveness of a prescribed drug is questionable, consult the physician, pharmacist, or dietitian.
- Patients with Parkinson's disease taking levodopa should be counseled to avoid foods and

- supplements high in pyridoxine, including fortified breakfast cereals.
- For patients on anticonvulsants, emphasize the importance of good dietary habits with adequate intake of vitamin D-containing foods.
- The nutritional status of patients on therapeutic agents should be monitored to ensure optimal handling and clearance of drugs and to diminish any resultant toxicity (Bidlack & Smith, 1984).

Effects of Nutrient-Drug Interaction on Excretion

Nutrient and drug excretion can be affected by altered reabsorption or transport of the drug. A drug can complex with a nutrient and cause it to be displaced from its binding site or replace a nutrient from its location, thus promoting excretion of the nutrient, which may or may not be accompanied by the drug.

Drugs may alter the kidneys' ability to reabsorb a nutrient. Increased sodium excretion precipitated by diuretics is desirable; however, loss of other electrolytes, potassium, magnesium, and zinc is an undesirable side effect (Table 22–11). Hypokalemia is associated with long-term therapy of thiazide and loop diuretics (except potassium-sparing diuretics such as triamterene and spironolactone). Not all patients on thiazide diuretics develop hypokalemia. Patients exhibiting hypokalemia have some of the following characteristics (Roe, 1981): (1) more than 65 years of age, (2) a diet low in potassium, (3) frequent diarrhea, and (4) other drug usage, e.g., laxatives or corticosteroids.

Corticosteroids, in addition to affecting metabolism, precipitate fluid and electrolyte disturbances. Urinary excretion of calcium, phosphorus, and potassium are increased, while sodium and water are retained.

A number of foods can affect drug excretion by changing the pH of the urine, which influences the ionization of drugs. A drug that has not been ionized will more readily diffuse from the urine back into the blood. A basic urinary pH increases tubular reabsorption of a weak-base drug, thereby decreasing renal elimination. An altered rate of drug excretion or retention may affect the expected drug action. As mentioned earlier, urine can be acidified with ascorbic acid, which increases urinary excretion of bases.

An alkaline urine decreases the excretion of quinidine, imipramine, and amphetamines, thereby increasing the duration of their action. Toxic symptoms have been reported in patients when the urine was alkalinized (Embil et al, 1976; Zinn, 1970). The pH of the urine will be alkalinized in patients taking antacids or diuretics, such as acetazolamide (Diamox) (Rodman, 1980).

Sometimes urinary pH may be altered to improve therapeutic efficacy. Methenamine mandelate (Mandelamine) for urinary tract infection is not effective unless the urine pH is 5.5 or less. Vitamin C, in the range of 2 to 3 gm, usually accompanies methenamine mandelate therapy to prevent alkalinization of the urine and to increase the therapeutic effectiveness of the drug (Visconti, 1977).

Table 22–11. Mineral Depletion Induced by Drugs*

Diuretics.	Calcium (not thiazides), potassium, magnesium, and zinc.
Laxatives (laxative abuse).	Potassium and calcium.
Glucocorticoids.	Calcium and potassium.
Chelating agents (penicillamine).	Zinc and copper.
Ethanol.	Potassium, magnesium, and zinc.
Antacids.	Phosphates.
Non-narcotic analgesics (aspirin, indomethacin).	Iron (by GI blood loss).

*From Roe, DA: Interactions between drugs and nutrients. *Medical Clinics of North America* 63(5):985, 1979.

Clinical Implications:

- Spironolactone (Aldactone) and triamterene (Dyrenium) alone, or in combination with thiazides (Aldactazide, Dyazide) are all potassium-sparing diuretics. Patients should avoid foods high in potassium content and potassium-containing salt substitutes because of possible retention.
- Hypokalemia in patients on potassium-depleting diuretics can be prevented by monitoring plasma potassium, encouraging a high-potassium diet (green leafy vegetables, citrus or fruit juices, tomato juice, bananas, dried apricots, raisins, potatoes, and milk). Patients should also be monitored for laxative abuse.
- An excellent high-potassium, low-calorie food supplement can be economically made by

combining vegetable scraps that are ordinarily discarded (e.g., carrot or potato peelings, celery stalks, outside pieces of lettuce, cabbage, and snipped ends from green beans). The use of parsley makes it especially high in potassium. These are covered with water and simmered for about one hour before being strained and seasoned to taste. It can be served hot or cold or substituted for water in many recipes.

- Calcium-rich foods, such as milk products, are recommended for patients on loop diuretics.
- Magnesium-rich foods include green leafy vegetables, legumes, and chocolate; zinc-rich foods include milk and red meats.
- Individuals on corticosteroids may require a sodium-restricted diet that is high in potassium and protein. The patient's weight should be closely monitored.
- Patients taking quinidine should be warned about creating a drug- or diet-induced alkaline urine (e.g., by consuming large amounts of antacids or citrus juices). Strict vegetarian diets or excessive eating of alkaline-ash foods can produce an alkaline urine (see Appendix D–6).

Health Application: Prevention of Food-Drug Problems

Nutrient depletion occurs gradually, but when drugs are taken over a long period of time, malnutrition may result. Drug-induced nutritional deficiencies occur most frequently in patients (1) taking multiple drugs; (2) with marginal nutritional status because of a poor diet, chronic disease, drug abuse, or physiological stress; or (3) with impaired metabolic or excretory functions. Deficiencies have been identified in those who abuse alcohol, drugs, or laxatives. Elderly persons are particularly at risk because of their need for many drugs combined with poor eating habits and a slow rate of drug metabolism.

Malnutrition caused by drug side effects is largely preventable. Health care professionals need to be aware of circumstances that could lead to problems and carefully monitor nutritional status, clinical signs, and laboratory reports of patients on long-term drug therapies. When an expected response to a planned therapeutic program does not occur, the possibility of interactions between the disease state, drugs, and food should be considered. Unless contraindicated, modification of the diet to include foods rich in the depleted vitamins and minerals is preferable to taking supplements. Supplemental vitamin and mineral mixtures can counter the effectiveness of certain drugs.

The requirement by the Joint Commission on Accreditation of Hospitals to provide patients with drug-nutrient information for medications they will be taking at home is a step in the right direction. Hopefully, the patient-care nurse, who is primarily responsible for this in most institutions, will also inquire about any over-the-counter medications and offer advice regarding potential interactions.

Unfortunately, individuals and groups most at risk are the hardest to reach and teach. The elderly, chronically ill, health faddists, abusers of over-the-counter drugs, and alcoholics require understanding and guidance (Roe, 1981).

Clinical Implications:

- The nursing assessment should list all the drugs the patient is taking, both prescription and nonprescription as well as any home remedies such as sodium bicarbonate or herbal teas.
- Teach the patient about the purpose of the drug and the proper time to take it.
- Advise against drastic modification of the diet or food "binges" without consulting the physician or pharmacist.

Summary

Interrelationships among drugs, diets, and diseases have complex interactions that require careful attention of the health care professional. Ensuring dietary adequacy in the face of long-term or multiple drug therapies is a difficult and complex task; the cooperation of the entire health care team is necessary. Efforts should be made to optimize the therapeutic effects of drugs and to minimize side effects by administering drugs at the optimal time. Drugs affect nutritional status by affecting taste, appetite, absorption, and metabolism of nutrients. In the same manner, food can affect therapeutic effectiveness of the drug. Nutrients most frequently involved in drug-food interactions are vitamins B_6 and B_{12} and folic acid. A summary of nutrients detrimentally affected by drugs is shown in the Appendix C-8. Clinical deficiencies of nutrients occur most frequently during extended periods of drug usage, when multiple drugs are used, or when the diet is inadequate or marginal.

Review Questions

1. In what ways can drugs decrease appetite?
2. Discuss the similarities and differences of food and drug absorption.
3. Why are some drugs given with food and some on an empty stomach?
4. What vitamins are most frequently implicated in drug-nutrient interactions? Discuss why this occurs. What clinical symptoms might you observe with deficiencies of each of these nutrients? (See Chapter 20.)
5. Discuss the commonplace use of antacids, laxatives, and analgesics. What are some dangers of these practices?

Case Study No. 1: A physician has ordered 35 ml of aluminum hydroxide gel (Amphojel) every two hours for an elderly gentleman with an ulcer. He ordinarily consumes one quart of milk daily. Because of urinary tract infection from *Escherichia coli* (which is susceptible to tetracycline), the physician also orders tetracycline, q.i.d. However, the urinary tract infection has shown no signs of abatement after four days of therapy. What might this be attributed to and what advice would you give the patient?

Case Study No. 2: An overweight woman with Type II diabetes mellitus has been on tolbutamide (Orinase) for three months. She is on no other medication but drinks about one six-pack of beer daily. Her three-month checkup reveals an elevated blood glucose level and 4+ urine. How would you counsel the patient?

Case Study No. 3: An 18-year-old high school student who has been placed on low-dosage tetracycline for acne is advised not to take the medication with dairy products. After several weeks of therapy, there is no appreciable improvement. When questioned further, she states that she never took the tetracycline with milk, but the capsule was taken each morning with her multivitamin and iron supplements.
1. Why was she advised not to take the medication with dairy products?
2. The nurse advised her to take the medication alone—not with the multivitamin and iron supplement. What is the rationale for this?
3. Are there other over-the-counter preparations that should not be taken with tetracycline?

Case Study No. 4: Mr. O. C. is a 63-year-old man whose wife died eight months ago. Since then, he has been depressed and talks about his own death. As his children become concerned, they convince him to see a physician, who prescribes tranylcypromine (Parnate), a monoamine oxidase inhibitor. Mr. O. C. is then referred for diet instruction.
1. What foods need to be eliminated from Mr. O. C.'s diet?
2. What is the rationale for their elimination?
3. What is the possible result of a combination of the medication and the foods to be restricted?

Case Study No. 5: Mrs. J. R. is an ovolactovegetarian who has been hospitalized for three weeks with deep vein thrombosis and pulmonary emboli. Following diet and medication instruction, she is to be discharged. The physician has ordered warfarin (Coumadin), 5 mg orally each day.
1. What additional data do you need?
2. What is the action of warfarin (Coumadin)?
3. What foods in Mrs. J. R.'s diet are of particular concern?
4. During the instruction, Mrs. J. R. states that she probably needs to take vitamins to improve her health after the hospitalization. What would be your response?

REFERENCE LIST

American Dietetic Association (ADA): *Handbook of Clinical Dietetics.* New Haven, Yale University Press, 1981.

American Medical Association Council on Scientific Affairs (AMA): Caffeine Labeling. *JAMA* 252(6):803, 1984.

Anderson, KE; Conney, AH; Kappas, A: Nutritional influences on chemical biotransformation in humans. *Nutr Rev* 40(6):161, 1982.

Baylis, EM; Crowley, JM; Preece, JM; et al: Influence of folic acid on blood phenytoin levels. *Lancet* 1(January 9):62, 1971.

Bidlack, WR; Smith, CH: The effect of nutritional factors on hepatic drug and toxicant metabolism. *J Am Diet Assoc* 84(8):892, 1984.

Brin, M; Roe, D: Drug-diet interactions. *J Fla Med Assoc* 66(4):424, 1979.

Clark, M; Dubowski, K; Colmore, J: The effect of chlorpromazine on serum cholesterol in chronic schizophrenic patients. *Clin Pharmacol Ther* 11(6):883, 1970.

Cohen, IK; Schechter, PJ; Henkin, RI: Hypogeusia, anorexia, and altered zinc metabolism following thermal burns. *JAMA* 223(8):914, 1973.

Commission for the Control of Epilepsy and its Consequences (CCEC): *Plan for Nationwide Action on Epilepsy*, volume 1. DHEW Publication No. (NIH) 78-276, 1977.

Conney, AH; Pantuck, EJ; Hsiao, KC; et al: Enhanced phenacetin metabolism in human subjects fed charcoal-broiled beef. *Clin Pharmacol Ther* 20(6):633, 1976.

Eisenstein, A: Effects of adrenal cortical hormones on carbohydrate, protein, and fat metabolism. *Am J Clin Nutr* 26(1):113, 1973.

Embil, K; Litwiller, DC; Lepore, RA; et al: Effect of orange juice consumption on urinary pH. *Am J Hosp Pharm* 33(12):1294, 1976.

Folks, DG: Monoamine oxidase inhibitors: Reappraisal of dietary considerations. *J Clin Psychopharmacol* 3(4):249, 1983.

Freedman, RB; Kindy, P, Jr; Reinke, JA: What to tell patients about weight loss methods. 2. Drugs. *Postgrad Med* 72(4):85, 1982.

Green, RF: Subclinical pellagra and idiopathic hypogeusia. *JAMA* 218(8):1303, 1971.

Hahn, TJ; Hendin, BA; Scharp, CR; et al: Effect of chronic anticonvulsant therapy on serum 25-hydroxycalciferol levels in adults. *N Engl J Med* 287(18):900, 1972.

Hambidge, KM; Hambidge, C; Jacobs, M; et al: Low levels of zinc in hair, anorexia, poor growth, and hypogeusia in children. *Pediatr Res* 6(12):868, 1972.

Harper, S; Higgins, W: Oral antibiotics and interference with meals in Kentucky hospitals. *J Am Diet Assoc* 83(3):330, 1983.

Hartshorn, EA: Food and drug interactions. *J Am Diet Assoc* 70(1):15, 1977.

Heaton, KW; Lever, JV; Path, RC; et al: Osteomalacia associated with cholestyramine therapy for postilectomy diarrhea. *Gastroenterology* 62(4):642, 1972.

Hodges, RE: Experimental vitamin A deficiency in man (abstract). In *Third Western Hemisphere Nutrition Congress Proceedings*. Edited by PL White, Mount Kisco, NY, Future Publishing Company, 1972, p 67.

Institute of Food Technologists' Expert on Food Safety and Nutrition (IFT): Caffeine. *Contemporary Nutr* 9(5), 1984.

Kappas, A; Alvares, AP; Anderson, KE; et al: Effect of charcoal-broiled beef on antipyrine and theophylline metabolism. *Clin Pharmacol Ther* 23(4):445, 1978.

Kater, RMH; Roggin, G; Tobon, F; et al: Increased rate of clearance of drugs from the circulation of alcoholics. *Am J Med Sci* 258(1):35, 1969.

Krondl, A: Present understanding of the interaction of drugs and foods during absorption. *Can Med Assoc J* 103(4):360, 1970.

Lecos, C: The latest caffeine scorecard. *FDA Consumer* 18(2):14, 1984.

Lindeman, RD: Minerals in medical practice. In *Quick Reference to Clinical Nutrition*. Edited by SL Halpern. Philadelphia, J. B. Lippincott Co, 1979, p 268.

Longenecker, JB; Basu, SG: Effect of cholestyramine on absorption of amino acids and vitamin A in man (abstract). *Fed Proc* 24(2):375, 1965.

Mars, H: Levodopa, carbidopa, and pyridoxine in Parkinson disease. *Arch Neurol* 30(6):444, 1974.

Mitchell, JF: Drug and food interactions: Oral medications that should not be crushed. *RD* 4(4):3, 1984.

Moore, AO; Powers, DE: *Food-Medicine Interactions*, P.O. Box 26464, Tempe, AZ 85282, 1982.

Moore, JR; Ball, EW: Folic acid replacement in folate deficient children on anticonvulsants. Arch Dis Child 47(252):309, 1972.

Pawan, GLS: Drugs and appetite. Proc Nutr Soc 33(3):239, 1974.

Phenylpropanolamine for weight reduction. *Med Letter Drugs Ther* 26(663):55, 1984.

Pinkerton, CR; Welshman, SG; Glasgow, JFT; et al: Can food influence the absorption of methotrexate in children with acute lymphoblastic leukaemia? *Lancet* 2(November 1):944, 1980.

Pozniak, PC: The carcinogenicity of caffeine and coffee: A review. *J Am Diet Assoc* 85(9):1127, 1985.

Reynolds, EH; Hallpike, JF; Phillips, BM; et al: Reversible absorptive defects in anticonvulsant megaloblastic anemia. *J Clin Path* 18(5):593, 1965.

Rodman, MJ: Drug therapy today: Drug interactions you can prevent. *RN* 43(2):137, 1980.

Roe, DA: Nutrient and drug interaction. *Nutr Rev* 42(4):141, 1984.

Roe, DA: Drugs and nutrient absorption. *Curr Concepts Nutr* 12:129, 1983.

Roe, DA: *Handbook: Interaction of Selected Drugs and Nutrients in Patients*. Chicago, American Dietetic Association, 1982.

Roe, DA: Dietary guidelines and drug therapies. *Compr Ther* 7(7):62, 1981.

Roe, DA: *Drug-Induced Nutritional Deficiencies*. Westport CT, AVI Publishing Co, 1976.

Rogers, HJ; Chir, B: Food and medicine incompatibility. *Royal Soc Health J* 102(1):24, 1982.

Rubin, E; Gang, H; Misra, PS; et al: Inhibition of drug metabolism by acute ethanol intoxication. A hepatic microsomal mechanism. *Am J Med* 49(6):801, 1970.

Safer, DJ; Allan, RR; Barr, E: Growth rebound after termination of stimulant drugs. *J Pediatr Pharm Therap* 86:113, 1975.

Safer, DJ; Allan, RR; Barr, E: Depression of growth in hyperactive children on stimulant drugs. *N Engl J Med* 287(5):217, 1972.

Smith, CH; Bidlack, WR: Dietary concerns associated with the use of medications. *J Am Diet Assoc* 84(8):901, 1984.

Spencer, H; Norris, C; Coffey, J; et al: Effect of small amounts of antacids on calcium, phosphorus, and fluoride metabolism in man (abstract). *Gastroenterology* 68(4):A-133/990, 1975.

Sriwatanakul, K; Weintraub, M: Understanding food-drug interactions. *Compr Ther* 9(4):6, 1983.

Stiel, JN; Liddle, GW; Lacy, WW: Studies on mechanism of cyproheptadine-induced weight gain in human subjects. *Metabolism* 19(3):192, 1970.

Stunkard, AJ: Anorectic agents lower a body weight set point. *Life Sci* 30(24):2043, 1982.

Trier, JS: Morphologic alterations induced by methotrexate in the mucosa of human proximal intestine. *Gastroenterology* 43(4):407, 1962.

Use of copper or zinc for taste loss. *Postgrad Med* 53(4):30, 1973.

Van Woert, MH: Low pyridoxine diet in Parkinsonism. *JAMA* 219(9):1211, 1972.

Visconti, JA: Food-drug interaction. *Nutrition in Disease*. Columbus, OH, Ross Laboratories, May 1977.

Waxman, S; Corcino, JJ; Herbert, V: Drugs, toxins and dietary amino acids affecting vitamin B_{12} or folic acid absorption on utilization. *Am J Med* 48(5):599, 1970.

Webb, DI; Chodos, RB; Mahar, CQ; et al: Mechanism of vitamin B_{12} malabsorption in patients receiving colchicine. *N Engl J Med* 279(16):845, 1968.

Wilson, CWM: Vitamins and drug metabolism with particular reference to vitamin C. *Proc Nutr Soc* 33(3):231, 1974.

Zallen, EM (ed): *Oklahoma Diet Manual*. Oklahoma Dietetic Association, 1979.

Zinn, MB: Quinidine intoxication from alkali ingestion. *Tex Med* 66(12):64, 1970.

Further Study

Bauwens, E; Clemmons, C: Foods that foil drugs. *RN* 41(9):79, 1978.

Black, CD; Popovich, NG; Black, MC: Drug interactions in the GI tract. *Am J Nurs* 77(9):1427, 1977.

Calesnick, B: What patients should know about alcohol and medications. *Consultant* 21(8):193, 1981.

Curatolo, PW; Robertson, D: The health consequences of caffeine. *Ann Int Med* 98(Part 1):641, 1983.

DiPalma, J: How you can prevent GI drug interaction. *RN* 40(7):63, 1977.

Giovannitti, C; Schwinghammer, T: Food and drugs: Managing the right mix for your patient. *Nursing* 11(7):26, 1981.

Hallal, JC: Caffeine. *Am J Nurs* 86(4):422, 1986.

Holmes, S: Drug-nutrient interactions. *Nurs Mirror* 160(12):43, 1985.

Keithley, JK; O'Donnell, J: Look out for these drug-nutrient interactions. *Nursing* 16(2):42, 1986.

Kemp, G; Kemp, D: Diuretics. *Am J Nurs* 78(6):1007, 1978.

Lehmann, P: Food and drug interactions. *FDA Consumer* 12(2):20, 1978.

Moseley, V: Medications and malnutrition, cause and effect. *J SC Med Assoc* 76(7):339, 1980.

Rodman, MJ: Drug therapy today: Drug interactions you can prevent. *RN* 43(2):137, 1980.

Roe, DA: Interactions between drugs and nutrients. *Med Clin North Am* 63(5):985, 1979.

Rosenberg, JM; Sangkachand, P: "Take with meals or not?" (Part I). *RN* 44(5):46, 1981.

Rosenberg, JM; Sangkachand, P: "Take with meals or not?" (Part II). *RN* 44(6):60, 1981.

Slawson, M; Slawson, S: Problem ingredients in OTCs. *RN* 48(4):53, 1985.

Food Exchange Lists

* Name the six food exchange lists.
* Describe the foods in each group.
* Assess the client's need for such a diet plan.
* Plan food intake for one day using the six exchange lists.

Fiber types
Food exchange lists

OBJECTIVES

TERMS TO KNOW

REASONS FOR FOOD EXCHANGE LISTS

Going on a trip? Where's the map? Food exchange lists are the guide for a person planning a controlled diet just as a map helps drivers get where they're going. Similar features shared by the two are:

1. Both are quick guides to follow a certain plan.
2. The total miles or kilocalories are easy to see.
3. The individual can select the most desirable of various routes to the same goal.

For a diet, these are remarkable qualities because the client can select favorite foods as well as different times to eat them. No more dreary unforgiving demands!

The exchange lists were developed primarily to provide optimum nutrition for the diabetic while counting carbohydrate intake. Presently, noninsulin-dependent diabetes mellitus (NIDDM) is the most common form of diabetes mellitus; it can be controlled completely by diet. People with insulin-dependent diabetes mellitus (IDDM) use the exchange list diet in addition to insulin. The dietary control of both types of diabetes mellitus is discussed in Chapter 29. Although the exchange lists were first developed for diabetics, health care professionals and the public soon realized that the lists are also an easy guide to a balanced diet for wellness and disease prevention. This diet meets the RDAs for all nutrients, with the exception of iron in women of childbearing age.

GOALS OF THE EXCHANGE LISTS

The exchange lists have found widespread use in the calculation of several therapeutic diet patterns, especially low-kilocalorie regimens. In fact, 90 percent or more of the individuals who develop diabetes mellitus exceed desirable body weight when diagnosed, which is usually after the age of 35. As a result, the exchange lists have become an extremely useful tool for all persons wishing to control weight as well as others interested in fighting cardiovascular disease. In fact, all persons who are overweight and live long enough are likely to face the problems of diabetes mellitus and/or cardiovascular disease.

Goals of the exchange lists include the following:

1. Improve the overall health of the patient by attaining and maintaining optimum nutrition.
2. Attain and/or maintain an ideal body weight.
3. Provide for normal physical growth in the diabetic child; provide adequate nutrition for the pregnant woman, her fetus, and lactation needs, if she chooses to breast-feed her infant.
4. Maintain plasma glucose as near the normal physiological range as possible.
5. Prevent and/or delay the development or progression of cardiovascular, renal, retinal, neurological, and other complications associated with diabetes, insofar as these are related to metabolic control.

The exchange lists divide food into six groups; within each group, all food items are approximately equal in kilocalories and in the amount of carbohydrate, protein, and fat. Therefore, foods in any one group can be traded, or exchanged, with other foods in the same group.

Table 23–1 shows the six major exchange lists and the calorie content as well as the carbohydrate, protein, and fat distribution for each exchange. The serving size varies so that one serving from any exchange is roughly equivalent to one serving of any other food in that group in energy nutrient content (protein, carbohydrate, and fat). Table 23–2 lists the foods within each exchange in order to provide information for planning meals. (Because of recent changes, when homogenized milk or high-fat meats are chosen, some fat servings must be omitted, as noted in Table 23–2.)

Additionally, there is a free food list. This list includes foods or beverages that contain less than 20 kcal per serving. Some items contain no calories; others could be considered low calorie and should be limited to two or three servings per day.

Foods are categorized somewhat differently than in the basic food groups. Instead of classifying all milk products together, the food exchange lists group cheese with the meats because of its low-carbohydrate, high-protein content. In the basic food groups, fruits and vegetables are in the same category. The exchange lists put vegetables with higher carbohydrate content in the bread exchange; only nonstarchy vegetables are in the vegetable exchange; and fruits are in a separate exchange.

SPECIAL CONSIDERATIONS

No special foods are required, but a predictable and regular intake is important for diet control. The American Diabetes Association, the American Dietetic Association, and the U.S. Pub-

Table 23–1. Major Exchange Lists

List	Exchange Group	CHO	Protein	Fat	Kcal
1	Starch/bread	15	3	0.9	80
2	Meat				
	Lean	–	7	3	55
	Medium-fat	–	7	5	75
	High-fat	–	7	8	100
3	Vegetable	5	2	–	28
4	Fruit	15	–	–	60
5	Milk				
	Skim	12	8	1	90
	Low-fat	12	8	5	120
	Whole	12	8	8	150
6	Fat	–	–	5	45

lic Health Service compiled the "Exchange System" more than 30 years ago. Recent modifications have updated the lists to reflect present concerns of controlling the fat content in the diet, increasing fiber, limiting the amount of sodium, recognizing the different types and percentages of fat in meats, and curbing the total cholesterol intake.

Fat. Many individuals with diabetes mellitus and other Americans have elevated serum levels of cholesterol and/or triglyceride. Fat is decreased from 40 percent to 20 to 30 percent, and cholesterol is limited to 300 mg/day to protect against heart diseases. The level of saturated fatty acids in the diet should be less than 10 percent of total kilocalories; 10 percent should be polyunsaturated fat; and the remainder of the fat is derived from monounsaturated sources. The use of fats such as eicosapentaenoic acid in fish may be desirable.

Because of this emphasis on lowering the total amount as well as distinguishing different types of fat and cholesterol, the exchange lists can also be used to provide a nutritionally adequate diet for persons who need to decrease their consumption of saturated fats and cholesterol, e.g., those with hypercholesterolemia or a family history of cardiovascular disease.

Carbohydrate. The recommendation for carbohydrate has recently been liberalized to include 55 to 60 percent of the total calories. The amount should depend on the individual's blood glucose levels, serum lipids, and food patterns. Unrefined carbohydrates are preferable because they supply required nutrients, including fiber. Modest amounts of refined sugars may be acceptable for some individuals, depending on metabolic control and body weight (Task Force, 1987). Typically, 10 to 15 percent of the carbohydrate kilocalories are derived from sugars—principally natural sugars. Carbohydrates given at mealtime produce lower plasma glucose responses than the same carbohydrates given alone, although insulin responses are similar (Jenkins et al, 1983). Simple saccharides offer less satiety, and hunger develops sooner than with polysaccharide-rich foods.

Fiber. Soluble fibers found in legumes, whole-grain cereals, green leafy vegetables, and fruits tend to lower plasma glucose concentrations (thereby decreasing glycosuria) and total cholesterol (especially low-density lipoprotein [LDL] cholesterol). The belief that higher fiber diets are beneficial is based on the theory that the rate at which food goes through the intestinal tract may decrease the amount of glucose absorbed (Nemchik, 1982). An increase of dietary carbohydrate without an increase of total kilocalories does not appear to increase insulin requirements in IDDM patients.

The average intake of dietary fiber in the United States is between 10 and 30 gm/day. Most individuals should double that amount gradually. Abdominal cramping, discomfort, diarrhea, and flatulence can be minimized if the fiber is increased gradually. An intake of up to 40 gm of fiber/day or 25 gm/1000 kcal appears to be beneficial (Task Force, 1987). Foods containing more than 3 gm of fiber per serving have been designated in the 1986 revised food exchange list.

Protein. The Task Force for the American Diabetes Association (1987) feels that Americans eat more protein than required for optimal nutrition (10 to 15 percent of the total kilocalories). With the exception of groups at risk of negative nitrogen

Text continued on page 445

Table 23–2. Food Lists[1]

Free Choices (Not more than 20 calories)

Beverages

Beef tea
Bouillon cube[2]
Broth
Clam juice: limit to ½ cup daily
Club soda, carbonated water, or mineral water
Cocoa, dry, unsweetened powder: limit to 1 Tbsp. daily
Coffee
Coffee lighteners: limit to 2 level tsp. daily
Consommé: limit to ½ cup daily
Decaffeinated coffee
Postum: limit to 3 rounded tsp. daily
Sauerkraut juice: limit to 1 cup daily
Soft drinks, sugar-free
Tea

Sauces and Relishes

Limit to 1 Tbsp. daily:
    A-1 or steak sauce
    Catsup
    Chili sauce
    Mustard
    Salad dressing, low-calorie
    Soy sauce[2]
    Tomato paste or puree
Horseradish, plain in vinegar: limit to 3 Tbsp. daily
Hot sauce
Pickle, unsweetened, dill or sour[2]
Pickle relish, sour or unsweetened
Pimiento
Salad dressing, low calorie: limit to 2 Tbsp.
Tabasco sauce
Taco hot sauce
Vinegar
Worcestershire sauce

Baking Aids

Baking powder, baking soda, cream of tartar
Flavoring extracts
Nostick pan spray
Yeast, baking

Seasonings

Herbs and spices
Monosodium glutamate
Pepper
Salt

Miscellaneous

Cranberries, cooked without sugar: limit to ½ cup daily
Gelatin, unflavored plain
Gum, sugar-free
Jams and jellies, artifically sweetened: limit to 2 level tsp. daily
Lemon or lime wedge; lemon or lime juice: limit to 2 Tbsp.
    daily

Pancake syrup, sugar-free: limit to 1–2 Tbsp.
Rennet tablets
Rhubarb unsweetened; limit to ½ cup daily
Umeboshi (pickled plums): limit to 2 daily
Wine, used in cooking: limit to ¼ cup daily
Yeast, brewer's: limit to 2 tsp. daily

Milk Choices: 8 gm protein, 12 gm carbohydrate, fat varies, calories vary

Skim/nonfat milk—no fat; 80 calories	
Skim or nonfat milk	1 cup
Alba 66 or Alba 77	1 envelope
Buttermilk made from skim milk	1 cup
Canned, evaporated skim milk	½ cup
Powdered nonfat milk (before adding water)	⅓ cup
Yogurt, plain, made from skim milk[3]	1 cup
Kefir	1 cup
1% milk—½ fat choice: 102 calories	
Lowfat milk	1 cup
Buttermilk made from lowfat milk	1 cup
2% milk—1 fat choice: 125 calories	
2% milk	1 cup
Acidophilus, 2% milk	1 cup
Yogurt, plain, made from partially skim milk[3]	1 cup
Whole milk—2 fat choices; 170 calories	
Whole milk	1 cup
Canned, evaporated whole milk	½ cup
Buttermilk made from whole milk	1 cup
Soy milk	1 cup
Yogurt, plain, made from whole milk[3]	1 cup

Fat Choices: 5 gm fat, 45 calories

Mostly Polyunsaturated	
Avocado	2 Tbsp.
Margarine	1 tsp.
Margarine, whipped or diet	1 Tbsp.

Table 23–2. Food Lists[1] Continued

Fat Choices: 5 gm fat, 45 calories

Mayonnaise	1 tsp.
Mayonnaise-type salad dressings	2 tsp.
Oil, vegetable	1 tsp.
Salad dressings, regular	
French	1 Tbsp.
Italian, Russian, Thousand Island	2 tsp.
Seeds: Pumpkin, sesame, squash, sunflower (no shells)	1 Tbsp.
Tahini, sesame butter	1 tsp.
Tartar sauce	2 tsp.
Nuts	
Almonds	6
Almonds, chopped	1 Tbsp.
Brazil	2 medium
Butternuts	2
Cashews	6 medium
Filberts (hazelnuts)	5
Hickory nuts	5 small
Macadamia nuts	3 medium
Peanuts, small Spanish type	20
Peanuts, large Virginia type	10
Pecans, large	5 halves
Pecans, chopped	1 Tbsp.
Pignolias	1½ tbsp.
Pinenuts	1 Tbsp.
Pistachio	1 tsp.
Walnuts, black, chopped	1 Tbsp.
Walnuts, English	4 halves
Mostly Saturated	
Achiote, prepared	1 tsp.
Butter	1 tsp.
Butter, whipped	2 tsp.
Bacon, thick sliced	½ strip
Bacon, thin or medium sliced	1 strip
Bacon fat	1 tsp.
Chicken fat	1 tsp.
Chitterlings, fried	2 Tbsp.
Coconut, fresh, grated not packed	2 Tbsp.
Cracklings, pork	1 rounded tsp.
Cream cheese	1 Tbsp.
Cream, light or half-and-half	2 Tbsp.
Cream, sour	2 Tbsp.
Cream substitute for coffee	see free list
Lard	1 tsp.
Olives, green or black, small size	5
Olives, green or black, large size	3
Olive oil	1 tsp.
Salad dressings, regular	
Blue cheese/Roquefort	2 tsp.
Salt pork or fat back	¾ inch cube
Sofrito	1 Tbsp.

Vegetable Choices: 2 gm protein, 5 gm carbohydrate, 28 calories[5]

Raw—up to 2 cups = 1 vegetable choice (less than 1 cup = free choice)

Alfalfa sprouts	Green pepper
Cabbage	Lettuce, all types
Chicory	Mushrooms
Chinese cabbage[4]	Parsley
Cucumber	Radishes
Endive	Spinach
Escarole	Watercress
Fennel	
Green onion	

Table continued on following page

Table 23–2. Food Lists[1] Continued

Vegetable Choices: 2 gm protein, 5 gm carbohydrate, 28 calories[5]

Raw or Cooked—1 to 2 cups = 1 vegetable choice (less than 1 cup = free choice)

Cauliflower
Celery

Summer squash

Raw or Cooked—½ cup = 1 vegetable choice

Artichoke, medium globe
Asparagus, 5–7 spears
Bamboo shoots
Bean sprouts, mung or soy
Beets, plain
Bittermelon
Borscht, beet, low calorie
Broccoli
Brussels sprouts
Cabbage, cooked
Carrots
Carrot juice, ¼ cup
Chayote
Cucumbers
Daikon
Eggplant
Greens, cooked
  Beet
  Collard
  Dandelion
  Kale
  Mustard
  Spinach
  Swiss chard
  Turnip
Green beans

Green pepper, cooked
Italian green beans
Jicama, medium
Kohlrabi
Leeks, 2 medium
Mushrooms, canned or cooked
Mustard cabbage
Okra
Onion
Pea pods or snow peas
Pimiento
Rhubarb, artificially sweetened
Rutabaga
Sauerkraut[2]
String beans or pole beans
Tomato catsup, 2 Tbsp.
Tomato, cherry, 6
Tomato juice[2]
Tomato, medium
Tomato paste, 2 Tbsp.
Tomato sauce, 2 Tbsp.
Turnips
Vegetable juice cocktail
Water chestnuts, 4 medium
Wax beans

Fruit Choices: 15 gm carbohydrate, 60 calories[6]

Fresh, Dried, Canned, Cooked or Frozen without Sugar or Syrup

Apple, small, 2 in. diameter	1	Kumquats, medium	3
Apple, diced	⅓ cup	Loquats	6
Applesauce	½ cup	Lychees	7
Apricots, medium	2	Lemon	1
Banana, small, 9 in.	½	Limes	2
Banana, sliced	⅓ cup	Mango	½
Berries		Mango, diced	⅓ cup
Blackberries (dewberries),[4] blueberries,[4]		Melon	
boysenberries, loganberries, mulberries,		Cantaloupe or muskmelon, 5 in. across	⅓
raspberries (red or black)[4]	¾ cup	Casaba, honeydew, medium	⅛
Cranberries	1 cup	Mixed melon balls or cubes	1 cup
Gooseberries	⅔ cup	Watermelon cubes	1¼ cup
Strawberries[4]	1¼ cup	Nectarine, 2½ in. diameter[4]	1
Cherries		Orange, small	1
Maraschino	4	Orange sections	½ cup
Sour, red	½ cup	Papaya, 5 in. long	⅓
Sweet, Bing, or Royal Anne	12	Papaya cubes	1 cup
Currants	1 Tbsp.	Peach, 2½ in.	1
Dates, whole, medium	2½	Pear, small	1
Fig, medium	1	Persimmon	2
Fruit cup or fruit cocktail	½ cup	Pineapple	2 slices or ¾ cup
Grapefruit, 3½ in.	½		
Grapefruit sections	½ cup	Plum	2
Grapes	20 small or 12 large	Plum, prune-type	2
		Pomegranate, medium[4]	½
		Prickly pear, medium	1
Guava, small	1	Prunes, medium[4]	3
Kiwi fruit, small	2	Raisins, uncooked	2 Tbsp.
		Tangelo, medium	1
		Tangerine, medium	2
		Ugli fruit	½

Drain the liquid from fruit canned in unsweetened fruit juice; ¼ cup of this liquid equals 1 fruit choice. Liquid from water-packed fruit does not need to be drained or counted separately.

Table 23–2. Food Lists[1] Continued

Fruit Drinks and Juices—Use unsweetened real fruit juice if possible because fruit drinks have added sugar.

1 cup = 1 fruit choice
Tomato juice | Vegetable juice cocktail

¾ cup = 1 fruit choice
Gatorade | Low-calorie cranberry juice
Low-calorie Hawaiian Punch drink

½ cup = 1 fruit choice
Blackberry juice | Lime juice
Grapefruit juice | Mixed citrus juice
Lemon juice | Orange juice

½ cup = 1 fruit choice
Apple juice | Hi-C fruit drinks
Cider | Pineapple juice
Del Monte fruit drinks | Tang instant breakfast drink, liquid (2 tsp. powder)
Grapefruit instant breakfast drink, liquid (2 tsp. powder) | Tangerine juice
Grape instant breakfast drink, liquid (2 tsp. powder)

⅓ cup = 1 fruit choice
Apricot nectar | Liquid drained from fruit canned in unsweetened fruit juice
Cranberry juice, regular | Peach nectar
Grape juice | Pear nectar
| Prune juice

Bread and Starch Choices: 3 gm protein, 15 gm carbohydrate, trace of fat, 80 calories

Breads
Bagel	½
Bialy	1
Biscuit, 2 in. baking powder (omit 1 fat choice)	1
Boston brown bread, 3 in. round × ½ in.	1 slice
Bread	
White, cracked-wheat, whole-wheat, rye, pumpernickel, raisin	1 slice
High-fiber or thinly sliced	1½ slices
Large or thickly sliced	½ slice
Italian, 3 in. across, 1 in. thick	1 slice
Cocktail rye	3 slices
Crumbs, dry grated	3 Tbsp.
Cubes or plain croutons	1 cup
Sticks, 7¾ in. long.	2
Sticks, 4¼ in. long	4
Cornbread, 2 in. square × 1 in. thick (omit 1 fat choice)	1 piece
Cornflake crums	3 Tbsp.
English muffin	½
Hamburger bun, 3½ in.	½
Holland rusk	2
Hot dog bun, 6 in.	½
Muffin, plain, 2 in. (omit 1 fat choice)	1
Pancake, 5 in. (omit 1 fat choice)	1
Pita or Syrian bread, 6 in.	¼
Popover, 2–3 in. (omit 1 fat choice)	1
Roll, dinner-type, 2 in.	1
Taco shell, ready-to-eat (omit 1 fat choice)	2
Tortilla, corn, not fried	1
Tortilla, flour, not fried	1
Waffle, 3½ in. × 4½ in. (omit 1 fat choice)	1

Dry Cereals
Bran cereals, not flake[4]	⅓ cup
Chex cereals	¾ cup
Flake cereals (corn, bran, rice, wheat)	¾ cup
Grapenuts	3 Tbsp.
Puffed cereals	1½ cup
Shredded wheat biscuit	1 regular
Shredded wheat, bite-size	16 pieces
Wheat germ, unsweetened[4]	¼ cup

Table continued on following page

Table 23–2. Food Lists[1] Continued

Bread and Starch Choices: 3 gm protein, 15 gm carbohydrate, trace of fat, 80 calories

Cereals and Grains, cooked unless otherwise specified

Barley, buckwheat (kasha), millet	½ cup
Bulgar, dry	2 Tbsp.
Chow mein noodles (omit 1 fat choice)	½ cup
Cooked breakfast cereals	½ cup
Cooked breakfast cereals, unsweetened instant	2 Tbsp.
Cornmeal or cracked wheat, dry	2 Tbsp.
Farfel, dry	3 Tbsp.
Grits, hominy	½ cup
Macaroni, noodles, spaghetti, and other pastas	½ cup
Rice, brown, regular, instant, wild	⅓ cup
Somen or Udon (noodles)	½ cup
Wheatberries	⅓ cup

Crackers and Snacks

Bacon-flavored crackers (omit 1 fat choice)	12
Cheese Nips (omit 1 fat choice)	20
Cheese Puffs (omit 1 fat choice)	1 cup
Cheese Tidbits (omit 2 fat choices)	28
Chipsters (omit 1 fat choice)	45
Chippers (omit 1 fat choice)	8
Corn chips (omit 2 fat choices)	½ cup
Cracker meal	3 Tbsp.
Goldfish (omit 1 fat choice)	45
Graham crackers	3
Korkers (omit 1 fat choice)	18
Matzo, 6 in. across	1
Melba toast, oblong	5
Melba toast, round	10
Oyster crackers	24
Popcorn, unpopped	1½ Tbsp.
Popcorn, popped, large kernel (popped without fat)	3 cups
Popcorn, popped with oil (omit 1 fat choice)	3 cups
Pretzels	
Dutch	1
Rods, 7½ in. long	1½
Three ring	6
Sticks, 3 in. long	25
Very thin sticks	60
Ritz crackers (omit 1 fat choice)	7
RyKrisp	3
Rye Thins (omit 1 fat choice)	10
Saltines, 2 in. square	6
Soda, regular, 2½ in. square	4
Triangle Thins (omit 1 fat choice)	15
Triscuit Wafers (omit 1 fat choice)	5
Tucs (omit 1 fat choice)	4
Vegetable Thins	13
Waverly Wafers (omit 1 fat choice)	6
Wheat Thins (omit 1 fat choice)	12
Zwieback	3

Starchy Vegetables

Baked beans, no pork[4]	¼ cup
Bonita, boiled	½ cup
Corn[4]	½ cup or 1 6" long cob
Chestnuts, roasted	4 large or 6 small
Lima beans (not dried)	½ cup
Malanga (dasheen tuber), boiled	½ cup
Onion rings, frozen (omit 1 fat choice)	2 ounces
Parsnips	½ cup
Peas, green[4]	½ cup
Potato, white	
Boiled or baked, 2 in.	1

Table 23–2. Food Lists[1] Continued

Bread and Starch Choices 3 gm protein, 15 gm carbohydrate, trace of fat, 80 calories

Chips, 2 in. (omit 2 fat choices)	15 or 1 oz. bag
Flakes, dry	⅓ cup
French fried (omit 1 fat choice)	10
Hash brown (omit 1 fat choice)	¼ cup
Mashed, plain	½ cup
Mashed, made from dry flakes according to box directions (omit 1 fat choice)	½ cup
Tater Tots (omit 1½ fat choices)	10
Sticks, canned (omit 2 fat choices)	¾ cup
Plantain, cooked[4]	½ cup
Pumpkin	½ cup
Squash: acorn, butternut, hubbard, winter	¾ cup
Succotash (corn and lima beans)	⅓ cup
Yam or sweet potato (not syrup packed)	⅓ cup
Yautia (tanier), boiled	½ cup
Yucca root (cassava), boiled	½ cup

Dried Peas, Beans and Lentils—

Black-eyed peas, cowpeas, chickpeas, garbanzo beans, Great Northern beans, kidney beans, lentils, navy beans, pinto beans, soy beans (all cooked)[4]	½ cup
Lima beans, mature dried, cooked[4]	½ cup

Flour (These are to level measures)

All-purpose flour	2½ Tbsp.
Buckwheat flour	3 Tbsp.
Carob flour	2 Tbsp.
Cornstarch	2 Tbsp.
Matzo meal	⅓ cup
Mochiko (glutinous rice flour)	2½ Tbsp.
Potato starch	2 Tbsp.
Rye flour	3 Tbsp.
Soy flour, defatted (omit 2 oz. lean/protein choice)	6 Tbsp
Tapioca, dry	2 Tbsp.
Whole-wheat flour	3 Tbsp.
Miso	3 Tbsp.

Bread Starch Choices High in Simple Sugars

Cake

Angel food, no frosting, 1½ in. cube	1 piece
Sponge cake, no frosting, 1½ in. cube	1 piece

Cookies

Animal Crackers	7
Arrow Root Biscuits	3
Brown Edged Wafers	3
Gingersnaps, medium	3
Lorna Doones (omit 1 fat choice)	3
Social Tea Biscuit	4
Vanilla Wafers	5

Doughnuts, Plain, No Glaze or Filling

Cake-type 2½ in. (omit 1 fat choice)	1
Yeast-type, 3¾ in. (omit 1 fat choice)	1

Frozen Deserts

Frozen yogurt on a stick, uncoated	1
Frozen yogurt, vanilla	½ cup
Ice cream, vanilla (not French or Deluxe) (omit 2 fat choices)	½ cup
Ice cream cone (no ice cream)	2 (1 cone = ½ bread/starch choice)
Ice milk, vanilla (omit 1 fat choice)	½ cup
Sherbet	¼ cup
Soft Serve ice cream (with cone)	1 very small
Soft Serve ice milk (without cone) (omit 1 fat choice)	½ cup

Table continued on following page

Table 23–2. *Food Lists[1] Continued*

Bread Starch Choices High in Simple Sugars

Other Deserts

Fruit-flavored gelatin (Jell-O)	½ cup
Ladyfingers	2
Malted powder, plain, dry	2 Tbsp.
Pudding, any flavor, regular	¼ cup

Low-Fat Meat/Protein Choices (each choice is 1 oz. unless otherwise stated)
7 gm protein, 3 gm fat, 55 calories

Beef
Beef shanks
Chipped beef
Cubed flank steak
Eye of round, roast or steak
Family steak
Filet mignon
Flank steak filet
Flip steaks, sandwich steaks
Jewish tenderloin
Kabob cubes

Loin steak, boneless
London broil
London grill steak
Rolled plate
Round steak
Rump roast
Rump steak
Skirt steak
Tenderloin tips
Top round roast

Lamb
Lamb cubes, lean
Shoulder roast

Sirloin roast
Square cut shoulder

Pork
Pig ears, 1 medium

Hog maw, stomach, ⅓ cup

Veal
Arm roast or steak
Blade roast or steak
Cutlet
Kidney chop

Loin roast or chop
Round steak or roast
Rump roast
Shank

Poultry
Capon
Chicken
Chicken, diced, ¼ cup
Cornish hen

Pheasant
Turkey
Turkey ham

Egg
Egg whites, 2

Organ Meats (all are high in cholesterol)
Heart
Kidney

Liver

Game
Opossum
Rabbit

Squirrel
Venison

Fish
Bass
Catfish
Cod
Flounder
Gefilte fish
Haddock
Halibut
Herring
Lox
Perch

Pike
Red snapper
Salmon
Scrod
Smelt
Sole
Sturgeon
Turbot
Whitefish

Clams, 4 cherrystones, 5–6 medium or ⅓ cup minced
Cod, dried, ¼ cup
Crab, lobster, or oysters, ⅓ cup
Frog legs, 3 medium
Mussels

Sardines, drained
Scallops
Shrimp
Squid
Tuna or salmon, canned and drained, ¼ cup[2]

Table 23–2. Food Lists[1] Continued

Low-Fat Meat/Protein Choices (each choice is 1 oz. unless otherwise stated)
7 gm protein, 3 gm fat, 55 calories

Cheese
Cottage cheese, creamed, 2%, 1%, or dry, ¼ cup
Pot cheese, ¼ cup[2]
Farmer cheese or pressed cheese from skim milk

Light 'n' Lively[2]
Tastee Loaf[2]
Weight Watchers[2]

Medium-Fat Meat Protein Choices (each choice is 1 oz. unless otherwise stated)
7 gm protein, 6 gm fat, 78 calories

Beef
Blade steak
Boston cut roast
Chuck steak or roast, well trimmed
Delmonico steak or roast
Eye of chuck roast
Ground beef, 85% lean, drained (½ cup = 3 oz.)

Ground round, 85% lean, cooked and drained
Liver (high in cholesterol)
Rib eye steak
Shoulder steak
Stew beef
Tongue
Chipped beef

Lamb
Lamb steak
Leg, roast or chop

Sirloin chop or roast

Pork
Breakfast chop
Butterfly chop
Canadian bacon, back bacon[2]
Crown roast of pork
Cutlets
Fresh butt
Ham, lean[2]

Loin roast
Pork cubes, lean
Sirloin chop
Smoked chop or roast
Tenderloin
Tongue

Veal
Breast
Crown roast

Rib chop or roast
Riblets

Fish
Anchovy fillets, drained, 9
Caviar, fish roe
Eel

Mackerel
Rainbow trout
Smelt

Cheese
American cheese spread[2]
Kraft Golden Image slices[2]
Mozzarella,[2] part skim

Neufchatel[2]
Ricotta,[2] partially skim milk, ¼ cup
Velveeta[2]

Other
1 egg (limit: 3 per week)

Egg substitute, ¼ cup
Tofu—4 oz.

Poultry
Duck, no skin

Squab (pigeon)

Luncheon Meats
Chicken franks[2]
Head cheese[2]
Olive loaf[2]

Pickle and pimiento loaf[2]
Veal franks[2]

High-Fat Meat/Protein Choices (each choice is 1 oz. unless otherwise stated)
7 gm protein, 8 gm fat, 100 calories

Beef
Brisket
Chuck stew beef
Club steak
Corned beef
Flank

Ground beef or chuck, 80% lean
Hamburger, 70% lean
New York strip steak
Plate beef
Porterhouse steak

Rib roast or steak
Ribs
Short ribs
Sirloin steak
T-bone steak

Table continued on following page

Table 23–2. Food Lists[1] Continued

High-Fat Meat Protein Choices (each choice is 1 oz. unless otherwise stated)
7 gm protein, 8 gm fat, 78 calories

Lamb

Breast	Crown roast	Saratoga chop
Chop	Riblets	Shoulder, rib or loin chop

Pork

Arm steak	Hock, smoked	Sausage, bulk patties or links[2]
Boston butt	Tail, 1	Shank
Boston blade roast	Pig's feet, ½ medium	Shoulder steak
Country ribs	Ribs (spareribs)	Smoked butt[2]

Organ Meats

Brains, ½ cup

Cheese[2]

Blue	Gouda	Swiss
Brick	Gruyere	Tilset
Brie	Gorgonzola	Pasteurized process:
Camembert	Limburger	American
Caraway	Monterey Jack	American cheese food
Cheddar	Mozzarella, whole milk	Cheese food
Cheshire	Muenster	Cold pack American
Colby	Parmesan	Pimiento
Edam	Port du Salut	Swiss
Feta	Provolone	Swiss cheese food
Fontina	Ricotta, whole milk	
	Roquefort	

Luncheon Meats[2]

Blood sausage	Deviled ham, canned	Pastrami
Bockwurst	Frankfurter or hot dog	Polish sausage
Bologna	Head cheese	Salami
Bratwurst	Knockwurst	Sausage links, canned or frozen
Braunschweiger	Liver sausage	Spam
Capicola	Liverwurst	Treet
	Mortadella	

Nuts (¼ cup = 1 choice and omit 2 fat choices)

Butternuts	Pumpkin, squash or sunflower seeds	Pinenuts
Cashews	(no shells)	Pistachios
Peanuts		Walnuts
Peanut butter, 1½ Tbsp.		
(omit 1 fat choice)		

Soup Choices[2]

Each can of the following soups provides three servings, so that one serving equals 7 oz. Approximate equivalents table is based on the addition of water to the concentrated soups. If milk is used to dilute the soup, subtract the amount used from the daily allowance.

Type	Brand		Approx. Equiv./7 Oz. Serving
	Campbell	*Heinz*	
Bean with Bacon		X	1 bread starch, 1 low-fat meat protein
Broth	X	X	free—limit to one serving day
Chicken Noodle	X		½ bread/starch, ½ fat
Chicken Noodle		X	1 bread/starch
Consommé (gelatin added)	X		free—limit to one serving/day
Consommé		X	free—unlimited amounts
Cream of Celery	X	X	½ bread/starch, 1 fat
Cream of Mushroom		X	1 bread/starch, 1 fat
Green Pea	X		1½ bread/starch
Split Pea with Ham	X		1 bread/starch, 1 medium fat meat/protein
Split Pea with Ham		X	1½ bread/starch
Tomato	X		1 bread/starch
Tomato		X	1 bread/starch, ½ fat
Vegetable	X		1 bread/starch
Vegetable w/Beef Stock		X	1 bread/starch

Table 23–2. Food Lists[1]

	Approx. Equiv./Serving (4 servings/package)
Lipton Mix[2]	
Onion	½ bread/starch
Cream of Mushroom	½ bread/starch
Chicken Noodle	½ bread/starch

[1]Adapted from Chicago Dietetic Association and South Suburban Dietetic Association of Cook and Will Counties: *Manual of Clinical Dietetics*, 2nd ed. Philadelphia, W. B. Saunders Co., 1981, with permission.
[2]Contains 400 mg or more of sodium per serving.
[3]Plain yogurt without added flavors or fruits. Commercially prepared, flavored, fruit, or frozen yogurts may have added sugar.
[4]Contains 3 gm or more of fiber per serving.
[5]Vegetables contain 2–3 gm dietary fiber.
[6]Fresh, frozen, and dry. Fruits have about 2 gm dietary fiber.

balance, protein should be restricted to the RDA (0.8 gm/kg for adults). Diabetic individuals are at risk of developing nephropathy; they might benefit from a lower protein level. If stress, strain, or an illness is present, 1.0 to 1.5 gm/kg should be allowed. During gestation, lactation, and periods of rapid growth, protein requirements are modestly increased.

Glycemic Index. Since factors other than the amount of carbohydrate affect the blood glucose profile, glycemic indexing of foods may be used as part of the exchange system. Since there are so many inconsistencies in glycemic effects, general application of this information is not appropriate. However, foods with low glycemic indices (see Table 7–3) may be tried to determine their overall effect in the diet of a particular individual (Task Force, 1987).

Sodium Intake. Although the exchange lists were not originally intended to control sodium intake, many persons with diabetes mellitus or heart disease may need to do so. Obviously, the exchange lists are not accurate for restricting sodium; one slice of bread may range from 125 to 250 mg of sodium. However, the 1986 revision of the exchange lists does identify foods containing more than 400 mg of sodium. (Most natural foods have less than 400 mg sodium; processed foods contain considerably more). It should also be noted that restriction may be harmful for persons with poorly controlled diabetes, postural hypotension, and fluid imbalances.

Alternative Sweeteners. Alternative sweeteners, both noncaloric (e.g., aspartame and saccharin) and caloric varieties (e.g., fructose and sorbitol), are not encouraged but acceptable in the diet (see Focus on Low Calorie Sweeteners in Chapter 14). The use of caloric sweeteners could perhaps undermine efforts to lose or maintain weight. They are not a substitute for noncaloric sweeteners.

It is recommended that a variety of non-nutritive sweeteners be used to minimize the potential risk from excessive consumption of any one type. Excessive use, of course, is not recommended (Task Force, 1987).

Alcohol. Alcohol consumption elicits different glycemic responses in the diabetic, depending on the individual's state of nutrition. The caloric value of alcohol is approximately 7 kcal/gm, but it has no other nutritional value. Alcohol is not converted into glucose but metabolized by the liver and does not require insulin.

Although alcohol is not recommended for diabetics, an IDDM individual may consume alcohol occasionally (not more than 2 oz. three times per week). They should not omit any food because the alcohol may cause hypoglycemia. A small amount of dry wine or brandy may be used in cooking since the alcohol evaporates but the flavor remains.

Since many dieters and NIDDM patients are concerned with maintaining or losing body weight, these superfluous calories become even more undesirable, interfering with the discipline required to stay on the prescribed diet. Alcohol can be substituted for an appropriate number of fat exchanges. One fat exchange should be omitted from the diet for every 45 kcal contained in the alcoholic beverage. The formula given in Table 8–5 can be used to calculate the number of kilocalories in alcohol. Table 23–3 shows the number of fat and bread exchanges for various alcoholic beverages. Sweet wine, liqueurs, beer, ale, and sweetened mixed drinks are high in sugar (increasing the caloric value) and may be counted as a bread exchange.

Determining Total Kilocaloric Intake

1. Generally, the number of calories an individual needs is based on his/her ideal body weight.

Table 23–3. *Alcoholic Beverages and Food Choices**

Alcohol	Grams Alcohol	Measure Ounces	Weight Grams	Approximate Equivalent
Ale, mild	8.9	8	240	½ bread, 1½ fat
Beer	13.3	12	360	1 bread, 2 fat
Brandy or cognac	10.5	1	30	1½ fat
Cider, fermented	9	6	180	1½ fat
Cordials, Anisette, Apricot brandy, Benedictine, Crème de Menthe, Curacao	7	⅔	20	½ bread, 1 fat
Daiquiri	15.1	3½	100	½ bread, 2 fat
Liquor: (80 proof) gin, rum, scotch, whiskey, vodka	15	1½	45	3 fat
Manhattan	19.2	3½	100	½ bread, 3 fat
Martini	18.5	3½	100	3 fat
Old Fashioned	24	4	120	¼ bread, 3½ fat
Port or Muscatelle wine	15	3½	100	1 bread, 2 fat
Tom Collins				
Regular mixer	21.5	10	300	½ bread, 3½ fat
Artificial sweetened	21.5	10	300	3½ fat
Sherry, dry	9	2	60	¼ bread, 1½ fat
Wines, dry table 12% alcohol, e.g., champagne, sauterne, claret, Chablis	10.5	3½	100	¼ bread, 1½ fat

*Nutritive Value of Foods. Home and Garden Bulletin No. 72. Washington, D.C., U.S. Department of Agriculture, 1970, p. 35, 36.
Note: Lite beers vary in calorie content and must be considered individually.

For adults, this can be calculated by using the formulas in *Focus On Calculating the Diabetic Prescription for Calories.* In some instances, it may be best to determine a "desirable" body weight rather than trying to force the client to adopt an unrealistic goal.

2. As a rule, the number of kilocalories needed for basal metabolism is the ideal weight multiplied by 10.
3. Since activity levels vary among individuals, the multiplication factor is adjusted to account for this (Step 2–B in *Focus on Calculating the Diabetic Prescription for Calories*).
4. To allow for weight gain or growth or for weight loss, add or subtract 500 kcal/day to the total caloric level (determined from the above steps) to allow for a weight gain or loss of one pound/week. For pregnancy, add 300 kcal/day to gain 23 lbs. in nine months; for lactation, 500 kcal/day should be allowed.
5. Children vary markedly in their kilocaloric needs depending or their rate of growth and level of activity. Energy needs can be determined by the guidelines in Step 2–A of *Focus on Calculating the Diabetic Prescription for Calories.*

Determining the Amount of Carbohydrate, Protein, and Fat

The percentage of carbohydrate, protein, and fat may be stipulated by the physician's diet order or may be determined after consideration of the client's normal eating pattern obtained from a diet history.

A realistic division of the total kilocalories utilizing the American Diabetes Association's guidelines would be 55 percent carbohydrate (CHO), 15 percent protein, and 30 percent fat. To determine the grams of protein, carbohydrate, and fat in the diet, multiply the percentage of each by the total number of calories and divide by the number of kilocalories per gram (4, 4, and 9, respectively), as shown in Step 2 (*Focus on the Mechanics of Food Exchange Lists*).

Determining the Servings from Each Exchange

1. Before determining the number of servings from each exchange list, an individual consultation with the client is imperative so that the diet will reflect his/her dietary patterns as closely as possible. Of course, some changes in the dietary pattern are to be expected, but the plan must be individualized for the client. For instance, if the client absolutely refuses to drink any type of milk or to eat yogurt, the milk group can be omitted. Instead, the client should be encouraged to eat cheeses and cottage cheese from the meat group and/or to take a calcium supplement.
2. Determine the number of servings from the milk group. Clients should be encouraged to use skim milk; however, if whole milk is usually preferred, recommend a gradual transi-

---

Step 1. Determine ideal weight for height.
   A. Children: Weight in pounds
   Height in inches
   (see Appendix C–6)
   B. Women: 100 lbs. for first 5 feet
   Add 5 lbs. for each additional inch
   Men: 106 lbs. for first 5 feet
   Add 6 lbs. for each additional inch
   C. For small frame, subtract 10%; for large frame, add 10%. (For other frame size estimates see Appendix C–2).

Step 2. Determine kilocalorie needs.
   A. Children: For children 1000 kcal for first year of life plus 100 kcal for each year of age up to 2000 kcal at age 11. From age 12 to 15, 100 kcal/year added for girls and 200 kcal per year for boys.†
   B. Adults: 10 × ideal weight in lbs. = kcal (obese or inactive person)
   13 × ideal weight in lbs. = kcal (over age 55 or sedentary)
   15 × ideal weight in lbs. = kcal (desirable weight or moderately active)
   20 × ideal weight in lbs. = kcal (thin or very active)

Step 3. Example for weight reduction: Since 3500 kcal are in each stored pound of fat, one should consume 500 fewer kcal/day than expended to lose 1 lb./week.

165	lb. desired weight
× 15	kcal/lb. for moderate activity/day
2475	kcal needed to maintain desired weight
− 500	kcal daily deficit to lose 1 lb./week.
1975	maximum daily calories

*Adapted from *Calculation of a Diabetic Diet Prescription.* Minneapolis, MN, International Diabetes Center.
†From Pricilla White, M.D., Joslin Clinic.

tion. Low-fat milk may help a person get used to skim milk.

3. Add the desirable number of servings from the vegetable and fruit groups and fill in the nutrient values for these choices.

4. Total the carbohydrate value of the milk, vegetables, and fruit. Subtract this from the total grams of carbohydrate prescribed. Divide this number by 15 (the carbohydrate value of one bread exchange). Use the nearest whole number of bread exchanges. Fill in the carbohydrate and protein values. Total the carbohydrate column. If the total deviates more than 3 or 4 gm from the prescribed amount, adjust the amounts of vegetables, fruits, or bread. Fractions of exchanges are usually awkward and are not usually used (Steps 3 and 4 in *Focus on the Mechanics of Food Exchange Lists*).

5. Consultation with the client is necessary to determine whether s/he normally eats low-, medium-, or high-fat meats. Meats in the high-fat group are high in saturated fat and cholesterol and should be used only three times a week. Of course, patients should be encouraged to choose more low-fat meats.

   Total the protein value of the milk, vegetable, and bread exchanges. Subtract this sum from the amount of protein prescribed. Divide the remainder by 7 (the protein value of one meat exchange). Use the nearest whole number of meat exchanges. Fill in the protein and fat values (Step 5 in *Focus on the Mechanics of the Food Exchange List*).

6. Total the fat values for milk and meat. Subtract this total from the amount of fat prescribed. Divide the remainder by 5 (the fat content of one fat exchange). Fill in the fat value and the number of exchanges (Step 6 in *Focus on the Mechanics of the Food Exchange List*).

7. Check the entire diet for the accuracy of the computations.

Suggested Division into Meals and Snacks

For all diabetics, the carbohydrates and energy should be divided evenly throughout the day to prevent hyper- or hypoglycemia and to maintain metabolic balance. The distribution depends on whether insulin is needed (and what type) and the patient's lifestyle.

For those with IDDM, it is especially impor-

FOCUS ON *THE MECHANICS OF THE FOOD EXCHANGE LIST*

Step 1. Determine the percent of CHO, protein, and fat either from the physician's order or by using the guidelines from the American Diabetes Association (ADA) and/or information from the client's diet history. This example uses the ADA guidelines—55% CHO, 15% protein, 30% fat—for planning a diet with a maximum of 1975 kcal/day.

Step 2. Determine the grams of CHO, protein and fat:

$$\frac{55}{100} \times 1975 \text{ kcal} \div 4 = 272 \text{ gm CHO (round off)}$$

$$\frac{15}{100} \times 1975 \text{ kcal} \div 4 = 74 \text{ gm protein (round off)}$$

$$\frac{30}{100} \times 1975 \text{ kcal} \div 9 = 66 \text{ gm fat (round off)}$$

Diet prescription: 1975 kcal, 272 gm CHO, 74 gm protein, 66 gm fat.

Step 3. Decide from the patient's diet history the desirable number of servings from the milk, vegetable, and fruit lists.

	Svgs	CHO	Protein	Fat
List 5: Milk, low-fat	2	24	16	10
List 3: Vegetables	2	10	4	—
List 4: Fruits	5	75	—	—
Subtotal A		109	20	10

Step 4. To determine the number of servings from the starch/bread list, subtract the total grams of CHO (109) from milk, vegetable, and fruit lists from the total grams of CHO (272). This amount (163) is divided by 15 to arrive at 11 servings from the starch/bread list.

	Svgs	CHO	Protein	Fat
Subtotal A		109	20	10
List 1: Starch/bread	11	165	33	10
Subtotal B		274	53	20

Step 5: To determine the number of servings from the meat list, subtract the total protein (53) from the milk, vegetable, and starch/bread lists from the total desired amount (74) and divide by 7.

	Svgs	CHO	Protein	Fat
Subtotal B		274	53	20
List 2: Meat, medium-fat	3	—	21	15
		—	—	—
Subtotal C		274	74	35

Step 6. To determine the number of servings from the fat list, subtract the total fat from the sum of the milk, starch/bread, and meat lists (31) from the total amount needed (65 gm) and divide by 5.

	Svgs	CHO	Protein	Fat
Subtotal C		274	74	35
List 6: Fat	6	—	—	30
Final total		274	74	65

---

tant to distribute kilocalories, particularly the carbohydrates, so they will be available for insulin activity. For intermediate-acting insulins taken in the morning, a snack is usually given in the after-noon or at bedtime, depending on the individual's schedule and lateness of the dinner hour. The daily total carbohydrate and kilocalories are divided as 2/7 for breakfast, 2/7 for lunch, 2/7 for dinner, and ½ for a bedtime snack. For labile insulin-dependent diabetics, particularly children, additional snacks are desirable and distribution may be ²/10 for breakfast, ¹/10 for midmorning, ³/10 for lunch, ¹/10 for midafternoon, ²/10 for supper; and ¹/10 at bedtime.

For the individual with NIDDM, food is usually divided into three meals per day with a bedtime snack, as desired, to comply with the client's normal lifestyle and the physician's prescription. The patient on a reduction diet usually prefers three light meals with several snacks for more satiety.

The number of servings for each exchange list is first determined and then divided into a meal pattern appropriate for the individual (see *Focus on Daily Distribution of Exchange Lists*). The client's schedule, physical exercise patterns, and usual diet pattern must also be considered. For instance, if the client is in a work or school situation where a snack is not appropriate or feasible, it should not be calculated. Additionally, the client's usual blood sugars may indicate a need for snacks throughout the day.

Utilizing the meal plan, it is wise to write down specific foods and their portion sizes for the client.

Client Consultation

Individuals with a diet prescription must participate directly in their own care for successful results. The plan must be customized and allow the person to make adjustments. In addition to understanding the diet, the patient must understand the advantages of the modifications and the reasons for the various strategies employed. The more clients know about the principles and specific details, the greater are their options, which make the regimen easier and more pleasant to follow. It is imperative that an appropriate family member also understand and be able to implement the daily meal plan, if necessary. Every effort should be made to work with family members

FOCUS ON DAILY DISTRIBUTION OF EXCHANGE LISTS

List	Food Group	Svgs	CHO	Protein	Fat
1	Starch/bread	11	165	33	10
2	Meat, lean	2	–	14	6
	Meat, medium	1	–	7	5
3	Vegetable	2	10	4	–
4	Fruit	5	75	–	–
5	Milk, low-fat	2	24	16	10
6	Fat	7	–	–	35

Daily Meal Pattern

Breakfast:

2 fruit exchanges	6 medium stewed prunes
2 starch/bread exchanges	½ cup Bran Flakes ½ English muffin
2 fat exchanges	2 tsp. corn-oil margarine
1 milk exchange	1 cup 2% milk

Lunch:

1 meat exchange, medium	¼ cup drained tuna stuffed in
1 vegetable exchange	1 whole tomato with
Free foods	2 Tbsp. low-calorie salad dressing
2 starch/bread exchanges	8 whole-wheat crackers (also uses 2 fat exchanges)
2 fat exchanges 2 fruit exchanges	1 banana

Dinner:

2 meat exchanges, lean 1 vegetable exchange 4 starch/bread exchanges	2 oz. baked fish ½ cup broccoli 2/3 cup blackeyed peas
Free food:	2 whole-wheat rolls
2 fat exchanges	Romaine lettuce salad
	2 Tbsp. regular salad dressing
2 fruit exchanges	1 cup cantaloupe cubes

Bedtime snack:

1 milk exchange 1 starch/bread exchange	1 cup 2% milk 3 cup popcorn with
1 fat exchange	2 Tbsp. diet margarine

so that the meal plan neither creates conflicts nor disrupts usual household activities.

In addition to explaining how the food exchange lists work and which foods are in each exchange, both the person who prepares the food and the client must be taught the importance of careful measurements. If 1 tbsp. of margarine is mistakenly used for 1 tsp., for example, the number of calories is tripled. Many people are not familiar with cooking measurements; measuring devices such as scales are useful teaching tools. Food models may also be used as a reference.

During the counseling process, it should be stressed that the diabetic diet should not be thought of as a diet but as a way of life. Foods need not be special, but attention must be given to the way they are prepared and to meal regularity. While some changes in meal patterns are inevitable, almost any food can be eaten occasionally.

West (1973) cites the following factors as important deterrents to successful diet therapy:
1. The recommended diet prescription may lack relevance to the patient's preferences and may not fit cultural or socioeconomic status.
2. An insulin-dependent diabetic may find frequent feedings and the balancing of exercise and carbohydrate intake inconvenient and unappealing.
3. The patient and family may misunderstand the general goals and priorities and/or the specifics of diet therapy.
4. The physician, dietitian, or nurse may have a poor understanding of the principles and methods of diet therapy.
5. The patient education system may be defective because of (a) limitations of professional enthusiasm and acumen, (b) limited teaching resources, (c) lack of economic incentives for either professionals or institutions to teach patients, (d) lack of systematic patient education efforts among health care professionals, or (e) underestimation of deficiencies in patients' understanding.

Clinical Implications:

- Reduction diets require regular spacing of food intake. At least three meals should be planned; four to six may often be more successful for satiety as well as nutrient utilization.
- Individuals should be discouraged from skipping meals or consuming all food at one meal.
- Consumption of complex carbohydrates

should be emphasized rather than simple carbohydrates.
- It is recommended that kilocalories be distributed as follows: 20 percent from protein, less than 30 percent from fat, and the rest from carbohydrates.
- Diets with 1200 kcal/day or greater can meet the RDAs for all nutrients, with the exception of iron in women of childbearing age.
- Alcohol is contraindicated for persons with hyperlipoproteinemia characterized by elevated serum triglycerides.

FALLACIES and FACTS

FALLACY: *When reducing, diets should contain no fat.*
- **FACT:** *Some fat is required for the utilization of fat-soluble vitamins, for satiety to prevent hunger pangs, and to furnish linoleic acid, an essential fatty acid. The fat intake should be carefully selected, but not eliminated.*

FALLACY: *Diabetics must eat as little carbohydrate as possible.*
- **FACT:** *Simple carbohydrates, such as candy, are not recommended, but complex carbohydrates (beans, whole-wheat breads, and cereals) and high-fiber foods (apples and broccoli) are beneficial as long as the total kilocaloric intake is limited to the prescribed amount.*

FALLACY: *No saturated fat should be eaten.*
- **FACT:** *Not true, nor is it even possible. Saturated fats are found in meats and various foods. Recommendations are to limit this intake to 10 percent of total kilocaloric intake.*

Summary

The exchange lists are designed to help all populations, whether diabetic, obese, cardiovascular, or even normal populations, to improve their quality of life by making wise food choices based on caloric content and/or energy nutrients. The basic parts of the diet involve: (1) increasing complex carbohydrates (50 to 60 percent) for higher fiber intake, (2) reducing total fat to 25 to 30 percent, and (3) limiting cholesterol to 100 to 300 gm/day. Diets planned by the exchange lists actually could be considered as plans for optimum wellness rather than menus for specific diseases.

Regular preplanned meals based on the exchange lists, exercise regimens, adequate rest, and systematic monitoring of glucose levels, lipids, and body weight are significant factors that contribute to vitality, energy, and good health.

Review Questions

1. How are the basic food groups different from the exchange lists? Cite three differences in classification other than those mentioned in the text.
2. Why are both of these food groupings useful?
3. Describe the type of client who needs to use the basic food groups. Who should follow the exchange lists?
4. Tally all the foods you eat for one day, then calculate the number of food exchanges. Can you see any changes in food choices that would be beneficial to you and why?
5. Why are complex carbohydrates especially important for the person using the exchange lists?
6. Plan three meals for one day to meet a diet prescription of 2500 kcal with 70 gm of protein, 364 gm of carbohydrate, and 85 gm of fat.
7. Why are some vegetables in the meat exchange and others in the bread exchange, instead of all being in the vegetable exchange?

Case Study: Sarah is 29 years old, single, works every day with little time for exercise programs. Since graduating from college, she has gained 22 lbs. and realizes that her energy level is lower and that her appearance is not as attractive with this additional weight.

Plan meals and snacks (including brown-bag lunches) for Sarah for three days using the exchange lists to provide a weight loss of 2 lbs./week by reduced dietary intake.

REFERENCE LIST

American Dietetic Association: *Handbook of Clinical Dietetics*. New Haven, Yale University Press, 1981.

Chicago Dietetic Association and South Suburban Dietetic Association of Cook and Will Counties (CDA & SSDA): *Manual of Clinical Dietetics*, 2nd ed. Philadelphia, W. B. Saunders Co, 1981.

Jenkins, DJA; Wolever, TMS; Jenkins, AL; et al: The glycaemic index of foods tested in diabetic patients: A new basis for carbohydrate exchange favouring the use of legumes. *Diabetologia* 24:257, 1983.

Nemchik, R: Diabetes today: A very different diet; a new generation of oral drugs. *RN* 45(11):41, 1982.

Task Force for the American Diabetes Association: Nutritional recommendations and principles for individuals with diabetes mellitus: 1986. *Diabetes Care* 10(1):126, 1987.

West, KM: Diet therapy of diabetes: An analysis of failure. *Ann Intern Med* 79(3):425, 1973.

Further Study

Benz, MM; Kohler, E: Baby food exchanges and feeding the diabetic infant. *Diabetes Care* 3:554, 1980.

Benz, MM; Pearson, RE: Sugar content of selected liquid medicinals. *Diabetes* 22:776, 1973.

Burgess, B; El-Beher, RB: Rationale for changes in the dietary management of diabetes. *J Am Diet Assoc* 8(3):258, 1982.

Davenport, RR; Ferguson, ED; Fitzpatric, EO; et al: Dietitians, nurses teach diabetic patients. *Hospitals* 48(December 1):81, 1974.

Kulkarni, K: Advice from the dietitians. Vegetarian diets. *The Diabetic Educator* 9(summer):35, 1983.

Lofquist, B: From hamburgers to haute cuisine. Guidelines for eating out. *Diabetes Forecast* (DF 303), 1979.

Midgley, W: On the fast food trail. *Diabetes Forecast* 32(4):20, 1979.

Maras, ML; Adolph, CL: Ethnic tailoring improves dietary compliance. *The Diabetic Educator* 11(winter):47, 1985.

Wedman, B: Solving the food label mystery. *Diabetes Forecast* 32(2):20, 1980.

Wyse, BW: Nutrient analysis of exchange lists for meal planning. *J Am Diet Assoc* 75(3):239, 1979.

Resources

For the visually impaired:
Order from: Volunteer Braille Services, Inc.
Exchange Lists for Visually Impaired
P.O. Box 1592
Houma, LA 70361

Spanish Language Material for People with Diabetes, 1981:
National Institutes of Health Publication No. 81-2180.
Order from: National Diabetes Information Clearinghouse
Westwood Building, Room 603
Bethesda, MD 20205

Oriental Cooking for the Diabetic, 1982:
Order from: Dorothy Revell, R.D.
P.O. Box 328
Fargo, ND 58107

Supplements to Exchange Lists for Meal Planning:
Jewish Cookery, 1978
Vegetarian Cookery, 1978
Oriental Cookery, Lists for Meal Planning, 1979
Indian Cookery, 1981
Directions for Recipe Calculations, 1978
Order from: American Diabetes Association
4405 East-West Highway, Suite 403
Bethesda, MD 20814.

Problems of Weight Control

24

THE STUDENT WILL BE ABLE TO:

- **Evaluate food intake and mobility of the patient to determine the future course of weight gain or loss.**
- **Discuss different food choices as well as activities to achieve desired weight.**
- **List psychological factors that influence weight control. Suggest alternate behavior patterns to support the patient in his/her program.**
- **Evaluate personal goals for optimum health and weight.**
- **Discuss ways to evaluate new and old fad diets in order to determine their degree of acceptability.**
- **Discuss harmful as well as helpful ways to increase the rate of recovery for the anorexia nervosa patient.**
- **Evaluate the use of surgery for the morbidly obese and discuss problems the patient may expect after surgery.**

Anorexia nervosa
Bulimarexia
Bulimia
Hyperplasia
Hypertrophy
Lean body mass (LBM)
Morbid obesity
Obesity
Overweight
Protein-sparing Modified
   Fast (PSMF)
Set-point theory
Very-low-calorie diet
   (VLCD)

OBJECTIVES

TERMS TO KNOW

"Why don't you lose weight?" This is the question asked of the obese as if it were their fault. On the other hand, thin persons are quizzed for their secret of being able to eat all they want without adding a pound. Others lose all rational thought to become victims of anorexia nervosa. Weight control is complicated with unlimited influences and no easy solutions (Fig. 24–1).

Unfortunately, 90 percent of Americans feel they weigh too much. Because of the lack of scientific data, one's ideal weight is somewhat hypothetical and may continue to change as knowledge increases. The Framingham studies claim that life expectancy is the worst for men in the lightest weight group. Increased weight does not have much effect on life expectancy unless it is more than 25 percent above normal. Among women, mortality rates are the highest for the lightest and the heaviest groups, but those in between have little correlation with mortality (Bennett & Gurin, 1982).

Obesity

DEFINITION

What is obesity? Overweight is identified as 10 to 20 percent above ideal weight; obesity is 20 percent above ideal weight; morbid obesity refers to more than 100 lbs. over ideal weight. For example, an individual weighing 163 lbs. with an ideal weight of 130 lbs. is about 25 percent overweight and may be called obese. The consensus of the National Institutes of Health is that a level of 20 percent or more above desirable body weight, although arbitrarily selected, is associated with sufficient risk to health to justify clinical intervention (Burton & Foster, 1985).

ANTHROPOMETRIC MEASUREMENTS

Many sophisticated methods determine the exact weight status; however, the simple ones, such as the Metropolitan height and weight tables, are actually fundamental measurements, give an immediate assessment, and are inexpensive (see Appendix C–1). Bone structure and fat distribution must also be considered when determining appropriate weight (see Table 20–2).

Skin-fold measurements with calipers indicate lean body mass (LBM) in relation to fat tissue (see Chapter 20). Many persons, although normal or below normal in weight, have excess amounts of fat stores, while some athletes, especially football players, are overweight because of increased muscles, not fat. Being overweight is not the same as being fat or obese. Additional muscle tissue aids body functions, but excessive fat tissue interferes with even normal body metabolism.

Etiology

The precise cause or causes of obesity are not clearly identified, but there are several influences.

HYPERPLASTIC VERSUS HYPERTROPHIC OBESITY

Obesity can be divided into two classifications—hyperplastic, which refers to increased numbers of fat cells, and hypertrophic, which refers to increased size of fat cells. Cell multiplication (or increased numbers of fat cells) occurs during peak growth periods: late infancy, early childhood (up to six years of age), adolescence, and pregnancy. The complexity and magnitude of obesity is more easily understood if overeating has occurred during any of these periods: As many as five times the number of body fat cells may develop (Stunkard, 1980). Adequate nutrition for growth during these stages without excessive amounts of energy is imperative.

Birth weights do not correlate with subsequent obesity in adult life. Obese infants do not necessarily become obese children. However, obesity may begin as early as age two for girls and age three for boys. Another period when obesity begins is from five to nine years old, which is before the normal child's growth spurts (Shapiro et al, 1984).

In hypertrophic obesity, the number of cells is limited, but they expand to increase body weight. This type of obesity may occur at any time throughout life but is frequently found in adults who gain weight.

HEREDITY

The definitive cause of obesity is not known, but heredity probably contributes to the condi-

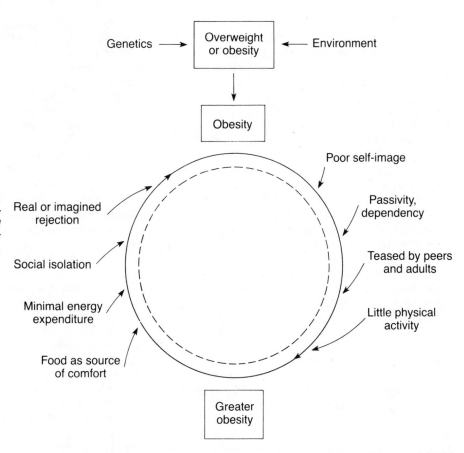

Figure 24–1. Factors that contribute to obesity. (Diagram by Betty Lucas, M.P.H., Nutritionist, Clinical Training Unit, Child Development and Mental Retardation Center, University of Washington, Seattle.)

tion. Heredity also dictates where fat is deposited in the body. Excessive stores may be located on the sides of the hips, across the buttocks or the abdomen, or around the waist. Excessive fat across the abdomen from whatever cause is an important predictor of the health hazards of obesity. High ratios of waist-to-hip circumference (simply measured with a tape) are associated with a higher risk for illness and decreased life span (Burton & Foster, 1985).

APPESTAT

The set-point theory (or appestat) proposes that a control system in each individual dictates how much fat s/he will have. For example, normal weight individuals stop eating sweetened or fatty foods sooner than the obese person (Gonzalez, 1983). This theory explains why it is as difficult for a thin person to gain weight as it is for an obese one to lose weight. The body adjusts the appetite for kilocaloric intake to maintain its set point. This set point changes at different stages of life.

While it is not clear as to what controls the appestat, the only way to lower the set point is through increased physical exercise. This can apparently help maintain weight loss as well.

HYPOTHROIDISM

Obesity caused by hypothyroidism occurs in fewer than one percent of overweight patients (Blackburn & Pavlou, 1983). In hypothyroidism, the basal metabolic rate (BMR) is lowered because of a deficiency in thyroid secretion. This results in excessive retention of calories which would normally be expended in basal metabolism. Thorough physical examinations are mandatory for optimum weight-control results.

TOTAL ENERGY EXPENDITURE

The basal metabolic rate (BMR) accounts for approximately 70 percent of daily energy expenditure (EE). The BMR depends principally on the amount of fat-free mass (muscle tissue). After the age of 25, BMR decreases. If food intake does not decrease accordingly, weight is gained.

A major component of overall EE is physical activity, which also usually decreases after the age of 25. Exercise can increase, decrease, or have no effect on food intake. This may be explained by differences in sex and age as well as the duration and intensity of the exercise. Since many obese persons are less active, fewer kilocalories are expended, which in turn, results in weight gain when the same amount of food is eaten. Decreased activity can also lead to an increase in food intake (Stunkard, 1980).

Increased activity may be required in order to achieve weight reduction. The BMR begins to decrease when energy is restricted. Within two weeks, the BMR can decrease more than 20 percent (Stunkard, 1980). This reduced kilocalorie expenditure can lessen weight reduction and become very depressing for the dieter.

PSYCHOLOGICAL FACTORS

The desire to eat frequently may be related to emotional factors. Greater weight usually means the individual is responding to feelings and emotions rather than actual hunger. Boredom triggers the desire to eat. The average housewife eats 18 times a day (Stunkard, 1976). Teenagers in particular do not eat when they are hungry as much as when they are bored (Winick, 1975).

Depression in obese persons results in crying, sulking, eating, and decreased activity. The non-obese person cleans house, reads, or contacts friends. Obese persons usually have difficulty developing relationships with other people.

Overeating at night can be caused by boredom, depression, loneliness, and anxiety. Obese people do not ordinarily sleep more than four to five hours per night. A night-eating pattern may occur in as many as 80 percent of obese patients (Stunkard, 1976).

Nutritional Care

MOTIVATION

Dieting should always be a serious undertaking, not a casual one. Before attempting a reduction program, an individual should be highly mo-

tivated to lose weight. This will increase the chances that s/he will stick with a diet until the weight is lost and will maintain the weight loss. Losing weight is relatively easy compared to maintaining weight loss. The weight loss program should have a high success rate.

Repeated cycles of weight loss and gain may have detrimental effects. Individuals who have lost weight only to put it back on are frequently unable to lose weight even on 800 kcal, take longer to lose the added weight, and regain the weight more rapidly. As previously mentioned, when energy intake decreases, BMR also decreases. Possibly, these weight cycles may make people more metabolically efficient, with the body interpreting these periods of low caloric intake as starvation. In other words, dieting may actually help to induce obesity in some people (Brownell, 1986). Repeated exchanges of gaining and losing weight may frequently result in the deposition of fatty cysts requiring surgical removal. When weight is regained, arterial plaque may be deposited at an accelerated rate, and the number and size of fat cells may increase.

Obesity contributes to many health problems. In some cases, understanding the physiological benefits can motivate patients to initiate a weight loss program. Physical conditions that can be expected to improve with weight loss include: shortness of breath, ease of tiring, fluid retention, gastric disorders, headaches, energy level, interest in sex, joint pains, muscle cramps, postnasal drip, pulse rate, restless sleep, urinary infection, and varicose veins (Casse & Tracy, 1983).

A 1976 survey by Stunkard revealed motivation is also affected by the amount of encouragement and support from family and friends. While husbands stated that: (1) their wives were heavier than when they got married, (2) they wanted their wives to lose weight, and (3) they were willing to help them, the husbands were also more likely to: (1) initiate conversations pertaining to food, (2) offer food, and (3) criticize rather than praise their wives' eating habits. It is easy to understand why obese persons in reduction programs lose more weight when their spouses attend meetings with them (Barlow & Tillotson, 1978). Support from family and friends is far more conducive to successful weight reduction than such sabotage techniques.

WEIGHT LOSS

A goal of 1 to 2 lbs. weight loss per week is safe for most persons. A 1 lb. (2.2 kg) weight loss requires a deficit of 3500 kcal. This can be accomplished by eating less, increasing activity, or a combination of both. When 2 lbs. (4.4 kg) per week are lost, the individual is more enthusiastic about the method of loss. Food intake with 500 kcal less than needed per day results in a 1 lb. loss per week. An additional energy expenditure of 500 kcal per day is recommended for the other pound of weight loss.

DIET PLAN

Diets may be planned from a general guide, such as the prudent diet (see Chapter 32) from the American Heart Association, or the guidelines suggested in the food exchange lists (see Chapter 23). Indispensible to any weight loss program is a preplanned food allotment with specified times throughout the day to lessen the deprivation syndrome of diets and eliminate excessive food intake. The total amount of foods should be divided into three or more feedings. Some "free" foods or beverages may be available for snack periods, but regular mealtimes are important.

Most overweight patients tend to eat the majority of their food in one meal, usually in the late afternoon or evening with little or no exercise before bedtime. Many of these people skip breakfast, eat a light lunch, and then consume most of their calories late in the day. Individuals who eat two meals per day tend to be more overweight than those eating three or four meals per day (Russ et al, 1984).

COMPOSITION OF THE DIET

The diet should be well balanced, nutritionally adequate, and based on the basic food groups. Foods from the accessory group should be minimized. A diet that totally eliminates one category or specific group of foods, e.g., fat or carbohydrate, is inadvisable because essential nutrients may be lacking. A minimum of 20 to 25 percent of fat in the diet increases satiety and provides for absorption of fat-soluble vitamins. Diets below 1500 kcal do not provide adequate amounts of vitamins and minerals; a mutivitamin-mineral supplement is advised.

Consumption of complex carbohydrates in meals and snacks has also been advised for weight loss. Complex carbohydrates maintain glycogen stores for optimum energy levels. Also, carbohydrate ingestion triggers a significant increase in brain serotonin followed by a decrease in the hunger impulse. Low serotonin levels encourage a person to eat more carbohydrates and less protein. If a faulty equalizing system such as this is present, the person might constantly crave carbohydrates. Therefore, all reduction diets should allow ample starchy foods to discourage binge eating (Wurtman, 1983).

Another strategy to increase satiety is through a high fiber intake (0.7 gm/kg of ideal body weight) that provides bulk with low caloric density foods.

The use of sugar substitutes is frequently a component of reduction diets. Their contribution to the dieter's success is questionable. The tongue perceives noncaloric sweeteners as food, but the rest of the body is not fooled. When sugars are eaten, chemical changes produce a satiated feeling; noncaloric sweeteners do nothing to appease the appetite, and may even stimulate the appetite (Blundell & Hill, 1986; Porikos et al, 1982).

Clinical Implication:

• Persons who are dieting should be warned not to consume unlimited amounts of beverages and/or foods sweetened with aspartame or any other artificial sweetener.

FASTING

Total fasting is extremely hazardous and is not recommended for more than three days unless in a hospital setting with adequate medical supervision. Factors such as underestimation of brief time periods, depression, concern with body size, lethargy, and anxiety change over a long-term fasting weight reduction plan. Short-term fasting apparently has no effect (Grinker, 1973).

VERY-LOW-CALORIE DIETS

Very-low-calorie diets (VLCD) containing less than 1000 kcal daily should be medically supervised. Meeting the RDAs requires more planning with less caloric intake, but the nutritive needs are still present. Multivitamin-mineral supplements with folate and at least 3 qt. of fluid daily are needed.

Very-low-calorie diets of 300 to 500 kcal/day should contain protein of high biological value (at least 55 gm) with adequate potassium supplementation and a reduced intake of carbohydrates and sodium. By including at least 50 gm of carbohydrate per day, the risk of ketogenesis can be reduced (Anderson et al, 1982). When kilocalories are inadequate, potassium depletion often occurs as well as the protein loss.

Weight loss averages 1.8 kg/week on these diets. However, the client does not learn how to choose foods wisely after going off of the diet. The extremely restricted diets are counterproductive since they seldom maintain weight reduction.

The VLCDs should be restricted to patients with severe obesity (30 to 40 percent above ideal weight) who are under medical supervision with appropriate cardiac evaluation in the initial screening and ongoing surveillance. Patients must be warned that these diets are potentially dangerous (Felig, 1984). Prolonged use of VLCDs may result in large losses of lean body mass in some individuals. Even small depletions may have unfortunate consequences if critical organs such as the heart are affected (Wadden et al, 1983).

FAD DIETS

With a national problem of about 88 million citizens considered overweight and 40 million clinically obese, Americans are still looking for the magic formula to lose weight (Fisher & Lachance, 1985). A fad diet is practiced with exaggerated zeal and usually does not have an authenic basis (Table 24–1). Such diets can be recognized instantly when they promise secret formulas to melt away fat without exercise while eating without limits and, of course, immediate results of several pounds lost. Miraculous promises are a good reason to run the other way.

Results of fad diets can be devastating and have even led to death. On the other hand, those immediate results, such as big weight losses due to low-carbohydrate diets, will disappear. The reduction in weight represents water loss instead of fat, so the previous weight returns when normal food intake resumes. Rapid weight loss is usually quickly regained (Lindner et al., 1981).

Most popular reduction diets do not provide 100 percent of the RDAs. Nutrients most often present in inadequate amounts are thiamin, vitamins B_6 and B_{12}, calcium, iron, zinc, and magnesium. Other nutrients are often lacking from some diets. While vitamin and mineral supplements may be taken with such diets, providing adequate amounts of all nutrients is questionable. Other dietary factors that may be excessive or lacking include sodium, P/S ratio, cholesterol, and fiber (Fisher & Lachance, 1985).

The severity of the diet may or may not be associated with success, even on a temporary basis. A diet that requires the least amount of change in dietary patterns will have the most acceptance and long-term success.

Because most obese patients regain their lost weight within three to four years, it is imperative that lifestyle considerations and increased self-understanding is included in reduction programs to decrease the chances for regaining the weight. Losing weight is only the first step; keeping it off may be even more difficult.

Clinical Implication:

- Clinical abnormalities among individuals on VLCDs include alopecia, hypercholesterolemia, normochromic anemia, and postural hypotension.

The Use of Drugs

Americans, always looking for a magic pill to cure ailments, will frequently use appetite depressants to lose weight. Indeed, $80 million was spent on appetite suppressants in one year.

Considerable controversy exists over the use of drugs for obesity. Some appetite suppressants are prescription drugs and some are available over-the-counter; bulk-forming agents, which fill the stomach or interfere with intestinal digestion and absorption, are also available over-the-counter.

ANORECTIC DRUGS

Prescription appetite suppressants include the amphetamines, such as Benzedrine, Dexedrine, Preludin, and Ionamin, and nonamphetamines, such as fenfluramine (Pondimin). These drugs depress the appetite by their stimulating action on the central nervous system, which results in increased motor activity.

The amphetamines have several other side effects: increased alertness, lowered fatigue, elevation of mood. The euphoriant effect of the amphetamines has led to their widespread abuse and dependency by some individuals. Common side effects include insomnia, restlessness, irritability,

Text continued on page 464

Table 24—1. Nutritional Analyses of Popular Diets*

Name of Diet	Kcal	Techniques Employed	Comments
1. *Kempner Rice Diet* or *Duke University Rice Diet,* from Mc-Call's Diet of the Month. Mc-Call's Magazine, April, 1970.	2200	Unspecified energy level, fixed menu; unbalanced energy sources (very low fat); low sodium; monotony; famous name; vitamin and mineral supplements required.	This diet consists of very large amounts of cooked rice, fruits and vegetables. It is virtually devoid of sodium and low in protein as well as vitamin A, riboflavin, calcium, and iron. No foods from the milk or meat groups of the Basic Four are permitted. The blandness and monotony are so great that most dieters on this diet fail to eat all the rice required and reduce their food intakes far below the 2200 kcal level. If this is done, then fat may be lost. Otherwise, early weight loss is likely to be due chiefly to shifts in water balance. This diet is inadequate unless vitamin-mineral supplements are added. The diet was originally formulated for persons who were removed from their usual environments and sent to live in a hospital setting. This diet is not necessarily approved by Duke University.
2. *Calories Don't Count,* from the book by the same name by H. Taller. Simon and Schuster, New York, 1961.	1800	Unspecified energy level, fixed menus; unbalanced energy sources (high fat); unsubstantiated claim for a scientific breakthrough, use of a famous name, special supplement of polyunsaturated vegetable oil required as well as food; one hour walk also specified; other specifications on eating; low sodium.	This diet is extremely high in fat and quite high in protein. Particular emphasis is paid to consuming large amounts of meat and milk products, avoiding sugars and starches including most fruits, breads, and cereals. The dieter must consume (or drink) approximately one third of a cup of vegetable oil high in polyunsaturated fat each day. Such a recommendation may be medically unwise for many reasons, not the least of which is the 800 kcal it contributes. Many commonly eaten foods are forbidden. Weight loss, if it occurs at all, is likely to be due in great measure to a temporary diuresis induced by the low carbohydrate/low sodium nature of the diet and the liberal use of black coffee, a weak diuretic.
3. *Stillman Diet,* also known as *The Doctor's Quick Weight Loss Diet* in book of that name by I. M. Stillman and S. Baker, Dell Publishing Company, New York, 1977.	2000	Unspecified energy level; unbalanced energy sources (very low carbohydrate); monotony; special conditions on eating (use of at least eight glasses of water a day); famous name.	Also known as the water diet, this is a perennial favorite at diet book counters. The diet works by specifying the types but not the amounts of foods which are permitted. Fails to meet the Basic Four for either fruits and vegetables or breads and cereals, since none of these foods are allowed. The diet consists of low fat cheeses, lean meat, fish, poultry, eggs and 8 glasses of water a day. Neither milk nor visible fats are permitted, but the contribution of the other foods makes the

Table continued on following page

Table 24–1. Nutritional Analyses of Popular Diets* Continued

Name of Diet	Kcal	Techniques Employed	Comments
			diet very high in fat, especially saturated fat, and protein and low in carbohydrate. Vitamins A, C, thiamine and iron are low in the diet. A multi-vitamin pill is suggested.
4. *Slim Chance in a Fat World,* from book by the same name by R. B. Stuart and B. Davis. Research Press, Champaign, Illinois, 1972. (See also *Act Thin, Stay Thin* by R. Stuart, W. W. Norton, New York, 1978).	Variable, depending upon the food plan chosen but usually 1200–1500 kcal for women, more for men.	Specified energy level; balanced energy sources; special conditions on eating (use of behavior modification techniques and environmental manipulation, record keeping); recommendations for exercise; famous name.	This diet can be highly recommended. It places heavy emphasis on behavior modification techniques, but includes a good deal of information on diet planning from the nutritional standpoint. If instructions are followed, nutrient needs other than energy will be met. Most patients using this diet will benefit from the simultaneous assistance of a health professional knowledgeable in behavior therapy and nutrition, since directions are many and rather complicated.
5. *Behavioral Control Diet,* from the book *Eating Is Okay* by H. A. Jordan L. S. Levitz, and G. M. Kimbrell, Rawson Associates Publishers, New York, 1976. (NOTE: Other excellent books outlining similar self-directed diet change methods include: *Permanent Weight Control: A Total Solution to the Dieter's Dilemma,* by M. & K. Mahoney, W. W. Norton, New York, 1976: *Habits, Not Diets: The Real Way to Weight Control,* by J. M. Ferguson, Bull Publishing Co., Palo Alto, 1976; *Learning to Eat: Behavioral Modification for Weight Control,* by J. M. Ferguson, Bull Publishing Co., Palo Alto, 1976; and *Take It Off and Keep It Off,* by D. B. Jeffrey and R. Katz, Prentice Hall, Englewood Cliffs, 1977).	Variable, but approximately 1500.	Unspecified energy level; balanced energy sources; special conditions on eating (keeping diet records, behavior modification); famous name; physical activity.	This diet can be highly recommended. It is actually a self-administered course in behavior modification rather than a diet per se, written by clinicians with extensive experience in the field. If the instructions are followed, all nutrient needs other than energy should be met, and the dieter will gain insight into how to plan eating styles over the long term to maintain reduced weights. Most patients will find that the assistance of a health professional knowledgeable in behavior therapy and nutrition will be helpful in following the directions.
6. *Pritikin Diet,* from *Live Longer Now: The First One Hundred Years of Your Life,* by N. Pritikin, Grosset and Dunlop. New York, 1974.	1400	Unspecified energy level; unbalanced energy sources (extremely low fat); special conditions on eating (portion size control); famous name; unsubstantiated scientific breakthrough; low sodium; prophylactic claims.	This diet is extremely low in fat (only about 10 per cent of total calories) and also quite low in salt and carbohydrate, especially sugar, Dr. Pritikin has popularized the regimen as a cure for heart disease, but after 5 years, evidence that this is the case is still lacking. The diet pattern forbids butter, margarine, oils, grain-fed beef, sugar and products containing them. While the types of foods allowed meet the Basic Four, particular emphasis is given to large amounts of fruits, vegetables, breads and cereals. Dairy products are forbidden unless they are made with skim milk. Slightly low in iron.

Table 24–1. Nutritional Analyses of Popular Diets* Continued

Name of Diet	Kcal	Techniques Employed	Comments
7. *The Fat Counter Guide,* from book by the name by R. M. Deutsch, Hawthorne Books and Bull Publishing Co., Palo Alto, 1978.	1300	Specified energy level, balanced energy sources; special conditions on eating (use of fat counter to plan menus and analyze choices).	With the help of the so-called fat counter table, which lists the percent of protein, fat and carbohydrate in foods, the would-be dieter analyzes his food intake. Using the Basic Four and the fat counter guide, the dieter then plans a diet with a 500 kcal deficit to his or her individual tastes which is somewhat lower in fat and higher in carbohydrate than usual, somewhat limiting the variety of foods. Written by one of the reputable popular writers in the diet field, the nutrition information presented is sound.
8. *Dietary Goals Diet* from the analysis by B. Peterkin, C. Shone and R. L. Kerr in Some diets that meet the dietary goals, J. Amer. Dietet. Assoc., 74:423, 1979.	1300	Specified energy level; fixed menus; balanced energy sources; monotony; use of a famous name.	This is a reducing diet based on the U.S. Dietary Goals. It meets Recommended Dietary Allowances but provides very large amounts of breads, cereals, fruits and vegetables and fewer servings from the meat and milk group than specified in the Basic Four. Variety of foods allowed is somewhat limited.
9. *Anti-Stress Diet* by Dr. Neil Solomon, Harper's Bazaar, August, 1976.	1300	Unspecified energy level (fixed menu); balanced energy sources; special conditions on eating; famous name; unsubstantiated scientific breakthrough.	This is a good reducing diet formulated by one of the more reputable physicians who write for the diet market. The novel feature of the diet is that it is to be followed only three days a week. Other than the unwarranted claim that protein and calcium are provided in abundance to assist in "high stress" situations, the diet is sensible. Simple relaxation techniques and exhortations to exercise to relieve stress are also included. Meets all nutrients needs.
10. *Wise Woman's Diet* in Redbook, June, 1979 (repeated each season).	1200	Specified energy level; set menus; balanced energy sources.	This diet is a good one which meets all of the Recommended Dietary Allowances and also the Basic Four guide. It is repeated with different menus several times a year in the same magazine along with behavior modification hints and a discussion of special problems dieters face. Some limited exchanges of one food for another are permitted.
11. *Protein Program Reducing Diet* from diet included with Health Brand Protein Powder, Republic Drug Co., Buffalo, New York.	1000	Unspecified energy level (fixed menu); balanced energy sources; special conditions on eating; famous name; unsubstantiated scientific breakthrough.	This diet cannot be recommended. It involves the use of a protein powder "supplement" at one or two meals a day in addition to a regular meal and snack. The powder contains a mixture of soy protein, casein and lactalbumin, along with brewer's yeast. While the protein sources are somewhat better than those found in liquid protein formula diets, directions

Table continued on following page

Table 24–1. Nutritional Analyses of Popular Diets* Continued

Name of Diet	Kcal	Techniques Employed	Comments
			about meals are ambiguous except for dinner, so some dieters may eliminate them as well. The diet is low in iron. It falls short of the Basic Four in the milk group and the breads and cereals group.
12. *Snack Diet or Wisconsin Diet* from article by the same name in McCall's, October 1970.	950	Unspecified energy level (fixed menu); unbalanced energy sources (low carbohydrate); special conditions on eating; famous name.	This diet cannot be recommended. It purports to be based on research conducted at the University of Wisconsin on the utility of frequent feedings, but the University does not endorse it. While an eating regimen of 6 small meals a day is stressed, it is the low calorie aspect of the diet which is crucial. The diet is ketogenic and relatively low in sodium, so that a diuresis would be likely to ensue in the first few days on the regime which would lead to rapid weight loss. The pattern recommended is lower in the milk group and breads and cereals group than the Basic Four, and the diet is low in calcium and iron.
13. *The Doctor's Metabolic Diet* from book of the same name by W. L. Kremer, Crown Publishers, New York, 1975.	900	Unspecified energy level (fixed menu alternating with a fast); unbalanced energy sources (low carbohydrate); special conditions on eating; famous name; unsubstantiated scientific claims; inadequate nutrients; low sodium.	This diet cannot be recommended. The most unusual features of this diet are that it insists on no food intake before lunch and only two meals per day, with one day a week devoted to a total fast. The diet is ketogenic, low in sodium, and recommends weak tea and coffee—all measures which are likely to induce a diuresis in the first few days and rather rapid weight loss at first. The claims that breakfast is "useless" and that carbohydrates should be eaten only at lunch are incorrect. Breads and cereals and the milk group fail to meet the Basic Four. The diet is low in riboflavin, thiamine, calcium and iron; the use of vitamin-mineral supplements is mentioned but not stressed. The very low calorie levels, periodic fasts, absence of a morning meal and lack of emphasis on selection of potassium-rich foods make this diet inappropriate for use without medical supervision.
14. *Scarsdale Diet*	750	Unspecified energy level; set or fixed menu; unbalanced energy sources (very low carbohydrate and fat); famous name; biochemical claims and hints of scientific breakthroughs; monotony; low sodium.	**This diet is dangerous to use without medical supervision.** This is one version of a popular new crash diet variously called the Scarsdale Diet and the Scarsdale Medical Group Diet which is to be used for 14 days only and is

Table 24–1. *Nutritional Analyses of Popular Diets* Continued

Name of Diet	Kcal	Techniques Employed	Comments
			"guaranteed" to cause a weight loss of 20 lb. Because of its low carbohydrate (about 50 gm) and energy content, this diet is ketogenic. Additional constraints on fluid intake, which is limited to black coffee or tea, both diuretics in themselves, and on salting, favor diuresis. Much of the weight lost on the diet is water, which will be promptly regained after the diet ceases. The diet is low in iron, vitamin A, calcium and riboflavin. The diet is low in the milk and bread and cereals groups. Danger of dehydration is high since fluid intakes are not specified.
15. *Last Chance Refeeding Diet,* from "The Last Chance Diet" by R. Linn, Bantam Books, New York, 1977.	500	Specified energy level; unbalanced energy sources (very low carbohydrate); special formula required as well as food; famous name; unsubstantiated claim for a scientific breakthrough.	**This diet is hazardous to use without medical supervision.** This diet follows the protein supplemented fast Dr. Linn advocates in his book. A high protein powder, called ProLinn, is suggested for the fast itself. Such fasts are dangerous in that they may induce ketosis, hypokalemia, and other complications when attempted by persons not under skilled medical supervision. During the fast, vitamin and mineral supplements, potassium and folic acid are also prescribed with at least 2 quarts of noncaloric fluids a day. Gradually food is introduced—this is called the refeeding phase and is detailed here. The ProLinn powder must still be consumed twice a day. Dangers of dehydration, hypokalemia, etc. are high if directions are not followed. Intakes of vitamin A, riboflavin, thiamine, iron, and calcium are inadequate as the diet is stated.
16. *Fasting Is a Way of Life,* from the book by the same title by L. Cott, Bantam Books, New York, 1977.	500	Specified energy level (fast followed by formula); unbalanced energy sources (low carbohydrate).	**The type of fasting described in this diet is extremely dangerous and may result in serious problems if done without medical supervision.** This book suggests a total fast followed by a very low calorie diet of liquid meals. The diet is very low in the meat group and breads and cereals compared to the Basic Four. It is lower than recommendations in protein, niacin, riboflavin, thiamine, calcium and iron. The diet is ketogenic because of the low carbohydrate levels.

*From Stunkard, AJ: Obesity. Philadelphia, W. B. Saunders Co., 1980, with permission.

tremor, excess perspiration, dry mouth, epigastric discomfort, constipation, and palpitations. They are contraindicated in coronary artery disease; in severe cases of hypertension, hyperthyroidism, and glaucoma; and in patients with a history of drug abuse. Amphetamines can become a crutch in a weight loss program; the FDA recommends that they should be prescribed by physicians only for a short period of time.

Fenfluramine is more effective as an appetite suppressant than the amphetamines; it apparently has a depressant effect on the central nervous system causing sedation rather than stimulation. It also has a mild hypotensive action independent of weight loss. Adverse side effects include dry mouth, drowsiness, lethargy, lightheadedness, and diarrhea. The effects of depressing or stimulating body metabolism 24 hours a day should be considered.

These appetite suppressants seem to become less effective with time. They will result in decreased appetite, which results in weight loss; however, weight loss is less difficult than keeping the weight off. Whenever these pills are prescribed, they should be used in combination with a calorie-restricted diet and a behavior modification program. The drugs alone are not an effective method of long-term weight control.

Phenylpropanolamine hydrochloride is widely available in over-the-counter preparations marketed for weight loss (Appedrine, Dexatrim, Dietac), as shown in Table 24–2. Many of these agents also contain caffeine, which slightly depresses the appetite. These drugs have adrenergic effects that may cause vasoconstriction, bronchodilation, and tachycardia. They are therefore contraindicated in pregnant or nursing mothers, in diabetics, and in patients with high blood pressure or with heart, kidney, or thyroid conditions. Dosage recommendations on the package should be followed.

Benzocaine, long known for its ability to numb pain, is marketed in candies and gum for use prior to meals to reduce food intake. The appetite is suppressed because of increased blood glucose level and a decreased ability to taste and

Table 24–2. Nonprescription Diet Aids*

Product	Example	Action	Comment
Candies to curb apetite	Ayds Fructose tablets	Suppress appetite by raising blood glucose levels.	Harmless; candies usually contain carbohydrate, fat, vitamins and minerals. Expensive, since fruit juice before meal could have similar effect.
Over-the-counter appetite suppressants	Appedrine Control Dexatrim Prolamine Dietac Dex-a-Diet II Anorexin	Most contain phenylpropanolamine (PPA) that reduces appetite temporarily. Many also contain caffeine.	PPA is mild stimulant, as is caffeine. PPA can be dangerous to those with heart disease, high blood pressure, diabetes or hyperthyroidism. CSPI, public interest group, has proposed banning PPA in diet aids.
Local anesthetics	Reducets Spantrol Diet-trim	Benzocaine, local anesthetic, is the active ingredient. Anesthetic presumably deadens taste buds.	No controlled studies demonstrate efficacy.
Bulking agents	Pretts Taper	Contain methylcellulose; due to affinity for water, increase in volume and supposedly trick stomach into feeling full.	Methylcellulose does not swell until in intestine, rather than in stomach, so limited effectiveness.
Diuretics	Diurex	Cause body to lose water and thus body weight reduces. Weight loss short-lived.	No loss of body fat. Can be dangerous in that it can cause dehydration and loss of potassium. Should be used only under direction of a physician.
Exotic and secret cures	Spirulina extract	Questionable action.	Not shown to be effective in controlled studies.
Amylase inhibitors	Calorex	*In vitro* inhibit action of pancreatic enzyme amylase and thus thought to prevent digestion and absorption of starch. *In vivo* cause diarrhea and GI distress.	Not shown to be effective. Banned from marketplace by FDA in 1982.

*Reproduced by permission from Mahan, L. K., and Reese, J. M.: *Nutrition in Adolescence.* St. Louis, The C. V. Mosby Co., 1984.

enjoy food. The dosage of two candies before each meal would result in 150 kcal/day. While this amount is not significant, the same effect could be obtained from the intake of a salad (with no-calorie dressing) or a large glass of tomato juice.

Clinical Implication:

- Persons taking phenylpropanolamine appetite suppressants should avoid the use of over-the-counter preparations for coughs, colds, and allergies that also contain phenylpropanolamine.

BULKING AGENTS

Bulk-producing agents such as methylcellulose and carboxymethyl cellulose sodium have been advocated to inhibit food intake. Taken before a meal, they create a feeling of fullness so that less food is ingested. While the theory sounds good, this practice has not proved effective in reducing the intensity of hunger feelings of patients trying to reduce. It is important that these agents be taken with large amounts of water.

Other bulk laxatives are advocated as digestion and absorption may be decreased; again, studies have not proved these effective in weight control.

DIURETICS

Diuretics are often combined with anorectic agents for weight loss. This results in loss of body fluid but not body fat. The use of diuretics is rarely indicated physiologically for obesity; however, the rapid weight loss it causes provides a psychological lift to patients. When patients are also on a low-calorie diet, the diuretics may aggravate the loss of electrolytes secondary to such regimens. This is an even greater problem when the individual is fasting.

THYROID

Early in the century, thyroid preparations were used for treatment of obesity. However, few overweight individuals have a decreased metabolic rate. Large doses of thyroid hormones induce a state of hypermetabolism that results in weight loss. The effects of this hypermetabolism are unknown.

THE ROLE OF DRUGS

While drugs may be used to suppress appetite, they are not the sole answer to the management of obesity. A weight reduction program can be a depressing experience; the psychological boost provided by the use of drugs may help some patients through a difficult situation. Anorectic drugs may be used if nondrug regimens fail to help the patient off to a good start with a weight control regimen. Drug therapy failed to produce more weight loss than that achieved by other means in an extensive review of outpatient obesity (Wing & Jeffrey, 1979). Combined therapy using drugs, diet, and behavior modification needs further evaluation.

Exercise

When physical exercise is increased while calories are restricted, lean body mass is maintained or increased, and fat loss is greater. Decreased physical activity can lead to an increase in food intake; moderately increasing the physical activity for about 1 hr/day is the preferred way to decrease food intake (Stunkard, 1980). Obese children and adults more often eat the same amount of food as (or even less than) their normal counterparts, but they exercise much less. Energy balance can be attained by food intake or energy output. An error of no more than 10 percent in either food intake or energy output can produce a 20 lb. change in body weight in one year. For example, energy saved by parking the car closer to walk less or watching television an extra half hour instead of a more active pursuit can easily cause a weight gain of 10 to 20 lb./yr (Fig. 24–2).

Even though exercise alone rarely produces more than a 5 percent weight loss (Brownell & Stunkard, 1980), it can be useful for other reasons. Exercise may have the following effects on weight control:

1. Decreases loss of lean body tissue and increases loss of fat tissue when combined with diet regimen.
2. Actually decreases appetite under certain circumstances (Brownell & Stunkard, 1980).
3. May provide an incentive to continue the diet or similar regimens (Glasser, 1976).
4. Reduces stress and alleviates depression.

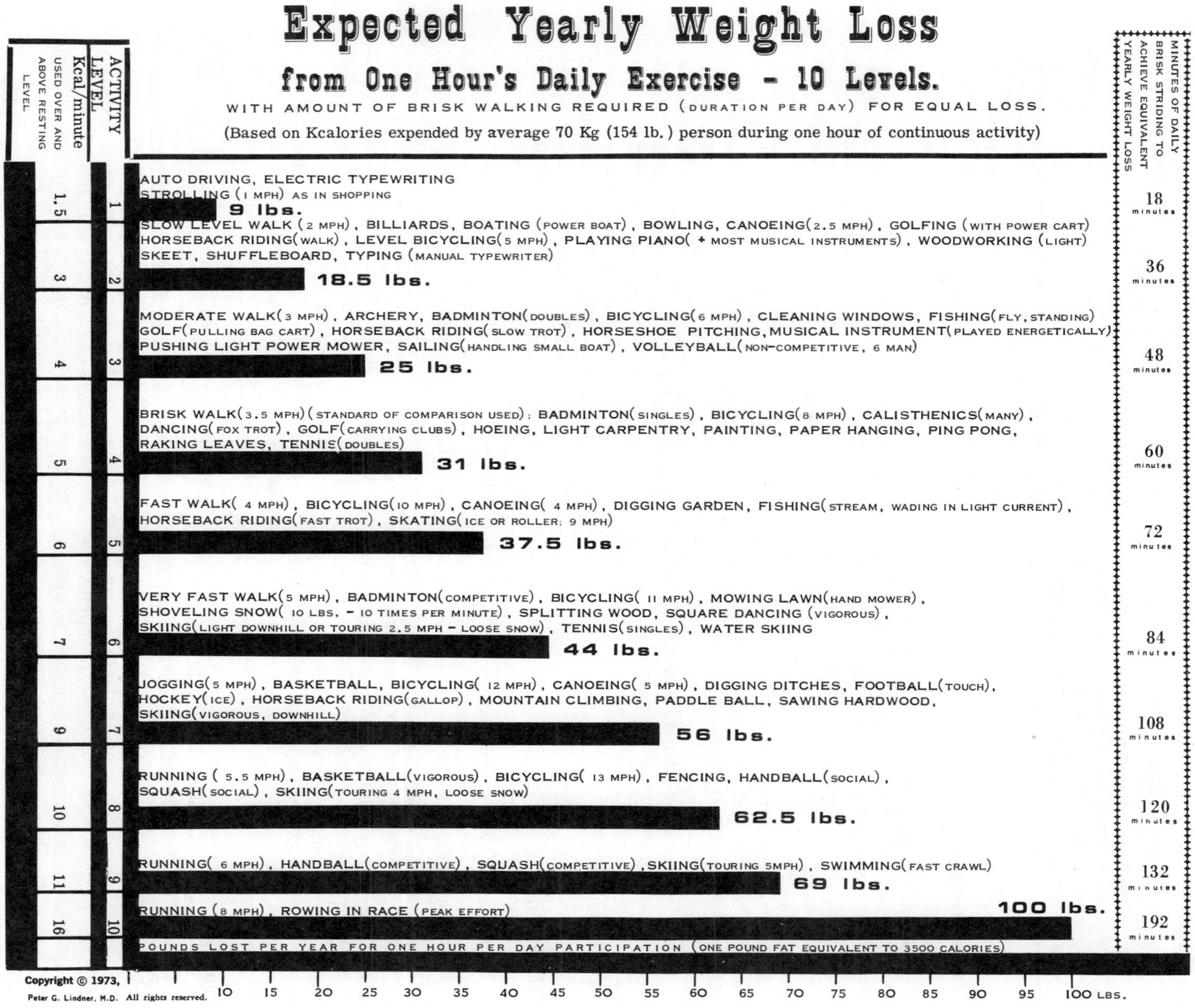

Expected Yearly Weight Loss
from One Hour's Daily Exercise – 10 Levels.

WITH AMOUNT OF BRISK WALKING REQUIRED (DURATION PER DAY) FOR EQUAL LOSS.

(Based on Kcalories expended by average 70 Kg (154 lb.) person during one hour of continuous activity)

MINUTES OF DAILY BRISK STRIDING TO ACHIEVE EQUIVALENT YEARLY WEIGHT LOSS

	minutes
	18 minutes
	36 minutes
	48 minutes
	60 minutes
	72 minutes
	84 minutes
	108 minutes
	120 minutes
	132 minutes
	192 minutes

Level 1 — 9 lbs.
AUTO DRIVING, ELECTRIC TYPEWRITING, STROLLING (1 MPH) AS IN SHOPPING

Level 2 — 18.5 lbs.
SLOW LEVEL WALK (2 MPH), BILLIARDS, BOATING (POWER BOAT), BOWLING, CANOEING (2.5 MPH), GOLFING (WITH POWER CART), HORSEBACK RIDING (WALK), LEVEL BICYCLING (5 MPH), PLAYING PIANO (+ MOST MUSICAL INSTRUMENTS), WOODWORKING (LIGHT), SKEET, SHUFFLEBOARD, TYPING (MANUAL TYPEWRITER)

Level 3 — 25 lbs.
MODERATE WALK (3 MPH), ARCHERY, BADMINTON (DOUBLES), BICYCLING (6 MPH), CLEANING WINDOWS, FISHING (FLY, STANDING), GOLF (PULLING BAG CART), HORSEBACK RIDING (SLOW TROT), HORSESHOE PITCHING, MUSICAL INSTRUMENT (PLAYED ENERGETICALLY), PUSHING LIGHT POWER MOWER, SAILING (HANDLING SMALL BOAT), VOLLEYBALL (NON-COMPETITIVE, 6 MAN)

Level 4 — 31 lbs.
BRISK WALK (3.5 MPH) (STANDARD OF COMPARISON USED), BADMINTON (SINGLES), BICYCLING (8 MPH), CALISTHENICS (MANY), DANCING (FOX TROT), GOLF (CARRYING CLUBS), HOEING, LIGHT CARPENTRY, PAINTING, PAPER HANGING, PING PONG, RAKING LEAVES, TENNIS (DOUBLES)

Level 5 — 37.5 lbs.
FAST WALK (4 MPH), BICYCLING (10 MPH), CANOEING (4 MPH), DIGGING GARDEN, FISHING (STREAM, WADING IN LIGHT CURRENT), HORSEBACK RIDING (FAST TROT), SKATING (ICE OR ROLLER: 9 MPH)

Level 6 — 44 lbs.
VERY FAST WALK (5 MPH), BADMINTON (COMPETITIVE), BICYCLING (11 MPH), MOWING LAWN (HAND MOWER), SHOVELING SNOW (10 LBS. – 10 TIMES PER MINUTE), SPLITTING WOOD, SQUARE DANCING (VIGOROUS), SKIING (LIGHT DOWNHILL OR TOURING 2.5 MPH – LOOSE SNOW), TENNIS (SINGLES), WATER SKIING

Level 7 — 56 lbs.
JOGGING (5 MPH), BASKETBALL, BICYCLING (12 MPH), CANOEING (5 MPH), DIGGING DITCHES, FOOTBALL (TOUCH), HOCKEY (ICE), HORSEBACK RIDING (GALLOP), MOUNTAIN CLIMBING, PADDLE BALL, SAWING HARDWOOD, SKIING (VIGOROUS, DOWNHILL)

Level 8 — 62.5 lbs.
RUNNING (5.5 MPH), BASKETBALL (VIGOROUS), BICYCLING (13 MPH), FENCING, HANDBALL (SOCIAL), SQUASH (SOCIAL), SKIING (TOURING 4 MPH, LOOSE SNOW)

Level 9 — 69 lbs.
RUNNING (6 MPH), HANDBALL (COMPETITIVE), SQUASH (COMPETITIVE), SKIING (TOURING 5 MPH), SWIMMING (FAST CRAWL)

Level 10 — 100 lbs.
RUNNING (8 MPH), ROWING IN RACE (PEAK EFFORT)

POUNDS LOST PER YEAR FOR ONE HOUR PER DAY PARTICIPATION (ONE POUND FAT EQUIVALENT TO 3500 CALORIES)

100 LBS. 95 90 85 80 75 70 65 60 55 50 45 40 35 30 25 20 15 10

ACTIVITY LEVEL	1	2	3	4	5	6	7	8	9	10
Kcal/minute USED OVER AND ABOVE RESTING LEVEL	1.5	3	4	5	6	7	9	10	11	16

Figure 24–2. Expected yearly weight loss from exercise. (From Asher WL: Treating the Obese. Copyright © 1974, Peter G. Lindner, M.D., reproduced by permission.)

5. Improves heart rate, circulation, breathing, and respiration.
6. Helps to maintain bone density.

The overall use of energy throughout the day is one of the most significant factors in caloric balance. Total body movement during an activity is more important than its degree of difficulty. Increasing the amount of walking and using the stairs rather than elevators are practical ways to use more kilocalories, and these habits are easy to maintain. If the exercise fits into one's lifestyle, it will more likely be repeated, while a formal exercise program is seldom continued (Brownell & Stunkard, 1980).

The obese may be easily embarrassed by routine exercise programs. They also suffer from physical strain and discomfort, so most exercise programs are eventually abandoned. Being able to achieve improved health through ideal weight seems too remote to be an effective stimulator for exercise programs. Frequent rewards, such as money or privileges, can be reinforcing. Even the recording of daily activities, feelings, and responses gives comfort and encouragement to increase confidence.

Psychological Treatment

BEHAVIOR MODIFICATION

A star was born when Richard Stuart and Barbara Davis at the University of Michigan School of Medicine began using behavioral control for overeating in 1967. Before then, almost none of the participants remained in a reduction program, and those who did immediately regained weight. Their book *Slim Chance in a Fat World* continues to be one of the leading guides to weight reduction. Behavior modification for weight control refers mainly to getting in touch with the reality of what the individual is actually eating, how much food, when, and why. Notes are taken to record food and feelings as well as the environment to understand what is occurring. Some of these techniques include:
1. Eat regularly in the same place.
2. Use smaller plates and containers.
3. Put down the utensils between each bite.
4. Do not watch television or read while eating.
5. Take at least 20 minutes to eat each meal.
6. Serve plates and store leftover food immediately to avoid returning for second helpings.

7. Buy only appropriate food to have available.
8. Arrange an attractive meal and serve it accordingly.

The most effective techniques used in behavior modification are the food, weight, and exercise records kept by the individual (Brownell & Foreyt, 1986; Johnson et al, 1986; Kayman, 1986). These records help the person to deal more directly with the weight problem, to gain new insights, and to devise strategies for dealing with it.

Another useful technique to get in touch with reality is to take a series of photographs showing weight at the beginning and during later stages of reduction (Fig. 24–3). Few overweight people have a true concept of their individual body size. When they can see themselves changing, new momentum is gained to continue on their weight reduction program.

These new self-discoveries can also demonstrate to individuals how a behavior affects themselves as well as others. For example, parents of obese children talk less to them during the meal, eat fewer meals together, and frequently watch television during meal time (Birch, 1981). Support, understanding, and praise from family and friends are also emphasized.

Among persons losing weight some generalities most often observed include (Adams et al, 1986):
1. Individuals who are more overweight tend to lose more weight.
2. The more diet programs previously tried, the less weight loss occurs.
3. Men lose weight more often in group sessions than individual sessions.
4. The more sessions attended, the greater the weight loss (but an extended number of sessions is not as influential as the frequency during one program series).
5. Eating more slowly results in greater weight loss.
6. Increasing age is associated with less weight loss.

Health Application: Prevention of Obesity

The more information gained about weight control, the more imperative preventing obesity becomes. The first step in preventing obesity is the early control of excessive weight during childhood. Ten percent of 10- to 14-year-old children are more than 20 percent over ideal weight for their age, height, and sex (Starke et al, 1981). The percentage of obese children who will become obese adults increases from 14 per-

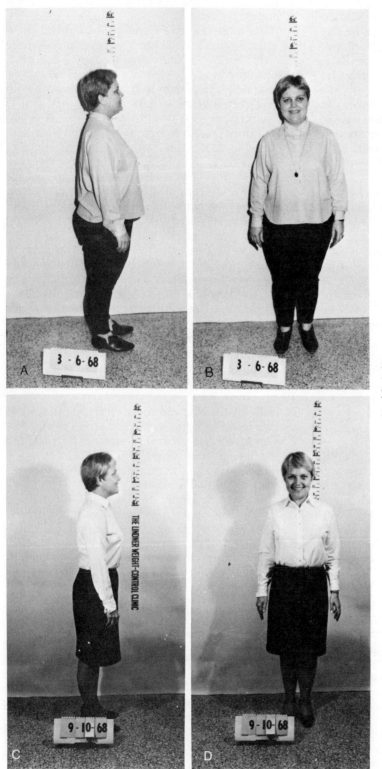

Figure 24–3. Progressive photographs enhance client's self-realization of actual weight and size and encourage further reduction. (From Asher WL: Treating the Obese. Copyright © 1974, Peter G. Lindner, M.D., reproduced by permission.)

cent during infancy (Charney et al, 1976) to 40 percent at age seven (Starke et al, 1981) and to 70 percent at ages 10 to 14 (Charney et al, 1976). The probability of an obese child attaining and maintaining normal weight as an adult is very low (Epstein et al, 1986).

Parents must be instigators of weight control among their children to avoid the problems of obesity as these children mature. Yet, most programs are geared toward weight reduction for the adult, who is less likely to be successful than the child. A problem with restricting food intake in children is that the demand for nutrients must be met to assure normal growth and development.

Many programs have been developed. A weight control program for children should utilize behavioral approaches to promote healthy eating and activity patterns (Epstein et al, 1986). Specific points for one program called Preschool Eating Patterns (PEP) include a traffic-light diet, shared exercise (usually parents walking with their children), and immediate praise for the desired behavior by hugging, verbal praising, and collecting stars for charts.

The traffic-light diet separates foods into green (go) less than 20 kcal/serving to be eaten in unlimited quantities; yellow foods (caution) are those within 20 kcal/serving; and red foods (stop) are those with more than 20 kcal/serving. Caloric limits are determined by subtracting 200 kcal/day from the child's normal intake, except that a lower limit of 900 kcal and an upper limit of 1300 kcal are set. Children can earn one star for each meal at which they avoid red foods and a bonus star if they do not eat a red food all day. Stars and praise are given after each meal.

Children are required to walk with parents six days a week with an objective of one mile per session. A star a day can be earned for their exercise chart for walking the required distance and is awarded immediately after the walk with praise.

Clinical Implications:

- Calcium and iron are most frequently below the RDAs for children on restricted diets. Choosing iron-fortified cereals and including a source of vitamin C can be useful to avoid deficiencies. Hematocrit levels rather than food records are more accurate assessments of iron levels (Epstein et al, 1986).
- Calcium levels may be maintained by carefully selecting adequate servings of allowed products high in calcium.

Surgery

A last resort for the morbidly obese is surgery. The jejunoileal bypass was the first surgical intervention developed. Because of disturbed metabolic complications in many jejunoileal bypass patients, this operation is being phased out in favor of gastric operations (Cegielski & Saporta, 1981). The four major types of gastric reduction operations are loop gastric bypass, Roux-en-Y gastric bypass, horizontal gastroplasty, and vertical banded gastroplasty (VBG) (Fig. 24–4) (Priddy, 1985). Currently, the VBG appears to be the preferred operation.

CANDIDATES

Different criteria are established to determine candidates for bypass surgery. Some physicians will perform surgery on individuals who are 100 lbs. overweight, while others require as much as 250 to 300 lbs. over normal weight. Older patients have more difficulty in adjusting to the consequences; therefore, few surgeries are performed on individuals over 50 years old.

Patients with a chronic condition, such as hypertension or diabetes mellitus, may be given a higher priority. No previous history of liver dysfunction, renal disease, serious myocardial disease, or bowel disease can be present (Miller, 1981). The person must be able to return to the physician regularly for follow-up visits for a couple of years and have close supervision by a qualified physician throughout life. Figure 24–5 shows a candidate before and after surgery.

PROGNOSIS

Such surgery always has complications, but the number and degree vary. Wound infections, incisional hernias, thrombophlebitis, hepatitis, renal failure, urinary tract infections, and cholelithiasis are frequently seen (Miller, 1981). Diarrhea is usually a complication following gastric surgery. Occasionally, these complications may require the surgery to be reversed or modified. The goal of gastric operations for morbid obesity is to return all patients to within 30 percent of ideal weight (MacLean et al, 1983). Weight loss following gastric bypass surgery results in favorable changes in

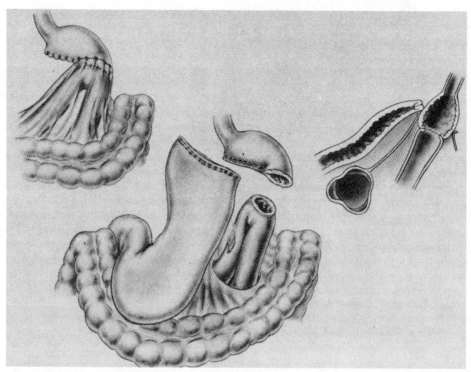

Figure 24—4. *Gastric bypass surgery. The upper pouch is small. A 2 cm opening is made along the greater curvature. The mesocolon is sutured to the stomach above the gastroenterostomy, and the proximal end of the excluded stomach is sutured to the anterior wall of the fundic pouch. (From Asher WL:* Treating the Obese. *Copyright © 1974, Peter G. Lindner, M.D., reproduced by permission.)*

lipoprotein metabolism, which may prevent or delay the development of atherosclerotic cardiovascular disease (Gonen et al, 1983).

Most subjects benefit from some psychotherapy. Behavior modification techniques start prior to surgery. If changes in eating habits are not effectuated, the small stomach pouch or the shortened intestinal tract may be stretched enough to eventually permit the client to return to the prior weight.

Not all people are happy with their new smaller bodies. Instead of having all their problems solved by weight reduction, these leaner persons are faced with new demands. More work is expected of them, more social life, more activity in general. They may not be able to handle such requests without psychological guidance.

NUTRITIONAL CARE

For stomach partitioning, the diet is restricted to liquids for the first eight weeks postoperatively. The staple line must be protected from disruption by controlling not only the consistency but also the volume of liquid and rate of ingestion

(Mojzisik & Martin, 1981). When the stomach is reduced to a pouch that holds a volume of 10 to 30 ml with a small stoma diameter of 10 to 12 mm, the patient must make drastic changes in eating behavior. A 30 ml medicine cup and a clock will help the patient realize how small a quantity can be eaten over a period of 30 minutes without drinking liquids (Priddy, 1985). A chemically defined formula may be used until regular liquids and pureed foods are tolerated.

Weight loss is very well tolerated among patients who remain normally nourished (with controlled intake). By contrast, those who become malnourished or who lose weight too rapidly after surgery are frequently found to be deficient in thiamin, folate, and vitamin B_{12}. Special attention should be given to the intakes of these nutrients.

Clinical Implications:

- Intake and output are recorded for one to three days postoperatively to assess renal function.
- Weight loss alone is not an accurate method to detect malnutrition after gastric operations. Laboratory values must be included in the assessments.

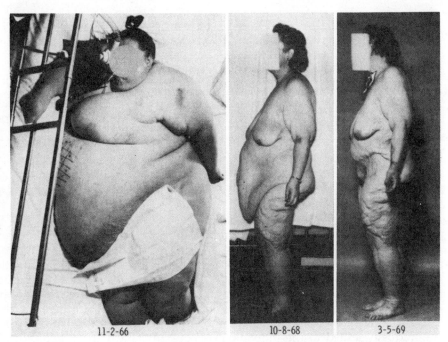

Figure 24–5. *This patient weighed more than 535 lb. and required respirator assistance for three months. Early in 1968, after her weight had been reduced to 330 lb. in the hospital, she had a gastric bypass. In 14 months, she weighed 212 lb. Her present weight is 229 lb., and she has had redundant skin removed from the lower abdomen, thighs, and arms. (From Asher WL: Treating the Obese. Copyright © 1974, Peter G. Lindner, M.D., reproduced by permission.)*

11-2-66   10-8-68   3-5-69

- Patients should be encouraged to eat foods and drink fluids high in potassium, such as oranges, potatoes, and bananas, to prevent hypokalemia.
- Patients must be cautioned to pay attention to feeling satisfied and eating moderate amounts.
- To help prevent thrombophlebitis, the legs and ankles should be rotated every two to three hours in the first 24 hours after surgery (Miller, 1981).
- Hypomagnesemia, hypokalemia, and hypocalcemia may occur immediately during the postoperative period or later. Discuss symptoms with the patient so complications can be recognized sooner.
- Malnutrition may be due to diarrheal losses or to malabsorption of nutrients. Vitamin supplements, vitamin B_{12} injections, and high-protein diets are needed for the impaired absorption of vitamins A, B_{12}, and E as well as amino acids.
- Patients often are not hungry after the small pouch replaces their normal stomach capacity. They must be cautioned about hypoglycemia and strongly encouraged to consume the chemically defined formula regularly to prevent hypoglycemia (Priddy, 1985).

BALLOON PROCEDURE

A new procedure to aid weight reduction without open surgery can be performed in about 10 minutes on an outpatient basis using local anesthesia. A flexible tube attached to a grapefruit-sized balloon is inserted through the patient's throat into the stomach. Then the balloon is inflated with air when in place and the tube removed. The floating balloon in the stomach causes a full feeling when small amounts of food are consumed (Balloon procedure, 1985).

This procedure can irritate stomach linings and has caused perforations and ulcers of the stomach and intestinal blockages. Even though the procedure is relatively simple, it should be used as a last resort, limited to patients with life-threatening morbid obesity.

Weight Gain

With so much attention given to obesity, few people recognize that there are people who need to gain weight. Underweight may be a symptom of disease and should be investigated medically. Illness may result in weight loss that should be restored.

The theory of an appestat or a set point gains favor among naturally thin individuals who cannot seem to change their weight no matter what they eat. It is as difficult for them to gain weight

Table 24–3. *Principles for Weight Gain*

1. Do not drink before a meal; minimize fluid intake with meals.
2. Include a large meal for supper and a snack before bedtime.
3. Increase the fat portion of the diet to 30 or 35 percent of total kilocalories.
4. Eat nutrient-dense foods first during a meal, then foods containing fewer calories (e.g., soup and salad).
5. Eat quickly, but chew the food well. Don't gulp the food down, but don't loiter.
6. Use sauces and gravies as well as embellishments such as nuts, olives, jams, jellies, margarine, and mayonnaise.
7. Don't engage in needless nervous activities, but exercise to stimulate appetite and build body muscle.
8. Snack frequently on energy-dense foods such as dried fruits and nuts. However, snacking should not interfere with meals.

and maintain it as it is for an obese person to lose weight without regaining it.

For thin individuals who want to gain weight, many of the tips for weight reduction can be reversed. However, the goal is to increase muscle mass as well as body fat. For this reason, exercise should be a vital part of the program. Nervous tension can utilize many calories and should be minimized as much as possible.

An allowance of 500 to 1000 kcal/day should be gradually added to the individual's caloric intake, based on present weight. The individual should ingest as much food as possible at mealtimes; supplemental feedings can be used to increase intake, but should not interfere with mealtime appetite. Other effective tips are given in Table 24–3.

Eating Disorders

"Fear of obesity" describes individuals who voluntarily restrict dietary intake because of intense social pressure against obesity but do not develop as drastic a disorder as anorexia nervosa. In children, this may result in short stature or delayed puberty. If corrected prior to fusion of the epiphyses, growth continues (Unwarranted dieting, 1984).

Many individuals go to extremes in restricting food intake. Fear of fatness is the basic core for all these eating disorders, except obesity. Such behaviors include a series of clinical syndromes with multiple variations exhibited by each individual. Females of all ages seem to be more vulnerable to these eating disorders than males. All of the syndromes may be associated with major psychiatric illnesses. Ultimately, people striving to be thin ignore most of the essential roles of nutrients; clinical deficiencies occur causing as much strife (or more) as obesity.

ANOREXIA NERVOSA

There are two basic categories of anorexia (from the Greek meaning "want of appetite") nervosa (from the Latin, meaning "nervous"). This illness appears chiefly in adolescent girls shortly after the onset of puberty. Weight loss is a result of zealous self-imposed dieting, continuing in spite of hunger, admonitions, and threats. This is frequently accompanied with excessive physical activity. Since these individuals deny that an illness exists, they will not seek professional or medical help on their own. Anorexia is not merely an illness of weight and appetite; it is a psychological problem relating to inner doubts and lack of self-confidence.

The typical anorectic may be described as a perfectionistic, achievement-oriented young woman (13 to 25 years old) who seeks to rule her life by controlling her body through refusing to eat. Compulsive behaviors may include trying to control bowel and bladder functions as well. These young women, generally surrounded with all the evidences of success, become, as Sir Richard Morton described in 1689, "skeletons only clad with skin" (Bruch, 1978), as shown in Figure 24–6.

The behavior of anorectics includes the traits listed in Table 24–4 as well as depression, diffi-

Table 24–4. *Characteristic Traits of Individuals with Anorexia Nervosa*

- Exhibit ideal behavior.
- Aways smiling.
- Rarely show anger.
- Outstanding student.
- Devoted to work and school.
- Enthusiastic athlete.
- Devise strenuous exercise schemes.
- Feelings of inferiority.
- Anxious about what others think about them.
- Lack of self-esteem.
- From upper- and middle-class backgrounds.

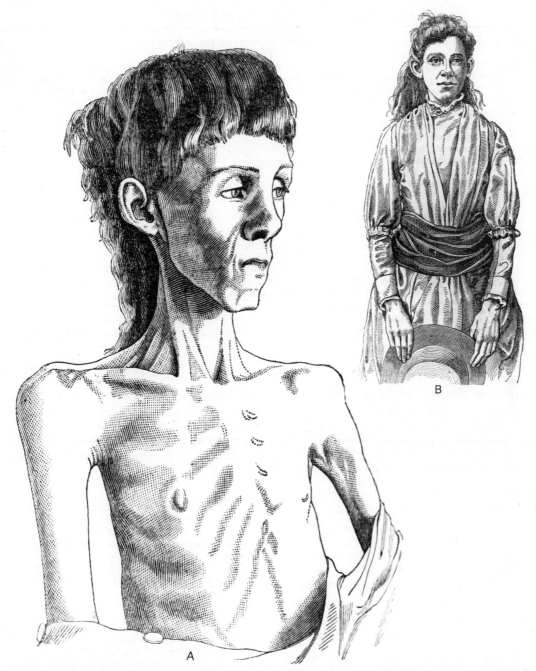

Figure 24–6. Wood engraving accompanying Sir William Gull's article "Anorexia Nervosa" in volume 1 of Lancet, 1888. A) View of young teenage girl with her emaciated chest draped with a sheet. B) The same patient recovered, six months later. (Courtesy of National Library of Medicine.)

culty in falling asleep, early morning waking, decreased pleasure in formerly enjoyable activities, amenorrhea, and decreased libido. Nearly one out of four anorectics attempt suicide, a signal of their disturbed condition (Potts, 1984). Criteria for a diagnosis of anorexia nervosa are shown in Table 24–5.

This disorder is frequently affected by family

Table 24–5. *Criteria for Diagnosis of Anorexia Nervosa**

Patients had to be between the ages of 10 and 40 and had to have had the onset of their illness between the ages of 10 and 30 years.

Patients had to have lost at least 25% of their original body weight and/or be 15% below a normal weight for their age and height (normal weights were obtained from the Metropolitan Life Insurance Policy Scales and the Iowa Growth Charts for Children).

Patients had to demonstrate a distorted attitude and behavior toward eating, food or weight which was represented by any one of the following:

a. Denial of illness with a failure to recognize nutritional needs.
b. Apparent enjoyment in losing weight.
c. A desired body image of extreme thinness.
d. Unusual hoarding or handling of food.

Patients had to have at least one of the following manifestations:

a. Lanugo (persistence of downy pelage)
b. Bradycardia (persistent resting pulse of 60 or less)
c. Hypothermia (36.1 C)
d. Periods of overactivity
e. Episodes of bulimia (compulsive overeating)
f. Vomiting (may be self-induced)

Amenorrhea of at least 3 months' duration unless illness occurs before onset of menses.

No known medical illness that could account for the anorexia and weight loss.

No other known psychiatric disorders which were excluded according to the Research Diagnostic Criteria (II). If during the course of the present illness but not prior to the present illness the patient met concurrently criteria 1 to 6 above and that of depression or of obsessive-compulsive neurosis she was considered to have anorexia nervosa.

*From Walker, J; Roberts, SL; Halmi, KA; Goldberg, SC: Caloric requirements for weight gain in anorexia nervosa. *American Journal of Clinical Nutrition* 32(7):1396, 1979. Copyright © *American Journal of Clinical Nutrition* and American Society for Clinical Nutrition, with permission.

interrelationships. Overachieving parents can influence the child's behavior in many ways. Regardless of whether the parents' goal is perfectionism in the child, a perfect child makes them look like ideal parents, which can develop into strong interdependent roles. The families are generally close-knit. Anorectics often take over the kitchen, cooking and feeding others, but not eating. They may become excellent gourmet cooks spending hours planning menus, finding special recipes, and shopping for exotic ingredients. Valuable information for health care personnel regarding these victims and their families may be found in the book *The Golden Cage* by Hilda Bruch.

BULIMIA

This eating disorder, by itself, is not associated with significant weight loss, and the individual might even be somewhat overweight. Bulimia is characterized by intentional, although not necessarily controllable, binges (periods of overeating). These are usually followed by purgation with laxatives, enemas, or vomiting (Table 24–6). However, some bulimics may severely restrict caloric intake.

Bulimics exhibit many of the same characteristics as anorectic patients, especially in their background and personality traits (Potts, 1984).

The bulimic is slightly older (18 to 29 years old) than the anorectic, is more sociable, and appears to be the ideal student, working woman, or wife. As many as 20 percent of college-age women may be affected by bulimia (Wooley & Wooley, 1982).

Table 24–6. *Diagnostic Criteria for Bulimia**

A. Recurrent eipsodes of binge eating (rapid consumption of a large amount of food in a discrete period of time, usually less than 2 hours).
B. At least three of the following:
   1. consumption of high-caloric, easily ingested food during a binge
   2. inconspicuous eating during a binge
   3. termination of such eating episodes by abdominal pain, sleep, social interruption, or self-induced vomiting, or use of cathartics or diuretics
   4. repeated attempts to lose weight by severely restrictive diets, self-induced vomiting, or use of cathartics or diuretics
   5. frequent weight fluctuations greater than 10 lb due to alternating binges and fasting
C. Awareness that the eating pattern is abnormal and fear of not being able to stop eating voluntarily.
D. Depressed mood and self-deprecating thoughts following eating binges.
E. The bulimic episodes are not due to anorexia nervosa or any known physical disorder.

*American Psychiatric Association. Diagnostic and Statistical Manual of Mental Disorders. 3rd ed. Washington, DC: APA, 1980. Reprinted with permission.

One of the problems with diagnosing bulimia is that it may occur in both men and women who are of normal weight and even in the elderly (Kirkley, 1986).

Bulimics have strong appetites and may binge several times a day with intakes ranging from 1200 to 11,500 kcal per episode. Binges usually involve a "forbidden" food—one that they believe to be high in calories. Binges may last from 15 minutes to several hours, may be planned or spontaneous, but ordinarily are related to stress (Kirkley, 1986).

These binges occur most often in the late afternoon or evening and end with self-induced vomiting—the main choice of purging (80 to 94 percent)—or laxative abuse (Potts, 1984). Vomiting may be induced by sticking a finger or other object down the throat. Some individuals apply external pressure to the neck. Eventually, most bulimics can vomit by merely contracting the abdominal muscles (Kirkley, 1986).

The bulimic has maladaptive attitudes such as a list of "bad" or fattening foods that have been eliminated from the diet. When these foods are eaten, self-control is abandoned and binging occurs. Unhappiness or emotional upsets precipitate binges since food offers the individual an immediate satisfying feeling of physical satiety and imagined feelings of being loved.

Psychological symptoms of bulimia include depression, irritability, feelings of gloom, and impaired concentration. Many bulimics also abuse alcohol and drugs. Drinking while binging reduces abdominal pain and discomfort as well as guilt. Compulsive stealing, of both food and the money to buy it, is another common characteristic (Potts, 1984).

Physiologic effects can lead not only to weight loss and dehydration, but also to more serious complications, such as urinary infections, renal failure, tetany, seizures, cardiac arrhythmias, and even death. Because of the low amount of calories available, the BMR is decreased. Frequent vomiting causes tooth enamel to erode and enlarged parotid glands, which are clinical signs of bulimia.

BULIMAREXIA

Bulimarexic individuals, while adhering to self-induced weight reduction schedules, are better able to recognize psychological problems, but may still refuse to work on the problem. Not only is the diet deficient in calories, but daily ritualistic purgation (vomiting or laxative abuse) is practiced. Anorectics who are unsuccessful at dieting may intensify their weight reduction efforts by vomiting and/or using laxatives (Wooley & Wooley, 1982).

TREATMENT

Anorexia nervosa and bulimia are primarily psychological illnesses in which bizarre eating behaviors result in serious medical consequences. Since successful treatment requires comprehensive treatment, a multidisciplinary team that addresses the psychiatric, nutritional, and medical problems is essential in promoting recovery. This team usually comprises a psychotherapist and/or psychiatrist, registered dietitian, nurses, social worker, and physician. The team must work together in avoiding replication of family dynamics, recognizing their own limitations, establishing open communications regarding patient progress, and collaborating without engaging in power struggles. This pooling of specialties provides more effective treatment as well as a support system for team members when difficult decisions are necessary or progress appears slow.

Psychological care is the most important aspect of these eating disorders. However, the patient's physiologic status must also be restored, and the person must be able to adequately control his/her eating behavior before psychological treatment is beneficial. The foundation of treatment includes outpatient psychotherapy utilizing individual, family, and group modalities. These modalities, tailored to individual needs, promote resolution of the underlying issues of identity, self-esteem, control, individuation, assertiveness, intimacy, conflict resolution, and perfectionism. Psychotropic medications can be helpful when mood fluctuations stem from biochemical abnormalities. Medical supervision is essential to determine the need for hospitalization, detect and treat intercurrent illness, and minimize health risks during outpatient treatment.

When patients are a danger to themselves or if their medical or psychiatric condition makes outpatient treatment ineffective, hospitalization is appropriate. The decision for hospitalization should include the patient, if at all possible. Upon admission, the patient's medical condition is evaluated and stabilized, followed by a nutritional assessment and development of a plan of care. Baseline data should include electrolyte abnormalities, electrocardiogram, blood pressure, and dentition. Daily monitoring may include weights, electrolytes, acid-base balance, liver enzymes, hematologic abnormalities, and mental acuity (Sanger & Cassino, 1984). Hospitalization time is kept to a minimum (one to two months). Once the patient is stabilized and nutritionally rehabilitated, outpatient therapy can be resumed.

Documentation of current weight and caloric intake is the most potent reinforcement in treating hospitalized anorectics (Agras et al, 1974). Realization of body size before and after weight reduction is extremely difficult. Photographs can assist the person to get in touch with his/her own physical reality.

While mortality is about 10 percent, periods of painful isolation and chronic invalidism persist through life (Bruch, 1978). The abnormal behaviors of bulimics may be improved by treatment; however, they are rarely given up completely (Smead, 1984).

NUTRITIONAL GOALS AND THERAPY

Major nutritional goals are refeeding for weight gain and normalization of eating habits. Additional goals are healthy family interactions concerning food, comfort in social eating, and ability to maintain weight within a safe range. Principles for dietary regimens are given in Table 24–7.

Nutritional counseling is an important part of therapy to correct nutritional beliefs and eating behavior. Food behaviors are entrenched as a result of the abnormal food behaviors exercised over an extended period of time and inability of the patient to differentiate food and nutrition truths from myths. While these subjects are aware of the caloric value of food, they do not understand the relationship between calories and nutrients for health and how to balance caloric intake with expenditure. Their false beliefs must be challenged by factual information. The registered dietitian is the most qualified person on the team to facilitate the patient's return to normal and healthy eating patterns. A dietitian generally provides patient counseling and education on topics such as normal nutrition and weight maintenance. Counseling should also involve the whole family by examining the eating patterns of each household member and the topics of conversation at mealtime.

In order to better understand the patient, a thorough diet history must be obtained, noting self-medicating practices (laxatives, over-the-counter diet aides, and caffeine), exercise routines, and unusual eating rituals.

Methods of accomplishing refeeding are individualized. During the initial recovery phase, the method of intake should try to minimize gastrointestinal disturbances. Options for renutrition include a regular diet, use of oral supplements (alone or in combination with food intake), tube feedings, or total parenteral nutrition. Considerable support from the dietitian and nurse is necessary to ease the transition from intravenous feedings in the hospital to supporting new eating patterns in an outpatient setting. Initially, a total liquid diet formula may serve a valuable purpose since the patient may consider this a medication or a low-calorie food and be more receptive to it (Claggett, 1980).

Goals for weight gain are established, usually an increase of ¼ lb./day or 1 kg (2.2 lbs.) weekly. The dehydration accompanying anorexia causes water retention and often edema when the strict dieting regime is broken (Wooley & Wooley, 1982). (Many patients become fearful that this weight gain is fat tissue.) Following initial weight gain, weight will plateau or drop as edematous fluid is lost prior to a steady, continuous rise in weight.

For accurate measurements, body weights are taken at the same time each day with the patient dressed in a hospital gown. Expectations of excessive weight gain or harsh punishments are ineffective.

Behavior modification techniques are generally unsuccessful. In some instances, they can be inappropriately coercive and are counterproduc-

---

Table 24–7. *Diet Principles for Patients with Anorexia Nervosa and Bulimia*

1. Encourage gradual increase in total caloric intake while maintaining a balanced intake of nutrients.
2. A specific set of dietary guidelines helps the patient maintain a feeling of control and assurance of adequate nutrition without weight gain.
3. Regularity in dietary habits should be encouraged to maintain weight stability and to minimize the likelihood of eating binges or long periods of fasting.
4. Diet information should specify appropriate quantities of food necessary for weight maintenance.

tive if someone else's will is imposed upon the patient.

Nursing staff or dietetic technicians maintain calorie counts to monitor intake. Because these patients are devious, close attention must be given to determine that food is actually eaten. Following feedings, patients may spend up to an hour in a social setting to reduce the chance of self-induced vomiting. A vital part of nutritional care involves teaching distractive activities to use when the desire to binge occurs. Walking, exercising, relaxation procedures, or talking to a friend may be effective strategies.

The current trend in treatment is to allow the patient to be in control of the food eaten and the subsequent weight gain. Rewards are personal privileges including use of television, telephone, or visitors.

Because of the reappearance of old eating patterns when hospitalized anorectics are fed family style, patients initially eat alone in their room with 30 minutes allowed for breakfast and 45 minutes each for lunch and dinner. However, total isolation may contribute to depression. When the patient progresses, dining room privileges are granted (Sanger & Cassini, 1984).

While food attitudes may be distorted in these patients, these patients have a higher percentage of food dislikes. These are related to differences in taste function. Taste sensations in the anorectic are altered because of zinc and copper deficiency. Normal acuity returns when eating patterns are normalized (Casper et al, 1980).

Clinical Implications:

- The minimum amount of weight required for rational thinking is about 90 lbs. for most teenage girls. This weight goal must first be achieved before psychological therapy is effective (Bruch, 1978).
- Lifesaving techniques such as hyperalimentation may help the patient feel less guilty about gaining weight, although solid food should be offered as well. Nutrient-dense beverages and foods are wise choices.
- Preparation of a meal considering patients' food preferences is better than asking them to do it, since they often bog down in trivial details.
- Ask patients questions and listen carefully to the answers. Do not overtly discuss making decisions for them even though you may be doing that.
- Do *not* trust anorectic or bulimic patients; monitor them closely at mealtime. They are fre-

quently guilty of (1) throwing away food but reporting they ate it, (2) vomiting when left alone, and (3) lying in order to be left alone.
- Treat each patient as an individual. All anorectics have their unique set of problems and beliefs. Improvement requires recognition by the person of being a unique, worthwhile individual.
- Bulimia is to be suspected in cases of unexplained poor control of diabetes; young diabetic women have frequently been known to skip their insulin treatments in order to binge and then purge (Hudson et al, 1983).
- As energy intake increases to a normal level, BMR also increases to a physiologically normal level so that weight gain may not be as significant as anticipated.
- Use of ipecac, an over-the-counter product that induces vomiting, may cause serious chronic medical complications and even death (primarily from the absorption of its principal alkaloid emetine). Reversible myopathy has been reported in bulimics with long-term abuse of ipecac (Palmer & Guay, 1985).
- Dieting is incompatible with bulimia because it can lead to binging and purging.

• FALLACIES and FACTS

FALLACY: *A remarkable natural food supplement, starch blockers, permits dieters to eat carbohydrate-rich foods without weight gain.*

• **FACT:** *Starch blockers is the popular name for the alpha-amylase inhibitors isolated from wheat or legumes (also known as phaseolin). However, this dieter's dream did not come true. These substances do not block starch digestion and, in addition, may contain enzymes that impair the uptake of nutrients in other ways. If they did block digestion of dietary starch, severe symptoms of gastrointestinal carbohydrate intolerance (flatulence and diarrhea) would occur. Besides, carbohydrates are essential to human metabolism (Hollenbeck et al, 1983; Starch blockers, 1985).*

FALLACY: *The larger a person is, the more food s/he needs.*

• **FACT:** *This is not necessarily true. While fat must have energy supplies, it does not burn energy like muscle tissue. Most of the time, the person is just not as active* *(by one sixth to one third as much). Those who are up to 30 percent overweight do not usually eat more than thinner people. This is the rule, not the exception (Stunkard, 1980).*

FALLACY: *If a child is obese, s/he should be required to follow a strict diet.*

• **FACT:** *Children are still growing and should not be severely limited in food intake because important nutrients may not be present in sufficient quantities. More physical activity is encouraged. Low nutrient density foods should be discouraged. Obese children should be checked for cholesterol and triglycerides to institute ambitious dietary regimens to reduce hyperlipidemia without severe kilocalorie restrictions.*

FALLACY: *The faster weight is lost, the better.*

• **FACT:** *Weight loss should not ordinarily be more than 1 to 2 lbs./week. Dramatic weight loss should be investigated. Sudden death has resulted from prolonged use of extremely low-calorie diets (approximately 300 to 400 kcal/day). Ventricular arrhythmias occurred after an average of five months using these diets, which were almost entirely protein (Sours et al, 1981).*

FALLACY: *The Zen macrobiotic diet can be used if you train your body to go through it step-by-step.*

• **FACT:** *The human body has its own metabolism that cannot be redesigned by whim. Necessary nutrients to sustain life are lacking in this diet, and death may be the ultimate result. The steps of eliminating foods to allow only brown rice and tea are not feasible to sustain life (Blackburn & Pavlou, 1983).*

FALLACY: *When the body goes into ketosis, fat is broken down into ketones and excreted as unused calories in the urine.*

• **FACT:** *The caloric value of these excreted ketones very rarely exceeds 100 kcal/day, so its contribution to weight loss is negligible. Water is lost; weight increases as soon as the diet is stopped owing to normal fluid retention (Blackburn & Pavlou, 1983).*

FALLACY: *Eating one meal a day, preferably at night, is a good way to lose weight.*

• **FACT:** *All the nutrients required for one day cannot be eaten in one meal. This is not*

healthy, and it could result in even more weight gain.

Summary

Obesity is a complex problem that causes great pain, misery, and ill-health. It is not a matter for jokes or ridicule. Obesity must be regarded as life-threatening. Being well-informed about obesity is most important to all people, whether fat or thin, because everyone has contact with someone who suffers from this problem, if not themselves.

Prevention of obesity begins early in life. Overfeeding young children and/or teenagers leads to increased numbers of fat cells (hyperplasia) throughout life. Excessive food intake later in life leads to increased size of fat cells (hypertrophy). The main emphasis for weight control should be prevention rather than cure.

Exercise is imperative, not merely physical exercise such as games and sports but being more active throughout the day. Most obese persons do not eat more than their lean counterparts but are less active.

Particularly with younger people, treatment should include reinforcement of positive behaviors, better grooming, and attempts to improve social skills. Psychological therapy for better self-understanding can produce excellent results for weight control as well as fuller, happier lives for all ages.

Food choices for recognized nutrition goals and desired weight are far more exciting than rigid dietary restrictions. Education is imperative to understand the importance of food to the body. The reinforcement of praise or love with candy, for example, should be discontinued and replaced with genuine caring. The dinner table should be recovered from the television trays and individual pursuits in order to introduce family and friends to the joy of fellowship and conversation that complements a delicious meal.

Review Questions

1. Outline a discussion with the mother of an obese child for future guidelines to achieve normal weight.

2. List some ways your friends might sabotage your reduction program if you were trying to lose weight.
3. Offer some tactics for persons to use as defense against such behavior.
4. Plan a 1200 kcal/day diet for a woman who works outside the home.
5. Suggest activities for persons 10, 25, 50, and 70 years old to lose 1 lb./week.
6. Utilizing a typical restaurant menu, tell how to keep the kilocalorie count down while participating in a dinner with friends.
7. Discuss techniques and behavior to be used by nurses while dealing with anorectics.

Case Study: Mrs. J. T. is a 38-year-old homemaker who has been referred for diet counseling. Her height is 156 cm and her current weight is 127 kg. She has been overweight since childhood and has tried a variety of diets with varying degrees of success; however, the weight loss has never been maintained. She states that with four children, two of whom are teenagers, it is difficult to cook low-calorie meals. She enjoys cooking and seems to spend much of her time involved with meal preparation.

Over the past two years, she has been less active and has been snacking throughout the day. She is frustrated by her weight problem and concerned about her health after hypertension was diagnosed at her latest physical examination.
1. Differentiate between juvenile and adult-onset obesity. Which is easier to treat?
2. What should be Mrs. J. T.'s ideal body weight for a medium frame?
3. What type of data do you need to collect for a nutritional assessment of this patient?
4. What nursing diagnoses can be developed for this patient? Identify appropriate goals.
5. Determine Mrs. J. T.'s daily caloric needs.
6. Outline a diet plan for one day for Mrs. J. T.
7. What complications are frequently found among patients who are chronically obese?

Case Study: Sally T. has been brought to the physician's office by her parents. She is 14 years old and a freshman in a private high school. Her parents are concerned about her weight loss over the past 15 months. She has lost 12 kg and has been progressively preoccupied with weight loss and food. They have also observed increasing irritability and resistance to their attempts to increase her food intake.

On examination, the physician notes brittle nails, dry skin and hair, subnormal temperature, and muscle wasting. She has experienced amenorrhea for the past five months. Her current height is 163 cm and her weight is 42 kg.

Both of Sally's parents teach at a local university and her older brother is a sophomore at a military academy. The family members are hard-working, disciplined, and achievement-oriented.

Sally states that she doesn't understand why everyone is so concerned about her weight because she still needs to lose a few more pounds.
1. Sally has a medium body frame. What is her ideal weight?
2. What signs of malnutrition are present?
3. What nursing diagnoses can you develop from this situation? List goals appropriate for each diagnosis.
4. The parents ask for a psychiatric referral for Sally; the physician states that therapy for Sally alone will not be effective. Why does the physician encourage family therapy?

Case Study: Shanna P. is a 13-year-old who was brought to the physician's office for a yearly physical examination. Her weight at this time is 90.7 kg and height is 174.8 cm.

Questions by the nurse indicate that Shanna has always been overweight but has gained approximately 25 lbs. since starting junior high school. She is a finicky eater and refuses many meat and vegetables dishes. She does not exercise except in physical education class and spends most of her time at home watching television. All lab work was normal, but her blood pressure was elevated (130/88).

Exogenous obesity with hypertension is diagnosed and the patient and her family are referred for dietary counseling.
1. Why are the early adolescent years so important for weight?
2. What other times in the life cycle is excess weight a particular problem?
3. What factors have prompted the development of this child's obesity?
4. What should she weigh?
5. What tentative nursing diagnoses could you develop?
6. List goals for this patient.
7. Develop a diet plan in your nursing care plan for Shanna.

REFERENCES

Adams, SO; Grady, KE; Wolk, CH; et al: Weight loss: A comparison of group and individual interventions. *J Am Diet Assoc* 86(4):485, 1986.

Agras, WS; Barlow, DH; Chapin, HN; et al: Behavior modification of anorexia nervosa. *Arch Gen Psychiatr* 30(March):279, 1974.

Anderson, L; Isaacson, PR; Jackson, TW; et al: Slow vs rapid weight loss programs. *Obesity Bariatr Med* 1(October/December):118, 1982.

Ashley, DVM; Fleury, MO; Golay, A; et al: Evidence for diminished brain 5-hydroxytryptamine biosynthesis in obese diabetic and non-diabetic humans. *Am J Clin Nutr* 42(December):1240, 1985.

Balloon procedure gives patients nonsurgical option for weight loss. *Hospitals* 59(December 1):48, 1985.

Barlow, DH; Tillotson, JL: Behavioral science and nutrition: A new perspective. *J Am Diet Assoc* 72(4):368, 1978.

Bennett, W; Gurin, J: Do diets really work? *Science* March:42, 1982.

Birch, LL; Marlin, LL; Kramer, L; et al: Mother-child interaction patterns and the degree of fatness in children. *J Nutr Ed* 13(2):17, 1981.

Blackburn, GL; Pavlou, K: Fad reducing diets: Separating fads from facts. *Contemporary Nutr* 8(7), 1983.

Blundell, JE; Hill, AJ: Paradoxical effects of an intense sweetener (aspartame) on appetite. *Lancet* 1(May 10):1092, 1986.

Brownell, KD: Behavioral and metabolic aspects of weight loss and gain. Presented at the American Dietetic Association Convention, Las Vegas, 1986.

Brownell, KD; Foreyt, JP: *Handbook of Eating Disorders: Physiology, Psychology and Treatment.* New York, Basic Books, 1986.

Brownell, KD; Stunkard, AJ: Physical exercise in the development and control of obesity. In *Obesity.* Edited by AJ Stunkard. Philadelphia, W.B. Saunders Co, 1980.

Bruch, H: *The Golden Cage: The Enigma of Anorexia Nervosa.* New York, Vintage Books, 1978.

Burton, BT; Foster, WR: Health implications of obesity: An NIH consensus development conference. *J Am Diet Assoc* 85(9):1117, 1985.

Casper, RC; Eckert, ED; Halmi, KA; et al: Bulimia: Its incidence and clinical importance in patients with anorexia nervosa. *Arch Gen Psychiatr* 37(9):1030, 1980.

Casse, RM: Tracy, GS: The physiological benefits of weight loss: A review of 92 patients in a private practice. *Obesity Bariatr Med* 12(April–June):48, 1983.

Cegielski, MM; Saporta, JA: Surgical treatment of morbid obesity: An update. *Obesity Bariatr Med* 10(March–April):44, 1981.

Charney, M; Goodman, HC; McBride, M; et al: Childhood antecedents of adult obesity: Do chubby infants become obese adults? *N Engl J Med* 295:6, 1976.

Claggett, MS: Anorexia nervosa: A behavioral approach. *Am J Nurs* 80(8):1471, 1980.

Epstein, LH; Valoski, A; Koeske, R; et al: Family-based behavioral weight control in obese young children. *J Am Diet Assoc* 86(4):481, 1986.

Felig, P: Very-low-calorie protein diets. *N Engl J Med* 310(March):589, 1984.

Fisher, MC; Lachance, PA: Nutrition evaluation of published weight-reducing diets. *J Am Diet Assoc* 85(4):450, 1985.

Foreyt, JP; Reeves, RS; Darnell, LS; et al: Soup consumption as a behavioral weight loss strategy. *J Am Diet Assoc* 86(4):524, 1986.

Gannon, MA; Mitchell, JE: Subjective evaluation of treatment methods by patients treated for bulimia. *J Am Diet Assoc* 86(4):520, 1986.

Glasser, W: *Positive Addiction.* New York, Harper & Row, 1976.

Gonen, B; Halverson, JD; Schonfeld, G: Lipoprotein-induced weight loss. *Metabolism* 32(5):492, 1983.

Gonzalez, ER: Studies show the obese may prefer fats to sweets. *JAMA* 250(7):579, 1983.

Grinker, J: Behavioral and metabolic consequences of weight reduction. *J Am Diet Assoc* 62(1):30, 1973.

Hollenbeck, C; Coulston, AM; Quan, R; et al: Effects of a commercial starch blocker preparation on carbohydrate diges-tion and absorption: in vivo and in vitro studies. *Am J Clin Nutr* 38(4):498, 1983.

Hudson, MS; Wentworth, SM; Hudson, JI: Bulimia and diabetes. *N Engl J Med* 309(7):431, 1983.

Johnson, KM; Dyer, JR; Hyg, MS; et al: Food records: A predictor of weight change in a long-term weight loss program. Presented at the American Dietetic Association Convention, Las Vegas, 1986.

Kayman, S: Maintaining weight loss—what works and what doesn't. Presented at the American Dietetic Association Convention, Las Vegas, 1986.

Kirkley, BG: Bulimia: Clinical characteristics, development, and etiology. *J Am Diet Assoc* 86(4):468, 1986.

Lindner, PG; Bistrian, BR; Gray, GA; et al: Roundtable: The great diet debate. *Obesity Bariatr Med* 10(May–June):72, 1981.

MacLean, LD; Rhode, BM; Shizgall HM: Nutrition following gastric operations for morbid obesity. *Ann Surg* 197(3):347, 1983.

Miller, BK: Jejunoileal bypass: A drastic weight control measure. *Am J Nurs* 81(3):564, 1981.

Mojzisik, CM; Martin, EW, Jr: Gastric partitioning: The latest surgical means to control morbid obesity. *Am J Nurs* 81(3):569, 1981.

Palmer, EP; Guay, AT: Reversible myopathy secondary to abuse of ipecac in patients with major eating disorders. *N Engl J Med* 313 (November 28):1457, 1985.

Porikos, K; Hesser, M; Van Itallie, T: Caloric regulation in normal-weight men maintained on a palatable diet of conventional foods. *Physio Behav* 29(2):293, 1982.

Potts, N: Eating disorders—the secret pattern of binge/purge. *Am J Nurs* 84(1):32, 1984.

Priddy, ML: Gastric reduction surgery: A dietitian's experience and perspective. *J Am Diet Assoc* 85(4):455, 1985.

Russ, CS; Ciavarella, PA; Atkinson, RL: A comprehensive outpatient weight reduction program: Dietary patterns, psychological considerations, and treatment principles. *J Am Diet Assoc* 84(4):444, 1984.

Sanger, E; Cassino, T: Eating disorders: Avoiding the power struggle. *Am J Nurs* 84(1):31, 1984.

Shapiro, LR; Crawford, PB; Clark, MJ; et al: Obesity prognosis: A longitudinal study of children from the age of 6 months to 9 years. *Am J Public Health* 74(9):968, 1984.

Smead, VS: Eating behaviors which may lead to and perpetuate anorexia nervosa, bulimarexia, and bulimia. *Women and Therapy* 3(2):37, 1984.

Sours, HE; Frattali, VP; Brand, CD; et al: Sudden death associated with very low calorie weight reduction regimens. *Am J Clin Nutr* 34(4):453, 1981.

Starch blockers do not block starch digestion. *Nutr Rev* 43(2):46, 1985.

Starke, D; Atkins, E; Wolff, DH; et al: Longitudinal study of obesity in the National Survey of Health and Development. *Br Med J* 283:12, 1981.

Story, M: Nutrition management and dietary treatment of bulimia. *J Am Diet Assoc* 86(4):517, 1986.

Stunkard, AJ: *The Pain of Obesity.* Palo Alto, CA, Bull Publishing Co, 1976.

Stunkard, AJ (ed): *Obesity.* Philadelphia, W.B. Saunders Co, 1980.

Unwarranted dieting retards growth and delays puberty. *Nutr Rev* 42(1):14, 1984.

Wadden, TA; Stunkard, AJ; Brownell, DK; et al: The Cambridge diet. More mayhem? *JAMA* 250(20):2833, 1983.

Walker, J; Roberts, SL; Halmi, KA; et al: Caloric requirements for weight gain in anorexia nervosa. *Am J Clin Nutr* 33(7):1396, 1979.

Wing, RR; Jeffrey, RW: Outpatient treatment of obesity: A comparison of methodology and clinical results. *Int J Obesity* 3:261, 1979.

Winick, M (ed): *Childhood Obesity*. New York, John Wiley & Sons, 1975.

Wooley, OW; Wooley, S: The Beverly Hills eating disorder. The mass marketing of anorexia nervosa. *Int J Eating Disorders* 1(1):57, 1982.

Wurtman, JJ: Obesity and the brain: A carbohydrate connection. *Prof Nutritionist* 15(spring):1, 1983.

Wurtman, RJ: Aspartame: Possible effect on seizure susceptibility. *Lancet* 2(October 5):1060, 1985.

Wurtman, RJ; Wurtman, JJ: Nutrients, neuro-transmitter synthesis, and the control of food intake. In *Eating and Its Disorders*. Edited by AJ Stunkard; E Stellar. New York, Raven Press, 1984.

Further Study

Brown, EK; Settle, EA; Van Rij, AM: Food intake patterns of gastric bypass patients. *J Am Diet Assoc* 80(5):437, 1982.

Bruch, H: *Eating Disorders: Obesity, Anorexia Nervosa and the Person Within*. New York, Basic Books, 1973.

Colvin, RH; Zopf, KJ; Myers, JH: Weight control among co-workers. Effects of monetary contingencies and social milieu. *Behav Modif* 7(1):64, 1983.

Dalvit-McPhillips, S: A dietary approach to bulimia treatment. *Physiol Behav* 33:769, 1984.

Fairburn, CA: A cognitive behavior approach to the treatment of bulimia. *Psychol Med* 11:707, 1981.

Farrell, MS; Layton, FF; Tervo, RC: Preventing obesity in spina bifida. *J Can Diet Assoc* 42(April):160, 1981.

Fenner, L: Cellulite: Hard to budge pudge. HHS Publ. No. (FDA) 80-1078, reprinted from *FDA Consumer*, May 1980.

Forbes, GB; Kreipe, RE; Lipinski, BA; et al: Body composition changes during recovery from anorexia nervosa: A comparison of two dietary regimes. *Am J Clin Nutr* 40(6):1137, 1984.

Garner, DM; Garfinkel, PE; Bemis, KM: A multi-dimensional psychotherapy for anorexia nervosa. *Int J Eating Disorders* 1(2):3, 1981.

Herzog, DB: Bulimia: Idiosyncrasy or psychiatric disorder? *Am J Nurs* 85(5):526, 1985.

Kirkley, BG; Agras, WS; Weiss, JJ: Nutritional inadequacy in the diets of treated bulimics. *Behav Therapy* 16:287, 1985.

LeShan, EJ: *Winning the Losing Battle. Why I Will Never Be Fat Again*. New York, Thomas Y. Crowell, 1979.

Lindner, PG; Bistrian, BR; Gray, GA; et al: Roundtable: The great diet debate. *Obesity Bariatr Med* 10(March–April):36, 1981.

Orr, J: Obesity. *J Adv Nurs* 10(1):71, 1985.

Polydextrose—new ingredient for reduced-calorie foods. *Food Eng* 53(6):140, 1980.

Rotatori, AF; Fox, R: *Behavioral Weight Reduction Program for Mentally Handicapped Persons*. Baltimore, MD, University Park Press, 1981.

Schwartz, RC: Barrett, MJ; Saba, G: Family therapy for bulimia. In *Anorexia Nervosa and Bulimia*. Edited by DM Garner; PE Garfinkel. New York, Guilford Press, 1985.

Stuart, RB: *Act Thin, Stay Thin*. New York, WW Norton, 1978.

Stuart, RB; Davis, B: *Slim Chance in a Fat World*. Champaign, IL, Research Press Company, 1972.

Trubo, R: Fad diets: Unqualified hunger for miracles. *Medical World News* 27(August 11):44, 1986.

Van Itallie, TB; Karl, JG: The dilemma of morbid obesity. *JAMA* 246(9):999, 1981.

Willis, J: About body wraps, pills and other magic wands for losing weight. HHS Publ. No. (FDA) 83-1096, reprinted from *FDA Consumer*, November 1982.

Resources

Boock, CA; Lowe, M: *Nutritional Guidelines Following Gastric Bypass Surgery*. Available (for a small charge) from:

Nutritional Services Dept of Milwaukee County Medical Complex, Box 127, 8700 W. Wisconsin Ave., Milwaukee, WI 53226.

Cancer Patients: Nutritional Support

25

THE STUDENT WILL BE ABLE TO:

- *Discuss the role of nutrition in the cancer patient.*
- *List common food aversions and suggest ways to enhance foods.*
- *Calculate the appropriate prescription for a dietary supplement.*
- *Describe dental and mouth hygiene.*
- *Suggest ways that the family and friends can care for the patient.*
- *List patient care to be handled by various medical team members.*

OBJECTIVES

Cacogeusia
Chemotherapy
Dysgeusia
Dysphagia
Heterogeusia
Hyposmia
Immunotherapy
Nitrogen trap
Pedal (pitting) edema
Phantogeusia
Protein-energy malnutrition (PEM)
Radiation
Xerostomia

TERMS TO KNOW

Prevalence of Cancer

How prevalent is cancer? Is the treatment different from other health problems? Why is the nurse one of the star performers on this medical team?

- Cancer will strike one in every three Americans (Trester, 1982).
- Cancer causes one out of every five deaths in the United States.
- Cancer kills more children 3 to 14 years of age than any other disease (American Cancer Society, 1985).

This year, more than eight million people around the world will discover that they have cancer. Almost seven million people die of this disease each year. Of those diagnosed with cancer in the United States, 45 percent can expect to live at least five years after treatment and 86 percent of that group can expect to live 20 years (Grundy, 1984).

Health Application: Cancer Prevention

Because of the extensive publicity studies indicating that certain kinds of cancers may have a dietary component, many Americans are "running scared," fearful that everything they put into their mouths may be carcinogenic. Can what we eat reduce or increase our chances of developing cancer? Unfortunately, that question is not simple to answer; cancer is not one disease, but a complex array of disorders with different etiologies and treatments. Epidemiology teaches coincidence; it does not teach cause and effect. However, epidemiological surveys indicate 60 percent of all cancers in women and 40 percent in men are associated with diet (Erickson, 1984).

Certain dietary factors are known carcinogens (such as aflatoxins); others are precarcinogens (such as nitrites). Approximately 16 naturally-occurring carcinogens have been identified in foods. This does not mean that if any of these items are eaten, a person will develop cancer. Normally, the body has mechanisms to cope with these substances; some dietary factors are natural inhibitors of carcinogenesis, such as the cruciferous vegetables.

It is presently thought that many dietary factors do not initiate cancer but instead act during the promotional stage of carcinogenesis as a modifier. Many studies implicate dietary fat as a promoter of carcinogenesis, although the mechanism is unknown.

Free radicals are potentially very destructive molecules that can damage the genetic material of cells. Damage from free radicals is thought to initiate and promote many cancers. Vitamin E interferes with this chain reaction of free radicals and may be a deterrent to carcinogenesis.

To live means we must eat. No one food has been identified that specifically causes cancer; if so, it would be banned from the food supply. It is the interaction of many different dietary factors that must be considered in assessing cancer risk. While certain nutrients have been implicated as the cause of tumors in specific areas, most individuals wish to avoid all types of cancer. In an effort to help Americans lower cancer risk, the American Cancer Society (1984) has issued the guidelines shown in Table 25–1. While scientific studies implicate many dietary factors in preventing cancer, vitamins A, C, and E and fiber are specifically beneficial; others are questionable and should be avoided, specifically alcohol and fat.

Although these guidelines cannot guarantee a reduction of cancer and are therefore rather controversial, they are consistent with good nutritional practices and are likely to reduce the risk of cancer. When a variety of foods is eaten, each contributes something the others lack. Figure 25–1 converts these guidelines into a practical plan for selecting foods.

Effects on Nutritional Status

Cancer, which is a multifaceted disease process, has no simple cause or cure. Rapidly-growing cell tissue competes with the host and deprives it of needed nutrients. The malignant tumor often parasitizes the host to meet unusual nutrient requirements. Cancer can be treated by surgical procedures, radiation therapy, chemotherapy, and immunotherapy. These therapies, used individually or in combination, affect some of the normal body cells as cancer cells are destroyed. Nutritional problems result from all therapies used to treat cancer as well as from the competition of the tumor tissue for nutrients. Nutritional status of the cancer patient is an important component within the interdisciplinary treatment plan. However, improved nutrition may be accompanied by increased tumor growth; therefore, it should be coordinated with one or more cancer therapies.

A comprehensive cancer treatment center must also provide three categories of nutritional

Table 25–1. Dietary Measures to Reduce Cancer Risk

1. Avoid obesity. Individuals 40 percent or more overweight increase their risk of colon, breast, prostate, gallbladder, ovary, and uterine cancers.

2. Cut down on total fat intake. A diet high in fat may be a factor in the development of certain cancers, particularly breast, uterus, colon, and prostate cancers.

3. Eat more high-fiber foods such as whole-grain cereals, fruits, vegetables. Diets high in fiber may help to reduce the risk of colon cancer.

4. Include foods rich in vitamins A and C daily. These foods may help lower the risk especially for cancers of the larynx, esophagus, stomach and the lung. They may protect against all types of cancer.

5. Include cruciferous vegetables in your diet. Cruciferous vegetables (e.g., Brussels sprouts, cauliflower, cabbage, and broccoli) have flowers with 4 leaves in the pattern of a cross. These vegetables apparently have their own unique protective characteristics, especially in the GI and respiratory tracts.

6. Eat moderately of salted, smoked and nitrate-cured foods. There is more incidence of cancer of the esophagus and stomach in areas of the world where these foods are eaten frequently. Vitamin C prevents the formation of carcinogens from nitrates and proteins; a source of vitamin C is advisable when nitrate-cured products are eaten. One should eat charcoal-grilled foods less often for the same reasons.

Liquid smoke can be used to replace hickory-smoked methods of cooking.

7. Keep alcohol consumption moderate, if you do drink. The heavy use of alcohol, especially when accompanied by cigarette smoking or smokeless tobacco, increases risk of cancers of the mouth, larynx, throat, esophagus, and liver.

*Adapted from American Cancer Society: Cancer Facts and Figures. New York, American Cancer Society, Inc, 1985.

care: (1) preventive care for those capable of maintaining their weight and of generally good nutritional status; (2) maintenance care for those undergoing aggressive chemotherapy, radiotherapy, or combined therapy with problems of anorexia and nausea and such potential nutritional consequences as stomatitis, xerostomia (dryness of the mouth), dysgeusia, dysphagia, constipation, and diarrhea; and (3) palliative care that contributes to the terminal patient's comfort by providing any desirable food in a tolerable form (Cantin, 1985).

The objective for preventive and maintenance care is for optimal nutritional status of the patient, which will:

1. Lessen the intensity of toxicities.
2. Induce a more favorable tumor response to treatment.
3. Increase immunocompetency with less infection.
4. Lessen physical and emotional insult from treatments.
5. Improve the sense of well-being.

ANOREXIA

A common problem among cancer patients is anorexia (lack of appetite). Decreased food intake may result in protein-energy malnutrition (PEM), which is the most common secondary diagnosis in cancer patients. PEM is a dangerous condition in which nutritional status is so poor s/he cannot fight either the cancer or any complications.

WEIGHT LOSS

Loss of appetite is accompanied with weight loss. Both are the result of cancer as well as its

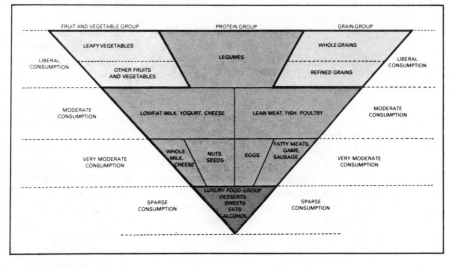

Figure 25–1. This food guide to lower cancer risk, as adapted by J.A.T. Pennington, is the basis for incorporating the "Dietary Guidelines to Lower Cancer Risk" into a variety of food patterns that meet individual food preferences and life styles. (From American Institute for Cancer Research Newsletter, 803 W. Broad Street, Falls Church, VA 22046, by permission.)

treatment. In starvation, the metabolic rate is low, but in cancer it is high. A majority of cancer patients experience weight loss during the course of their illness; however, this weight loss is different from that of a healthy person on a reduction diet losing fat tissue. Muscle wastage in the cancer patient results in progressive fatigue, weakness, and inactivity (DeWys, 1980).

Weight can be used to a limited extent to evaluate nutriture of the cancer patient. However, edema or dehydration may interfere with accurate assessments. As much as 10 lbs. of fluid in the lower extremities, or pedal edema, may accumulate before the condition is recognized as pitting edema. Fluid restriction is not recommended and may be counterproductive when the cause of edema is not from cardiac or renal pathology. Usually, the diet is modified for protein, sodium, and potassium (Maxwell, 1982).

CACHEXIA

Cachexia (kah-kek'-se-ah) is a very frequent accompaniment of advanced cancer, affecting one third to two thirds of cancer patients (Costa & Donaldson, 1979). This complex metabolic problem of uncertain etiology is characterized clinically by marked anorexia, early satiety, weight loss, wasting, and weakness (Fig. 25–2). In patients with advanced malignant disease, it is the predominant cause of mortality (Fuller, 1986).

Cachexia caused by cancer is not the same as uncomplicated starvation. Decreased levels or adaptations of hormones observed in uncomplicated starvation accompany metabolic adaptations of specific nutrients. Energy needs are frequently increased in cachexia because of tumor metabolic requirements while necessary therapies interfere with the patient's ability to eat.

Nutrition Assessment

Severe cachexia is easily recognized, but it is vital to recognize it in the moderately malnourished cancer patient, so nutritional support may be implemented. The patient may quickly become dehydrated and cachectic after radiation treatment to the abdominal cavity or head and neck region. Specific assessments are essential not only to prescribe optimum treatments for the patients but to

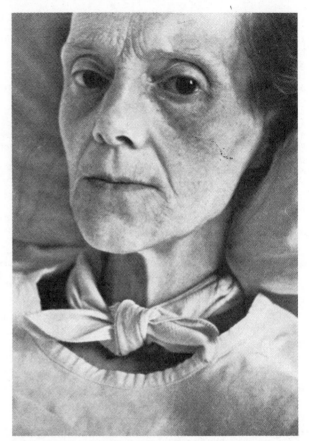

Figure 25–2. *A woman with cancer. (From* Nutrition Today *16(3), 1981. Reproduced with permission of* Nutrition Today *Magazine, P.O. Box 1829, Annapolis, MD.)*

correctly classify the condition for maximum Diagnosis-Related Group (DRG) reimbursement.

NUTRITIONAL STATUS TESTS

Particularly in cancer patients, laboratory values reflect the disease state as much as the nutritional state (Carter et al, 1983). Malnutrition is almost invariably a part of the diagnosis for cancer patients even at the beginning of treatment.

The following three assessment tools (see Chapter 20) should be used to determine nutritional status:
1. Weight change over time (indicates the severity of nutritional depletion).
2. Creatinine-height index from a 24-hour urine collection (reflects the status of the skeletal muscle mass).
3. Blood serum proteins (albumin, prealbumin, transferrin).

A more expensive test is the total peripheral lymphocyte count. When any of these values is less than 80 percent of normal, nutritional status may be compromised; a comprehensive nutritional status review is in order.

Clinical Implications:

- Histamine is excreted in the urine in most patients with systemic mastocytosis and in some patients with carcinoid tumors. These patients should be warned not to eat or drink foods that are high in histamine content, e.g., spinach, red wine, and eggplant as well as Parmesan, blue, and Roquefort cheese, on the days of urine collection (Feldman, 1983).
- Elevated serum calcium occurs in a significant number of patients with malignant diseases. It is critical for these patients to be treated because hypercalcemia often precipitates and aggravates renal failure (Gupta et al, 1981).
- Immunocompetence (the degree of ability to fight infection) can suggest subtle but distinct changes in immune response preceding the occurrence of frequent infections and decreases in growth velocity (Chandra & Scrimshaw, 1980).

WEIGHT CHANGE

Even though anthropometric measures lack the precision attained by biochemical analysis of blood and urine samples, they are inexpensive, noninvasive, and easily obtained.

Since weight fluctuates more with the fluid content of the body, measurements such as arm circumference (see Chapter 20) may be more accurate assessments (Dixon, 1985). However, weight changes still are significant assessments.

The weight prior to illness should be compared to the present one and evaluated at least weekly throughout the treatment period. More than a 10 percent weight loss within two to three weeks reflects fluid balance rather than protein or fatty tissue loss. Weight loss is an important prognostic factor in the patient with cancer. In a study of 3000 patients, DeWys (1980) found that the median survival of patients who experienced weight loss before chemotherapy was approximately half that of patients who had not lost weight. (An exception was gastric and pancreatic cancer, in which patients had short-term survival with or without weight loss.)

Radiation patients who lose more than five percent of their pretreatment weight (about two thirds of all radiation patients) suffer dysphagia,

mouth and throat pain, dysgeusia, and xerostomia more severely and for a longer period of time than other patients (Johnston et al, 1982).

Types of Therapy

Malignancies may be treated by one or more types of therapy.

RADIATION

When rapidly-growing neoplastic cells are treated with radiation therapy, fast-growing normal cells (e.g., hair follicles, bone marrow, and gastrointestinal mucous membranes) are also usually affected. Radiation therapy may last for one month to one year. The effect of treatment may last for several weeks or longer after the last dose.

The patient's nutriture will be affected especially in the area of treatment. Without nutritional intervention, 88 to 92 percent of the patients receiving high-dose radiation experience significant weight loss (Costa & Donaldson, 1979).

Common problems seen as a result of therapy are general loss of appetite, nausea and vomiting, and diarrhea caused by malabsorption from mucosal damage. Food intake is affected because of a loss of taste sensation, decreased salivation, difficulty in swallowing, and a burning sensation in the mouth when the larynx or pharynx area is irradiated. If food becomes tasteless, appearance and aroma become even more important. The diet order may read high protein, high calorie with six feedings. The challenge is to identify optimal eating times and determine foods that are acceptable to the patient. Dental problems and loss of teeth may also become a dietary problem.

Radiation damage to the small and large bowel alters intestinal function; this may result in malabsorption, diarrhea, obstruction, or fistulas. A low-residue, low-fat diet with adequate fluid intake may be required.

Clinical Implications:

- High-dose radiation to the abdomen almost invariably causes acute radiation enteritis. In addition to diarrhea and malabsorption, rapid weight loss occurs as well as vitamin deficiencies, lactose intolerance, and steatorrhea. But these signs of radiation enteritis may not occur until 10 years after radiation exposure and can easily be confused with other entities, including tumor recurrence (Fuller, 1986).

SURGICAL INTERVENTION

The effects of surgery may be varied and numerous. Frequently, the patient may be subjected to surgery more than once. Information given in Chapter 21 on surgical patients is equally applicable to cancer patients.

Radical surgery in the oropharyngeal area may present problems in chewing and swallowing and decreased taste sensations. Tube feedings may be indicated.

Esophagectomy and vagotomy may result in decreased absorption of fat, gastric stasis, and diarrhea (see Chapter 27). Steatorrhea can be improved by the use of medium-chain triglycerides.

Gastrectomy results in clinical problems proportionate to the extent of the resection. Dumping syndrome, hypoglycemia, steatorrhea, and lack of intrinsic factor are common problems necessitating nutritional intervention.

Massive small-bowel resection presents very serious and long-term problems in maintaining adequate nutrition, including water and electrolytes (see Chapter 27). When the distal ileum has been resected, vitamin B_{12} cannot be absorbed. Lactase, the enzyme necessary for the breakdown of milk sugar, may be removed causing intolerance to milk.

CHEMOTHERAPY

The treatment of disease by chemical agents is known as chemotherapy. Drugs are used to destroy malignant cells without destroying an excessive number of normal cells in patients with cancer. Chemotherapy has more widespread effects on the body than either radiation or surgical treatment. Table 25–2 lists some of these effects.

Most chemotherapeutic agents, while effective against malignancies, adversely affect food intake as a result of anorexia, nausea, vomiting, stomatitis, oral ulcerations, and to a lesser extent diarrhea. Drugs commonly used having these side effects are actinomycin D, methotrexate, vinblastine, cytarabine, and hydroxyurea (Visconti, 1977).

Anorexia usually begins on the day of treatment and lasts for several days. If the chemotherapeutic agent is administered monthly, the patient will have several weeks without anorexia

Table 25–2. *Alimentary Tract Effects of Cancer Chemotherapeutic Agents*

EFFECT / AGENT	Adriamycin	Asparaginase	BCNU	Bleomycin	Busulfan	Cyclophosphamide	Cytarabine	Dactinomycin	Daunorubicin	CDDP ("Cis-Pt")	Hydroxyurea	Methotrexate	Mithramycin	Procarbazine	Vinblastine	Vincristine
Anorexia	•	•	•		•		•	•	•			•	•	•		
Nausea	•	•	•		•	•	•	•	•	•	•	•	•	•		
Diarrhea						•				•		•				
Mucositis	•		•			•	•	•		•	•					
Abdominal Pain				•		•					•					•
Obstipation																•
Intestinal Ulceration						•						•	•			
Vomiting	•	•	•		•	•	•	•	•	•		•		•		

From Shils ME: Nutrition and neoplasia. In Goodhart RS, Shils ME: *Modern Nutrition in Health and Disease*, 6th ed. Philadelphia, Lea & Febiger, 1980, by permission.

when high-protein and high-calorie foods should be eaten.

Adrenocortical steroids, which exert immunosuppressive activity, are a well-known cause of protein, calcium, and potassium losses. They cause increased gastric mucosal vulnerability to hydrochloric acid, which can be prevented by giving antacids or histamine antagonists with the drug (Trester, 1982). Since edema is common, body weight is inaccurate.

Antimetabolites, such as methotrexate, are folic acid antagonists. Treatment with the drug should be alternated with folic acid supplements (Shils, 1980). Methotrexate, 5-fluorouracil, and actinomycin D affect the gastrointestinal mucosa, precipitating a condition similar to sprue. Since the absorption of all nutrients is decreased, increased intake as well as supplementation is required (Shils, 1980).

Vincristine, vinblastine, and hydroxyurea therapy may result in constipation (Visconti, 1977). Increasing the fluid and fiber intake may relieve this problem. Vincristine may cause acute jaw pain. High-protein supplements and fluids may be accepted by straw when jaw pain is present.

In patients receiving 5-fluorouracil, the bone marrow may become megaloblastic resembling pernicious and other megaloblastic anemias (Shils, 1980). Mithramycin, an antibiotic frequently used in cancer patients, may precipitate hypocalcemia. Milk and cheese products as well as calcium supplements can offset the calcium loss.

IMMUNOTHERAPY

Although still in the developmental stage, immunotherapy is a form of cancer treatment being used in which the tumor is altered and antibody production is increased to enhance the host's immune response. The host may be injected with irradiated tumor cells or antigens prepared from tumor cells. Such augmentation of the general immune response can cause tumor destruction. However, its side effects include anorexia, changes in taste sensations, nausea, heart failure, vomiting, gastrointestinal abnormalities, and mucosal ulcerations. Immunotherapy normally complements surgery, radiation, and chemotherapy, since even under optimal conditions, the general immune response cannot deal with large amounts of tumor.

Another type of immunotherapy involves improving nutritive status or inducing certain deficiencies in an effort to slow tumor growth or reduce tumor size. For example, some tumors may respond to selective starvation of their specific amino acid supply (Munro, 1977). The main problem with the latter is that the whole body might lose its nutritive status, which frequently precipitates infections that may prove fatal (Rundles, 1982).

The "nitrogen trap" concept proposes that the tumor is favored over the host for certain nutrients. If there is a shortage, the tumor will use it before the host can. Situations during cancer therapy that lead to host starvation may possibly favor tumor survival at the expense of host depletion (Goodgame et al, 1979).

Nutritional Support

BENEFITS

Nutritional support benefits the patient's overall health. Research shows that high-risk cancer patients given nutritional support before surgery have half as many complications, half as many infections, and one third as many major septic events. They are also only one third as likely to die (Smale et al, 1981). Women with advanced ovarian cancer receiving total parenteral nutrition (TPN) were compared to a group not receiving TPN, but who were younger and had less extensive disease. The group without TPN had longer hospitalization (24 versus 20 days), larger weight loss (15 lbs. versus none), more major complications (seven versus three), and more deaths (two versus none) (Fuller & Griffiths, 1979).

Nutrition support does not cure cancer, but recovery rates are definitely related directly to patients' receiving optimal nutritional support.

PROBLEMS

No matter what medicines or treatments are used, the body must have protein, calories, vitamins, and minerals to repair the damage and to grow new tissues. Food *is* therapy to the cancer patient. Cancer has a devastating effect first upon the nutritional status, which is in turn reflected throughout the body. The condition requires much attention to maintain body weight; a high-protein, high-energy diet is usually prescribed. While the importance of adequate food intake cannot be overemphasized, measures must be taken to tempt patients' appetites. It is the responsibility of team members to use ingenuity and different strategies to increase food acceptance. Because of the complexity of cancer, patients with the same symptoms may respond very differently. The diet must be tailored for the individual.

Preparing attractive trays and providing a pleasant environment at mealtime are very important to achieve the goal of increased food acceptance. The setting should be calm, not rushed. The patient may need to keep the tray longer than usual. Timing of the meal can also be very important. Patients should be encouraged to eat when their appetite is good. This frequently means a large breakfast with smaller feedings throughout the day. When hospitalized patients eat together, they gain increased peer support.

Various feeding techniques must be implemented when feeding cancer patients. Whenever possible, oral feedings are preferred. Tube feedings can be used if only chewing and swallowing are impaired. Elemental diets can be used if digestion is impaired, but absorption is intact.

TPN may be appropriate when the patient cannot or will not eat or when the gastrointestinal tract is temporarily unable to handle nutrient intake. TPN provides sources of nitrogen, amino acids, calories, electrolytes, vitamins, and minerals (see Chapter 27). However, because of the dangers of the procedures and possibility of infections, it is not normally initiated, unless used for periods of more than 10 days. A well-trained nutrition support team is desirable. While TPN therapy is very expensive, it is the most effective therapy for patients who have lost more than six percent of their pre-illness weight (Brennan, 1981). Ultimately, decisions about methods of feeding depend upon the patient's prognosis.

GUIDELINES FOR NUTRITIONAL SUPPORT

Because of the various types of cancer, there are many different effects upon the resting metabolic rate (basal metabolic rate or basal energy expenditure, BEE). Beside the extremely large tumor burden, the daily energy needs of cancer patients are at least 1.5 times their predicted BEE and possibly as much as 1.7 to 2.0 times. For patients confined to bed, 20 percent above BEE is recommended (Long et al, 1982).

In nutritionally-depleted patients, the goal is restoration of lean tissues with concomitant restoration of fat. Information for caloric requirements for hypercatabolism is provided in Chapter 26. Decreased utilization of vitamins and minerals require individual assaying and possible supplementation.

NAUSEA, VOMITING, AND EARLY SATIETY

Cancer patients may unknowingly decrease their food intake because of a full feeling after eating small amounts. A diet diary can help to determine just how much the patient is eating. Carbohydrates are easier and faster to digest, which helps prevent early satiety. Small frequent meals are beneficial in the management of nausea and vomiting in order to increase food intake.

Antiemetics are most effective if started the night before chemotherapy and continued at six-hour intervals as long as nausea persists. Favorite foods should be avoided while the stomach is upset. If vomiting occurs, those foods may lose their popularity.

Hyposmia (abnormally decreased sensitivity to odors) frequently limits the appetite, too. Some smells may be perceived as unpleasant. Patients should avoid cooking foods or being in the area while food is prepared. Cold foods, which have fewer aromas, are often preferred.

Clinical Implications:

- Abrupt movements frequently provoke nausea; allow about an hour for rest after food intake.

- Encourage deep breaths of fresh air for nausea.
- The nauseated patient should be encouraged to remain in an upright position. If the patient must lie down, the head should be at least four inches above the feet.
- Withhold liquids and foods until vomiting is arrested; then begin with clear liquids or crushed ice.
- Apple juice, iced tea, dry crackers or dry toast, and gelatin are especially suitable initially. Then, clear cold beverages or juices are followed by small quantities of easily-digested foods, as tolerated.
- Limit fluids during mealtimes. Some patients may tolerate liquids one hour before or after the meal.
- Cold foods or foods at room temperature are better tolerated than hot ones.
- Highly spiced and acidic foods are poorly tolerated.
- Avoid any fried, greasy, or fatty foods or excessive fat with food, e.g., margarine and sour cream with baked potato.
- Always have snacks available; waiting even for a few minutes may lessen the desire to eat.
- Evaluate discomfort as a possible side effect of drug therapy, e.g., nausea in a patient taking digitalis may indicate drug toxicity, especially in the elderly (Smith & Bidlack, 1984).
- Encourage the patient to eat slowly, taking small bites and chewing thoroughly.
- Offer small amounts of easily digestible food frequently.
- Aromas from hot foods may aggravate nausea.
- If nausea occurs at consistent times of day, reschedule mealtimes.

DIARRHEA, CRAMPS, AND OTHER INTESTINAL UPSETS

When diarrhea is severe, food intake may have to be withheld. Beverages low in sugar are first introduced. The diarrhea may be checked by a low-residue diet. If the diarrhea is caused by resection of the ileum, medium-chain triglycerides may be necessary.

If diarrhea and flatulence are caused by the lack of lactase in the gastrointestinal tract, milk and milk products will have to be limited or removed completely from the diet. Yogurt can be helpful since the fermentation process alters the lactose. Also, beneficial intestinal tract bacteria, frequently destroyed by the cancer treatment, are replaced by eating yogurt.

Constipation in the cancer patient may be due to medications (see Chapter 27).

Clinical Implication:

- Monitor all patients for typical variations of the medication prescribed, e.g., the frequency and characteristics of bowel movements. Constipation is one of the earliest signs of vincristine toxicity (Rothweiler, 1983).

IMMUNE RESPONSE

Reduced immune response makes the patient more susceptible to infection. Sterile diets are difficult as well as being unappetizing for the patient. Foods that are not cooked and sanitized, such as lettuce and fresh fruits, can carry germs, precipitating an infection. To reduce the chances of infection, salads and fresh fruit may be eliminated, especially in patients with granulocytopenia (Pizzo, 1981). Dietary departments can also pay special attention to their sanitation control.

Clinical Implication:

- Protective or reverse isolation may be used.

Dysgeusia

A common complaint of cancer patients is a distorted sense of taste (dysgeusia). Taste aversions are related more to the extent of the disease rather than the type of cancer or treatment, except chemotherapy (Carson & Gormican, 1977). Weight loss, decreased appetite and early satiety are precipitated by food aversions in many patients (Nielsen et al, 1980).

There are three types of dysgeusia: (1) cacogeusia, an abhorrent or obnoxious taste produced by foods or beverages that normally taste pleasant; (2) heterogeusia is a consistently inappropriate taste produced by all foods or beverages; and (3) phantogeusia is a usually unpleasant taste perceived in the absence of any taste stimulus (Markely et al, 1983). Hypogeusia (decreased taste acuity) and hyposmia (decreased smell acuity) also interfere with normal food patterns for the cancer patient. Loss of taste and smell do not influence energy intake directly; in fact, weight gain may result as patients continue to eat (Mattes-Kulig &

Henkin, 1985). But dysgeusia usually results directly in weight loss.

Often, an entire food group will be eliminated from the diet when only one food tastes distorted. When this occurs, serious nutritional deficiencies are likely to follow.

Patients who eat favorite foods before chemotherapy treatment sometimes find they have lost the enjoyment of that food after treatment. To avoid food aversions, patients should limit intake to small amounts of one or two foods prior to chemotherapy (Bernstein et al, 1982). When the tumor regresses, the dysgeusia is reversed (DeWys, 1979).

TASTE BLINDNESS

The most frequent types of mouth or taste blindness (a combination of the above types of dysgeusia), in which there are changes in sense of taste include: (1) sweetness is harder to taste, (2) bitter tastes become stronger (Gallagher & Tweedle, 1983), (3) salt is harder to taste, and (4) a metal taste is present in the mouth.

Most high-protein foods, especially red meats, cereal products, and sweet foods are generally less palatable to patients (Vickers et al, 1981). Poultry and fish are usually preferred to beef and pork (DeWys, 1980). Often eggs, cheese, and custard are preferred protein sources. Coffee is the most commonly taste-distorted beverage (Markely et al, 1983).

Many drugs used in therapy, especially 5-fluorouracil, may produce some changes in taste acuity. Decreased serum zinc or copper levels may be responsible for some alterations in taste and odor sensations. Oral zinc sulfate has been effective in improving these sensations (Shils, 1981).

Clinical Implications:

- To achieve as much flavor as possible from their foods, cancer patients should be encouraged to chew well and to switch from one food to another as they eat, which minimizes sensory adaptation.
- As much protein and as many calories as possible should be included in each snack.
- If foods taste bitter, avoid foods cooked in metal pans. Instead, use plastic utensils and glass pots and pans (Fuller, 1986).
- Breakfast is usually the most important meal for cancer patients since their appetites are better in the morning.

- Variety of texture can be pleasant when tolerated (Schiffman, 1983).
- Sugar may be added to make foods more palatable and to increase calorie intake. Increasing the number of mildly sweet foods is more likely to improve the palatability of food for the anorectic (Trant et al, 1982).
- Well-stocked unit kitchens may help to increase intake.
- For anorectic patients: (1) decrease fluid intake during meals, (2) encourage the family to suggest favorite foods, and (3) decrease stress at meal times by encouraging rest and quiet before and after meals and utilizing relaxation techniques (Rothweiler, 1983).
- Food may be tolerated better if time of treatment can be changed; if not, alter mealtimes to coincide with the patient's appetite.
- Usually, several small meals or snacks are preferred. Eating more often can compensate for reduced meal size (Trant et al, 1982).
- If patients lose their taste for coffee and tea, they may need assistance in identifying other beverages they like so their fluid intake is not decreased. Frozen slushes of fruits, juices, or milk may be welcomed.
- Sipping beverages like sugarless ginger ale, or chewing gum, or sucking sugarless hard candies will improve cacogeusia (bad taste) in the mouth (Schiffman, 1983).
- Alcohol, such as a glass of wine, may be used to stimulate appetite but should be avoided during chemotherapy (Trester, 1982).
- Cold foods are better accepted than hot foods.
- Spices may make foods more palatable.
- Pain medication may be given before meals.

Dysphagia

Difficulty in swallowing (dysphagia) is a common problem. To retrain patients, remind them to (1) inhale, (2) swallow, and (3) exhale. This is the normal swallowing sequence, but the patient usually is frightened and tense. Positive support and encouragement are vital to their progress. Most of these patients swallow better in a semireclining position with the head and back on the same level. The effects of gravity will be maximized without increasing aspiration (Fleming et al, 1977). Clinical implications for dysphagia are in Chapter 27.

Laryngectomy

Supraglottic laryngectomy causes some degree of dysphagia in patients. Liquids are usually most difficult to swallow without aspiration, as these spill into the laryngeal inlet. Nonsticky custard and pureed fruits or vegetables are suitable. Foods with varying consistency are more difficult to handle, e.g., vegetable soup.

Supplemental Feedings

Suggesting a supplement is not enough. Specific directions should be given and monitored for a successful regimen. A prescription will state the amount of supplement to be taken; the actual amount should be recorded by the patient or nurse. The appropriate prescription is determined by the physician, nurse, dietitian, and patient.

PRESCRIPTION

The nurse observes food and beverages consumed. A current caloric and nutrient intake is determined by a dietitian or dietetic technician from a 24-hour dietary recall or a three-day diet diary or by checking the patient's tray. The caloric needs are then calculated based on body weight using the following formula:

Caloric need = weight in kg × 20 + 1100 kcal

Subtracting the caloric intake from the calculated caloric need yields the volume of the supplement to be prescribed (this switch from calories to volume is valid, since most of the supplements contain 1 kcal/ml) (DeWys, 1980).

The patient's taste preference is the paramount factor in determining acceptance of any supplement. Many liquid and powdered supplements as well as those in the form of puddings are commercially available (see Appendix A-2). The main concern is to utilize types that will be consumed by the patient and are economical for the patient at home. Ready-to-serve liquids are usually more convenient.

Clinical Implications:

- A tasting tray containing 1 oz. each of several supplements permits patients to identify their preferences (DeWys, 1980).
- Relaxation training by nurses improves weight gain and arm muscle circumference in many cancer patients. It can be as vital a component in the nutritional well-being of these individuals as supplementation is (Dixon, 1984).
- The liquid supplement should be lactose-free if the patient is lactose-intolerant.
- By supplementation of snacks, energy value can be increased as much as 700 kcal.
- If high-calorie liquid formulas are used, they should be placed in the patient's room to encourage intake.

Oral-Dental Care

Cancer therapy can cause a maze of bewildering side effects in the mouth. Oral-dental care is mandatory. A dental oncologist or hygienist should be a member of the team to assist with these problems.

PREVENTION

Ideally, everyone should be under the continuous care of a dentist. This would prevent the simultaneous occurrence of malignancy and extensive dental work. In either case, an immediate trip to the dentist at the first indication of neoplasm can prevent serious complications and intense pain that might be precipitated later.

COMPLICATIONS

In young patients (10 to 12 years old), a beam of radiation passing through developing permanent teeth will arrest the formation of the roots as well as the expansion of the jaws.

Since drugs may cause oral lesions and chemotherapy may impair immunity, benign dental disease can escalate to become serious. For example, gingivitis, a minor complaint, becomes difficult to manage in patients with leukemia. Diffi-

culty in cleaning teeth and gums may increase periodontal disease.

PATIENT RESPONSIBILITY

An informed patient is usually more attentive to oral care and should be encouraged to assume as much responsibility as possible. A strict protocol of oral hygiene must be established by the dentist, nurse, and patient. A very soft toothbrush or a toothette can be tolerated. Short horizontal strokes for at least three to four minutes with a fluoridated toothpaste are suggested. Rinsing with a topical fluoride mouthwash after brushing has proven beneficial for the cancer patient.

Clinical Implications:

- If a Water Pik is used, it must be adjusted to the lowest pressure possible to avoid injury to gums and tissue.
- A fluoride rinse is not meant to replace brushing teeth. Both are necessary for optimum care.

MOUTHWASH

Commercial mouthwashes are not recommended because they usually contain alcohol, which is painful to open lesions and causes surfaces to become even drier. Also, they may eliminate normal, healthy flora, which could result in a yeast infection. Solutions used to control superimposed infection of mucosa by frequent oral irrigations include any of the following:

1. One tablespoon of peroxide in an 8 oz. glass of water.
2. A half teaspoon of baking soda in an 8 oz. glass of water.
3. Weak saline solution.

These will reduce the pain caused by dryness and lubricate the tissues.

XEROSTOMIA

Dryness of mouth from lack of normal secretion (xerostomia) is one of the greatest immediate complaints among patients receiving therapy. Even though water does not replace saliva, patients are encouraged to drink large amounts of fluids. Artificial salivas may be used as desired, but their effects are transitory. They buffer the acidity in the mouth and lubricate the mucous membranes.

When the mouth has sores, soft foods or foods covered with sauces, gravies, or salad dressing may be better tolerated. Cream soups and milk beverages are usually palatable. Cold foods have a numbing effect, making them acceptable; however, extremely hot foods should be avoided.

Clinical Implications:

- Soak foods like toast in coffee or milk.
- Fruit nectars are better tolerated than acidic beverages when the mouth is inflamed.
- Very salty foods, hot spices, and coarse, rough foods are not well tolerated.
- It may be easier to swallow liquids through a straw.
- Encourage fluids throughout the meal to provide additional moistness.
- Lidocaine (Xylocaine) may be used as a mouthwash to numb the pain (Toth & Hoar, 1982).
- A humidifier in the room may be useful.
- Tilting the head either back slightly or forward may ease swallowing.

---

and should grow within themselves while supporting each other.

Such a philosophy of living, caring, and dying can only materialize when each team member inwardly explores his/her own beliefs and reads valid references for new expansions of his/her ideas. To help the health care professional as well as patients and their families to form their own philosophy about death and dying, excellent bibliographies and references are available (Luckmann & Sorensen, 1980). Quiet time is essential for this growth process, and the rewards are ongoing and most worthwhile.

Nurses with constant responsibility of the cancer patient can help the patient and family cope with the situation by:
- Learning as much as possible about cancer.
- Forming a personal philosophy about negative and positive results.
- Allowing the patient to express his/her feelings and concerns.
- Maintaining calmness and reinforcing the patient's hopes.
- Guiding the family and friends in beneficial ways of patient care.
- Informing patients and family of hospice care in the community and the "I Can Cope" groups, a program sponsored by the American Cancer Society for education and support of families of cancer patients (Rothweiler, 1983).

Caring for the Dying Patient

Few conditions can be as demanding as cancer for the patient, the family, and the health care staff. Psychological counseling may be needed by each of these persons. One of the primary goals is alleviation of discomfort, including loneliness and despair, which frequently are overlooked while attempting to alleviate the discomfort of pain, nausea, vomiting, and insomnia. For optimum care, the holistic team approach must be expanded to include a wide variety of persons with different areas of expertise.

While cancer and death are becoming less synonymous terms, death is certainly prevalent among cancer patients. The health care team, particularly the nursing staff, must develop a concrete philosophy to enable them to nurture the patient throughout the course of events without draining the strength and joy of living from their own individual lives. All persons involved can

• FALLACIES and FACTS

Sidney L. Arje and Lois V. Smith in The Health Robbers *(1976) state:*

Cancer quackery is big business, with an estimated yearly income in the billions. It is also cruel business, for its customers come in desperate fear. Those customers who come while also undergoing good medical care will buy only empty promises. But those ... who delay or abandon medicine's best, will purchase death.

The best advice is to first consult the oncologist to avoid delay in treatment.

FALLACY: *High doses of vitamin C will cure cancer.*

- **FACT:** *High amounts of vitamin C do not cure patients with advanced cancer (Rossman et al, 1980). Nor is high-dose vitamin C therapy effective against ad-*

vanced malignant disease even if the patient has had chemotherapy (Moertel et al, 1985).

FALLACY: Vitamin E will cure cancer.

- **FACT:** Vitamin E is not a miracle cure for cancer or any other health problem. Vitamin E seems to inhibit carcinogenesis, which might help prevent the start of tumorigenesis. It has been reported to enhance radiation-induced tumor killing in studies with rats, but this does not mean that vitamin E results in longer survival rates for humans (Ellison, 1982).

FALLACY: Marijuana relieves nausea and pain.

- **FACT:** Marijuana may offer patients with prior experience relief, but for those who have not had this, no advantages of marijuana over codeine are observed. In fact, marijuana carries the risk of unacceptable side effects of sedation, thought impairment, and depersonalization reactions (Anderson, 1982).

FALLACY: Laetrile will cure cancer.

- **FACT:** Laetrile, sometimes referred to as vitamin B_{17}, is extracted from the kernels of peaches, apricots, and apple seeds. Laetrile contains the chemical amygdalin, which breaks down into a toxic cyanide. There is no medically or nutritionally recognized vitamin B_{17}. Laetrile supporters have not been able to prove that it can control cancer in animals; other independent laboratory experiments have also been negative (Arje & Smith, 1976).

FALLACY: Teeth may as well be extracted before chemotherapy begins because of the caries that follow.

- **FACT:** Preventive dentistry and regular cleaning care of the teeth can protect them during therapy.

FALLACY: A macrobiotic diet will detoxify the body.

- **FACT:** The reasoning behind this theory is that cancer is caused by an "imbalance" in the body or by accumulated "poisons" or "impurities" and that the body will be "purified" by a proper diet. This reasoning can only interfere with the adequate nutrient intake that is critical for the cancer patient. Eating an unbalanced diet could result in reduced protein intake and, in turn, increase rather than prevent malnutrition (Cassileth, 1982).

The promoters of this diet claim that the cancer should not be treated by any therapy other than diet. While this is an essential part of the cancer program, it is never used as the only form of treatment.

The diet recommends that 50 percent of each meal consist of whole grains. This would reduce the intake of other essential nutrients, might be difficult to swallow because of fiber, might not contain all the essential amino acids and adequate calories, and might interfere with absorption of minerals. There is no valid justification for such a diet at this time.

Summary

In spite of the commonalities among cancer patients, each patient should be viewed as an individual with his/her own likes and dislikes. These patients have such a variety of needs that a broad multidisciplinary team approach is essential for cancer treatment. Management of nutritional status should be an important component of the health care plan.

Nutritional status is a prime goal because of its direct relationship to mortality and morbidity; it is related to improved survival and less relapse among cancer patients. Nutritional care should be optimized in the early states of cancer, before patients become malnourished or the disease spreads. It is as significant as the treatment itself in the final balance of success. Nutrition is not a cure-all for cancer, but it is a critical aspect of cancer treatment that may prolong life and improve the response to different therapies.

Nutrients are essential to restore immunocompetence, lessen toxicity, improve results of other therapeutic treatments, and provide optimum body weight. Recovery (if possible), reduced hospital stays, fewer infections and complications, and improved quality of life are the goals for cancer patients.

Review Questions

1. How does a tumor compete with the overall nutrition of the patient?

2. Differentiate between PEM and cachexia.
3. List four reasons why nutritional status in the cancer patient is important.
4. What assessment tools should be used to screen cancer patients?
5. Since radiation therapy affects rapidly-growing cells, what normal cells are frequently affected by nutrition?
6. What flavors are commonly affected by taste blindness?
7. List ways to increase food intake in the anorectic patient.
8. Why would cancer patients feel tired? What could be done to improve their feelings?
9. What are some ways that cancer patients can help themselves get well?
10. How can family members help patients be more comfortable as well as improve their general condition?

Case Study: Elizabeth, 38 years old, was rushed to the hospital emergency room with symptoms of shock and a blood glucose level of 20/100 mg/dL. After many tests, an abdominal tumor was identified as pressing against the pancreas.

An internist, endocrinologist, oncologist, and three surgeons consulted before, during, and after surgery to evaluate the case. Removal of the cancer through the abdominal cavity was not possible because the tumor was too extensive.

Relatives came to be with Elizabeth and stay with her husband Michael and their two children, Ashley, age 13, and Jeremy, age 12. Members of Elizabeth's church furnished ample food to the visiting relatives at home. Flowers, cards, and phone calls expressed love and prayers for her.

Then, Elizabeth was transferred to the state medical center 250 miles away for further assessment. Michael arranged to be away from his work to go with her, but extra funds were not available to take their children with them. A suggestion to call the social services office at the medical center resulted in a retired couple within walking distance of the hospital who offered their home.

Chemotherapy treatments were started to continue treating the cancer. Before Elizabeth lost her hair, her mother went to the American Cancer Society office to choose two free wigs. One was natural hair to allow for various styles; the other wig was synthetic for easy wash-and-wear care during periods when Elizabeth would have less energy. Her mother also borrowed a friend's pattern for turban-scarf caps. Shopping for fabrics and sewing the caps offered her relief from the grief and anxiety during this period.

The dietitian discussed the use of the food exchange lists to plan menus that would include Elizabeth's food preferences and help prevent the recurring hypoglycemic attacks. Each time a meal or snack would be delivered to her, the nurse would explain to Elizabeth and members of her family which foods were complex carbohydrates and other features of the exchange lists to curb hypoglycemia.

When they returned home, Ashley decided to plan their meals by the exchange lists for her project in homemaking class. Each one in the family chose meals to prepare.
1. Plan meals and snacks for Elizabeth for one day using the food exchange lists (see Chapter 23).
2. Prepare a list of altered serving sizes and additional foods necessary to meet the needs of each family member. (See the RDA list on the findsheets for different members' needs.)
3. What effect do you think that planning and shopping for foods and preparing the meals will have upon each member of this family?
4. What foods might Elizabeth choose during periods of taste changes and anorexia from the chemotherapy?
5. Make a list of professionals and nonprofessionals who might help Elizabeth and her family. Mention specific ways or activities that family members could use to offer Elizabeth emotional support.

REFERENCE LIST

American Cancer Society: Cancer Facts and Figures. New York, American Cancer Society, Inc., 1985.

Anderson, JL: Nursing management of the cancer patient in pain: A review of the literature. Cancer Nurs 5(1):33, 1982.

Arje, SL; Smith LV: The cruelest killers. In The Health Robbers. Edited by S Barrett; G Knight. Philadelphia, George F. Stickley, 1976.

Bernstein, I; Webster, MM; Bernstein, ID: Food aversions in children receiving chemotherapy for cancer. Cancer 50(12):2961, 1982.

Brennan, M: Total parenteral nutrition in the cancer patient. N Engl J Med 305(7):375, 1981.

Cantin, L: An approach to the provision of nutrition services in a cancer treatment centre. J Can Diet Assoc 46(spring):51, 1985.

Carson, JS; Gormican, A: Taste acuity and food attitudes of selected patients with cancer. J Am Diet Assoc 70(4):361, 1977.

Carter, P; Carr, D; Van Eys, J; et al: Nutritional parameters in children with cancer. J Am Diet Assoc 82(6):616, 1983.

Cassileth, BR: After Laetrile, what? N Engl J Med 306(24):1482, 1982.

Chandra, RK; Scrimshaw, NS: Immunocompetence in nutritional assessment. AM J Clin Nutr 33(12):2694, 1980.

Costa, G; Donaldson, SS: Current concepts in cancer: Effects of cancer and cancer treatment on the nutrition of the host. N Engl J Med 300:1471, 1979.

DeWys, WD: Changes in taste sensation and feeding behaviour in cancer patients: A review. J Human Nutr 32(6):447, 1979.

DeWys, WD: Nutritional care of the cancer patient. JAMA 244(4):374, 1980.

Dixon, JK: Validity and utility of anthropometric measurements: A survey of cancer outpatients. J Am Diet Assoc 85(4):439, April, 1985.

Ellison, NM: Relationship between vitamin E and cancer—facts, not fancy. Cancer Bulletin 34:43, 1982.

Erickson, KL: Dietary fat and tumorigenesis in laboratory animals. *Food Nutr News* 56(2):1, 1984.

Feldman, JM: Histaminuria from histamine-rich foods. *Arch Intern Med* 143(11):2099, 1983.

Fleming, SM; Weaver, AW; Brown, JM: The patient with cancer affecting the head and neck: Problems in nutrition. *J Am Diet Assoc* 70(4):391, 1977.

Fuller, AF; Griffiths, CT: Ovarian cancer cachexia—surgical interactions. *Gynecol Oncol* 8:301, 1979.

Fuller, E: How cancer affects nutritional status. *Patient Care* 20(11):80, 1986.

Gallagher, P; Tweedle, DE: Taste threshold and acceptability of commercial diets in cancer patients. *JPEN* 7(4):361, 1983.

Goodgame, JT; Lowry, SF; Reilly, JJ; et al: Nutritional manipulations and tumor growth. 1. The effects of starvation. *Am J Clin Nutr* 32(11):2277, 1979.

Grundy, S: Nutrition and cancer: A preliminary report. *Nutr Health News* 1(2):1, 1984.

Gupta, MM; Singh, H; Christian, S: Hypercalcaemia of malignancy. *J Indian Med Assoc* 76(1–2):9, 1981.

Johnston, CA; Keane, TJ; Prudo, SM: Weight loss in patients receiving radical radiation therapy for head and neck cancer: A prospective study. *JPEN* 6(5):399, 1982.

Long, CL; Merrick HW: Dennis, RS; et al: Energy requirements for cancer patients. *Cancer Bulletin* 34(4):155, 1982.

Luckmann, J; Sorensen, KC: *Medical-Surgical Nursing: A Psychophysiologic Approach*, 3rd ed. Philadelphia, W.B. Saunders Co., 1987.

Markley, EJ; Mattes-Kulig, DA; Henkin, RI: A classification of dysgeusia. *J Am Diet Assoc* 83(5):578, 1983.

Mattes-Kulig, DA; Henkin, RI: Energy and nutrient consumption of patients with dysgeusia. *J Am Diet Assoc* 85(7):822, 1985.

Maxwell, MB: Pedal edema in the cancer patient. *Am J Nurs* 82(8):1225, 1982.

Moertel, CG; Fleming, TR; Creagen, ET; et al: High dose vitamin C versus placebo in the treatment of patients with advanced cancer who have had no prior chemotherapy: A randomized double-blind comparison. *N Engl J Med* 312(3):137, 1985.

Munro, HN: Tumor-host competition for nutrients in the cancer patient. *J Am Diet Assoc* 71(4):380, 1977.

Nielsen, SS; Theologides, A; Vickers, ZM: Influence of food odors on food aversions and preferences in patients with cancer. *Am J Clin Nutr* 33(11):2253, 1980.

Pizzo, RA: Bacteria in food. *N Engl J Med* 304(24):1495, 1981.

Rossman, ML; Brostoff, WS; Cameron, E; et al: Vitamin C for cancer. *N Engl J Med* 302(5):298, 1980.

Rothweiler, TM: Coping with the complications of cancer. *RN* 46(9):56, 1983.

Rundles, SC: Effects of nutritional status on immunological function. *Am J Clin Nutr* 35(Suppl 5):1202, 1982.

Schiffman, SS: Taste and smell in disease. *N Engl J Med* 308(22):1337, 1983.

Shils, ME: How to nourish the cancer patient. *Nutr Today* 16:4, 1981.

Shils, ME: Nutrition and neoplasia. In *Modern Nutrition in Health and Disease*, 6th ed. Edited by RS Goodhart; M Shils. Philadelphia, Lea & Febiger, 1980, p 1153.

Smale, AF; Mullen, J; Busby, G; et al: The efficacy of nutritional assessment and support in cancer surgery. *Cancer* 47(10):2375, 1981.

Smith, CH; Bidlack, WR: Dietary concerns associated with the use of medications. *J Am Diet Assoc* 84(8):901, 1984.

Toth, B; Hoar, RE: Oral/dental care of the pediatric oncology patient. *Cancer Bulletin* 34:66, 1982.

Trant, AS; Serin, J; Douglass, HO: Is taste related to anorexia in cancer patients? *Am J Clin Nutr* 36(1):45, 1982.

Trester, AK: Nursing management of patients receiving cancer chemotherapy. *Cancer Nurs* 5(3):201, 1982.

Vickers, ZM; Neilsen, SS; Theologides, A: Food preferences of patients with cancer. *J Am Diet Assoc* 79(4):441, 1981.

Visconti, JA: Drug-food interactions. *Nutrition in Disease*. Columbus, OH, Ross Laboratories, 1977.

Further Study

Butler, JH: Nutrition and cancer: A review of the literature. *Cancer Nurs* 3(2):131, 1980.

Calcium and vitamin D intakes influence the risk of bowel cancer in men. *Nutr Rev* 43(6):170, 1985.

Colditz, GA; Branch, LG; Lipnick, RJ; et al: Increased green and yellow vegetable intake and lowered cancer deaths in an elderly population. *Amer J Clin Nutr* 41(1):32, 1985.

Creasey, WA: *Diet and Cancer*. Philadelphia, Lea & Febiger, 1985.

Crosley, MA: Watch out for nutritional complications of cancer. *RN* 48(3):22, 1985.

Dixon, J: Effect of nursing interventions on nutrition and performance status in cancer patients—nutrition supplementation and relaxation training. *Nurs Res* 33(6):330, 1984.

Fleming, TJ: Dental care for cancer patients receiving radiotherapy to the head and neck. *Cancer Bull* 34:63, 1982.

Fuller, E: Is nutrition a weapon against cancer? *Patient Care* 20(11):52, 1986.

Gormican, A: Influencing food acceptance in anorexic cancer patients. *Postgrad Med* 68(2):145, 1980.

Gregory-Addesa, G: Helping your patient when nausea goes with the treatment. *RN* 49(4):43, 1986.

Groer, M; Pierce, M: Guarding against cancer's hidden killer: Anorexia cachexia. *Nursing* 11(6):39, 1981.

Hearne, BE; Dunaj, JM; Daly, JM; et al: Enteral nutrition support in head and neck cancer: Tube versus oral feeding during radiation therapy. *J Amer Diet Assoc* 85(6):669, 1985.

Kokal, WA: The impact of antitumor therapy on nutrition. *Cancer* 55(1 suppl):271, 1985.

Lum, LLQ: Nutrition and the cancer patient: A cooperative effort by nursing and dietetics to overcome problems. *Cancer Nurs* 7(6):469, 1984.

Purtilo, DT; Cohen, SM: Diet, nutrition, and cancer. *Postgrad Med* 78(1):193, 1985.

Shizgal, HM: Body composition of patients with malnutrition and cancer. Summary of methods of assessment. *Cancer* 55(1 suppl):250, 1985.

Showdon, CA: Diet and ovarian cancer. *JAMA* 254:356, 1985.

Silberman, H: The role of preoperative parenteral nutrition in cancer patients. *Cancer* 55(1 suppl):254, 1985.

U.S. Dept. of Health and Human Services: *Eating Hints: Recipes and Tips for Better Nutrition During Cancer Treatment*. Bethesda, MD, National Institutes of Health, 1982.

U.S. Dept. of Health and Human Services: *Young People with Cancer*. Bethesda, MD, National Cancer Institute, 1982.

Vininga, KS: Improving nutrition in children with cancer. *Pediatr Nurs* 11(1):18, 1985.

Walsh, TD; Bowman, KB; Jackson, GP: Dietary intake of advanced cancer patients. *Hum Nutr Appl Nutr* 37A:41, 1983.

Williams, LT; Peterson, DE; Overholser, C: Acute periodontal infection in myelosuppressed oncology patients: Evaluation and nursing care. *Cancer Nurs* 5(6):465, 1982.

Yen, PK: Feeding the patient who has cancer. *Geriatric Nurs* 2(1):68, 1981.

Dietary Management of Patients with Physiological Stress

26

THE STUDENT WILL BE ABLE TO:

- *List metabolic changes in the body caused by stress that affect nutritional status.*
- *Discuss dietary nutrients affected by stress.*
- *State the usual diet order for stressed patients.*
- *Identify patients and types of surgery that may result in malnourishment.*
- *Discuss nutritional care for surgical and burn patients.*
- *Explain the effect of fever and infection on nutritional requirements.*

Bulk
Catabolic
Curling's ulcer
Hypercapnia
Hypermetabolic
Hyperosmolar
Hypoxemia
Paralytic ileus
Respiratory acidosis
Respiratory quotient
Stress
Trauma

Physiological stress can be identified as any condition or stimulus that threatens the body's homeostasis or a person's well-being. Fear and anxiety, as experienced during illnesses or hospitalization, are simple stress factors. Physiological stress is a general term that includes surgical procedures and anesthesia (even though they are life-saving and under controlled circumstances), burns, trauma, fever, and infections. All of these types of stresses elicit similar hypermetabolic and hypercatabolic responses in the body to reestablish body homeostasis.

Hypermetabolism indicates an increased expenditure of resting energy. Hypercatabolism is characterized by a marked loss of tissue substances with negative nitrogen balance and large amounts of sulfur, phosphorus, potassium, magnesium, and zinc excreted. Increased urinary nitrogen, which is caused by the utilization of protein for energy, is not specifically related to the site of infection or trauma, but represents a generalized catabolism of skeletal muscle (Aulick & Wilmore, 1979) and redistribution of body proteins (Fig. 26–1).

However, each person reacts to stress differently. The magnitude of the physiological response is related to the type, duration, and severity of the condition, and treatments are slightly different depending on these three variables.

Metabolic Responses to Stress

EBB PHASE

A physiological stress activates the sympathetic nervous system. The initial response is an increase of hormones and catecholamines, which causes an elevated heart rate, increased respiratory rate, oliguria, and bronchial dilatation.

Increased catecholamines and hormones result in hyperglycemia. Glycogen is broken down to glucose (glucogenesis); proteins and fats are also broken down to elevate blood sugar levels (gluconeogenesis) in an attempt to regain homeostasis.

Increased glucagon levels reduce sensitivity of the peripheral tissues to insulin causing a pseudo-diabetic state and also increasing the glycemic level.

Increased glucocorticoids and antidiuretic hormone (ADH) increase fluid and sodium retention and increase potassium excretion. This physiological response expands intravascular volume as a safeguard to maintain blood volume.

Sympathetic nerve stimulation increases digestive juices and decreases peristalsis. These are accompanied by anorexia, nausea, vomiting, and abdominal distention. The elevated blood glucose also contributes to decreased appetite.

Since available glucose cannot be used for energy, branched-chain amino acids (BCAA) in the muscle tissues are utilized by the muscle for energy. This demonstrates how the stress response protects and defends the body by attempting to maintain circulating energy substrates, resulting in muscle-wasting and weakness. Because of the presence of insulin (which leads to a decrease in lipolysis), the body is not well-adapted to oxidize fatty acids and ketones during the initial response to stress. This ebb phase may last for two to four days after a major stress (Table 26–1).

FLOW PHASE

In the flow phase, which follows the ebb phase, hypercatabolism is being resisted, even though the body remains hypermetabolic to cope with the stress.

Catecholamines and hormonal secretions causing gluconeogenesis decrease, resulting in lower glucose levels and increased fatty acid levels. The important feature in this phase is that the body utilizes fatty acids and ketone bodies for energy so that less skeletal protein is catabolized. If the body is unable to make this adaptation, it becomes overwhelmed and may reach a state of exhaustion; death may occur. Hyperthermia in addition to hypermetabolism are characteristic of this phase.

Adequacy of the metabolic responses to stress is affected by the body's ability to satisfy energy requirements imposed by the catabolism without excessively depleting its protein reserves even during kilocalorie deprivation.

Nutritional support is of primary importance during hypermetabolic stress. The goal is to restore anabolism by furnishing nutrients to meet increased demands and to replace lost tissue protein. Nitrogen equilibrium can be achieved and at times positive nitrogen balance obtained in otherwise catabolic patients given adequate calories and protein. In most situations, the state of anabolism should be established by the seventh to tenth day after the stress or trauma (Metheny & Snively, 1983).

Figure 26–1. Alterations in protein metabolism with injury create a functional redistribution of proteins from skin, gut, and muscle to aid increased synthetic activity of the viscera and healing wound. (From Molnar JA, Wolfe RR, Burke JR: Burns: Metabolism and nutritional therapy in thermal injury, in Schneider HA, Anderson CE, Coursin DB (eds): Nutritional Support of Medical Practice, 2nd ed. Philadelphia, Harper & Row, 1983, p 263, by permission. As adapted from Benotti R, Blackburn GL: Protein and calories or macronutrient metabolic management of the critically ill patient. Critical Care Medicine 7(12):520, 1979.)

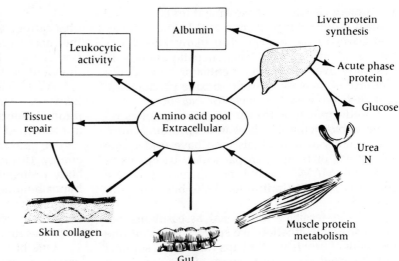

Clinical Implications:

- Since gluconeogenesis occurs in the liver, patients with liver disease may have problems coping with the acute phases of stressful conditions.
- Diabetic patients are especially susceptible to stressful conditions because of their inability to increase insulin production in response to hyperglycemia.
- A cachectic or malnourished patient has a poor tolerance for stressful situations.
- Fluids being given to the hypermetabolic person should be closely monitored. Because of the abnormal fluid-electrolyte balance, potassium depletion and fluid overload are potential hazards.
- During hypercatabolism, potassium is released from the cells, and an abnormal physiological response (hyperkalemia) may occur unless the kidneys are functioning normally. Adequate renal function should be established before giving high potassium foods (Metheny & Snively, 1983).

Nutritional Assessment for the Hypermetabolic Patient

Nutritional assessments serve to establish baseline data. The metabolic rate, nonprotein energy intake, nitrogen intake, and the metabolic state should be evaluated when considering nutritional needs since they affect nitrogen balance and

Table 26–1. Phases of Response to Trauma*

	Ebb Phase	Flow Phase		
				→Convalescence
		Acute Phase	Adaptive Phase	
DOMINANT FACTORS: SYMPTOMS:	Inadequate circulation Hyperglycemia Hyperlactic	Catecholamines Hyperglycemia	Glucocorticoid Hyperglycemia	
		Low insulin	High insulin	
	Hyperacidemia			
When compared to equivalent *Food Deprivation WITHOUT Trauma:*				
Fat Mobilization is:		Activated	Curtailed	
Nitrogen Losses:		May be less	Increased	

*From Blackburn, GL; Bistrian, BR: Nutritional care of the injured or septic patient. *Surgery Clinics of North America* 56(5):1195, 1976, with permission.

net protein utilization. Assessment for energy and protein requirements is important to prevent further harm to the patient. Too many kilocalories can result in hyperglycemia, hepatic abnormalities, fatty liver infiltration, ventilator dependence (because of increased carbon dioxide production), and elevated waste products for excretion.

Anthropometric measurements are not as reliable as biochemical indices in determining nutritional status of individuals who have undergone some form of trauma. In particular, triceps skinfold and MAMC cannot be utilized if severe edema is present (Indicators, 1986; Bencich et al, 1986).

Where feasible, nutritional assessments before a stressful situation like surgery will alert one to potential problems. Perhaps nutritional support can be used to correct some of the problems thereby preventing occurrence of major ones. For instance, if anergy is identified before an operation, nutritional support can be initiated for repletion. However, it may require two to three weeks to restore debilitated patients to a satisfactory status. Three to seven days of nutritional support for critically ill patients can only replete hepatic glycogen stores and correct the blood volume (Holter & Fisher, 1977). To prevent possible infection in an emergency situation, more aggressive treatment may be adopted, such as utilizing aseptic techniques or antibiotics to reduce bacteria (McLean & Meakins, 1981).

Nutritional Requirements for Physiological Stresses

During the flow phase, energy demands are initially met by the release of fatty acids from adipose tissue. Therefore, immediate concern for energy requirements are not of primary importance. The effect of initiating nutritional support before the flow phase is detrimental because: (1) The metabolism of large amounts of protein results in increased urea synthesis, or (2) excessive kilocalories result in lipogenesis (Maini et al, 1976).

Nutritional support is more effective and should be initiated when the body moves into the adaptive phase (see Table 26–1), when the strong catabolic effects of hormones and catecholamines have subsided. The adaptive phase can be identified by a decreased blood glucose level, normal BUN, ketosis, ketonuria, and less excretion of urea nitrogen. A fall in the blood glucose level is the most significant factor. In contrast, when intravenous (IV) dextrose solutions are being given, the identification of this phase is not apparent.

As a general rule, nutritional support of patients in stressful situations—be it surgery, trauma, infection, burns, or fractures should be implemented within five days to prevent an excessive amount of body proteins being utilized for energy (Kudsk et al, 1981). With depletion of body proteins, weakness, immunoincompetence, hypoalbuminemia, decreased wound healing, decreased synthesis of enzymes and plasma proteins, infection, and pressure sores further increase morbidity and mortality.

One of the primary goals for nutritional support is to decrease the amount of weight lost. Weight loss may approach 20 to 30 percent if nutritional support is not promptly implemented (Wilmore et al, 1974); this will result in high risk of mortality or severe complications such as infections. A weight loss of more than 40 to 50 percent is generally fatal (Wilmore & Kinney, 1981).

The mode of nutritional therapy in anticipation of or following a hypermetabolic stress condition can be any one or a combination of enteral and parenteral feedings, as appropriate (see Chapter 21). Consideration of the requirements to attain positive nitrogen balance may influence the method of nutritional support. For patients with greater requirements whose oral intake is inadequate to meet these needs, a combination of oral supplements, such as polymeric formulas, tube feeding, or parenteral nutrition may be required. In general, the hypermetabolic state induced by physiological stress causes increased requirements of *all* nutrients. Some individuals will be unable to orally consume adequate amounts of food because of the sizable requirements. Early feedings utilizing the gastrointestinal tract result in a reduced hypermetabolic response (Alexander, 1985).

The diet order may frequently read "high-energy, high-protein." While the order may not state increased minerals and vitamins, it is generally assumed that larger amounts will also accompany the protein and kilocalories. A sample menu pattern and analysis is shown in Table 26–2.

Communication is vital when ordering the high-energy, high-protein diet. By stating the purpose of the diet, confusion can be minimized. Frequently, a specific number of kilocalories and grams of protein will be stated (according to calculations presented later) to assure the adequacy of energy and protein. A diet specifying 3000 kcal

Table 26–2. High-Energy, High-Protein Diet and Its Nutrient Values

Protein: 15%   Carbohydrate: 49%   Fat: 36%

Sample Menu	Nutrient	Daily Total	Percent RDA†
Breakfast	Kilocalories	3457	172
1 cup Pineapple juice	Protein	132 gm	300
1 Scrambled egg with milk	Carbohydrate	440 gm	–
2 slices Bacon	Fat	141 gm	–
2 slices Whole wheat toast	Fiber	7.04 gm	–
1 Tbsp. Margarine	Cholesterol	557 mg	–
2 Tbsp. Jelly	Saturated fatty acids	46.9 gm	–
Midmorning Snack	Oleic fatty acids	49.7 gm	–
1 cup Homogenized milk	Linoleic fatty acids	25.2 gm	–
4 Crackers	Sodium	3132 mg	–
1 Tbsp. Peanut butter	Potassium	4760 mg	–
Lunch	Magnesium	473 mg	157
Sliced roast beef sandwich:	Iron	15.8 mg	87
2 oz. Lean, cooked roast beef	Zinc	17.2 mg	114
2 leaves Butterhead lettuce	Vitamin A	4457 IU	111
2 slices Tomato	Vitamin D	236 IU	117
1 Tbsp. Mayonnaise	Vitamin E	47.4 mg	592
1 cup Ice cream	Vitamin C	128 mg	213
Midafternoon Snack	Thiamin	3.01 mg	301
8 oz. Fruit-flavored yogurt	Riboflavin	3.3 mg	275
Dinner	Niacin	24.1 mg	185
3 oz. Broiled pork loin chop	Vitamin B_6	2.14 mg	107
1 medium Baked potato with 2 Tbsp. margarine	Folacin	346 mcg	86
½ cup Lima beans	Vitamin B_{12}	6.93 mcg	231
½ cup Gelatin salad with sliced peaches	Pantothenic acid	9.14 mg	166
2 Cloverleaf rolls with 2 tsp. margarine	Calcium	1829 mg	228
1 piece Gingerbread cake	Phosphorus	2377 mg	297
Evening Snack			
1 cup Homogenized milk			
4 Fig bar cookies			

Coffee and tea are allowed with sugar and cream, as desired.

*Nutrient values and percent RDA were determined by computer software Nutritionist II, Silverton, Oregon.
†Percent RDA for a female, 23 to 50 years old.

and 150 gm of protein may be interpreted as a diabetic diet, and the patient might receive three or four slices of bread instead of any sugar or apple pie à la mode. By prescribing the same diet and specifying that it is for a burn patient, the intention will be clear. The dietitian should be given special notification for prompt consultation.

The dietitian and nurse should try to provide the types of food the patient normally enjoys, which are more likely to be eaten. Regardless of the diet prescription, the nurse can encourage the patient to maintain a well-balanced intake consisting of selections from all food groups.

Anorexia is frequently present in stressed patients, significantly decreasing the amount of food eaten. The nursing challenge is to persuade the patient to consume the required nutrients. Every effort should be made to get the patient to eat the high-energy, high-protein diet composed of easily-digested foods. Six daily feedings are recommended to increase intake. Foods should be served appetizingly and special attention given to individual food preferences or tolerances. Polymeric formulas left in a chilled container and accessible to the patient can be taken over a period of time; their nutrient content is substantial.

FLUID-ELECTROLYTE BALANCE

In addition to normal fluid losses, the stressed patient may have increased fluid requirements because of losses from exudates, hemorrhage, vomiting, diuresis, and fever. Initially, adequate replacement of fluid loss is of paramount importance. These losses may be complicated by the patient's inability to consume enough beverages and foods to supply even the normal amounts of fluids. Intravenous infusions are used to maintain hydration and to correct electrolyte imbalances. However, stress may lead to renal shutdown. Renal function must be monitored by fluid output as well as intake. Oral intake should begin as soon as possible.

ENERGY

When the body is rebuilding tissue, adequate nonprotein kilocalories must be supplied for energy to reserve protein for tissue rebuilding. Positive nitrogen balance cannot be established with a negative kilocalorie intake. The energy can be supplied by carbohydrate and/or fat. Carbohydrates will maintain glycogen stores in the liver. Fats, while they should not be excessive and may be poorly tolerated, are a concentrated source of energy so that less volume is necessary.

As shown in Figure 26–2, the energy requirement depends on the percent of change in metabolic activity caused by the catabolic condition. The degree of catabolism has been categorized by Rutten and colleagues (1975) by measuring the amount of urinary nitrogen excreted. Energy requirements are increased directly proportional to urine urea nitrogen (UUN) Using Table 26–3, a rough estimate of energy requirements can be determined. If the patient is suffering from more than one of the catabolic conditions (for instance, both sepsis and multiple fractures), energy requirements are additive; the requirement for energy may increase 70 to 100 percent over the BEE (see Chapter 9).

Because of variations among individuals, energy requirements are difficult to determine. Energy levels are also influenced by the type of nutritional support. For anabolism to occur under hypermetabolic conditions, Paauw and colleagues (1984) have found that between 25 and 35 kcal/kg accurately predicts energy needs. For most hospitalized patients, 2000 to 3000 kcal meet these maintenance requirements; however, burn patients may need 4000 to 7000 kcal daily. Frequent weights should be taken; the patient should gain about 1/2 lb./day. More than this indicates water retention; less suggests inadequate kilocalorie intake.

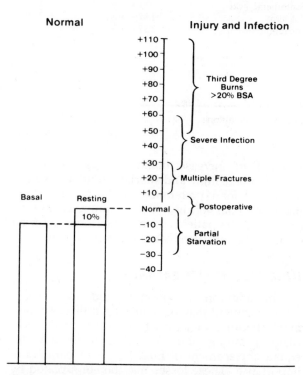

Figure 26–2. Effects of injury, sepsis, and starvation on resting energy expenditure. (From Elwyn DH: Nutritional requirements of adult surgical patients. Critical Care Medicine 8(1):9, 1980, by permission. As adapted from Kinney JM, Duke JH Jr, Long CL, et al: Tissue fuel and weight loss after injury. Journal of Clinical Pathology 4(suppl):65, 1970.)

PROTEIN

A disproportionately high ratio of protein to calories is necessary to provide sufficient amounts for the increased requirements and to maintain optimal immunological response (Alexander, 1985). If protein intake is inadequate, as much as 1 lb. of tissue protein per day may be catabolized. In addition to protein losses from tissue breakdown (from sepsis, fever, infection, or trauma), exudates, discharges, or hemorrhaging can cause nitrogen losses. Depletion of body protein can result in serious complications, since it is important for many physiological functions (Table 26–4).

Protein can only be synthesized after the nonprotein kilocalorie requirements have been met. This represents 16 percent of the total energy intake.

Protein requirements can also be calculated as follows:

Moderate stress = 1.0 to 1.5 gm/kg body weight

Severe stress   = 1.5 to 2.0 gm/kg body weight

Therefore, for a stressed individual weighing 70 kg, 100 to 140 gm of protein may be needed. To determine protein adequacy, nitrogen balance should be measured in the critically ill patient (see Chapter 20).

Table 26–3. Classification of Catabolism*

Clinical Situation	Degree of Catabolism	Urea=N (gm/day)	Increase of Resting Metabolic Rate Over BMR (%)	Total Caloric Requirement† (kcal)
Person in bed	1° (Normal)	<4	None	1800
Uncomplicated surgery	2° (Mild)	5–10	0–20	1800–2200
Multiple fractures or trauma	3° (Moderate)	10–15	20–50	2200–2700
Acute major infections or major burns	4° (Severe)	>15	50–125	2700–4000 or more

*Classification of patients according to the following: (1) obligate nitrogen loss expressed in gm urea-N per 24 hr; (2) energy expenditure expressed as per cent increase of the resting metabolic expenditure over calculated basal energy expenditure.

†This total caloric resting metabolic requirement includes the amount needed for activity, about 20 percent since these patients usually are not active, and 10 percent for specific dynamic action. This is a rough estimate for a 70 kg man and depends on the patient's size.

From Krause, MV; Mahan, LK: *Food, Nutrition and Diet Therapy*, 7th ed. Philadelphia, W. B. Saunders Co, 1984, with permission.

Monomeric formulas and parenteral protein solutions enriched with 35 percent branched-chain amino acids (BCAA) have been advocated for use in hypercatabolic patients since serum BCAA levels (of leucine, isoleucine, and valine) are decreased. The theory is that these amino acids, which are not readily used by the liver for glucose production, could be metabolized by skeletal muscle. Presently, 20 to 25 percent BCAA is recommended, which is the amount found in normal proteins. To date, studies using BCAA have not shown any difference in outcome or length of hospital stay even though positive nitrogen balance was achieved earlier (Andrassey et al, 1985; Maksoud & Tannuri, 1984). If patients can tolerate high-protein intakes (1.5 to 2.0 gm/day/kg), BCAA-enriched formulas should not be necessary. BCAA are currently recommended when positive nitrogen balance has not been achieved within a reasonable period of time after receiving standard feeding or formulas supplying adequate protein and energy (Skipper, 1984).

LIPIDS

Intravenous feedings normally consist of glucose for energy, amino acids to replace protein, and vitamins and minerals. Lipids used in these feedings can be beneficial. In addition to supplying essential fatty acids, they prevent side effects frequently seen with large amounts of intravenous glucose. Stress-related hypermetabolic hormones stimulate lipid catabolism. If lipids are used in the intravenous feeding, the plasma insulin level is reduced, allowing peripheral amino acids to be used for synthesis of critically needed visceral proteins (Gilder, 1986).

VITAMINS

While requirements for all vitamins are increased during stress, a few play vital roles in the patient's recovery (Table 26–5). If possible, these should be obtained from foods; reliance on multivitamin supplements can be risky since they may contain only 10 to 12 nutrients instead of the 40 or more needed. Minor surgery would not necessitate supplementation; however, patients fasting longer than four days, on routine intravenous or parenteral therapy require a therapeutic source of vitamins.

Vitamin C. Ascorbic acid has long been recognized for its role in wound healing and collagen formation. Urinary excretion is increased during stress (Effect of infection, 1983). Oral or parenteral supplements may be prescribed for extensive tissue regeneration.

Vitamin A. Tissue regeneration is dependent on Vitamin A. Low plasma retinol levels have been observed in fracture patients after surgery and usually correspond with decreased zinc levels. Since corticosteroid medications can lower serum vitamin A levels, it is felt that the effect of

Table 26–4. Physiological Functions of Protein as Related to Stress

Enhances	Prevents
Tissue synthesis for wound healing	Hypovolemia shock
Bone healing	Edema
Resistance to infection	Fatty deposits in the liver
Replenishing lost hemoglobin	Loss of muscular strength

Table 26–5. *Role of Vitamins and Minerals During Stress*

Nutrient	Physiological Role in Stress
Vitamin A	Required for tissue integrity and collagen formation; maintains immune function (lymphocytes, macrophages, and lysozymes).
Vitamin C	Enhances capillary formation, collagen synthesis, tissue integrity, and antibody production (phagocytes and neutrophils).
Folic acid	Needed for nucleic acid metabolism and protein synthesis; maintains immune function (lymphocytes and macrophages).
Vitamin B_{12}	Required for protein synthesis; maintains immune function (lymphocytes and macrophages).
Thiamin	Necessary in energy metabolism; maintains immune function (lymphocytes and macrophages).
Vitamin K	Needed for coagulation.
Biotin	Required for antibody production.
Vitamin B_6	Necessary in amino acid metabolism; maintains immune function (lymphocytes and macrophages) and white blood cell formation.
Riboflavin	Necessary for energy metabolism; maintains immune function (lymphocytes and macrophages).
Niacin	Necessary in energy metabolism; maintains immune function (lymphocytes and macrophages) and tissue integrity.
Vitamin E	Maintains immune function (lymphocytes and macrophages) and protects cellular lysosomes.
Zinc	Necessary for retinol-binding protein (RBP) and wound repair (cell mitosis and cell proliferation).
Copper	Part of ceruloplasmin (copper-binding protein); enhances host defensive mechanisms and collagen formation.
Iron	Required for collagen synthesis; enhances bactericidal activity of leukocytes; transports oxygen to the wound.
Phosphates	Needed for energy transfer.
Sulfates	Maintain protein structure.

stress can also precipitate this effect (Dickerson, 1981).

B Vitamins. When energy and protein intake is high, B vitamin requirements are also increased for metabolism. Many are required for antibody formation and white blood cell function.

ELECTROLYTES

Iron, calcium, magnesium, manganese, copper, and especially zinc have important roles in tissue repair. While their exact role in wound healing is not known, wounds in patients with clinical deficiencies return to normal healing rates with dietary supplementation. Large doses of zinc have no therapeutic value beyond that of correcting frank deficiency. Zinc is excreted in the urine; patients with renal dysfunction must be monitored to prevent high plasma concentrations (Elwyn, 1980).

Special Nutritional Concerns for Trauma Victims

Trauma, such as fractures or gunshot and stab wounds, causes protein losses through direct destruction of tissues. Unlike elective surgery, there is no time to replenish the body nutrition-

ally. However, most trauma victims are under 38 years of age and are basically healthy before the injury (Kudsk et al, 1981). Nutritional therapy should prevent deterioration of body cell mass, treat any specific complications, and restore the individual to an active normal functioning life.

Trauma imposes stress, and within moments after the event, the metabolic changes (explained earlier) will occur. In addition to protein catabolism caused by the stress reaction, protein-rich fluid may accumulate at the injury site, further increasing protein losses. Available energy will preferentially be used to feed the healing wound. Fortunately, a patient in good health before the incident has significant stores to initially offset catabolic effects.

Energy requirements are increased from the stress reaction and the need to reestablish metabolic processes (see Fig. 26–3). Vigorous nutritional therapy supplying the elevated requirements should be implemented for stressed patients to achieve positive balance.

Special Nutritional Concerns for Pulmonary Patients

Patients with chronic obstructive pulmonary disease (COPD) and acute respiratory failure are

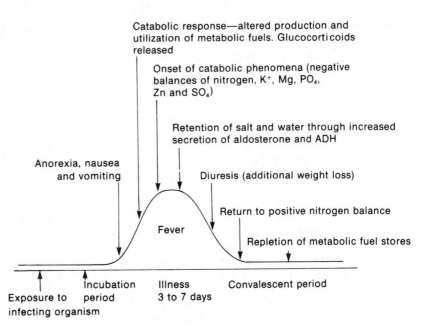

Figure 26–3. Timing of catabolic response to infection. (From Krause MV, Mahan LK: Food, Nutrition and Diet Therapy, 7th ed. Philadelphia, W. B. Saunders Co, 1984. As adapted from Beisel WR: The influence of infection or injury on nutritional requirements during adolescence, in McKigney JL, Munro HN (eds): Nutritional Requirements in Adolescence. Cambridge, Mass, MIT Press, 1976, p 259. Copyright © 1976 by The Massachusetts Institute of Technology.)

often malnourished, increasing their susceptibility to infections and adversely affecting hypoxic ventilatory response, respiratory muscle function, and lung structure. Additionally, the intensive care needs of mechanically-ventilated patients may take priority over nutritional requirements, interfering with the ability to wean the patient from the ventilator. Patients with respiratory disease must maintain a delicate balance between obtaining adequate oxygen and eliminating carbon dioxide. These manifestations of COPD indicate specific nutritional needs.

PHYSIOLOGICAL PROBLEMS

Respiratory muscle fatigue, hypoventilation, carbon dioxide retention, and oxygen depletion (hypoxemia) are common because of the patient's inability to regulate oxygen and the carbon dioxide content of the blood. In contrast to healthy individuals who breathe in response to elevated carbon dioxide levels, breathing is a response to hypoxia in patients with respiratory failure. Carbohydrate metabolism results in significantly more carbon dioxide production than other substrates (fat or protein). Normally, ventilation increases with greater carbohydrate intake, but patients with COPD are already breathing at their maximum, and patients on mechanical ventilators have a fixed ventilatory response. Hypercapnia (i.e., an elevated partial pressure of carbon dioxide) and respiratory acidosis may ensue if excessive energy is provided or if carbohydrate is the

primary energy source (Covelli et al, 1981). Because of its low respiratory quotient, fat is considered the best fuel for patients with respiratory disease.

The caloric requirement for breathing may be as high as 430 to 720 kcal/day in the patient with COPD, in contrast to 36 to 72 kcal for the normal individual (Brown & Light, 1983). Inadequate nutrient intake and increased caloric utilization from the work involved in breathing causes depleted nutritional status (Braun et al, 1984). However, hyperalimentation of calories, especially in the form of carbohydrate, may contribute to respiratory failure (Covelli et al, 1981; Askanazi et al, 1980).

NUTRITIONAL CARE

For patients with respiratory problems, BEE should be closely calculated to determine energy needs. The goal is to achieve a calorie-nitrogen balance. Dietary manipulation of energy substrates is beneficial for the patient with carbon dioxide retention because of hypoventilation. Carbohydrate is used to furnish some of the energy needs (a maximum of 40 to 50 percent) to help decrease metabolic rate; substituting fats for some carbohydrate will reduce carbon dioxide production. As much as 30 to 60 percent of the energy can safely be provided as fats. Excessive amounts of protein are avoided since it may increase ventilatory drive in patients with limited alveolar reserve. Specialized enteral formulas such as

Pulmocare (Ross) have been developed for pulmonary patients. Fluid intake is carefully controlled since there is an increased tendency to retain fluid (Kinney et al, 1984).

Special Nutritional Concerns for Burn Patients

The severely burned patient has all of the typical characteristics of the hypermetabolic state, and nitrogen losses exceed any other type of stress or trauma. The amount of protein wasting and weight loss is generally proportional to the extent and severity of the injury. Hypermetabolism increases with the size of burn area, peaking at about 2 to 2.5 times above the normal metabolic rate for burns involving as much as 40 percent of the body surface (Weinsier & Butterworth, 1981).

When the skin surface is destroyed, the body's first line of defense against infection is lost. Loss of skin also results in increased water and heat loss; the larger the burned area, the greater the loss of water vapor and heat. Approximately 2.5 to 4.0 L/day of water vapor may be lost from a major burn wound. The burned surface allows leakage of a protein-rich fluid, containing approximately two thirds as much protein as plasma (Metheny & Snively, 1983).

A diabetic-type glucose intolerance is frequently observed in burn patients. Hyperglycemia is due to insulin insufficiency resulting from increased secretion of catecholamines.

FLUID AND ELECTROLYTE REPLACEMENT

Large losses of fluids and electrolytes make their replacement the major concern during the first 12 to 24 hours to maintain circulatory volume and prevent acute renal failure; large amounts of waste products (such as nitrogen and potassium) must be excreted by the kidney. Fluids are required to keep these wastes in solution. The use of a balanced electrolyte solution, such as lactated Ringer's, is used by many physicians during the first 24 hours to correct metabolic acidosis associated with burns (Metheny & Snively, 1983). Intravenous feedings, blood transfusions and plasma or albumin are in order. At this time, no attempt is made to meet nutritional requirements.

Burns are accompanied by an increased desire for fluids. However, plain water should be limited in the seriously burned patient because of the possibility of water intoxication. Oral electrolyte fluids for the burn patient are usually recommended. A suitable solution consists of 1 tsp. of sodium chloride and 1/2 tsp. of sodium bicarbonate in 1 L of water. This may be more palatable chilled or in the form of ice chips or flavored with lemon juice (Metheny & Snively, 1983).

NUTRITIONAL CARE

After the period of fluid resuscitation, aggressive nutritional support should be implemented. This may be between 48 and 72 hours after the burn.

Enteral intake may have to be delayed for as long as five to seven days because of paralytic ileus, gastric dilatation, nausea, disorientation, narcotic medications, facial burns, associated injuries, or the need for respiratory support, but parenteral feedings may be implemented.

Burn patients do not eat well because of pain, generalized discomfort, and depression. Additionally, many are anorectic and unable to consume a sufficient number of kilocalories to satisfy energy requirements. Nurses must accept the challenge of encouraging these patients to eat and explain the role of nutrition in their healing process. In many cases, parenteral or tube feedings used in addition to oral feedings may be lifesaving.

Curling's ulcer, or acute ulceration of the stomach or duodenum, is frequently observed in burn victims. Large amounts of vitamin A can reduce the incidence of stress ulcer (Chernov et al, 1972). Antacid therapy is another preventive measure. Table 26–6 summarizes the nutritional care of burn patients.

Energy and Protein. Roughly twice the predicted BMR is adequate to prevent significant weight loss (Bell et al, 1986), but the formula shown in Table 26–6 is a more accurate determination of energy requirements. The rate of protein breakdown and gluconeogenesis is reflected in the rate of urine urea nitrogen (UUN). When 2 to 3 gm of protein/kg/day is supplied, positive nitrogen balance is maintained. The efficient use of nitrogen requires simultaneous availability of potassium, which is excreted heavily after a burn. A potassium-to-nitrogen ratio of 6:1 has been recommended (Weinsier & Butterworth, 1981).

Even with the daily administration of more

Table 26–6. Care of Burn Patients

Important Concerns	Recommendations
Environment	Keep temperature around 32° C with 20 to 30 percent humidity.
Fluids	Cover wounds to prevent fluid loss. Provide oral electrolyte fluids in adequate amounts.
Energy	(25 × IBW) = (40 × burned surface area)
Protein allowance	2 to 3 gm protein/kg/day. Calorie-to-nitrogen ratio of approximately 100:1.
Potassium	Adequate potassium with a potassium-to-nitrogen ratio of 6:1.
Vitamins and minerals	Supplement with vitamins and minerals, with special attention given to vitamin C (5 to 10 times the RDA)* and zinc (2 times the RDA).*
Gastric integrity	Give antacids or vitamin A and frequent feedings to prevent development of Curling's ulcers.
Mode of nutritional support	Give oral feedings with oral supplements, tube feedings, and/or parenteral nutrition to provide an adequate nutrient intake.
Daily documentation	Record fluid intake and output daily. Weigh daily. Record kilocalorie and protein intake daily.

*Bell, SJ; Wyatt, J: Nutritional guidelines for burned patients, *J AM Diet Assoc* 86(5):648, 1986.

than 5000 kcal by combining IV and oral feedings, actual weight gain is seldom attained in the first few weeks after the burn. However, weight stabilization is possible and usually precedes definitive wound closure and is considered to reflect diminishing metabolic demands (Newsome et al, 1973).

Vitamins and Minerals. Efforts should be taken to see that all other nutrients are supplied in adequate amounts. Normally, burn patients are given 1 to 2 gm of vitamin C daily.

Twenty percent of the body's stores of zinc are in the skin. Large amounts of zinc are lost when skin is destroyed and through exudates and urinary excretion. As much as 40 to 50 mg of zinc are lost daily as compared to 2 to 2.5 gm normally present in the entire body. Sanstead (1977) recommends 100 to 150 mg orally or 10 to 30 mg parenterally. Pharmacological doses have not been proven beneficial; adequate zinc replacement for amounts lost is needed, but megadoses are not indicated (Molnar et al, 1983).

Clinical Implications:

- The first priority is restoring electrolytes, fluids, and blood volume.

- The environment for burn patients should be warm (32°C) and dry to prevent further increase in convective heat loss. The rate of protein catabolism is increased in cooler conditions in order to maintain normal body temperature (Davies et al, 1969).
- When implementing central-vein TPN in burn patients, precautions must be taken in giving hyperosmolar solutions because the plasma osmolality may already be increased. Isotonic solutions of fat emulsions are recommended.
- Since burn victims often have paralytic ileus and reduced gastrointestinal tolerance, enteral feedings should be initiated only after normal bowel sounds have returned; tube feedings should be started at a rate of 20 cc/hr and doubled every eight hours, barring complications such as gastric retention or diarrhea (Weinsier & Heimburger, 1985).
- Orange juice and other high-potassium foods should be withheld until renal function is established.
- Record the patient's weight and caloric and protein intakes daily.
- The psychological state of the patient will greatly affect his/her attitude towards food.
- Burn victims often experience grief and anger over body disfigurement and the many painful treatments necessary. Constant emotional support and encouragement is vital. Encourage patients to talk about their feelings, wants, and needs.

Special Nutritional Concerns Associated with Infections and Fever

Nutritional status influences patient susceptibility to infections; additionally, an infection can deplete nutrient stores. Diets low in protein and blood serum levels low in vitamins A and C, pyridoxine, thiamin, and folic acid have been implicated in increasing vulnerability to infection. Iron, zinc, copper, and selenium also affect the immune functions (see Table 26–5), which can modulate the patient's responses to infectious agents (Keusch, 1982). While several researchers have postulated that vitamins can help prevent infections, evidence does not support an enhanced immunologic effect by taking an excess of vitamins. Defense mechanisms needed to fight infection are highly dependent on adequate protein synthesis to support phagocytic and lymphoid cell activity and immunoglobulin production (Tayek & Blackburn, 1984).

INFECTION AND NUTRITIONAL CHANGES

Overall metabolic responses to infection can be similar in spite of many different types of infectious organisms. Fevers are accompanied by metabolic and hormonal responses similar to those encountered by stress. Infections can cause some nutrients to be lost directly via secretion or excretion and others to be lost as a result of accelerated or functionally-altered metabolic processes (Beisel, 1980).

The acute infectious process is characterized by increased metabolic rate, weight loss, and wasting of body protein. Additionally, anorexia accompanied by a negative nitrogen balance is closely correlated with losses of potassium, phosphorus, magnesium, sulfur, and zinc (Beisel, 1983). Catabolic processes in relation to an infection are summarized in Figure 26–3. The catabolic period associated with an infectious disease is likely to last for several days; the anabolic period of increased nitrogen retention is generally twice as long (Gordon & Scrimshaw, 1970). Catabolic losses are associated with the febrile phase of infection. The amount of energy utilized increases when temperature deviates in either direction to generate heat and because of the increased enzymatic activity associated with elevated temperature (Keusch, 1982). The use of antipyretic drugs reduces energy requirements produced by a fever.

NUTRITIONAL CARE

For centuries, fevers were treated by fasting, sometimes with even withholding of water. Each degree Fahrenheit of elevated temperature increases metabolic demands by seven percent (13 percent for each degree Celsius). However, with extensive infections, such as peritonitis or cellulitis, metabolic rates may range from 25 to 50 percent above BMR. Energy adequacy can be determined by body weight changes.

Fluid and electrolyte balance is of concern since fluid imbalances caused by the infection can range from severe overload to severe dehydration. As much as 3 to 4 L of fluids may be required to replace water lost from the fever and to help eliminate the products of catabolism. Reten-

tion of sodium and chloride are influenced more by hormones than by diet.

Since defensive mechanisms to fight infection are ultimately dependent on protein-synthesizing capabilities, an increased amount of protein is required for visceral protein synthesis. But energy intake must first be adequate. Exact protein requirements have not been determined. In general, the protein allowance should be 1.5 gm/kg/day for febrile adults and 3 gm/kg/day for children.

Plasma concentrations of iron and, to a lesser extent, zinc are greatly diminished during acute infections (Wannemacher, 1983). However, while the infection is active, oral or parenteral doses of iron, folate, and vitamin B_{12} are ineffective in reversing anemia caused by the infection (Beisel, 1983).

Vitamins C, A, and the B complex (including folate, B_6, and B_{12}) all have a part in the immune function to fight off the invasive organisms. In general, it is felt that the RDAs for vitamins should be available throughout the course of an infection, or at most, doses should be doubled or tripled to replace those excreted or needed during hypermetabolism (Beisel, 1983).

Clinical Implications:

- Fluid intake and output (I & O) records should be maintained to assure adequate intake in order to prevent dehydration; insufficient output may indicate fluid overload.
- When evaluating weight changes, weight loss can be masked by the retention of salt and water.

SEPSIS

McLean and Meakins (1981) have defined sepsis as an "invasive infection characterized by a positive blood culture and evidence of an infective focus." Weight loss, marked reduction in muscle mass, progressive hypoalbuminemia, and increased urea excretion are part of the classic metabolic effects of ongoing sepsis. Septic patients are unable to efficiently utilize major energy reserves, i.e., lipids. Long (1977) has estimated an energy requirement of 42 kcal/kg in septic patients. In the average-sized male (70 kg), approximately 3000 kcal are needed. Because of decreased ability to ingest and digest foodstuffs, it may be necessary to utilize tube or parenteral feedings for part of the kilocalories.

During infection, iron is deposited in the liver

in the form of hemosiderin and other unavailable storage forms. This causes the anemia frequently seen; however, it must be corrected by administration of red blood cells (McLean & Meakins, 1981).

Special Nutritional Concerns of Surgery

Surgical procedures are usually "planned" or "induced" trauma; they produce an extraordinary stress on the body. Nutritional needs are increased by this stress, yet they are often ignored.

PREOPERATIVE NUTRITIONAL CARE

Good nutritional status before surgery enables a patient to withstand postoperative catabolic stresses of negative nitrogen balance and several days of "starvation" without seriously hampering recovery. More efficient and faster wound healing is another benefit. As previously discussed, morbidity and mortality are related to nutritional status.

For elective surgery, nutritional repletion can be made over a period of time. Since obesity presents a risk during surgery, weight reduction is usually advisable.

Preoperative nutritional therapy is implemented to lessen possible risks postoperatively; problems are more prevalent in certain types of patients. Patients over 40 years old and children generally experience preoperative apprehension and anxiety or stressful preoperative preparation. Patients may have become depleted as a result of vomiting, diarrhea, or bleeding. Also, patients with a chronic or neoplastic disease have usually experienced significant weight loss. Frequently, protein-energy malnutrition is present in surgical patients with gastrointestinal tract diseases (Roe, 1979). These surgical interventions are discussed in Chapter 27.

Whenever necessary and possible, surgical intervention can be delayed in order to replenish body stores by implementing a high-energy, high-protein diet. An increased amount of nutrients can be ingested if six small feedings are offered. Liquid supplements between meals can increase the kilocalorie and total nutrient content. This diet, if utilized long enough, will correct deficiencies and provide optimum reserves for surgery as well as for the "starvation" period following it.

When emergency surgery must be performed, correction of fluid and electrolyte imbalances must be frequently initiated immediately before surgery. Whole blood transfusions will raise hemoglobin and hematocrit levels.

The stomach should be empty during surgery and before administering any general anesthesia; no food is allowed for at least six hours before surgery. Food in the stomach may be aspirated during the induction of anesthesia or in the recovery period. The general procedure is a light dinner with fluids allowed until midnight for surgery scheduled the following morning.

Clinical Implication:

- Preoperatively, the patient's appetite may be diminished from psychological and/or mental stress, especially if she or he is malnourished. Failure to eat adequate amounts should be reported.

POSTOPERATIVE NUTRITIONAL CARE

Many patients may not eat at all for a few days or may eat very little following an operation, thereby inducing a starvation effect. This causes a negative nitrogen balance with increased mobilization of amino acids for energy and increased potassium excretion. Dextrose and electrolyte fluids are generally given intravenously during this period to prevent dehydration and electrolyte imbalances. The dextrose provides energy for the brain and other vital organs; a minimum of 100 gm of dextrose prevents ketosis.

Foods can normally be tolerated when peristalsis returns. This function can be determined by the presence of bowel sounds or the passage of flatus or stools. While postoperative nutrition should be initiated as soon as possible, if oral feedings are started before the resumption of normal functioning of the gastrointestinal tract, nausea, and the possibility of intestinal obstruction may occur. Most adults have nutrient reserves that enable them to endure three or four days of semistarvation without detrimental effects.

To avoid excessive amounts of muscle protein being utilized for energy, adequate nourishment of the adult should be implemented within five days. If the patient is unable to ingest adequate amounts of calories in a short period of time, other types of nutritional support must be considered.

As described in Chapter 19, patients are first put on a clear-liquid diet, and progress, as foods are tolerated, to a regular diet or the one they had before surgery. In general, the diet after surgery should contain plenty of energy-containing, nutrient-dense foods. If adequate amounts of nutrients and kilocalories cannot be taken, oral supplemental feedings may be necessary.

Clinical Implications:

- Postoperatively, many patients are disturbed by intestinal gas. Ambulation is a better therapy than seltzer or carbonated beverages for intestinal gas pains (Kirsner et al, 1985).
- During the postoperative period in which there is a temporary inability to ingest nutrients, a weight loss of 1/2 lb./day reflects muscle and fat catabolism; a weight gain of more than this indicates fluid retention.
- Accurate I & O records are essential postoperatively to determine fluid balance.

Complications Associated with Physiological Stresses

Other complications can result from the prolonged period of bedrest resulting from a physiological stress. Muscle-wasting is a serious problem. In addition to adequate nutrition, the nurse can encourage range of motion (ROM) exercises and ambulation according to the physician's orders to maintain dynamic equilibrium.

IMMOBILIZATION

Patients immobilized by fractures or paralysis and those with prolonged bedrest excrete large amounts of calcium. Serum levels of calcium and phophorus are elevated during bedrest. Mineral losses occur to a greater extent in the weight-bearing bones; the process is apparently reversible. These changes in mineral metabolism can be reversed by quiet standing for two or more hours daily (Page & Clibon, 1982). While this demineralization could result in osteoporosis, large amounts of dietary calcium are not wise since serum calcium levels are already elevated. This problem is not due to calcium intake but is precipitated by a lack of weight-bearing activity. Corticosteroids are frequently prescribed to reduce calcium absorption; a low-calcium diet has been recommended by some physicians.

PRESSURE SORES

Bedfast patients frequently have poor appetites and may become nutritionally depleted because of poor intake. Pressure sores (decubitus ulcers) occur primarily in patients with protein-energy deficiencies. The exudate from a draining decubitus ulcer is high in protein and can greatly increase protein requirements. At least 100 gm of protein are needed to promote healing. Oral supplements between meals can be given; tube feedings may be necessary. An adequate intake of zinc is also important. Pressure sores usually respond well to 500 mg of vitamin C supplements given twice daily (Taylor et al, 1974). However, hemoglobin levels must be at least 10 gm/dl for healing to occur as well as for relief of the constant pressure on the tissues.

Clinical Implications:

- Large amounts of fluids should be taken by immobilized patients to prevent the formation of renal stones from elevated serum calcium. Mobility of these patients should be attempted as soon as possible.
- Increasing the protein and kilocalorie intake of the patient with pressure sores is as important as turning the patient frequently and properly medicating the ulcer.

• FALLACIES and FACTS

FALLACY: *Everyone should take Stresstabs for our stressful lifestyle.*
- **FACT:** *Although physiological stress necessitates increased nutrient requirements, emotional stress does not have the same effect. Emotional stresses may produce physiological changes by increasing vitamin excretion, especially vitamin C. A balanced diet is the best insurance for maintaining a good nutritional status, which will provide nutrient stores when needed. For usual stresses encountered in daily living, nutrient intakes higher than a supplement which*

contains 100 percent of the RDAs in addition to the diet are unnecessary.

FALLACY: Vitamin E is important for wound healing and supplements should be given for surgery and trauma.

• **FACT:** Vitamin E suppresses collagen synthesis, making new repair tissue weaker. While the diet should contain adequate amounts of vitamin E, supplements should be avoided as a postoperative therapy (Pollack, 1979).

Summary

During physiological stress, the body is generally thrown into a hypermetabolic state with increased catabolism. Combined supportive treatment modalities are essential for optimal outcome; nutritional support is an important aspect of the treatment. An individual's well-being can be severely threatened with any stress or trauma. The rate of recovery will be affected by the nutritional status prior to the stress, which can be determined by a nutritional assessment.

The extent of the trauma and the expected duration of recovery should be evaluated, and along with consideration of the patient's nutritional status, an appropriate diet should be prescribed. In general, the patient needs liberal amounts of all the nutrients. Energy and protein are of primary concern; when nutrient-dense foods are ingested in sufficient quantities to provide energy and protein, increased amounts of vitamins and minerals will accompany them.

Anorexia, prevalent during periods of stress, interferes with adequate intake. Inventive efforts must be made to increase the intake of patients who have increased dietary needs. Between-meal feedings or oral supplements can be used to increase intake. In some instances, other modes of nutritional support may be implemented to avoid nutritional depletion and accompanying risks.

Review Questions

1. What are the nutritional implications of the metabolic changes caused by stress?
2. State reasons why it is important: (a) to maintain I & O records in physiologically stressed patients, (b) to provide adequate kilocalories, and (c) to provide adequate protein.
3. Why is it difficult for stressed patients to get adequate intake? List some ways of increasing their intake.
4. Why might a patient with emphysema using a ventilator be given a low-carbohydrate, moderate-protein, high-fat diet or tube feeding?

Case Study: Mrs. I. M. is an 85-year-old woman who has been in a nursing home following a cerebrovascular accident (CVA) six years ago. Since the CVA, she has experienced difficulty with chewing and swallowing and has required increasing staff time to be fed. She has been virtually bedfast and now has decubitus ulcers over the sacrum and greater trochanter of the left femur. Her serum hemoglobin is 7.4 gm/dl, hematocrit is 22 gm/dl and her total serum protein is 4.8 gm. An aggressive ulcer care program was implemented. Despite the care, the ulcers show no sign of healing.

1. What additional information would you need to determine why healing is not occurring?
2. List two nursing diagnoses for this patient and a goal for each.
3. How many grams of hemoglobin are considered minimal for healing to occur?
4. What measures may be necessary to ensure that healing is possible?

Case Study: Ms. J. T. is a 20-year-old college student. While returning to school after a holiday, she is involved in a multi-car accident in which her car bursts into flame. She sustains deep partial- and full-thickness burns over 35 percent of her body surface area. One week after the original injury, her vital signs have stabilized, but her serum glucose remains consistently above 130 mg/dl. She is placed on a high-calorie, high-protein diet with vitamin and mineral supplements.

1. Before the accident, her weight was 120 lbs. and her height was 5'6". What should her daily protein allowance be at this time? Caloric requirements?
2. Why does her blood glucose remain elevated one week after her injury?
3. What are the possible complications of a persistently elevated serum glucose?
4. What is the rationale for the high-calorie, high-protein diet for this patient?
5. What vitamin and mineral supplements would you expect for the burn patient?

REFERENCE LIST

Alexander, JW: Immunity, nutrition and trauma: An overview. *Acta Chir Scand* (Suppl) 522:141, 1985.

Andrassey, RJ; DuBois, T; Page, CP; et al: Early postoperative nutritional enhancement utilizing enteral branched-chain amino acids by way of a needle catheter jejunostomy. *Am J Surg* 150(6):730, 1985.

Askanazi, J; Elwyn, DH; Silverberg, PA; et al: Respiratory distress secondary to a high carbohydrate load: A case report. _Surgery_ 89(5):596, 1980.

Aulick, LH; Wilmore, DW: Increased peripheral amino acid release following burn injury. _Surgery_ 85(5):560, 1979.

Beisel, WR: Infectious diseases. In _Nutritional Support of Medical Practice,_ 2nd ed. Edited by HA Schneider; CE Anderson; DB Coursin. Philadelphia, Harper & Row, 1983, p 443.

Beisel, WR: Effects of infection on nutritional status and immunity. _Fed Proc_ 39(13):3105, 1980.

Beisel, WR: Magnitude of host nutritional response to infection. _Am J Clin Nutr_ 30(8):1236, 1977.

Bell, SJ; Molnar, JA; Krasker, WS; et al: Weight maintenance in pediatric burned patients. _J Am Diet Assoc_ 86(2):207, 1986.

Bencich, J; Twyman, D; Fierke, A; et al: Failure of anthropometry as a nutritional assessment tool in ICU patients. Presented at the annual meeting of the American Dietetic Association, Las Vegas, NV, October 1986.

Braun, SR; Keim, NL; Dixon, RM; et al: The prevalence and determinants of nutritional change in chronic obstructive pulmonary disease. _Chest_ 86(4):558, 1984.

Brown, SE; Light, RW: What is now known about protein-energy depletion: When COPD patients are malnourished. _J Respir Dis_ 4(5):36, 1983.

Chernov, MS; Cook, FB; Wood, M; et al: Stress ulcer: A preventable disease. _J Trauma_ 12(10):831, 1972.

Covelli, HD; Black, JW; Olson, MW; et al: Respiratory failure precipitated by high carbohydrate loads. _Ann Intern Med_ 95(5):579, 1981.

Davies, JWL; Liljedahl, SO; Birk, G: Protein metabolism in burned patients treated in a warm (32°C) or cold (22°C) environment. _Injury_ 1(1):43, 1969.

Dickerson, JWT: Vitamins and trace elements in the seriously ill patient. _Acta Chir Scand_ 507(suppl):144, 1981.

Elwyn, DH: Nutritional requirements of adult surgical patients. _Crit Care Med_ 8(1):9, 1980.

Gilder, H: Parenteral nourishment of patients undergoing surgical or traumatic stress. _JPEN_ 19(1):88, 1986.

Gordon, JE; Scrimshaw, NS: Infectious disease in the malnourished. _Med Clin North Am_ 54(6):1495, 1970.

Holter, AR; Fisher, JE: The effects of perioperative hyperalimentation on complications in patients with carcinoma and weight loss. _J Surg Res_ 23(1):31, 1977.

Indicators of surgical risk. _Lancet_ 1(June 21):1422, 1986.

Keusch, GT: Nutrition and infections. _Compr Ther_ 8(5):7, 1982.

Kinney, JM; Weissman, C; Askanazi, J: Influence of nutrients on ventilation. _Nutr Abst Rev_ 54(11):917, 1984.

Kirsner, JB; Sawyers, JL; Crow, S: Postoperative gas pains. _JAMA_ 253(5):705, 1985.

Kudsk, KA; Stone J; Sheldon, GF: Nutrition in trauma. _Surg Clin North Am_ 61(3):671, 1981.

Long, CL: Energy balance and carbohydrate metabolism in infection and sepsis. _Am J Clin Nutr_ 30(8):1301, 1977.

McLean, APH; Meakins, JL: Nutritional support in sepsis. _Surg Clin North Am_ 61(3):681, 1981.

Maini, B; Blackburn, GL; Bistrian, BR; et al: Cyclic hyperalimentation: An optimal technique for preservation of visceral protein. _J Surg Res_ 20(6):515, 1976.

Maksoud, JG; Tannuri, U: Effects of branched-chain amino acids and insulin on postinjury protein catabolism in growing animals. _JPEN_ 8(3):416, 1984.

Metheny, N; Snively, W: _Nurses' Handbook of Fluid Balance,_ 4th ed. Philadelphia, J. B. Lippincott Co, 1983.

Molnar, JA; Wolfe, RR; Burke, JF: Burns: Metabolism and nutritional therapy in thermal injury. In _Nutritional Support of Medical Practice,_ 2nd ed. Edited by HA Schneider; CE An-

derson; DB Coursin. Philadelphia, Harper & Row, 1983, p 260.

Newsome, TW; Mason, AD; Pruitt, BA: Weight loss following thermal injury. _Ann Surg_ 178(8):215, 1973.

Paauw, JD; McCamish, MA; Dean, RE; et al: Assessment of calorie needs in stressed patients. _J Am Coll Nutr_ 3(1):51, 1984.

Page, C; Clibon, U: A method of enterally feeding defined formula diets. _Am J IV Ther Clin Nutr_ 9(1):9, 1982.

Pollack, S. W.: Wound healing: A review. _J Dermatol Surg Oncol_ 5(8):615, 1979.

Roe, DA: _Clinical Nutrition for the Health Scientist._ Boca Raton, FL, CRC Press, 1979.

Rutten, P; Blackburn, GL; Flatt, JP; et al: Determination of optimal hyperalimentation rate. _J Surg Res_ 18(5):477, 1975.

Sandstead, HH; Myers, ML; Telander, RL; et al: Nutrition in trauma and burns. _Dialogues in Nutrition_ 2(1):1, 1977.

Skipper, A: Enteral nutrition: Feeding by tube, specialized formulas. Presented at the ADA Annual Meeting, October, 1984.

Tayek, JA; Blackburn, GL: Goals of nutritional support in acute infections. _Am J Med_ 76(5A):81, 1984.

Taylor, TV; Dymock, IW; Torrance, B: The role of vitamin C in the treatment of pressure sores in surgical patients. _Br J Surg_ 61(11):921, 1974.

Wannemacher, RW, Jr: Effect of infection on nutrient metabolism. _Nutrition and the MD_ IX(1):1, 1983.

Weinsier, RL; Butterworth, CE: _Handbook of Clinical Nutrition._ St. Louis, C. V. Mosby Co, 1981.

Weinsier, RL; Heimburger, DC: Nutritional support of the burned patient. _Nutrition and the MD_ XI(9):1, 1985.

Wilmore, DW: Nutrition and metabolism following thermal injury. _Clin Plast Surg_ 1(4):603, 1974.

Wilmore, DW; Kinney, JM: Panel report on a nutritional support of patients with trauma or infection. _Am J Clin Nutr_ 34(suppl 6):1213, 1981.

Wilmore, DW; Long, JM; Mason, AD; et al: Catecholamines: Mediator of the hypermetabolic response to thermal injury. _Ann Surg_ 180(4):653, 1974.

Further Study

Apelgren, KN; Wilmore, DW: Nutritional care of the critically ill patient. _Surg Clin North Am_ 63(2):4907, 1983.

Braun, SR; Keim, NL; Dixon, RM; et al: The prevalence and determinants of nutritional changes in chronic obstructive pulmonary disease. _Chest_ 86(4):558, 1984.

Buchanan, RT; Levine, NS: Nutritional support of the surgical patient. _Ann Plast Surg_ 10(2):159, 1983.

Cerrato, PL: Is your patient really ready for surgery? _RN_ 48(6):69, 1985.

Forlaw, L: The critically ill patient: Nutritional implications. _Nurs Clin North Am_ 18(1):111, 1983.

Holli, BB; Oakes, JB: Feeding the burned child. _J Am Diet Assoc_ 67(9):240, 1975.

Irwin, MM; Openbrier, DR: A delicate balance: Strategies for feeding ventilated COPD patients. _Am J Nurs_ 85(3):274, 1985.

Irwin, MM; Openbrier, DR: Feeding ventilated patients—safely. _Am J Nurs_ 85(5):544, 1985.

Keim, NL; Luby, MH; Braun, SR; et al: Dietary evaluation of outpatients with chronic obstructive pulmonary disease. _J Am Diet Assoc_ 86(7):902, 1986.

Keithley, JK: Nutritional assessment of the patient undergoing surgery. _Heart Lung_ 14(5):449, 1985.

Keithley, JK: Infection and the malnourished patient. _Heart Lung_ 12(1):23, 1983.

Luterman, A; Adams, M; Curreri, PW: Nutritional management of the burn patient. *Crit Care Quarterly* 7(3):34, 1984.

Marcineck, MB: Stress in the surgical patient. *Am J Nurs* 77(11):1809, 1977.

National Dairy Council: Nutritional demands imposed by stress. *Dairy Council Digest* 61(6):31, 1980.

Palmer, PN: Malnutrition: Reversing the trend in the surgical patient . . . home study program. *AORN J* 40(3):347, 1984.

Phipps, M; Bauman, B; Berner, D; et al: Staging care for pressure sores. *Am J Nurs* 84(8):999, 1984.

Rhoads, JE: The impact of nutrition on infection. *Surg Clin North Am* 10(1):41, 1980.

Rosequist, CC; Shepp, PH: Burn care: The nutrition factor. *Am J Nurs* 85(1):45, 1985.

Salmon, SW: Trauma and fracture: Meeting your patient's nutritional needs. *Orthop Nurse* 3(4):27, 1984.

Schumann, D: Symposium on wound healing. Preoperative measures to promote wound healing. *Nurs Clin North Am* 14(6):683, 1979.

Specialized Nutrition for Pulmonary Patients. Columbus, OH, Ross Laboratories, December 1984.

Dietary Management of Gastrointestinal Disorders

27

THE STUDENT WILL BE ABLE TO:

- *Discuss the treatment for hiatus hernia.*
- *Plan a progressive dietary program for a patient with a peptic ulcer.*
- *Explain the outmoded Sippy diet and tell why it was used previously and why it is not recommended today.*
- *List foods included on high-fiber diets and discuss low-fiber dietary regimens.*
- *Define and discuss diverticulosis.*
- *Explain the steps and precautions for the nutritional care of a colostomy patient.*

Achalasia
Bland diet
Dumping syndrome
Gliadin
Gluten
Gluten-sensitive
  enteropathy (GSE)
Hiatus hernia
Irritable bowel syndrome
  (IBS)
Peptic ulcer disease
Pyrosis

OBJECTIVES

TERMS TO KNOW

Gastrointestinal disorders can be particularly devastating because the GI tract is the only natural way of providing nutriment for the body. When functions of the gastrointestinal tract are compromised, digestion and/or absorption may be compromised. One out of nine Americans is affected by some type of digestive disorder, which is the leading cause of hospitalization (Given & Simmons, 1984).

Upper Gastrointestinal Tract

DYSPHAGIA

Numerous mechanical, neuromotor, or even cardiovascular abnormalities may cause dysphagia (i.e., difficulty in swallowing). Symptoms range from problems initiating swallowing to completing the activity. Pain and a feeling of fullness are frequently present.

Nutritional Care. To maintain nutritional status, special attention is given to help patients eat and drink safely so that foods are not aspirated or regurgitated. Observance of types of foods and conditions best tolerated (e.g., hot or cold, solid or liquid, whether the patient eats alone or with company) not only results in improved food intake but can help the physician identify the problem (Luckmann & Sorensen, 1980). Tips for feeding the dysphagic patient (Rombeau & Caldwell, 1984) include:

1. Proper positioning during eating is important. The patient should sit up if at all possible.
2. Special equipment, such as plate guards and built-up spoons, may need to be used.
3. Sufficient time for eating must be allowed, especially in the elderly person. The patient should not be hurried while eating.
4. Small bites of food or sips of liquid should be taken, allowing sufficient time to hold food in the mouth. Food should not be washed down with liquids, as the food may be aspirated.
5. When the patient is ready to swallow, he should hold his head slightly forward and hold his breath.
6. If the patient needs to be fed:
   a. Watch the thyroid cartilage (Adam's apple) to see if the patient has swallowed.
   b. Allow the patient to indicate when he is ready for the next mouthful.
   c. Converse with the patient only in regard to his condition. Communication may be distracting for patients with pseudobulbar dysphagia, but others may actually need verbal direction for eating.
7. Certain medications may affect swallowing. For example, atropine may cause the mouth to be dry, making swallowing difficult. Excessive drooling or salivation will also cause problems.
8. Some foods can be more difficult to manage than others:
   a. Milk and ice cream (i.e., uncooked milk) may produce phlegm. Cream soups and puddings are acceptable, however.
   b. Sticky foods such as mashed potatoes, fresh bread, and bananas are difficult to swallow.
   c. Dry foods (crackers) need to be moistened. Gravy can be added to potatoes and meat.
   d. Slippery foods are easier to swallow but may be difficult to control in the mouth for mastication.
   e. Puréed foods provide insufficient texture for stimulation and may be aspirated.
   f. Liquids or solid foods without flavor, or with flavors that the patient is insensitive to, will cause problems. For example, the patient may be able to drink orange juice but not water.
   g. The temperature of foods may affect the stimulation required for swallowing.

Dysphagia is a real challenge to nursing and cannot be covered in depth in this discussion. The article by Buckley and colleagues (1976) is highly recommended.

Clinical Implications:

- Position the patient in a comfortable upright position with the head in an upright position, slightly tilted forward.
- Textured foods that require chewing stimulate a better swallow, e.g., toast instead of bread or a boiled potato instead of mashed potatoes.
- Offer juices diluted with water at first, and use flexible straws if the patient has sucking capabilities.
- Mildly sweetened and salted foods are generally favored. Foods should be close to room temperature. Avoid acid or bitter flavors and sticky foods (e.g., soft bread, bananas, or peanut butter).
- Make consistency adjustments according to the patient's tolerance. Liquids can be used to moisten foods for individuals with decreased saliva production.
- Adapt the diet to the patient's need and gradually upgrade it as feeding skills improve.

GASTROESOPHAGEAL REFLUX

One of the most common problems encountered in clinical practice is gastroesophageal reflux (heartburn or pyrosis). Because many people assume heartburn is normal, they do not report it to their physician.

Pathophysiology. Heartburn, or severe burning sensations under the sternum, is the main symptom of gastroesophageal reflux, but it is also accompanied by a feeling of fullness or regurgitation. It can masquerade as a chest pain or pulmonary disorder, especially in children (Richter & Castell, 1982). This reflux of gastric contents into the esophagus occurs most frequently about a half hour to one hour following a meal.

Acidity, alkalinity, pepsin, or bile may be damaging to the esophageal mucosa. The acidity from the stomach is quite destructive. The lower esophageal sphincter (LES), a special muscle between the stomach and the esophagus, usually keeps the stomach's caustic juices from refluxing (coming back up) into the esophagus. If the pressure is reduced, juices reflux into the esophagus and cause pain. If the condition is not treated, esophagitis may result.

Heartburn in pregnant women is common. Sphincter pressures are progressively decreased during pregnancy, in women taking birth control pills containing progesterone, and even in the late stage of normal menstrual cycles. Increased levels of serum progesterone are correlated with increased gastroesophageal reflux (Richter & Castell, 1982).

Pharmacological Treatment. Alkalinization by antacids has been used as a treatment for gastrointestinal reflux. Antacids (1) increase LES pressure, (2) decrease reflux, and (3) neutralize gastric acidity. Magnesium hydroxide (milk of magnesia) is almost perfect as an antacid, except for people with kidney disease who have an impaired ability to eliminate magnesium. For heartburn, only 1 to 3 tsp. is required instead of the 6 tsp. for laxative results. Aluminum hydroxide is also a safe and effective antacid. (Fein, 1980). However, it may lead to constipation and phosphorus depletion with constant use. Tables 27–1 and 27–2 compare many antacids, their content and acid-neutralizing capacity. Antacids differ not only in duration and strength but also in their side effects (e.g., inducing constipation or acting as laxative). Alternating the intake of various antacids may be recommended.

Anticholinergic drugs relieve the symptoms of reflux by decreasing acid production, which reduces antacid medication. These drugs have few side effects and do not affect the LES, esophageal peristalsis, or gastric emptying.

Nutritional Care. Sphincter muscle tone varies considerably during the day. Foods may affect the LES pressure or increase acid secretion. Intake of fat, alcohol, chocolate, and some medications (anticholinergics and sedatives) as well as smoking can lower the pressure.

Table 27–1. Electrolyte Content of Leading Antacid Suspensions*

Product (Manufacturer)	Aluminum hydroxide (mg/5 ml)	Magnesium hydroxide (mg/5 ml)	Calcium carbonate (mg/5 ml)	Other Ingredients (mg/5 ml)	Sodium (mg/5 ml)	Acid neutralizing capacity (mEq/5 ml)
Alternagel (Stuart)	600				<2.0	16.0
Aludrox (Wyeth)	307	103			1.15	14.0
Aluminum Hydroxide Gel (Roxane)	350				8.5	†
Amphojel (Wyeth)	320				<7.0	6.5
Gelusil (Parke-Davis)	200	200		Simethicone (25)	0.7	12.0
Maalox (Rorer)	225	200			1.35	13.5
Maalox Plus (Rorer)	225	200		Simethicone (25)	1.35	13.5
Maalox T.C. (Rorer)	600	300			0.8	28.3
Mylanta (Stuart)	200	200		Simethicone (20)	0.68	12.7
Mylanta II (Stuart)	400	400		Simethicone (30)	1.14	25.4
Riopan (Ayerst)				Magaldrate (540)	<0.1	15.0
Riopan Plus (Ayerst)				Magaldrate (540) Simethicone (20)	<0.1	15.0
Titralac (3M)			1000		11.0	19.0

*From Cantrell, MD: Drug and food interactions: Coordinating diet and antacid intake. *RD* 5(3):4, 1985.
†Information not available.

Table 27–2. Electrolyte Content of Leading Antacid Tablets*

Product (Manufacturer)	Aluminum hydroxide (mg/tab)	Magnesium hydroxide (mg/tab)	Calcium carbonate (mg/tab)	Magnesium trisilicate (mg/tab)	Other ingredients (mg/tab)	Sodium (mg/tab)	Acid neutralizing capacity (mEq/tab)
Aludrox (Wyeth)	233	83				1.6	11.5
Gaviscon (Marion)	80			20	Alginic acid, sodium bicarbonate†	19.0	†
Gaviscon-2 (Marion)	160			40	Alginic acid, sodium bicarbonate†	36.8	†
Gelusil (Parke-Davis)	200	200			Simethicone (25)	0.8	11.0
Gelusil-II (Parke-Davis)	400	400			Simethicone (30)	2.1	21.0
Gelusil-M (Parke-Davis)	300	200			Simethicone (25)	1.3	12.5
Lo-Sal (Glenbrook)		120	585			<0.14	†
Maalox #1 (Rorer)	200	200				0.84	8.5
Maalox #2 (Rorer)	400	400				1.84	18.0
Maalox Plus (Rorer)	200	200			Simethicone (25)	1.0	8.5
Mylanta (Stuart)	200	200			Simethicone (20)	0.77	11.5
Mylanta II (Stuart)	400	400			Simethicone (30)	1.3	23.0
Riopan (Ayerst)					Magaldrate (480)	0.1	13.5
Tempo (Vicks)	133	81	414		Simethicone (20)	2.5	14.0
Titralac (3M)			420			<0.3	7.5

*From Cantrell, MD: Drug and food interactions: Coordinating diet and antacid intake. *RD* 5(3):4, 1985.
†Information not available.

Carminatives, the volatile oils of plant extracts used in food seasonings, flavorings, and liqueurs, produce hypotension of the LES. Some of these include spearmint, peppermint, garlic, and onions.

Caffeine, coffee, protein, and calcium stimulate acid secretion (Feldman et al, 1981). Alcohol seems to indirectly increase acid after its absorption (McArthur et al, 1982). Other foods that increase acid secretion include red peppers, colas, citrus juices, and tomato products (Richter & Castell, 1982).

A high-protein, low-fat diet helps to increase sphincter pressure. The following are recommendations for treating gastrointestinal reflux and hiatus hernia:

1. Achieve and maintain ideal body weight to improve mechanical and postural status (except pregnant women, who should not try to lose weight).*
2. Increase protein and reduce fat intake.
3. Avoid foods that decrease LES pressure: chocolate, alcohol, peppermint, coffee, and carbonated drinks.
4. Avoid foods that may irritate and cause spasms: citrus juices, tomatoes, and tomato sauce.
5. Stop smoking, if that is a habit.
6. Eat small meals four times a day.
7. Eat a larger meal at noon with a lighter meal in the evening. Finish the evening meal at least two to four hours before bedtime. Avoid late evening snacks.

*The problem may be resolved with no further treatment if weight is reduced.

8. Wear loose clothing.
9. Use gravity for prevention:
   a. Raise the head of the bed at least six inches, or use a wedge-shaped pillow to elevate the head while sleeping.
   b. Avoid lying down or bending over immediately after eating food.

HIATUS HERNIA

A protrusion (herniation) of a portion of the stomach above the diaphragm through the esophageal opening into the chest is called a hiatus hernia (Fig. 27–1). Most hiatus hernias are a sign of aging (weakness of tissue), too little roughage in the diet, or the sudden impact from penetration or compression. However, an increase in abdominal pressure can also cause herniation through the hiatus, such as obesity and chronic cough. One of the main symptoms of a hiatus hernia is gastric reflux, resulting in gastroesophageal reflux or heartburn (see preceding recommendations). Some people suffer none of these symptoms of hiatus hernia, while others require surgery.

Clinical Implications:

- Cimetidine (Tagamet) and antacids should not be taken together; antacids inhibit the absorption of cimetidine (Steinberg et al, 1982).

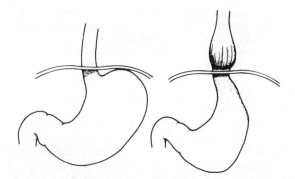

Figure 27–1. Hiatus hernia showing displacement of cardia of stomach through diaphragm into thoracic cavity. (From Given BA, Simmons SJ: Gastroenterology in Clinical Nursing, 4th ed. St. Louis, The C. V. Mosby Co, 1984, by permission.)

- A heart attack and simple indigestion can be so similar that detection is difficult. Distinguishing features of a heart attack include a sensation of chest pressure or tightness rather than burning, sometimes radiating to the arms, neck, or jaw, and sweating. Weakness and shortness of breath may also be present (How to choose, 1983).
- Inform patients about ways to prevent reflux and the particular symptoms to watch for.
- If antacids are not given, the acidic gastric content can further damage the esophageal lining to cause inflammation, severe pain, difficulty in swallowing, and even bleeding and anemia (Fein, 1980).
- Counseling for pregnant patients should include management of heartburn due to reduced LES pressure.
- Cimetidine (Tagamet) may interfere with vitamin B_{12} absorption, so monitoring is important (Anderson et al, 1982).
- Aluminum-containing antacids may increase excretion of calcium during a low-calcium intake (about 250 mg/day), but not when calcium intake is more than 800 mg/day (Spencer et al, 1982).
- Many persons become obese by eating food instead of taking medicine for gastric acidity.

PEPTIC ULCER

A peptic ulcer may occur in any part of the gastrointestinal tract from the lower part of the esophagus, stomach, duodenum, or jejunum. Stress ulcers are so common from trauma (burns, major illness, or injuries) that antacids are often given prophylactically.

Pathophysiology. The fundamental cause of peptic ulcer is not clear. Whenever the mucosa is eroded to allow exposure to the gastric juices, an ulcer may develop. Secretion of hydrochloric acid increases after a meal in order to help digest the food and activate enzymes. In some instances, too much hydrochloric acid is secreted with or between meals; the mucosal lining of the stomach is not sufficiently protected; or the motility of the digestive tract is reduced, allowing acidity to remain in the tract longer than usual. Any of these abnormalities may precipitate an ulcer.

A duodenal ulcer refers to a peptic ulcer in the duodenum. Either name may be used correctly. In the patient with a duodenal ulcer, excessive production of acid and pepsin may be the main factor, whereas decreased tissue resistance may be more important in the patient with peptic ulcer (Given & Simmons, 1984).

Ordinarily, burning pain similar to heartburn occurs in the epigastrium, but some ulcers are discovered by hemorrhage or melena (tarry stools). Other symptoms that occur before meals include aching, burning, gnawing, and boring sensations. Pain occurs one to four hours after a meal or in the middle of the night when the stomach is empty.

Lifestyle. The ulcer personality is well known; movements and secretions of the gastrointestinal tract are directly affected by tensions and strains. A basic component of treatment involves modifying the individual's lifestyle and personality toward a more relaxed and slower pace with less strain and pressure.

Dietary Management. Bertram Sippy used dietary and medicinal treatments to control gastric activity. The Sippy diet consisted of frequent milk and cream feedings to coat the stomach lining. This diet has fallen into disfavor because of its excessive fat and cholesterol content. Additionally, constipation and scurvy accompanied the diet.

Currently, milk is *not* used as a therapy since large amounts of calcium and protein are potent stimulants of gastric acid secretion (McArthur et al, 1982). This does not mean milk must be eliminated, but frequent feedings of milk are not advisable. Skim milk is quite acceptable as part of the dietary regimen. It does, however, destroy the old concept of milk as the major treatment.

In spite of many different diets for ulcers, the therapeutic effect of such diets is unknown. There is much disagreement about which foods to include or exclude. Research shows that a bland diet does not decrease gastric acid secretion or increase the rate of healing.

A bland diet is now considered a transitional diet to be used for severe inflammation. It is designed to avoid chemical, thermal, and mechanical irritations of the gastrointestinal tract and to decrease peristalsis. Fried and raw foods are usually excluded. Small feedings are given hourly throughout the day. When pain disappears, intervals between feedings may be lengthened, and larger amounts of food eaten. While the bland diet is safe, it is not a requirement for the patient with a peptic ulcer.

Contrary to earlier beliefs, most condiments do not cause gastric irritation, with the exception of black pepper, chili powder, caffeine (coffee, tea, or cocoa), alcohol, and drugs (particularly salicylates). If tolerated, caffeine-containing beverages may be taken with or near mealtime even though they may increase gastric acid production.

Increased dietary fiber has been used in the management of ulcers with less recurrence (Rydning et al, 1982; Malhotra, 1978). It has been postulated that the fiber delays gastric emptying. Adequate chewing is important for any ulcer patient, but even more so for the fiber-rich diet.

However, a study by Rydning and colleagues (1986) indicated that a high-fiber diet was not effective in relieving ulcer symptoms or healing. A low-fiber diet may result in constipation, which is frequently a problem when antacids are the principal form of therapy.

Symptoms of intolerance are related more to individual response than to intake of specific foods or the presence of disease; the individual is the best person to decide which foods are to be eliminated, if any. A person with an ulcer may continue on a normal diet or a diet as tolerated. However, the individual should maintain a regular eating schedule, eating moderately and in a relaxed atmosphere.

Milk-Alkali Syndrome. In the past, when large amounts of milk and absorbable alkalis were given for the treatment of ulcers, milk-alkali syndrome was frequently seen. Characterized by hypercalcemia and hypercalciuria, it is caused by excessive intake of calcium. It can result in metastatic calcification, nephrocalcinosis, and renal calculi, which can produce renal insufficiency, and azotemia. With current ulcer treatments using nonabsorbable antacids and less milk, this condition is prevented (or corrected).

Clinical Implication:

- Uncompromising food restrictions have no place in the dietary management of peptic ulcer. Assure the patient of your support and offer an environment dedicated to his/her well-being to encourage healing.

ACHALASIA

Lack of peristalsis and excessive lower esophageal sphincter (LES) constriction prevent the normal flow of food into the stomach, resulting in esophageal dilatation, dysphagia, and/or regurgitation (Fig. 27–2). Usually, dilation of the LES relieves this, but the motor ability for it to close may be lost, so that reflux occurs. Patients are encouraged to relax and live with this condition (Luckmann & Sorensen, 1980). Dysphagia is dealt with as previously discussed. Prior to dilation or surgery, liquid or blenderized foods may be used, or tube feedings may be necessary. Fluids may help wash down soft foods.

HYPOCHLORHYDRIA

When hydrochloric acid secretion is insufficient, protein denaturation (which normally occurs in the stomach) is incomplete so that complete hydrolysis of amino acids in the intestine is incomplete. Since resistance to bacterial agents is reduced, problems with putrefaction may occur. Dietary measures include low milk intake (to maintain low bacterial count) and minimal fat intake. (See Chapter 28 for calculations of fat content.)

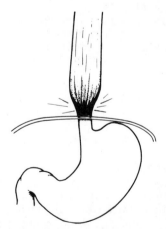

Figure 27–2. Achalasia showing dilatation of esophagus above stricture at cardia. (From Given BA, Simmons SJ: Gastroenterology in Clinical Nursing, 4th ed. St. Louis, The C. V. Mosby Co, 1984, by permission.)

Lower Gastrointestinal Disorders

Even though the colon is not essential, it helps to recycle nutrients for a more efficient digestive system. The small intestine is crucial to nutrient absorption. Without the large intestine, many essential electrolytes as well as a large volume of fluid are lost (Phillips & Stephen, 1981).

DIARRHEA

Abnormal frequency and liquidity of stools in diarrhea result in significant losses of sodium and potassium. The goals of therapy are to replace fluid plus electrolytes and to decrease the number and frequency of stools. Without fluid replacement, dehydration or death may result.

Nutritional Care. For the first few hours, nothing by mouth may serve to relieve the digestive tract. In severe cases, intravenous (IV) therapy may be required to replace fluids and electrolytes. Fluids should be used that will help replace the sodium and potassium losses. For simple diarrhea, commercial preparations of glucose-electrolyte solutions (Pedialyte, Lytren, or Gatorade) are available; root beer, cola, ginger ale, and other carbonated beverages are weaker, with about 1/10 of the sodium (no potassium) of the special preparations designed for diarrhea or dehydration. These beverages should be allowed to become decarbonated before use. In contrast, apple juice is high in potassium with little sodium. Applesauce is particularly useful since the pectin binds free water and improves consistency of the stools. Saltine crackers are a source of sodium, and ripe bananas may be eaten as a source of potassium (see Chapter 12). No food containing fat should be consumed.

Frequently, lactose intolerance is experienced after abnormal digestive problems. Milk may delay gastric emptying, so it should be withheld for at least six hours after the last episode of diarrhea.

Travelers' Diarrhea. Poor sanitation may result in foods being contaminated with a variety of infectious agents (*Escherichia coli* is the most common). Travelers' diarrhea may be called "turista," "Montezuma's revenge," or "green-apple two-step." This untimely illness is usually not severe; high fever, vomiting, or bloody stools occur in only a minority of cases.

The most important measure is prevention; foods and beverages likely to promote diarrhea should be avoided. Improperly-handled, cooked or uncooked foods may be implicated. Raw vegetables, raw meat, and raw seafood are especially risky foods. Other items associated with increased risk of travelers' diarrhea include tap water, ice, unpasteurized milk and dairy products, and unpeeled fruits. Only canned or bottled carbonated beverages using water that has been boiled or chemically treated are safe. Little can be done to relieve the symptoms or shorten its course, but suggestions for diarrhea in general may be followed. Drugs can be used to reduce the severity of the diarrhea, as discussed in the article by Weber and Lefrock (1985); prophylactic antimicrobial drugs are not recommended.

Clinical Implications:

- Fluids must be replaced to avoid dehydration; solids should be gradually added as tolerated. A low-residue diet may be in order to decrease the intake of fibrous materials.
- Evaluate the use of foods that may contribute to diarrhea, especially those high in fiber, caffeine, and alcohol.
- Encourage juices high in potassium.
- Remove milk products from the diet if there is a possibility of lactose intolerance.
- Bananas, grated raw apples, or cooked applesauce contain pectin, which helps bind the fluid and retard its transit time.
- Extremely hot or cold foods increase peristalsis and may aggravate diarrhea.

CONSTIPATION

Prolonged retention of feces in the colon resulting in small volume and difficult evacuation of hard, dry stools is constipation. Infrequency does not mean constipation. A normal elimination pattern may be only two or three times per week. Possible causes include: (1) not eating food with enough fiber, (2) too little fluid intake, (3) too little exercise, (4) not responding to defecation urges, or (5) habitual use of laxatives or enemas.

The dietary prescription should include (unless contraindicated by other conditions) sufficient fluids (at least six to eight glasses daily), and foods with fiber such as raw fruits and vegetables, whole-grain cereals, and bran breads.

Bran may be added to a wide variety of foods and is cost-effective. In a study conducted by Hull and colleagues (1980) at a geriatric center, 6 to 8 gm of bran was added to hot cereal. This increase of 25 to 50 percent of the total dietary fiber eliminated constipation in 60 percent of the residents. Since many had previously required laxatives, this resulted in an annual savings of $44,000 for laxatives. In addition, nurses appreciated the fewer enemas and disimpactions necessary.

Clinical Implications:

- Ask patients about their use of cathartics or laxatives.
- Gradually increase the amount of fiber or bulk in the diet (raw vegetables and fruits, whole-grain breads, and cereals).
- Force fluid intake; drink at least the equivalent of six to eight glasses of water a day.
- Dried fruits, especially prunes, contain natural laxatives.
- Any hot beverage upon arising, such as coffee, tea, or lemon water, may stimulate peristalsis because duodenal-ileal or gastric colic is strongest in the morning. Breakfast is also important and should contain some fiber.
- Encourage activity and relaxation as much as possible; allow sufficient time for bowel habits.
- The use of docusate sodium (Colace) may not be an effective treatment for constipation (Chapman et al, 1985)

FLATUS

Swallowed air from eating with the mouth open, certain foods digesting in the gut, and intestinal bacteria can produce flatus (gastrointestinal gas). Aerophagia (air swallowing) is the main source of intestinal gas (60 to 80 percent). Gulping food or fluids, sipping through a straw, air whipped into food, and frequent sucking of hard candy or chewing gum with the mouth open are reasons for aerophagia. Even some foods contain gas; e.g., apples have a gas volume of 25 percent (Given & Simmons, 1984).

Treatment. Anxiety, nervousness, or breathing problems from asthma can cause some persons to be chronic aerophagics. Once aware of the problem, the behavior can be modified. Gas-forming foods (e.g., beans and cabbage) contain nonabsorbable oligosaccharides, which remain in the bowel, increasing bacterial action and forming gas. These foods can be eliminated (Table 27–3). Since fats produce carbon dioxide, their intake may be reduced.

Clinical Implications:

- Discourage drinking with straws.
- Avoid foods that produce gas. (This is a highly individual matter, one in which the patient must be observant.) In many persons, dried beans, peas, and foods from the cabbage family (e.g., broccoli and Brussels sprouts) cause problems.
- Decrease the amount of fat in the diet.
- Encourage the patient to chew food slowly, closing the mouth.
- Discourage the intake of carbonated beverages.
- Malabsorption syndromes, peptic ulcers, and cholelithiasis are disorders that cause excessive flatulence; these treatable disorders must be excluded by conventional means (Van Ness & Cattau, 1985).

Table 27–3. *Possible Causes of and Solutions to Mild Gas Problems**

Possible Cause	Solution
carbonated beverages	herb teas, fruit juices, water
gulping or swallowing air	relax, take small sips and bites
beans and peas	smaller portions: try different variety
cabbage family (sulfur-containing vegetables, i.e., cabbage, broccoli, Brussels sprouts, cauliflower)	Cook *without* placing a lid on the pot
excess bulk	reduce added bran (if used) or amounts of salad-type vegetables and/or fruits
intolerance to milk sugar	smaller portions of milk, yogurt, and cheese; omit when discomfort is persistent.
specific sensitivity	omit *on a trial basis* any one (at a time) of the following: carrots, raisins, bananas, apricots, prune juice, pretzels, bagels, wheat germ, pastries, potatoes, eggplant, apples, citrus fruits and bread.

*From Nelson, M: Dietary Guidelines. *Nutrition and Health* 5(3):3, 1983.

GLUTEN-SENSITIVE ENTEROPATHY (GSE)

GSE and gluten-induced enteropathy (GIE) are the terms most often used for a variety of conditions including nontropical sprue, celiac disease, and idiopathic steatorrhea. Celiac disease appears in familial clusters, implicating a hereditary factor. It is often diagnosed in adults 20 to 30 years of age, but symptoms can usually be traced to early childhood. The infantile and adult forms are now thought to be the same.

Pathophysiology. This malabsorption syndrome involves pathological changes in the structure of the absorbing cells in the intestine. In many cases, this is due to an abnormal sensitivity to the dietary protein gluten. Symptoms include diarrhea or foul-smelling, frothy, bulky stools; bloating; anorexia; muscular wasting; anemia; chronic fatigue; crampy abdominal pain; and dermatitis herpetiformis. Projectile vomiting, a bloated abdomen, and growth failure are seen in children. Infants with celiac disease are asymptomatic until cereals are introduced, at which time they become irritable, refuse to eat, and develop the above symptoms.

Nutritional Care. When damage occurs to the lining of the small intestine, many nutrients cannot be digested and absorbed. The small intestine will repair itself when gliadin-containing foods are totally removed from the diet. Since protein, fat, and carbohydrates are poorly absorbed, weight loss is common. Nutrients that are often deficient include fat-soluble vitamins, vitamins B_6 and B_{12}, trace elements, iron, and folate.

Actually, only the gliadin part of the gluten causes mucosal damage in susceptible individuals, with the other part of gluten, glutenin, not involved. Gluten is found mainly in wheat, with less in rye and still lower amounts in oat and barley flours. Dietary management of primary GSE requires elimination of wheat and rye from the diet for life; however, if GSE is secondary to another condition, symptoms may not recur.

Wheat flour can be replaced with corn flour or meal and potato and rice flour (Table 27–4). All products using wheat, rye, oats, and barley must be eliminated from the diet, which means labels must be carefully read for cereal, starch, flour, thickening agents, emulsifiers, gluten, and stabilizers (Table 27–5). (Since the gluten has been removed from wheat starch, it is acceptable.) Lists of gluten-free products may be obtained from food companies (CDA, 1981). Recipes are available substituting rice and other flours in most traditional wheat-flour products.

Table 27–4. Substitutions for Wheat Flour*

Special cookbooks may be helpful. Many other recipes can be modified by the following substitutions.
1 cup of wheat flour may be replaced by:
  1 cup of wheat starch
  1 cup of corn flour
  1 scant cup of fine cornmeal
  3/4 cup of coarse cornmeal
  5/8 cup (10 tbsp) of potato flour
  7/8 cup (14 tbsp) of rice flour
  1 cup of soy flour plus 1/4 cup of potato flour
  1/2 cup of soy flour plus 1/2 cup of potato flour
1 tablespoon of wheat flour may be replaced by (for thickening)
  1/2 tbsp of cornstarch, potato flour, rice starch, or arrowroot starch
  2 tbsp of quick-cooking tapioca

Temporary intolerance to lactose is common in GSE patients and may also involve fats. After a few months on a gluten-free diet, many gastrointestinal villi will return to normal and more lactase is produced. When sufficient amounts of lactase are made, dairy products can be tolerated again. When diarrhea and steatorrhea are present, special emphasis should be given to replace nutrients lost (especially magnesium, calcium, and vitamins A, D, E, and K).

The diet should initially be low in fiber because the mucosal villi are flattened in patients with GSE. Gradually, fiber content can be increased. Medium-chain triglycerides are usually well tolerated. Since fat absorption is decreased, fat-soluble vitamins should be given in water-miscible forms.

Foods that may need to be excluded because of intolerance (but that are not readily recognized as containing wheat, rye, oats, and barley) include: creamed soups and vegetables, ice cream, cakes, cookies, breads, spaghetti, macaroni and other pastas, mixed infant and junior dinners, malted milk, processed cheese, commercial salad dressings, Postum, and Ovaltine.

Clinical Implications:

- Grain products containing gliadin may be added in food processing (e.g., hot dogs and luncheon meats) or in staple foods, such as vinegar (cider and wine are acceptable). Reading the label is a *must* to avoid these products.
- Malt and malt flavoring may be derived from barley or corn.

Table 27–5. Sample Menu for Gluten-Restricted Diet*

Breakfast	Lunch	Dinner
1/2 cup orange juice	6 oz. vegetable soup	1/2 cup tomato juice
1/2 cup Cream of Rice	2 oz. beef patty	3 oz. broiled chicken
8 oz. milk (whole or low-fat)	2 slices gluten-free bread	1/2 cup mashed
1 poached egg or egg	Sliced tomato and lettuce	potatoes
substitute	French dressing	1/2 cup peas
2 slices broiled bacon or	Catsup, mustard	1/2 cup fruited JellO
bacon substitute	3 apricot halves	salad
1 slice gluten-free bread	2 rice wafers	1/2 cup orange sherbet
1 tsp. butter or margarine	8 oz. milk (whole or low-fat)	1 slice gluten-free bread
1 Tbsp. jelly		1 tsp. butter or
1 cup coffee		margarine
1 oz. cream or nondairy		1 cup coffee
creamer		1 oz. cream or nondairy
4 tsp. sugar		creamer
		2 tsp. sugar

Approximate Nutritive Value of Sample Menu

Protein	97 gm	Riboflavin	2.015 mg
Fat	100 gm	Thiamine	1.429 mg
Carbohydrate	268 gm	Calcium	962 mg
Calories	2360 (MJ 9.9)	Phosphorus	1534 mg
Vitamin A	10,976 IU	Iron	15 mg
Vitamin C	150 mg	Sodium	3639 mg
Niacin	24.5 mg NE	Potassium	3218 mg

*Chicago Dietetic Association: *Manual of Clinical Dietetics.* Philadelphia, W. B. Saunders Co, 1981, with permission.

- Hydrolyzed vegetable protein may be from soybeans, corn, wheat, or a mixture of these; vegetable protein may include soybeans, corn, wheat, rye, oats, and/or barley.
- When starch is listed as an ingredient on a product made in the United States, it is corn starch.
- Glucocorticoids may produce remission in celiac disease even on a regular diet; their long-term use is not advisable because of other associated risks (Response, 1982).
- Because of a long history of malabsorption before diagnosis, patients with celiac disease are at greater risk of developing nutrient deficiency–related disorders, such as osteoporosis. Calcium supplements may be needed to reverse bone demineralization.
- Helping these individuals become familiar with products and recipes using allowable foods will improve their dietary compliance, especially in children.
- Since the major grain sources used in this diet are refined and unenriched, a multivitamin and mineral supplement is recommended.
- Strict, lifelong adherence to a gliadin-free diet is essential; the disease is not outgrown.
- Gluten-containing foods can cause severe villi damage in persons with celiac disease, even in those who do not have symptoms.

CROHN'S DISEASE (REGIONAL ENTERITIS)

One of the two types of inflammatory bowel disease (IBD) is Crohn's disease. This inflammatory process primarily affects the ileum and the proximal colon (though it can affect any part of the alimentary tract). Crohn's disease affects mainly children and young adults. Currently, there is no medical treatment totally effective in curing Crohn's disease.

Inadequate nutrient intake, even for short periods, produces morphological and functional changes that may further increase malabsorption and depress the body's ability to heal (Walker, 1980). Frequently, inadequate energy intake is responsible for protein-energy malnutrition in the early stages of Crohn's disease (Gee et al, 1985). Reduced intakes of vitamins A, B_6, and B_{12}, folate, riboflavin, thiamin, calcium, and iron have been found in assessments of patients with Crohn's disease. Whether or not these nutrient deficiencies are contributing factors to the incidence or results of this disease is unknown (Hodges et al, 1984).

Pathophysiology. Crohn's disease involves ulcerations through all layers of the mucosa and submucosa with a characteristic cobblestone appearance. It is a slow, progressive, inflammatory process with affected areas scattered among normal sections, so some absorption is maintained. Symptoms include cramping, abdominal pain, diarrhea, and weight loss. Scarring, thickening, and narrowing of the intestinal wall restricts nutrient absorption and causes a thick, narrowed lumen with intestinal obstruction. Steatorrhea may result (Hoppe et al, 1983).

Nutritional Care. Nutritional deficiencies are related to the extent, severity, and location of the ulcerations. Malnutrition is caused by inadequate intake, anorexia, malabsorption, and intolerance to many different food components (fat, lactose, and fiber). Adequate nutritional support is a challenge. Because of the effects of foods, patients are finicky and apprehensive about eating. Spontaneous food intake will not usually maintain or increase weight in these patients.

Patients with acute Crohn's disease may require total parenteral nutrition (TPN) or elemental diets to rest the bowel and improve healing and closure. This will curtail drainage and induce remission (Ostro et al, 1985). However, it is generally felt that TPN has no significant advantage over oral feedings in most situations, and its widespread use is discouraged (Heatley, 1984).

When foods are reintroduced, corticosteroids are used to maintain remission. Jones and colleagues (1985) were able to prolong remission by detecting and eliminating foods not tolerated by the patient. Initially, liquid diets are given, followed by low-residue foods. Seasonings and chilled foods may be poorly tolerated.

Foods high in kilocalories, protein, vitamins, and minerals are needed to replenish depleted stores; small frequent meals are better tolerated. Even though the patient can tolerate some foods, supplementation may be necessary to augment nutrient intake. A team approach in the treatment of this condition is vital.

In patients with Crohn's disease of the distal ileum or an ileal resection, a low-fat diet (40 gm/day) is required to prevent the possibility of oxalate stone formation and to control diarrhea.

Anemia may result from bleeding or inadequate intake of iron, folic acid, and vitamin B_{12}. Therapeutic doses of sulfasalazine, used to treat bowel disease, interfere with folate absorption. Taking medication between meals can improve the utilization of folates. Folic acid supplementation may also be needed. Most multivitamin supplements omit folic acid. Parenteral vitamin B_{12} should be administered every three months to all patients with extensive involvement or resection

of the ileum in Crohn's disease (Codini & Rosenberg, 1981).

Clinical Implications:

- During bouts with diarrhea, sources of potassium intake should be increased.
- Multivitamin and mineral supplements are frequently recommended.

ULCERATIVE COLITIS

The second type of inflammatory bowel disease, ulcerative colitis, is an inflammation of the colon, sometimes extending into the rectum (Fig. 27–3). The two diseases are so similar that they are often hard to distinguish. However, in ulcerative colitis, the mucosa becomes very fragile and bleeds easily. It is usually continuous along the intestinal tract, while Crohn's disease affects only segments. Other symptoms include fever, diarrhea, edematous colonic mucosa, abdominal pains, anorexia, and weight loss.

Causes of nutritional problems in inflammatory bowel disease may be seen in Table 27–6. Nutritional deficiencies are similar for both of these conditions with losses of water, sodium, potassium, chloride, bicarbonate, vitamins, and other minerals (Table 27–7). Diarrhea, occurring when scar tissue fills in ulcerations of the mucosa and destroys the absorptive areas of the colon, is the most critical factor (Hoppe et al, 1983).

As with other gastrointestinal disorders, the psychological aspects are significant. Psychotherapy for depression, relaxation, and biofeedback can benefit these patients (Goldsmith & Patterson, 1985).

Nutritional Care. Elemental formulas have become a key therapy for patients with acute inflammatory bowel disease; total parenteral nutrition (TPN) is used when fistulas, obstruction, or abscesses are present. Bowel rest, positive nitrogen balance, and repletion of nutritional deficits can be achieved by the use of elemental formulas or TPN. Such treatment can result in 60 to 80 percent remission without surgical intervention (Hoppe et al, 1983).

Counseling is extremely important to help the patient understand the reasons for dietary intervention. Abdominal discomfort with expectations of diarrhea cause the patient to become reluctant to eat. Fever may also occur with the disease itself

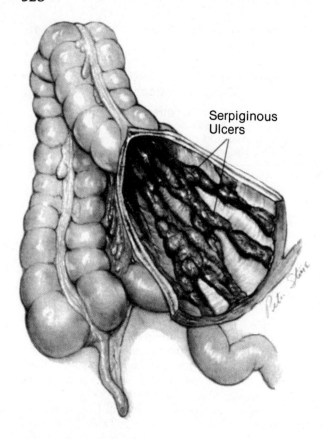

Serpiginous
Ulcers

Figure 27–3. *Ulcerative colitis is characterized by widespread inflammation of the colon. Less severe cases fluctuate between episodes of exacerbations and remissions. In the fulminating type, the patient may die within a short time from intestinal and systemic complications. (From Phillips SF, Stephen AM: The structure and function of the large intestine. Nutrition Today 16(6):4, 1981. Reproduced with permission of Nutrition Today Magazine, P.O. Box 1829, Annapolis, MD 21404.)*

or secondary infections. Diarrhea and malabsorption, caused by bacterial overgrowth within the lumen of the bowel, create deficiencies of nutrients and trace elements. Exacerbations often follow emotional upsets, illness, or dietary indiscretions involving milk and fried or fatty food. When symptoms are under control, a low-residue diet, high in protein and energy, is initiated. Irritating foods such as nuts, seeds, legumes whole grains and fresh fruits and vegetables are excluded.

As the patient progresses, fiber supplementation should be started and increased to a high-fiber diet. Soluble fibers, or guars and pectins are especially helpful because of their water-retaining capacity. Exercise is an important adjunct (Goldsmith & Patterson, 1985).

Table 27–6. *Causes of Nutritional Problems in Inflammatory Bowel Disease**

Mechanism	Contributing Factors
Decreased nutritional intake	Anorexia, nausea, pain, malaise, restrictive/unbalanced diet.
Increased nutritional requirements	Inflammation, fever, infection, cell proliferation.
Increased nutritional losses	Malabsorption secondary to mucosal disease, intestinal resection (short bowel), bacterial overgrowth, bile salt deficiency, drugs.
	Diarrhea.
	Bleeding.
	Protein-losing enteropathy.
	Intestinal lymphangiectasia.
Nutritional interference by drugs	Corticosteroids, sulfasalazine, cholestyramine.

*From Given, BA; Simmons, J: Gastroenterology in Clinical Nursing, ed. 4. St. Louis, 1984, The C. V. Mosby Co.

Table 27–7. Nutritional Deficiencies in Inflammatory Bowel Disease*

Protein-calorie malnutrition	Trace metal deficiencies
	Zinc
Vitamin deficiencies	Iron
Vitamins A, D, E, K	Copper
Vitamin C	Cobalt
Folate	Manganese
Vitamin B_{12}	
Mineral deficiencies	
Calcium	
Magnesium	

From Given, Barbara A., and Simmons, Sandra J.: *Gastroenterology in Clinical Nursing*, ed. 4, St. Louis, 1984, The C. V. Mosby Co.

Clinical Implications:

- Patients with severe diarrhea or steatorrhea should be monitored for magnesium, which is usually deficient in chronic inflammatory bowel disease (Phillips & Garnys, 1981).
- Low serum zinc levels are prevalent among children with chronic inflammatory bowel disease. Response to zinc intake is abnormal and growth is retarded (Nishi et al, 1980).
- The use of azulfidine requires a daily intake of eight to ten cups of fluid.

IRRITABLE BOWEL SYNDROME (IBS)

This common disorder accounts for over half of all referrals to gastroenterologists and is a major cause of absenteeism (Burns, 1980). IBS is as "common as the common cold" and the most frequent problem seen by physicians (Robins, 1982). This disorder in motility of the small and large intestine may be a reaction to psychological stress, hormones, drugs, or food intolerance. Diarrhea, sometimes with pain, usually causes the patient to consult the physician.

Nutritional Care. For an acute form of IBS, an elemental formula or minimal fiber diet may be indicated. As the condition improves, soft nonirritating foods are used with a high-fluid intake. Gradually, fiber is added. A high-fiber diet is the ultimate goal in order to avoid constipation and produce bulkier stools with less tension in the walls of the colon. Other therapeutic measures include patient education and reassurance, hydrophilic mucilloids, anticholinergics, and antispasmodic agents (as needed), occasional use of antidiarrheal agents, increased exercise for patients with constipation, postprandial rest periods for patients with diarrhea, and operant conditioning for biofeedback training (Burns, 1980).

Clinical Implications:

- Patients with irritable bowel syndrome must be tested for lactose intolerance or malabsorption before further treatment is started (Goldsmith & Patterson, 1985).
- Hydrophilic mucilloids necessitate large amounts of fluid intake.

DIVERTICULAR DISEASE

Almost 50 percent of the elderly develop diverticula (Almy & Howell, 1980). A protrusion of the intestinal mucosa through the muscular coat is called a diverticulum of the colon. Diverticulosis (Fig. 27–4) is the term used when inflammation is not present in the protruding pouches; diverticulitis refers to inflammation that occurs because of inadequate drainage or impacted feces. Diverticulosis is thought to be precipitated by constipation, with hard, dry stools causing increased intraluminal pressures. The mucosal layer herniates through the muscular layer; abdominal pain and fever result. A low dietary fiber intake is common among individuals with diverticulosis (Manousos et al, 1985).

Nutritional Care. A gradual and deliberate increase in fiber intake may prevent the formation of diverticula and also offer relief from pain and bowel dysfunction in uncomplicated diverticular disease (Almy & Howell, 1980). An elemental diet may be required during severe inflammation, progressing to a bland diet (i.e., eliminating spices, fiber, nuts, seeds and fibrous vegetables that may accumulate in sacs). As the inflammation subsides, efforts should be directed toward increasing fiber to reduce strain during defecation. Insoluble fibers from grains and unrefined cereals are beneficial because they reduce transit time and increase stool weight. At first, bran intake may result in flatulence, but this will subside. Initially, 1 tsp. of bran daily is added to foods. Recommendations generally are for 2 tsp. of bran three times daily (10 gm of dietary fiber), with modifications according to individual needs. A high intake of fluid should be emphasized.

HEMORRHOIDS

When enlarged veins protrude into the anal canal or the anal orifice, they are called internal

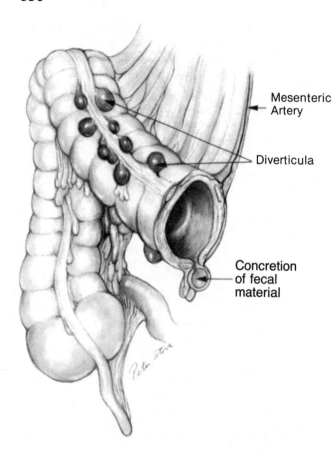

Mesenteric Artery

Diverticula

Concretion of fecal material

Figure 27–4. *Diverticulosis. (From Phillips SF, Stephen AM: The structure and function of the large intestine.* Nutrition Today *16(6):4, 1981. Reproduced with permission of* Nutrition Today *Magazine, P.O. Box 1829, Annapolis, MD 21404.)*

hemorrhoids; external hemorrhoids lie distal to the pectinate line and are covered with modified skin of ectodermal origin (Fig. 27–5). The problem becomes more serious as malignant degenerations occur after many years (Phillips & Stephen, 1981). Pregnancy, straining to defecate, infiltrating carcinoma, or portal hypertension may cause hemorrhoids. The position while sitting on the toilet impairs blood flow and puts added pressure on anal vessels; time spent in this position should be minimal (Given & Simmons, 1984).

Nutritional Care. The same fiber modifications as listed for diverticula also apply to hemorrhoids. Highly seasoned foods or relishes may not be well tolerated. Strong laxatives are irritants and should be avoided.

MODIFIED FIBER DIETS

Fiber. As discussed in Chapter 7, crude fiber refers to the cellulose content of food; dietary fiber refers to all indigestible fibers (see Appendix D–1). Residue is the total amount of solids in feces including undigested or unabsorbed food and metabolic and bacterial products. There is confusion among these terms, and they are frequently misused. One confusing example is prune juice, which yields no residue upon chemical digestion but is classified as a high-residue food because it contains a laxative that indirectly increases the volume of the stool (ADA, 1981).

FIBER-RESTRICTED OR LOW-FIBER DIETS

The purpose of this diet is to help prevent the formation of an obstructing bolus in a narrowed intestinal or esophageal lumen and to rest the gastrointestinal tract. In acute phases of ulcerative colitis, diverticulosis, or infectious enterocolitis, a fiber-restricted diet lessens the pain and stress of defecation by decreasing the weight and bulk of the stool and delaying intestinal transit time. Continued use of a low-fiber diet high in refined carbohydrates is believed to cause diverticular disease of the colon. Reduced bulk causes the colonic lumen to narrow.

The low-fiber diet contains approximately 2 gm of crude fiber. Foods included are refined

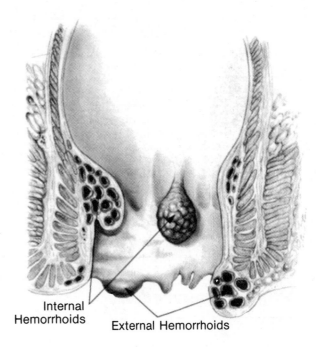

Figure 27–5. Hemorrhoids are varicosities of branches of hemorrhoidal veins. A variety of factors have been brought forward to explain hemorrhoid formation ranging from man's erect posture to anatomic configuration. (From Phillips SF, Stephen AM: The structure and function of the large intestine. Nutrition Today 16(6):4, 1981. Reproduced with permission of Nutrition Today Magazine, P.O. Box 1829, Annapolis, MD 21404.)

Internal Hemorrhoids   External Hemorrhoids

bread and cereal products, cooked fruits and vegetables that are low in fiber, and juices. Nuts, seeds, legumes, and whole-grain bread and cereal products are restricted.

MINIMAL FIBER DIET

To further decrease residue, strained fruit and vegetable juices and white potatoes without skins may be used. Milk is limited to 2 cups/day as it indirectly contributes to fecal residue even though it contains no fiber.

HIGH-FIBER DIET

A high-fiber diet contains increased amounts of foods containing cellulose, hemicellulose, lignin, and pectin, and reduced amounts of refined carbohydrates. Insoluble fibers (cellulose, hemicellulose) increase volume and weight of the residue to maintain the normal size of the colonic lumen and increase gastrointestinal mobility. Soluble fibers, such as gums and pectins, reduce the rate of intestinal absorption, altering the metabolic effects. High-fiber intake necessitates increased fluids. A high-fiber menu is provided in Table 27–8.

Table 27–8. High-Residue, High-Fiber Sample Menu*

Breakfast	Lunch	Dinner
1/2 cup orange juice	6 oz. vegetable soup	1/2 cup tomato juice
1/2 cup All-Bran	2 oz. beef patty	3 oz. broiled chicken
8 oz. milk (whole or low-fat)	2 slices whole-wheat bread	1/2 cup mashed potatoes
1 poached egg or egg substitute	Sliced tomato and lettuce	1/2 cup peas
2 slices broiled bacon or bacon subsitute	French dressing	Sliced avocado on lettuce with lemon wedge
1 slice whole-wheat toast	Catsup, mustard	1 slice whole-wheat bread
1 tsp. butter or margarine	4 apricot halves, dried, stewed	1 tsp. butter or margarine
1 Tbsp. jam	8 oz. milk (whole or low-fat)	1/2 cup canned blackberries
1 cup coffee		1 cup coffee
1 oz. cream or nondairy creamer		1 oz. cream or nondairy creamer
1 tsp. sugar		1 tsp. sugar

*From Chicago Dietetic Association: Manual of Clinical Dietetics, 2nd ed. Philadelphia, W. B. Saunders Co, 1981, with permission.

Clinical Implications:

- Certain individuals should not be encouraged to increase the amount of fiber in their diet. Those who have had gastric surgery (Billroth I and II, vagotomy, pyloroplasty, or Roux-en-Y) and some diabetics with gastroparesis diabeticorum have less gastric acid secretion or decreased gastrointestinal motility and may encounter bezoar formation (i.e., a compacted mass that does not pass into the intestine).
- The high-fiber diet has been recommended in the treatment or prevention of dumping syndrome, hyperlipidemia, gallstones, diabetes, and many other diseases.

Surgical Intervention

Individuals undergoing gastrointestinal surgery are at greater nutritional risk because of the longer periods of abstinence from food both pre- and postoperatively. Lowered serum albumin levels and total lymphocyte counts have been associated with the incidence of postoperative complications and death. Using these parameters, preoperative nutritional support is indicated in patients (Winters & Lieder, 1983).

When surgery involves the gastrointestinal tract, a minimal residue diet may be used for two to three days to minimize intestinal residue. An elemental formula is appropriate because all nutrients are easily absorbed, leaving no residue.

MOUTH OR ESOPHAGUS

After surgery involving the mouth, throat, or neck, the patient may not be able to chew or swallow. Other methods of obtaining the necessary nutrients may be needed; tube feedings are most likely to be indicated (see Chapter 21). Since these may be used for prolonged periods, it is essential that adequate nutrients be provided.

When the ability to chew food is interrupted because of pain or physical immobility for more than one week, the patient should receive nutritional counseling to avoid weight loss and to optimize wound healing. Frequently, these patients are hospitalized for only two or three days; this group may easily be overlooked by the dietitian unless a specific request is made for a consultation visit.

When the patient's condition improves, several guidelines* should be followed for reestablishing oral feedings:

1. The patient will initially be apprehensive about taking foods orally.
2. Begin with soft, moist foods—for example, gradually advance from nonirritating liquids to ground or blenderized foods followed by soft foods.
3. Serve appetizing foods in small frequent feedings.
4. Liquids of thick consistency are better tolerated than thin fluids.
5. Serve only foods that are moist and nonirritating:
   a. Serve meats with gravies and sauces unless contraindicated.
   b. Hard foods such as toast or cookies can be softened by dunking in a beverage.
6. If adequate nutrients cannot be ingested initially, tube feedings can be given simultaneously.
7. Initially, milk may need to be avoided because it tends to coat the mucous lining of the mouth and increases phlegm production.

This diet will be low in fiber.

TONSILLECTOMY

The diet used after a tonsillectomy is usually referred to as *T & A* (tonsillectomy and adenoidectomy). The purpose of the diet is to offer foods that are chemically, mechanically, and thermally nonirritating in order to protect the very sensitive throat. Although the diet is not nutritionally adequate, the convalescent period is relatively short.

Foods allowed are generally the same as the full-liquid diet, omitting citrus fruit juices and hot foods (soups, hot chocolate, or coffee). Milk, fruit nectars, punches, Popsicles, and plain gelatin desserts are given during the first 24 hours. Some physicians prefer that milk be omitted for the first 12 to 24 hours to avoid excessive mucus production. As tolerated, warm foods (strained soups and cereals) and soft foods (soft-cooked eggs and mashed potatoes) are added. The patient gradually returns to a normal diet within a week.

GASTRIC SURGERY

After gastric surgery, many individuals become underweight and malnourished because of nutritional problems. This, of course, depends on

---

*Data from Blackburn, GL; Maini, BS; Bistrian, BR; et al: Surgical nutrition. In *Quick Reference to Clinical Nutrition.* Edited by SL Halpern. Philadelphia, J. B. Lippincott Co, 1979.

Table 27–9. Effects of Gastric Surgery on Digestive Functions with Nutritional Implications

Type Gastric Surgery	Digestive Alterations	Nutritional Implication
Vagotomy Billroth I Billroth II Total gastrectomy	Decreased amount of gastric juices.	Protein digestion occurs in the small intestine. Intrinsic factor reduced or missing. Iron not converted to its absorbable form.
Total gastrectomy Billroth II	No "holding" area; food is dumped into the jejunum instead of being gradually released.	Dumping syndrome; individuals are not able to eat adequate amounts of food.
All types of gastric surgery	Less mixing of foods.	Fats not well mixed with digestive juices. Anemia caused by decreased availability of absorbable iron.
Vagotomy	Stomach becomes atonic.	Food may ferment and cause flatus and diarrhea.
Billroth II	Pancreatic and bile insufficiency.	Malabsorption of fats and proteins.

the type of gastric surgery and the individual's response. The nutritional effects of these physiological changes are summarized in Table 27–9.

Postoperative Period. Immediately following surgery, the patient will be NPO (nothing by mouth) for 24 to 48 hours, with intravenous feedings given until peristalsis returns (determined by the return of bowel sounds and passing of flatus). Edema and swelling must also have subsided enough for fluids to pass the surgical area. When clear water is tolerated, small amounts of liquids will be given hourly, gradually progressing to soft foods and a regular diet of five or six small feedings per day. Progressions may take as much as two weeks following surgery but are determined by the patient's progress and tolerance. If the diet order is written "as tolerated," the progression is determined by the nurse and patient. As tissue heals and becomes stronger, it will gradually expand. Within a year, some patients are able to eat three regular meals daily. Total gastrectomy patients may need to eat several small meals a day for the rest of their lives.

Dumping Syndrome. After gastric resection, dumping syndrome may occur as the patient begins to eat foods in larger quantities and variety. The condition is precipitated by large amounts of the partially digested food being propelled rapidly into the jejunum without being well mixed.

Five minutes to a half hour after a meal, the individual may complain of abdominal cramping and fullness, nausea, cold sweating, and dizziness. This occurs in the patient who has had a total gastrectomy but may also occur if more than two thirds of the stomach has been removed.

This hyperosmolar syndrome occurs when nutrients in the jejunum are hydrolyzed, producing a hypertonic solution. Water is drawn from the blood into the intestine, decreasing vascular fluids and causing vasomotor disturbances. About two hours later, the concentrated carbohydrate solution is absorbed. Blood glucose rises, stimulating an overproduction of insulin, thereby precipitating hypoglycemia.

Nutritional Care. The rationale of diet modification for gastric surgery is to provide the functioning gastrointestinal tract with easily digested, low-bulk foods in small amounts that will not cause discomfort. The objective is not to restrict but to restore nutritional status by minimizing complications. The diet is referred to as the "dumping syndrome diet," which includes the following nutritional guidelines:

1. Meals should be eaten slowly in a relaxed atmosphere.
2. Provide five or six small meals daily; portion sizes depend on the patient's tolerance.
3. A high-protein, moderately high-fat diet helps to maintain weight and rebuild tissue. (Medium-chain triglycerides can be used for steatorrhea.)
4. Complex carbohydrates (bread, rice, and vegetables) are used in moderation since they are not rapidly absorbed.
5. No liquids with a meal or for one hour before or after; low-carbohydrate fluids are provided between meals to retard gastric emptying.
6. No concentrated sweets or sugars, including candy, desserts, and sweetened beverages.
7. Sodium content is moderate (3 gm).
8. The patient should lie down for one hour after eating.
9. Extremely hot or cold food increases gastric motility and should be avoided.

10. Temporary lactose intolerance may be a problem. Proceed slowly when introducing milk-containing items and observe their effect.
11. Frequently check with the patient regarding responses to foods and portions. Adjust the diet to suit the patient's tolerances.

Because only small amounts of food can be tolerated, six small feedings a day are given. Each feeding should contain protein of high biological value and some fat, which delay gastric emptying time.

Foods high in protein and fat are better tolerated. Simple carbohydrates are rapidly digested and are kept to a minimum. Complex carbohydrates are more slowly digested, and a moderate amount is allowed. (The food exchange list in Chapter 23 identifies foods containing various types of carbohydrate.)

Fluids are taken between meals (30 minutes before or after the meal) to delay gastric emptying. Very cold foods or ice may be poorly tolerated. Since sodium draws fluid into the duodenum, it should be moderately restricted. Milk may or may not be tolerated. Tolerance should be established by starting with puddings or custards. These should be homemade because commercial varieties contain more sugar.

Because of some distressing reactions that may accompany food intake, many postgastrectomy patients become frustrated and do not eat adequate amounts of food. Alexander (1975) has devised a supplement made of casein and soy to increase the protein and kilocalories for those who do not eat well. Frequently encountered problems such as dumping syndrome should be explained to the patient when the diet is discussed.

Clinical Implications:

- By eating in a semirecumbent position and lying down following a meal, food will remain longer in the stomach pouch.
- Iron absorption (from food or oral preparations) can be improved by efforts to delay gastric emptying time (such as lying down after eating).
- Guar gum and pectin (gel-forming vegetable fibers) have been used to slow gastric emptying time, eliminating dumping symptoms and increasing tolerance to foods (Harju & Larmi, 1983; Leeds et al, 1981).
- Since the amount of gastric mucosa is reduced, intrinsic factor may be significantly reduced and, in turn, may affect B_{12} absorption. Vitamin B_{12} injections are usually necessary in patients following total gastrectomy. Others should be observed for macrocytic anemia.
- Folate deficiency has been attributed to general malabsorption from gastric surgery.

INTESTINAL SURGERY

An ileostomy or colostomy may be performed to treat Crohn's disease, colonic cancer, intestinal lesions or obstruction, or for severe ulcerative colitis or trauma to the bowel. The affected section of the intestine is removed and the remaining end is attached through an opening in the abdominal wall for defecation. For an ileostomy, the ileum is brought through an artificial outlet in the abdomen; for a colostomy, some section of the colon is brought through the abdominal wall (Fig. 27–6). Because of the different stages of absorption of chyme between the ileostomy and colostomy, nutritional problems and management are somewhat different.

Ileostomy. The waste material from an ileostomy will be fluid and irritating to the skin. An ileostomy may drain almost continuously. Because of the large amount of intestinal resection, nutrient losses are great. Fluid, sodium, potassium, and vitamin B_{12} absorption are reduced or absent.

Colostomy. Because some water is reabsorbed from the chyme, the fecal material is mushy to fairly well formed. Bowel regularity can be established by some patients. A greater percentage of the electrolytes are reabsorbed.

Nutritional Care. Most patients who are candidates for ileostomy are in a poor state of nutrition; therefore, nutritional repletion is important. Diet will be a primary concern of ostomy patients. The consistency of the stool and presence of flatus depend on the types of food eaten. Following the postoperative intravenous feedings and clear-liquid period, a low-residue diet is usually prescribed. The diet should progress to a general diet. However, roughage, fresh fruits, prunes, and other laxative or bulk-forming foods may be limited to prevent diarrhea. A high-protein, high-carbohydrate intake is advisable. Foods may be added one at a time to determine their effect. Milk may not be tolerated by these patients; carbonated beverages and acidic foods cause increased peristalsis and may need to be excluded. Patients must observe their own tolerances regarding food and bowel movements and then eat appropriately.

Another concern of these patients is odor. Foods that seem to produce a malodorous stool are alcohol (especially beer), onions, beans, cab-

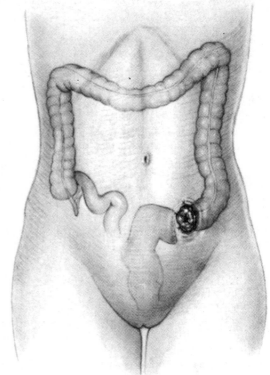

Figure 27–6. A colostomy in the lower left quadrant. (From Phillips SF, Stephen AM: The structure and function of the large intestine. Nutrition Today 16(6):4, 1981. Reproduced with permission of Nutrition Today Magazine, P.O. Box 1829, Annapolis, MD 21404.)

bage, turnips, radishes, cucumbers, highly spiced foods, fish, and some antibiotics. Commercial deodorants placed in the bag may be preferred to eliminating those foods.

Flatus is another problem because these patients have no control over its expulsion and no sensations to indicate when it will pass (Luckmann & Sorensen, 1980). Each person has to learn by trial and error which foods are tolerated. Frequently implicated gas-forming foods are nuts, cabbage, sauerkraut, broccoli, corn, cauliflower, and legumes. Simethicone and activated charcoal can be used to decrease flatus.

Clinical Implications:

- Because less fluid in the gastrointestinal tract is reabsorbed, liberal fluid intake is needed.
- If permitted by the physician, Lomotil may be used to decrease odor and thicken excreted wastes.
- Patients should be encouraged to chew food well to avoid obstructions (Sorensen & Luckmann, 1986). Whole-kernel corn, peas, celery, nuts, and popcorn have been known to block stoma.
- Chlorophyll (Complex Perles) and foods such as parsley, dark green leafy vegetables, buttermilk, and yogurt are intestinal deodorizers (Sorensen & Luckmann, 1986).

- Bismuth subgallate is a medication that has a deodorizing effect; however, it may be constipating.

SMALL BOWEL RESECTION

Since most nutrients are absorbed in the small intestine, nutritional status can be seriously affected by this surgery, especially if more than two thirds of the small bowel is removed. An understanding of nutrient absorption in the gastrointestinal tract is necessary to implement nutritional support (see Chapter 4). Short bowel syndrome is the result of surgical resection of large amounts of the small intestine. The condition is characterized by significant malabsorption, diarrhea, severe malnutrition, and weight loss. The severity of the syndrome is dependent on how much of the small intestine is removed (less than 50 percent is best), what section is removed (resection of jejunum is better tolerated than the ileum), and the condition of the remaining bowel. The prognosis is also better if the ileocecal valve remains. Some adaptation of the remaining small intestine will occur.

Protein and glucose are generally well absorbed. However, fats are poorly absorbed, which decreases the absorption of fat-soluble vitamins (as well as calcium and magnesium). Since vitamin B$_{12}$ is absorbed only in the ileum, if it has been removed, parenteral injections are necessary.

In addition to malabsorption problems, there are several other gastrointestinal complications (MacFadyen et al, 1983):

1. Hypersecretion of gastric acid damages the mucosa and inactivates pancreatic lipase and trypsin, which may affect protein and fat absorption. Cimetidine (Tagamet) is usually given to decrease hyperacidity.
2. Gastrointestinal motility and peristalsis are increased, decreasing the length of time chyme is present for absorption. Most patients receive drugs such as Pro-Banthine, Lomotil, and others, as necessary to decrease intestinal transit time.
3. Large amounts of bacteria in the gastrointestinal tract (of unknown etiology) increase the risk of viral gastroenteritis.

Nutritional management of these patients is complicated, involving a combination of individually tailored oral and parenteral feedings for a period of two years or more. Initially or during the first month, the goal is to control fluid and electrolyte abnormalities and infections. Nutritional support is through parenteral feedings.

If 20 to 30 percent of the small bowel remains, oral isotonic fluids may be offered after about one month. The oral intake of food stimulates the release of gastrointestinal hormones, which, in turn induces the remaining small intestine to increase its absorptive surface area (MacFadyen et al, 1983). Therefore, it is important to encourage oral intake as soon as possible. If liquids are tolerated, the patient can very slowly increase oral intake to a normal diet. Although elemental diets may be used, they are rather unpalatable and may cause diarrhea. They should be diluted so they are not hyperosmolar (Taylor, 1983). As oral intake increases, parenteral therapy can be decreased (see Chapter 21).

Foods are introduced gradually until adequate oral intake is reached. Small frequent meals are tolerated best. Patients need to be aware of their tolerance for various foods; a food diary will help.

Fats are usually poorly tolerated and are restricted to about 40 to 60 gm of fat. It is thought that the low-fat intake reduces steatorrhea and increases the absorption of energy nutrients and divalent cations (e.g., calcium and magnesium).

However, the necessity for this restriction is controversial (Woolf et al, 1983; Young, 1983).

Alcohol and caffeine are discouraged because they stimulate gastrointestinal activity. Large amounts of all the nutrients are required to maintain weight. Up to 175 gm of protein and 5000 kcal may be necessary with daily supplements of vitamins (especially fat-soluble ones) and minerals (particularly calcium and magnesium), as indicated by laboratory data.

RECTAL SURGERY

A clear-liquid or nonresidue diet may be indicated following rectal surgery, such as hemorrhoidectomy, to permit healing and to decrease the risk of wound infection. A minimal-residue diet or monomeric formula can be used. The foods allowed on a minimal residue diet are almost completely digested and absorbed in the intestine, resulting in nominal feces. A normal diet is resumed when tolerated, after which the patient should consume a high-fiber diet.

• FALLACIES and FACTS

FALLACY: *"For heartburn, digestive enzyme tablets should be taken. Good health starts with good digestion. This most complete digestion aid is available for only $19.98."*

• FACT: *Heartburn is not caused by food that has not been digested. However, it may be aggravated by certain foods. Whenever a claim is made for products (particularly in health food stores), the labels should be carefully read. In this case, the assumption is that heartburn may be eliminated if food is digested thoroughly. Also, if this product is composed of enzymes, the words should end with "-ase" because each enzyme is named accordingly; i.e., the enzyme lipase acts on lipids, lecithinase on lecithin (see Chapter 4). Instead, such words as the names of organs in the body might be found, e.g., whole dried pancreas, duodenum, or liver. A few minutes spent reading labels can quickly show most readers these fallacies.*

FALLACY: *Pure dietary fiber in tablet form can alleviate constipation.*
  • **FACT:** *The quantity of fiber found in tablets cannot be large enough to significantly contribute to the diet for this purpose. "Pure" is a word that can be applied to ordinary food and is not restricted to manufactured products.*
FALLACY: *A special blend of herbs will insure an internal cleansing if six tablets are taken daily.*
  • **FACT:** *Such cleansing is unnecessary; if normal elimination is not occurring, suggestions given in the section on constipation can be tried.*

Summary

Gastrointestinal disorders may be caused directly or indirectly by a number of things. Personality characteristics may be one of the biggest factors of the cause as well as the cure. Generalized therapy necessary for the healing process in gastric disorders includes small, frequent feedings to minimize irritation while maintaining nutritional status; and reduction of stress, anxiety, and frustration in the patient's life. In many cases, the last part is the key to successful treatment. In other cases, medical and surgical procedures are necessary. All gastrointestinal patients need personal attention and an individualized plan of nutritional care to correct and maintain their nutritional status.

Review Questions

1. Discuss ways to treat heartburn.
2. How do the symptoms vary for a heart attack and heartburn?
3. What is the one factor that, if achieved, could prevent the symptoms of heartburn in most cases?
4. What are some special nursing strategies for the peptic ulcer patient?
5. What types of products should be eliminated from the diet of a patient with celiac disease?
6. List conditions requiring a low-fiber diet and state reasons for its use; list conditions requiring a high-fiber diet and state reasons for its use.
7. Why are individuals undergoing gastric or intestinal surgery at a greater nutritional risk than other surgical patients?

Case Study: Mrs. A.B. is a 60-year-old personnel director who has complained of increasing indigestion following meals, particularly after her evening meal. Her usual schedule is to work until 7 PM, then eat a heavy meal and retire by 10 PM. The heartburn following her evening meals is so severe, she cannot lie down at night and sleeps propped up by pillows in a sitting position. Following a physical evaluation, her physician diagnoses hiatus hernia. Six small feedings are ordered, plus elevating the head of the bed on 4- to 6-inch blocks.
  1. What is the effect of caffeine and nicotine on the lower esophageal sphincter?
  2. What foods have the same effect?
  3. What nursing diagnoses could you develop from the data? Develop goal(s) for each.
  4. As you plan Mrs. A.B.'s nursing interventions, what would you teach her regarding: lying down after meals, tight belts and foundation garments, and meal spacing?
  5. If antacids are added to the therapeutic regimen, when is the best time for them to be administered?
  6. If she were on a bland diet, what foods should be restricted?

Case Study: Ms. S.J. is a 26-year-old secretary who is the sole support of her four-year-old son. She has been diagnosed with ulcerative colitis for the past three years. During the latest flare-up of her disease, she lost 10 lbs. She now weighs 97 lbs., and her height is 64 inches. After discharge from the hospital, she is referred to a nutritionist for diet counseling. Her physician orders a 2500 kcal low-residue diet with vitamin and mineral supplements.
  1. What dietary restrictions are imposed during the acute phase of the disease?
  2. Why are foods with lactose often restricted?
  3. Why do long-chain triglycerides often cause steatorrhea in ulcerative colitis patients? What substitutions are possible?
  4. Plan a low-fiber diet for one day.
  5. In counseling the patient about her diet, what activities will help to avoid episodes of diarrhea?

REFERENCE LIST

Alexander, HC: A protein dietary supplement for the severe dumping syndrome. *Surg Gynecol Obstet* 141(6):863, 1975.
Almy, TP; Howell, DA: Diverticular disease of the colon. *N Engl J Med* 302(6):324, 1980.

American Dietetic Association (ADA): *Handbook of Clinical Dietetics.* New Haven, Yale University Press, 1981.

Anderson, L; Dibble, MV; Turkki, PR; et al: *Nutrition in Health and Disease,* 17th ed. Philadelphia, J. B. Lippincott Co, 1982.

Buckley, JE; Addicks, CL; Manniglia, J: Feeding patients with dysphagia. *Nurs Forum* 15(1):69, 1976.

Burns, TW: Colonic motility in the irritable bowel syndrome. *Arch Intern Med* 140(2):247, 1980.

Chapman, RW; Sillery, J; Fontana, DD; et al: Effect of oral dioctyl sodium sulfosuccinate in intake-output studies of human small and large intestine. *Gastroenterology* 89:489, 1985.

Chicago Dietetic Association and South Suburban Dietetic Association of Cook and Will Counties (CDA): *Manual of Clinical Dietetics.* Philadelphia, W. B. Saunders Co, 1981.

Codini, RT; Rosenberg, IH: Nutritional therapy in inflammatory bowel disease. *Current Concepts Gastroent* 6(3):8, 1981.

Fein, HD: Nutrition in diseases of the stomach. In *Modern Nutrition in Health and Disease,* 6th ed. Edited by RS Goodhart; ME Shils. Philadelphia, Lea & Febiger, 1980, p 892.

Feldman, EJ; Isenberg, JI; Grossman, MI: Gastric acid and gastrin response to decaffeinated coffee and a peptone meal. *JAMA* 246(3):248, 1981.

Gee, MI; Grace, MGA; Wensel, RH; et al: Protein-energy malnutrition in gastroenterology outpatients: Increased risk in Crohn's disease. *J Am Diet Assoc* 85(11):1146, 1985.

Given, BA; Simmons, SJ: *Gastroenterology in Clinical Nursing,* 4th ed. St. Louis, C. V. Mosby Co, 1984.

Goldsmith, G; Patterson, M: Irritable bowel syndrome: Treatment update. *Am Fam Physician* 31(1):191, 1985.

Harju, E; Larmi, TKI: Efficacy of guar gum in preventing the dumping syndrome. *JPEN* 7(5):470, 1983.

Heatley, RV: Nutritional implications of inflammatory bowel disease. *Scand J Gastroenterol* 19(8):995, 1984.

Hodges, P; Gee, M; Grace, M; et al: Vitamin and iron intake in patients with Crohn's disease. *J Am Diet Assoc* 84(1):52, 1984.

Hoppe, MC; Descalso, J; Kapp, SR: Gastrointestinal disease: Nutritional implications. *Nurs Clin North Am* 18(1):47, 1983.

How to choose an antacid. *Consumer Reports* 48(8):417, 1983.

Hull, C; Greco, RS; Brooks, DL: Alleviation of constipation in the elderly by dietary fiber supplementation. *J Am Geriatr Soc* 28(9):410, 1980.

Jones, VA; Dickinson, RJ; Workman, E; et al: Crohn's disease: Maintenance of remission by diet. *Lancet* 2(July 27):177, 1985.

Kirsner, JB: Crohn's disease. *JAMA* 251(1):80, 1984.

Leeds, AR; Ralphs, DNL; Ebied, F; et al: Pectin in the dumping syndrome: Reduction of symptoms and plasma volume changes. *Lancet* 1(May 16):1075, 1981.

Luckmann, J; Sorensen, KC: *Medical-Surgical Nursing,* 2nd ed. Philadelphia, W. B. Saunders Co, 1980.

McArthur, K; Hogan, D; Isenberg, JI: Relative simulatory effects of commonly ingested beverages on gastric acid secretion in humans. *Gastroenterology* 83(1):199, 1982.

MacFadyen, BV; Copeland, EM, III; Dudrick, SJ: Surgery and oncology. In *Nutritional Support of Medical Practice,* 2nd ed. Edited by HA Schneider; CE Anderson; DB Coursin. Philadelphia, Harper & Row, 1983, p 611.

Malhotra, SL: A comparison of unrefined wheat and rice diets in the management of duodenal ulcer. *Postgrad Med* 54(1):6, 1978.

Manousos, O; Day, NE; Tzonou, A; et al: Diet and other factors in the aetiology of diverticulosis: An epidemiological study in Greece. *Gut* 26(6):544, 1985.

Nishi, Y; Lifshitz, F; Bayne, MA; et al: Zinc status and its relation to growth retardation in children with chronic inflammatory bowel disease. *Am J Clin Nutr* 33(12):2613, 1980.

Ostro, MJ; Greenberg, GR; Jeejeebhoy, KN: Total parenteral nutrition and complete bowel rest in the management of Crohn's disease. *JPEN* 9(3):280, 1985.

Phillips, GD; Garnys, VP: Trace element balance in adults receiving parenteral nutrition. *JPEN* 5(1):11, 1981.

Phillips, SF; Stephen, AM: The structure and function of the large intestine. *Nutr Today* 16(6):4, 1981.

Response of gluten-sensitive enteropathy to corticosteroids. *Nutr Rev* 39(3):132, 1981.

Richter, JE; Castell, DO: Gastroesophageal reflux: Pathogenesis, diagnosis, and therapy. *Ann Intern Med* 97(1):93, 1982.

Robins, AH: *The Irritable Bowel Syndrome.* Richmond, VA, A. H. Robins Co, 1982.

Rombeau, JL; Caldwell, MD: *Enteral and Tube Feeding,* vol. 1. Philadelphia, W. B. Saunders Co, 1984.

Rydning, A; Berstad, A; Aadland, E; et al: Prophylactic effect of dietary fibre in duodenal ulcer disease. *Lancet* 2(October 2):736, 1982).

Rydning, A; Weberg, R; Lange; et al: Healing of benign gastric ulcer with low-dose antacids and fiber diet. *Gastroenterology* 91(1):56, 1986.

Sorensen, KC; Luckmann, J: *Basic Nursing: A Psychophysiologic Approach,* 2nd ed. Philadelphia, W. B. Saunders Co, 1986.

Spencer, H; Kramer, L; Norris, C; et al: Effect of small doses of aluminum-containing antacids on calcium and phosphorus metabolism. *Am J Clin Nutr* 36(1):32, 1982.

Steinberg, WM; Lewis, JH; Katz, DM: Antacids inhibit absorption of cimetidine. *N Engl J Med* 307(7):400, 1982.

Taylor, KB: Gastroenterology. In *Nutritional Support of Medical Practice,* 2nd ed. Edited by HA Schneider; CE Anderson; DB Coursin. Philadelphia, Harper & Row, 1983, p 352.

Van Ness, MM; Cattau, EL, Jr: Flatulence: Pathophysiology and treatment. *Am Fam Physician* 31(4):198, 1985.

Walker, WA: Cellular and immune changes in the gastrointestinal tract in malnutrition. In *Nutrition and Gastroenterology.* Edited by M Winick. New York, John Wiley & Sons, 1980.

Weber, SJ; Lefrock, JL: Health advice for the international traveler. *Am Fam Physician* 32(6):165, 1985.

Winters, JO; Leider, ZL: The value of instant nutritional assessment in predicting postoperative complications and death in gastrointestinal surgical patients. *Am Surg* 49(10):533, 1983.

Woolf, GM; Miller, C; Kurian, R; et al: Diet for patients with a short bowel: High fat or high carbohydrate? *Gastroenterology* 84(4):823, 1983.

Young, EA: Short bowel syndrome: High-fat versus high-carbohydrate diet. *Gastroenterology* 84(4):872, 1983.

Further Study

Bell, L; Hoffer, M; Hamilton, JR: Recommendations for foods of questionable acceptance for patients with celiac disease. *J Can Diet Assoc* 42(2):143, 1981.

Bengoa, JM; Sitrin, MD: Nutritional aspects of inflammatory bowel disease. *Ann Rev Nutr* 5:463, 1985.

Breckman, BE: Role of the nurse specialist in stoma care. *J Human Nutr* 33(5):383, 1979.

Consensus Conference: Travelers' diarrhea. *JAMA* 253(18): 2700, 1985.

Fenner, L: When digestive juices corrode, you've got an ulcer. *FDA Consumer,* 18(6):20, 1984.

Gray, DS: Short bowel syndrome. *Am Fam Physician* 30(9):227, 1984.

Hartwig, MS: Sticking to a gluten-free diet. *Am J Nurs* 83(9):1308, 1983.

Hecht, A: The colon goes up, over, down and out. *FDA Consumer* 18(5):28, 1984.

Henry, CL: Patient's view of a gluten-free diet. *J Human Nutr* 34(1):50, 1979.

Hoppe, MC; Descalso, J; Kapp, SR: Gastrointestinal disease: Nutritional implications. *Nurs Clin North Am* 18(1):47, 1983.

Jenkins, DJA; Jenkins, AL; Wolever, TMS; et al: Fiber and starchy foods: Gut function and implications in disease. *Am J Gastroenterol* 81(10):920, 1986.

Loustau, A; Lee, KA: Dealing with the dangers of dysphagia. *Nursing* 15(2):47, 1985.

Navab, F; Texter, EC: Gastroesophageal reflux. *Arch Intern Med* 145(2):329, 1985.

Rados, B; Hopkins, H: Laxatives overused in the quest for "regularity." *FDA Consumer* 19(4):12, 1985.

The patient with a gastrostomy. *RN* 49(3):33, 1986.

Watts, V; Madick, S; Pepperney, J; et al: When your patient has jaw surgery. *RN* 48(10):44, 1985.

Resources

Ener-G Goods, Inc.
P.O. Box 64487
Seattle, WA 98124-5787

Gluten-free flours and flour mixes. Variety of baked products, pasta, and crackers available.

Gluten Intolerance Group
P.O. Box 23053
Seattle, WA 98102-0353

Variety of publications dealing with celiac sprue.

Dietary Management of Disorders of Accessory Gastrointestinal Organs

28

OBJECTIVES

THE STUDENT WILL BE ABLE TO:

- *Relate the pathophysiological conditions of the liver and pancreas to nutritional status.*
- *Recognize the role of protein in liver disease.*
- *Identify nutritional problems associated with alcoholism.*
- *State the role of fat in gallbladder disease.*
- *Explain dietary management of pancreatitis.*
- *Assist clients in planning adequate diets for cystic fibrosis.*
- *Modify a normal diet to meet the requirements for a patient with each of these conditions: hepatitis, cirrhosis, hepatic encephalopathy, gallbladder disease, pancreatitis, and cystic fibrosis.*

TERMS TO KNOW

Aromatic amino acids
Ascites
Branched-chain amino acids (BCAA)
Cholecystitis
Cholecystokinin
Cholelithiasis
Cirrhosis
Common bile duct
Dyspepsia
Encephalopathy
Endocrine
Esophageal varices
Exocrine
Fibrosis
Hemochromatosis
Hypochloremic alkalosis
Hypoalbuminemia
Lipotropic
Necrosis
Pancreatitis
Steatosis

Since digestion of all foodstuffs is accomplished by the actions of enzymes, bile salts, and other substances secreted into the gastrointestinal tract, an alteration in their availability will affect digestion and, ultimately, absorption of nutrients. The liver and pancreas produce important digestive substances to facilitate absorption; the gallbladder stores, concentrates, and releases bile on stimulation. Additionally, the liver has many other physiological functions that affect health and well-being; it can be adversely affected by ingested substances.

Liver

FUNCTIONS OF THE LIVER

As discussed in Chapter 4, the liver is the chemical governor of the body, storing and regulating the release of most of the body's nutrients. All digested substances, except long-chain fatty acids, are transported directly to the liver. From

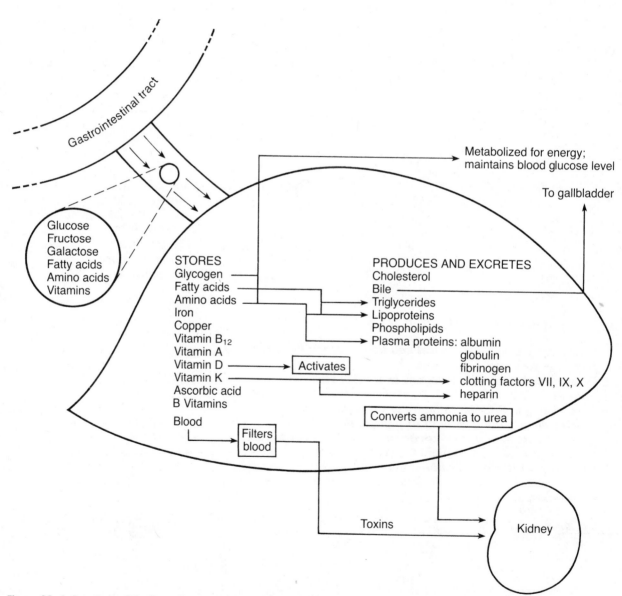

Figure 28–1. *Functions of the liver affecting nutritional status. The liver is the chemical governor for the body; any damage to the liver may affect nutritional status.*

Table 28–1. Implications of Common Liver Function Tests

Diagnostic Test	Alteration due to Liver Damage	Significance
Serum/urine bilirubin	Elevated	Bile formation and excretion.
Albumin, globulin, total protein	Decreased	Inability to synthesize protein or decreased protein intake.
Prothrombin time	Decreased	Prothrombin and fibrinogen production reduced.
Urea	Decreased	Liver cannot produce urea to remove ammonia, or too much ammonia is entering the bloodstream from action of colonic bacteria.
Ammonia	Elevated	
Urine N, total		Measures the amount of nitrogen required (from the diet).
Cholesterol (total or ester)	Elevated	Cholesterol not being converted to bile acids.
Bromsulphalein (BSP)	Elevated	Liver is unable to filter at normal rate.
Serum glutamic-oxaloacetic transaminase (SGOT) or aspartate transaminase (AST)	Elevated	Reflects enzyme production.
Serum glutamic-oxaloacetic transaminase (SGOT) or aspartate transaminase (AST)	Elevated	Reflects enzyme production.
Serum glutamic-pyruvic transaminase (SGPT) or alanine transaminase (ALT)	Elevated	Reflects enzyme production.
Alkaline phosphatase	Elevated	Increase indicates deterioration.
Transferrin	Decreased	Failure of liver to synthesize.

there, they may be altered before distribution to the rest of the body. Not only are nutrients handled in this manner, but ingested poisons, medications, antigens, and possibly some bacteria are detoxified or destroyed for excretion. Thus, the liver changes nutrients into a utilizable form for the body and stores some nutrients until they are needed (Fig. 28–1). Various liver function tests are invaluable and reflect the functions and changes as they occur during therapy (Table 28–1).

Alcohol

"Alcoholism is the most common form of drug abuse in the United States," Halsted (1980) commented in a symposium on alcoholism. He estimates that 10 million people suffer from the effects of excessive drinking and can be classified as alcoholics. Alcoholism can be defined as the intermittent or continual ingestion of alcohol leading to dependence or harm (Davies, 1979). Alcohol intake has a major impact on our society, causing social and personal upheavals that affect the entire family and society, not just the alcohol-addicted individual.

Alcohol consumption has become very common for social affairs and special occasions as well as for routine use by many individuals. It is consumed regularly by about one third of the U.S. population (an average of 3 drinks/week) with one third of the population consuming more than four drinks/week (Eckardt et al, 1981); the average intake is 25 gm/day for adults who drink (Walser,

1984). Alcohol is a drug that can produce deleterious effects on virtually every organ in the body; health care professionals should be aware of problems that can result from excessive drinking.

Most people underestimate their alcohol consumption. Generally, if a person states he/she has two or three drinks a day, this means at least three drinks. A generous 2 oz. of 86-proof whiskey would amount to 120 gm of alcohol a day. The *chronic* effects of alcohol abuse are not related to intoxication, but rather to the amount and duration of alcohol consumption (Rubin, 1982).

ALCOHOL EFFECTS ON NUTRITIONAL STATUS

Unlike regular foodstuffs, alcohol contains few nutrients other than calories; therefore, the alcoholic's intake of nutrients may readily become insufficient. Alcohol also has some direct effects upon the gastrointestinal tract, resulting in maldigestion and malabsorption of essential nutrients. Several factors associated with increased alcohol intake contribute to malnutrition (Fig. 28–2).

1. Appetite is suppressed and diet is poor.

2. Alcohol may damage the stomach and bowel, compromising absorption and digestion, frequently resulting in nausea, diarrhea, impaired water and electrolyte absorption, and ulceration. Absorption of thiamin, vitamin B_{12}, folic acid, and glucose is decreased; iron absorption is increased.

3. Alcohol may damage the liver and interfere with the transport, activation, catabolism, utilization, and storage of almost every nutrient studied.

4. Vitamin requirements, particularly for the B complex, are higher in alcoholics than in nonalcoholics.

Additionally, the chronic alcoholic may prefer to spend his/her resources on alcohol, contributing to reduced consumption of nutrient-rich foods, particularly those containing protein. Therefore, alcoholism remains one of the major causes of nutritional deficiency, even in societies that have adequate food supplies. However, nutritional deficiencies are more frequently marginal than overt (Smith, 1979). The alcohol-derived nutritional deficiency may result in suboptimal health and contribute to frequently seen conditions such as anemia, convulsions, and small-bowel malfunction.

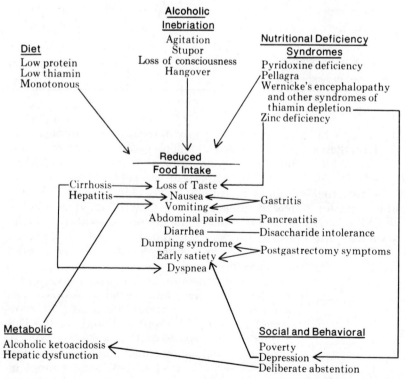

Figure 28–2. Summary of factors contributing to reduced food intake. (From Roe DA: Alcohol and the Diet. Copyright © 1979 by AVI Publishing Co, Westport, CT.)

Table 28-2. Clinical Deficiencies in the Alcoholic

Clinical Symptoms	Pathophysiology and Nutritional Implication
Wernicke-Korsakoff syndrome	Thiamine deficiency.
Shuffling gait (motor weakness), polyneuropathy	Chronic blood loss; folic acid and iron deficiencies.
Generalized weakness	Decreased folate stores.
Macrocytic anemia	Protein deficiency; increased loss with ascitic fluid.
Edema, fatty liver, hypoalbuminemia, anemia	Niacin deficiency.
Photosensitive dermatitis, stomatitis, gastritis, diarrhea, peripheral neuropathy	
Dermatitis, stomatitis, cheilosis	Riboflavin deficiency.
Alcoholic withdrawal convulsions, mild ataxia, skin lesions, irritability, insomnia	Pyridoxine deficiency.
Delirium tremens	Increased magnesium excretion; decreased intake of magnesium (must be replenished parenterally).
Cardiac myopathies	Potassium deficiency due to decreased intake, poor absorption, and increased urinary losses.
Night blindness	Increased zinc excretion and/or vitamin A deficiency.
Osteomalacia and fractures	Vitamin D deficiency.
Increased prothrombin time	Vitamin K deficiency.

Several neurological complications of alcoholism, such as polyneuropathy and Wernicke-Korsakoff syndrome, are now recognized as vitamin deficiencies resulting primarily from an inadequate thiamin intake (Korsten & Lieber, 1979). Night blindness, which responds to administration of vitamin A (sometimes with zinc supplements), is commonly found in chronic alcoholics (Roe, 1981). Other signs of malnutrition include muscle wastage; raw, beefy tongue; scurvy; pellagra; cheilosis; cardiomyopathy; and other symptoms (see Table 28-2).

Experimental, clinical, and epidemiological studies indicate that even with adequate diets, these toxic effects on the digestion, absorption, and activation of nutrients contribute to malnutrition; relatively small amounts of alcohol may have cirrhogenic potential (Korsten & Lieber, 1979).

ALCOHOL AS A NUTRIENT

Nutrition and alcohol interact at many levels. Alcoholic beverages are themselves nutrients, theoretically providing energy (7.1 kcal/gm). However, alcohol is a relatively inefficient source of calories, particularly at high consumption levels. In experimental studies of both animals and humans, isocaloric replacement of other calories by alcohol (50 percent of total calories) in a balanced diet results in weight loss. Additionally, when alcohol is added as supplemental calories, weight gain is less than for calorically equivalent foods

(Pirola & Lieber, 1972). While it is recognized that the metabolism of ethanol is an energy-wasteful process, the reason is not fully understood. Alcohol consumed in excess of 50 gm/day provides less than 7 kcal/gm, but it is not known whether this is true at lower levels of intake.

RATE OF ABSORPTION

Alcohol delays gastric emptying (Barboriak & Meade, 1970). When food and alcohol are consumed together, absorption of alcohol is delayed and decreased. Peak levels of alcohol in the blood are similarly delayed (Shultz et al, 1980). Soluble carbohydrate causes a greater delay in alcohol absorption than either protein or fat (Sedman et al, 1976).

ALCOHOL METABOLISM

More than 90 percent of the alcohol consumed is metabolized by the liver (see Chapter 8). In nonalcoholics, the rate of metabolism is fairly constant, but a chronic alcoholic develops a supplemental system for metabolism, and the rate may double (Spritz, 1979). A 70 kg individual may metabolize from 10 to 25 gm of alcohol per kilogram per hour. The *maximum* amount of alcohol that could be metabolized in a 24-hour period is about 340 gm (Walser, 1984). The amount of alcohol in beverages is shown in Table 28-3.

Table 28–3. *Ethanol Content of Some Common Beverages**

Beverage	Source	% Ethanol, v/v	Serving Size (oz)	Ethanol Content per Serving (g)	Nonintoxicating No. of Servings†		
					50 KG	70 KG	90 KC
Beer	Cereals	4	12	11	3	4	5
Table wine	Grapes	10–14	4	9–13	3	4	5
Whiskey	Cereals	40–45	1½	14–16	2	3	3½
Rum	Molasses	40–45	1½	14–16	2	3	3½
Gin	Grain	40–45	1½	14–16	2	3	3½
Vodka	Grain	40–45	1½	14–16	2	3	3½
Brandy	Wine	40–45	1½	14–16	2	3	3½

*From Walser, M: Alcohol. In *Nutritional Management.* Edited by M Walser; AL Imbembo; S Margolis; et al. Philadelphia, W. B. Saunders Co, 1984, with permission.

†"Nonintoxicating" is defined here as a quantity just *insufficient* to induce a blood alcohol level of 0.1 percent in a person of average fatness/leanness (body water 60 percent of body weight), even if ingested over a short time span. Nondrinkers or young persons become intoxicated at lower blood levels.

Health Application: Hazards of Alcohol

Heavy alcohol consumption results in various toxic effects. Alcohol misuse has a potentially detrimental effect on the body from its point of entry throughout the gastrointestinal tract; its most striking effects are on the brain and liver, but the pancreas is also frequently affected. Hepatitis and cirrhosis are the two most common hepatic complications of alcoholism. In 1975, cirrhosis was the seventh most common cause of death in the United States (Eckardt et al, 1981).

Whereas in the past, it was felt that a fatty liver was due to improper eating habits, Lieber and colleagues (1968, 1983) produced fatty livers in animals and humans with a nutritionally adequate diet. Fatty infiltration of the liver is a consequence of ethanol metabolism mainly caused by an increased synthesis and decreased degradation of fatty acids (Mezy, 1980). If the patient abstains from alcohol, fatty liver and alcoholic hepatitis are reversible, but cirrhosis is not. Once signs of portal hypertension are present, cessation of alcohol intake seems to have little impact on the progression of cirrhosis (Spritz, 1979).

Alcohol consumption is closely associated with a wide range of other health disorders. These include hematological abnormalities, cardiomyopathy, high blood pressure, peripheral neuropathy, acute and chronic muscle disorders, central nervous system degeneration (particularly of the cerebellum and cortex), chronic pulmonary disease, certain malignancies (particularly involving the tongue, mouth, oropharynx, esophagus, larynx, and liver) intestinal malabsorption, hypertriglyceridemia, hyperuricemia, gout, and increased susceptibility to infection (Gruchow et al, 1985; Spritz, 1979). Discussions of these problems are found in the article by Eckardt and colleagues (1981). Alcohol abuse is a risk factor in adverse fetal outcome (see Chapter 15).

Usually, heavy drinkers are considered more at risk of sustaining these adverse health consequences, but even drinking in moderation may present problems to some individuals because of genetic and other biological factors that may predispose the individual to specific conditions (Eckardt et al, 1981).

BENEFICIAL EFFECTS OF ALCOHOL

With low doses of alcohol, a feeling of well-being occurs, which subsequently changes to sedation and hypnotic effects as the blood alcohol level rises. For these reasons, alcohol is used for its psychological effects; it is also used for various effects in medications.

Low levels of alcohol may be protective against coronary heart disease. In numerous studies, a negative association was found between alcohol intake and myocardial infarction (Willett et al, 1980; Hennekens et al, 1978; Castelli et al, 1977). A Honolulu study found that coronary heart disease was less likely to occur in Japanese men who drank alcoholic beverages than in abstainers and that the risk was lowest for moderate drinkers (2 oz./day of wine) (Yano et al, 1977). Turner and colleagues (1981) have summarized the results of these studies.

This negative association between alcohol consumption and coronary heart disease may be at least partially explained by an alcohol-related increase in high-density lipoprotein (which is a protective factor against myocardial infarction) and a decrease in low-density lipoprotein (which is atherogenic). However, caution is advisable when interpreting or applying these data: (1) The benefits are weak when compared with the possible health hazards, and (2) the benefits are associated with very *low levels* of consumption. Abstinence is recommended for pregnant women or those who might become pregnant and for persons taking certain drugs.

There is little information on how much alcohol can be consumed without risk of liver damage. In the average-sized woman (not pregnant), 20 gm/day is probably safe, but 60 gm/day is not. In the average-sized man, 40 gm/day is probably safe, but 80 gm/day is not (Walser, 1984).

Liver Disorders

The liver can be injured from infections, parasites, nutritional deficiencies, metabolic disorders, obstructions, toxins, and malignancies. Degenerative processes can lead to fatty infiltration, necrosis, and fibrosis. Diseases of the liver are often accompanied by anorexia, nausea, vomiting, and food intolerance; a variety of dietary measures have been advocated in their management.

Dietary treatment is aimed at relieving disease symptoms; in most instances, a modified diet will not cure the underlying disease. A diet for a liver condition should be as pleasant and tolerable as possible (Bateman, 1979). Nutritional care should maintain or improve nutritional status by providing adequate kilocalories, protein, fluids, and other nutrients and allow the liver to "rest" as much as possible. Depending on the extent of liver damage, various nutrients are tolerated in different amounts, as compared in Table 28–4.

HEPATITIS

This condition is an inflammation of the liver, which can result in destruction of liver cells. Generally, the liver can regenerate destroyed cells, but when excessive amounts of liver tissue are wasted, the liver cannot perform its functions normally.

Pathophysiology. In hepatitis, the hepatotoxic agent is usually caused by microorganisms. Type A (infectious hepatitis) is transmitted through drinking water, food, or sewage (via the fecal-oral route). The Centers for Disease Control (CDC) advocates injections of immune serum globulin as a prophylactic measure against hepatitis A both before exposure (especially for international travelers) and postexposure (Recommendations, 1985).

Type B (serum hepatitis) can be transmitted through blood transfusions, improperly sterilized medical instruments, and body fluids such as tears, saliva, and semen. Hepatitis can also be caused by chemical toxins such as chloroform, carbon tetrachloride, or alcohol. Alcoholic hepatitis is the earliest (and completely reversible) stage of liver damage.

Common clinical symptoms for the disease may interfere with food intake: anorexia, nausea, vomiting, fever, abdominal discomfort, and diarrhea. Weight loss may be great, and jaundice may develop. A recently developed vaccine for hepatitis B is considered safe and recommended by the CDC for health care personnel, especially those who handle blood or routinely treat high-risk patients (Grady, 1986; Francis et al, 1986).

Nutritional Care. All types of hepatitis are treated in the same manner. Currently, no medication is available to cure hepatitis; the major components of therapy are bed rest and dietary management to prevent further injury to the liver and to allow or hasten healing and regeneration of damaged cells.

Table 28–4. *Comparison of Dietary Guidelines for Liver Disease*

Nutrients	Hepatitis	Cirrhosis	Encephalopathy
Kilocalories	3000 or more	2000 to 3000 kcal	1800 kcal minimum
Carbohydrate	300 to 400 gm	300 to 400 gm	450 gm
Protein	High: 1.5 to 2.0 gm/kg (100 to 150 gm)	Moderate: 1.0 gm/kg (70 gm)	Low: 0.5gm/kg (20 to 40 gm)
Fat	Moderate: 35% of kcal	Low: 25 to 30% of kcal	Initially none: increase as tolerated 25 to 30% of kcal
Other	Vitamin supplement including folic acid	Vitamin supplement	Vitamin supplement

FOCUS ON   SAMPLE DIET FOR HEPATITIS AND CIRRHOSIS

Hepatitis		Cirrhosis
Serving Size	**Breakfast**	*Serving Size*
1/4	Cantaloupe	1/4
1	Poached egg	1
2 oz.	Sliced ham	–
2 slices	Raisin toast	2 slices
2 tsp.	Margarine	1 tsp.
	Midmorning	
4	Graham crackers	4
1 cup	Low-fat milk (1%)	–
	Apple juice	1 cup
	Lunch	
4 oz.	Sliced turkey	2 oz.
1 medium	Candied sweet potato	1 medium
1/2 cup	Green beans	1/2 cup
1/2 cup	Spinach salad	1/2 cup
2 Tbsp.	Italian salad dressing	1 Tbsp.
1	Whole-wheat bread	1
1 tsp.	Margarine	–
1/12	Boston cream pie	1/12
1 cup	Lemonade	1 cup
	Midafternoon	
1 cup	Low-fat mlk (1%)	1/2 cup
1	Bran muffin	1
1 tsp.	Margarine	1 tsp.
	Dinner	
1 cup	Vegetable beef soup	1 cup
4	Crackers	4
1 slice	Sliced pineapple with	2 slices
3/4 cup	cottage cheese (2% low-fat)	1/2 cup
1 cup	Tapioca cream pudding	–
1 cup	Lemonade	1 cup
	Bedtime	
1 cup	Ice cream	–
2	Oatmeal cookie with raisins	2
	Fruit juice	1 c
	This diet furnishes the following amounts of nutrients:	
3000	Kilocalories	2200
140 gm (19%)*	Protein	73 gm (14%)*
356 gm (47%)*	Carbohydrate	341 gm (63%)*
117 gm (35%)*	Fat	59 gm (25%)*

*Percent of total kcal.

During the initial stage of anorexia and vomiting, intravenous solutions of dextrose are given. If prolonged parenteral feedings are indicated, protein hydrolysates should be added. Polymeric formulas can also be given via tube feeding or orally, as the condition permits.

As soon as the patient is able to tolerate food orally, persistent and persuasive efforts are implemented to assure the patient's intake of a nutritionally adequate diet. Even though the patient may feel hungry, nausea may be experienced after eating only a few bites. Small frequent feedings are better tolerated. Attractively served foods are important to stimulate appetite.

Energy intake should be 3000 kcal or more, with at least 40 percent beng furnished from carbohydrates (300 to 400 gm) to promote glycogen synthesis and to spare protein (see Table 28–3). Protein intake should be relatively high (100 to 150 gm) to maintain positive nitrogen balance, as liver function tests permit. When protein is supplied from both animal and vegetable sources (meats, fish, eggs, dairy products, legumes, and cereals), adequate amounts of lipotropic agents (e.g., choline, inositol, and methionine) accompany these foods to prevent further development of fatty liver. Additionally, fluid intake should be very high.

In the past, a low-fat diet was ordered, especially when jaundice was present. There is no reason to restrict dietary fat below the normal level of about 35 percent of total energy intake unless fat is not well tolerated (Bateman, 1979). Fats increase the diet's palatability and also decrease the enormous volumes of food necessary to consume when a 3000 kcal, low-fat diet is imposed. Fats in dairy products and eggs are usually better tolerated than fried foods and fatty meats (*Focus on Sample Diet for Hepatitis and Cirrhosis*).

In hepatitis, the plasma prothrombin level is reduced, but in most cases, it does not respond to vitamin K therapy since it is a result of impaired liver function. On the other hand, if intrahepatic biliary obstruction occurs, parenteral or oral, water-miscible vitamin K will increase prothrombin levels (Davidson, 1980).

Complications. Sometimes the condition deteriorates with increased fatty infiltration and impending hepatic coma. This condition requires a lower quantity of protein and is discussed under hepatic encephalopathy.

Clinical Implications:

- Alcohol is toxic and forbidden during the illness and for four to six months after recovery.
- Precautions must be taken to prevent further spread of the infectious form of the disease: (1) Disposable dishes should be used and disposed of in the patient's room. (2) Visitors shoud not eat foods from the patient's tray.
- Because of decreased hepatic protein synthesis and hypoalbuminemia, patients are especially susceptible to pressure sores.
- Adequate fluid intake is necessary to replace losses and prevent dehydration: At least 3000 ml/day are needed.

CIRRHOSIS

More severe liver damage has occurred from cirrhosis than hepatitis. Cirrhosis is characterized by prolonged fatty degeneration with fibrous connective tissue replacing destroyed liver cells. It may be caused by improperly treated hepatitis or toxic or viral hepatitis, but it is usually associated with chronic alcoholism.

Primary treatments are alcohol abstinence, bed rest, and nutritional support. Effective management of nutritional problems depends on nutritional status (determined by clinical assessment) and level of liver function.

Nutritional Care. The goal of diet therapy in the cirrhotic patient is to (1) provide adequate kilocalories, nutrients, and vitamins; (2) correct nutritional deficiencies; (3) enhance tissue repair; and (4) prevent endogenous protein catabolism. Recovery is enhanced by a high-energy, normal-protein, normal-fat, and vitamin-enriched diet. (See Table 28–3 and previous sample diet.)

The energy requirement is approximately 2000 to 3000 kcal/day with a recommended protein intake of 1 gm/kg of body weight. Protein intake must be adequate to prevent nitrogen wasting. High-protein diets do not appear to be indicated, and excessive amounts can precipitate encephalopathy. When the diet is adequate in protein, supplementation with choline and methionine is not necessary.

Vitamin deficiencies are seldom limited to one vitamin. Water-soluble vitamins are usually supplemented two to three times the RDAs (without known harmful effects) for the first week or two of therapy or until the patient is able to eat adequately (Shaw & Lieber, 1980). Precursor blood cells in the bone marrow can be damaged by alcohol, which increases the requirements for vitamins utilized in the maturation of red and white blood cells. This includes folacin and vitamins B_6 and B_{12}. Initially, vitamin supplements are used to correct deficiencies and for repletion but are not necessary once the patient is eating well. Guidelines for vitamin-mineral therapy are given in Table 28–5.

Alcoholism may be accompanied by pancreatic insufficiency and alterations in bile salt metabolism; fat must be used judiciously to prevent steatorrhea. Dietary fat may need to be lowered to constitute 25 percent of the energy level, or 50 gm of fat. Emulsified fats (homogenized milk and eggs) decrease the demand for bile. The fat content of the diet should be as high as possible for greater palatability of food given to the anorectic

Table 28–5. Protocol for Vitamin-Mineral Therapy Required by Alcoholics in Acute Care Units[1]

1. If signs and laboratory studies permit diagnosis of defined avitaminoses, treat by administration of individual micronutrients at therapeutic dosage levels.[2]

2. When evidence for specific deficiencies is unclear or incomplete, proceed to the following routine:

    a. On admission, give a single intramuscular dose of 100 mg of thiamin (thiamin hydrochloride USP solution, 100 mg/ml).

    b. If macrocytic (megaloblastic) anemia is present, check vitamin B_{12} status before prescribing folic acid greater than RDA.

    c. Give daily water-soluble and fat-soluble vitamins in hospital mixture based on approximately the following dosages: thiamin mononitrate, 15 mg; riboflavin, 15 mg; pyridoxine hydrochloride, 25 mg; niacinamide, 100 mg; cyanocobalamin, 5 mcg; folic acid, 1.5 mg; ascorbic acid, 200 mg; vitamin A, 5000 IU; vitamin D, 400 IU; and vitamin E, 30 IU.[3]

    d. Correct electrolyte imbalance and magnesium deficiency by intravenous mineral solutions.

    e. If zinc deficiency is clearly present or suspected, give zinc sulfate, 300 mg daily.

[1]From Roe, DA: *Alcohol and the Diet.* Copyright © 1979 by MAVI Publishing Co, Westport, CT.
[2]Phytonadione (vitamin K_1) may be required to treat vitamin K deficiency with hypoprothrombinemia prior to surgery. Usual preparation can be AquaMEPHYTON, 2.5–25 mg.
[3]Proprietary therapeutic vitamin preparations do not conform with the composition of recommended mixture. Acceptable commercial formulations of water-soluble vitamins are Berocca tabs (Roche) or Larobec (Roche), which should be given (1 tab daily) with a fat-soluble vitamin preparation such as decavitamin U.S.P.

patient but low enough so as not to precipitate steatorrhea. The use of medium-chain triglycerides (MCT) has resulted in reduced fatty accumulation while supplying necessary energy (Lieber & Spritz, 1977).

Patients with malabsorption problems, those with clinical symptoms of vitamin A and K deficiency, and those receiving lactulose or antibiotics will need fat-soluble vitamin supplements. Antibiotics, such as neomycin or ampicillin, are instituted to decrease colonic bacteria, which produce ammonia from protein, thereby decreasing the amount of nitrogenous wastes in the blood. These drugs, however, cause malabsorption. Lactulose (a synthetic nonabsorbable disaccharide) will reduce the absorption of ammonia and increase peristalsis. When prothrombin levels are low, the importance of foods high in vitamin K (green, leafy vegetables) can be emphasized. Therapeutic supplementation of the fat-soluble vitamins, especially vitamin A, is complicated by the fact that

they can be especially toxic to the alcohol-damaged liver (Leo et al, 1982).

Dilated veins are frequently seen in cirrhotics because of increased portal pressure, which causes a back flow (increased pressure) in the collateral veins, producing dilated esophageal, umbilical, and rectal veins. This condition, due to portal hypertension, is known, for example, as an esophageal varix. Low-sodium antacids or anticholinergics may be needed. Other gastrointestinal irritants, such as caffeine and spices, should be avoided; foods that are smooth in texture may be indicated to prevent the danger of rupture. Another complication frequently seen is an intolerance to glucose, which indicates the necessity of a diabetic-type diet (see Chapter 29).

While the diet ordered by the physician and the diet planned by the dietitian may be important, it is the food eaten by the patient that will affect the condition. The provision of six small daily feedings generally results in an increased total intake. Therefore, nursing's role is to encourage and support the patient, especially if alcohol withdrawal is part of the treatment.

Because poor appetite is associated with cirrhosis, ingenuity is needed to prepare food attractively. Efforts to furnish patients with foods they feel they can eat can be frustrating; patients may become nauseated after eating only a few bites of their favorite dish. These attempts may, however, entice the patient to try to eat. They also offer an opportunity to stress the importance of diet. As the patient's condition improves, appetite will also improve. The diets for hepatitis and cirrhosis are the same; only the amounts are different.

Behavior Modification. Nutritional care is more complex than mere nutritional replenishment, which may be corrected while the individual is in the hospital. A typical alcoholic exhibits many self-abusive behaviors. The individual is not interested in food and has little appetite. This is usually associated with excessive coffee consumption, heavy smoking, and heavy use of prescription and over-the-counter drugs. Counseling is used to overcome personal and situational factors that contribute to these problems and to deal with anxiety and depression with a motivational approach.

Behavior modification techniques are an innovative attempt to change habits; other methods have not had a long-lasting effect. Rewards are given for desired behavior. Nutrition education is integrated into therapy sessions, focusing on long-term rehabilitation of the alcoholic. Older chronic alcoholics are less likely to be motivated to change food habits than young alcoholics; their participation in therapy is irregular, frequently reverting to excessive alcohol intake (Roe, 1979).

Ascites. Increased intrahepatic pressure results from large quantities of fluid that accumulate in the abdomen. This complication of cirrhosis is called ascites. It may be caused by obstruction of the damaged liver, decreased osmotic pressure from hypoalbuminemia, sodium retention, or impaired water excretion. A diet low in sodium is important.

The level of sodium restriction depends on whether the physician simultaneously orders a diuretic, the patient's tolerance, and the rate of diuresis. Sodium restriction may be as low as 32 mEq (730 mg). Since this severe restriction is not well received by patients, it may be utilized for only three to four days (Barthel & Butt, 1983).

When the sodium content of the diet is severely restricted, protein foods must necessarily be limited. Low-sodium milk, such as Lonalac, and low-sodium breads can be used. Because the patient already has a depressed appetite, these substitutions may not be well received (see Chapter 32). Sodium intake is gradually liberalized as the rate of diuresis increases.

Some salt substitutes are not advisable for the cirrhotic patient. Ammonia chloride salts increase the high ammonia levels caused by the liver disease and should not be used. Potassium chloride salts can be used if the potassium level is normal.

Sodium restriction is not without risks; unless fluid intake is restricted, severe symptomatic hyponatremia may occur (Barthel & Butt, 1983). Fluid intake may be restricted to 1000 to 2000 ml/24 hours. (Helpful hints for easing the patient's discomfort are listed in *Focus on Facilitating Fluid Intake Restriction* in Chapter 5.) This limitation may be followed by oliguria, which may not be noticed for several days without accurate recording of intake and output.

Clinical Implications:

- Cirrhotic patients have a better appetite earlier in the day; nausea tends to increase as the day progresses.
- Decreased motility and increased intraabdominal pressure secondary to ascites contributes to poor appetite.
- Daily dietary intake should be charted.
- Patients with ascites should be weighed and their abdominal girth measured daily in addition to intake and output charting (Barthel & Butt, 1983).

- Supplements of methionine, choline, and liver extract do not have any special benefits and may sometimes be dangerous because of the additional nitrogen load they impose (Davidson, 1980).
- Thiamin deficiency in alcoholics is common because of inadequate consumption and malabsorption. Severe deficiency (contributing to amnesia and personality changes) is known as the Wernicke-Korsakoff syndrome.
- Since most vitamin supplements omit folic acid, attention should be given to the vitamin B supplement used in cirrhosis; folic acid should be included in the mixture (Davidson, 1980).
- Hypervitaminosis may be encountered in alcoholics who self-medicate in the belief that it will prevent damage to the liver (Roe, 1981).
- Development of alcoholic liver disease (fatty liver, hepatitis, or cirrhosis) cannot be prevented by supplements of a nutrient or a combination of nutrients. On the other hand, if alcohol intake is terminated, liver functions return toward normal if promoted by nutritional support.
- Serum iron levels are normal in alcoholics unless there is bleeding.
- Hyperabsorption of iron in genetically predisposed alcoholics will cause hemochromatosis (Karcioglu & Hardison, 1978). These patients should be cautioned not to eat iron-fortified foods (Dextrose, 1978).
- Patients with ascites may try to "diet away" the added weight by not eating all the foods sent to them. Explain that the additional pounds are due to water retention or the ascites; the weight will be lost by diuresis or removal of ascitic fluid.
- A low-sodium diet is not easy to follow, but can be made reasonably palatable; most patients will accept this restriction as preferable to the discomfort of severe ascites.

HEPATIC ENCEPHALOPATHY

Advanced liver disease or hepatic encephalopathy is reflected in disturbance of consciousness that can readily progress into deep coma (hepatic coma). Portal blood circulation is decreased with development of collateral circulation. This allows blood to bypass the liver, and toxic substances are not eliminated. In addition, amino acids are not metabolized normally.

Clinical symptoms include abnormal mental state, including confusion, apathy, personality changes, and intellectual deterioration. While the exact cause has yet to be determined, it is known that although the patients need protein for recovery, they cannot tolerate it!

Ammonia. Intestinal flora break down dietary protein and blood (from gastrointestinal bleeding) into ammonia, which is absorbed. Ammonia not converted to urea by the damaged or bypassed liver accumulates in amounts that are toxic to the central nervous system.

Ammonia levels can be lowered in several ways: drugs, including antibotics and lactulose, a low-protein diet, and/or specifically limiting foods that induce higher ammonia levels. Foods that can cause hyperammonia include many cheeses, buttermilk, chicken, salami, ground beef, ham, peanut butter, potatoes, onions, and gelatin (Rudman et al, 1973).

Branched-Chain Amino Acids (BCAA). In hepatic diseases (including cirrhosis), abnormalities of amino acid metabolism are typical. Serum branched-chain amino acids (leucine, isoleucine, and valine) are decreased, and aromatic amino acids (phenylalanine, tyrosine, and tryptophan) and methionine are increased. Since BCAA can be metabolized by muscles, they are probably catabolized for energy. On the other hand, aromatic amino acids depend primarily on the liver for their catabolism. These aromatic amino acids may bypass the liver or cannot be catabolized by the diseased liver; their increase in the circulation also affects the central nervous system. These amino acids are precursors of neurotransmitters (norepinephrine). High levels of aromatic amines function as "false neurotransmitters" (Fischer & Baldessarini, 1971), which are involved in the pathogenesis of hepatic coma and other neurological and cardiovascular problems.

Studies have been conducted to normalize plasma concentrations of amino acids by providing increased amounts of BCAA and to minimize the amount of aromatic amino acids given (Fischer & Bower, 1981). The amount of BCAA is 35 percent, compared with 22 percent present in most foods and amino acid mixtures. Several studies support the theory that BCAA-enriched diets have greater protein tolerance and less severe encephalopathy (Rossi-Fanelli et al, 1981; Freund et al, 1981, 1979; Nasrallah & Galambos, 1980).

Vegetarian diets can also be used to improve encephalopathy. Plant proteins contain less methionine and aromatic amino acids, and more BCAA than animal proteins. The use of vegetable proteins has been shown to lower blood serum levels of tryptophan, phenylalanine, and tyrosine (Greenburger et al, 1977) and results in less nitrogen excretion (Bruijn et al, 1983). Shaw and asso-

ciates (1983) have found, however, that vegetable proteins do not promote positive nitrogen balance as well as animal proteins. Also, the diet, which contains large amounts of food and causes gaseous abdominal distention, may not be well received by the anorectic patient (Uribe et al, 1982). Additionally, when sodium restriction is necessary, palatability is decreased.

Nutritional Care. While metabolism of all nutrients in hepatic failure is abnormal, intolerance to protein limits nutritional support. The basic objectives of diet therapy in hepatic coma are to (1) remove the sources of excess ammonia (dietary and pharmacological), (2) furnish adequate amounts of energy to prevent hypoglycemia and excessive tissue catabolism, and (3) balance fluids and electrolytes and promote regeneration of liver tissue. Initial therapy for encephalopathy is focused on decreasing absorption of toxic materials (especially ammonia) from the gastrointestinal tract by utilizing poorly-absorbed antibiotics.

If drugs are not effective in improving the condition, protein intake will be modified. The amount of protein allowed is regulated according to the patient's level of consciousness or tolerance. A very low-protein diet (20 to 30 gm) is associated with improvement in the encephalopathic patient's mental condition. The narrow range of protein tolerance, however, makes therapy treacherous. With an excess of protein, coma may occur; without enough, the illness will be prolonged. Therefore, the diet may progress from 20 gm of protein, which is increased in 10 gm increments every few days, to a total of 50 gm, as tolerated and as the patient's condition improves.

For rough calculations of protein levels, the amounts of protein from the food exchange lists can be used (see Chapter 23). Thirty grams of protein can be provided, as shown in Table 28–6. Maximum amounts of high-biological-value protein are incorporated into the diet, but complex carbohydrates also provide some protein that cannot be ignored. (They are necessary to increase energy content of the diet for their protein-sparing role). For maximum utilization, the daily pro-

Table 28–6. *Using Diabetic Food Exchanges to Calculate 30 Grams Protein*

Food Item	Protein (gm)
2 oz. of meat	14
8 oz. of skim milk	8
2 servings of bread/cereal	6
2 servings of vegetables	2
Total	30

tein content is equally distributed between the three meals.

Protein increases are implemented as soon as possible for tissue regeneration. Avoidance of ammonia-producing foods is wise. By modifying amino acid mixtures and thereby improving protein tolerance in hepatic encephalopathy, liver protein synthesis is stimulated (Freund et al, 1981). While natural foods cannot be manipulated to increase the BCAA proportions, several BCAA preparations are available for enteral feedings—Travasorb Hepatic (Travenol), and Hepatic Aid (McGaw) or, for parenteral use, Hepatamine (McGaw). Patients with hepatic encephalopathy in poor nutritional status and who are intolerant of regular protein are candidates for BCAA to reestablish positive nitrogen balance. BCAA have also been used successfully in chronic hepatic encephalopathy (Freund et al, 1979).

As protein is being increased and is better tolerated, up to 40 to 50 gm of fat can also be gradually added (20 to 25 percent of the kilocalories). At least 1800 kcal are necessary to prevent catabolism.

Comatose patients are only given intravenous glucose solutions without any protein until some response is seen. As soon as signs of recovery are observed (or the level of consciousness increases), protein can be instituted in 10 gm increments, progressing as previously discussed. While 0.5 gm/kg/day promotes nitrogen balance in patients with advanced liver disease, the ultimate goal is 1 gm/kg/day (Roe, 1979).

Clinical Implications:

- Protein tolerance can be enhanced by giving antibiotics and lactulose.
- BCAA formulas are not nutritionally complete; supplementation with vitamins and electrolytes is necessary.
- Monitor patients carefully for adherence to the low-protein diet or low ammonia-containing foods and for any gastrointestinal bleeding.
- Monitor mental status and motor function for alterations (confusion, apathy, drowsiness, slurred speech, asterixis or flapping tremor, or fetor hepaticus) and correlate with serum ammonia levels.
- Since serum levels of aromatic amino acids are high in patients with liver disease, the use of the sweetener aspartame (an aromatic amino acid) is not currently recommended (Uribe, 1982).
- When the diet is adequate in energy, nitrogen equilibrium can be maintained with 30 to 40 gm of protein of high biological value.

Gallbladder

FUNCTIONS

The gallbladder receives bile produced by the liver, concentrates it by reabsorbing water and electrolytes, and stores it. When fats enter the duodenum, the hormone cholecystokinin is secreted, which signals the gallbladder to contract and release bile. The bile then travels through the common bile duct to the duodenum where it emulsifies fats so they can be hydrolyzed and absorbed. This aids in the digestion and absorption of the fat-soluble vitamins and activates enzymes.

PATHOPHYSIOLOGY

Common diseases of the gallbladder are cholelithiasis and cholecystitis, which occur more frequently in obese women over 40 years of age, particularly those with previous multiple pregnancies.

In both conditions, when the gallbladder contracts, it causes pain. Stones, composed of cholesterol, calcium, bilirubin, and inorganic salts, form in the gallbladder, causing a condition called cholelithiasis. Several conditions are associated with an increased incidence of gallstones, including hemolytic disorders, obesity, diabetes, familial hypercholesterolemia, cardiovascular disease, multiple pregnancies, and use of oral contraceptives.

Most gallstones are about 85 percent crystallized cholesterol. Cholesterol saturation of bile is only one of the multiple factors leading to formation of gallstones. When bile is supersaturated with cholesterol, it is precipitated, beginning the core of a cholesterol stone (LaMorte et al, 1981). Accumulation of layers of cholesterol and calcium increases the size of the stone. Although stones mainly contain cholesterol, evidence does not support the conjecture that a low-cholesterol diet will decrease the amount of cholesterol in bile. Capron and colleagues (1981) associated longer periods of time between eating and fasting (specifically, time between the evening meal and the first meal of the next day) with increased risks of gallstone formation in younger women. An intake of at least 2 cups of water taken on awakening will induce emptying of the gallbladder. This routine might be effective in preventing gallstone formation in persons who refuse to eat breakfast (Taylor, 1986).

An inflammation of the gallbladder is called cholecystitis. Gallstones are the most common cause of cholecystitis in which the cystic duct between the gallbladder and the common bile duct is obstructed (Thorpe & Caprini, 1980).

DIAGNOSTIC TESTING

In the past, a fat-free meal before a cholecystographic examination for gallstones was recommended. Mauthe (1974) challenged this and found that x-ray films were actually clearer in patients receiving a regular diet than in those who received the no-fat diet. No specific diet is required before gallbladder testing.

METHODS OF THERAPY

Chenodeoxycholic acid (CDCA) can be used to dissolve small stones, but it is a slow process and must be taken daily for at least six months (Pimstone & Mok, 1981). Its use is contraindicated in patients with liver disease or obstructed bile ducts. The usual therapy is to surgically remove stones or the gallbladder. If inflammation is present or the patient is obese, the physician may postpone surgery, and nutritional therapy is implemented during this period.

NUTRITIONAL CARE

The goal for nutritional care in both conditions is the same: to minimize discomfort by decreasing fat-induced gallbladder contractions. Patients usually quickly learn which foods cause distress. While a low-fat diet for gallbladder is a traditional therapy, some physicians have questioned its validity. Mogadam and associates (1984) found that the action of the gallbladder is independent of a meal's fat content.

Acute Gallbladder Attacks. In acute gallbladder attacks, a low-fat, clear-liquid diet is used with intravenous fluids and electrolytes to replace losses and to rest the gallbladder. In some cases, a minimal-fat, full-liquid diet may be given. Skim milk supplies protein, and fruit juices and gelatin supply carbohydrate. As soon as possible, the patient can progress to soft foods, very restricted in fats (20 to 30 gm), with foods similar to those shown in *Focus on Sample Menu for 30 and 50 gm Low-Fat Diets.*

Chronic Gallbladder Problems. Patients awaiting gallbladder surgery as well as those with chronic gallbladder problems are treated with a diet limited to 50 gm of fat. Foods are prepared simply—not fried and without added fats or fat-laden sauces and gravies. Fatty meats, cream, and rich desserts are avoided. This diet contains approximately 80 gm of protein and 50 gm of fat; the carbohydrate and kilocalories are limited only by the amount the patient eats. If weight reduction is necessary, sugar, juices, and other "accessory" foods can be limited. By reducing fat intake, weight loss can usually be accomplished since fat is the most concentrated source of energy.

The American Health Foundation has devised a system for tracking total fat intake but allowing for flexibility and versatility, according to the individual's desires (Boyar & Loughridge, 1985). The Fat Portion Exchange List (Table 28–7) is a partial list that groups fat-containing foods according to food type (dairy products, meat and poultry, etc.). Each food item used in the portion size listed provides 5 gm of fat and constitutes one fat portion. The system is very simple: for a diet with 50 gm of fat, 10 fat portions would be allowed daily. Patients can determine how to "spend" their fat portions.

Clinical Implications:

- When a low-fat diet is used for prolonged periods, water-soluble supplements of the fat-soluble vitamins may be needed.
- Fried foods are the worst offenders and should be avoided, even if the patient is on a normal diet.
- Many patients with gallbladder disorders may not be able to tolerate strongly flavored or gas-forming vegetables (onions, sauerkraut, cabbage, radishes, turnips, or cucumbers) or spicy foods (chili or curry). These need not be restricted unless they cause problems.

Postoperative Cholecystectomy. Following a cholecystectomy, clear liquids will be initiated within 24 to 48 hours. The patient gradually progresses toward resumption of a regular diet. Postoperatively, bile enters the small intestine continually rather than being secreted in response to fat intake. Whether or not fat is controlled in this progressive diet depends on the patient's tolerance and the physician's preferences. There is little reason to restrict the diet beyond one month following surgery (Spiro, 1983).

Some patients have less distress on a low-fat

FOCUS ON SAMPLE MENU FOR 50 AND 30 GM LOW-FAT DIETS				
	50 gm Fat		**30 gm Fat**	
	Portion	*Amt*	*Portion*	*Amt*
Breakfast				
Stewed prunes	1/2 cup	0.5	1/2 cup	0.5
Poached egg	1	6.0	1	6.0
Whole-wheat toast	2	2.0	2	2.0
Margarine	2 pats	8.0	0	0
Jelly (packets)	2	0	2	0
Midmorning				
Cranberry juice	6 oz.	0	6 oz.	0
Lunch				
Sandwich made with				
Whole-wheat bread	2 slices	2.0	2 slices	2.0
Sliced chicken	3 oz.	10.0	2 oz.	6.6
Salad dressing (mayonnaise type)	1 Tbsp.	6.0	(Use low-calorie)	
Celery and carrot sticks	3 each	0	3 each	0
Vanilla pudding (made with skim milk)	1/2 cup	2.0	1/2 cup	2.0
topped with fresh strawberries	1/4 cup	0.25	1/4 cup	.25
Skim milk	1 cup	0	1 cup	0
Midafternoon				
Banana	1 medium	0	1 medium	0
Dinner				
Baked bluefish with butter	3 oz.	4	3 oz.	4
Brown and wild rice with mushrooms	1/2 cup	0	1/2 cup	0
English peas	1/2 cup	0	1/2 cup	0
Sliced tomato on lettuce leaf	2 slices	0	2 slices	0
Pumpernickel bread	1 slice	0	1 slice	0
Margarine	1 tsp.	4	0	
Sherbet	1/2 cup	2	1/2 cup	2
Bedtime				
Skim milk	1 cup	0	1 cup	0
Graham crackers	2	1	2	1

diet for the first several weeks after surgery. Diarrhea after a cholecystectomy indicates a dietary intolerance. Spicy foods, such as Mexican food, may also cause diarrhea. Six small feedings are better tolerated and may let these patients increase their nutrient intake.

Clinical Implication:

- Patients may gain considerable weight after a cholecystectomy, enjoying many fatty foods previously not tolerated (Houghton et al, 1984).

Pancreas

FUNCTION

The pancreas secretes enzymes for digestion of proteins, fats, and carbohydrates (exocrine function) and manufactures insulin (endocrine function). While these enzymes are normally inactive until they reach the duodenum, an obstruction can block their flow, causing a reflux. The duct that carries pancreatic secretions to the gas-

Table 28–7. Fat Portion Exchange List[1]

Food	Amount Equal to 1 Fat Portion
Fats and Oils	
Margarine, diet	1 Tbsp.
Margarine, soft	1 tsp.
Mayonnaise, diet	1 Tbsp.
Mayonnaise, regular	1 1/2 tsp.
Avocado	2 Tbsp.
Bacon fat, lard	1 tsp.
Eggs	
Egg yolk	1
Whole egg	1
Dairy Group	
Evaporated whole milk	1/4 cup
1% Milk, buttermilk	2 cups
Whole milk, regular, homogenized	1/2 cup
Cream cheese	1 Tbsp.
Heavy cream, fluid	1 Tbsp.
Egg nog	1/4 cup
Ice cream	1/3 cup
Ice milk	1 cup
American, blue, brick, Colby cheese	1/2 oz.
Meat and Poultry[2]	
Beef, lean (choice grade cooked, boneless, trimmed of all fat)	3 oz. (most lean)
Beef, rib roast, or steak	1 oz.
Canadian bacon	2 oz.
Chicken breast without skin	1 breast (5 to 6 oz.)
Chicken breast with skin	1/4 to 1/3 breast
Ham, cured, extra lean	3 oz.
Ham, cured, regular	1 1/2 oz.
Pepperoni	1/2 oz. (1/2 slice)
Turkey ham	4 oz.
Veal (except breast)	3 oz.
Fish and Seafood[3]	
Cod, flounder, grouper, haddock, scallops, shrimp, lobster, sole	Unlimited[4]
Pike, pollack, turbot	16 oz.
Tuna, canned in oil	2 oz.
Protein Alternatives	
Legumes, cooked, lima beans, split peas	6 cups
Tofu (soybean curd)	2 to 3 oz.
Canned Soups (made with water)	
Chicken noodle	2 1/2 cups
Cream of celery, chicken, or mushroom	3/4 cup
Tomato	2 1/2 cups
Bread and Starch (high-fat snacks and desserts)	
Baked custard	1/2 cup
Cheesecake, pie	1/3 average piece
Corn bread	1 piece (2" by 3" square)
Corn chips, potato chips	1/2 oz. (1/2 small bag)
Croissant, Danish	1/3 of one whole
Pancakes, waffles, Poptarts, muffins	1
Sweets	
Caramel, peanut brittle	2 oz. (6 small caramels)
Cocoa powder, unsweetened	6 Tbsp.
Fudge	1 oz.

[1]From Boyar, AP; Loughridge, JR: The fat portion exchange list: A tool for teaching and evaluating low-fat diets. Copyright Boyar/Loughridge AHF 1985. Reprinted by permission from *Journal of the American Dietetic Association,* 85(5):589, 1985.

[2]Weight after cooking; no fat added.

[3]Raw weight.

[4]All fish and seafood for which the amount is unlimited contain so little fat that if they are prepared without any added fat, the fat content is negligible.

trointestinal tract joins the common tube through which bile is also carried to the duodenum (see Chapter 4).

PANCREATITIS

Blocked pancreatic enzymes somehow become activated and begin to digest pancreatic cells. The extent of this enzyme autodigestion may be limited to a small area or may be generalized throughout the gland. It may sometimes even move out of the pancreas and affect surrounding tissue.

Pancreatitis can be caused by gallbladder diseases, mumps, tumors, or bacterial infections, but it is usually related to excessive use of alcohol. Pancreatitis can be acute, relapsing acute, chronic relapsing, or chronic. Acute pancreatitis may or may not progress to chronic pancreatitis.

An inflammatory state of the pancreas with decreased amounts of pancreatic enzymes can result in the following problems:

1. Fluid and electrolyte imbalances, particularly hypocalcemia and dehydration.

2. Impaired acid-base balance, particularly hypochloremic alkalosis (decreased chloride).

3. Malabsorption of nutrients, especially fats and fat-soluble vitamins.

4. Impaired utilization of nutrients.

5. Impaired growth, healing, and resistance.

Digestion is impaired depending on the availability of pancreatic secretions. Insulin-dependent diabetes mellitus will also be present when the islets of Langerhans are destroyed. Inadequate digestion may be accompanied by malabsorption of fat-soluble vitamins and vitamin B_{12}. Steatorrhea will result in increased calcium excretion.

Methods of Therapy. Primary objectives of care are to reduce pancreatic secretions and provide rest, yet provide "optimal" nutritional support and fluid-electrolyte balance. Pancreatic enzymes are secreted in response to food or alcohol. In order to rest the organ, alimentary feedings may be withheld for a time, or the types of foods modified, depending on the severity of the condition.

Antacids are diluted and given half an hour before meals to neutralize gastric secretions and decrease pancreatic stimulation. Anticholinergics can also be given to reduce pancreatic secretions; they will enhance the effects of antacids by allowing them to remain in the stomach longer.

Enzyme replacements (Pancreatin, Pancrease) are commercially available to aid in digestion. These enzymes are contained in the core of enteric-coated tablets or in the form of acid-resistant granules, so they will not be hydrolyzed by the gastric acid. They are utilized best when given with or immediately after meals. Their effectiveness can also be improved when given with antacids (Dhar et al, 1980). They should be swallowed whole; the protective coating will be destroyed if the medication is crushed or given with hot foods or liquids.

Nutritional Care. Proper nutritional support is essential and often difficult. During acute pancreatitis, intravenous feedings are given in order to rest the gastrointestinal tract. Rehydration should be closely monitored as well as repletion of sodium, potassium, and calcium lost from vomiting and steatorrhea. This period usually lasts for two or three days and may also include the use of nasogastric suction and anticholinergics. In the case of a pancreatic abscess, oral feedings must be withheld longer and total parenteral nutrition may be implemented (Kirby & Craig, 1985). TPN may also be necessary if the patient has a decreased appetite and cannot eat.

When oral feedings can be instituted, clear liquids are given to determine tolerance. Since proteins and fats stimulate pancreatic secretion, carbohydrates are the best initial source of energy. Elemental protein feedings can be utilized, but they are hydrolyzed or "predigested" and do not increase pancreatic secretions. Since larger amounts of protein can be given to increase the total amount of proteins absorbed, undigested dietary fat causes flatulence and diarrhea.

A low intake of fat is continued until there is no evidence of steatorrhea. Medium-chain triglycerides (MCT) can be utilized in patients with pancreatic insufficiency to relieve steatorrhea and to help restore weight. The level of fat is gradually increased to promote weight gain and absorption of fat-soluble vitamins until the patient's limit is reached, as indicated by steatorrhea.

A high-fiber diet may increase steatorrhea in patients with pancreatic insufficiency on pancreatic enzyme therapy. This may be related to a reduction in the enzyme activity by the dietary fiber (Dutta & Hlasko, 1985).

Most patients with acute pancreatitis exhibit an impaired glucose tolerance (Porte & Halter, 1981). This is controlled with a carbohydrate-restricted diet similar to diabetic management.

As the patient improves, a bland, low-fat diet with six feedings a day is instituted. A high-protein (120 gm), high-carbohydrate (450 gm), low-fat (50 gm) diet is also used for chronic pancreatitis (*Focus on High-Protein, High-Carbohydrate,*

FOCUS ON *HIGH-PROTEIN, HIGH-CARBOHYDRATE, LOW-FAT DIET*

Breakfast
1/2 cup Stewed prunes
1 Poached egg
2 slices Whole-wheat toast
1 tsp. Margarine and 2 Tbsp. Jelly
1 cup Skim milk (protein-fortified)
Decaffeinated coffee or tea

Midmorning
1 cup Cranberry juice

Lunch
4 oz. Sliced chicken in broth
1/2 cup Cooked carrots
1/2 cup Congealed salad with fruit
1 slice Whole-wheat bread with 1 Tbsp. Jelly
1 cup Vanilla pudding (made with skim milk)
topped with 1/4 cup sliced strawberries
1 cup Skim milk (protein-fortified)

Midafternoon
1 Banana

Dinner
3/4 cup Pineapple juice
4 oz. Bluefish, baked with butter
1/2 cup Brown and wild rice with mushrooms
1/2 cup Green peas
2 slices Tomato on lettuce leaves
2 slices Pumpernickel bread
1 cup Sherbet
1 cup Skim milk (protein-fortified)

Bedtime
1 cup Skim milk (protein-fortified)
4 Graham crackers

This menu provides approximately 2700 kcal, 130 gm protein, 450 gm carbohydrate, and 50 gm fat. Nutrient data and calculations by Nutritionist II software, Silverton, OR.

Low-Fat Diet). Patients are usually anorectic and nauseous; efforts should be made to provide foods that the patient prefers and can tolerate.

Clinical Implications:
- Alcohol is completely eliminated from the diet.
- Large meals are to be avoided; small feedings low in fat are needed.
- Gastric stimulants, including coffee, tea, spices, and condiments, should be avoided.
- The patient must understand the diet and its importance in order to comply with it at home and to prevent future attacks.

- Though the cause is not known, vitamin B_{12} is not absorbed in patients with pancreatitis and must be given parenterally.
- Enzyme replacements are the primary treatment for steatorrhea; a low-fat diet may bring additional benefits.

CYSTIC FIBROSIS

Today, cystic fibrosis (CF) is the most lethal congenital disease of childhood, but most of those affected survive into adolescence, and some into adulthood. This chronic disease affects the exocrine glands, with excessively thick and viscid mucus and abnormal secretion of sweat and saliva. The viscous pancreatic secretions may obstruct the pancreatic and bile ducts. The condition is characterized by pancreatic insufficiency, gastrointestinal malabsorption, recurrent respiratory infections, and excessive losses of sodium and chloride in the sweat. Treatment involves controlling respiratory symptoms and infections (asthma-like attacks, recurrent pneumonia, and sinusitis) and maintaining nutritional status.

Nutritional Concerns. Nutritional deficiencies occur frequently during infancy and childhood when nutritional demands are great because of increased growth rates (Farrell & Hubbard, 1983). Deficits of body fat and muscle mass implicate chronic catabolic stress (Shepherd et al, 1984). The degree of malabsorption will affect the nutritional requirement and severity of malnutrition.

Almost all nutrients are affected by CF, including the energy requirement, protein, fat, fat-soluble vitamins, and several minerals (Table 28–8). The use of pancreatic enzyme supplements (previously discussed in the pancreas section) with each meal enhances the intestinal absorption of fat and protein.

Nutritional Care. Routine monitoring of nutritional status and the amount of energy absorbed is recommended. Total energy requirement for CF is 50 to 100 percent over the RDAs for the age group (Table 28–9) because (1) malabsorption results in energy nutrients not being absorbed, (2) labored breathing requires extra energy, and (3) frequent infections and fever increase basal metabolic rate. Additionally, intake

Table 28–9. Nutrient Guidelines for Children with Cystic Fibrosis*

Age, years	Kilocalories (kilojoules)
Infants (to 1)	150–200 kcal/kg/day (630–840 kJ/kg/day)
Children (1–9)	130–180 kcal/kg/day (545–755 kJ/kg/day)
Males (9–18)	100–130 kcal/kg/day (420–545 kJ/kg/day)
Females (9–18)	80–110 kcal/kg/day (335–460 kJ/kg/day)

Age	Protein
Infants	4 gm/kg/day
Older children	3 gm/kg/day
Young adults	2½–3 gm/kg/day

*From *Guide to Diagnosis and Management of Cystic Fibrosis.* Cystic Fibrosis Foundation, 6000 Executive Blvd, Suite 309, Rockville, MD 20852, 1974.

is compromised because of fatigue from breathing, chest physical therapy, and chronic coughing, which leads to anorexia and vomiting.

Protein deficiencies in cystic fibrosis are frequently seen during the first year of life and early childhood, as reflected by a stunted growth rate. Protein requirement is high; 15 to 20 percent of the total daily energy intake should be furnished by protein (Farrell, 1983).

Simple sugars are better tolerated than complex starches; concentrated sweets are not tolerated well. Fats are not well tolerated either, and they are usually low in the diet; this compromises energy intake, inhibiting growth and development. It is felt that, because of its importance in improving the palatability of the diet and providing essential fatty acids, the fat content should be as high as the patient can tolerate without discomfort from abdominal cramps. Most authorities recommend that 40 to 50 percent of the total calories be provided by fats (Farrell, 1984; Roy et al, 1984). Medium-chain triglycerides (MCT) are better absorbed and can be used to decrease the characteristic steatorrhea. They are most appropriately used as a dietary additive or partial replacement of long-chain fatty acids. To prevent fatty acid deficiency, an absorbable form of linoleic acid should be supplied.

Fat-soluble vitamins are of concern because of fat malabsorption. Water-miscible forms of these vitamins are better absorbed. Vitamin A deficiencies have been observed, and 2000 IU of a water-soluble preparation is recommended. Bone demineralization is seen frequently (Mischler et al, 1979), but no additional supplementation of vita-

Table 28–8. Major Nutritional Concerns in Cystic Fibrosis*

Energy (calories)	Increased requirement because of malabsorption, respiratory disease and other complications
Protein	Appropriate quantity and quality are needed especially during infancy
Fat	Provides an important source of calories, as well as essential fatty acids
Fat-soluble vitamins (A, D, E, and K)	All may be deficient in CF patients
Miscellaneous minerals	Sodium, calcium, iron, zinc, and selenium

*From Farrell, PM; Hubbard, VS: Nutrition in cystic fibrosis: vitamins, fatty acids, and minerals. In *A Textbook of Cystic Fibrosis.* Edited by JD Lloyd-Still. Boston, John Wright, PSG, Inc., 1983, p 265.

min D over the 400 IU present in a multivitamin supplement is recommended. Vitamin E supplementation of a water-soluble preparation should contain 50 IU/day for infants or 200 IU/day for adults. While vitamin K deficiency is not a common problem, a daily dose of 50 to 100 mcg or 2.5 to 5.0 mg/week is recommended.

Calcium intake is especially important; because many patients with CF are lactase-deficient, calcium supplements are necessary. Lactose-free polymeric formulas are available containing MCT oil. These can be utilized for supplementation or during an acute phase of the disease (Dhar et al, 1980).

The sodium content of sweat is abnormally high; salt depletion is hazardous. While patients with cystic fibrosis need two to four times the amount of sodium required normally, patients with CF do not need sodium supplements unless they are exposed to conditions inducing profuse sweating (exercise or fever) for extended periods. In this case, it is better to recommend salt tablets than to encourage overly salted foods (Farrell & Hubbard, 1983).

In general, the diet should be high in protein and energy with the fat content as high as tolerated to improve the growth rate and prognosis. Supplementation of all vitamins is needed; two multivitamin supplements daily are advised (Farrell & Hubbard, 1983). Foods high in fat or containing concentrated carbohydrates and heavily spiced foods may cause distress. Patients should be encouraged to eat slowly. Small frequent feedings are better tolerated.

Clinical Implications:

- Appetite stimulants may be used occasionally in patients with CF (Hunt, 1976).
- Any food that causes distress should be omitted.
- Cholesterol levels in these patients are normally low; patients are encouraged to eat eggs for their protein content.
- Introduce new foods gradually; observe the patient for any distress.
- Dietary restrictions make the child feel different; keep dietary manipulations to a minimum by utilizing enzyme preparations.
- Required kilocalorie intake for children with CF is frequently more than that for normal children.
- Adequate nutritional support should be provided during and after each episode of pulmonary disease, which adversely affects protein-energy balance (Holt et al, 1985).
- The nutritional status of patients with CF can be improved (as evidenced by increased body

fat) by nutrition counseling at frequent intervals (not just at the time of diagnosis) (Luder & Gilbride, 1985).

• FALLACIES and FACTS

FALLACY: *Spicy foods and citrus fruits cause the yellow color present with jaundice; they should be omitted from the diet.*

  • **FACT:** *There is no basis for this. Citrus fruits should be included for a person with liver disease for the vitamin C content. Spices should be avoided only if they cause gastrointestinal discomfort.*

FALLACY: *Wine makes "strong blood."*

  • **FACT:** *No individual food or beverage is responsible for the production of blood.*

FALLACY: *Beer is not as damaging to the liver as hard liquor.*

  • **FACT:** *Alcohol is hepatotoxic; enough of any type of alcohol can cause problems.*

FALLACY: *Caffeine will help "sober up" after a hangover.*

  • **FACT:** *A hangover is caused by high serum levels of alcohol and/or other pharmacologically active molecules found in alcoholic beverages. Enzymes present in the liver metabolize alcohol. Alcohol will be metabolized as fast as these enzymes can handle it. No food substance can increase this enzymatic process.*

FALLACY: *One can prevent liver damage by taking lipotropic agents, such as methionine and choline.*

  • **FACT:** *While these substances do protect the liver against fatty infiltration in normal circumstances, the amounts produced by the body when a well-balanced diet is eaten are adequate. Even the best of diets cannot protect the liver against damage when excessive amounts of alcohol are consumed (Appel & Briggs, 1980).*

Summary

The accessory gastrointestinal organs—namely, the liver, gallbladder, and pancreas—all have special functions affecting digestion and absorption of foods. When they are unable to function properly, malabsorption results, negatively affecting nutritional status. In most cases, nutritional care is imperative to restore health; it is not a cure for the disease.

When the liver is diseased, protein is crucial for its healing. Since protein can only worsen a severe condition, the amount of protein allowed depends on the amount of damage to the liver (as measured by various laboratory tests).

Nutritional care for patients with gallbladder disease may involve control of total dietary fat to minimize discomfort. Diseases affecting the pancreas, including pancreatitis and cystic fibrosis, will affect the digestion and absorption of all nutrients because of pancreatic insufficiency. Large amounts of all nutrients except fat are required.

Review Questions

1. Why is protein important in liver disease? Discuss the different amounts of protein recommended for initial treatment of hepatitis, cirrhosis, and encephalopathy. Discuss the reasons for the different levels.
2. Explain why branched-chain amino acids may be well tolerated and hasten recovery in a patient with liver disease.
3. When is sodium restriction necessary for liver disease?
4. Why might a patient with gallbladder disease choose to eliminate potato chips, mayonnaise, and chocolate cake from his diet?
5. Why would an elemental diet be better tolerated than a bland diet by a patient with pancreatitis?
6. Plan a menu for a seven-year-old school child with cystic fibrosis who carries her lunch to school. She weighs 18.1 kg and should have at least 3000 kcal, 50 gm of protein, and 50 gm of fat.

Case Study: Three weeks following ingestion of contaminated oysters, Mr. C.M., a 26-year-old accountant, showed signs of hepatitis A. At the physician's office, he complains of weight loss, right upper abdominal quadrant tenderness, anorexia, nausea, and a loss of taste for cigarettes. His skin and sclerae are slightly jaundiced. After his admission, he is placed on a high-calorie, high-protein diet with vitamin supplements.

1. Why is a high-calorie, high-protein diet indicated for this patient?
2. What precautions must be observed in caring for this patient, particularly concerning food left on his tray?

3. What alterations should be made in meal times and the quantity of food served at each meal?
4. Is a soft diet indicated for this patient?

Case Study: Dr. B.D. has consumed an increasing amount of alcohol over the past five years. Staff members have noted his decreasing ability to function in the office. Over the past two months, they have also noted discoloration of the skin and sclerae, increasing size of his abdomen, and ankle edema. On his admission to the hospital, tests reveal serum albumin, 2.5 gm/dl; prothrombin time, 25 seconds; and elevated serum ammonia. He is confused, irritable, and uncoordinated and has fetor hepaticus. He is placed on a soft diet of 20 gm of protein and 1000 mg of sodium.

1. Why is the protein restriction deemed necessary at this time?
2. What is the physiological basis for the sodium restriction?
3. In planning Dr. B.D.'s care, prepare a meal plan for the protein and sodium restrictions.
4. Are vitamin supplements indicated for this patient?
5. Why is magnesium an important electrolyte for the patient with alcoholic cirrhosis?
6. Why is a soft diet often indicated for this type of patient?

REFERENCE LIST

Appel, JA; Briggs, GM: Choline. In *Modern Nutrition in Health and Disease*, 6th ed. Edited by RS Goodhart; ME Shils. Philadelphia, Lea & Febiger, 1980, p. 286.

Barboriak, JJ; Meads, RC: Effect of alcohol on gastric emptying in man. *Am J Clin Nutr* 23(9):1151, 1970.

Barthel, JS; Butt, JH, II: Ascites. *Am Fam Physician* 27(3):248, 1983.

Bateman, EC: Dietary management of liver disease. *Proc Nutr Soc* 38(3):331, 1979.

Boyar, HP; Loughridge, JR: The fat portion exchange list: A tool for teaching and evaluating low-fat diets. *J Am Diet Assoc* 85(5):589, 1985.

Bruijn, KM de; Blendis, LM; Zilm, DH; et al: Effect of dietary protein manipulations in subclinical portal-systemic encephalopathy. *Gut* 34(1):53, 1983.

Capron, JP; Delamarre, J; Herve, MA; et al: Meal frequency and duration of overnight fast: A role in gall-stone formation? *Br Med J* 293(Nov 28):1435, 1981.

Castelli, WP; Doyle, JT; Gordon, T; et al: Alcohol and blood lipids: The cooperative lipoprotein phenotyping study. *Lancet* 2(July 23):152, 1977.

Davidson, CS: Nutrition in diseases of the liver. In *Modern Nutrition in Health and Disease*, 6th ed. Edited by RS Goodhart; ME Shils. Philadelphia, Lea & Febiger, 1980, p. 962.

Davies, DL: Preventing alcoholism. *Royal Soc Health J* 99(5):196, 1979.

Dextrose, phosphorus, and iron metabolism in alcoholism. *Nutr Rev* 36(5):142, 1978.

Dhar, P; Zamcheck, N; Broitman, SA: Nutrition in diseases of the pancreas. In *Modern Nutrition in Health and Disease*, 6th ed. Edited by RS Goodhart; ME Shils. Philadelphia, Lea & Febiger, 1980, p 953.

Dutta, SK; Hlasko, J: Dietary fiber in pancreatic disease: Effect of high fiber diet on fat malabsorption in pancreatic insufficiency and in vitro study of the interaction of dietary fiber with pancreatic enzymes. *Am J Clin Nutr* 41(3):517, 1985.

Eckardt, MJ; Harford, TC; Kaelber, CT; et al: Health hazards associated with alcohol consumption. *JAMA* 246(6):648, 1981.

Farrell, PM: Nutrition in cystic fibrosis. *ASDC J Dent Child* 50(5):385–388, 1984.

Farrell, PM: Nutrition in cystic fibrosis. *Contemporary Nutr* 8(8), 1983.

Farrell, PM; Hubbard, VS: Nutrition in cystic fibrosis: Vitamins, fatty acids, and minerals. In *A Textbook of Cystic Fibrosis*. Edited by JD Lloyd-Still. Boston, John Wright, PSG, Inc, 1983, p 263.

Fischer, JE: Baldessarini, RJ: False neurotransmitters and hepatic failure. *Lancet* 2(July 10):75, 1971.

Fischer, JE; Bower, RH: Nutritional support in liver disease. *Surg Clin North Am* 61(3):653, 1981.

Francis, DP; Feorino, PM; McDougal, S; et al: The safety of the hepatitis B vaccine. *JAMA* 256(7):869, 1986.

Freund, HR; James, JH; Fischer, JE: Nitrogen sparing mechanisms of singly-administered branched-chain amino acids in the injured rat. *Surgery* 90(2):237, 1981.

Freund, HR; Yoshimura, N; Fischer, JE: Chronic hepatic encephalopathy. Long-term therapy with a branched-chain amino acid–enriched elemental diet. *JAMA* 242(4):347, 1979.

Grady, GF: The here and now of hepatitis B immunization. *N Engl J Med* 315(4):250, 1986.

Greenberger, NJ; Carley, J; Schenker, S; et al: Effect of vegetable and animal protein diets in chronic hepatic encephalopathy. *Am J Dig Dis* 22(10):845, 1977.

Gruchow, HW; Sobocinski, KA; Barboriak, JJ: Alcohol, nutrient intake, and hypertension in US adults. *JAMA* 253(11):1567, 1985.

Halsted, CH: Alcoholism and malnutrition. Introduction to the symposium. *Am J Clin Nutr* 33(12):2705, 1980.

Hennekens, CH; Rosner, B; Cole, DS: Daily alcohol consumption and fatal coronary heart disease. *Am J Epidemiol* 107(3):196, 1978.

Holt, TL; Ward, LC; Francis, PF; et al: Whole body protein turnover in malnourished cystic fibrosis patients and its relationship to pulmonary disease. *Am J Clin Nutr* 41(5):1061, 1985.

Houghton, PWJ; Donaldson, LA; Jenkinson, LR; et al: Weight gain after cholecystomy. *Br Med J* 289(November 17):1350, 1984.

Hunt, MM: Dietary care of patients with cystic fibrosis. *Dietetic Currents* 3(3):11, 1976.

Karcioglu, GL; Hardison, JE: Iron-containing plasma cells. *Arch Intern Med* 138(1):97, 1978.

Kirby, DF; Craig, RM: The value of intensive nutritional support in pancreatitis. *JPEN* 9(3):353, 1985.

Korsten, MA; Lieber, CS: Nutrition in the alcoholic. *Med Clin North Am* 63(5):963, 1979.

LaMorte, WW; Matolo, NM; Birkett, DH; et al: Pathogenesis of cholesterol gallstones. *Surg Clin North Am* 61(4):765, 1981.

Leo, MA; Arai, M; Sato, M; Lieber, CS: Hepatotoxicity of vitamin A and ethanol in the rat. *Gastroenterology* 82(2):194, 1982.

Lieber, CS; Jones, DP; Mendelson, J; et al: Fatty liver, hyperlipemia, hyperuricemia produced by prolonged alcoholic consumption despite adequate dietary intake. *Trans Assoc Am Physicians* 76:289, 1963.

Lieber, CS; Rubin, E: Ethanol: A hepatoxic drug. *Gastroenterology* 54(4):642, 1968.

Lieber, CS; Spritz, LM: Study of agents for the prevention of the fatty acid produced by prolonged alcohol intake. *Gastroenterology* 50(3):316, 1977.

Luder, E; Gilbride, J: The effect of nutrition counseling on growth, weight gain and pulmonary function in cystic fibrosis patients. Unpublished paper presented at the American Dietetic Association, New Orleans, October 1985.

Mauthe, H: The low fat meal in gallbladder examinations. *Radiology* 112(1):5, 1974.

Mezey, E: Alcoholic liver disease: Roles of alcohol and malnutrition. *Am J Clin Nutr* 33(12):2709, 1980.

Mischler, EH; Chesney, J; Chesney, RW; et al: Demineralization in cystic fibrosis. *Am J Dis Child* 133(6):632, 1979.

Mogadam, M; Albarelli, J; Ahmed, SW; et al: Gallbladder dynamics in response to various meals: Is dietary fat restriction necessary in the management of gallstones? *Am J Gastroenterol* 79(10):745, 1984.

Nasrallah, SM; Galambos, JT: Aminoacid therapy of alcoholic hepatitis. *Lancet* 2 (December 13):1276, 1980.

Pimstone, NR; Mok, HYI: Current status of medical treatment of gallstones. *Surg Clin North Am* 61(4):865, 1981.

Pirola, RC; Lieber, CS: The energy cost of the metabolism of drugs, including ethanol. *Pharmacology* 7(3):185, 1972.

Porte, D; Halter, JB: The endocrine pancreas and diabetes mellitus. In *Textbook of Endocrinology*, 6th ed. Edited by RH Willams. Philadelphia, W. B. Saunders Co, 1981, p 716.

Recommendations for protection against viral hepatitis. *JAMA* 254(1):29, 1985.

Roe, DA: Nutritional concerns in the alcoholic. *J Am Diet Assoc* 78(1):17, 1981.

Roe, DA: *Alcohol and the Diet*. Westport, CT, AVI Publishing Co, 1979.

Rossi-Fanelli, F; Angelico, M; Cangiano, C; et al: Effect of glucose and/or branched chain amino acid infusion on plasma amino imbalance in chronic liver failure. *JPEN* 5(5):414, 1981.

Roy, CC; Darling, P; Weber, AM: A rational approach to meeting macro- and micronutrient needs in cystic fibrosis. *J Pediatr Gastroenterol Nutr* 3(suppl):S154, 1984.

Rubin, E: The "social" drinker. *JAMA* 248(17):2179, 1982.

Rudman, D; Smith, RB, III; Salam, AA; et al: Ammonia content of food. *Am J Clin Nutr* 26(5):487, 1973.

Sedman, A; Wilkinson, P; Sakmar, E; et al: Food effects on absorption and metabolism of alcohol. *J Stud Alcohol* 37(9):1197, 1976.

Shaw, S; Lieber, CS: Nutrition and alcoholism. In *Modern Nutrition in Health and Disease*, 6th ed. Edited by RS Goodhart; ME Shils. Philadelphia, Lea & Febiger, 1980, p. 1220.

Shaw, S; Worner, TM; Lieber, CS: Comparison of animal and vegetable protein sources in the dietary management of hepatic encephalophy. *Am J Clin Nutr* 38(1):59, 1983.

Shepherd, RW; Holt, TL; Thomas, BJ; et al: Malnutrition in cystic fibrosis: The nature of nutritional deficit and optimal management. *Nutr Abs Rev* (Series A) 54(12):1009, 1984.

Shultz, J; Weiner, H; Westcott, J: Retardation of ethanol absorption by food in the stomach. *J Stud Alcohol* 41(9):861, 1980.

Smith, JC, Jr: Marginal nutritional states and conditioned deficiencies. In *Alcohol and Nutrition*. Edited by TK Li; S Schenker; L Lumeng. National Institute on Alcohol Abuse and Alcoholism Research Monograph 2. Washington, DC, Government Printing Office, 1979, 23.

Spiro, HM: *Clinical Gastroenterology*, 3rd ed. New York, Macmillan, 1983.

Spritz, N: Appraisal of alcohol consumption as a causative factor in liver disease and atherosclerosis. *Am J Clin Nutr* 32(suppl 12):2654, 1979.

Taylor, KB: Diet and gallstone formation. *Nutr & the MD* 12(6):1, 1986.

Thorpe, CJ; Caprini, JA: Gallbladder disease: Current trends and treatments. *Am J Nurs* 80(12):2181, 1980.

Turner, TB; Bennett, VL; Hernandez, H: The beneficial side of moderate alcohol use. *John Hopkins Med J* 148(2):53, 1981.

Uribe, M: Potential toxicity of a new sugar substitute in patients with liver disease. *N Engl J Med* 306(3):173, 1982.

Uribe, M; Marques, MA; Ramos, GG; et al: Treatment of chronic portal-systemic encephalopathy with vegetable and animal protein diets. A controlled crossover. *Dig Dis Sci* 27(12):1109, 1982.

Walser, M: Alcohol. In *Nutritional Management.* Edited by M Walser; AL Imbembo; S Margolis; et al. Philadelphia, W.B. Saunders Co, 1984.

Willett, W; Hennekens, CH; Siegel, AJ; et al: Alcohol consumption and high-density lipoprotein cholesterol in marathon runners. *N Engl J Med* 303(20):1159, 1980.

Yano, K; Rhoads, GG; Kagan, A: Coffee, alcohol and risk of coronary heart disease among Japanese men living in Hawaii. *N Engl J Med* 297(8):405, 1977.

Further Study

Baghurst, KI: The effect of high alcohol intake on nutritional status and health outcome. *Aust Fam Physician* 11(4):259, 1982.

Brodsley, L: Avoiding a crisis: The assessment. *Am J Nurs* 82(12):1865, 1982.

Cohn, L: The hidden diagnosis. *Am J Nurs* 82(12):1862, 1982.

Davies, DL: Preventing alcoholism. *Royal Soc Health J* (5):196, 1979.

Eckardt, MJ; Harford, TC; Kaelber, CT; et al: Health hazards associated with alcohol consumption. *JAMA* 246(6):648, 1981.

Editorial: Supplementary nutrition in cystic fibrosis. *Lancet* (February 1):249, 1986.

Eisenstein, AB: Nutritional and metabolic effects of alcohol. *J Am Diet Assoc* 81(3):247, 1982.

Fraser, CL; Arieff, AI: Hepatic encephalopathy. *N Engl J Med* 313(14):865, 1985.

Fredette, SL: When the liver fails. *Am J Nurs* 84(1):64, 1984.

Heinemann, E; Estes, N: Assessing alcoholic patients. *Am J Nurs* 76(5):785, 1976.

King, D: How to give your portal hypertension patient a fighting chance. *RN* 46(7):31, 1983.

Lieber, CS: Alcohol-nutrition interaction. *Contemporary Nutr* 8(12), 1983.

Schoenfield, LJ: Gallstones and other biliary diseases. *Clin Symp* 34(4):2, 1982.

Shenkin, A: Assessment of nutritional status: The biochemical approach and its problems in liver disease. *J Human Nutr* 33(5):341, 1979.

Simmons, S; Given, B: Acute pancreatitis. *Am J Nurs* 71(5):934, 1971.

Tomaiolo, PP: Nutritional problems in the alcoholic. *Compr Ther* 7(7):24, 1981.

Truswell, AS: Nutritional advice for other chronic diseases. *Br Med J* 291(July 20):197, 1985.

Visocan, BJ: Nutritional management of alcoholism. *J Am Diet Assoc* 83(6):693, 1983.

Woodell, WJ: Alcoholism and health. Liver disease in alcohol-addicted patients. *Fam Comm Health* 2(2):13, 1979.

Dietary Management of Diabetes Mellitus

29

THE STUDENT WILL BE ABLE TO:

- *Discuss the role of diet in the treatment of diabetes mellitus.*
- *Explain the basic dietary principles of managing diabetes to patients.*
- *Discuss the clinical symptoms of diabetes mellitus.*
- *Discuss the importance of a specific amount of calories in diabetes mellitus.*
- *Compare the roles of simple versus complex carbohydrates (including fiber) in the diabetic diet.*
- *List the recommendations of the American Diabetic Association for the amount of carbohydrate in the diet.*
- *Explain why the diabetic diet is relatively low in fat.*
- *Explain the role of insulin and how the meal plan varies according to the type of insulin prescribed.*
- *Discuss the role of oral hypoglycemic agents and their effect on diet.*
- *State the causes, symptoms, and treatment for hyperglycemia and hypoglycemia.*
- *Discuss the effect of exercise on insulin and dietary requirements.*
- *Plan a liquid and semisoft diabetic diet for one day.*

Asthenia
Chemical control
Clinical control
Diabetes mellitus
Dietetic
Euglycemia
Gestational diabetes mellitus
Glycemia
Microangiopathy
Neuropathy
Oral hypoglycemic agent
Polydipsia
Polyphagia
Polyuria
Renal threshold
Somogyi effect

OBJECTIVES

TERMS TO KNOW

Many body functions are regulated by hormonal secretions of the endocrine glands. Hormones are "messengers" produced by a group of cells that stimulate or retard the functions of other cells. Hormones principally control different metabolic functions that affect growth and secretions. Deviations in the amount of secretions will affect normal mental and physiological functions. Hormones are influential in regulating nutrient metabolism, i.e., carbohydrates, protein, fat, minerals, and electrolytes. Dietary management is sometimes effective in alleviating general discomfort, maintaining metabolic balance, rehabilitating the patient, or preventing further complications.

Other endocrine disorders are also frequently considered to be metabolic problems because altered hormonal levels affect body metabolism (see Chapter 30).

Diabetes Mellitus

Diabetes is first noted in an Egyptian medical treatise around 1500 B.C. (about the time of Moses). The Ebers Papyrus prescribed grains, grapes, honey, and berries for a condition described as "too great emptying of urine." Diabetes was referred to as "polyuria without pain but with emaciation and danger" by Celsus (30 B.C. to A.D. 50). During the second century A.D., Aretaeus, a Greek physician, named the condition "diabetes," which means "a siphon." Diabetes was described by a physician as a disease of thirst after observing a patient drink 10 quarts of water a day. Ants were attracted to the urine of patients suffering from the condition. During the seventeenth century, "mellitus," meaning "honeyed," was added to the name to better describe the condition in which sugar was found in the urine. (Hence, the term used by lay people "sugar diabetes" is a literal translation of the medical terminology.)

Even though the cause remained unknown for centuries, it was treated by diet or a semistarvation "cure." Patients lived very short lives. In 1921, Banting and Best discovered "insulin." Kilocalories and carbohydrate were allowed more liberally. Progress toward identifying the cause of the disease with its many complications has greatly increased our understanding of body metabolism. While much progress has been made, it is a complex condition about which there is much more to learn.

Diabetes mellitus has been defined by Friedman (1980) as "an hereditary disease of metabolism in which there is an inadequate supply of effective insulin, characterized by disturbances of carbohydrate, fat, and protein." Diabetes mellitus may also be a result of damage to the pancreas, which inhibits insulin production. In some patients the amount of insulin present is insufficient for the body's needs; in others, insulin cannot be utilized by the tissues. The condition is specifically related to endocrine secretions of the pancreas but involves the entire endocrine system. The main manifestation of diabetes mellitus is hyperglycemia. However, glucose homeostasis is a very complex network of many hormones (see Fig. 7–5).

Diabetes mellitus is presently one of the most common diseases. The incidence of diabetes mellitus is increasing worldwide, affecting as much as five percent of the population of the United States (RNCD, 1976) and with less than half of the conditions being diagnosed (West, 1983). In addition to diabetics being prone to blindness, kidney disease, gangrene, and heart disease, their life expectancy is one third less than that of the general population (RNCD, 1976).

PANCREATIC ROLE

The pancreas has cells that produce the hormones glucagon and insulin. Beta cells in the islets of Langerhans produce insulin, which is important in transporting glucose into cells and aids in converting glucose to glycogen or fat tissue. The overall effect is to decrease serum glucose.

Pancreatic alpha cells secrete another hormone, glucagon, which works in opposition to insulin. It causes the blood glucose level to increase by glucogenesis in which glycogen is broken down to glucose; as such, it is a counterbalance to insulin by increasing the hypoglycemic level. It also causes adipose tissue to release free fatty acids and glycerol that can be utilized for energy.

Normally, both of these secretions are controlled by the glycemic (blood glucose) level. When the blood sugar level is high, insulin is secreted, which causes the blood sugar level to decrease. Glucose combined with a carrier substance is transported through the cell membrane at specific places where insulin is attached onto insulin receptor sites. In diabetes mellitus, insulin is absent, deficient, or ineffective; glucagon is present in excessive amounts. These problems then precipitate clinical manifestations.

CLASSIFICATIONS

In 1978, the National Institutes of Health outlined classifications of diabetes and other categories of glucose intolerance (NDDG, 1979), as summarized in Table 29–1. The two types of diabetes mellitus have different basic metabolic defects (Arky, 1978) and can appear to be very different conditions (Table 29–2).

Type I, or Insulin-Dependent Diabetes Mellitus (IDDM)

Type I is distinguished by little or no endogenous insulin production. This condition most commonly manifests itself in young people but can occur at any age. Onset is sudden with all the clinical symptoms associated with the condition. The individual is ketosis-prone and must receive exogenous insulin.

About five to ten percent of the cases in the United States are IDDM (Fig. 29–1); life expectancy is only about half the normal life expectancy (West, 1983). "Tight control" is the best method of preventing or alleviating the many complications—retinal, renal, neuropathological, and cardiovascular (Nemchik, 1982).

Type II, or Noninsulin-Dependent Diabetes Mellitus (NIDDM)

About 90 percent of the cases of diabetes in the United States are NIDDM (Fig. 29–1). It is diagnosed most frequently in overweight individuals over 40 years of age; only about 10 percent are not obese. This type of diabetes develops more slowly; clinical symptoms are mild. In most of these cases, insulin is secreted in adequate or higher-than-normal amounts; body cells are glucose-intolerant. Obesity associated with this form of diabetes mellitus is thought to trigger metabolic resistance to insulin. During stress or infection, ketosis may occur, even though patients are normally not prone to ketosis. Vascular complications and degenerative changes are common.

Type II diabetes mellitus is more genetically

Table 29–1. Sorting Out the Old and the New*

Clinical Categories

New Names	Old Names	Clinical Characteristics
Type I: Insulin-dependent diabetes mellitus (IDDM)	Juvenile diabetes (JD) Juvenile-onset diabetes (JOD) Ketosis-prone diabetes Brittle diabetes	Patients have little or no endogenous insulin and need injections to preserve life. New patients may be of any age but are usually young; they often have islet-cell antibodies. Scientists believe causes may be genetic, environmental, or acquired, probably involving abnormal immune responses.
Type II: Noninsulin-dependent diabetes mellitus (NIDDM)	Adult-onset diabetes (AOD) Maturity-onset diabetes (MOD) Ketosis-resistant diabetes Stable diabetes Maturity-onset diabetes of youth (MODY)	Except during infection or other stress, patients rarely develop ketosis. They vary in amount of endogenous insulin and may need injections to avoid hyperglycemia. New patients may be of any age but are usually over 40. Most are obese. NIDDM is thought to be caused by genetic susceptibility plus environmental factors.
Diabetes mellitus associated with other conditions or syndromes	Secondary diabetes	These patients' diabetes is accompanied by conditions known or suspected to cause the disease, including pancreatic or hormonal disease, drug or chemical toxicity, abnormal insulin receptors, or certain genetic syndromes.
Impaired glucose tolerance (IGT) Type a: nonobese Type b: obese	Asymptomatic diabetes Chemical diabetes Subclinical diabetes Borderline diabetes Latent diabetes	Glucose levels are between those of normal people and those of diabetics. Patients have above-normal susceptibility to atherosclerotic disease. Renal and retinal complications generally do not become clinically significant.
Gestational diabetes mellitus (GDM)	Gestational diabetes	This classification is retained for women whose diabetes begins (or is recognized) during pregnancy. They have an above-normal risk of perinatal complications. Their glucose intolerance may be transitory, but it frequently recurs.

*From Nemchik, R: Diabetes today: A startling new body of knowledge. *RN* 45(10):31, 1982. Published in *RN* the full-service nursing journal. Copyright©1982, Medical Economics Company, Inc, Oradell, NJ. Reprinted by permission.

Table 29-2. Comparison of Type I and Type II Diabetes*

	Type II (NIDDM)	Type I (IDDM)
Age of onset	Frequently over 35	Most frequently during childhood or puberty
Type of onset	Usually gradual	Sudden
Family history of diabetes	Usually positive	Frequently positive
Nutritional status at time of onset	Usually obese	Frequently undernourished
Symptoms	Frequently none	Polydipsia, polyphagia, polyuria
Hepatomegaly	Uncommon	Rather common
Stability	Blood sugar fluctuations are less marked	Blood sugar fluctuates widely in response to changes in insulin, dose, exercise, and infection
Control of diabetes	Easy, especially if a diet is followed	Difficult
Ketosis	Uncommon except in the presence of unusual stress or moderate-to-severe sepsis	Frequent
Plasma insulin	Plasma insulin may be low, but not absent, or high.	Negligible to zero.
Vascular complications and degenerative changes	Frequent	Occurs after diabetes has been present for about five years
Diet	Diet therapy may eliminate the need for hypoglycemic agents	Required
Insulin	Used for a few patients	Necessary for all patients
Oral agents	Effective	Not suitable

*Adapted from *Diabetes Mellitus*, 8th ed. Indianapolis, Eli Lilly & Co, 1980.

related than IDDM, as evidenced by a closer association of familial occurrence. Type II also includes diabetes mellitus that is secondary to other conditions or syndromes (frequently triggered by illness, trauma, or toxins).

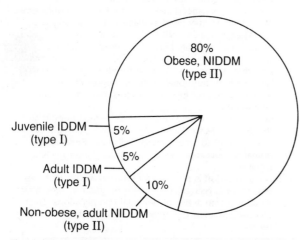

Figure 29-1. *The incidence of various types of diabetes mellitus. (Data from* Diabetes Mellitus, *8th ed. Indianapolis, Eli Lilly & Company, 1980.)*

DIAGNOSTIC TESTS

Diabetes mellitus is diagnosed by laboratory tests; the classification of diabetes affects how the condition will be treated. Normally, the fasting blood glucose level is 60 to 110 mg/dl. Fasting blood sugar (FBS) levels will be elevated (over 120 mg/dl) in diabetics.

The oral glucose tolerance test (OGTT) may be ordered to confirm a diabetic diagnosis. This test measures blood glucose levels at specific intervals after glucose is given. The diabetic response results in a higher glycemic level that returns to normal more slowly than in a nondiabetic (Fig. 29-2). In order to get an accurate response, for three days prior to the test the patient should eat a high-carbohydrate diet and discontinue the use of hormones, hypoglycemic agents, diuretics, and salicylates. Additionally, the patient is NPO (except for water) for 12 hours prior to testing.

A new diagnostic test is the hemoglobin A_{1C} (glycosylated form of hemoglobin). Hemoglobin A_{1C} is produced when glucose molecules attach to normal hemoglobin in a high-glucose environment. Since it reflects an average of blood sugar

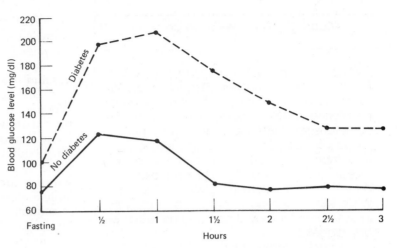

Figure 29-2. Glucose tolerance test curves. (From McFarland MB, Grant MM: Nursing Implications of Laboratory Tests. New York, copyright © 1982 John Wiley & Sons, Inc. Reprinted by permission of John Wiley & Sons, Inc.)

levels for two to three months (hemoglobin has a life span of 120 days), it can be used as a long-term indicator of glycemic levels or to determine if the patient's condition has been well managed during the past two to three months. Hemoglobin A_{1C} levels are double the amounts found in nondiabetics. No restriction on sampling time is required. Besides being a more accurate reflection of the patient's metabolic control, the test can be used as a motivational tool: Patients are given more incentive in their self-management (Johny, 1984; White & Miller, 1983).

Urine specimens can be tested to determine total urine volume (for a 24-hour period), specific gravity, glucose, and ketone bodies. Glucose in the urine does not necessarily denote diabetes mellitus, but this test was previously used by diabetics to determine daily management. Certain drugs can cause false-negative or false-positive reactions in testing for glycosuria; also renal thresholds for glucose will vary among individuals and from numerous other factors. Because urine testing does not accurately reflect current blood sugar levels (especially if they are lower than the renal threshold), most physicians and diabetics rely on blood sugars. Ketonuria (ketones in the urine) indicates that excessive amounts of fats are being metabolized; this requires an immediate adjustment of diet and insulin.

In 1982, the American Diabetes Association indicated that self-monitoring of glycemia is "preferable to urine testing in any insulin-requiring diabetic patient." Determinations of glucose levels can accurately be measured by a relatively new technique using visual blood glucose testing sticks or glucose monitoring instruments (Pecoraro et al, 1986) (Focus on Self-Monitoring of Glucose). It

can be used to effectively control blood sugar levels if patients use the test results properly. Glucose monitoring is essential for insulin pump therapy. Unfortunately, primary care physicians are not implementing this type of diabetic management as much as diabetologists or endocrinologists (Bergman & Felig, 1984).

CLINICAL SYMPTOMS

Type I diabetes is characterized by many clinical symptoms. In Type II, symptoms are less obvious or not apparent, necessitating a diagnosis by laboratory testing. Symptoms are secondary to insulin deficiency.

Insulin deficiency results in hyperglycemia. Because glucose cannot be transported into the cell or converted into glycogen, blood glucose level rises, increasing osmotic pressure within the vessels and pulling fluid out of cells. This results in cellular dehydration. When blood sugar exceeds the kidney's ability to reabsorb glucose (the renal threshold is usually about 180 mg/dl), sugar is excreted in the urine.

Hyperglycemia results in glycosuria. Glycosuria, or sugar in the urine, increases the osmotic pressure of the urine, preventing water reabsorption, which results in excessive amounts of water being excreted.

Glycosuria results in polyuria. Along with the excretion of large amounts of water, sodium (from the extracellular fluid) and potassium (from the intracellular fluid) are also excreted.

Polyuria results in polydipsia, or increased thirst, which is symptomatic of fluid depletion.

Insulin deficiency results in polyphagia and asthe-

New technology has made it possible for diabetics to monitor their own blood sugar levels frequently anywhere. Home monitoring is very popular, as evidenced by numerous reagents, equipment, and meters available. In addition to being more accurate than urine testing, a record can be maintained to evaluate diet and exercise and to effect optimum glycemic control. While self-monitoring is more important with insulin pump therapy, it can also be used by any diabetic.

A prick sample of blood is placed on a reagent strip, which is then visually compared with a color chart to determine blood sugar level. Or a different reagent strip can be used with a reflectance meter, which gives a specific glycemic reading (Fig. 29-3). The article by Orzeck (1984) is recommended for its discussion and list of various blood glucose-measuring products available. While timing and techniques are important, both are very simple procedures.

Blood sugar level determinations are important at seven different times of the day (before and after each meal and before bedtime); however, many physicians recommend that blood sugar be monitored one or two times daily, at least once for each of the seven ideal times during a one-week period for stable diabetic conditions. This glycemic information can be used to adjust food, exercise, and insulin to control blood glucose. Guidelines for adjusting insulin to control blood glucose can be found in the excellent article written by Skyler and colleagues (1981).

With the use of blood glucose monitoring, the trend is to adjust insulin dosage to suit the diet. The benefits of a nutritionally well-balanced, regular meal plan should be emphasized. The advent of self-monitoring allows diabetics to have more control over their health and daily schedules, thereby achieving a greater sense of independence (Bergman & Felig, 1984).

---

nia. Because cells are unable to utilize available glucose, they have no source of energy. The individual will have asthenia, or a lack of energy. The starved state also results in an increased appetite,

or polyphagia. Additionally, muscle protein and adipose tissue will be broken down to supply energy needs.

Catabolization of muscle tissue results in weight loss and negative nitrogen balance.

Catabolization of fatty tissue results in ketosis. When excessive amounts of fatty acids are being broken down, muscles cannot utilize them fast enough and the liver will change them into ketone bodies. Excretion of ketone bodies in the urine is accompanied by excretion of sodium, which is drawn from the extracellular fluid. With large amounts of acidic or ketone bodies and loss of sodium ion (having a basic pH), a state of metabolic acidosis can occur.

Ketosis can result in diabetic acidosis. Poorly controlled diabetics in a state of diabetic acidosis have fruity-smelling breath. If this is not corrected, hypovolemia will result, which leads to diabetic coma and death.

So, as can be seen, diabetes is not just an abnormality of carbohydrate metabolism but also involves metabolism of protein, fat, and fluid and electrolyte balance.

COMPLICATIONS

Because of metabolic alterations secondary to diabetes mellitus, treatment should be implemented as soon as possible after diagnosis. It is felt by most diabetic authorities that early control of diabetes can postpone and minimize many of the severe complications, which should be explained to the diabetic patient.

Diabetics have problems with slow wound, healing, frequent abscesses, skin irritations, pruritus, numbness and tingling of the extremities, and visual problems. These are generally associated with vascular problems.

In diabetes, vascular changes, which are thought to result from chronic hyperglycemia and hyperlipidemia, are seen (Solomon, 1979). Atherosclerosis develops at an earlier age in diabetics than in nondiabetics. Microangiopathy is unique to diabetes. It can be identified as a thickening of the capillary basement membrane. These changes result in renal complications (leading to renal failure), obstruction of circulation in the extremities (leading to gangrene), and progressive blood vessel damage in the retina of the eye (leading to blindness).

Peripheral vascular degenerative changes accompanying atherosclerosis are associated with dietary intake of total fat and cholesterol; decreased intake of fats and cholesterol is recom-

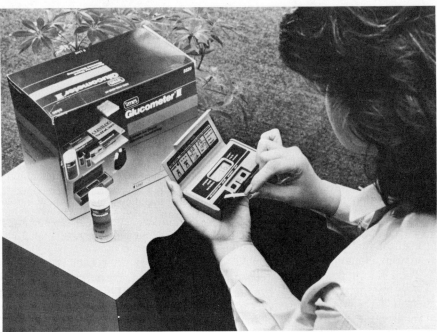

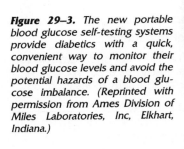

Figure 29–3. *The new portable blood glucose self-testing systems provide diabetics with a quick, convenient way to monitor their blood glucose levels and avoid the potential hazards of a blood glucose imbalance. (Reprinted with permission from Ames Division of Miles Laboratories, Inc, Elkhart, Indiana.)*

mended in diabetics in order to attempt to prevent these complications.

Neuropathy, or deterioration of nervous tissue, is also frequently seen in the diabetic. Impaired sensations attributable to diabetic neuropathy are a contributing factor in gangrene.

OTHER ETIOLOGICAL FACTORS

While heredity and diabetes mellitus are related, the genetic mechanisms are poorly understood. Since the incidence has been elevated in different societies, the rates were thought to be attributed to racial factors. However, it is now felt that environmental factors have an influence on its prevalence (West, 1983).

In Type II diabetes, diet may play an important role. The prevalence of diabetes in adults is closely related to adiposity throughout several populations (West, 1978). Precisely how diet contributes to diabetes other than overconsumption of energy-containing nutrients, which produces obesity, is unknown. Several conclusions have been made. High starch consumption is negatively correlated with the incidence of diabetes (West, 1978). (This does not mean that starch prevents diabetes, but that eating a diet high in complex carbohydrates is not associated with diabetes.) While sugar consumption has been suspected, most epidemiologic evidence has found

no relationship between sugar consumption and the prevalence of diabetes (Bierman, 1979; Keen, 1979; West, 1978). In societies where the incidence of diabetes mellitus has increased remarkably, sugar and fat consumption have concurrently increased, accompanied by a decrease in exercise and an increase in obesity (West, 1983).

Excessive consumption of iron results in hemochromatosis, which is a major cause of diabetes in some African nations (West, 1983). Zinc deficiency is associated with decreased glucose tolerance in rats (Quarterman & Florence, 1972). Whether the reduced zinc levels frequently observed in diabetics are a causative factor or a consequence of diabetes is not known.

Infectious diseases, trauma, and stressful conditions may precipitate diabetic symptoms. These conditions increase catecholamine secretions, incuding hyperglycemia.

METHODS OF TREATMENT

Therapeutic measures should be implemented to enable the patient to lead a normal life, to minimize clinical symptoms (especially fluctuating blood glucose levels and ketosis), and to minimize the onset of degenerative complications. These are accomplished by maintaining a fine balance between exercise, diet, and use of insulin or oral hypoglycemic agents.

Several conditions important in the treatment of both types of diabetes meet the above goals:

1. Weight should be close to the suggested desirable range for age, body structure, and height. This will involve controlling energy intake to maintain normal growth rate (more applicable to Type I and gestational diabetes) and to maintain ideal body weight or decrease body weight (especially in Type II diabetes). Increased size of the fat cells results in decreased proportions of insulin receptor sites.
2. The mealtime schedule should be regular, with food intake coinciding with insulin therapy.
3. Diet should include all the nutritional requirements, with proportions of carbohydrate, protein, and fat as prescribed. Different factors important for diabetes treatment with or without insulin are compared in Table 29–3.
4. Total fat intake is restricted; polyunsaturated fats are increased, while saturated fats and cholesterol are decreased because of increased incidence of vascular problems.
5. An oral hypoglycemic compound (for Type I) or insulin (for Type II) is used concurrently with diet therapy to control hyperglycemia.
6. Routine exercise on a regular basis is an important part of management. Activity facilitates glucose entry into the cells, decreasing blood sugar, and may alter the insulin requirement, especially in Type II. (While exercise will lower blood glucose levels in well-controlled diabetics, this is not necessarily true for poorly controlled cases.)

Clinical Implication:

- Diet is important in both Type I and II diabetes, regardless whether insulin or oral hypoglycemics are taken or even if diet alone controls blood sugar.

PRINCIPLES OF DIET THERAPY FOR DIABETES

Diet is regarded by many physicians as the cornerstone for treatment of diabetes mellitus. This opinion has not gone unchallenged (Dorchy et al, 1981; Henry et al, 1981; Abraira et al, 1980). However, the consensus supports the role of diet therapy as being beneficial in preventing hyper- and hypoglycemia as well as decreasing complications (Simpson et al, 1979; Olefsky et al, 1974).

Because of different philosophies regarding diabetic control, physicians differ in their ap-

Table 29–3. *Dietary Strategies for the Two Main Types of Diabetes**

Dietary Strategy	Type II (NIDDM)	Type I (IDDM)
Decrease calories	Yes	No
Protect or improve beta cell function	Very urgent priority	Seldom important because beta cells are usually extinct
Increase frequency and number of feedings	Usually not†	Yes
Day-to-day consistency of intake of calories, carbohydrates, protein, and fat	Not crucial if average caloric intake remains in low range	Very important
Day-to-day consistency of the ratios of carbohydrate, protein, and fat for each of the feedings‡	Not crucial	Desirable
Consistency of timing of meals	Not crucial	Very important
Extra food for unusual exercise	Not usually appropriate	Usually appropriate
Use of food to treat, abort, or prevent hypoglycemia	Not necessary	Important

*From West, KM: Diet therapy of diabetes: An analysis of failure. *Annals of Internal Medicine* 79(3):425, 1973.
†There are some theoretical advantages in dividing the diet into four or five feedings even in mild diabetes *if* this can be done without increasing caloric consumption. However, because limitation of calories has highest priority in obese diabetics, there are some potential disadvantages in providing extra feedings. Giving fat people an opportunity to eat at bedtime is particularly "risky" if weight reduction is the prime goal.
‡The total daily insulin requirement is apparently not much affected when dietary constituents are changed *under isocaloric conditions.* But insulin requirement *immediately* after a high-carbohydrate meal is higher than immediately after a low-carbohydrate meal, even if the meal is isocaloric.

proach to diet therapy. A patient may be allowed to eat anything so long as s/he does not have any clinical symptoms (no ketosis or hypoglycemia) and maintains or gains weight as appropriate. Glycosuria and hyperglycemia are permitted. Insulin dosages are adjusted frequently. This approach is known as clinical control.

Chemical control utilizes a measured diet and a level amount of insulin to control the blood sugar within normal limits and allowing only small amounts or no glucose to spill into the urine.

Dietary requirements and recommendations for diabetics are based on sound principles of nutrition—the same as for nondiabetics. A diabetic diet is a healthful way to eat; this fact should be stressed to new diabetics and the family food providers. It helps them recognize that the whole family benefits by eating in a similar manner.

One of the most important considerations of a diabetic diet is that it should be flexible in allowing wide choices of foods and adaptable to specific needs and individual preferences. It should also cause minimal disruption in the patient's lifestyle. Increased flexibility is associated with improved compliance. Additionally, the diet must be economical; half the diabetics in the United States are in a low-income bracket (Friedman, 1980). Special foods are not necessary; the foods can be the same as those purchased for the rest of the family.

Successful programs for diabetic management use a team approach, utilizing the skills and expertise of the physician, dietitian and nurse. Some programs include a physical therapist for the exercise component. Diet therapy is ineffective unless it is enthusiastically endorsed and supported by all members of the team. The most important factor in a team approach is the patient's input.

Priorities and objectives of the diet are determined based on endogenous and exogenous insulin, weight, age, activity level, and the presence of any special requirements, such as pregnancy or hyperlipoproteinemia. Then, the patient's attitudes, dietary preferences, usual feeding patterns, and capacity for self-discipline are assessed. Differences in schedules and activity levels over the weekend versus weekdays should be considered and discussed with the patient. Motivation is important in patient compliance. Family involvement and understanding are also important in motivating and supporting adherence to the diet.

Diabetics who are happy with their regime are more likely to follow it regularly (West, 1983). Compliance is better if the prescription begins with the patient's normal diet and effects minimal modifications to meet essential requirements of the metabolic disorder. In order to gain patient compliance, a thorough understanding and realization of its importance is necessary.

Energy. The most important objective in nutritional care of the diabetic is total energy intake (ADA, 1977). The kilocalories should be sufficient to achieve or maintain ideal body weight. (Usually, the minimum level of the average range of weight for height is advisable.) When the kilocalorie content is controlled, all foods containing carbohydrate, protein, fat, and alcohol are restricted to some degree. All these sources of energy are potential sources of glucose (58 percent from protein; 10 percent from fat). Recommendations for the distribution of kilocalories represented by carbohydrate, protein, and fat have been changed, as shown in Table 29–4.

Table 29–4. *Distribution of Major Nutrients in Normal and in Diabetic Diets (as percentages of total calories)*[1]

	Starch and Other Polysaccharides[2] (%)	Sugars[3] and Dextrins (%)	Fat (%)	Protein (%)	Alcohol (%)
Typical American diet	25–35	20–30	35–45 P/S ratio 1:3[6]	12–19	0–10
Traditional diabetic diets	25–30	10–15[4]	40–45	16–21	0
Newer diabetic diets	35–45[5]	5–15[4]	<30[5] P/S ratio 1:1[6]	12–20	0–6

[1]Adapted from West, KM: Diabetes mellitus. In *Nutritional Support of Medical Practice*, 2nd ed. Edited by HA Schneider; CE Anderson; DB Coursin. Philadelphia, Harper & Row, 1983.
[2]Almost all of these calories are starch, but complex carbohydrates also include cellulose, hemicellulose, pentosans, and pectin.
[3]Monosaccharides and disaccharides, mainly sucrose, but also includes fructose, glucose, lactose, and maltose.
[4]Almost exclusively natural sugars, mainly in fruit and milk (lactose).
[5]The ideal diet is probably even higher in starch and lower in saturated fat, but in typical affluent Western societies it is usually not feasible to achieve higher ratios of starch to fat than shown on the bottom line of this table.
[6]Polyunsaturated : saturated (fatty acids).

The total amount of energy needed is based on the ideal body weight (kg) and activity. This can be determined as described in *Focus on Calculating the Diabetic Prescription for Calories* in Chapter 22.

Carbohydrate. Little priority is given to starch restriction except as it affects the energy level. Contrary to earlier opinions, high-starch diets are very well tolerated (Simpson et al, 1979), and the American Diabetes Association (1979) has endorsed a proportionately high-carbohydrate diet (50 to 60 percent of total kilocalories) with most coming from complex carbohyrates, in the absence of carbohydrate-induced hypertriglyceridemia type IV (see Chapter 32). As shown in Table 29-4, the recommended carbohydrate content is similar to the typical American diet.

A high-carbohydrate diet actually increases the sensitivity of peripheral tissues to both endogenous and exogenous insulin. This improves glucose tolerance and lowers the requirement for exogenous insulin (Chait, 1984; Cole & Camerini-Davalos, 1979). Another plus for the high-carbohydrate diet is that with more energy being furnished from carbohydrate, fewer kilocalories are needed from fat sources. The high-carbohydrate diet in IDDM may lower lipoprotein cholesterol concentration (Simpson et al, 1981; 1979).

Many studies have recently focused attention on blood glucose responses to different sugars and complex carbohydrate foods (Wheeler, 1983). As shown in Table 7-3, blood glucose responses to various carbohydrates overlap so that simple and complex carbohydrates cannot be distinguished as separate groups having different glycemic responses.

These varied responses are apparently related to digestibility of the starch components, energy nutrient components in the food, and other factors related to food handling, as discussed in Chapter 7. In addition to elements within a food that affect glucose response, other foods consumed simultaneously may affect glucose responses. Some studies indicate that the glycemic response may not be as dramatic when various carbohydrates are given as part of a mixed meal instead of by themselves. A recent study by Hallenbeck and colleagues (1985) supports the theory that variation in relative proportions of naturally occurring complex and simple carbohydrates will have no deleterious effects on the glycemic effect in patients with NIDDM.

From the data currently available, the American Diabetes Association Council on Nutrition (1984) made the following recommendations:

1. Blood glucose and lipid levels are primary objectives of dietary treatment without compromising overall nutritional status.
2. Modest amounts of sucrose are acceptable, contingent on maintenance of metabolic control.
3. Carbohydrate-containing foods that produce the smallest rise in blood glucose should be emphasized.

At this time, the use of these different glycemic responses is not widely practiced because of many unanswered questions. While definite recommendations cannot be made on the basis of known information, several facts have been established: (1) Starchy foods do not all have the same effect, and (2) minimally processed and leguminous carbohydrates generally have lower glycemic effects.

Glycemic responses fail to consider the nutrient density of a food or other factors important in controlling diabetes mellitus and should not be used as the only criterion for food choices. Other factors such as total energy, fiber, saturated fat and cholesterol content, and nutrient density should be considered.

Self-monitoring of blood glucose allows a diabetic to test individual responses to specific foods or food combinations. The glycemic index can be used to interpret unexpected blood glucose variations, and thereby fine-tune the diet by emphasizing foods from the individual groupings that have lower glycemic responses (Wolever & Jenkins, 1985, 1986). While there is no longer any reason to prohibit foods containing simple sugars, habitual use of simple carbohydrates (sugar, candy, honey, or soft drinks) is discouraged, especially when other nutrients are not present.

Fiber. High-fiber diets offer several advantages for the diabetic: (1) They prevent other conditions such as diverticulosis, hyperlipoproteinemia, and colon cancer (Smith & Hamburger, 1983); (2) they help reduce kilocalorie intake (Dodson et al, 1981); (3) they may diminish postprandial surges of hyperglycemia and decrease glycosuria (Kinmonth et al, 1982; Asp et al, 1981; Dodson et al, 1981); (4) they may reduce insulin requirements (Harold et al, 1985; Anderson & Ward, 1979); and (5) they increase tissue sensitivity to insulin (Friedman, 1980). An increase in dietary fiber is more likely to improve serum glucose levels if total carbohydrate intake is high (Manhire et al, 1981; Jenkins et al, 1980). It is felt that the high-fiber, high-carbohydrate diet results in increased insulin binding to its receptors and insulin sensitivity of peripheral tissues (Anderson & Bryant,

1986). While purified fibers like guar gum and pectin are effective in controlling glucose and cholesterol levels (Smith & Hamburger, 1983), their availability and palatability are limited. As much as possible, natural foods containing unrefined carbohydrate with fiber should be substituted for highly refined carbohydrates. Dietary fiber intake is increased gradually, with a goal of about 45 gm of fiber daily (Task force, 1987). Adequate amounts of fluid should be ingested with a higher fiber intake.

Protein. The amount of protein required by diabetics is the same as for individuals with normal hepatic and renal status; the RDA for protein is 0.8 gm/kg for adults. Although diabetic recommendations have emphasized protein in the past, it is now felt that protein intake should be reduced in individuals who are identified at risk for or who have clinical evidence of nephropathy (Task force, 1987). For most diabetics, about 15 percent of the kilocalories are supplied by protein. By incorporating vegetable sources of protein (dried beans and peas) to maintain the protein level, less high-fat meats (which increase the level of dietary fat) can be used, and the fiber content of the diet is increased.

Fat. Since atherosclerosis and other vascular complications are the leading causes of death in diabetics, a diet that favors the reduction of serum cholesterol and triglycerides is wise. Triglycerides are controlled by multiple factors, including the amount of carbohydrate, the proportion of saturated fat, weight control, and energy intake.

The American Diabetes Association (ADA) Committee on Food and Nutrition (1979) states, "Although it is not certain that restriction of dietary saturated fat and cholesterol and replacement with unsaturated fat will slow the progression of atherosclerosis, it is a reasonable expectation." The 1986 ADA task force (1987) recommends that a maximum of 30 percent of the total kilocalories be in the form of fat: Saturated fat is limited to less than 10 percent, and polyunsaturated fat is increased to 10 percent. Cholesterol should be limited to 300 mg/day.

Vitamins and Electrolytes. Supplemental vitamins and minerals are not ordinarily required. However, patients with poorly controlled diabetes, infection, malabsorption, or other complications may require supplements. Additionally, Type I diabetics with recent weight loss may initially benefit from vitamin supplements since growth and development might have been compromised before diagnosis. Patients consuming very low energy levels (below 1200 kcal) should receive a multivitamin supplement. Vitamin supplements, including thiamin and vitamin B_{12}, have been given to prevent diabetic neuropathy but have not been proved to be effective (West, 1983).

Since diabetic individuals are frequently hypertensive, a moderate restriction of salt intake (not more than 3 gm daily) should be considered in well-controlled diabetes mellitus. For hypertensive diabetic individuals, sodium may be restricted to 1000 mg/1000 kcal (Task force, 1987). If the diabetes is poorly controlled, diuresis may produce deficits of water, sodium, potassium, and chloride. Large doses of insulin produce hypoglycemia and will lower blood potassium (Friedman, 1980).

Alcohol. While alcohol intake has several disadvantages in the diabetic, it is possible for the diabetic to occasionally have an alcoholic beverage without compromising blood glucose control. Alcohol is primarily metabolized by the liver and does not require insulin (see Chapter 8). Alcohol is high in energy (7 kcal/gm) and its metabolism is similar to that of fats. Large quantities of alcohol have been associated with hyperglycemia, especially in malnourished diabetics. Conversely, diabetics are actually more vulnerable to hypoglycemic effects from alcohol, which may develop up to several hours after the ingestion because of reduced gluconeogenesis in the liver; this is especially a problem when ingestion follows a fasting period (12 to 36 hours) in which glycogen reserves are depleted or if alcohol is taken with readily absorbed carbohydrate (Conner & Marks, 1985). Therefore, Type I diabetics should not omit any food from their diet to replace the calories from alcohol.

Moderate alcohol intake by a controlled diabetic does not have a deleterious effect on glucose homeostasis when a mixed meal is consumed simultaneously (Avogaro et al, 1983). Alcohol is incorporated into the diet as two to three saturated fat exchanges or a combination of bread and fat exchanges, as shown in Table 23–3.

Clinical Implications:

- Diabetic patients should be warned against excessive alcohol consumption without eating some type of food or when taking some of the oral hypoglycemic medications.
- The quantity of alcohol should be limited to one or two drinks in the course of an evening.
- Hypoglycemic symptoms may be obscured by the cerebral effects of alcohol (Connor & Marks, 1985).

- Patients with peripheral neuropathy should limit alcohol intake to one drink daily since excessive amounts may aggravate the condition (Conner & Marks, 1985).
- Hypoglycemia or Antabuse-like reactions may occur in patients taking first-generation sulfonylurea drugs.

DIABETIC DIETS

Diabetes mellitus is a chronic, lifelong disease. No one dietary plan can be appropriate for all people with different personalities and lifestyles. The objective of a diet is to enable the individual to maintain good control of the diabetes. Handing someone a diet does not necessarily help in the self-management of their disease.

While the food exchange lists are by far the most widely used (see Chapter 23), alternative diets are used with comparable diabetic control. Some of the options are basic food groups; healthy food choices; U.S. dietary guidelines; high-carbohydrate, high-fiber (HCHF) diet; calorie counting, total available glucose (TAG), and the point system. The structured diets (food exchange lists, HCHF diet, calorie counting, and point system) are best for those who require structure and consistency in a diet. The TAG system is appropriate for those who want maximum glucose control, but it is generally reserved for the most compliant patients because it requires so much planning.

Ideally, the patient's personality and lifestyle are assessed before determining the appropriate type of diet. Since proper treatment is definitely a matter of self-management, input from the patient regarding the type of diet preferred may result in better compliance.

Exchange System

The food exchange lists allow flexibility of the diet in addition to achieving a reasonable constancy of carbohydrate, protein, fat, and energy. It is extremely important to teach both the patient and person who prepares the meals how to use the exchange lists.

A diabetic diet prescription can be written by the physician in a number of ways:

- 1500 kcal diabetic diet
- 1500 kcal diet (220-60-40)
- 1500 kcal diabetic diet (60% CHO, 15% protein, 25% fat)
- Diabetic diet 220-60-40

The three sets of numbers written together, such as the 220-60-40, means the diet should contain 200 gm of carbohydrate, 60 gm of protein, and 40 gm of fat. (The larger number indicates the amount of carbohydrate; the amount of fat is always written last.) If this specific breakdown is not ordered by the physician, the standard American Diabetic Association recommendation will be followed.

The diet order may also state the number of feedings or snacks per day. Unless the order specifically states a snack or snacks, the total amount of kilocalories allowed will be somewhat equally divided between the three meals, or it may provide for an evening snack with the following distribution: 1/6, 1/3, 1/3, 1/6.

As explained in Chapter 23, the total food allotment is divided into the number of exchanges from each group allowed for the day. Then, they are divided between the number of feedings, so the food (especially the carbohydrate) is distributed equally throughout the day or to coincide with insulin activity.

When the exchange system is first implemented, it is advisable for foods to be measured (or meats may be weighed on ounce scales) until the individual (and the one who prepares the food) becomes visually accustomed to the appropriate amounts. Food models may also be used to demonstrate correct portions. Foods are measured after cooking.

While foods within an exchange list are interchangeable, it is not permissible to exchange food from one list for another because each group contains different amounts of carbohydrate, protein, and fat. Any interchange between groups could disrupt the balance. Foods cannot be saved from one meal and eaten at another, but with the permission of the physician, a food from one list can be "saved" for a later snack. However, if the snack is a regular habit, it should be calculated as such into the meal plan.

Lacto- and ovolactovegetarian diets can be utilized by the diabetic since they are nutritionally adequate. It is advisable that both milk and egg products be eaten. Meat, fish, and poultry from the meat group are omitted; and peas, lentils and legumes, peanut butter, eggs, and nonfat or low-fat cheese make up the meat exchange list. Two plant sources are selected (see Chapter 6) to supply complementary proteins at each meal. Whole grains and legumes help in meeting zinc requirements (Kulkarni, 1983).

MEAL TIMING

The total diet prescription should be eaten regularly at meals that are evenly spaced throughout the waking hours (every four to five hours). In IDDM and, to a lesser extent, in NIDDM controlled by oral hypoglycemic agents, precautions regarding the amount, distribution, and timing of food intake are important to avoid inordinate swings in glycemic levels.

A typical diet prescription provides 10 to 30 percent of the energy in breakfast, 25 to 35 percent in lunch and dinner, and sometimes zero to 25 percent for between-meal snacks. A sample menu is shown in *Focus on Meal Planning for a Noninsulin-Dependent Diabetic*. This distribution must take into account the patient's preferences and lifestyle. Meals should not be delayed or omitted. Good control of diabetes is based on regularity; however, that may be the most difficult aspect, especially in children and adolescents.

FOCUS ON *MEAL PLANNING FOR A NONINSULIN-DEPENDENT DIABETIC*

Diet Prescription: 1200 kcal* (125 gm of carbohydrate; 70 gm of protein; 45 gm of fat)†
Mealtime Division: Equally divided between three meals

Total Daily Division of Food into Exchanges:

Food Exchange List	Number of Exchanges
Milk, nonfat	1
Vegetables	2
Fruits	4
Bread	5
Meat (medium fat)	4
Fats	3

Sample Menu Plan

Sample Menu

Breakfast

Fruit	1	3 Stewed prunes
Bread	2	1/2 cup Flaked bran cereal
		1 slice Toast with
Fat	1	1 tsp. Polyunsaturated margarine
Milk, nonfat	1/2	1/2 cup Skim milk

Lunch

Meat	1	Sandwich made with:
		1 oz. Sliced ham
Vegetable	Free	Lettuce and tomato
Bread	2	2 slices Bread
Fat	1	1 tsp. Mayonnaise
Fruit	1	1 Fresh nectarine
Milk, nonfat	1/2	1/2 cup Skim milk

Dinner

Meat	3	3 oz. Lean roast beef
Vegetable	2	1/2 cup Steamed broccoli
		1/2 cup Cooked carrots
		Lettuce wedge with no-calorie dressing (free)
Bread	1	1 slice Pumpernickel bread
Fruit	2	2/3 cup Pineapple, canned in juice
Fat	1	1 tsp. Polyunsaturated Margarine

Coffee, tea, and artificially sweetened beverages are allowed as desired.
*Supplement with multivitamin supplement and calcium.
†Percentage of total Kcal: 52% carbohydrate, 18% protein, 30% fat.

Table 29–5. *Guidelines for Carbohydrate Distribution Based upon Peak Action and Duration of Insulin Categories**

Insulin	Morning Percent	Midmorning Percent	Noon Percent	Midafternoon Percent	Evening Percent	H.S. Percent
Rapid-acting	25	10	30	—	25	10
Intermediate-acting	20	—	30	10	30	10
Slow-acting	20	—	25	—	35	20
Combinations (rapid/intermediate)	20	10	30	10	20	10

*From Chicago Dietetic Assoc. and South Suburban Dietetic Assoc. of Cook and Will Counties: *Manual of Clinical Dietetics*, 2nd ed. Philadelphia, W. B. Saunders Co, 1981, with permission.

MEAL TIMING WITH INSULIN

Timing and constancy of food intake for patients on insulin is the most important consideration (Table 29–5), but both diet and insulin intake must be tailored for the patient's lifestyle. For instance, if an individual becomes nauseated when forced to eat breakfast, insulin and meal patterns should take this into consideration. In other words, familiarity with the individual's routine eating patterns will influence the insulin prescription. The insulin given is proportional to the amount of food eaten. Carbohydrate should be available when the level of circulating insulin is high. If glucose is insufficient relative to the amount of insulin present or if a meal is omitted, hypoglycemia may occur.

Several types of insulin are available; their action is different with regard to onset, peak, and duration of activity (Table 29–6). Regular, quick-acting insulin is used for immediate effects—surgery or ketoacidosis in diabetics. It may be used in Type I diabetes to give a more balanced level of blood sugar. Because of the number of injections needed daily, it is seldom used on a regular basis by itself.

Insulin can have a prolonged action, such as protamine zinc insulin. Its activity lasts approximately 24 hours. When this type is used, a bedtime feeding is essential. The carbohydrate distribution may be divided into three meals and a snack, as follows: 20 percent at breakfast, 25 percent at lunch; 35 percent at dinner, and 20 percent at bedtime.

Intermediate-acting insulins are presently the most popular because their action is more inter-

Table 29–6. *Insulin Preparations Commercially Available in the United States, Classified According to Approximate Duration of Action**

Classification	Insulin Preparation†	Action		
		Onset	Peak	Duration
Rapid	Regular (neutral)	IV:‡ immediate	15–30 min	1–2 hr
		IM: 5–30 min	30–60 min	2–4 hr
		SC: 30 min	1–2 hr	5–10 hr
	Semilente (insulin zinc suspension prompt)	SC: 1 hr	3–4 hr	10–16 hr
Intermediate	Globin zinc insulin	SC: 2 hr	6–8 hr	12–18 hr
	NPH (isophane insulin suspension)	SC: 2 hr	8–14 hr	18–24 hr
	Lente (insulin zinc suspension)	SC: 2 hr	8–14 hr	18–24 hr
Slow	Protamine zinc insulin suspension	SC: 6 hr	16–20 hr	24–30 hr
	Ultralente (insulin zinc suspension extended)	SC: 6 hr	18–29 hr	30–36 hr
Combinations	Regular + NPH	SC: 30 min	2–10 hr	18–24 hr
	Regular + Lente	SC: 1 hr	2–10 hr	18–24 hr
	Semilente + Lente	SC: 1 hr	4–10 hr	18–24 hr
	Semilente + Ultralente	SC: 1 hr	2–24 hr	30–36 hr

*Adapted from Owen, O; Boden, G; Shuman, CR: Managing insulin-diabetic patients. *Postgraduate Medicine* 59(1):127, 1976.
†Insulins are available as beef-pork insulin mixtures and as special monospecies insulins made exclusively from beef or pork pancreas or as "synthetic" human insulin.
‡IV, IM, and SC denote intravenous, intramuscular, and subcutaneous routes of administration.

Diet Prescription: 2000 Kcal (264 gm of carbohydrate; 64 gm of protein; 74 gm of fat)*

Mealtime Division: 20% Breakfast
30% Lunch
10% Midafternoon snack
30% Dinner
10% Bedtime snack

Total Daily Division of Food into Exchanges:

Food Exchange List	Number of Exchanges
Milk, nonfat	2
Vegetables	3
Fruits	8
Bread	7
Meat (medium fat)	3
Fats	10

Sample Menu Plan		Sample Menu
Breakfast		
Fruit	1	1/2 cup Orange juice
Bread	2	1 slice Toast
		1/2 cup Oatmeal
Fat	3	2 tsp. Polyunsaturated margarine
Milk, nonfat	1	1 cup Skim milk
Lunch		
Meat, medium fat	1	1/4 cup canned tuna (drained)
Free Food		Lettuce, tomato, pickle
Bread	2	2 slices Whole Wheat bread
Vegetable	1	1 cup Spicy-Hot V8 juice
Fats	2	2 tsp. Mayonnaise (for sandwich)
Fruit	1	15 Fresh grapes
Milk, nonfat	1	1 cup Skim milk
Snack		
Fruit	2	1 large Fresh apple
Fat	1	20 small Peanuts
Dinner		
Meat, medium fat	2	2 oz. Baked loin pork chop
Vegetable	2	1/2 cup Steamed yellow squash
		1/2 cup Steamed cauliflower with
		1 tsp. Bacon-flavored bits
Bread	2	2 Whole wheat rolls
Fruit	2	1-1/4 cup Fresh strawberries
		1/2 cup Apple juice
Fats	3	3 tsp. Polyunsaturated margarine
Bedtime Snack		
Bread	1	1 Bran muffin
Fruit	1	4 oz. Pineapple juice
Fat	1	(Used in bran muffin)

Coffee, tea, and artificially sweetened beverages are allowed as desired.
*Percentage of total Kcal: 52% Carbohydrate, 13% Protein, 33% Fat.

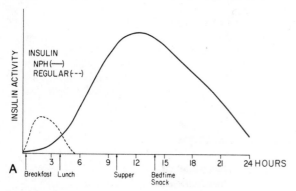

Figure 29—4A. *Time-course of action of one injection of insulin per day before breakfast. (Reprinted by permission of the* Western Journal of Medicine. *From Davidson MB: The case for control in diabetes mellitus.* Western Journal of Medicine *129 (September):193, 1978.)*

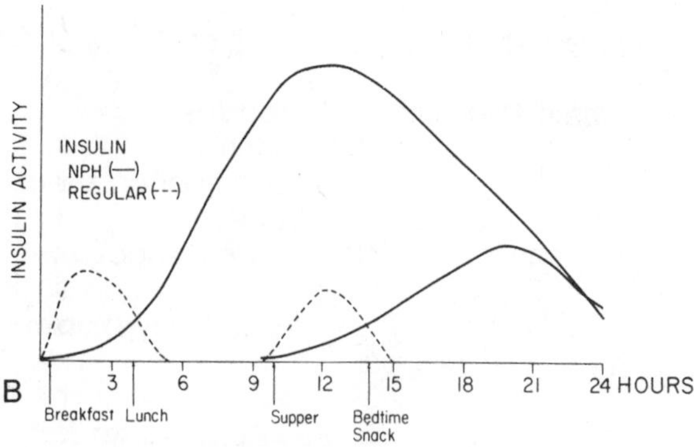

Figure 29—4B. *Time-course of action of two injections of insulin—one before breakfast and one before supper. (Reprinted by permission of the* Western Journal of Medicine. *From Davidson MB: The case for control in diabetes mellitus.* Western Journal of Medicine *129 (September):193, 1978.)*

mediate in duration and intensity; they are injected once or twice daily. Examples include globin zinc insulin, NPH, or lente. A bedtime snack is usually given. The breakdown of food exchanges and a sample menu is provided in *Focus on Meal Planning for an Insulin-Dependent Diabetic Using an Intermediate-Acting Insulin.*

The type, dosage, and frequency of insulin are tailored for the patient, depending upon the stage of growth, physical state, and activity. Types of insulin can be mixed to approximate glycemic equilibrium and to fit into the lifestyle. For instance, a farmer who enjoys a large breakfast might be given a combination of regular and protamine zinc insulin. Carbohydrate distribution would then be divided to provide a larger breakfast (30 percent), smaller lunch (30 percent) and dinner (20 percent), with midafternoon and bedtime snacks each consisting of 10 percent of the total kilocalories.

Food intake should be spaced so that it takes into account the type of insulin (and the period of peak action), as shown in Figure 29–4 A and B. (For more effective care, the dietitian planning the diabetic's diet should be aware of the type of insulin being used.) Physical activity should also be considered in relation to meal scheduling and insulin dosage to avoid hypoglycemia. Regularity of food intake and exercise are of paramount importance.

IDDM patients are more effectively treated when several snacks are allowed to avoid hypoglycemia. However, these snacks should be planned to suit the circumstances under which the patient is supposed to consume them. Snacks that fit into the patient's regular schedule become

a pleasant habit and a dependable element of their therapeutic program.

Patients who utilize the insulin pump can enjoy a more flexible meal schedule *(Focus on Continuous Subcutaneous Insulin Infusion).* The patients have a great advantage to control the timing and amount of insulin appropriate for the time and size of the meal. The glucometer monitors blood sugar more accurately, and insulin injections are adjusted appropriately (Skyler, 1981).

Clinical Implications:

- Patients receiving long-acting insulin should have a bedtime feeding to prevent nocturnal hypoglycemia (Friedman, 1980).
- The patient's tray should be checked after each meal to be certain the patient is eating well. If an IDDM patient does not eat everything, substitutions should be made to prevent hypoglycemia. In addition to the replacement of actual carbohydrate, potential glucose available from protein (58 percent) and fat (10 percent) should be replaced.
- Any diet restriction containing less than 1200 kcal requires vitamin supplementation.
- Patients may react more favorably to the term "meal plan" or "eating pattern" than to "diet" (Flood, 1979).
- A nutritionally-balanced diet is important; fad diets should be avoided.
- Diabetic control may be improved by increasing fiber intake.
- To prevent ketosis in adult diabetics, at least 80 gm of carbohydrate must be consumed daily.
- Regularity of food intake is as important as total kilocalorie intake. Diabetics should be advised to consult with a dietitian or physician for suggestions dealing with irregular schedules,

---

FOCUS ON CONTINUOUS SUBCUTANEOUS INSULIN INFUSION

Type I diabetics may now have a chance to achieve something close to euglycemia by using a continuous subcutaneous insulin infusion, or insulin pump. Insulin pumps can dramatically improve the diabetic's ability to maintain a stable and satisfying life. However, pumps are only suitable for the highly compliant patient.

The *closed-loop system* means that the system is self-contained, detecting blood sugar levels and infusing the proper amount of insulin. This system, currently too large to be portable, is used in hospitals.

The *open-loop system* infuses a preprogrammed amount of insulin. Insulin is injected automatically every few minutes (basal infusion) with the individual manually infusing larger (bolus) doses before meals. About half of the daily insulin is given in the basal infusion with the remainder in bolus infusions. Self-monitoring of glucose is essential.

Because the individual sets the time of his/her premeal bolus, greater flexibility of mealtime is possible. The individual is no longer "bound" to the insulin dosage taken early in the morning, which forces him/her to eat according to a preplanned schedule.

These pumps are small and lightweight, and fit nicely on a belt or in a pocket. The infusion pump has four parts: a battery, a programmable microchip, an electric motor and drive mechanism, and a syringe. Insulin from the syringe flows through tubing and into the body via a needle inserted subcutaneously. The pump is worn all the time unless the individual is engaged in an activity that might damage the pump (e.g., swimming, bathing, or contact sports). Most pumps have alarms that warn of various problems.

The pump is effective in controlling glycemia with insulin doses that are usually 10 to 20 percent lower than previous insulin requirements. Blood sugar level is maintained between 80 and 140 mg/dl. While euglycemia has been achieved in some studies utilizing insulin pumps, normal glycohemoglobin values are not as easily achieved as predicted (Brink & Stuart, 1986). The method of insulin delivery may not be as important as the patient having a thorough understanding of the management of his/her diabetic condition so that the blood sugar, insulin, and diet are balanced (Coustan et al, 1986; Thorp, 1986).

Because of this new flexibility, dietary habits may not be as good as before; this may have harmful effects. The constant insulin infusion makes it necessary for snacks to be eaten to prevent hypoglycemia. The practice of eating larger meals or additional snacks may be compensated by additional insulin. An increase in fat intake will not be reflected in the glycemic level. High-fat, low–complex-carbohydrate diets are atherogenic and may increase serum cholesterol levels (Kirkpatrick et al, 1984). Also, patients frequently experience a weight gain during pump treatment (Capper et al, 1985). Because increasing weight may create additional health problems, the need for careful dietary management should be reinforced. While there are risks and problems with the use of this relatively new device, most patients are highly motivated to maintain good glycemic control.

---

for instance, being a guest in another's home or traveling that results in jet lag.

- Insulin injections result in the lowest frequency of hypoglycemia and the most acceptable pattern of glucose concentrations if the meal is delayed for 45 minutes after the injection (Lean et al, 1985).
- If blood sugar is above 140 mg/dl, it is almost impossible to make a patient hypoglycemic within one hour after a subcutaneous insulin injection (Lean et al, 1985).
- Before changing the evening insulin dose, the 3 to 4 AM blood glucose level should be checked.

Special Considerations in the Insulin-Dependent Diabetic

While IDDM may occur in adulthood, it usually begins in childhood or adolescence. Whenever diabetes is diagnosed, it is a problem the individual will have to live with on a day-to-day basis forever. It often requires that the individual radically change his/her eating habits and lifestyle overnight. Therefore, every effort should be made to achieve a happy, healthy, and full life for the child and to support normal growth and development. Sensible and careful management of the disease is needed, as opposed to exact or carefree management.

Insulin production may be present when the condition is first diagnosed, but it becomes nonexistent within a few years. Vascular degenerative changes do not usually develop until the disease has been present for five years (Friedman, 1980).

Diet therapy for Type I diabetes is to provide adequate kilocalories for growth and weight gain and to help avoid wide fluctuations in glycemic levels. Several factors should be considered when planning a diet for these individuals (ADA, 1979): (1) meal timing, (2) diet composition, (3) energy content of the diet, and (4) amount of physical activity.

Treatment of Type I diabetes demands a multidisciplinary approach. The team should teach patients and their families about the disorder and the usual complications and provide guidance about daily management as well as some insight into problems they may face (Clothier, 1979). Additionally, teachers and the school nurse must be aware of the situation. While degenerative changes usually seen in diabetes should not be ignored, a positive approach is helpful. As the child grows, insulin dosages will increase. This should be explained to parents so they do not interpret it as a deteriorating condition. During stable periods, the amount of insulin may be adjusted downward.

For individuals taking insulin, regularity and consistency of food intake, including the amounts and distribution of carbohydrate, protein, and fat, are imperative for maintaining good metabolic management. Glycemic equilibrium is basically managed by diet and insulin control. Other factors, such as variation in physical activity and emotional stresses, are more difficult to control. It is important to consider lifestyle and physical activity when establishing the type and amount of insulin and distribution of nutrients for these patients. A timetable for eating becomes tiresome and tedious but, if ignored, can cause the unpleasant consequences of hypoglycemia. For most people, unavoidable problems, such as airport delays and traffic jams, are annoying; for the diabetic on insulin without access to food, such problems become frightening and even dangerous. Whereas most people never consider it, diabetics must always think about going from fed to fasted states because their insulin secretions do not automatically react.

The diet composition should be in the percentages recommended earlier. Protein allowances for juvenile diabetics should be on the generous side because of requirements for growth and development. After severe infections or episodes of ketoacidosis, protein needs are increased to replenish protein catabolized during the stressful situation.

Energy needs for these patients are the same as for nondiabetics. Growth spurts and hormonal changes influence energy requirements. Since many are thin when first diagnosed, energy allowances should be adequate for normal growth and development in order to attain a desirable body weight. Physical activity is erratic in most people, but it has profound effects on the insulin needs of diabetics. Variations in exercise patterns may require adjustments in food intake. Exercise is rarely contraindicated in these patients, and active sports should be encouraged since exercise facilitates glucose transport into the cell without insulin.

To adhere to the life long commitment of the diabetic regime takes a great deal of discipline, and occasional deviations from the diet should be put into the perspective of overall control rather than trying to elicit guilt. The psychological implications of a child never having a birthday cake may be worse than the effects of sucrose in the cake. Contrary to previous opinions, diabetics can utilize moderate amounts of sugar in a mixed meal (Crapo & Olefsky, 1983). When possible, sugar substitutes should be used, which is especially advisable when the total amount of kilocalories is limited for weight control.

Health care personnel who work with children and adolescents should understand the behaviors and stages of growth and development. They should also have an acute awareness of the everyday challenges to parents as well as to the child or adolescent. The preschool child must eat meals on time, take injections, and be protected against hypoglycemia. Later, the child must cope with school activities and lunches and hypoglycemia at school or parties and during the other usual activities of childhood. For adolescents, being different is not the "in" thing; efforts should be made to normalize the diet as much as possible. There may be increased requirements for insulin, instability of the diabetes, accidents, and the usual stresses as the adolescent searches for independence.

Exchange lists for fast foods are available from the American Diabetes Association and may help these children and adolescents fit in more with peers while still following their diets.

Special Considerations of the Noninsulin-Dependent Diabetic

Most cases of noninsulin-dependent diabetes are secondary to excessive kilocaloric intake and resultant obesity; weight loss alone (to within about 15 percent of ideal weight) is often all that is necessary to produce an acceptable blood glucose. There is no relationship between the amount of weight lost and the improved insulin response. Every pound counts! While ideal body weight may be the goal, blood sugar level is improved with any weight loss.

A fat cell response to insulin is inversely proportional to its size; the larger the cell, the less responsive it is to insulin. Abnormal glucose tolerance is found even though plasma insulin level is high. This suggests that patients are insensitive to their own insulin (Friedman, 1980) or that they have inadequate cell receptors.

ROLE OF DIET

Patients can frequently be managed successfully with diet alone or with a combination of diet and oral compounds. The basic objectives of diet therapy in NIDDM are to provide adequate nutrition at regular intervals, maintain the patient's ideal body weight, and prevent secondary complications of retinopathy, neuropathy, nephropathy, and macrovascular disease. A blood sugar less than 180 to 200 mg/dl will respond better to diet intervention.

The goal for overweight individuals is to achieve ideal body weight (IBW) or to be on the low side of IBW for their height. Weight reduction can be accomplished by reducing total energy intake to levels below energy expenditure and increasing activities.

The diet should provide adequate nutrients with appropriate kilocaloric intake to cause weight loss. Because weight loss is not an easy task, a diet program requires incentive, vigor, and skill on the part of all involved. The patient should have an appreciation of the beneficial effects of weight reduction on the course of the disease. The rate of weight loss is slow; a single eating binge may undo several weeks of successful dieting efforts. It is felt that by restricting energy, glucose tolerance is improved via several mechanisms:

1. Fat cell size is decreased.
2. Available insulin increases the rate of glucose metabolism.
3. More fatty acids are synthesized from glucose.

Weight loss is successful in lowering blood sugar, cholesterol, and triglycerides. Additionally, by following the previously discussed American Diabetes Association's recommendations to decrease the amount of fat in the diet, risks of degenerative processes should be lessened.

Simple sugars are normally avoided because of their kilocalorie content. As long as simple sugars are avoided, high levels of carbohydrate intake do not increase blood glucose. Complex carbohydrate and fiber intake should be high. Carbohydrate restriction can increase insulin resistance.

Meals should be regular, and the relationship of meals to physical activity is important. However, this requirement is less important than decreased energy intake. Meals are normally distributed equally with one third of the carbohydrate being given at each meal. Snacks are usually discouraged to allow the blood sugar to return to normal.

ORAL HYPOGLYCEMIC AGENTS

If diet and exercise are ineffective for metabolic control, pharmacologic intervention is appropriate. Oral hypoglycemic agents increase the cell's sensitivity to insulin in response to glucose. They are only effective if the pancreas is able to produce insulin. They include tolbutamide (Orinase), tolazamide (Tolinase), chlorpropamide (Diabinese), acetohexamide (Dymelor), glipizide (Glucotrol), and glyburide (DiaBeta) (Table 29–7). Pharmaceutical studies suggest that glipizide and glyburide (second-generation sulfonylureas) may elicit insulin secretion only when hyperglycemia is present. These drugs are more potent (weight-for-weight basis) than the first generation sulfonylureas in insulin-releasing capacity. On the other hand, with equally potent doses, there is no evidence these drugs are more effective than the others (Baker & Campbell, 1985).

These drugs are popular with patients because the necessity for dieting is often not emphasized. Insulin is not recommended for obese patients because of the large amounts that must be given to normalize their blood glucose. In these large doses, appetite may be increased along with decreased insulin utilization. This results in increased food intake, weight gain, and the need for

Table 29–7. Pharmacokinetics of the Oral Hypoglycemics*

Drug	Equivalent Therapeutic Dose (mg)	Usual Minimum and Maximum Daily Dose	Mean Half-Life	Duration of Activity	Metabolism and Excretion
First-generation sulfonylureas					
Acetohexamide (Dymelor)	500	0.25–1.5 gm single or divided doses	1.5 hr parent; 6 hrs, metabolites	12–18 plus hr	Metabolite's activity greater than parent drug; excreted, in part, via kidney
Chlorpropamide (Diabinese)	250	0.1–0.5 gm single dose	35 hr	24–72 hr	Extensive metabolism to compounds with unknown activity; 20% excreted unchanged, which may vary widely
Tolazamide (Tolinase)	250	0.1–1.0 gm single or divided doses	7 hr	10–16 plus hr	Some metabolites have weak activity; excreted via kidney
Tolbutamide (Orinase)	1000	0.5–2.0 gm divided doses	7 hr	6–12 hr	Totally metabolized to compounds with negligible activity
Second-generation sulfonylureas					
Glyburide (DiaBeta) (Micronase)	5	1.25–20 mg single or divided doses	10 hr	24 hr	Metabolized to compounds, one of which may be weakly active
Glipizide (Glucotrol)	5	2.5–40 mg single or divided doses	4 hr	16–24 hr	Metabolized to inactive compounds

*From Baker, DE; Campbell, RK: The second generation sulfonylureas: Glipizide and glyburide. *Diabetes Educator* 11(3):29, 1985.

even more insulin. Additionally, insulin, an anabolic hormone, may increase fat deposits and fluid retention. Therefore, insulin should be given only as a last resort or for specific conditions such as ketoacidosis or pregnancy (Prosser, 1982).

Clinical Implications:

- Oral sulfonylureas are only used with Type II diabetics. They should be used in conjunction with reduction diets and exercise.
- Oral hypoglycemics are not advisable for patients with other diseases, such as liver or kidney disorders, or during pregnancy.
- About one week is necessary for the metabolic processes to stabilize when oral sulfonylureas are given; doses should not be changed too quickly.
- Prescribing insulin for Type II diabetics should be limited to those who are not obese.
- Obese patients with NIDDM will experience less hyperglycemia and glucose intolerance if they lose weight.
- Some Type II diabetics will require insulin to control glucose levels; inappropriately high levels of insulin will cause polyphagia leading to increased weight.

Abnormal Blood Glucose Levels

Since the glycemic level is not normally regulated in either type of diabetes, hyperglycemia and hypoglycemia are both common problems. Whenever the delicate balance between exercise, diet, and medication is upset by any one of these factors (or even uncontrollable ones such as stress), the glycemic level may be detrimentally affected. Either situation can be life-threatening.

While uncontrolled Type II diabetics may have incredibly high blood sugar levels that may result in coma, Type I diabetics using insulin are vulnerable to hypoglycemic shock. It is important to be able to recognize the different symptoms of each and to treat them (Table 29–8).

HYPERGLYCEMIA

Hyperglycemia may develop when patients do not take their medication, omit their regular exercise, or do not follow their diet. Physiological stress will also flood the bloodstream with sugar because stress releases hormones that are insulin

Table 29–8. Warning Signs for Diabetic Reactions*

Hypoglycemic Reaction (Insulin Reaction)	Warning Signs	Hyperglycemic Reactions (Diabetic Coma)
Sudden	ONSET	Gradual
Pale, moist, perspiring	SKIN	Flushed, hot, dry
Excited, nervous, trembling, weak, irritable, confused, faint, blurred vision	BEHAVIOR	Drowsy, weak
Normal	BREATH	Fruity odor (acetone)
Normal to rapid shallow	BREATHING	Deep, labored
Absent	VOMITING	Present with nausea
Moist, numb, tingling	TONGUE	Dry
Present	HUNGER	Absent
Absent	THIRST	Present (dehydration)
Headache	PAIN	Abdominal
Normal, slight sugar	URINE	Frequent with large amounts of sugar; ketones present
Unconsciousness	CONSCIOUSNESS	Unconsciousness leading to coma
Too much insulin	CAUSE	Not enough insulin
Undereating		Overeating
Vomiting or diarrhea		Infection
Delayed meal		Illness
Excessive exercise		Surgery
		Stress
		Nausea or vomiting
Orange juice (100 ml)	TREATMENT	Check urine
Coke		Go to bed
Hard candy (Lifesavers, 4–5)		Keep warm
Glucagon if unconscious		Force fluids
		Take usual or increased dose of insulin
		Call doctor

*From Green, ML; Harry, J: *Nutrition in Contemporary Nursing Practice.* New York, copyright©1981, John Wiley & Sons, Inc. Reprinted by permission of John Wiley & Sons, Inc.

antagonists. A high blood sugar will cause blurred vision, drowsiness, weakness, confusion, increased urinary output and thirst, warm dry skin, and deep labored breathing with a fruity acetone odor.

The situation is precipitated when there is a deficiency of insulin to reduce the glucose level. The situation can lead to ketosis, ketoacidosis, and then diabetic coma. Nonketotic hyperosmolar coma may be seen in NIDDM. The syndrome, called hyperosmolar hyperglycemic nonketotic coma (HHNKC), may develop in elderly patients, most of whom also have cardiovascular or renal disease. Hyperglycemia develops without ketoacidosis because the patient has enough insulin present to inhibit excessive fat mobilization and development of ketonemia, but not enough to prevent hyperglycemia. Dehydration develops rapidly. HHNKC frequently follows severe stress: burns, pulmonary emboli, or intercurrent infections.

Either type of coma must be treated promptly. Treatment consists of insulin to bring the blood glucose level down, and administration of electrolytes and fluids to replace the fluids and to correct the ac-

idosis. Blood sugar must be lowered gradually. When glucosuria and hyperglycemia begin to drop, glucose may be added in the form of intravenous dextrose to prevent too rapid a drop in the glycemic levels. As soon as fluids can be taken orally, the patient is given fruit juices, gruels, regular ginger ale, tea, and broth to correct fluid and electrolyte imbalances. (An excellent review of the two types of hyperglycemia can be found in Murray, 1983.)

INSULIN REACTION

Hypoglycemic reactions precipitated by the action of insulin, exercise, or lack of food intake are physically and emotionally upsetting and can cause damage to the central nervous system since brain cells can only use glucose for energy. Symptoms include headaches, nervousness, sweating, trembling, confusion, and incoordination. Immediate treatment is essential; a readily available source of glucose, such as dextrose tablets, sugar, or fruit juice, is given.

Hypoglycemia can appear at any time, even

during a meal. Special activities, even a simple outing, can cause hypoglycemic reactions. The needed boost in blood sugar can be supplied by any of the usual sugar-containing foods that are not usually allowed. The amount of carbohydrate may not be known, but one cannot be certain about the amount of energy expended in the activity either.

A dextrose tablet contains 3 or 5 gm of glucose, depending on the brand, and can be given to counter an insulin reaction. Brodows and associates (1984) have shown that a 3 gm tablet of D-glucose raises the blood sugar 15 mg/dl without rebound hypoglycemia in adults. At least four tablets should be taken immediately, with more being given if symptoms do not subside shortly. (Or, for better accuracy, blood glucose testing can be used to determine how much should be given.)

Instant glucose is also available; it can be squeezed into the cheek if the diabetic is semiconscious. Because of its rapid absorption, the individual soon becomes alert enough to take additional carbohydrate orally.

A patient on regular insulin will have a rapid reaction that requires immediate recognition and treatment. When the reaction is from too much long-acting insulin, additional carbohydrates may be needed for several hours because of the duration of the insulin effects. For this type of reaction, some complex carbohydrates may be given along with a simple sugar, such as bread and jelly or milk. This food is not subtracted from the daily carbohydrate intake.

SOMOGYI EFFECT

This is a pattern of swings from hypoglycemia to hyperglycemia in the body's effort to correct hypoglycemia caused by overinsulinization. It may be present in Type I diabetes. Subclinical hypoglycemia is followed by spontaneous hyperglycemia and ketonuria. Insulin doses may be increased in an effort to alleviate hyperglycemia, but the glycemic levels increase. The body's normal defense mechanisms overreact to hypoglycemia caused by overinsulinization and secrete large amounts of epinephrine, glucocorticoids, glucagon, and pituitary hormone. This causes a skyrocketing blood sugar and poor control of the condition. By increasing insulin, the problem is compounded. Correction of the problem is to *decrease* insulin to the point at which it no longer triggers the *rebound* effect. If the problem occurs in the evening or during the night, a redistribution

of meals and snacks can increase the amount of the evening feeding. This effect may be precipitated by stressful situations, such as pregnancy or surgery. Occasionally, the Somogyi effect will be diagnosed when the problem is a deviation from the diet.

Clinical Implication:

- To prevent hypoglycemia, the following must be stressed: meal and snack regularity, injection of the correct amount of insulin, and regularity of exercise and daily activity.

Special Considerations for Exercise

Diabetics should fully understand the benefits of exercise. Type I diabetic children should be encouraged to participate in active sports, e.g., soccer or basketball. They should also have an understanding of the effects of exercise on insulin usage. Consistent, regular exercise is more beneficial than sporadic and taxing workouts. Muscular exercise has a blood sugar–lowering effect and increases the uptake of free fatty acids. It may even decrease the body's insulin requirements (though it does not replace insulin) (Richter et al, 1985). Diabetics should exercise when the blood sugar is between 100 and 200 mg/dl (soon after a meal) rather than when the insulin or oral hypoglycemic dose is at its greatest. If the blood sugar is over 300 mg/dl, glucose uptake by the cell is decreased and glucose production by the liver is increased (Franz, 1985).

Short periods of exercise of modest intensity

Table 29–9. *Foods to Provide 10 Grams of Carbohydrate*

1 fruit exchange
1/2 cup (4 oz.) carbonated beverage (regular)
1/2 cup orange juice
3/4 cup Tang
1/4 cup grape juice
1 cup Gatorade
1/2 twin Popsicle bar
2 tsp. corn syrup or honey
2 1/2 tsp. sugar
1/4 cup sweetened gelatin
6 Life Savers
1 bar of Hershey milk chocolate (1.45 oz.)

do not require additional feedings. When a diabetic anticipates an extensive special exercise, additional carbohydrate is needed. A typical allowance might include 10 to 15 gm/hr for moderate exercise, such as playing golf, or 20 to 30 gm/hr for a vigorous exercise such as playing soccer or digging (West, 1983).

Diabetic patients active in sports or vigorous activities can increase their food intake earlier in the day. A large meal just prior to *vigorous* activity is discouraged, and the diabetic might be better advised to eat a snack, which should contain carbohydrate to maintain the glycemic level until the next regular meal.

Clinical Implications:

- Hypoglycemia may occur during exercise and for up to 24 hours after strenuous exercise (Franz, 1985).
- To avoid unexpected hypoglycemia, the IDDM should not inject insulin in an area that will soon be exercised.
- One hour before moderate exercise, the Type I diabetic should eat a 15 gm carbohydrate snack, which could be a fruit exchange or equivalent (Table 29–9). This does not need to be counted as part of the daily allowance.
- The NIDDM diabetic not receiving insulin or oral agents does not require extra food for exercise, which helps decrease insulin resistance.

Special Considerations for Illness

Special measures are required for IDDM patients when illness decreases the appetite or interferes with eating habits. Even though the patient is ill, insulin is necessary because insulin requirements increase during febrile illnesses.

An illness such as diarrhea that may be minor for most persons may become complicated in the diabetic. The physician should be notified if vomiting or diarrhea occurs, because of rapid loss of fluid and electrolytes. Acetone or blood sugar levels are monitored frequently.

Liquids should be consumed hourly to help replace losses. Carbohydrate is necessary to prevent ketosis; 50 to 75 gm every six to eight hours is usually sufficient. When sickness impairs appetite and digestion, simple sugars in the form of liquids and semiliquids are used to replace the normal carbohydrate value of solid foods (see Table 29–9). Small, frequent, high-carbohydrate feedings can be used to prevent hypoglycemia. If the patient cannot eat, the protein and fat allowances may not be replaced. These foods may be used on an emergency basis for a three-day period. If used longer, the physician should be consulted. To replace sodium, potassium, and water lost from vomiting and diarrhea, salty foods such as crackers and broth should be included. If the illness is not gastrointestinal, semiliquid foods such as dairy foods and soft-cooked eggs or custards are desirable. Table 29–10 shows an example of a replacement meal. The amounts can be taken in small frequent amounts, rather than as a meal. The dietary carbohydrate portion can be met on a clear-liquid diet; the entire carbohydrate, protein, and fat can be met on a full-liquid diet.

Special Considerations for Pregnancy

A diabetic may have a healthy, normal pregnancy and a healthy normal infant if the diabetes

---

Table 29–10. Replacement Meal for Illness

Usual Meal Pattern	Carbohydrate	Replacement Carbohydrates	
3 meat exchanges	0	2 cups broth	0
2 bread exchanges	30	1 cup ginger ale	20
2 fat exchanges	0	1/2 cup Jell-O	20
1 fruit exchange	15	1/3 cup grape juice	15
1 milk exchange	12	Hot tea (no sugar)	0
Total	57	Total	55

is well controlled throughout the pregnancy. If diabetes is controlled, fertility of diabetic women is normal, and maternal mortality is almost negligible (Levin et al, 1986). Fetal survival rate (97 percent) approaches that of nondiabetics (98 to 99 percent), but without strict control of the diabetes the rate of birth defects is three to four times higher (Hare & Solomon, 1981). Most of these malformations occur in the seventh week of pregnancy (Pederson, 1979).

Metabolic control of diabetes before pregnancy is crucial to normal development of the fetal organs. If the diabetes is not well controlled, the patient may be hospitalized immediately for stabilization and education. Avoiding hyperglycemia and ketones is critical during the first few weeks of pregnancy because the baby's organs are just developing. This may occur even before the woman is aware of the pregnancy; therefore, the great concern is for prepregnancy counseling with control of the diabetic condition before conception.

As a consequence of metabolic changes, insulin requirements vary during pregnancy. Insulin dosage must be reduced early in pregnancy when the mother tends to become hypoglycemic, but the dose may be doubled or tripled later with a leveling off by about the eighth month (Hare & Solomon, 1981). Ketosis is associated with a high incidence of intrauterine fetal deaths (Levin et al, 1986) and has been known to retard brain development. Rapid proliferation of neural tissue occurs between the 16th and 20th week of pregnancy.

Babies of diabetic mothers are usually large. These babies are subjected to hyperglycemia in utero (glucose crosses the placenta). Since insulin does not cross the placenta, the infant produces increased amounts of insulin in response to the high glucose level. Insulin is the "growth" hormone for the developing fetus. These high insulin levels are also implicated in the hypoglycemia that frequently occurs shortly after birth. Newborn infants may present other problems such as respiratory difficulties, hypocalcemia, and/or jaundice (Hare & Solomon, 1981).

Team management during pregnancy to minimize possible congenital abnormalities may include an internist (diabetologist), obstetrician (perinatologist), pediatrician (neonatologist), nurse-educator, dietitian, and social worker. Perinatal complications can be reduced by intense efforts to control the diabetes by means of hospitalization, bed rest, and tight supervision by specialized team members (Freinkel et al, 1985).

NUTRITIONAL CARE

Desired weight gains and protein allowances are the same as for nondiabetics (see Chapter 15). To ensure the 1.5 gm/kg of protein, protein levels in the prescription may need to be raised.

Adequate nutrients for a normal pregnancy plus avoidance of hyperglycemia and insulin reactions are the goals for the pregnant diabetic. Maintaining maternal glucose levels below 100 mg/dl at all times in both pregestational and gestational diabetics is imperative to maintain normal fetal weight and reduce perinatal mortality. Home glucose monitoring is necessary. An evening snack is always included, and the recommended carbohydrate intake is usually not less than 200 gm. No meal, especially breakfast, should be omitted.

GESTATIONAL DIABETES MELLITUS

Pregnancy is a potentially diabetogenic condition; most of the hormones that support a pregnancy have an anti-insulin effect. During pregnancy, carbohydrate intolerance may occur, as evidenced by high blood sugars (see Table 29–1). Gestational diabetes is probably caused by the stress of pregnancy; it disappears after delivery unless the diabetes is actually a preexisting mild condition first discovered during pregnancy. Periodic checkups are suggested since there is an increased risk for developing diabetes later in life. The predominant risk is large babies. Pregestational diabetes is usually controlled by diet alone. By merely restricting the amount of simple carbohydrates, the incidence of infant macrosomia and hypoglycemia is decreased (Lieberman & Chan, 1986).

Clinical Implications:

- Reassure diabetic mothers that an increased need for insulin in the second trimester is not harmful, that this normal response of a healthy developing pregnancy is due to the insulin's antagonistic effects on the placental hormones (Riblett, 1983).
- Hospitalization during the last four weeks is not uncommon for the diabetic with edema.
- The diabetic newborn may remain in the hospital to be monitored for blood sugar levels, and particularly to determine respiratory adequacy (Riblett, 1983).
- Oral glycemic agents should be discontinued even before conception, if possible, because they tend to produce fetal deformities (Riblett, 1983).

Special Food Considerations

DIETETIC PRODUCTS

One of the special benefits of utilizing the food exchange lists is that the diabetic can more easily select readily available foods at home or in a restaurant. Regular foods are utilized on the diabetic diet. No special low-carbohydrate foods are required. Several special products may, however, be used, such as fruits canned without sugar. Those canned in their own juice may be more economical than those labeled "dietetic" and packed with artifical sweeteners. The use of egg substitutes can add variety to the diet. *Some dietetic products can actually be hazardous;* dietetic ice cream may contain more sugar than the real thing.

SUGAR SUBSTITUTES

Artificial sweeteners have been developed because of inborn desires for sweetness. As much as possible, the diabetic should be encouraged to eat foods without added sweeteners. Several artificial sweeteners have been developed that can be used by the diabetic and are considered safe in *moderation*. By using a variety of non-nutritive sweeteners, the possibility of excessive consumption of a single agent is lessened.

Saccharin is a suitable sugar replacement for some individuals. While it has been questioned as being carcinogenic, the evidence is weak, and it is still available as a nonprescription drug and in food and beverage products.

Fructose has been recommended for use in the diabetic diet. It is considerably sweeter than sucrose, so that a smaller quantity is needed for the same amount of sweetening. Initially, it does not require insulin for its metabolism. Fructose has much less impact on blood glucose levels. However, the liver changes much of the fructose into glucose; fructose contains the same number of kilocalories as other sugars. For these reasons, fructose could cause diabetics who are on insulin or trying to reduce their weight some problems. When fructose is substituted for sucrose in the well-controlled diabetic, fructose is better tolerated (lower hyperglycemia and insulin response) than sucrose (Crapo et al, 1982). Its use should be limited (less than 75 gm/day) so that the diet can still be nutritively adequate (Powers & Crapo, 1982). It is not advised for cases of poorly controlled diabetes.

Aspartame, being a combination of two amino acids, should be well utilized by the diabetic and may prove to be the optimal sweetener for diabetics. While it provides 4 kcal/gm as do all disaccharides, it is 180 to 200 times as sweet as sucrose. The same sweetness of one teaspoon of sugar can be supplied by one tenth of a calorie of aspartame. It is relatively new on the market; studies regarding its use by diabetics are not available.

Sorbitol is a popular sugar substitute in dietetic foods. It is slowly absorbed and does not require insulin initially but, like fructose, is eventually converted to glucose. It contains the same number of kilocalories and is 60 percent as sweet as sucrose. When consumed in large amounts, it may cause diarrhea. It is not usually recommended by diabetologists (Vaaler et al, 1980). Other sweeteners not usually recommended include xylitol and mannitol; they also cause diarrhea.

Clinical Implications:

- Because of the liberal amount of carbohydrate allowed, diabetic diets are not necessarily more expensive than a regular diet. Dietetic foods are not necessary or desirable.
- Special foods are not required, except perhaps sweeteners.
- "Dietetic" or "sugar-free" may not be synonymous with "noncaloric."
- Patients need to be able to distinguish between "dietetic" and "diabetic." Some dietetic products are intended for salt-restricted or other types of diets. Labels must be read carefully.

Education of the Diabetic

When an individual is diagnosed as a diabetic, many adjustments must be made that affect emotional well-being and lifestyle. It is a matter of adjusting to a condition that must be given constant attention every day. Initially, the patient will be overwhelmed and very anxious; basic information is introduced to help him/her to "cope." The patient will be responsible for learning many new things about the condition and caring for it. This education process will take time; Jovanovic and Peterson (1984) have determined that approximately 35 hours are needed. A patient cannot be expected to learn everything in one session. (S/He should not even be expected to learn everything about the diet in one session).

A team approach is necessary for teaching the patient about the many facets of self-care for which s/he will be responsible. S/He must be taught about the disease, the diet, and the type of medication (insulin or oral hypoglycemics). The patient will comply better with these regimens if s/he believes that the benefits exceed the disadvantages.

S/He must also be taught how to assess the daily status of the condition (glucose testing) as well as how to avoid hypo- and hyperglycemia and diabetic acidosis and what to do when they do occur. The effect of exercise must be explained.

While individual counseling is important, studies have shown that a series of group instruction classes are more effective for the patients (Jovanovic & Peterson, 1984) as well as more economical for the hospital. These are taught by several specialists—nurses, dietitians, physical therapists, and physicians. Many visual teaching aids are available that can help explain all facets of the disease.

Hospital patients who are able should be started on an educational program regarding diabetes as soon as possible, not at the time of discharge. While all aspects of the condition are important, a study at the University of Michigan Medical School determined that diet and diet-related issues constituted the most difficult problem (Lockwood et al, 1986). Recognizing this problem, the ADA task force (1987) has developed a simplified meal planning tool (entitled "Health Food Choices") for the initial education of diabetic individuals. Its simplified approach has planned stages for further teaching as appropriate. Initially, patients are counseled on how they can use less salt, sugar, and fat and increase dietary fiber. In the second stage, foods are divided into six groups by approximate portion sizes and calories. The nutritional counselor offers specific suggestions for the individual to follow.

Diabetics should eventually learn to calculate and plan the diet. They also need to know what may happen when they do not adhere to the diet. Changing the diet may be very difficult; sticking to a set regimen can be even more upsetting for some people. The diabetic should understand the important distinction between the short-term effect of occasional overconsumption and the more harmful effects of persistent dietary noncompliance. For a successful continuing education program, children should be seen for nutritional counseling at least every three to six months;

adults may only need to be seen one or two times a year.

There is so much for the patient to learn that it is virtually impossible for him/her to comprehend it all while in the hospital. S/He needs to know whom to call when s/he has problems putting it all into action. The hospital may have regular meetings for the diabetic. The American Diabetes Association has local chapters in most communities that can function as a support group and furnish reading and reference materials.

───────────────────────────────

• *FALLACIES and FACTS*

FALLACY: *Diabetes mellitus is the consequence of lower-than-normal insulin production.*

• ***FACT:*** *That was a good explanation until many Type II diabetics were found to have higher insulin levels in addition to an elevated glucose level.*

FALLACY: *Vascular and neurological degenerative complications are inevitable consequences of the diabetic disease process.*

• ***FACT:*** *By maintaining blood glucose at relatively normal levels, such complications can be prevented or delayed (Nemchik, 1982).*

FALLACY: *A diabetic who is ill and not eating should omit his/her insulin to prevent hypoglycemia.*

• ***FACT:*** *Because of the stress reaction that occurs during fevers and infection, insulin therapy is still necessary. It is important for the patient to eat some foods to supply the carbohydrate needed.*

FALLACY: *Honey is a natural sugar and can be eaten by diabetics.*

• ***FACT:*** *Honey is a concentrated source of fructose and other sugars with the same amount of kilocalories as all carbohydrates. In ordinary amounts, it has no extra nutritional value; and no advantages have been demonstrated for its use. Like sugar, it is not appropriate for diabetics and should be used in limited quantities.*

FALLACY: *Diabetics who exercise a lot and eat foods containing fiber do not need insulin.*

• ***FACT:*** *It is true that exercise and high-fiber foods may decrease the need for insulin, but rarely do they eliminate the need. Even though exercise is advisable, before beginning an exercise pro-*

gram, the diabetic should consult his/her physician.

FALLACY: *Diabetic diets are very expensive.*
- **FACT:** *Since the new recommendations increase the starch content of the diet, this is no longer true. No special foods need to be purchased.*

FALLACY: *Ice cream is all right for diabetics.*
- **FACT:** *Nathan and colleagues (1984) found blood sugar levels could be controlled when a modest amount of ice cream was given to weight-maintaining IDDM patients with a small injection of rapid-acting insulin. However, this study does not consider the overall effect of simple sugars in the diabetic diet. The amount of fat, cholesterol, and other nutrients has long-term complications in diabetics. Emphasis is still on complex carbohydrates with low intake of simple sugars and fats.*

Summary

Diabetes mellitus is a complex disorder that requires a regimen of insulin, diet, and exercise. The most important objective of the diet is control of total kilocalorie intake to attain ideal body weight. Obesity is diabetogenic. Meals must be eaten on a regular schedule. A flexible approach that takes into consideration the patient's lifestyle, socioeconomic and ethnic factors, food preferences, and eating habits will result in better compliance.

Review Questions

1. Describe the clinical symptoms seen in diabetes mellitus.
2. Why are the current dietary recommendations for diabetes high in carbohydrate and fiber and low in fat?
3. Why are polyunsaturated fats stressed on the diabetic diet?
4. Your patient is on a 2000 kcal diabetic diet with protamine zinc insulin. What important facts should you stress to him about his diet? Discuss the total management of the patient's medication, exercise, and diet.
5. What would you advise your diabetic patient to do in order to avoid having a hypoglycemic reaction?

6. Why is it important for the obese NIDDM patient to reduce?
7. What are the effects of pregnancy on the diabetic condition? What changes would patients expect with regard to diet and insulin?
8. Your insulin-dependent diabetic patient is ill with strep throat. She is on an 1800 kcal diabetic diet (210-95-70). Plan her diet to include her carbohydrate allowance using foods she will most likely be able to tolerate.

Case Study: Mr. M.P. is a 63-year-old postal worker currently undergoing his annual physical examination. The physician notes hypertension, a weight gain of 15 lbs. since the last examination (current weight 194 lbs.), and elevated serum glucose, cholesterol, and triglycerides. Following a glucose tolerance test, the diagnosis of adult-onset diabetes is made. He is started on tolbutamide (Orinase) and referred to the nutritionist for dietary counseling.

Since his son and daughter-in-law have moved out of his house into a home of their own eight months ago, Mr. M.P. has been eating frequently at restaurants. When he eats at home, he uses prepackaged food.

1. What additional assessment data do you need?
2. List at least two nursing diagnoses that can be derived from the history.
3. List a goal for each diagnosis.
4. Why is it important to reduce his serum glucose?
5. Calculate Mr. M.P.'s caloric requirements with the proportions of carbohydrate, protein, and fat.
6. What lifestyle factors should be considered when planning his diet plan?
7. As you are evaluating the effectiveness of the diet counseling, Mr. M.P. states, "Well, if I can't eat the proper foods every day, can't I just take an extra pill?" What should you say?

Case Study: Mrs. S.M. is a 42-year-old female who has been an insulin-dependent diabetic for 19 years. She has a family history of diabetes (mother and maternal grandfather). She has been admitted to the hopsital twice in the past two years for ketoacidosis.

On examination, her height is 165 cm and her weight is 77.8 kg; she is of medium frame. Mrs. S.M. also demonstrates diabetic retinopathy. Laboratory studies reveal a fasting serum glucose of 310 mg/dl, 4+ urine glucose, 4+ urine protein, negative urine acetone, and a serum creatinine of 2.3 mg/dl. Her blood pressure is 158/92.

She has been receiving NPH insulin U-100 42 units and regular insulin U-100 8 units each morning. With further questioning, Mrs. S.M. admits to straying frequently from her 1500 kcal diet. She is again referred to the center for diabetic education classes and individual dietary counseling.

1. What additional dietary information is needed before a plan of care can be developed?

2. Identify two nursing diagnoses (include relevant supporting data) and appropriate goals for each.
3. What is Mrs. S.M.'s ideal weight?
4. What is the desirable range for her blood glucose?
5. Outline a meal plan for a 1500 kcal diet (220-60-40) and a distribution of 1/6, 1/3, 1/3, 1/6.
6. What is the dietary treatment for hypoglycemia?
7. What insulin adjustments would be made if Mrs. S.M. were to increase her level of physical activity? If she were to develop a systemic infection?

REFERENCE LIST

Abraira, C; de Bartolo, M; Myscofski, JW: Comparison of unmeasured versus exchange diabetic diets in lean adults. Body weight and feeding patterns in a two-year prospective pilot study. *Am J Clin Nutr* 33(5):1064, 1980.

American Diabetes Association (ADA): *A Guide for. Professionals: The Effective Application of Exchange Lists for Meal Planning.* New York, American Diabetes Association, Inc, 1977.

American Diabetes Association Ad Hoc Committee on Therapeutic Modalities: Indications for use of continuous insulin delivery systems and self-measurement of blood glucose. *Diab Care* 5(2):140, 1982.

American Diabetes Association Committee on Food and Nutrition (ADA): Principles of nutrition and dietary recommendations for individuals with diabetes mellitus. *Diabetes* 28(11):1027, 1979.

American Diabetes Association Council on Nutrition: Glycemic effect of carbohydrates. *Diab Care* 7(6):607, 1984.

Anderson, JW; Bryant, CA: Dietary fiber: Diabetes and obesity. *Am J Gastroenterol* 81(10):898, 1986.

Anderson, JW; Ward, K: High-carbohydrate, high-fiber diets for insulin-treated men with diabetes mellitus. *Am J Clin Nutr* 32(11):2312, 1979.

Arky, RA: Diet and diabetes mellitus: Concepts and objectives. *Postgrad Med* 63(6):72, 1978.

Asp, NG; Agardh, CD; Dencker, I; et al: Dietary fibre in type II diabetes. *Acta Med Scand* 656(suppl):47, 1981.

Avogaro, A; Duner, E; Marescotti, C; et al: Metabolic effects of moderate alcohol intake with meals in insulin-dependent diabetics controlled by artificial endocrine pancreas (AEP) and in normal subjects. *Metabolism* 32(5):463, 1983.

Baker, DE; Campbell, RK: The second generation sulfonylureas: Glipizide and glyburide. *Diab Ed* 11(3):29, 1985.

Bergman, M; Felig, P: Self-monitoring of blood glucose levels in diabetes. *Arch Intern Med* 144(10):2029, 1984.

Bierman, EL: Carbohydrates, sucrose, and human disease. *Am J Clin Nutr* 32(suppl):2712, 1979.

Brink, SJ; Stewart, C: Insulin pump treatment in insulin-dependent diabetes mellitus. *JAMA* 255(5):617, 1986.

Brodows, RG; Williams, C; Amatruda, JM: Treatment of insulin reactions in diabetics. *JAMA* 252(24):3378, 1984.

Capper, AF; Headen, SW; Bergenstal, RM: Dietary practices of persons with diabetes during insulin pump therapy. *J Am Diet Assoc* 85(4):445, 1985.

Chait, A: Dietary management of diabetes mellitus. *Contemporary Nutr* 9(2), 1984.

Clothier, C: Dietary management of diabetic children. *Proc Nutr Soc* 38(3):359, 1979.

Cole, HS; Camerini-Davalos, R: New concepts of the diet therapy of diabetes mellitus. In *Quick Reference to Clinical Nutrition.* Edited by SL Halpern. Philadelphia, J. B. Lippincott Co, 1979, p 235.

Connor, H; Marks, V: Alcohol and diabetes. *Hum Nutr Appl Nutr* 39A(December):393, 1985.

Coustan, DR; Reece, A; Sherwin, RS; et al: A randomized clinical trial of the insulin pump vs intensive conventional therapy in diabetic pregnancies. *JAMA* 255(6):631, 1986.

Crapo, PA; Olefsky, JM: Food fallacies and blood sugar. *N Engl J Med* 309(1):44, 1983.

Crapo, PA; Scarlett, JA; Kolterman, OG: Comparison of the metabolic responses to fructose and sucrose sweetened foods. *Am J Clin Nutr* 36(2):256, 1982.

Diabetes and fiber. *Nutr and the MD* X(7):3, 1984.

Dodson, PM; Stocks, J; Holdsworth, G; et al: High-fibre and low-fat diets in diabetes mellitus. *Br J Nutr* 46(2):289, 1981.

Dorchy, H; Mozin, MJ; Loeb, H: Unmeasured diet versus exchange diet in diabetics. *Am J Clin Nutr* 34(5):964, 1981.

Flood, TM: Diet and diabetes mellitus. *Hosp Pract* 14(2):61, 1979.

Franz, M: Diabetes and exercise; benefits and precautions. Presented at the American Dietetic Association's 68th Annual Meeting, New Orleans, October 1985.

Freinkel, N; Dooley, SL; Metzger, BE: Care of the pregnant woman with insulin-dependent diabetes mellitus. *N Engl J Med* 313(2):96, 1985.

Friedman, GJ: Diet in the treatment of diabetes mellitus. In *Modern Nutrition in Health and Disease,* 6th ed. Edited by RS Goodhart; ME Shils. Philadelphia, Lea & Febiger, 1980, p 977.

Hare, JW; Solomon, EK: Giving birth. *Diabetes Forecast* 34(1):26, 1981.

Harold, MR; Reeves, RD; Guthrie, RA; et al: Effect of dietary fiber in insulin-dependent diabetics: Insulin requirements and serum lipids. *J Am Diet Assoc* 85(11):1455, 1985.

Henry, CL; Heaton, KW; Manhire, A; et al: Diet and the diabetic: The fallacy of a controlled carbohydrate intake. *J Human Nutr* 35(2):102, 1981.

Hollenbeck, CB; Coulston, AM; Donner, CC; et al: The effects of variation in percent of naturally occurring complex and simple carbohydrate on plasma glucose and insulin response in individuals with NIDDM. *Diabetes* 34(2):151, 1985.

Jenkins, DJA; Wolever, TMS; Bacon, S; et al: Diabetic diets: High carbohydrate combines with high fiber. *Am J Clin Nutr* 33(8): 1729, 1980.

Johny, A: Glycosylated hemoglobin test as an educational and motivational tool. *Diab Ed* 10(3):37, 1984.

Jovanovic, L; Peterson, C: Comparison of eight educational programs. *Diab Ed* 10:40, 1984.

Keen, H; Thomas, BJ; Jarrett, RJ; et al: Nutrient intake, adiposity, and diabetes. *Br Med J* 1(March 10):655, 1979.

Kinmonth, AL; Angus, RM; Jenkins, PA; et al: Whole foods and increased dietary fibre improve blood glucose control in diabetic children. *Arch Dis Child* 57(3):187, 1982.

Kirkpatrick, J; Kulkarni, K; Smithgall, J: Advice from the dietitians: Insulin pumps, self-blood glucose monitoring and dietary compliance. *Diab Ed* 10(1):58, 1984.

Kulkarni, K: Advice from dietitians. Vegetarian diets. *Diab Ed* 9(2):35, 1983.

Lean, MEJ; Ng, LL; Tennison, BR: Interval between insulin injection and blood glucose control in adult diabetics. *Br Med J* 290(January 12):105, 1985.

Levin, ME; Rigg, LA; Marshall, RE: Pregnancy and diabetes: Team approach. *Arch Intern Med* 146(3):758, 1986.

Lieberman, DA; Chan, MM: The relationship of dietary compliance to outcome of pregnancy in gestational diabetes. Presented at the annual American Dietetic Convention, Las Vegas, October, 1986.

Lockwood, D; Frey, ML; Gladish, NA; et al: The biggest problem in diabetes. *Diab Ed* 12(1):30, 1986.

Manhire, A; Henry, CL; Hartog, M; et al: Unrefined carbohydrate and dietary fibre in treatment of diabetes mellitus. *J Human Nutr* 35(2):99, 1981.

Murray, P: Diabetes today: When hyperglycemia goes critical. *RN* 46(3):56, 1983.

Nathan, DM; Godine, JE; Gauthier-Kelley, C; et al: Ice cream in the diet of insulin-dependent diabetic patients. *JAMA* 251(21):2825, 1984.

National Diabetes Data Group (NDDG): Classification and diagnosis of diabetes mellitus and other categories of glucose intolerance. *Diabetes* 28(12):1039, 1979.

Nemchik, R: Diabetes today: A startling new body of knowledge. *RN* 45(10):30, 1982.

Olefsky, J; Reaven, GM; Farquhar, JW: Effect of weight reduction on obesity: Studies of lipid and carbohydrate metabolism in normal and hyperlipoproteinemic subjects. *J Clin Invest* 53(1):64, 1974.

Orzeck, EA: Consumer's guide to blood testing. *Diab Forecast* 37(2):25, 1984.

Pecoraro, RE; Koepsell, TD; Chen, MS; et al: Comparative clinical reliability of fasting plasma glucose and glycosylated hemoglobin in non–insulin-dependent diabetes mellitus. *Diabetes Care* 9(4):370, 1986.

Pederson, J: Congenital malformation in newborns of diabetic mothers. In *Carbohydrate Metabolism in Pregnancy and the Newborn*. Edited by HW Sutherland; JM Stowers. New York, Springer-Verlag, 1979, p 264.

Powers, MA; Crapo, PA: The fructose story. *Diab Ed* 7(4):22, 1982.

Prosser, PR: Diabetes mellitus: Diet therapy for the noninsulin-dependent patient. *Consultant* 22(2):209, 1982.

Quarterman, J; Florence, E: Observations on glucose tolerance and plasma levels of free fatty acids and insulin in zinc-deficient rats. *Br J Nutr* 28(1):75, 1972.

Report of the National Commission on Diabetes to the Congress of the United States (RNCD). Volume 1. DHEW Pub. No. (NIH) 76-1018, 1976.

Riblett, B: Insuring a safe pregnancy for your diabetic patient. *RN* 46(2):50, 1983.

Richter, EA; Ploug, T; Galbo, H: Increased muscle glucose uptake after exercise: No need for insulin during exercise. *Diabetes* 34(10):1041, 1985.

Simpson, HC; Simpson, RW; Lousley, S; et al: A high carbohydrate leguminous fibre diet improves all aspects of diabetic control. *Lancet* 1(January 3):1, 1981.

Simpson, RW; Mann, JI; Eaton, J; et al: High-carbohydrate diets and insulin-dependent diabetic. *Br Med J* 2(September 1):523, 1979.

Skyler, JS; Skyler, DL; Siegler, DE; et al: Algorithms for adjustment of insulin dosage by patients who monitor blood glucose. *Diab Care* 4(2):311, 1981.

Smith, E; Hamburger, S: Diabetes and fiber. A review. *Missouri Med* 80(2):76, 1983.

Solomon, YC: Diabetic retinopathy and carbohydrate metabolism. *Proc Nutr Soc* 38(3):351, 1979.

Task force for the American Diabetes Association: Nutritional recommendations and principles for individuals with diabetes mellitus: 1986. *Diab Care* 10(1):126, 1987.

Thorp, FK: Insulin pump therapy reconsidered. *JAMA* 255(5):645, 1986.

Vaaler, S; Hansen, KF; Aagenaes, O: Sucrose and sorbitol as sweeteners in the diet of insulin-dependent diabetics. *Acta Med Scand* 207(5):371, 1980.

West, KM: Diabetes mellitus. In *Nutritional Support of Medical Practice*, 2nd ed. Edited by HA Schneider, CE Anderson, DB Coursin. Philadelphia, Harper & Row, 1983, p 302.

West, KM: *Epidemiology of Diabetes and Its Vascular Lesions*. New York, Elsevier Science Publishing Co, 1978.

Wheeler, ML (ed): *Diabetes Mellitus and Glycemic Responses to Different Foods: A Summary and Annotated Bibliography*. Chicago, American Dietetic Association, 1983.

White, NE; Miller, BK: Glycohemoglobin: A new test to help the diabetic stay in control. *Nursing* 13(8):55, 1983.

Wolever, TMS; Jenkins, DJA: Application of glycemic index to mixed meals. *Lancet* 2(October 26):944, 1985.

Wolever, TMS; Jenkins, DJA: The use of the glycemic index in predicting the blood glucose response to mixed meals. *Am J Clin Nutr* 43(1):167, 1986.

Further Study

American Journal of Nursing: Programmed Instruction: Controlling diabetes mellitus. *Am J Nurs* 80(10):1827, 1980.

Anderson, JW; Chandler, C: High fiber diet benefits for diabetics. *Diabetes Ed* 7(2):34, 1981.

Borgatti, RS: Patient education: Helping diabetics learn control habits. *Patient Care* 14(15):120, 1980.

Cook, KA: Diabetics can be vegetarians. *Nursing* 9(10):70, 1979.

Crapo, PA: Complex carbohydrates in the diabetic diet. *Diab Ed* 7(3):37, 1981.

Criegler-Meringola, D: Making life sweet again for the elderly diabetic. *Nursing* 14(4):61, 1984.

Criegler-Meringola, D; Ryan, D: The diabetic who takes a drink. *Diab Ed* 9(4):27, 1984.

Friedman, EA: Living with kidney disease. *Diabetes Forecast* 33(3):34, 1980.

Fuller, E: Diet programs for diabetes. *Patient Care* 20(11):115, 1986.

Guthrie, DW: Control in an adolescent. *Diab Ed* 7(3):48, 1981.

Guthrie, DW; Guthrie, RR: *Nursing Management of Diabetes Mellitus*. St Louis, C. V. Mosby Co, 1982.

Guthrie, DW; Guthrie, R; Hinnen, D: Urine tests—still useful after all these years. *Diabetes Forecast* 38(2):43, 1985.

Heins, JM: Dietary management in diabetes mellitus. A goal-setting process. *Nurs Clin North Am* 18(4):631, 1983.

Hopper, SV: Meeting the needs of the economically deprived diabetic. *Nurs Clin North Am* 18(4):813, 1983.

Kaplan, RM; Davis, WK: Evaluating the costs and benefits of outpatient diabetes education and nutrition counseling. *Diab Care* 9(1):81, 1986.

Klosiewski, M: Hypoglycemia—what does the diabetic experience? *Diab Ed* 10(3):18, 1984.

McCarthy, JA: The continuum of diabetic coma. *Am J Nurs* 85(8):878, 1985.

McFadden, HE: The ups and downs of diabetes. *Am J Nurs* 85(8):881, 1985.

Nemchik, R: Diabetes today: The new insulin pumps. *RN* 46(5):52, 1983.

Nemchik, R: Diabetes today: The news about insulin. *RN* 45(12):49, 1982.

Nemchik, R: Diabetes today: A very different diet—a new generation of oral drugs. *RN* 45(11):41, 1982.

Richardson, B: The real world of diabetic non-compliance. *Nursing* 12(1):68, 1982.

Robertson, C: How to teach patients to monitor blood glucose. *RN* 8(12):24, 1985.

Sacks, SR: Diabetes therapy: Caring for patients with type II diabetes. *Patient Care* 14(5):146, 1980.

Smith, D: Outpatient care of the diabetic. *J Ger Nurs* 9(8):422, 1983.

Smokvina, G; Givens, R: Hyperglycemia in the aged. *J Ger Nurs* 9(8):449, 1983.

Villeneuve, ME; Murphy, JA; Mazze, RS: Evaluating blood glucose monitors. *Am J Nurs* 85(11):1258, 1985.

Wedman, B: Nutrition for the amputee. *Diab Ed* 8(4):29, 1983.

Dietary Management of Endocrine and Genetic Disorders

30

THE STUDENT WILL BE ABLE TO:

· **Identify endocrine disorders that respond to nutritional care.**
· **Discuss the prevention and treatment of phenylketonuria.**

OBJECTIVES

Addison's disease
Addisonian crisis
Aminoacidopathy
Corticosteroids
Cretinism
Cushing's syndrome
Goiter
Graves' disease
Hypercortisolism
Myxedema
Phenylketonuria (PKU)

TERMS TO KNOW

Metabolism includes all the chemical processes to build and maintain the body. When the activity of a hormone, enzyme, or cofactor is abnormal (i.e., excessive, absent, or reduced), the metabolism of that compound and the entire body is detrimentally affected. Most metabolic disorders are hereditary traits, such as diabetes mellitus (see Chapter 29).

Hormones secreted by the pancreas, adrenal cortex, thyroid gland, and parathyroid glands are very potent; imbalances (too much or too little) of these hormonal secretions have a direct effect on how the body handles nutrients. With modern technology, the most effective treatment is hormonal replacement. Nutritional care is used in the therapy of some of these metabolic problems during the acute phase and to restore nutritional balance.

A genetic disorder, also called an inborn error of metabolism, is a physiological problem caused by an inherited defective gene in which a metabolic block is produced by an enzymatic defect. Pathological consequences may be manifest soon after birth or later in life. Nutritional care for these problems usually involves preventing the accumulation of the substrate, which becomes toxic in excessive amounts, and/or replacing the deficient product.

While early detection and diagnosis of metabolic disorders by the physician are important, effective treatment involves active participation of the nurse and dietitian to plan and implement effective nutritional care and to teach the family to understand the disorder and to follow the frequently rigid guidelines.

Pancreatic Dysfunction

HYPOGLYCEMIA

Hypoglycemia is not a distinct disease but rather symptomatic of problems involving insulin secretion and carbohydrate metabolism. The symptoms are similar to those of a diabetic hypoglycemic reaction: weakness, shakiness and trembling, blurred vision, dizziness, hunger, tachycardia, and agitation. Hypoglycemia occurs when excessive amounts of insulin are secreted in response to carbohydrate intake or when excessive amounts of glucose are removed from the blood. It can be the result of serious disorders of the nervous system, liver, intestinal tract, or endocrine glands. It can also be indicative of early diabetes.

Normally, after food is eaten, the blood glucose level rises, and the pancreas secretes insulin to normalize blood sugar levels. In hypoglycemia, excessive amounts of insulin are secreted causing blood glucose to fall to below-normal levels within two to four hours after eating. Early diabetic stages have a delayed secretion of insulin, allowing high blood glucose levels to remain longer, followed by hypoglycemia.

Hypoglycemia was a popular diagnosis during the 1970s for symptoms similar to those previously mentioned. This diagnosis may have been given when it was caused by emotional or psychological factors. A statement issued by the American Diabetes Association, the Endocrine Society, and the American Medical Association (Statement, 1973) recommended that a diagnosis of hypoglycemia be given only if: (1) low levels of glucose are demonstrated, (2) the patient has symptoms, and (3) the symptoms are relieved by food or carbohydrate intake.

A low blood glucose level is normally diagnosed with a five-hour oral glucose tolerance test (OGTT) that demonstrates a circulating glucose of less than 45 mg/dl. However, in most cases, this glucose level does not necessarily correlate with the symptoms (Johnson et al, 1980). Studies questioning the value of the OGTT in diagnosing hypoglycemia have led investigators at the Fitzsimmons Army Medical Center and the Mayo Clinic to conclude that patients with hypoglycemic symptoms should be evaluated using mixed meals rather than liquid oral glucose (Hogan et al, 1983; Charles, et al, 1981).

Organic or Fasting Hypoglycemia. An oversecretion of insulin will result in organic hypoglycemia. Symptoms appear eight or more hours after a meal. Known causes include insulinoma or other tumors, endocrine deficiency, overadministration of insulin or sulfonylureas, liver damage, and starvation.

Reactive Hypoglycemia. Experienced two to four hours after eating, reactive hypoglycemia is the same type of hypoglycemia seen after a gastrectomy (see Chapter 27) and may also be associated with certain inherited metabolic disorders.

Nutritional Care. The purpose of nutritional support for hypoglycemia is to provide a more even release of glucose; carbohydrate causes hypoglycemia in those with reactive hypoglycemia (Lavine, 1979). The most common diet recommended is low in carbohydrate and high in protein with frequent feedings. Six feedings help to maintain euglycemia. Three high-protein snacks are provided in addition to three meals daily, as shown in *Focus on Sample Menu for Hypoglycemia.*

Since proteins and fats are digested and ab-

FOCUS ON	SAMPLE MENU FOR HYPOGLYCEMIA*

Breakfast
¾ cup Tomato juice
2 oz. Canadian bacon
½ slice Whole-wheat toast
1 pat Margarine
½ cup Homogenized milk

Midmorning Snack
⅓ cup Smoked almonds

Lunch
Tomato stuffed with ¾ cup cottage cheese
Tossed salad with 2 Tbsp. French dressing
10 Seedless Thompson grapes

Midafternoon Snack
2 oz. Cheddar cheese cubes
4 Saltine crackers

Dinner
3 oz. Ribeye steak
Mushrooms sauteed in 2 Tbsp. Margarine
½ cup Cooked spinach with Bacon Bits
½ cup Grated carrots with 2 Tbsp. Fresh pineapple cubes
and 2 Tbsp. mayonnaise
½ cup Sugar-free flavored gelatin

Bedtime Snack
Celery sticks stuffed with 2 Tbsp. peanut butter

Decaffeinated coffee or tea or artificially sweetened, caffeine-free beverages can be used as desired.

The protein and fat content of this diet are adjusted according to individual needs for appropriate kilocaloric intake. This diet provides approximately 2000 kcal, 100 gm of protein, 90 gm of carbohydrate, and 129 gm of fat.

---

*Nutrient data and calculations from Nutritionist II software, Silverton, OR.

---

sorbed more slowly and stimulate less insulin secretion, thereby providing a delayed source of glucose, they are better tolerated. All forms of sugar-sweetened desserts and concentrated sweets are avoided. The food exchange lists (see Chapter 23) are utilized to calculate the diet and to help patients limit their consumption of carbohydrates.

Total energy intake should meet the individual's requirements. Carbohydrate content of the diet is generally 80 to 100 gm to prevent ketosis. Carbohydrates are spread equally between the feedings throughout the day. Protein is usually 20 percent of the kilocalories (100 to 125 gm) and should also be distributed equally. The remainder of the kilocalories is provided by fat.

Three examples of high-protein snacks are cheese, nuts, or cottage cheese. The diet will usually reduce the symptoms of hyperglycemia; however, a careful diagnosis, utilizing endocrine and metabolic testing procedures, may determine a correctable cause. As stated by Danowski and colleagues (1975), "It is a disservice to such patients to limit treatment to diet manipulations without seeking the origins of the hypoglycemia."

Clinical Implications:

- When milk intake is low (because of its carbohydrate content), monitor the diet for calcium and riboflavin adequacy. Supplementation may be necessary.
- Alcohol can potentiate hypoglycemia by decreasing gluconeogenesis; it should be avoided.
- Caffeine can also lower blood glucose levels and should be avoided.
- Meals and snacks should be taken with regularity.
- Because of limited intake of fruits and vegetables, emphasis should be given to vitamin C–rich foods.
- An increase in dietary fiber will decrease carbohydrate absorption and prevent hypoglycemic symptoms (Ensinck & Williams, 1981).

Adrenal Dysfunction

ADDISON'S DISEASE

Insufficient production of one or more hormones by the adrenal glands results in Addison's disease. It is a long-term and rare metabolic disorder. Most cases are idiopathic; approximately one third of the cases are caused by tuberculosis, histoplasmosis, or other infectious diseases (Molitch & Dahms, 1983). The adrenal medulla (inner portion) secretes epinephrine and norepinephrine; the cortex (outer portion) secretes aldosterone, the glucocorticoids, and androgenic hormones. In Addison's disease, the medulla functions normally, but cells in the cortex may be damaged, interfering with hormonal production.

Addison's disease is characterized by anorexia, weight loss, weakness, loss of body hair in women, and abnormal skin pigmentation. When insufficient amounts of aldosterone are secreted, sodium absorption is decreased, precipitating excessive sodium and fluid losses. Extracellular volume is decreased; acidosis develops; serum potassium levels are increased; and cardiac output

decreases. If the disease is untreated, blood volume falls, precipitating the addisonian crisis. Glucocorticoid deficiencies cause decreased conversion of fats and proteins to glucose; hypoglycemia is a frequent occurrence.

Treatment. Replacing the deficient adrenal cortex hormones is the major therapy. Hormones are given to lower the serum potassium and to decrease the amount of salt and water excreted. If the medication is taken regularly, the individual can lead a normal life.

Nutritional Care. A modified diet may be used in conjunction with drug therapy; this decreases the drug requirement. Depending on the hormones administered, additional salt (4 to 6 gm/day) is often advised. Several salt tablets may be given along with high-salt foods. If a sodium-retaining hormone is given, salt intake is not increased.

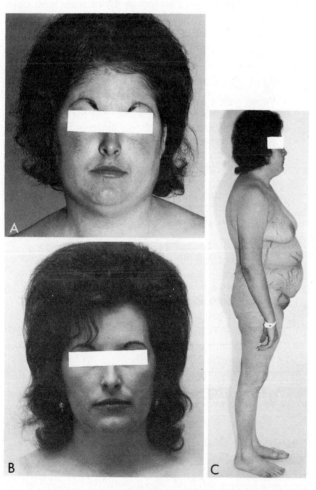

Figure 30–1. A & B A patient with Cushing's syndrome before treatment. C, One year after treatment (removal of an adrenal adenoma). (From Tyrrell JB, Baxter JD: Endocrine and reproductive diseases, in Wyngaarden JB, Smith LH Jr (eds): Cecil Textbook of Medicine, 17th ed. Philadelphia, W. B. Saunders Co, 1985, by permission.)

A high-protein, moderate-carbohydrate diet is used to prevent hypoglycemia (as described earlier). Six feedings, each containing some protein, are given with a substantial bedtime feeding to prevent nocturnal hypoglycemia. Simple sugars are avoided. Because of an increased metabolism associated with the disease management, vitamin B complex and C supplements may be needed.

Blood chemistries are important; both hypo- and hyperkalemia can be a problem. On the basis of laboratory data, advice can be given whether to avoid or increase potassium-containing foods.

Clinical Implications:

- Large amounts of fluids are needed to prevent dehydration.
- Corticosteroids should be taken with milk or antacids to minimize gastric irritation.
- Meals should not be skipped; fasting is not well tolerated.
- The patient should always carry a high-protein snack.

CUSHING'S SYNDROME AND CORTICOSTEROID THERAPY

Pharmacological use of glucocorticoids and endogenous secretion of excess cortisol, as seen in Cushing's disease, results in a state of hypercortisolism. Both conditions can be considered together. Increased amounts of glucocorticoids affect carbohydrate, protein, and lipid metabolism. Glucocorticoids increase protein catabolism, and patients may exhibit signs of muscle wasting, thin skin and subcutaneous tissues, poor wound healing, and dissolution of the vertebral bone matrix. Subcutaneous fat is lost in the arms and legs with excessive fatty deposits in the trunk and neck areas (Fig. 30–1). Growth retardation is a common finding among children.

Mineralocorticoid-like effects may be seen, even though aldosterone levels are not significantly elevated. Fluid and sodium retention are characterized by "moon face." Potassium depletion will cause weakness.

Nutritional Care. Nutritional support for Cushing's disease or patients on corticosteroid therapy should include an adequate amount of kilocalories, high levels of protein (100 gm), and moderate amounts of carbohydrate (200 to 300 gm). Concentrated sugars are normally eliminated to prevent hypoglycemic reactions. Sodium restriction may be used to decrease fluid retention. Ascorbic acid supplementation is advised because ACTH depletes adrenal tissue of vitamin C.

When corticosteroids are given for a prolonged period, vitamin D (50,000 IU, three times a week) plus calcium (500 to 1000 mg/day) should be given to prevent steroid-induced osteopenia (Hahn, 1978). In some cases of glucocorticoid therapy, oral supplements of zinc have been used because of zinc depletion, and this may improve wound healing (Molitch & Dahms, 1983).

Thyroid Dysfunction

Hormones secreted by the thyroid affect many metabolic processes in the body. Iodine supplied by the diet is an important constituent of these hormones. Two hormones, thyroxine (T_4) and triiodothyronine (T_3), control the rate of biochemical processes. They increase oxidation of active cells (increasing calorigenic activity), stimulate the quantity and rate of enzymatic activity, increase glucose absorption and utilization, and regulate vitamin requirements because of their role in enzymatic functions. They are needed for normal growth and mental acuity. Since these hormones increase anabolism and catabolism, an overabundance or deficiency will affect the metabolism of all energy nutrients—carbohydrate, protein, and fat. The enlargement of the thyroid gland is termed a goiter and may be associated with either hypo- or hyperthyroidism (Fig. 30–2).

HYPERTHYROIDISM OR GRAVES' DISEASE

This condition, caused by excess secretion of thyroid hormones, results in an increased basal metabolic rate (BMR) and weight loss in spite of increased food intake. Graves' disease is characterized by nervousness, exophthalmos (protruding eyes), hyperexcitability, emotional instability, increased peristalsis, sweating, and heat intolerance. In addition to increased requirements for all nutrients because of an elevated metabolism, bone demineralization can be a complication if left untreated.

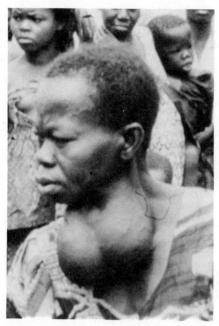

Figure 30–2. *Goiter resulting from iodine deficiency. (Courtesy of Food and Agricultural Organization of the United Nations. Photo by Marcel Ganzin.)*

Treatment. Several methods of treatment are used to decrease the amount of hormonal secretion: (1) antithyroid drugs, (2) surgery, or (3) radioiodine therapy. Iodine has been given for hyperthyroidism; its major action is to inhibit hormonal release. Antithyroid drugs, which inhibit the biosynthesis of hormones, are currently the mode of treatment (Ingbar & Woeber, 1981).

Nutritional Care. A very high kilocalorie diet is indicated. There is no limitation on the energy needs, but the diet should contain at least 3000 kcal. Liberal amounts of protein are needed to offset the negative nitrogen balance. Carbohydrates and fats can be used liberally to increase the kilocalorie content of the diet. Snacks are usually beneficial in increasing the amount of food eaten.

Enhanced cellular metabolism increases requirements for thiamin, riboflavin, ascorbic acid, pyridoxine, and vitamins A, B_{12}, D, and E. Supplements are usually advisable.

Clinical Implications:

- Readily accessible foods should be available for patients in the hospital; "constant nibbling" is acceptable.
- Since the patient is already overstimulated, caffeinated beverages, tobacco, and alcohol are limited or avoided because of their stimulating effect.
- Large amounts of fluid are encouraged to offset excessive losses from sweating and heavy breathing.
- Milk consumption is encouraged to compensate for calcium losses.
- The patient should be encouraged to relax and eat in quiet and pleasant surroundings.
- High-fiber foods may need to be limited because of increased peristalsis.
- Glucose intolerance may be a problem, as evidenced by hyperglycemia.
- After hyperthyroidism is controlled, appetite does not always decrease. Patients should be advised about the possibility of obesity, if food intake is not altered.

HYPOTHYROIDISM

Thyroxine activity is decreased in hypothyroidism; BMR is decreased. The condition may be related to: (1) inadequate consumption of iodine, (2) high intake of goitrogens, or (3) an inborn error of metabolism. Patients may gain weight despite a decreased appetite, exhibit an intolerance to cold, and have a decreased basal body temperature. Lipid metabolism is decreased in relation to its synthesis, resulting in increased serum triglycerides and cholesterol.

While the United States has practically eliminated goiter caused by iodine deficiency with the use of iodized salt, some groups of people in Kentucky have a high prevalence of goiter in spite of sufficient iodine intake. These goiters occur mainly in children 12 to 13 years old. Apparently, environmental and immunological factors play a role in the goiter endemic of this area (Ziporyn, 1985).

Cretinism. The childhood disease cretinism develops as a result of hypothyroidism. This condition affects brain development, usually causing mental retardation. The child shows a depressed growth rate and bone maturation. Lethargy and an increased susceptibility to respiratory infections are also observed.

Myxedema. Hypothyroidism in adults is known as myxedema, which develops frequently after treatment for hyperthyroidism. Puffiness of the face and eyelids are clinical symptoms.

Nutritional Care. Hormonal therapy and regulation of the diet are generally corrective measures. Kilocalories should be limited for patients who are overweight. The amount allowed should be determined by the degree of overweight and the metabolic rate. High-fiber foods and natural laxatives, such as bran and prunes, are encouraged in order to stimulate peristalsis. Plenty of fluids should also be encouraged for constipation. Iodized salt is important. A daily intake of 100 to 150 mcg of iodine is recommended; this can be supplied by approximately 1 tsp. of iodized salt daily.

Goitrogenic substances naturally present in some foods can interfere with iodine uptake by the thyroid (Table 13–1). If hypothyroidism is induced by goitrogenic foods, one should encourage thorough cooking to inactivate the goitrogens in the following foods: cabbage, rutabagas, turnips, cauliflower, Brussels sprouts, and soybeans.

Parathyroid Dysfunction

The parathyroid glands function to maintain a constant serum calcium level, which is necessary for blood coagulation, cardiac and skeletal muscle contraction, and nerve function. Their secretion is inversely proportional to serum calcium level. Calcium absorption and phosphorus excretion are controlled by the parathyroids.

TETANY

Tetany is caused by an imbalance of calcium and phosphorus and is characterized by convulsions, cramps, or muscle twitching. Hypocalcemic tetany is the result of parathyroid hypofunction associated with rickets, osteomalacia, pregnancy, hypermagnesia, steatorrhea, and renal insufficiency. Alkalotic tetany may be caused by hyperventilation or vomiting, or injection of alkaline salts. Total plasma calcium may be as low as 4 mg/dl (normally 8.5 to 10.5 mg/dl). Tetany resulting from alkalosis is treated with large doses of an acid-producing salt, frequently ammonium chloride.

Nutritional Care. The usual treatment is to increase calcium levels with a high-calcium diet. At least 1 to 1 1/2 qt. of milk daily are advisable. (Milk contains the most utilizable form of calcium.) Vitamin D supplementation (25,000 to 200,000 IU/day) enhances calcium absorption

(Molitch & Dahms, 1983). However, patients must be monitored for hypervitaminosis D. For patients who are lactose-intolerant, calcium citrate may be used. When phosphate levels are high, aluminum salts are used to decrease absorption of dietary phosphorus.

Clinical Implication:

Tetany may be caused by conditions other than hypocalcemia; the underlying factors should be diagnosed. A prescription for quinine sulfate tablets (Quinamm) alleviates only the symptom, not the condition.

HYPERCALCEMIA

Elevated serum calcium levels accompanied by hypophosphatemia are seen with many disorders including hyperthyroidism, bone disorders, and hyperparathyroidism. Hypercalcemia is observed in vitamin A and D intoxication and in the milk-alkali syndrome (see Chapter 27). Hypercalcemia is not due to overconsumption of calcium-containing foods. This metabolic disorder causes calcium to be extracted from skeletal tissue and decreases the integrity of the bone.

Nutritional Care. Since hypercalcemia is only a symptom, the underlying disorder is usually treated. However, several nutritional factors can be implemented until effective medical treatment can be established. A high level of fluid intake is needed to prevent formation of kidney stones. An acid-ash diet may be prescribed to produce an acidic urine and prevent calcium stone formation (see Appendix D–6). Intravenous phosphate solutions promote deposition of calcium into skeletal tissue, thereby lowering serum calcium levels. However, the patient should be carefully monitored to prevent metastatic calcification and acute renal failure.

Inborn Errors of Metabolism

The discovery of many inborn errors of metabolism has increased dramatically recently, even though their occurrence is relatively rare. The development of successful therapeutic nutritional interventions has resulted from many studies. Success is varied with the type of disease and the ease with which dietary modifications can be achieved. While this text only discusses one inborn error of metabolism (phenylketonuria), there are other less-prevalent conditions that respond only to diet therapy, e.g., maple syrup urine disease (MSUD), tyrosinemia, and galactosemia. Because of the specialized diagnostics and treatments required for controlling these conditions, only large medical facilities are equipped to handle them.

Aminoacidopathy is an inborn error of metabolism in which a particular step in the utilization of an amino acid is blocked. Unless the offending amino acid is restricted, excessive amounts of the amino acid or its derivatives will accumulate in body fluids; on the other hand, adequate amounts must be provided for growth. Careful monitoring must continue in order to maintain such delicate balances.

PHENYLKETONURIA (PKU)

Phenylketonuria (PKU) is an inborn error of metabolism in which the enzyme, phenylalanine hydroxylase, is either absent or present in trace amounts. So, the amino acid phenylalanine is not converted to tyrosine in a normal manner (Fig. 30–3), and phenylalanine accumulates while tyrosine is inadequate. High levels of circulating phe-

nylalanine affect brain development. Infants in whom the condition is detected early and treatment initiated before six weeks of age are not retarded. Approximately one in every 70 persons in the United States is a carrier of phenylketonuria, an autosomal recessive disorder.

If an infant is not identified by testing, the first conspicuous sign of PKU is an inability by the child to sit unassisted at the normal age. Marked irritability, severe vomiting, eczema, seizures, and a musty odor are other typical characteristics. Untreated PKU infants may not walk until early childhood or may never learn to walk. Motor development is slow, and electroencephalographic abnormalities are common in these blond, blue-eyed children.

Screening Tests. Screening for PKU in the newborn is mandatory in most states even though some controversy still exists about this requirement (Annas, 1982). A serum phenylalanine concentration of 20 mg/dl or greater implies a potential PKU case. For tests performed soon after birth, the cutoff level may be between 2 and 6 mg/dl. Urine testing at four to six weeks of age may be conducted in the physician's office.

Two blood phenylalanine determinations of 20 mg/dl or higher with tyrosine concentrations of less than 5 mg/dl should be obtained before treatment is started. A small percentage of those will develop the ability to convert phenylalanine to tyrosine during the first year of life; the special diet should be challenged with milk about three

Metabolic Defect in Phenylketonuria

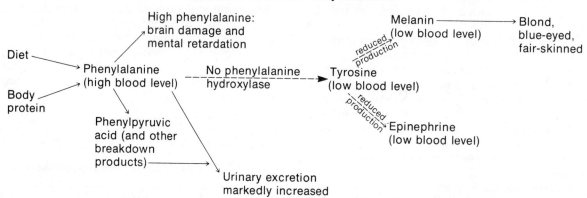

Figure 30–3. Absence of the enzyme phenylalanine hydroxylase prevents conversion of phenylalanine to tyrosine. Blood samples reveal high phenylalanine and low tyrosine. Urine samples show excessive phenylalanine and its breakdown products. Production of melanin and epinephrine is decreased. Mental retardation develops owing to the toxic character of high levels of phenylalanine in the brain. (From Sorensen KC, Luckmann J: Basic Nursing: A Psychophysiologic Approach. Philadelphia, W. B. Saunders Co, 1979, by permission.)

months after the start of therapy. If the dietary restrictions are lifted, laboratory tests are used to verify phenylalanine restriction is not needed.

Nutritional Care. The only effective method of treatment of PKU is dietary control of the amount of dietary phenylalanine. Enough must be consumed to allow for growth but the accumulation of excessive amounts of phenylalanine must be prevented. Phenylalanine, an essential aminoacid, is contained in all foods at a remarkably constant and relatively large amount—about five percent of the protein fraction (Lynch, 1968). The diet can be modified by utilizing protein hydrolysates to limit the phenylalanine and supplement tyrosine. As shown in Table 30–1, recommended intakes of phenylalanine gradually decrease (based on body weight) throughout infancy and childhood, to 3 to 4 mg/kg/day by adulthood (Holt et al, 1960).

Initially in infancy, all the protein requirements can be met from a minimal phenylalanine formula such as Lofenalac (Mead Johnson), Phenyl-Free (Mead Johnson), PKU-Aid (Milner), and PKU-2 (Milupa). Lofenalac may be considered a balanced and complete formula for PKU infants. Natural protein can be added to provide the minimum requirement of phenylalanine and additional protein when plasma phenylalanine falls to 6 mg/dl. Early warning signs of phenylalanine deficiency are lethargy, anorexia, fever, and vomiting (Lynch, 1968). The mother must be instructed how to calculate the composition of feedings to allow proper amounts of protein, phenylalanine, and fluid provided by the formula as the infant grows and increases intake (Table 30–2).

Because of too vigorous application of dietary therapy, profound malnutrition and even deaths during the first year have occurred (Hanley et al, 1970). As a primary preventive measure, serum phenylalanine levels are measured once or twice a week during the first year; serum protein and hemoglobin levels as well as height and weight are measured to determine adequacy of protein and energy intake. In spite of the restrictions, the diet must be well balanced; mineral and vitamin intakes are below the recommended levels in a surprisingly large number of PKU patients (Acosta et al, 1982, 1977).

For older children with PKU, an appropriate diet consists of a low-phenylalanine or phenylalanine-free protein substitute, some phenylalanine-containing foods, and many low-protein products. Consistent with the diet during infancy, foods must provide nutrients necessary for growth, development, and general well-being but prevent the accumulation of excess phenylalanine. Low-protein products produced commercially and low-protein recipes are used to incorporate variety; fruits, vegetables, and small amounts of other foods are added to provide adequate amounts of phenylalanine. The phenylalanine, protein, and caloric content of the vegetables, fruits, breads, and cereals used in the phenylalanine-restricted diet is important; the mother should calculate the child's intake of phenylalanine daily.

There is much debate over when these

Table 30–1. Recommended Phenylalanine, Protein, and Energy Intakes for Children with Phenylketonuria

Age	Phenylalanine Intake*†	Protein Intake	Energy Intake
Months	*mg/kg/day*	*mg/kg/day**	*kcal/kg/day**
0–3	40–70	4.2	120
4–6	25–55	3.0	115
7–9	25–50	2.5	110
10–12	25–50	2.5	105
Years		*Total mg/day‡*	*kcal/day‡*
1–2	20–40	23.0	1300
2–3	20–40	23.0	1300
3–4	20–40	23.0	1300
4–6	10–40	30.0	1700
6–8	10–40	34.0	2400
8–10	10–40	34.0	2400

*Data from Acosta, PB; Wenz, E; Williamson, M: Nutrient intake of treated infants with phenylketonuria. *Am J Clin Nutr* 30(2):198, 1977.

†Individual variations due to tolerance for phenylalanine, growth patterns, and activity should be considered.

‡Data from National Research Council, National Academy of Sciences. Recommended Dietary Allowances, 1980.

Table 30–2. Sample Prescription and Calculation
of Low-Phenylalanine Diet Utilizing Lofenalac*

Prescribe and calculate a diet for a 3.4 kg. 1-month-old infant recently diagnosed as having phenylketonuria.

1. Using Table 30-1 determine the phenylalanine, protein, water, and energy allowances:
   3.4 kg × 120 kcal/kg/day = 408 kcal/day
   3.4 kg × 150 ml water/kg/day = 510 ml water/day
   3.4 kg × 88 mg phenylalanine/kg/day = 299.2 mg phenylalanine/day
   3.4 kg × 2.5 gm protein/kg/day = 8.5 gm protein/day
2. Determine the amount of Lofenalac to be used:

$$408 \text{ kcal} \times \frac{\text{oz. Lofenalac}}{20 \text{ kcal}} = 20.4 \text{ oz. Lofenalac (rounded off to 20 oz.)}$$

3. Determine whether the minimum fluid requirement is met, by the following formula:

$$20 \text{ oz. formula} \times \frac{30 \text{ ml}}{\text{oz.}} = 600 \text{ ml fluid}$$

The infant requires 510 ml, so the formula satisfies this requirement.

4. Determine the amount of phenylalanine provided by the formula, then calculate the amount of milk needed to satisfy the patient's phenylalanine requirement:
   a. 20 oz. Lofenalac × 3.6 mg phenylalanine/oz. Lofenalac = 72 mg phenylalanine
   b. 299 mg phenylalanine required − 72 mg phenylalanine from Lofenalac = 227 mg phenylalanine needed from additional milk

   c. $227 \text{ mg phenylalanine} \times \dfrac{1 \text{ oz. milk}}{53 \text{ mg phenylalanine}} = 4.3 \text{ oz. milk}$

Rounding off to the nearest half ounce gives 4.5 oz. whole milk.

5. Check the protein content of the following formula:
   20 oz. Lofenalac × 0.65 gm protein/oz. = 13 gm protein
   4.5 oz. whole milk × 1 gm protein/oz. = 4.5 gm protein

Total protein given by the formula is thus 17.5 gm protein, which is in excess of that required.

6. Convert the formula prescription to packed measures of Lofenalac powder and ounces of water:

   1 packed measure Lofenalac powder and 2 oz. of water make 2⅛ oz. of formula. 20 oz. formula divided by 2⅛ oz. gives approximately 9.5 packed scoops. Add 19 oz. of water to this to give approximately 21.5 oz. formula.

7. Check the caloric, fluid, phenylalanine, and protein content of the total formula:

	Amount	Phenylalanine (mg)	Protein (gm)	Energy (kcal)
Lofenalac	9½ scoops	71.2	13.3	408
Water	19 oz.	0	0	0
Whole milk	4.5 oz.	238	4.5	90
Total	26 oz. (approximately)	309	17.8	498

8. Monitor infant and adjust prescription as needed.

*From Valle, DL: Dietary management of inborn errors of metabolism. In *Nutritional Management.* Edited by M Walser; AL Imbembo; S Margolis; et al: Philadelphia, W. B. Saunders Co, 1984, p 312, with permission.

dietary restrictions may be modified; hasty changes made too early in life can be harmful. About two thirds of the 90 clinics treating PKU in the United States now recommend indefinite continuation of a low-phenylalanine diet (Schuett & Brown, 1984). Holtzman and colleagues (1986) advocate that phenylalanine restriction should continue after the age of eight in order to avoid adversely affecting the child's IQ.

Other adverse consequences of liberalizing the diet too early are thought to be responsible for behavior patterns that interfere with normal mental functioning. Short attention span, poor short-term memory, impaired visual-motor perception, and defective motor coordination may result when serum phenylalanine levels are allowed to increase (Schuett et al, 1985; Hunt et al, 1985; Brunner et al, 1983). Although plasma phenylalanine levels below 8 mg/dl have been considered acceptable, Dobson and colleagues (1977) found higher IQ scores in children with PKU in whom phenylalanine levels were kept below 5.5 mg/dl as compared with those having higher levels (between 5.5 and 10 mg/dl).

The diet restrictions are costly—as much as $5000 to $7000/year or more for a teenager or young adult (Yankauer, 1982). Health care professionals should assist clients with economic hardships to obtain financial aid.

A PKU child must be treated as normally as possible, even though rigid dietary regulations are required, and should not be babied or infantilized in his/her attitude or behavior. Because of social interactions, after two years of age, it becomes increasingly difficult to maintain a restricted diet. Positive attitudes regarding the diet must be initiated and cultivated during the toddler period and continued through early childhood and adolescence. The parents often discover these dietary restrictions more difficult than the PKU child. Parents must have a sincere commitment and considerable patience to keep the child on this special diet; the struggles involved may place a serious emotional burden on them. An experienced multidisciplinary health care team can offer support and guidance at the time of diagnosis and during difficult periods.

As the child grows and matures, s/he must increasingly take responsibility for self-management of the diet. By seven or eight years of age, the child is taught how to make the formula. By 12 years of age, the child should be calculating the phenylalanine content of the food (Caballero, 1985). A major goal of the health care team is to encourage the child's independence.

Pregnancy. Increasingly, healthy and intelligent women with PKU are reaching childbearing age and presenting new challenges for health care professionals. While PKU mothers may have healthy, normal infants, the risks of pregnancy and alternatives such as birth control and sterilization must be explained to all women with PKU considering marriage and a family (Caballero, 1985). A fetus exposed to elevated levels of phenylalanine, which crosses the placenta, is likely to develop congenital anomalies and profound mental retardation. Low birthweight and congenital heart disease are other possible outcomes (Yankauer, 1982). Untreated pregnant women with blood phenylalanine concentrations of 20 mg/dl or higher have a 95 percent chance of having at least one mentally retarded child (Lenke & Levy, 1980).

When a PKU woman wants to become pregnant, she should begin a low-phenylalanine diet before conception. Within a few weeks of concep-tion, fetal damage has already occurred, resulting in reduced brain growth, microcephaly, and cardiac malformations (Summer & Frazier, 1983). However, good dietary control of phenylalanine levels throughout pregnancy can result in normal fetal development and the birth of a healthy infant.

The diet, begun before conception, is manipulated to keep the plasma phenylalanine around 8 mg/dl. Lofenalac and Product 3229 (Mead Johnson) can be used to help provide the nutritional requirements for pregnant PKU women. These formulas are used in conjunction with fruits and vegetables and low-protein grain products to allow some variety in the diet (Kromrower et al, 1979). Additionally, women with PKU should be closely monitored from the onset of pregnancy.

Clinical Implications:

- Low-protein products such as pastas and bread can be used to supplement the food pattern.
- Aspartame, a high-intensity sweetener, contains phenylalanine and another amino acid. Any product that contains aspartame is contraindicated for PKU patients and pregnant PKU carriers (Guttler & Lou, 1985).

Summary

Dietary management in endocrine disorders can help alleviate symptoms. Nutritional care may be used in conjunction with drugs for an extended period of time or temporarily until other therapies can correct the endocrine dysfunction.

Inborn errors of metabolism, such as PKU, need prompt diagnosis and proper attention to prescribe exact dietary intakes and to avoid problems such as mental retardation and abnormal motor function.

Review Questions

1. Explain how and why the hypoglycemic diet differs from the diabetic diet.
2. What type of diet might be ordered for hypothyroidism, and why?
3. What is tetany, and what foods should be encouraged for a patient with tetany?

4. How is phenylketonuria identified, and what dietary measures are taken to provide for normal growth? What are the consequences if the diet is not controlled?

Case Study: Following a normal pregnancy, Mrs. A. J. delivers a 7 lb. 6 oz. full-term infant. In compliance with state requirements, the baby is screened for PKU. After the initial tests, more definitive studies are ordered. These also are positive. Mr. and Mrs. A. J. are angry and confused as they begin counseling for their son's dietary management.

1. What is the physiological basis of phenylketonuria?
2. What signs will the son demonstrate in the first month without dietary modification?
3. What are the complications if the condition is left untreated?
4. Outline a diet plan for the first year.
5. Will the timing of the introduction of pureed and finger foods differ in the child with PKU compared to a child without it?
6. What factors would cause the phenylalanine intake to be altered?
7. What are the names of commercially-available milk substitutes?
8. Mrs. A. J. asks, "Won't he ever be able to eat normally?" What should you say to her?
9. What are some of the foods allowed as desired?
10. As the child grows, should s/he use the artificial sweetener aspartame?

REFERENCE LIST

Acosta, PB; Fernhoff, PM; Warshaw, HS; et al: Zinc status and growth of children undergoing treatment for phenylketonuria. *J. Inherited Metab Dis* 5:107, 1982.

Acosta, PB; Wenz, E; Williamson, M: Nutrient intake of treated infants with phenylketonuria. *Am J Clin Nutr* 30(2):198, 1977.

Annas, GJ: Mandatory PKU screening: The other side of the looking glass. *Am J Public Health* 72(12):1401, 1982.

Brunner, RL; Jordan, MK; Berry, HK: Early-treated phenylketonuria: Neuropsychologic consequences. *J Pediatr* 102(6):831, 1983.

Caballero, B: Dietary management of inborn errors of amino acid metabolism. *Clin Nutr* 4(3):85, 1985.

Charles, MA; Hofeldt, F; Shackelford, A; et al: Comparison of oral glucose tolerance tests and mixed meals in patients with apparent idiopathic postabsorptive hypoglycemia. *Diabetes* 30(6):465, 1981.

Danowski, TS; Nolan, S; Stephan, T: Hypoglycemia. *World Rev Nutr Diet* 22:288, 1975.

Dobson, JC; Williamson, ML; Azen, C; et al: Intellectual assessment of 111 4-year-old children with phenylketonuria. *Pediatrics* 60(6):822, 1977.

Ensinck, JW; Williams, R: Disorders causing hypoglycemia. In *Textbook of Endocrinology*, 6th ed. Edited by RH Williams. Philadelphia, W. B. Saunders Co, 1981.

Guttler, F; Lou, H: Aspartame may imperil dietary control of phenylketonuria. *Lancet* 1(March 2):525, 1985.

Hahn, TJ: Corticosteroid-induced osteopenia. *Arch Intern Med* 138(May 15):882, 1978.

Hanley, WB; Linsao, L; Davidson, W; et al: Malnutrition with early treatment of phenylketonuria. *Pediatr Res* 44:318, 1970.

Hogan, MJ; Service, FJ; Sharbrough, FW; et al: Oral glucose tolerance test compared with a mixed meal in the diagnosis of reactive hypoglycemia. *Mayo Clin Proc* 58(8):491, 1983.

Holt, LE, Jr; Gyorgy, P; Pratt, EL; et al: *Protein and Amino Acid Requirements in Early Life.* New York, New York University Press, 1960.

Holtzman, NA; Kronmal, RA; Doorninck, W; et al: Effect of age at loss of dietary control on intellectual performance and behavior of children with phenylketonuria. *N Engl J Med* 314(10):593, 1986.

Hunt, MM; Berry, HK; White, PP: Phenylketonuria, adolescence and diet. *J Am Diet Assoc* 85(10):1328, 1985.

Ingbar, SH; Woeber, KA: The thyroid gland. In *Textbook of Endocrinology*, 6th ed. Edited by RH Williams. Philadelphia, W. B. Saunders Co, 1981, p 117.

Johnson, DD; Dorr, KE; Swenson, WM; et al: Reactive hypoglycemia. *JAMA* 243(11):1151, 1980.

Kromrower, GM; Sardharwalla, IB; Coutts, JMJ; et al: Management of maternal phenylketonuria: An emerging clinical problem. *Br Med J* 1(May 26):1383, 1979.

Lavine, R: How to recognize and what to do about hypoglycemia. *Nursing* 9(4):52, 1979.

Lenke, RR; Levy, HL: Maternal phenylketonuria and hyperphenylalaninemia: An international survey of the outcomes of untreated and treated pregnancies. *N Engl J Med* 303(21):1202, 1980.

Lynch, HD: Phenylketonuria. Evansville, IN, Mead Johnson Laboratories, 1968.

Molitch, ME; Dahms, WT: Endocrinology. In *Nutritional Support of Medical Practice*, 2nd ed. Edited by HA Schneider, CE Anderson, DB Coursin. Philadelphia, Harper & Row, 1983, p 328.

Schuett, ME; Brown, ES: Diet policies of PKU clinics in the United States. *Am J Public Health* 74(5):501, 1984.

Schuett, VE; Brown, ES; Michals, K: Reinstitution of diet therapy in PKU patients from twenty-two U.S. clinics. *Am J Public Health* 75(1):39, 1985.

Statement on hypoglycemia. *JAMA* 223(6):682, 1973.

Summer, GK; Frazier, DM: Inborn errors of metabolism. In *Nutritional Support of Medical Practice*, 2nd ed. Edited by HA Schneider, CE Anderson, DB Coursin. Philadelphia, Harper & Row, 1983, p 421.

Yankauer, A: Maternal PKU: Control of an emerging problem. *Am J Public Health* 72(12):1320, 1982.

Ziporyn, T: For many, endemic goiter remains a baffling problem. *JAMA* 253(13):1846, 1985.

Further Study

Acosta, PB; Wenz, E: Diet management of PKU for infants and preschool children. DHEW Pub. No. (HSA) 77-5209, 1977.

Armstrong, MD; Tyler, FH: Restricted phenylalanine intake in phenylketonuria (Nutrition Classics). *J Clin Invest* 34(4):565, 1955.

Justice, P; Smith, GF: PKU-phenylketonuria. *Am J Nurs* 75(8):1303, 1975.

Kindt, E; Motzfeldt, K; Halvorsen, S; et al: Protein requirements in infants and children: A longitudinal study of children treated for phenylketonuria. *Am J Clin Nutr* 37(5):778, 1983.

Lenke, RR; Levy, HL: Maternal phenylketonuria results of dietary therapy. *Am J Obstet Gynecol* 142(5):548, 1982.

Marino, MA: Developing and testing a programmed instruction unit on PKU. *J Am Diet Assoc* 76(1):29, 1980.

Nelson, RL: Hypoglycemia: Fact or fiction? Mayo Clinic Proceedings 60(2):844, 1985.

Pueschel, SM; Hum, C; Andrews, M: Nutritional management of the female with phenylketonuria during pregnancy. *Am J Clin Nutr* 30(7):1153, 1977.

Pueschel, SM; Yeatman, S; Hum, C: Discontinuing the phenylalanine-restricted diet in young children with PKU. *J Am Diet Assoc* 70(5):506, 1977.

Schuett, VE; Gurda, R; Yandow, JL: Treatment programs for PKU and selected other metabolic diseases in the United States: A survey. DHEW Pub. No. (HSA) 82-5296, 1982.

University of Colorado Health Sciences Center: *Living with PKU*. Evansville, IN, Mead Johnson & Company, 1984.

Williamson, ML; Koch, R; Azen, C; et al: Correlates of intelligence tests results in treated phenylketonuric children. *Pediatrics* 68(2):161, 1981.

Dietary Management of Disorders of the Musculoskeletal System

31

THE STUDENT WILL BE ABLE TO:

- **List dietary measures that might help an arthritic person and be able to distinguish fact from fallacy among the many "cures."**
- **Name some foods high in purines.**
- **List dietary recommendations to prevent osteoporosis.**
- **Recommend special devices to aid the handicapped person consume beverages and food.**
- **Name some techniques to help feed an infant with a cleft palate.**

Hyperuricemia
Osteoarthritis
Osteoporosis
Purines

OBJECTIVES   TERMS TO KNOW

Skeletal or muscular disability may present problems in eating and therefore affect nutritional status. If the disability is the result of trauma, techniques and equipment to aid feeding are important. Either temporary or permanent handicaps may exist that interfere with the ability to feed oneself or prevent food preparation. Physical or occupational therapy, special devices, and pertinent nutritional information may reduce problems and maintain optimum nutrition.

Neuromuscular Feeding Problems

ETIOLOGY

Interruption or interference in normal development related to eating behavior directly influences food consumption. Most handicapped children do not attain the physical growth norms of the general population. Nutrient deficiencies are common. Food intake usually supplies an insufficient amount of kilocalories, resulting in underweight, but it may provide too many, resulting in obesity instead.

PATHOPHYSIOLOGY

Neuromuscular defects may make it difficult for patients to achieve adequate nutrient intake because of the inability to suck, bite, chew, or swallow. When the tongue and throat muscles are involved in the handicap, feeding is most difficult. Reversal of the swallowing wave results in masticated food being lifted from the throat and pushed onto the rear of the tongue when the individual tries to swallow. The possibility of choking compounds the problem of food consumption.

NORMAL AND ABNORMAL FEEDING SKILLS

Normal development of oral reflexes and feeding skills are discussed in Chapter 16. Often, the handicapped child does not want (nor is able) to progress like the normal child. S/He may be reluctant to relinquish the sucking reflex to learn finger-feeding or spoon-feeding skills, thereby postponing the transition to solid foods. Flacid musculature and lack of control of the head and upper trunk impede self-feeding. Involuntary tongue and lip movements make it most difficult to control food in the mouth. Encouragement to progress toward normal feeding stages may require certain strategies during the eating process (Table 31–1).

ADAPTIVE EQUIPMENT

Special equipment to ease the problems of feeding oneself can increase the self-respect, independence, dignity, and happiness of the handicapped individual besides improving the food intake. Self-feeding improves one's morale and allows more social contact. Many persons of all ages may benefit from such devices either temporarily or permanently. These problems may result from a variety of birth defects or illnesses such as cerebrovascular disease, multiple sclerosis, Parkinson's disease, and Alzheimer's disease or simply the aging process.

Special equipment not only makes food easier to handle but may also help patients avoid positions and stress that are immediately painful and prevent future harm to their joints. Figure 31–1 shows typical hold on a fork and another more relaxed position to benefit the handicapped individual. Combination fork-spoon or fork-knife utensils simplify food service. Angled knives can be gripped strongly with a straight wrist, thus requiring less strength and strain on joints. A deeper bowl on the spoon holds more food and resists spills.

Utensils with built-up handles can improve grasp function. Adjustable swivel utensils may overcome a patient's inability to turn his/her wrist. Knives and forks designed for the right or left hand may be combined as well as the curvatures of handles to facilitate use. Superlightweight utensils may have long handles for better control, which may help an adult feed the child whose grasping technique is erratic or may assist the individual with limited range of motion control. For those persons with less strength, a wrist support may prove useful (Fig. 31–2).

An inner lip plate or a round scoop dish can allow blind people or stroke victims to feed themselves and help prevent food spillage. Nonskid mats or suction cups prevent plates from sliding (Fig. 31–3). Insulated or heated equipment protects the temperature allowing more time for the eating process while the food is still warm.

For easier drinking, an unbreakable, dishwasher-safe plastic glass has a cutout for the nose so a person can drink without tipping the head

Table 31–1. Suggested Strategies for Developing Feeding Skills*

Areas of Concern	Strategies	
1. Inability to suck, chew, and swallow	Suck:	• Use cold substances around lips to stimulate sucking. • Use a cloth soaked with water for the child to suck. • Try different types of nipples. • As child begins to improve in ability, change to nipple with smaller holes.
	Chew:	• Place a small amount of food between back teeth and move jaw up and down. A mirror may help demonstrate and point out various body parts. • Wash with tongue—place foods such as peanut butter on lips, to allow tongue to be used. Gradual transition from pureed foods to solid foods (sprinkle crackers in soup, etc.).
	Swallow:	Swallowing easiest when mouth closed. • Close jaw and lips of child together. • Stroke throat upward under chin. • Offer next bit of food only after child swallows. • Demonstrate—let child feel *you* swallow.
2. Inability to grasp; hand-mouth coordination	To assist grasping coordination:	• Allow child to finger food. • Guide child in exploring mouth. • Cut food into small pieces. • Place your hand over child's hand and help him or her grasp spoon. • Use adaptive equipment (plastic spoon, etc.). • Make sure bowl is stabilized (suction, tape). • Use plates with high straight sides, or build higher edge using aluminum foil.
	Develop activities which will help child with coordination:	• Pour sand, etc. • Play with ball. • Push-pull objects. • Study body parts with child.
	Visually impaired:	• Place meats and vegetables consistently in same areas of plate so child can find.
3. Caloric problems: (Overweight/Underweight)	Obtain medical examination and evaluate growth. Provide variety of foods.	
	Overweight:	• Cut down snacks and high-calorie foods. • Refrain from rewarding with food. • Increase exercise and leisure-time activities.
	Underweight:	• Increase number of meals per day. • Include high-calorie foods, especially liquid supplements. • Proper exercise is important.
4. Lack of nutrition education	Work with families:	• Stress importance of proper nutrition for *all* family members. • Teach proper feeding environment (good eating habits, eating positions). • Provide nutrition-instruction materials.

*From *Ross Timesaver: Dietetic Currents.* Columbus, OH, Ross Laboratories, May–June 1977.

back or extending the neck. Snorkel lids are available that allow liquid to be sucked out by placing a finger over a hole; with the hole uncovered, liquid flows in a steady stream. Handles on both sides of a cup, no-tip cup holders, and tilting glass holders offer patients a wide variety of beverage containers (Fig. 31–4).

Some automatic feeders are available to enable patients to feed themselves at their own speed without the use of arms. These may be manipulated by a battery-controlled device that attaches to the forehead or chin (Fig. 31–5).

Other devices are available for persons preparing food. Some of these resources are listed at the end of this chapter.

Not to be ignored is the cost-effectiveness of adaptive equipment. With brief training, the individual may achieve enough success to need little or no help in eating. Nurse's aides use less than five minutes to set up a tray, as opposed to 30 minutes to feed a person (Shinnar, 1983). For patients who are not referred to physical or occupational therapists or dietitians, nurses may be the only source of such information.

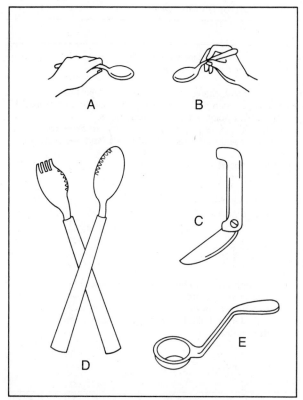

Figure 31–1. Hand position on silverware. A) Palmer grasp. B) Conventional grasp. C) Angled knife. D) Combination cutlery. E) Bent handle.

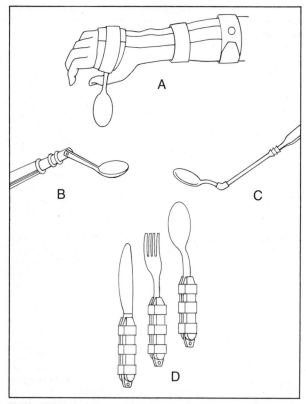

Figure 31–2. Variations on silverware. A) Wrist support. B) Swivel spoon. C) Spoon extension. D) Built-up handles.

MEALTIME ENVIRONMENT AND BEHAVIOR

A physical or occupational therapist can help teach the handicapped child and caretaker some exercises and procedures to improve eating abilities. The child and therapist should be relaxed and rested. The child should be positioned securely without fear of falling. Bibs may be used to cover the child, and newspaper or plastic drop cloths can protect the floor. This is not a time to be concerned with neatness. Food should not be wiped from the chin or mouth while the training is in progress, as this introduces other stimuli.

Disruptive behavior may be handled in a variety of ways, but consistency is very important for successful control. Many parents find it effective to remove the child from the table as soon as disruptive behavior begins. The child should go to another room in the house, where no adult attention is received until after the meal. No food (only water) is offered until the next meal. Of course, when appropriate behavior occurs, encouragement must be given to increase the desired con-

duct. The child should not be forced to eat. Sincere praise must be given whenever appropriate. Progress may be recorded; other procedures should be investigated if progress does not occur.

FOOD INTAKE

The main goal is to encourage as much independence as possible in the handicapped child. Patience and ingenuity are demanded. When children learn to feed themselves, they eat better and improve their social behavior (Pipes, 1981).

To provide sufficient food for children with cerebral palsy and similar neuromuscular disorders, special modifications are necessary in the selection of foods. Nutrient-dense foods are advised in order to provide as much energy and nutrients as possible with the least effort.

Liquids and soft foods are easier to handle. New textures should be introduced as soon as the child has mastered the appropriate skills. Firmer-textured foods to improve movements are then initiated. To develop biting and chewing abilities,

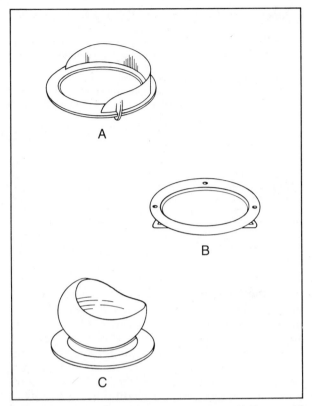

Figure 31–3. Bowls and plates for easier eating. A) Plate guard. B) Suction plate. C) Scooper bowl.

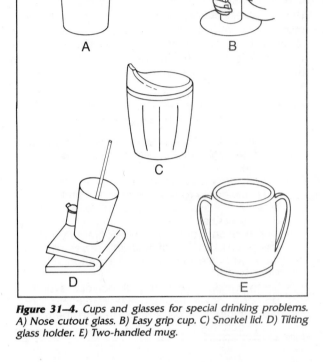

Figure 31–4. Cups and glasses for special drinking problems. A) Nose cutout glass. B) Easy grip cup. C) Snorkel lid. D) Tilting glass holder. E) Two-handled mug.

the individual must be challenged to chew. Games and activities can enhance feeding skills by developing hand-to-mouth movements.

Impaired oral and hand movements are related to insufficient energy intake, but special foods that require less chewing and are easy to swallow can be prepared. In a psychogeriatric unit, more rewarding eating experiences resulted when a variety of soft-textured foods (e.g., soft sandwiches, tomato wedges, sardines, French fries, hard-cooked eggs, ground meat, and casserole dishes) replaced traditional mechanical and pureed diets. These patients had poor hand and finger coordination, tremors, flailing, dysarthria, poor dentition, a high degree of distractibility, and limited concentration (Nangeroni & Pierce, 1984).

WEIGHT CONTROL

The problem observed in physically handicapped persons is most often weight control. Being underweight or overweight is usually related to excessive (spastic) or insufficient (immobile) activity levels as well as types and quantities of food intake. In excessive weights, the ability to walk or to participate in activities is severely restricted, leading to further obesity. Children with spastic-

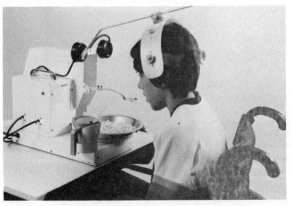

Figure 31–5. Automatic feeder. (Courtesy of Maddak Inc., Pequannock, NJ.)

ity (hypertonia) frequently become overweight even while consuming low-calorie intakes for their ages. In spite of the spasticity, their basal energy expenditure is half that of a normal person (Drum et al, 1981).

Athetoid syndrome, a major complication of cerebral palsy, involves involuntary motor activity that increases energy needs. For example, an athetotic 17-year-old boy needs 6000 kcal to maintain ideal weight for height, but a boy the same age with spastic palsy only needs 1500 kcal. A healthy boy requires 3000 kcal/day (Calvert & Davies, 1977).

Clinical Implications:

- Never use breakable utensils for handicapped children; lightweight articles are easier to handle.
- Parents of handicapped children are particularly vulnerable to persons selling vitamin supplements. Education is imperative to offset these pressures.
- Constipation among developmentally-delayed children is not unusual, especially in those who are hypertonic or hypotonic (see Chapter 27).
- Some children with central nervous system damage never express hunger. Setting an alarm clock can be used to remind them to eat (Pipes, 1981).

Cleft Palate

In the United States, one infant out of every 700 (some 5000 children) is born with a cleft lip or palate each year. "Cleft" describes a split where parts of the upper lip or palate fail to grow together. Scientists believe that any number of factors such as malnutrition, drugs, disease, or heredity may cause this condition (March of Dimes, 1985).

Feeding the infant with a cleft palate, with or without a cleft lip, presents unique problems. It is difficult for a baby to suck, and food backs up through the nose causing choking. Unless the infant is breast-fed, special equipment will be needed. In the beginning a special feeder (like a medicine dropper) may be required. As soon as possible, a bottle should be used; the feeding schedule should be as close to normal as possible. Infants should be held in a sitting position to help prevent the formula from entering the nose.

Table 31–2. Suggestions for Feeding an Infant with Cleft Palate*

- Enlarge the hole in the nipple of the baby's bottle to enable him or her to get milk more easily.
- Boil new nipples prior to use to soften them.
- Thin pureed foods (fruits, vegetables, meats) should be mixed with milk or broth so that they may be fed from a bottle with a nipple with an enlarged hole.
- Frequent burping aids in releasing excessive air intake.
- To prevent regurgitation, the older child should be taught to eat slowly and to take small bites.
- Using a straw helps some children to take liquids more easily.
- Since feeding the child with a cleft palate takes longer than feeding a normal child, the mother needs to allow the necessary time. Fatigue on the part of the parent may interfere with the child's receiving adequate nourishment.

*From Nizel, AE: *Nutrition in Preventive Dentistry Science and Practice*, 2nd ed. Philadelphia, W. B. Saunders Co, 1981.

Patience is required, and extra time for feeding must be provided to assure adequate amounts of nutrients. Parents ordinarily require constant support and reassurance that these children will indeed survive. After surgical repair, the infant needs to be encouraged to catch up with normal chewing development (Nizel, 1981). Table 31–2 offers some suggestions for feeding these infants.

Muscular Dystrophy

Muscular dystrophy affects muscles of the shoulders and face, which may make eating difficult. Decreased levels of potassium and vitamin E are found in these patients. Diet therapy may be directed toward including high intakes of these nutrients; however, dietary measures do not alleviate the course of the condition.

Paraplegics and Amputees

Nutritional guidelines for a paraplegic patient suggest that, just after injury, 15 percent of the usual weight is often lost. A loss of appetite often occurs for about six weeks and may be accompanied by clinical depression. For nonambulatory patients, kilocaloric requirements are 10 to 15 percent less.

Patients with above-the-knee amputations require 25 percent more energy than a normal person walking at the same speed (Wedman, 1983). Energy requirements are higher if the injury is recent or the patient is septic or has decubitus ulcers.

Adequate intake of fluid is essential for the spinal injury patient because urinary infections and/or kidney stones are common. To prevent these problems, patients should have a urinary volume of at least 1500 or 2000 ml/day. To ensure this volume, an intake of 3000 to 4000 ml of fluid is required (Ainsley & Blackburn, 1982).

Osteoporosis

Each year, more than half a million American women develop osteoporosis; 200,000 osteoporotic women over the age of 45 fracture one or more bones; 40,000 die of complications from their injuries; and thousands become seriously disabled for the rest of their lives. Osteoporosis and its complications are the 12th most common cause of death in the United States, and in women, it must be considered a major fatal disease (Winick, 1984). Many different factors may be responsible for osteoporosis (Table 31–3).

Prevention of osteoporosis is an ideal goal that is unattainable for many individuals. For too many women, their future includes decreased height, curved spine, and porous bones (Fig. 31–6). Women are affected more often than men, but all older persons may be susceptible. Resulting fractures can interfere with food purchasing, preparation, and consumption.

NUTRITIONAL CARE AND SUPPLEMENTAL THERAPY

The most important dietary guidelines should begin at birth. All through life, some bone tissue is being formed, particularly calcium stores. However, the largest deposits occur during adolescence, yet few young people realize how important their food intake is for optimal health the rest of their lives. Successful treatment of osteoporosis lies in prevention, so dietary guidelines to decrease its risk are extremely important (Table 31–4).

Calcium. Osteoporosis is a complex, multifactorial disorder related primarily to calcium intake and other influential absorption factors (Parfitt, 1983). An elemental calcium intake of 1000 to 1500

Table 31–3. Risk Factors for Osteoporosis*

Risk Factor	Effects
Sex	Women are 10 times more likely to suffer from severe osteoporosis than men.
Menopause	The earlier menopause occurs the greater the risk. Twenty-five percent of women undergoing natural menopause exhibit osteoporosis in later life. Fifty percent of women having their ovaries removed before natural menopause develop osteoporosis.
Family history	The greater the history of fractures among elderly relatives, especially of the hip and vertebrae, the greater the risk.
Ethnic background	Those of British, Northern European, Chinese, or Japanese extract are at the highest risk. Jewish women are at moderate risk, and Black women are at low risk.
Body build	The smaller the build, the greater the risk.
Body weight	The thinner the person, the higher the risk.
Oral contraceptives	Lower the risk.
Pregnancy	Women who have never been pregnant have an increased risk.
Smoking	Increases the risk.
Alcoholism	Increases the risk.
Cortisone	Increases the risk.
Anticonvulsants	Increase the risk.
Antacids	Antacids containing aluminum increase the risk.
Illness	Hyperparathyroidism, hyperthyroidism, Cushing's syndrome, diabetes, rheumatoid arthritis, kidney disease, and gastrointestinal problems that impair absorption—all increase the risk.

*Courtesy of The Institute of Human Nutrition, Columbia University, New York, NY.

mg/day is considered safe in all persons except those with sarcoidosis, active tuberculosis, or other absorptive hypercalciuric syndromes (Consensus Conference, 1984). Bone mass peaks at about 35 years of age in men and slightly earlier in women (Fish & Dons, 1985). Unless optimum intakes of calcium are available through that period, maxium storage cannot result. Later, intake is provided to maintain bone mass.

Vitamin D. Since vitamin D deficiency contributes to the pathogenesis of hip fractures and other osteoporotic problems, special attention should be given to subjects most likely to need supplementation, i.e., housebound persons or those with malabsorption, gall bladder, gastric resection, or liver problems. Patients recovering

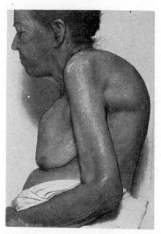

Figure 31—6. *Kyphosis is often a consequence of advanced osteoporosis. (From Delp MH, and Manning RT: Major's Physical Diagnosis, 9th ed. Philadelphia, W. B. Saunders Co, 1981 by permission.)*

from a hip fracture require an average hospital stay of 24 days and have a predicted first-year mortality rate of 20 percent (Fish & Dons, 1985). Calcium absorption requires an adequate supply of vitamin D. The minimum RDA (400 IU) is sufficient early in life, but the vitamin D requirement increases with age, and a supply of 600 to 800 IU (15 to 20 mcg) is recommended later (Dattani et al, 1984).

Estrogen. Estrogen enhances absorption of calcium (Heaney, 1982) and prevents accelerated bone loss occurring after menopause. Yet, the controversy over the influence of estrogen supplementation increasing the risk of endometrial cancer reappears from time to time. The present consensus recommends 0.625 mg/day of conjugated equine estrogen (Premarin) taken cyclically for 25 days and five days without. A small percentage of women are advised to take the conjugated equine estrogen from Day 1 through Day 25 with the addition of progestational agents, such as medroxy-

progesterone acetate (Amen and Provera), to induce endometrial shedding from Day 16 through Day 25 (Fish & Dons, 1985; Heaney, 1982).

Fluoride. Fewer fractures have occurred in several communities that fluoridate the water supply. Controversy exists over additional supplementation of fluoride. If it is included in the prescription for the susceptible osteoporotic patient, 40 to 60 mg/day of sodium fluoride is advised (Heaney et al, 1982). Toxic reactions from fluoride are not well understood, but gastrointestinal complaints and rheumatic symptoms are the most common problems. Even more important, since increased fluoride results in faster bone replenishment, spurs may occur. At this time, fluoride supplementation above the levels in fluoridated water is not recommended.

Clinical Implications:

- Excessive vitamin D intake may result in hypercalcemia and extraosseous calcification, particularly in the kidney, leading to chronic renal failure. Significant hypercalcemia is highly variable between individuals, but it rarely results from less than 1000 IU/day of vitamin D (Parfitt et al, 1982).
- Though a low-fat, high-fiber diet reduces risks of heart disease and certain cancers, the risk of osteoporosis may increase (Risk of bone disease, 1984).
- Adequate amounts of calcium and vitamin D are required throughout life to prevent osteoporosis even though restrictive diets (weight reduction) are consumed (Lee et al, 1981).

Table 31—4. *Principles of a Diet Designed to Lower Risks of Osteoporosis**

- Adequate calories to attain and/or maintain ideal weight.
- A calcium intake of 1 gm (1000 mg) per day (1500 mg during periods of high calcium need such as adolescence, pregnancy, and lactation).
- A relatively low phosphorus intake.
- A relatively low protein intake.
- Avoidance of excess dietary sodium.
- Adequate but not excessive amounts of vitamin D (not over 400 IU).

*Courtesy of The Institute of Human Nutrition, Columbia University, New York, NY.

Common Types of Rheumatic Disease

Arthritis has been called "everybody's disease" because it will affect everyone directly or indirectly, sooner or later. The word arthritis literally means joint inflammation (*arthron*, joint; *-itis*, inflammation) and refers to more than 100 related rheumatic diseases.

Arthritis is America's number one crippling disease affecting one in seven people, or one in every three families. A million people develop arthritis each year. Arthritis is second only to heart problems as the cause of disability payments (Arthritis Foundation, 1984).

Of the various forms of arthritis that belong to the larger group of rheumatic diseases, only three have nutritional implications—rheumatoid arthritis, osteoarthritis, and gout.

RHEUMATOID ARTHRITIS

Rheumatoid arthritis is an autoimmune, systemic disease involving chronic inflammation and destruction that begins in the synovial membrane of the joints and spreads to other joints (Fig. 31–7). These outgrowths of the inflamed tissue may invade and damage the cartilage and deform the shape of the joints. Using adaptive equipment is especially beneficial for these persons to protect their bodies against pain and further destruction.

Nutritional Care. Renewed interest in dietary factors in arthritis has occurred because of reports that some patients appear to have alleviated their symptoms by means of diet (Ratner et al, 1985). The role of food in the management of rheumatoid arthritis is controversial and has not been defined at this time. However, studies are being conducted to explore this possibility. Significant improvement, e.g., a reduced number of tender joints and shorter duration of morning stiffness, appears among many patients who follow specific regimens for weight loss (Coughlan & Hazleman, 1986).

Some patients have improved on diets high in polyunsaturated fat supplemented with eicosapentaenoic acid similar to the diet for cardiovascular disease (Kremer et al, 1985). Other studies refute this theory, even though their subjects' pain assessment worsened when they returned to their usual diet (Hart, 1985).

One of the most popular notions restricts foods that might cause allergic reactions, which in turn, would aggravate the arthritis. Universally, subjects have significantly improved during the fasting periods at the beginning of these regimens (Darlington, et al, 1986), but then the results vary. Foods most likely to cause allergies are introduced one at a time for observations. Typical foods such as eggs, milk, beef, and wheat as well as fruits and vegetables from the nightshade family (tomatoes, eggplants, potatoes, and peppers) have been implicated.

At this time, there is no specific valid diet for patients with the various forms of arthritis, but the goals are to: (1) maintain ideal body weight, (2) consume balanced diets for the best quality of life, and (3) preserve the integrity of immune responses. Vitamin E and zinc are of primary importance in this last regard, yet they are often be-

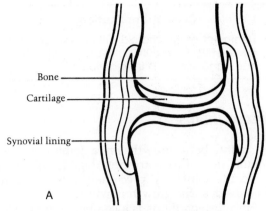

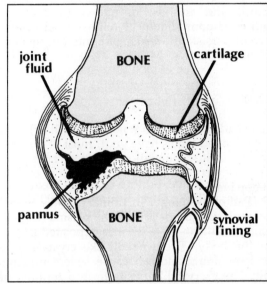

Figure 31–7. Normal joint and joint pathology in rheumatoid arthritis. A) Normal joint. B) The joint inflamed: Cartilage, which protects bone ends in a joint, is eaten away and destroyed in the area of inflammation by enzymes from various sources, and by substances released from cells (pannus). (From Arthritis Medical Information Series, Osteoarthritis, Arthritis Foundation, by permission.)

low the RDAs in patients with rheumatoid arthritis, an immunologically-mediated disease (Panush, 1983).

Surveys have found that many patients with arthritis consume diets at least marginally inadequate in several other essential nutrients, e.g., folacin, vitamin B_6, pantothenic acid, calcium, magnesium, and carbohydrate (Kowsari et al, 1983). The disabilities and chronic diseases of these patients probably interfere with their nutritional status because of physical limitations and even depressed emotions.

Clinical Implication:

- Treatment of rheumatoid arthritis with massive doses (150,000 to 500,000 IU/day) of vitamin D has led to vitamin D intoxication.

OSTEOARTHRITIS

Painful bony growths in a joint may be a common sign of osteoarthritis (Fig. 31–8). An injury to the joint may precipitate this. After the pain subsides, the growth remains.

Since osteoarthritis is a combination of osteoporosis and arthritis, nutritional guidelines for both conditions should be followed. Also, avoidance of persistent overuse of joints can be beneficial in prevention.

GOUT

Nearly two million (eight out of 1000) people in the United States have gout, most of whom are men (Arthritis Foundation, 1983). Women rarely have this very painful form of arthritis until after menopause.

Pathophysiology. In primary gout, excessive accumulation of uric acid in the plasma (hyperuricemia) results in urate crystals deposited throughout the body. These needle-like crystals irritate the joint lining and can cause severe inflammation. These crystal deposits form a tophus, or a nodular deposit (Fig. 31–9). The joint in the big toe is affected in three out of four people, but any

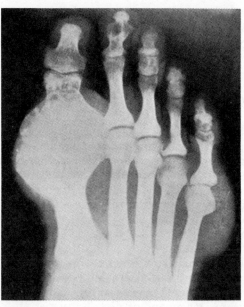

Figure 31–9. Deposit of sodium urate crystals from tophi in the big toe. Gouty involvement of the bones of the first metatarsophalangeal joint simulating a bone tumor. (Bondy PK, Rosenberg LE: Metabolic Control and Disease, 8th ed, Philadelphia, W. B. Saunders Co, 1980, by permission.)

joint may be involved (Arthritis Foundation, 1983).

Uric acid is the end product of purine (a nucleic acid) metabolism, which is normally passed through the kidneys into the urine. About 10 to 20 percent of gout patients have uric acid kidney stones (Luckmann & Sorenson, 1980).

The objectives of treatment include prevention of acute attacks, progressive disability from erosion of bone and joint cartilage, and progressive renal dysfunction. In patients with chronic gout, progressive renal dysfunction is the greatest threat to life (Luckmann & Sorenson, 1980).

Nutritional Care. Gout is the only rheumatic disease that has been helped by avoiding certain foods, yet this is a controversial matter. However, the single, most important dietary recommendation is for the patient to drink large volumes of fluids.

Drug therapy is the main treatment for gout, but in cases where the drug is less effective, diet may be important. Serum uric acid levels generally decrease from 0.5 to 1.5 mg/100 ml in patients on diets permitting up to 1 gm of protein per kilogram of ideal body weight (Talbott & Yu, 1976).

A purine-restricted diet may be prescribed in certain instances. Foods highest in purines are or-

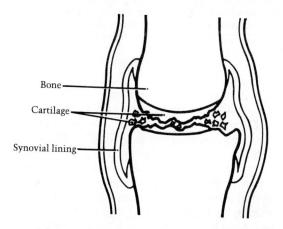

Figure 31–8. Joint with osteoarthritis. (From Arthritis Medical Information Series, Osteoarthritis, Arthritis Foundation, by permission.)

Bone

Cartilage

Synovial lining

Table 31–5. Dietary Guidelines for the Treatment of Gout

1. The diet should be low in fat; a high-fat diet increases the frequency of acute attacks.
2. Obese patients should follow a nutritionally-balanced weight reduction program. The course of their gout may be favorably influenced by a slow steady weight loss. Fasting is recognized as a precipitating factor of acute attacks and should be avoided since it produces a metabolic situation comparable to that of a high-fat diet.
3. A high intake of liquids will lessen the incidence of kidney stones and prevent the dehydration associated with anti-gout medications. A minimum of 2 qt./day of water and fruit juices is advised.
4. Purine and protein intakes are not rigidly restricted, but a high-protein diet does accelerate gout. Limiting protein to 50 to 75 gm/day with most of it in the form of plant and dairy products is often recommended.

gan meats, anchovies, sardines, meat extracts, gravy, broth, and bouillon. Severe limitations on protein and purine content are rarely necessary or even of value.

Diet is less effective than it might be because it decreases only exogenous sources of nucleoproteins, which account for less than half the uric acid found in the blood. It does not appreciably affect the endogenous production of uric acid from available compounds such as carbon dioxide, ammonia, and glycine, which may also be synthesized into uric acid (ADA, 1981).

Excessive drinking of alcoholic beverages may precipitate attacks of gout. Large quantities of alcohol result in accumulation of lactic acid, which inhibits the renal secretion of urates (Salmon et al, 1982). When fasting is added to the increased alcoholic intake, the effects are multiplied. Yet, alcohol diluted with water and taken in moderation (not more than 100 gm/day) with food is acceptable. Complete abstinence is not required (Table 31–5).

Clinical Implications

- Hyperuricemia is correlated to alcohol abuse in male subjects (Drum et al, 1981).
- Acute medical or surgical illnesses may necessitate involuntary fasting for gout patients. Under these conditions, a high-carbohydrate intake is important as well as adequate fluids, even if parenteral fluids are necessary.
- Three-day diaries may help identify those who could benefit from more stringent dietary measures. Kilocalories, protein, purine, and oxalate content can be evaluated in hyperuricosuria (ADA, 1981).

• FALLACIES and FACTS

FALLACY: A person with gout should not drink coffee, tea, or cocoa because they contain the methylxanthines, theobromine, theophylline, and caffeines.
- **FACT:** Formerly, it was believed that the methylxanthines were converted to uric acid. Further investigation has shown that they are metabolized to methyl urates, not urates, and are not deposited in the gouty tophus. They may be included in the diet for a patient with gout (ADA, 1981).

FALLACY: Gout is a special kind of arthritis caused by "high living" with too much food and drink.
- **FACT:** Gout is an inherited defect in body chemistry. Overeating and over indulgence in alcohol can trigger attacks, but they are not the basic cause.

FALLACY: Wear copper bracelets to cure arthritis.
- **FACT:** This is a popular gimmick that has no scientific basis.

Summary

Individuals who are physically handicapped either temporarily or permanently face unique obstacles each time they eat. Independence in caring for oneself increases self-esteem and pride. Food intake is improved. Many types of apparatuses are available to help in food preparation and eating. Not only can this equipment improve food intake, but the use of it can delay further harm to joints and tissues. Less pain is present with utensils that avoid pressure and strain.

Nutritional education is important to allow these individuals to maintain their own physical well-being. Nutrient intake should be close to normal within the related restrictions.

Maintaining ideal body weight reduces strain on joints, but some handicapped persons may find this difficult.

Often the time and energy required for meal preparations are enormous, yet special attention should be given to making mealtimes pleasant.

Satisfaction of hunger should be accompanied by enjoyment of interpersonal relationships.

Review Questions

1. What dietary recommendations would you offer a person who has gout?
2. Define osteoporosis, osteomalacia, and osteoarthritis.
3. Describe various equipment available to help the handicapped person eat without assistance.
4. List suggestions to develop feeding skills for persons unable to suck, chew, and swallow.
5. List suggestions to develop feeding skills for persons unable to grasp and who are uncoordinated in hand-to-mouth motions.

Case Study: Mrs. S.T., a 78-year-old female, suffered a cerebrovascular accident (CVA) three months ago. Her condition was stabilized, and she is being transferred to a long-term care facility. She is noted to have impaired control over the muscles needed for chewing, swallowing, and movement of the tongue. She also has a decreased visual field. Her dominant hand is on the affected side, and her nondominant hand has limited movement because of osteoarthritis. Mrs. S. T. chokes and coughs during the meal. She has lost an effective gag reflex and aspirates food and saliva. Over the past few weeks, Mrs. S.T. has appeared increasingly frustrated with her eating difficulties and her inability to communicate effectively with staff members.

1. What effect does the diminished visual field and tactile sensation have on swallowing?
2. What additional information should you gather from the family members?
3. Identify a nursing diagnosis and a goal for this patient.
4. What are some of the mechanical devices appropriate for this patient?
5. As you plan Mrs. S.T.'s care, what nursing interventions will facilitate feeding and reduce the incidence of complications?
6. Why is oral hygiene so important for this patient?

REFERENCE LIST

Ainsley, BM; Blackburn, GL: Nutritional needs of paraplegic patients. *JAMA* 248(17):2180, 1982.

American Dietetic Association (ADA): *Handbook of Clinical Dietetics*. New Haven, Yale University Press, 1981.

Arthritis: A Serious Look at the Facts. Atlanta, Arthritis Foundation, 1984.

Arthritis Basic Facts. Atlanta, Arthritis Foundation, 1983.

Calvert, A; Davies, F: Nutrition of children with handicapping conditions. *Dietetic Currents* 4(3), 1977.

Consensus Conference: Osteoporosis. *JAMA* 353(6):799, 1984.

Coughlan, RJ; Hazleman, BL: Dietary manipulation in rheumatoid arthritis. *Lancet* 1(February 22):442, 1986.

Darlington, LG; Ramsey, NW; Mansfield, JR: Placebo-controlled, blind study of dietary manipulation therapy in rheumatoid arthritis. *Lancet* 1(February 1):236, 1986.

Dattani, JT; Exton-Smith, AN; Stephen, JML: Vitamin D status of the elderly in relation to age and exposure to sunlight. *Hum Nutr Clin Nutr* 38C(2):131, 1984.

Drum, De; Goldman, PA; Jankowski, CB: Elevation of serum uric acid as a clue to alcohol abuse. *Arch Intern Med* 141(3):477, 1981.

Fish, HR; Dons, RF: Primary osteoporosis. *Am Fam Physician* 31(1):216, 1985.

Hart, FD: Dietary fatty acids and rheumatoid arthritis. *Lancet* 1(March 23):699, 1985.

Kowsari, SKF; Finnie, SK; Carter, RL; et al: Assessment of the diet of patients with rheumatoid arthritis and osteoarthritis. *J Am Diet Assoc* 82(6):657, 1983.

Kremer, JM; Michalek, AV; Lininger, L; et al: Effects of manipulation of dietary fatty acids on clinical manifestations of rheumatoid arthritis. *Lancet* 1(January 26):184, 1985.

Lee, CJ; Lawler, GS; Johnson, GH: Effects of supplementation of the diets with calcium and calcium-rich foods on bone density of elderly females with osteoporosis. *Am J Clin Nutr* 34(5):819, 1981.

Luckmann, J; Sorensen, KC: *Medical-Surgical Nursing: A Psychophysiologic Approach*, 2nd ed. Philadelphia, W.B. Saunders Co, 1980.

March of Dimes: *Cleft Lip and Palate*. Birth Defects Foundation 5, 1985.

Nangeroni, JB; Pierce, PS: Development of a geriatric diet through behavioral observation of feeding behaviors of regressed and severely demented patients. *J Nutr Elderly* 3(2):25, 1983.

Nizel, AE: *Nutrition in Preventive Dentistry Science and Practice*, 2nd ed. Philadelphia, W.B. Saunders Co, 1981.

Panush, RS; Carter, R; Katz, P; et al: Diet therapy for rheumatoid arthritis. *Arthritis Rheum* 26(4):462, 1983.

Parfitt, AM: Dietary risk factors for age-related bone loss and fractures. *Lancet* 2(November 19):1181, 1983.

Pipes, PL: *Nutrition in Infancy and Childhood*. St Louis, C.V. Mosby Co, 1981.

Ratner, D; Eshel, E; Schneeyour, A; et al: Does milk intolerance affect seronegative arthritis in lactase-deficient women? *Israel J Med Sciences* 21:532, 1985.

Risk of bone disease with low fat, high fiber diets. *J Am Diet Assoc* 84(5):531, 1984.

Salmon, SE; Schrier, RW; Smith, LH: Hyperuricemia pathogenesis and treatment. *Calif Med* 116(6):38, 1982.

Shinnar, SE: Use of adaptive equipment in feeding the elderly. *J Am Diet Assoc* 83(3):321, 1983.

Talbott, JH; Yu, TF: *Gout and Uric Acid Metabolism*. New York, Stratton Intercontinental Medical Book Corp, 1976.

Watkin, DM: Nutrition for the aging and the aged. In *Modern Nutrition in Health and Disease*, 6th ed. Edited by RS Goodhart; ME Shils. Philadelphia, Lea & Febiger, 1980, p. 781.

Wedman, B: Nutrition for the amputee. *Diab Ed* 8(4):29, 1983.

Winick, M: Osteoporosis. *Nutr Health* 6(1), 1984.

Resources:

Albanese, AA; Calcium in the prevention and management of osteoporosis in the elderly. *J Nutr Elderly* 3(3):57, 1984.

Davidson, A; Van Der Weyde, MB; Fong, H; et al: Red cell ferritin content: A re-evaluation of indices for iron deficiency in the anaemia of rheumatoid arthritis. *Br Med J* 289(September 15):648, 1984.

Davies, R; Saha, S: Osteoporosis. *Am Fam Physician* 32(5):107, 1985.

Do It Yourself Again: Self-Help Devices for the Stroke Patient. Dallas, American Heart Association.

Horsman, A; Jones, M; Francis, R; et al: The effect of estrogen dose on postmenopausal bone loss. *N Engl J Med* 309(23):1405, 1983.

Jones, AM: Overcoming the feeding problems of the mentally and the physically handicapped. *J Human Nutr* 32(5):359, 1978.

Lockshin, MD: The unproven remedies committee. *Arthritis Rheum* 24(9):1188, 1981.

Notelovitz, M; Ware, M: *Stand Tall: The Informed Woman's Guide to Preventing Osteoporosis.* Gainesville, FL, Triad Publishing, 1982.

Panush, RS; Carter, R; Katz, P; et al: Diet therapy for rheumatoid arthritis. *Arthritis Rheum* 26(4):462, 1983.

Pensis, NT; Maloney, MA: *Mealtimes for People with Handicaps: A Guide for Parents, Paraprofessionals, and Allied Health Professionals.* Springfield, IL, Charles C. Thomas, 1983.

Robinson, WD: Nutrition and rheumatoid diseases. In *Textbook of Rheumatology.* Edited by WN Kelley; ED Haria; S Ruddy; et al. Philadelphia, W.B. Saunders Co, 1980.

Selley, WG; Boxall, J: A new way to treat sucking and swallowing difficulties in babies. *Lancet* 1 (May 28):1192, 1986.

Wainwright, H: Feeding problems in elderly disabled patients. *Nurs Times* 34(13):542, 1978.

Weber, B: Eating with a trach. *Am J Nurs* 74(8):1439, 1974.

Resources:
Arthritis Foundation
1314 Spring
Atlanta, GA 30309

Nutrition and Feeding Techniques for Handicapped Children
Developmental Disabilities Program
California Department of Health
Sacramento, CA 95814

Adaptive equipment available from:
Abbey Medical Catalog
13782 Crenshaw Blvd.
Gardena, CA 90249

Maddak, Inc.
Pequannock, NJ 07440-1993

Fred Sammons, Inc.
Bissel Healthcare
145 Tower Drive
Burr Ridge, IL 60521

Swedish Rehabilitation Products Corp.
17 Briar Cliff Drive
Scotch Plains, NJ 07076

Dietary Management of Cardiovascular Disease

32

THE STUDENT WILL BE ABLE TO:

- *Identify and discuss the dietary management of all five types of hyperlipoproteinemia.*
- *Plan a day's menus using the recommendations for a Prudent Diet.*
- *Identify methods of reducing cholesterol in the body.*
- *Name factors that modify the high-density lipoproteins in the blood.*
- *List guidelines for managing hypertension without drugs.*

TERMS TO KNOW

Apoprotein
Arteriosclerosis
Atherosclerosis
Cardiovascular disease
Cholesterol/saturated-fat index (CSI)
Coronary heart disease (CHD)
Eicosapentaenoic acid (EPA)
High-density lipoproteins (HDL)
Hypercholesterolemia
Hyperlipidemia
Hyperlipoproteinemia
Hypertriglyceridemia
Ischemia
Myocardial Infarction
National Heart, Lung, and Blood Institute (NHLBI)
Very low-density lipoproteins (VLDL)
Xanthoma

Cardiovascular disease is still the leading cause of death in the United States. Its major form is coronary heart disease (CHD); other cardiovascular disorders include stroke, hypertension, peripheral vascular disease, rheumatic heart disease, and congenital heart disease. Nearly one fourth of all persons who die from cardiovascular disease are under age 65.

As many as 1.5 million Americans may have a heart attack this year and about 550,000 of them will die (American Heart Association, 1985). Approximately $60 billion are spent on direct and indirect costs from CHD in the United States each year (Lowering blood, 1985). Yet, nutritional intervention can play a significant role in alleviating some of these problems.

Coronary Heart Disease

The cause of CHD is atherosclerosis, which is caused by an accumulation of fatty materials (such as cholesterol) within and upon the smooth inner walls of the medium and larger arteries (Fig. 32–1). Atherosclerosis occurs particularly in the coronary arteries. As this plaque thickens, the artery becomes progressively narrow and rough, and the flow of blood, which carries oxygen and nutrients, may be disrupted. Arteries afflicted with atherosclerosis may gradually become thickened and less elastic, a condition called arteriosclerosis.

An artery may become blocked from atherosclerosis or thrombosis (a blood clot); damage occurs from the lack of oxygen to the part of the body supplied by the blocked artery (ischemia). In the heart, this results in a sudden chest pain (angina pectoris); complete occlusion leads to myocardial infarction, and sometimes death. If it occurs in an artery supplying the brain, a stroke results. Occlusion of a leg artery causes claudication (pain and lameness) and gangrene. Occlusion of the renal arteries may cause hypertension and poor renal function.

Risk Factors. Certain risk factors cannot be eliminated, but some may be changed to significantly reduce the incidence of CHD. Since the United States has 10 times the rate of CHD as Japan, modifying risk factors may be the key to prevention (NHLBI, 1979), as shown in Figure 32–2. The three most important risk factors are hypertension, cigarette smoking, and elevated serum cholesterol. Heredity is a risk factor that cannot be

controlled; however, individuals from families in which heart disease is common can follow a preventive diet. Other risk factors include diabetes mellitus, hypertriglyceridemia, obesity, a sedentary lifestyle, and stress. Diet can be manipulated to alter several of the risk factors: obesity, hypercholesterolemia and hypertriglyceridemia, and hypertension. Basic dietary interventions may include: (1) weight reduction via kilocalorie restriction and exercise, (2) modification of fat intake either by type or percentage, and/or (3) sodium restriction among salt-sensitive patients.

ELEVATED SERUM LIPIDS AND CHD

Hypercholesterolemia. Clinical atherosclerosis seldom occurs with lifelong serum cholesterol concentrations below 200 mg/dl. Generally, hypercholesterolemia is a serum cholesterol in excess of 260 mg/dl. At a serum cholesterol level of 260 mg/dl, the risk for developing CHD is about twice that of persons with a serum level lower than 210 mg/dl (Kannel et al, 1971). Normal ranges for serum cholesterol and other forms of cholesterol are shown in Table 32–1. Ideally, total blood cholesterol should be determined on all children before adulthood to prevent CHD (Paige, 1983).

An elevated serum cholesterol has been implicated in CHD for many years. Even though hypercholesterolemia is considered one of the three most significant risk factors for CHD, other factors may play more important roles. Only one fourth of all high-risk persons have increased total cholesterol levels; other diseases, particularly diabetes and hypertension, apparently are more influential than hypercholesterolemia (Hager, 1983).

Many studies, including the Framingham Study (Dawber, 1980), have proved that hypercholesterolemia is a good predictor of the development of atherosclerosis. The Multiple Risk Factor Intervention Trial (MRFIT) found that controlling certain risk factors (hypertension and cigarette smoking) and lowering blood cholesterol through dietary intervention did not reduce CHD mortality for many individuals (MRFIT Research Group, 1982).

Results from a 10-year study called the Lipid Research Clinic's Coronary Primary Prevention Trial (LRC-CPPT) determined that CHD can be reduced in men at high risk for CHD by reducing serum total cholesterol using diet and drugs. Therefore, the Consensus Development Panel (1985) concluded that (1) individuals with high and moderate-risk blood cholesterol levels should be treated intensively by diet and/or drugs, and (2) all Americans should be advised to change dietary habits to lower blood cholesterol levels. This conclusion is in line with the recommendations from the American Heart Association.

This conclusion has stirred considerable controversy in the scientific community. Since the study involved men 35 to 59 years old with very high cholesterol levels, it is questionable whether the benefits observed in this study can be expected for men, women, and children with lower plasma cholesterol levels (two thirds of the population) (Ahrens, 1985).

Hypertriglyceridemia. Current data do not prove that treatment of hypertriglyceridemia is always effective in reducing CHD. Elevated triglyceride levels can be reached or normalized by dietary means and/or medication.

When evaluating triglyceride levels, other lipid values are important. If cholesterol levels are normal, then mild elevations of plasma triglyceride levels do not necessarily increase CHD risk. Triglyceride levels less than 250 mg/dl do not necessarily increase the risk of CHD if serum cholesterol is normal. Triglyceride levels in the range of 250 to 500 mg/dl indicate patients who are at increased risk and need specific therapy (Consensus Conference, 1984). Hypertriglyceridemia is almost always associated with reduced HDL and often with increased plasma cholesterol. If dietary management is not successful, drugs are prescribed.

CLASSIFICATION OF HYPERLIPIDEMIA

Four different types of lipoproteins transport lipids in the blood; each contains triglycerides,

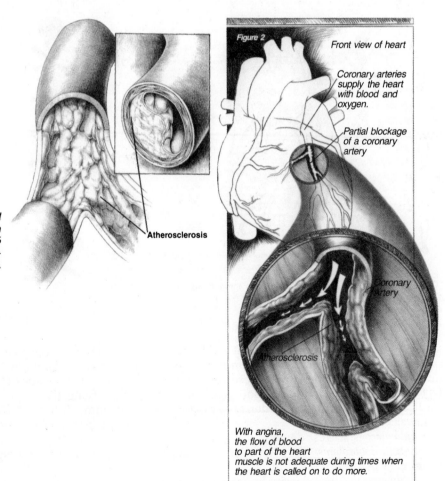

Figure 32–1. Diagram of the natural history of atherosclerosis. (From American Heart Association: 1986 Heart Facts. American Heart Association, National Center, Dallas, TX, 1985, by permission.)

Atherosclerosis

Figure 2

Front view of heart

Coronary arteries supply the heart with blood and oxygen.

Partial blockage of a coronary artery

Coronary Artery

Atherosclerosis

With angina, the flow of blood to part of the heart muscle is not adequate during times when the heart is called on to do more.

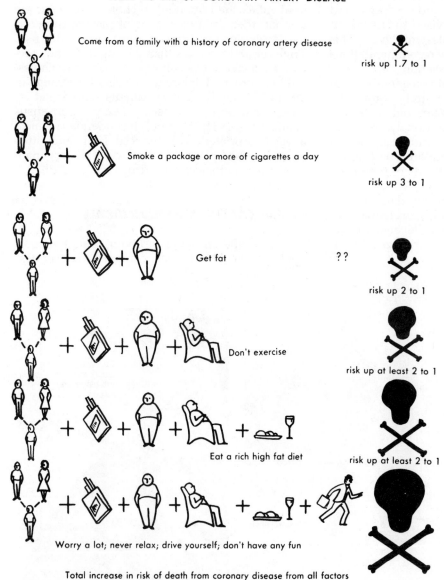

Figure 32–2. Risk factors in coronary artery disease. (From Griffith GC, Phibbs B: Coronary artery disease, in Phibbs B (ed): The Human Heart, 4th ed. St. Louis, The C. V. Mosby Co, 1979, by permission.)

HOW TO DIE OF CORONARY ARTERY DISEASE

Come from a family with a history of coronary artery disease — risk up 1.7 to 1

Smoke a package or more of cigarettes a day — risk up 3 to 1

Get fat — ?? — risk up 2 to 1

Don't exercise — risk up at least 2 to 1

Eat a rich high fat diet — risk up at least 2 to 1

Worry a lot; never relax; drive yourself; don't have any fun

Total increase in risk of death from coronary disease from all factors at least 10 to 1 (may be more like 30 to 1)

phospholipids, and cholesterol that are bound to protein. The ratio of lipid to protein in the serum lipoprotein varies widely, and these variations affect their density. Therefore, lipoproteins may be classified according to their density, ranging as follows:

1. *Chylomicrons:* lowest density.
2. *Pre-beta-lipoproteins:* very low-density lipoproteins (VLDL).
3. *Beta-lipoproteins:* low-density lipoproteins (LDL).
4. *Alpha-lipoproteins:* high-density lipoproteins (HDL) with the largest amount of protein.

Hyperlipoproteinemia is the term used for abnormal levels of any of the lipoproteins. Fredrickson and colleagues (1967) developed a system for classifying five types of hyperlipoproteinemia to distinguish the individual causes and identify the appropriate treatment. Table 32–2 summarizes the characteristics of these types of hyperlipoproteinemic disorders, and Figure 32–3 shows planar xanthomas in hyperlipidemia.

Chylomicrons, formed in the intestine to transport absorbed dietary fat, carry some cholesterol, and 90 percent of the triglycerides. Hyper-

Table 32–1. Normal Limits for Fasting Cholesterol,
Triglycerides, and LDL and HDL Cholesterol*

| | Age (yrs) | Cholesterol (mg/dl) | | | Triglycerides (mg/dl)† |
		Total†	LDL†	HDL‡	
Males (white)	10–14	202	132	37	125
	15–19	197	130	30	148
	20–24	218	147	30	201
	25–29	244	165	31	249
	30–34	254	185	28	266
	35–39	270	189	29	321
	40–44	268	186	27	320
	45–49	276	202	30	327
	50–54	277	197	28	320
	55–59	276	203	28	286
	60–64	276	210	30	291
Females (white)	10–14	201	136	37	131
	15–19	200	135	35	124
	20–24	216	136	37	131
	25–29	222	151	37	145
	30–34	231	150	38	151
	35–39	242	172	34	176
	40–44	252	174	33	191
	45–49	265	187	33	214
	50–54	285	215	37	233
	55–59	300	213	36	262
	60–64	297	234	36	239

*From U.S. Department of Health and Human Services. Public Health Service, National Institute of Health, Lipid Metabolism Branch, NHLBI: The Lipid Research Clinics. Population Studies Data Book, Vol 1. Bethesda, NIH Publication No. 80-1527, 1980. Normal ranges for blacks have not been defined.
†95th percentile.
‡5th percentile.

chylomicronemia is a natural phenomenon dependent upon the fat content of each meal. Normally, hyperchylomicronemia peaks three to four hours after the intake of fat and is cleared within 12 to 14 hours unless more fat is consumed. However, in the Type I disorder, the body is unable to clear chylomicrons normally from the blood. Type I is extremely rare and familial.

Most of the remainder of the triglycerides (and some cholesterol) are found in the VLDL. It is felt that these are the endogenous triglycerides being transported from the liver. VLDL will release their triglycerides to the tissues and the remainder is LDL. LDL, after releasing their triglycerides, are principally cholesterol. Cholesterol transported by LDL may infiltrate the arterial intima and contribute to the atherosclerotic process.

The most important but smallest group of lipoproteins are the HDL. They contain moderate amounts of cholesterol. However, this cholesterol is being transported to the liver for catabolism and excretion, and may have a protective effect (Mat-

tective effect (Matter et al, 1980). Thus, it is felt that elevated levels of HDL and low levels of LDL and serum cholesterol are the best preventive measures for coronary heart disease.

DIETARY FACTORS AFFECTING SERUM LIPIDS

Several dietary factors may be used to lower serum cholesterol and triglyceride levels. The amount and type of fat and fiber content may be particularly significant factors to consider. Weight reduction may also be effective.

Cholesterol. Modifying fat intake has a greater effect upon lowering hypercholesteremia than lowering dietary cholesterol. In a study with normolipemic healthy subjects, the addition of three eggs (1500 mg of cholesterol) to their normal diet did not significantly affect serum cholesterol levels (Flynn et al, 1986).

If a high intake of cholesterol (300 mg/1000 kcal) is reduced by half, only a slight reduction in

Table 32–2. Classification of Hyperlipidemia*

Type and Prevalance	Appearance of Plasma on Overnight Refrigeration	Major Fraction Elevated		Clinical Manifestations (Signs and Symptoms)	Risk of Coronary Artery Disease	Other Features
		Lipid†	Lipoprotein			
I: Familial hyperchylomicro-nemia—rare	Creamy layer over clear infranatant	TG	Chylomicrons	Bouts of abdominal pain, hepatosplenomegaly, eruptive xanthomas; recurrent pancreatitis.	Normal	Deficient lipoprotein lipase activity causes inability to utilize dietary fat. Symptoms begin in infancy or childhood.
IIA: Familial hypercholesterolemia—common	Clear	CH	LDL	Tendinous and tuberous xanthomas; corneal arcus, xanthelasma.	Very high	A small fraction of these individuals have a genetic form, familial hypercholesterolemia, which is inherited as an autosomal dominant trait and can be diagnosed at birth.
IIB: Familial combined hyperlipidemia—common	Clear or cloudy	CH TG	LDL and VLDL			
III: Familial combined hyperlipidemia—uncommon	Clear or cloudy	CH TG	LDL; abnormal "broad beta" lipoprotein	Palmar xanthomas; risk of peripheral vascular disease is high.	Very high	Obesity and abnormal glucose tolerance are common. Abnormal conversion of VLDL to LDL.
IV: Familial endogenous hyper-triglyceridemia—common	Clear or grossly cloudy	TG	VLDL		Uncertain	Obesity and abnormal glucose tolerance are common. Usually not manifested until early adulthood.
V: Mixed hyperlipidemia—uncommon	Creamy layer over cloudy infra-natant	TG	Chylomicrons and VLDL	Bouts of abdominal pain, hepatomegaly, eruptive xanthomas; recurrent pancreatitis.	Normal	Sensitive to dietary fat. Obesity and abnormal glucose tolerance are common. Symptoms begin in adult life.

*Walser, M; Imbembo, AL; Margolis, S; et al: *Nutritional Management: The Johns Hopkins Handbook.* Philadelphia, W. B. Saunders Co, 1984, with permission.

†TG = Triglycerides; CH = cholesterol.

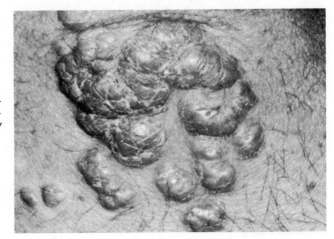

Figure 32–3. *Planar xanthomas in patient with Type III hyperlipidemia. (From Rifkind BM, Levy RI:* Hyperlipidemia Diagnosis and Therapy. *New York: Grune & Stratton, 1977, p 142, by permission.)*

total serum cholesterol occurs. But, if saturated fatty acid intake is reduced by half (from 18 percent of total kilocalories) and if these calories are replaced with carbohydrates, cholesterol is reduced by one third. If both cholesterol and fat intakes are lowered, serum cholesterol will decrease even more.

Type of Fat. The level of saturated fats should be decreased to about 10 percent of the total kilocalories and polyunsaturated fatty acids (PUFA) should supply about 10 percent. (Excessive intakes of PUFA have been linked to cancer.) A 2:1 (or 2:2) P/S ratio is recommended. Even small changes in the P/S ratio may have a general cholesterol-lowering effect (Jackson et al, 1984).

The remainder of the ingested fat is derived from monounsaturated sources, such as olive, canola, and peanut oils, which have previously been considered neutral in CHD. However, recent studies indicate monounsaturated fats may be significant in lowering cholesterol and in protecting against harmful blood clots (Mattson & Grundy, 1985).

Cholesterol/Saturated-Fat Index (CSI). To understand the combined hypercholesterolemic and atherogenic effects of cholesterol and saturated fat in the diet, a new index called cholesterol/saturated-fat index (CSI) has been calculated (Connor et al, 1986). By adding both of these factors together, each food is given a number to express its total effect. Lower numbers denote less atherogenicity of the food.

For example, shellfish (shrimp, crab, and lobster) are high in cholesterol but low in saturated fat. Shellfish have a low CSI index because the saturated fat content is very low, despite a high cholesterol content. Using this method, shellfish with a CSI of six are the same as poultry; beef, ranging from a CSI of 9 to 18, is less preferable than shellfish. Even though salmon has a higher fat content than shellfish, it is lower in cholesterol, so it has a CSI of five. Thus salmon has a lower hypercholesterolemic and atherogenic potential than red meat. Table 32–3 shows the CSI and kilocalorie content of selected foods. Traditional menus can be modified to reduce saturated fat and cholesterol levels, as shown in Table 32–4.

Fiber. Some plant fibers, especially the soluble carbohydrates (pectin and guar gum) found in apples, citrus fruit, legumes, oats, and barley, can have significant hypocholesterolemic effects (Hodges & Rebello, 1985). It is felt that these substances may bind with bile acids, causing the cholesterol to be excreted or converted into bile acids. Patients consuming about 140 gm of beans and 41 gm of oat bran per day not only have reduced serum cholesterol concentrations but also lowered LDL cholesterol and raised HDL concentrations (Anderson et al, 1984). Earlier studies with dried beans only lowered serum cholesterol, without as much effect on the low- or high-density lipoprotein cholesterol levels (Jenkins et al, 1983).

Triglyceride levels are also consistently lower among populations who habitually consume approximately two thirds of their calories as carbohydrates. The Japanese with over 65 percent and the Tarahumara Indians in Mexico with 75 percent of total calories as carbohydrates prove that these diets can be nutritionally adequate in every respect (Hodges & Rebello, 1985).

Garlic. There is a cholesterol-lowering mechanism in garlic (Qureshi et al, 1983). However, the

Table 32–3. *Cholesterol/Saturated-Fat Index (CSI) and Kilocalorie Content of Selected Foods**

Food	CSI	kcal
Fish, poultry, red meat (100 gm cooked):		
Whitefish (snapper, perch, sole, cod, halibut, &c), shellfish (clams, oysters, scallops), water-pack tuna	4	91
Salmon	5	149
Shellfish (shrimp, crab, lobster)	6	104
Poultry, no skin	6	171
Beef, pork, and lamb:		
10% fat (ground sirloin, flank steak)	9	214
15% fat (ground round)	10	258
20% fat (ground chuck, pot roasts)	13	286
30% fat (ground beef, pork, and lamb-steaks, ribs, pork and lamb chops, roasts)	18	381
Cheeses (100 gm):		
2% fat cheeses (low-fat cottage cheese, pot cheese), tofu (bean curd)	1	98
5–10% fat cheeses (cottage cheese, low-fat cheese slices)	6	139
25–30% fat cheeses†	6	317
11–20% fat cheeses (part skimmed milk)	12	256
32–38% fat cheeses (gruyere, cheddar, cream cheese)	26	386
Eggs:		
Whites (3)	0	51
Egg substitute (equivalent to 2 eggs)	1	91
Whole (2)	29	163
Fats (¼ cup, 4 tablespoons or 55 gm):		
Peanut butter	5	353
Most vegetable oils	8	530
Mayonnaise	10	431
Soft vegetable margarines	10	432
Hard stick margarines	15	432
Soft shortenings	16	530
Bacon grease	23	541
Very hydrogenated shortenings	27	530
Butter	37	430
Coconut oil, palm oil, cocoa butter (chocolate)	47	530
Frozen desserts (1 cup):		
Water ices, sorbet (193 gm)	0	245
Frozen yogurt, low-fat (166 gm)	2	144
Sherbet (193 gm)	2	218
Frozen yogurt‡ (166 gm)	4	155
Ice milk (141 gm)	6	214
Ice cream, 10% fat (141 gm)	13	272
Rich ice cream, 16% fat (141 gm)	18	349
Specialty ice cream, 22% fat (214 gm)	34	684
Milk products (1 cup, 240 ml):		
Skimmed milk (0–1% fat) or skimmed milk yogurt	<1	88
1% milk, buttermilk	2	115
2% milk or plain low-fat yogurt	4	144
Whole milk (3–5% fat) or whole milk yogurt	7	159
Sour cream	37	468
Imitation sour cream	43	499

*Connor, SL; Artaud-Wild, SM; Classick-Kohn, DJ; et al: The cholesterol/saturated-fat index: An indication of the hyper-cholesterolaemic and atherogenic potential of food. *Lancet* 1 (May 31):1229, 1986.

†Cheeses made with skimmed milk and vegetable oils.

‡Made with added cream.

amount required demands that capsules of the oil (with the odor removed) be consumed. The role of garlic will have to be examined further.

Coffee. A daily intake of six or more cups of boiled black coffee increases the serum cholesterol concentration (Arneson et al, 1984).

Alcohol. As discussed in Chapter 28, moderate alcohol consumption is associated with an increase in HDL (Willett et al, 1980). On the other hand, high alcohol intake raises triglyceride levels.

Weight Reduction. The most important determinant of serum cholesterol is body weight (Kromhout, 1983). Overweight men and women have higher total serum cholesterol, serum triglycerides, and VLDL cholesterol levels and usually a higher LDL cholesterol level than those within their ideal weight (Matter et al, 1980). Even children who weigh more than normal are at increased risk for CHD later in life. A reduction in weight is accompanied by lower serum cholesterol and triglyceride levels.

Omega-3 Fatty Acid. Eicosapentaenoic acid (EPA) and omega-3 fatty acid are names for this important fish lipid that is a significant discovery for decreasing serum triglycerides in a majority of problem patients (Ackman, 1986). It also lowers total cholesterol and blood pressure and increases the proportion of HDL. Eicosapentaenoic acid and related very long-chain marine polyunsaturated fats are the most potent inhibitors of CHD found in ordinary diets (Truswell, 1985), as evidenced by the low incidence of CHD among Eskimos (Harris, 1985; Woodcock et al, 1984; Lorenz et al, 1983). While all deep-sea, cold-water species of fish and some that live in cold fresh water have some EPA, the amounts vary with the seasons and diet of the fish (Table 32–5).

Mollusks and crustaceans contain significant amounts of cholesterol; however, the presence of omega-3 fatty acids apparently offsets the presence of cholesterol. From the studies with EPA, three meals weekly containing fish and shellfish with high levels of EPA are recommended. When planning menus, foods containing cholesterol may be eaten in moderation if foods with omega-3 fatty acids are regularly selected.

Clinical Implications:

- During pregnancy, serum lipids are increased markedly. Serum cholesterol levels should be monitored and prophylactic measures enacted to maintain the level close to 220 mg/dl.

Table 32–4. *Cholesterol/Saturated-Fat Index (CSI) of Sample Intake at 2000 kcal for the Western Diet and a Low-Fat Diet[1]*

Western diet[2]	Sat fat	Cholesterol	CSI	Low-fat diet[3]	Sat fat	Cholesterol	CSI
Breakfast:				*Breakfast:*			
1 slice white toast	0.2	0	0.2	2 slices whole wheat toast	0.2	0	0.2
1 tsp. (5 gm) soft margarine	0.7	0	0.7	1 tsp. (5 gm) soft margarine	0.7	0	0.7
1 cup (240 ml) orange juice	0.0	0	0.0	1 tbsp. (15 gm) jam	0.0	0	0.0
				½ pink grapefruit	0.0	0	0.0
				Snack:			
				1 cereal bran muffin[4]	0.8	1	0.9
Lunch:				*Lunch:*			
Sandwich:				1 cup (250 gm) navy bean soup[4]	0.1	0	0.1
2 slices rye bread	0.0	0	0.0	2″ × 4″ piece cornbread[4]	1.1	1	1.2
1 tbsp. (15 gm) mayonnaise	2.0	10	2.5	1 tsp. (5 gm) soft margarine	0.7	0	0.7
2 oz. (57 gm) turkey	0.6	49	3.1	9 carrot sticks	Trace	0	0.0
Tomato slices	0.0	0	0.0	Celery sticks	Trace	0	0.0
2 lettuce leaves	0.0	0	0.0	1 cup (150 gm) fresh strawberries	Trace	0	0.0
1 oz. (28 gm) potato chips	2.6	0	2.6	4 gingersnaps	0.7	0	0.7
1 large apple	0.0	0	0.0				
Dinner:				*Dinner:*			
5 oz. (143 gm) grilled filet mignon	11.6	119	17.7	Flank steak florentine (87 gm)[4]	2.8	71	6.4
1 large baked potato	Trace	0	0.0	1 large baked potato	Trace	0	0.0
¼ cup (60 gm) sour cream	6.4	20	7.5	¼ cup (60 gm) mock sour cream[4]	0.7	5	1.0
1 cup (55 gm) lettuce salad	0.0	0	0.0	1 cup (55 gm) lettuce salad	0.0	0	0.0
2 tbsp. (30 gm) blue cheese dressing	3.2	18	4.1	2 tbsp. (30 gm) Western dressing[4]	0.6	2	0.7
3″ × 3″ × 1″ chocolate fudge cake	7.9	52	10.6	1 cup (155 gm) broccoli	0.0	0	0.0
				3 pieces whole wheat french bread	0.1	0	0.1
				2 tsp. (10 gm) soft margarine	1.3	0	1.3
				3″ × 3″ piece cocoa cake[4]	1.6	0	1.6
				Snack:			
				3 cups (18 gm) air-popped popcorn	Trace	0	0.0
				1 tsp. (5 gm) soft margarine	0.7	0	0.7
Totals	35.2	268	49.0	Totals	12.1	80	16.3

[1]From Connor, SL; Artaud-Wild, SM; Classick-Kohn, DJ; et al: The cholesterol/saturated-fat index: An indication of the hyper-cholesterolaemic and atherogenic potential of food. *Lancet* (May 31):1229, 1986, with permission.
[2]2053 kcal, 14% protein, 44% fat, 41% carbohydrate, 15% saturated fat.
[3]2117 kcal, 15% protein, 24% fat, 61% carbohydrate, 5% saturated fat.
[4]Fat and cholesterol modified.

Careful food choices can ensure nutrient needs.

- Even when one uses fasting blood determinations, cholesterol values fluctuate. For an accurate assessment, several blood samples should be checked. The time of sample collection must be constant as cholesterol levels follow a circadian rhythm. Highest values are at midnight and lowest at noon, if not influenced by food intake. High-fat meals result in high values.

NONDIETARY FACTORS AFFECTING SERUM LIPIDS

Vigorous endurance-type exercise can lower the risk of CHD by increasing HDL and lowering plasma triglyceride concentrations. About 1000 kcal/week of moderate-intensity endurance-type exercise, or walking and/or jogging 9 to 15 miles each week is sufficient to produce these changes (Haskell, 1984; Rauramaa et al, 1984).

Health Application: Nutritional Recommendations for Preventing Heart Disease

Several dietary factors may be used to prevent CHD. The amount and type of fat and fiber content may be particularly significant factors to consider. Weight reduction may also lower serum cholesterol. In general, following the Prudent Diet recommended by the American Heart Association is the first step (Table 32–6).

All Americans who are at high risk of developing CHD (except children less than two years of age) should be encouraged to adopt a cholesterol-lowering diet. A low-fat diet may be detrimental in other ways to children who need a full complement of lipids for neurological development (Fuller, 1986).

NUTRITIONAL RECOMMENDATIONS FOR HYPERLIPOPROTEINEMIA

Originally, there was a diet prescription for each of the five types of hyperlipoproteinemias. However, these have been condensed into a single basic diet, or the alternative diet. This diet is implemented in stages, as warranted by the type of hyperlipidemia. The Prudent Diet, which is low in total fat, saturated fat, and energy (if weight loss is necessary), is a beginning point. If hyperlipidemia is not effectively altered, further restrictions may be implemented utilizing the alternative diet. This basic diet is low in cholesterol and total and saturated fat, high in complex carbohydrates and fiber, and relatively low in calories (less fat, sugar, and alcohol). It can also be used to achieve and maintain ideal body weight (Connor & Connor, 1982). Familial hyperchylomicronemia (Type I) and mixed hyperlipidemia (Type IV) are very rare conditions; more appropriate measures for them are geared to alter the specific faulty hyperlipidemia.

The Alternative Diet. In this diet, dietary cholesterol is reduced to 100 mg/day to lower total plasma and LDL cholesterol (Table 32–7). Dietary fat is lowered to 20 percent of total calories; this has a beneficial effect on all forms of hyperlipidemia. Most of the reduction is in saturated fat content to about five percent of total calories. The PUFA content is only increased slightly, to six to eight percent of total calories. Omega-3 fatty acids may also be used to lower plasma lipids.

In the alternative diet plan, the reduction of dietary fat is replaced by complex carbohydrate from grains, beans, and vegetables. This larger amount of complex carbohydrates means the diet is high in fiber. Sugars are reduced to about 10 percent of total calories. The protein content of the diet is adequate, even though there is a shift from animal to vegetable proteins. A comparison of the nutrients of the alternative diet as compared to the American diet is shown in Table 32–8.

Reduction of excess body weight is usually the crucial measure for hypertriglyceridemia. This diet is lower in caloric intake than most American diets just because of its composition. The lower fat intake almost automatically decreases calories. The increase in carbohydrate content increases the bulk of the diet considerably and induces satiety sooner per unit of calories and helps to promote weight loss. This diet meets all nutritional requirements (Connor & Connor, 1982).

Since the effects of alcohol upon the plasma lipid and lipoprotein levels are variable, advice concerning alcohol intake must be individualized.

People do not make abrupt dietary changes that are lasting, therefore, this diet is implemented in phases. In phase I, the foods high in cholesterol and saturated fats are reduced. In phase II, the amount of meat and cheese consumption is reduced to 6 to 8 oz./day. In phase III, the cholesterol content of the diet is reduced to 100 mg/day and the saturated fat lowered to five to six percent of the total calories. Meat and cheese intake are severely curtailed. A summary of the diet with ways to implement it is shown in Table 32–9.

Familial Hyperchylomicronemia. Chylomicrons and serum triglycerides are elevated in this disorder. The goals of treatment are to reduce plasma triglyceride levels to between 400 to 1000 mg/dl.

During the acute stage, when hepatomegaly or acute pancreatitis is present, the diet is virtually fat-free to permit the clearance of chylomicrons. A rice-fruit diet is frequently used.

After these symptoms subside, the fat content is kept extremely low (25 to 35 gm/day). It may be inadequate in fatty acids, iron, and fat-soluble vitamins (Frederickson et al, 1973a). Cho-

Table 32–5. Eicosapentaenoic Acid (EPA) Content of Fish*

Species	Grams per 4-ounce serving
Chinook salmon	3.6
Albacore tuna	2.6
Sockeye salmon	2.3
Mackerel	1.8–2.6
Herring	1.2–2.7
Rainbow trout	1.0
Whiting	0.9
King crab	0.6
Shrimp	0.5
Cod	0.3

*Reprinted with permission from *Harvard Medical School Health Letter.* May, 11(7):8, 1986.

Table 32—6. *The Prudent Diet*

Fat

1. *Reduce the amount of fat from current 40 percent to below 35 percent with 10 percent PUFA, 10 percent saturated, and 10 percent monosaturated fats (e.g., peanut or olive oils).*

    Polyunsaturated fat should not exceed eight percent of the *total* kilocaloric intake (Connor et al, 1986). Choose margarines that list liquid vegetable oil as the first ingredient on the label. Prepare salad dressings with oils high in linoleic acid (e.g., safflower, corn, or sunflower).

2. *Limit cholesterol intake to no more than 300 mg/day.*

Eggs

Eggs should not exceed four per week for adults, four to six per week for children.

Milk

Two cups of low-fat milk (less than one percent fat); low-fat plain yogurt may be substituted for milk.

1 oz. of hard cheese may occasionally be substituted for 2 oz. of lean meat.

2 to 4 cups of milk for children (2 cups whole milk daily for children under two years of age); milk in excess of two cups should be low-fat.

Fish, Poultry, Lean Meat

Two servings daily—choose from these with about equal frequency.

Limit portion sizes to 2 or 3 oz. cooked.

Substitute liver for meat one to two times a month.

Limit salty varieties of meat (ham, smoked meat, and smoked fish) to small amounts.

Of the fish meals, at least two should be from fish high in EPA (e.g., herring, mackerel, pompano, salmon, whitefish, shad, albacore, trout, flounder, sardines, tuna, or sole, but those with less total fat should be chosen more often (e.g., sole and flounder).

Frozen fish should be rinsed under cold running water because frozen fish is often kept in a diluted salt solution.

Fresh fish will keep well for two days if it is placed in a heavy plastic bag and refrigerated promptly and iced down.

Remove skin from poultry.

3. *Increase carbohydrate intake to 55 or 60 percent of total kilocalories.*

Grains

Include one or more of these at each meal: breads, cereals, rice, oats, cornmeal, pasta, grits, buckwheat, wholewheat. Preferred items include oats, rice, pasta, pumpernickel, and barley.

Dried Legumes and Nuts

Combine dried beans or peas with smaller servings of meat, fish, poultry.

Balance legumes, nuts, and grains with complementary foods to complete protein content as vegetarians do.

Select nuts for meals or snacks frequently (e.g., almonds, walnuts, pecans, sunflower and sesame seeds, or peanuts)

Fruits and Vegetables

Include at least four servings daily with as many as possible being fresh to provide more fiber as well as nutrients.

Choose at least one source high in vitamin C (e.g., citrus fruits, tomatoes, cantaloupe, or strawberries).

Include sources high in pectin frequently (apples, citrus fruits).

Select a source high in vitamin A at least four times a week (dark leafy green vegetables or deep yellow or orange ones, such as carrots, spinach, squash, and sweet potatoes).

4. *Limit the use of refined sugar, salt, coffee, and alcohol.*

5. *Combine foods for the lowest cholesterol/saturated-fat index (CSI) possible.*

lesterol intake is not restricted. Low-fat seafoods (shellfish and fish), skim milk, egg white, and dried cottage cheese may be utilized. The lack of fat in the diet is a serious detriment to its palatability and acceptance. Medium-chain triglycerides may be used to enhance these diets because they are not incorporated into chylomicrons. Without the use of medium-chain triglycerides, no other fat or oil can be used (ADA, 1981). Studies with the omega-3 fatty acids have shown further enhancement of triglyceride decreases (Nestel, 1986).

Table 32–7. *Changes in Certain Dietary Constituents: Effects upon the Plasma Lipids and Lipoproteins**

Reduction of dietary cholesterol to 100 mg per day	*Decreases* Total plasma cholesterol LDL Remnants (IDL) VLDL (slightly) HDL (slightly) LDL/HDL ratio
Reduction of total fat to 20 percent of total calories and saturated fat to 5 percent of total calories	*Decreases* Chylomicrons Total plasma cholesterol LDL Remnants VLDL (slightly) LDL/HDL
Caloric reduction (if adiposity present)	*Decreases* Plasma triglyceride VLDL Remnants LDL and total cholesterol
	Increases HDL

*From Connor, WE; Connor, SL: The dietary treatment of hyperlipidemia: Rationale, technique and efficacy. Medical Clinics of North America *66(2):485, 1982, with permission.*

When a patient has lost excessive weight, the plasma triglyceride concentration will occasionally approach normal; the fat content of the diet can be gradually increased to 20 percent so that the alternative diet plan can be used.

Familial Hypercholesterolemia or Combined Hyperlipidemia. In these conditions, serum cholesterol and triglycerides are elevated. The majority of patients may control their serum cholesterol and triglyceride levels using the alternative diet (Kane & Malloy, 1982).

Dietary cholesterol is kept to a minimum (100 to 200 mg/day); the type of fat is modified to maintain a P/S ratio of 1.0 or higher. For each ounce of meat in the diet, 1 tsp. of PUFA is consumed. In order to keep the total fat content low, lean meat, especially fish and poultry (without skin), is recommended. A 3 oz. portion of beef, lamb, ham, or pork is allowed three times a week. Skim milk must be used.

Weight reduction is usually a primary concern. Concentrated sweets are restricted. If serum lipids are not controlled, complex carbohydrates may be limited by using the food exchanges.

Since iron may be inadequate in this diet, the patient's iron nutriture should be periodically as-

sessed and iron supplements provided as needed in order to prevent iron deficiency anemia (Frederickson et al, 1973b).

Mixed Hyperlipidemia. Chylomicrons and VLDL are elevated with corresponding hypertriglyceridemia; serum cholesterol may also be raised. Metabolic disorders, such as diabetic acidosis, alcoholism, nephrosis, and pancreatitis as well as a genetic tendency, aid in the diagnosis of this condition. Abdominal pain may occur before an appropriate amount of fat is consumed.

The cholesterol level is kept as low as possible. The amount of fat is kept very low (25 to 30 percent) to reduce chylomicrons by recommending a high ratio of polyunsaturated to saturated fats. With weight reduction and a maintenance diet limited in simple carbohydrates, plasma triglyceride ranges may be below 300 to 600 mg/dl. Alcohol is not recommended.

Clinical Implications:

- Family members with all types of hereditary hyperlipoproteinemias, especially Type II, should be screened for premature CHD and encouraged to adopt preventive treatment early in life.
- Extremely low-fat diets decrease not only LDL but also HDL. Therefore, they may not be desirable (Walser et al, 1984).

Congestive Heart Failure

Pathophysiology. In heart failure, the heart is unable to maintain adequate circulation to supply the body's needs. Decreased cardiac output results in less blood flow through the kidney. Tubular resorption of sodium is increased and more water is retained.

To compensate for inadequate cardiac output, the body enlarges the pumping chambers of the heart so they can hold a larger volume of blood. This leads to fluid overload within the vascular system and in all of the body's fluid compartments. Fluids accumulate in the tissue spaces, causing edema.

Additionally, the heart increases its muscle mass so it can contract better. This ventricular hypertrophy results in a larger oxygen demand that the coronary arteries will eventually not be able to meet. Heart failure and myocardial infarction may

Table 32–8. Chemical Composition of the Present American Diet and the Alternative Diet*

Nutrient	American Diet		Alternative Diet (Phase III)	
Cholesterol, mg/day	500		100	
Fat, percent of total calories	40		20	
Saturated fat, percent calories		15		5
Monounsaturated fat, percent calories		16		8
Polyunsaturated fat, percent calories		6		7
P/S value		0.4		1.3
Iodine number		63		99
Vegetable fat, percent fat		38		75
Animal fat, percent fat		62		25
Protein, percent calories	15		15	
Vegetable protein, percent protein		32		56
Animal protein, percent protein		68		44
Carbohydrate, percent calories	45		65	
Starch, percent calories		22		40
Sucrose (added to food), percent calories		15		10
Fructose, glucose, sucrose, lactose, maltose, percent calories (naturally present in foods)		8		15
Dietary fiber, gm	10–12		48–60	
Sodium, mEq	200–300		75–100	
Potassium, mEq	30–70		120–150	

*From Connor, WE; Connor, SL: The dietary treatment of hyperlipidemia: Rationale, technique and efficacy. *Medical Clinics of North America* 66(2):485, 1982.

result. Bed rest, diuretics and drugs (e.g., digitalis) are prescribed to increase the force and velocity of contraction in the heart.

Nutritional Care. Restricting sodium intake reduces the work load for the heart by decreasing extracellular fluids. In severe conditions, the sodium restriction may be 20 mEq in a hospital setting. As the edema is controlled, the sodium restriction may be raised until a level of 90 mEq is reached prior to the patient's dismissal from the hospital (Pemberton & Gastineau, 1981).

Caffeine and alcohol are prohibited because they may provoke cardiac arrhythmia, a common hazard under these conditions. Temperatures of food and beverages should not be extremely hot or cold immediately following a myocardial infarction.

Several small meals should be served to avoid excessive stress and exertion by the body. Caloric restriction to 1000 to 1200 kcal is in order and also lessens the quantity of food consumed. Ordinarily, weight reduction is a priority; strict dietary restrictions are necessary because of inactivity.

Recent tests show that the uncomplicated patient may tolerate more "typical" meals than the previously recommended ones which were more stringent in the postinfarction period without undue hemodynamic stress (Bagatell & Heymsfield,

1984). Dietary prescriptions by the physician and the institution may vary accordingly.

Hypertension

Etiology. Hypertension is one of the high risk factors for CHD; it may also result in stroke and congestive heart failure. For every increment of blood pressure above normal levels, there is a commensurate increase in risk. Hypertension is defined as a persistent elevation of a systolic blood pressure above 140 mmHg and diastolic pressure above 90 mmHg. Mild hypertension refers to a diastolic blood pressure of 90 to 100 mmHg (Kaplan, 1985). Table 32–10 shows the upper limits of normal blood pressure by age groups.

Between the ages of 65 and 74 years, three of every four Americans have definite or borderline high blood pressure. Even though it is far less common, hypertension can strike youths and even infants. Women develop hypertension more frequently than men but are less dramatically affected by a sustained elevation of blood pressure. Persons living in stressful urban environments and those frequently subjected to emotional

Table 32–9. *Summary and Implementation of the Alternative Diet*

Phase I: *Avoid foods very high in cholesterol and saturated fat.*
Implementation:
1. Egg yolk, butterfat, lard, and organ meats are eliminated.
2. Some products are substituted for products containing saturated fats and cholesterol: soft margarine for butter, vegetables oil and shortening for lard, skim milk for whole milk, egg whites for whole eggs, low-fat cheese for regular cheese, and yogurt for sour cream. Many cookbooks on the market have altered popular recipes so the product contains less cholesterol and saturated fats.
3. Products such as egg substitutes, soy meats, and frozen yogurt may be used.
4. Two egg whites can be substituted for one whole egg in making cakes, cookies, custards, and potato salad without changing their quality.
5. Lean, well-trimmed meats will help decrease the amount of cholesterol and saturated fat. The skin should be removed from poultry.
Phase II: *Gradual transition from using up to 16 oz./day of meat to no more than 6 to 8 oz./day, with further reductions of total dietary fat.*
Implementation:
1. Meat is allowed only once a day (6 to 8 oz./day).
2. High fat meats, such as luncheon meats, bacon, sausage, hot dogs, and spareribs should only be eaten occasionally.
3. Broiling, baking, steaming, braising, or stir-frying can be used instead of frying.
4. Since 1 oz. of whole-milk cheese replaces 3 oz. of lean meat, cheese made partly or wholly from skim milk is suggested.
5. Foods that are principally meat or high-fat dairy products need to be replaced with items that use greater amounts of grains, legumes, vegetables, and fruits.
Phase III: *Meats are used primarily as condiments; complex carbohydrates are used generously.*
Implementation:
1. The total meat, shellfish, and poultry content allowed is 3 to 4 oz./day.
2. Meat, fish, and poultry are used as condiments rather than the main attraction.
3. Poultry contains less saturated fat and should be stressed.
4. Fish that contains omega-3 fatty acids is allowed in amounts up to 6 oz./day.

Data from Connor, WE; Connor, SL: The dietary treatment of hyperlipidemia: Rationale, technique and efficacy. Medical Clinics of North America 66(2):485, 1982.

trauma become hypertensive far more frequently than persons who live in rural or relaxed environments. Hypertension is about twice as common in blacks as in whites (Fig. 32–4).

Pathophysiology. The major characteristic of hypertensive heart disease is hypertrophy of the left ventricle, which eventually leads to congestive heart failure. Left ventricular hypertrophy results from increased work load as the heart attempts to pump blood into constricted, narrowed vessels. There are two major types of arterial hypertension:
1. Essential hypertension, also known as primary or idiopathic hypertension, constitutes 90 percent of all cases and is of unknown origin.
2. Secondary hypertension develops secondarily from eclampsia or results from primary disease of the cardiovascular system, renal system, adrenal glands, or neurological system (Luckmann & Sorensen, 1980).

Persons taking antidepressants that contain monoamine oxidase (MAO) inhibitors and who are currently ingesting food substances that contain large amounts of tyramine are likely to develop hypertension (see Chapter 22).

Factors Related to Hypertension. Blood pressure is the result of an exceedingly complex interplay of multiple hereditary, constitutional, and environmental factors. Many factors have been implicated in hypertension.

Exercise. Numerous studies have found that physically active individuals report less hypertension (Kannel, 1984; Paffenbarger et al, 1983) and hypertensive individuals can lower their blood pressure by regular exercise (Krotkiewski et al, 1979).

Relaxation. Behavioral stress and certain social factors are often considered to have a contributing effect on hypertension (Anderson, 1984); however, experimental results have been inconsistent. The prevalence of hypertension is considerably higher among rural Southern blacks than among blacks living in large U.S. cities. Muscular relaxation has been noted to lower the blood pressure in many hypertensives both during relaxation and for prolonged periods thereafter (Peled-Ney et al, 1984).

Genetics. There is strong evidence that elevated arterial pressure may have roots early in life. Many factors have been implicated including

Table 32–10. Age Variations of Blood Pressure*

Age	Mean Blood Pressure (mmHg)
Newborn	75/50
1–6 months	80/46
6–12 months	96/65
1–2 years	99/65
2–4 years	100/60
4–6 years	110/60
6–8 years	105/60
8–10 years	110/60
10–12 years	110/60
12–14 years	118/60
14–16 years	120/65
16–18 years	120/65
Adult	127/76

*Notes: Sources differ in their values for normal vital signs. Be sure to establish baseline measurements for each individual. Also find out if the facility for which you work has established ranges to use for comparisons.

Adapted and reprinted with permission of Ross Laboratories, Columbus, OH 43216, from *Children Are Different*, 2nd ed. Copyright 1978 Ross Laboratories.

genetic and hereditary influences, body stature, dietary salt intake and other dietary components, racial predisposition, and environmental and psychosocial factors. Hofman and associates (1983) claim that hypertension may be preventable if infants are given half as much sodium as usual for the first six months of life.

Weight. Although a relationship between body weight and hypertension is well established in the United States, such a correlation does not seem to be true in many populations. Excessive weight has been a more consistent factor in predicting hypertension as well as an accompanying symptom. Lean hypertensives are more likely to gain weight than normotensives. The frequency of hypertension is about two times higher in obese than in nonobese persons (Havlik et al, 1983). Ordinarily, an increase of 3 mmHg in diastolic pressure may be expected for every 10 kg increase in body weight. When people are put on calorically-restricted diets, blood pressure drops before weight loss is significant. It is estimated that about half of all cases of hypertension could be prevented entirely with weight control (Silverberg, 1980).

Sodium. Hypertension is not found in societies where low sodium intake and excretion are universal. Unlike no-salt cultures, the blood pressures of all populations that use salt rises with age. Likewise, individuals originally from populations with low blood pressure who have become acculturated to Western civilization often develop higher blood pressure as they age.

While studies *between* different groups and salt intake show a positive linear relationship, the same is not always true *within* the groups. The Framingham Study failed to find any correlation between blood pressure and daily salt intake (Dawber, 1980). In other words, all subjects who consume the same amount of salt would not have the same probability of developing hypertension because of variations in individual biological responsiveness.

About 9 to 20 percent of the U.S. population is genetically susceptible to developing essential hypertension by the time they reach middle age. If a person is genetically resistant to hypertension, s/he can eat as much as 200 mEq of sodium chloride daily.

Potassium. Many investigators feel that a high-potassium intake has a protective effect against hypertension; indeed, a low-potassium intake, particularly when sodium consumption is high, may contribute to high blood pressure. The usual high-sodium, low-potassium diet consumed

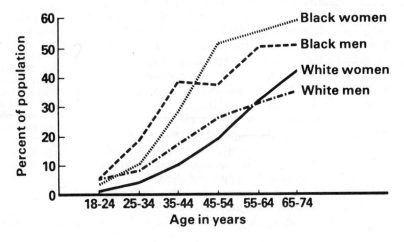

Figure 32–4. Prevalence of hypertension uncontrolled by diet or medication increased rapidly with age. It was twice as great among black adults as among white adults—an age-adjusted figure of 30% compared with 17%. (From Simopoulos AP: Overview of nutritional status in the United States. Progress in Clinical and Biological Research 67:237, 1981, by permission.)

when most foods are highly processed may be detrimental to normal blood pressure regulation (Meneely & Battarbee, 1976).

Calcium. According to McCarron and colleagues (1984a), calcium plays a more active role in blood pressure regulation than either sodium or potassium. By decreasing dairy product consumption in order to lower sodium intake, a backlash effect occurs. Higher intakes of calcium and potassium are associated with lower mean systolic blood pressure and lower absolute risk of hypertension in the general population. In fact, a lack of calcium and not an excess of sodium is related to high blood pressure in certain individuals. Hypocalcemia seems to correlate more with elevated blood pressure than sodium (McCarron et al, 1984a). Many hypertensive persons consume less sodium than those with normal blood pressure and significantly less calcium, potassium, and vitamins A and C (McCarron et al, 1984b).

Fiber. In societies whose diet is high in fiber, blood pressure is lower than in Western cultures. Vegetarians also maintain lower blood pressures. A recent study comparing a high-fiber, hypocaloric diet to a liquid hypocaloric diet resulted in the same amount of weight loss, but the high-fiber diet was more effective in decreasing blood pressure. While the mechanism for this effect remains unclear, fiber may provide an important effect (Anderson & Tietyen-Clark, 1986).

Vitamins A and C. Fruits and vegetables are often encouraged not only because they usually have less sodium than other foods, but because many of them contain vitamins A and C. Decreased levels of vitamin C are frequently found in people who have died from CHD, particularly among younger age groups in which hemorrhagic stroke is more prevalent than ischemic stroke (Vollset & Bjelke, 1983).

Alcohol. Small amounts of alcohol appear to protect against CHD, but even moderate intake may elevate the blood pressure (Kaplan, 1985). Therefore, its merits are controversial. More than 2 oz. or 60 ml/day raises the blood pressure. Alcohol may be the most prevalent cause of reversible hypertension and is responsible for at least 10 percent of hypertension in men and one percent in women (MacMahon et al, 1984).

Heavy drinkers have higher blood pressures than light drinkers or abstainers. This effect starts to be consistent above about four drinks per day and continues to rise with larger intakes. When alcoholics are institutionalized for detoxification, their average blood pressure falls by about 20 mmHg systolic and stays down. If alcohol intake is resumed, it rises again (Truswell, 1985).

Water Supply. Total cardiovascular mortality has generally been found to be lower in areas where the drinking water is hard (containing more calcium, magnesium, and other minerals). Persons in hard water areas would benefit by not installing water softeners for their drinking water.

NUTRITIONAL CARE FOR HYPERTENSION

Nondrug treatments of mild hypertension (Table 32–11) should be used frequently because they may sufficiently lower the blood pressure of many patients to a safe level (Kaplan, 1985). Diet therapy should be the first consideration for the hypertensive patient; it may be required to reduce weight and for sodium restriction. Six weeks is a suitable period to determine if diet alone can control this problem, unless the condition is critical enough to require drugs immediately (Walser et al, 1984). Medications may be prescribed if diet therapy is not adequate at that time.

An initial step in treating hypertension is to advise overweight people to lose weight by reducing their intake of kilocalories and increasing physical exercise. Depending on the degree of excessive weight at the time of diagnosis, moderate weight loss (about five or six percent of body weight) influences blood pressure more or less uniformly (Wilber, 1982). If hypertensive obese patients lose 5 kg, the blood pressure typically falls 10 mmHg systolic and 5 mmHg diastolic (Truswell, 1985).

However, weight loss without sodium restriction may be discouraging; a lower blood pressure

Table 32–11. *A Practical Prescription for Nondrug Management of Hypertension**

1. For the overweight person, weight reduction should be the primary goal.
2. For all hypertensives, dietary sodium intake should be restricted to 2 gm/day, with caution not to reduce the consumption of low-fat, low-sodium milk and cheese products in order to maintain calcium intake.
3. More fiber and less saturated fat are beneficial for other reasons and may also help lower the blood pressure.
4. Alcohol should be limited to 2 oz./day.
5. Regular isotonic exercise should be encouraged.
6. Potassium intake need not be specifically increased because it will rise with a lowered sodium intake.
7. Supplemental magnesium and calcium should be given only to those who are deficient until additional evidence of their efficacy is available.
8. Those who are willing and able should be encouraged to do some type of relaxation therapy.

*From Kaplan, NM: Non-drug treatment of hypertension. *Annals of Internal Medicine* 102:359, 1985.

is observed when sodium intake is restricted in sodium-sensitive hypertensives (Reisin et al, 1978). In addition to consuming more food, heavier people consume more sodium (Connor et al, 1984). By losing weight, sodium intake is decreased and potassium intake increases.

Some level of sodium restriction is appropriate; this is determined by the condition and the patient's ability to follow a diet. Potassium chloride may be partially substituted for sodium chloride in cooking and at the table unless renal disease is also present or unless a potassium-sparing diuretic is ordered (Kaplan, 1985).

Patients should also be encouraged to increase their intake of fresh fruits and vegetables. These items are not only low in calories and high in fiber (beneficial for weight reduction) but also high in potassium. By including more fresh foods and less processed foods, fewer high-fat, high-sodium foods are consumed. Additionally, adequate amounts of dairy products should be included in the diet. If a patient cannot tolerate dairy products, calcium supplements of 1 gm/day may reduce blood pressure (Henry et al, 1985).

SODIUM RESTRICTIONS

Some people with high blood pressure do not benefit from a sodium restricted diet. For these people and for those who are not salt-sensitive (particularly athletes), a sodium reserve is important.

Restriction of dietary sodium is indicated for two major pathological processes: hypertension and edema. About one third of the mild cases of hypertension can be controlled with mild salt restriction (Silverberg, 1980). The severity and type of condition determines the degree of sodium restriction as shown in Table 32–12.

When sodium is restricted, all potential sources of sodium should be considered. Most foods naturally contain it; animal foods such as meat, saltwater fish, eggs and dairy products, and some vegetables (beets, carrots, celery, spinach, and other dark-green leafy vegetables) contain appreciable amounts of sodium. These may need to be restricted depending on the level of restriction. A listing of the sodium and potassium content of foods is in Appendix D–3.

Additionally, salt or sodium compounds may be added in food processing. Sodium bicarbonate and other sodium products are used as leavening agents; sodium benzoate is a preservative in margarine and relishes, sodium citrate and monosodium glutamate are both flavor enhancers used in gelatin desserts, beverages, and meats. It is important to read labels to determine the amount of sodium added.

Many low-sodium products are available. A product can be considered low in sodium if it contains no more than 10 mg per serving.

"No Added Salt." The stipulation of no extra salt may be significant, especially for patients who have excessive intakes. An intake of 4 gm or 170 mEq of sodium per day can be achieved by avoiding salty foods and by not adding salt to food at the table; small amounts may be used in cooking. Suggestions for no-extra-salt diets are listed in Table 32–13.

Mild Sodium Restriction. Approximately 2 to 3 gm of sodium (87 to 130 mEq) is allowed on a mild sodium restriction. Salt is not added at the table, but foods can be lightly salted in cooking. Foods high in salt are omitted: pickles, olives, bacon, ham, chips, canned soups, salted nuts, and crackers.

Moderate Sodium Restriction. Generally, moderate sodium restriction is achieved by removing most high-sodium foods from the diet and adding no extra salt at the table or in cooking. This diet is more difficult for many persons to follow because many canned or processed foods (vegetables and meats) containing added salt are omitted. Four servings of regular bread are allowed (salt-free bread is not limited). Vegetables and other foods containing naturally high amounts of sodium are restricted; meat and milk

Table 32–12. Levels of Dietary Sodium Restriction

	Condition	Sodium Content	
		mEq/day	mg/day
No added salt	Mild hypertension; mild fluid retention	174	4000
Mild restriction	Hypertension; cirrhosis with ascites	87	2000
Moderate restriction	Congestive heart failure	43	1000
Severe restriction	Congestive heart failure; cirrhosis with massive ascites	22	500

Table 32–13. Suggestions for No-Extra-Salt Diets*

The sodium content of the no-extra-salt diet varies according to the calorie level; the usual range is 90 to 150 mEq. Guidelines for this diet are as follows:

1. Do not add salt to food at the table.
2. Use only limited amounts of salt in food preparation: 1/4 tsp. of salt per pound of meat; 1/8 tsp. of salt per serving of cooked cereal, potatoes, potato substitutes, and cooked vegetables.
3. Avoid the following foods:
   - Salt-cured meats; salted canned, or processed meats, fish, and fowl; bacon; ham; dried beef; corned beef; frankfurters; processed cold cuts; sausages; sardines; salted cheese and cheese foods; salted peanuts; commercial casserole mixes; frozen dinners.
   - Commercially prepared salted salad dressings (except mayonnaise and mayonnaise-type salad dressing); commercial gravy and gravy mixes; salt pork.
   - Salted snack foods; salted crackers; salted popcorn; pretzels; potato chips; corn chips; salted nuts; canned soups; dried soup mixes; broth; bouillon (except salt-free).
   - Sauerkraut; pickled vegetables; commercially frozen vegetable mixes with sauces.
   - Seasoning salt; seasoning mixes; meat tenderizer; monosodium glutamate; catsup; prepared mustard; prepared horseadish; soy sauce; bottled meat and barbecue sauce, olives; pickles.
   - Cultured buttermilk; cocoa mixes; cocktail beverage mixes; club soda; Gatorade.
4. Limit the following foods:
   - Organ meats (such as liver, heart, and kidney), shellfish (such as shrimp, clams, and lobster), or peanut butter to two servings per week. Additional servings of salt-free peanut butter may be used.
   - Tomato juice or vegetable juice cocktail to 1/2 cup per day. Additional servings of salt-free tomato juice or salt-free vegetable juice cocktail may be used.

(Foods not listed here are allowed on the no-extra-salt diet.)

*From Pemberton, CM; Gastineau, CF (Eds): *Mayo Clinic Diet Manual.* Philadelphia, W. B. Saunders Co, 1981, with permission.

products are used in moderation. Although this diet is more difficult for an individual to follow at home, it has a greater rate of compliance than diets with more severe restrictions.

Severe Sodium Restriction. This severe restriction, or about 33 mEq (500 mg) of sodium may be impractical for patients to achieve and may limit both the antihypertensive and potassium-sparing effects of moderate sodium restriction (Ram et al, 1981). In addition to items that must be omitted, milk is limited to two cups/day, meat to a total of 5 or 6 oz., and no more than one egg. Salt-free margarine is used, and high-sodium vegetables are omitted.

Occasionally, a patient in the hospital needs an even greater sodium restriction (11 mEq or 250 mg). Such a diet is extremely unpalatable and may not be nutritionally adequate. As soon as the patient's condition permits, the level of sodium is increased. Meat is limited to 4 oz./day plus one egg. Low-sodium milk may be used instead of regular milk, but very few patients will drink it. Distilled water must be used.

Other Sources of Sodium. Because water may account for up to 10 percent of an individual's daily sodium consumption, the sodium content of the public water supply is important for patients on severe sodium-restricted diets. Approximately 42 percent of the nation's water sup-

plies contain sodium in excess of the optimal level (Korch, 1986). A maximum of 20 mg of sodium per liter or quart of water is advisable for persons who require a low-sodium diet because of heart or kidney diseases. If a person on a 1000 mg sodium diet consumes about 2 L of water containing as much as 270 mg/L of sodium, s/he is ingesting 540 mg sodium from this basic fluid. Bottled water may be required in such cases.

Medications may contain sodium and add significant amounts to the diet, particularly when taken regularly and frequently such as antacids (see Tables 27–1 and 27–2). Laxatives and cough medicines may also contain significant amounts of sodium. A pharmacist can help the patient choose products low in sodium.

Sodium Intake and Diuretics. Diuretics commonly used in the treatment of hypertension may be classified into two groups by their effect on potassium excretion: thiazide or loop diuretics, which cause potassium excretion, and other less potent diuretics, which cause relative potassium retention. Frequently, a combination of the two types of agents is used to maintain potassium balance. A potassium-sparing diuretic, a potassium chloride supplement, or a salt substitute containing potassium chloride plus foods high in potassium may be selected.

With the potassium-wasting diuretics, the

amount of sodium excretion is dependent on the amount of potassium excreted. The more sodium the patient consumes, the more potassium is lost (Wilber, 1982). Reduction of sodium intake, by making less sodium available at the distal tubules for exchange with potassium, reduces the degree of potassium wastage, at least during the first month or two of treatment. An intake of less than 60 mEq/day of sodium enhances the effect of all antihypertensive drugs in patients with established hypertension.

Since both hypo- and hyperkalemia can be life-threatening, monitoring potassium levels while using diuretics is imperative (Wilber, 1982). Renal, muscle, and cardiac function may be affected by reduced blood levels of potassium.

When patients use salt substitutes, this source of potassium can be significant and should be considered to prevent hyperkalemia. One teaspoon per day of a salt substitute supplies approximately 60 mEq of potassium. This is within the range of potassium supplementation usually prescribed for outpatients taking potassium chloride preparations. Sometimes, if patients dislike the supplement prescribed, they may prefer 1/3 to 1/2 tsp. of Adolph's Salt Substitute, for example, which contains 20 to 30 mEq of potassium and less than 1 mEq of sodium.

Compliance and Palatability. In spite of low-sodium diets being used so frequently, they are difficult to follow. The chief complaint is that they are bland and tasteless. People are accustomed to higher amounts of salt on foods; additionally, they are unaware of the myriad of spices other than salt (*Focus on Suggestions for Reduction of Sodium Intake*). If a high-salt intake has been established, the sodium intake can gradually be decreased. The preferred salt level will decrease after about three months of moderately lowered intake (Beauchamp et al, 1983).

Nurses are vital to a successful hypertensive program. Since sodium restriction is so widespread (even if the restriction is moderate), there are not enough dietitians available for the desired consultation and monitoring. An informed nurse can honestly compliment patients on even a modest reduction in weight or sodium intake. This feedback can be most encouraging and a prime motivating factor in a successful program.

Sodium output closely reflects sodium intake. A 24-hour urinary sodium measurement is useful for monitoring intake. Reporting this sodium value to hypertensive patients is a very effective way to motivate them to limit their salt intake (Nugent et al, 1984).

FOCUS ON	SUGGESTIONS FOR REDUCTION OF SODIUM INTAKE

1. **Seasonings:** Other seasonings to use during sodium restriction are in many cookbooks and offer a variety of new enjoyable experiences for the person willing to experiment. Shakers that contain mixtures of spices and herbs can be most useful.

   Adding lemon juice, for example, to tomato juice increases the salty taste (Little & Brinner, 1984). Lemon juice can enhance the flavor of many foods.

2. **Unknown Sources:** Cutting down on table salt is one of the first recommendations; however, this is not enough. It is easy to consume as much sodium as in 2 tsp. of salt without adding salt to foods. Processed foods, particularly soups, ketchup, and soy sauce can ruin a regimen without the person realizing what is happening.

   Labels must be read to determine hidden as well as obvious sources of sodium. Flavor enhancers such as monosodium glutamate and sodium citrate and preservatives such as sodium benzoate are sources of sodium. Low-sodium products should contain no more than 10 mg of sodium per serving (Pemberton & Gastineau, 1981).

   Sodium content may vary greatly from the fresh source as opposed to the canned source. For example, a small serving of cooked fresh salmon contains 116 mg of sodium while the canned equivalent has 522 mg (Crocco, 1982).

3. **Water Supply:** The sodium content should be determined by asking the local water company for this analysis. When sodium exceeds 40 parts per million (2 mEq or 40 mg of sodium per liter), distilled water is appropriate for a 20 mEq/day restriction (Pemberton & Gastineau, 1981). If a water softener is needed at home, it should be attached only to the hot water lines.

4. **Economy:** The cost of following a low-sodium diet is expensive if special low-sodium products are purchased. However, with home preparation of mayonnaise, soup, ketchup, peanut butter, bread, and cake, the diet can be most appetizing yet economical (Kris-Etherton,

1982). A simple and economical method of rinsing foods with water can significantly reduce the sodium content of such items as canned green beans, tuna, and cottage cheese (Vermeulen et al, 1983).

Clinical Implications:

- A 24-hour urine specimen of an individual on moderate salt restriction will contain 90 to 120 mEq of sodium; with no sodium restriction, the specimen will contain over 200 mEq (Silverberg, 1980).
- Patient experimentation with salt substitutes should be anticipated and the life-threatening risks of hypo- or hyperkalemia discussed before a problem develops.
- Patients receiving potassium-sparing diuretics and/or similar medications should be warned that they are likely to store potassium and not excrete it appropriately (Riccardella & Dwyer, 1985).
- Medications and beverages containing caffeine should be used in moderation for the hypertensive patient because caffeine has been reported to increase blood pressure.
- While a high-potassium diet probably inhibits the pressure-raising effect of sodium, a high-potassium intake poses a definite risk for those with compromised renal function (Altschul et al, 1984).
- Sodium depletion should not result from dietary restriction alone but may occur in combination with excessive losses due to vomiting, diarrhea, surgery, or profuse perspiration from exercise, or fever. Symptoms include lethargy, weakness, oliguria, azotemia, and abdominal cramps (Pemberton & Gastineau, 1981).
- When caring for patients with heart disease, watch carefully for the following signs of edema:
  1. Sudden weight gain, which may precede the appearance of edema.
  2. Puffiness of the ankles and hands in ambulatory patients.
  3. Swelling of tissues over the sacrum, buttocks, and posterior thighs in bedridden patients (Luckmann & Sorensen, 1987).
- Elderly patients may be more vulnerable to abrupt dietary sodium withdrawal than younger persons.
- Severe sodium restriction may precipitate or aggravate shock by complementing the extensive loss of salt occurring as a result of profuse diaphoresis immediately following myocardial infarction (Christakis & Winston, 1973).
- Diets that are very low in sodium must be used with caution because they can deplete the body's sodium stores. Too little sodium in the diet can produce muscle cramps, convulsions, hypovolemia, and hypotension.

- The progesterone derivatives in birth control pills can stimulate the production of renin. The vast majority of women who take birth control pills experience a slight increase in blood pressure, and approximately two percent actually develops hypertension (Luckmann & Sorensen, 1987).
- The patient taking diuretics for hypertension should be informed of the beneficial effects of reducing sodium intake (Wilber, 1982):
  1. A modest but definite reduction of elevated blood pressure can be expected.
  2. The patient may not have to take potassium supplements or relatively expensive potassium-sparing diuretic.
  3. The antihypertensive effect of the diuretic is enhanced.

• FALLACIES and FACTS

FALLACY: *Restricting calcium intake will effect the same antihypertensive response as the drugs known as calcium channel blockers.*

- **FACT:** *Calcium by itself exerts actions similar to those of the channel blockers. There is also the potential problem of hypertensive patients restricting dairy products because of the fat and sodium content. Calcium is sodium-dependent, so caution should be exercised in reducing dietary levels of sodium, or the efficacy of calcium may be diminished or lost. Low-fat milk products may be chosen to lower fat content (Parrott-Garcia & McCarron, 1984).*

FALLACY: *All sources of sodium must be restricted in cases of hypertension.*

- **FACT:** *Until recently, it has been assumed that the problems with sodium chloride relate to the sodium ion. Recent animal studies have shown that sodium in other forms, e.g., sodium bicarbonate (Whitecarver et al, 1984) or bicarbonate and ascorbate (Kurtz & Morris, 1983) did not raise the blood pressure, but sodium chloride did. Therefore, it is prudent to give special attention to the reduction of dietary sodium chloride (Kaplan, 1985).*

FALLACY: *Eat garlic to cure hypertension.*

- **FACT:** *The amount of garlic necessary to affect hypertension is too great to be incorporated into a practical diet. Garlic extract has a potent, though transient, antihypertensive effect in animal studies,* *but no controlled trials of its use in humans have been reported (Foushee et al, 1982).*

Summary

Dietary control of hyperlipoproteinemia is one of the most promising ways to treat coronary heart disease (CHD) and to help prevent it in those genetically at risk. The three basic goals of any preventive program for cardiovascular disease include:

1. Limiting total dietary fat to not more than 30 percent and to equally divide it among polyunsaturated (especially linoleic acid as well as omega-3, saturated, and monosaturated fatty acids).
2. Restricting cholesterol to 300 mg/day or less.
3. Increasing the intake of complex carbohydrates.

The recommended dietary approach for reducing hypertriglyceridemia is to achieve or maintain normal weight, to reduce dietary fats (especially saturated fats) and increase the intake of fish high in omega-3 fatty acid, to choose more complex carbohydrates over simple sugars, and to restrict alcohol intake.

Hypertension is characterized by deficiencies as well as excesses. Reduced consumption of calcium and potassium may result from a diet for hypertension that restricts intake of the dairy products food group in an effort to lower sodium. Diets too low in sodium may even raise blood pressure because calcium and potassium are usually found in the same kinds of foods that are often restricted. When persons with low calcium levels then increase their sodium intake, blood pressure is elevated more than usual.

Relaxation therapy and a calm lifestyle can reduce hypertension. An exercise program is highly recommended for any type of cardiovascular problem, not only to reduce tension but also for weight control. Excessive weight increases the chances for hyperlipoproteinemia; loss of weight is recommended for all of these patients.

Review Questions

1. How can cholesterol levels be reduced in the body?
2. List the sodium levels for various restricted diets.
3. Define high-density lipoproteins and discuss factors that influence their levels.
4. When are low-sodium diets ineffective?
5. What are the three phases of diets for hyperlipoproteinemia?

Case Study No. 1: Mr. A.C. is a 43-year-old bank vice president who has been experiencing chest pain for the past five years. His family history is positive for coronary heart disease; his father died at age 58 of a myocardial infarction, and his brother, who is in his early forties, has had two myocardial infarctions. He is approximately 22 kg overweight and smokes two packs of cigarettes per day.

At his yearly physical examination, the physician noted a blood pressure of 168/100. All laboratory findings were within normal limits except for the serum cholesterol (305 mg/dl) and serum triglycerides (176 mg/dl).

1. What risk factors for coronary artery disease does Mr. A.C. have?
2. Is it important that the type of hyperlipoproteinemia be identified before diet counseling?
3. What would be the impact of weight loss on Mr. A.C.'s serum cholesterol and triglycerides?
4. What is the range of cholesterol intake allowed for the patient with familial combined hyperlipoproteinemia?
5. What is the P/S ratio desirable for this patient?

Case Study No. 2: On physical examination, Mr. H.G., a 63-year-old postal worker, was found to have a blood pressure of 192/114. There were no other significant findings, except for his being 25 lbs. overweight. After an unsuccessful trial of hygienic measures (weight reduction, increased exercise, and decreased salt intake), the physician prescribed a thiazide diuretic, continuation of the hygienic measures, and increased intake of foods high in potassium.

1. Why were weight reduction and increased activity initially prescribed for Mr. H.G.?
2. Why is the increased potassium intake necessary?
3. Prepare a list of at least 10 foods that are high in potassium.
4. What prepared snacks are particularly high in sodium and should be avoided?
5. What prepared snacks are lower in sodium and should be suggested to Mr. H.G.?
6. What flavoring agents should be recommended to replace salt?

REFERENCE LIST

Ackman, R: New studies in fish oils: Molecular nutrition research. *J Am Oil Chemists' Society* 63(1):58, 1986.

Ahrens, EH: The diet-heart question in 1985: Has it really been settled? *Lancet* 1(May 11): 1085, 1985.

Altschul, AM; McPherson, RA; Burris, JF: Dietary sodium, the ratio Na$^+$/K$^+$ and essential hypertension. *Nutr Abst Rev* 54(10):823, 1984.

American Dietetic Association (ADA): *Handbook of Clinical Dietetics.* New Haven, Yale University Press, 1981.

American Heart Association: *1986 Heart Facts.* Dallas, American Heart Association, 1985.

Anderson, DE: Interactions of stress, salt, and blood pressure. *Ann Rev Physiol* 46:143, 1984.

Anderson, E; Hellstrom, P; Karlander, SG, et al: Effects of a rice-rich versus a potato-rich diet on glucose, lipoprotein, and cholesterol metabolism. *Am J Clin Nutr* 39(4):598, 1984.

Anderson, JW; Tietyen-Clark: Dietary fiber: Hyperlipidemia, hypertension, and coronary heart disease. *Am J Gastroenterol* 81(10):907, 1986.

Arnesen, E; Forde, OH; Thelle, DS: Coffee and serum cholesterol. *Br Med J* 288(June 30):1960, 1984.

Bagatell, CJ; Heymsfield, SB: Effect of meal size on myocardial infarction diet. *Am J Clin Nutr* 39(3):421, 1984.

Beauchamp, GK; Bertino , M; Engelman, K: Modification of salt taste. *Ann Intern Med* 98(5):763, 1983.

Christakis, G; Winston, M: Nutritional therapy in acute myocardial infarction. *J Am Diet Assoc* 63(3):233, 1973.

Connor, SL; Artaud-Wild, SM; Classick-Kohn, CJ; et al: The cholesterol/saturated-fat index: An indication of the hypercholesterolaemic and atherogenic potential of food. *Lancet* 1(May 31):1229, 1986.

Connor, SL; Conner, WE; Henry, H; et al: The effects of familial relationships, age, body weight, and diet on blood pressure and the 24-hour urinary excretion of sodium, potassium and creatinine in men, women, and children of randomly selected families. *Circulation* 70(1):76, 1984.

Connor, WE; Connor, SJ: The dietary treatment of hyperlipidemia: Rationale, technique and efficacy. *Med Clin North Am* 66(2):485, 1982.

Consensus Conference: Treatment of hypertriglyceridemia. *JAMA* 251(9):1196, 1984.

Consensus Development Panel: Lowering blood cholesterol to prevent heart disease. *JAMA* 253(14):2080, 1985.

Crocco, SC: The role of sodium in food processing. *J Am Diet Assoc* 80(1):36, 1982.

Dawber, TR: *The Framingham Study: The Epidemiology of Atherosclerotic Disease.* Cambridge, MA, Harvard University Press, 1980.

Dawber, TR; Kannel, WB; Kagar, A; et al: Environmental factors in hypertension. In *The Epidemiology of Hypertension.* Edited by J Stamler; R Stamler; TN Pullman. New York, Grune & Stratton, Inc, 1967, p. 255.

Flynn, MA; Nolph, GB; Sun, GY; et al: Serum lipids and eggs. *J Am Diet Assoc* 86(11):1541, 1986.

Foushee, DB; Ruffin, J; Banerjee, U: Garlic as a natural agent for the treatment of hypertension: A preliminary report. *Cytobios* 34:145, 1982.

Frederickson, DS; Levy, RI; Bonnell, M; et al: *Diet I: For the Dietary Management of Hyperchylomicronemia (Type I Hyperlipoproteinemia).* Washington, DC, Government Printing Office, 1973a.

Frederickson, DS; Levy, RI; Bonnell, M; et al: *Dietary Management of Hyperlipoproteinemia: A Handbook for Physicians and Dietitians.* Washington, DC, Government Printing Office, 1973b.

Frederickson, DS; Levy, RI; Lees, RS: Fat transport in lipoproteins—an integrated approach to mechanisms and disorders. *N Engl J Med* 276:34, 1967.

Fuller, E: The diet-heart connection. *Patient Care* 20(11):26, 1986.

Hager, T: High-risk 'heart' families. A genealogical look. *JAMA* 250(13):1663, 1983.

Harris, WS: Health effects of omega-3 fatty acids. *Contemporary Nutr* 10(8), 1985.

Haskell, WL: Exercise-induced changes in plasma lipids and lipoproteins. *Preventive Med* 13(1):23, 1984.

Havlik, RJ; Hubert, HB; Fabsitz, RR; et al: Weight and hypertension. *Ann Intern Med* 98(5):855, 1983.

Henry, HJ; McCarron, DA; Morris, CD; et al: Increasing calcium intake lowers blood pressure: The literature reviewed. *J Am Diet Assoc* 85(2):183, 1985.

Hodges, RE; Rebello, T: Dietary changes and their possible effect on blood pressure. *Am J Clin Nutr* 41(5):1155, 1985.

Hofman, A; Hazebroek, A; Valkenburg, HA: A randomized trial of sodium intake and blood pressure in newborn infants. *JAMA* 250(3):370, 1983.

Jackson, RL; Kashyap, ML; Barnhart, RL; et al: Influences of polyunsaturated and saturated fats on plasma lipids and lipoproteins in man. *Am J Clin Nutr* 39(4):589, 1984.

Jenkins, DJA; Wong, GS; Patten, R; et al: Leguminous seeds in the dietary management of hyperlipidemia. *Am J Clin Nutr* 38(4):498, 1983.

Kane, JP; Malloy, MJ: Treatment of hypercholesterolemia. *Med Clin North Am* 66(2):537, 1982.

Kannel, WB: Cardiovascular consequences of physical inactivity. *Primary Cardiol* 10(4):74, 1984.

Kannel, WB; Castelli, WP; Gordon, T; et al: Serum cholesterol lipoproteins and the risk of coronary heart disease: The Framingham study. *Ann Intern Med* 74(1):1971.

Kaplan, NM: Non-drug treatment of hypertension. *Ann Intern Med* 102(3):359, 1985.

Korch, GC: Sodium content of potable water: Dietary significance. *J Am Diet Assoc* 86(1):80, 1986.

Kromhout, D: Body weight, diet and serum cholesterol in 871 middle-aged men during 10 years of follow-up (the Zutphen study). *Am J Clin Nutr* 38(4):591, 1983.

Krotkiewski, M; Mandroukas, K; Sjostrom, L; et al: Effects of long-term physical training on body fat, metabolism, and blood pressure in obesity. *Metabolism* 28(6):650, 1979.

Kurtz, TW; Morris, RC Jr: Dietary chloride as a determinant of "sodium-dependent" hypertension. *Science* 222(December 9):1139, 1983.

Little, AC; Brinner, L: Taste responses to saltiness of experimentally prepared tomato juice samples. *J Am Diet Assoc* 86(9):1022, 1984.

Lorenz, R; Spengler, U; Fischer, S; et al: Platelet function, thromboxane formation and blood pressure control during supplementation of the Western diet with cod liver oil. *Circulation* 67(3):504, 1983.

Lowering blood cholesterol to prevent heart disease. *Nutr Reviews* 43(9):283, 1985.

Luckmann, J; Sorensen, KC; *Medical-Surgical Nursing: A Psychophysiologic Approach,* 3rd ed. Philadelphia, W. B. Saunders Co, 1987.

MacMahon, SW; Blackett, RB; MacDonald, GJ; et al: Obesity, alcohol consumption and blood pressure in Australian men and women: The National Heart Foundation of Australia risk factor prevalence study. *J. Hypertension* 2(1):85, 1984.

McCarron, DA; Morris, C: Oral Ca^{2+} in mild to moderate hypertension: a randomized, placebo-controlled trial. *Clin Res* 32(2):335A, 1984.

McCarron, DA; Morris, CD; Henry, HJ; et al: Blood pressure and nutrient intake in the United States. *Science* 224(June 29):1392, 1984.

Mattson, FH; Grundy, SM: Comparison of effects of dietary saturated, monounsaturated and polyunsaturated fatty acids on plasma lipids and lipoproteins in man. *J Lipid Research* 26(February):194, 1985.

Matter, S; Weltman, A Stamford, BA: Body fat content and serum lipid levels. *J Am Diet Assoc* 77(2):149, 1980.

Meneely, GR; Battarbee, HD: High sodium–low potassium environment and hypertension. *Am J Cardiol* 38(6):768, 1976.

MRFIT Research Group: Multiple risk factor intervention trial: Risk factor changes and mortality results. *JAMA* 248(12):1465, 1982.

National Heart, Lung and Blood Institute (NHLBI): *Working Group Report on Heart Disease Epidemiology.* U.S. Department of Health, Education, and Welfare Publication No. (NIH) 79-1667, 1979.

Nestel, PJ: Fish oil attenuates the cholesterol induced rise in lipoprotein cholesterol. *Am J Clin Nutr* 43(5):752, 1986.

Nugent, CA; Carnahan, JE; Sheehan, ET; et al: Salt restriction in hypertensive patients. Comparison of advice, education, and group management. *Arch Intern Med* 144(6):1415, 1984.

Paffenbarger, RS, Jr; Wing, AL; Hyde, RT; et al: Physical activity and incidence of hypertension in college alumni. *Am J Epidemiol* 117(3):245, 1983.

Paige, DM (ed): *Manual of Clinical Nutrition.* Pleasantville, NJ, Nutrition Publications, Inc, 1983.

Parrott-Garcia, M; McCarron, DA: Calcium and hypertension. *Nutr Rev* 42(6):205, 1984.

Peled-Ney, R; Silverberg, DS; Rosenfield, JB: A controlled study of group therapy in essential hyertension. *Isr J Med Sci* 20(1):12, 1984.

Pemberton, CM; Gastineau, CF (eds): *Mayo Clinic Diet Manual.* Philadelphia, W. B. Saunders Co, 1981.

Qureshi, AA; Din, ZZ; Abuirmeileh, N; et al: Suppression of avian hepatic lipid metabolism by solvent extracts of garlic: Impact on serum lipids. *J Nutr* 113(9):1746, 1983.

Ram, CV; Garrett, BN; Kaplan, NM: Moderate sodium restriction and various diuretics in the treatment of hypertension: Effects of potassium wastage and blood pressure control. *Arch Intern Med* 141(7):1015, 1981.

Rauramaa, R; Salonen, TJ; Kukkonen-Harjula, K; et al: Effects of mild exercise on serum lipoproteins and metabolites of arachidonic acid: A controlled randomised trial in middle aged men. *Br Med J* 288(February 18):603, 1984.

Reisin, E; Abel, R; Modan, M; et al: Effect of weight loss without salt restriction on the reduction of blood pressure in overweight hypertensive patients. *N Engl J Med* 298(1):1, 1978.

Riccardella, D; Dwyer, J: Salt substitutes and medicinal potassium sources: Risks and benefits. *J Am Diet Assoc* 85(4):471, 1985.

Silverberg, DA: Treating hypertension with diet. *Consultant* 20(7):115, 1980.

Truswell, AS: Diet and hypertension. *Br Med J* 291(July 13):125, 1985.

Vermeulen, RT; Sedor, FA; Kimm, SYS: Effect of water rinsing on sodium content of selected foods. *J Am Diet Assoc* 82(4):392, 1983.

Vollset, SE; Bjelke, E: Does consumption of fruit and vegetables protect against stroke? *Lancet* 2(September 24):742, 1983.

Walser, M; Imbembo, Al; Margolis, S; et al: *Nutritional Management: The Johns Hopkins Handbook.* Philadelphia, W. B. Saunders Co, 1984.

Wilber, JA: The role of diet in the treatment of high blood pressure. *J Am Diet Assoc* 80(1):25, 1982.

Willett, W; Hennekens, CH; Siegel, AJ; et al: Alcohol consumption and high-density lipoprotein cholesterol in marathon runners. *N Engl J Med* 303(20):1159, 1980.

Woodcock, BE; Smith E; Lambert, WH; et al: Beneficial effect of fish oil on blood viscosity in peripheral vascular disease. *Br Med J* 288 (Feb 18):592, 1984.

Further Study

Ackley, S; Barrett-Conner, E; Suarez, L: Dairy products, calcium, and blood pressure. *Am J Clin Nutr* 38(3):457, 1983.

American Heart Association: *Dietary Guidelines for Healthy American Adults: A Statement for Physicians and Health Professionals by the Nutrition Committee.* Dallas, TX, ADA National Center, 1986.

Anderson, JW; Story, L; Sieling, B; et al: Hypocholesterolemic effects of high-fibre diets rich in water-soluble plant fibres. *J Can Diet Assoc* 45(April):140, 1984.

Blair, SN; Goodyear, NN; Gibbons, LW; et al: Physical fitness and incidence of hypertension in healthy normotensive men and women. *JAMA* 252(4):487, 1984.

Council on Scientific Affairs: Dietary and pharmacologic therapy for the lipid risk factors. *JAMA* 250(14):1873, 1983.

Dyckner, T; Wester, PO: Effect of magnesium on blood pressure. *Br Med J* (Clin Res) 286:1847, 1983.

Fagerberg, B; Andersson, OK; Issakson, B; et al.: Blood pressure control during weight reduction in obese hypertensive men: Separate effects of sodium and energy restriction. *Br Med J* 288(January 7):11, 1984.

Fujita, T; Noda, H; Ando, K: Sodium susceptibility and potassium effects in young patients with borderline hypertension. *Circulation* 69(3):468, 1984.

Haskell, WL: Exercise-induced changes in plasma lipids and lipoproteins. *Prev Med* 13(1):23, 1984.

King, DE: How to give your portal hypertension patient a fighting chance. *RN* 46(7):31, 1983.

Kirkendall, WM; Hammond, JJ: Hypertension in the elderly. *Arch Intern Med* 140(9):1155, 1980.

Kris-Etherton, PM; Kisloff, L; Kassouf, RA; et al: Teaching principles and cost of sodium-restricted diets. *J Am Diet Assoc* 80(1):55, 1982.

Lipid Research Clinics Program: The Lipid Research Clinics coronary primary prevention trial results. *JAMA* 251(3):351, 1984.

Loustau, A; Blair, BJ: A key to systematic teaching to help hypertensive patients. *Nursing* 81(2):84, 1981.

Moore, M; Guzman, MA; Schilling, PE; et al: Dietary atherosclerosis study on deceased persons. *J Am Diet Assoc* 79(6):668, 1981.

Moser, M: Sodium restriction, diuretics and potassium loss. *Arch Intern Med* 141(7):983, 1981.

Raymond, J; DeVries, WC; Joyce, LD: Nutrition for the first total artificial heart patient: Implications for future patients. *J Am Diet Assoc* 84(5):532, 1984.

Shank, FR; Park, YK; Harland, BF; et al: Prospectives of food and drug administration on dietary sodium. *J Am Diet Assoc* 80(1):29, 1982.

Singer, P; Jaeger, W; Wirth, M; et al: Lipid and blood pressure–lowering effect of mackerel diet in man. *Atherosclerosis* 49(1):99, 1983.

Dietary Management of Renal and Urinary Tract Disorders

33

OBJECTIVES

THE STUDENT WILL BE ABLE TO:

- **Discuss the complications of renal dysfunction.**
- **Explain reasons for the modifications of protein, sodium, and potassium in renal disease.**
- **Discuss nutrient supplements that are usually required with renal disorders.**
- **List the types of kidney stones, their causes, and the recommended dietary interventions.**

TERMS TO KNOW

Acute glomerulonephritis
Anephric
Anuria
Azotemia
Continuous ambulatory peritoneal dialysis (CAPD)
Chronic renal failure (CRF)
Cystinuria
Giordano-Giovanetti diet
Glomerular filtration rate (GFR)
Hyperuricosuria
Lithotripsy
Low-phosphorus, low-nitrogen (LPLN) diet
Massive proteinuria
Nephrolithiasis
Nephrotic syndrome
Nocturia
Oliguria
Osteodystrophy
Protein catabolic rate (PCR)
Renal osteodystrophy
"Sand" (or "gravel")
Uremia

Physiology of the Kidney

The functional unit of the kidney is the nephron in which blood from the renal artery enters into a cluster of tiny capillaries called a glomerulus (Fig. 33–1). Each kidney contains about one million of these nephrons, which are the filtering system. Filtrates pass through the glomerulus into the surrounding double-walled, funnel-like Bowman's capsule leading to a series of collecting tubes. Within the loop of Henle, further reabsorption occurs. Substances reabsorbed are glucose, amino acids, electrolytes, and vitamins.

Urine, which is about 96 percent water, is continuously produced by the kidney and collected in the bladder. The kidneys have a remarkable flexibility to conserve water output (urine) especially if the intake is low. Other constituents of urine are the nitrogenous end products of protein metabolism, i.e., urea, nitrogen, uric acid, creatinine, ammonium salts, and electrolytes. These waste products are eliminated in significant amounts only through the kidneys. The kidneys filter and reabsorb fluids at the rate of about 125 ml/minute or 180 L/day, yet only 1 to 2 L/day are normally excreted. Minimal renal excretory capacity is maintained as long as the kidney has 10 percent functioning tissue (Burton & Hirschman, 1983).

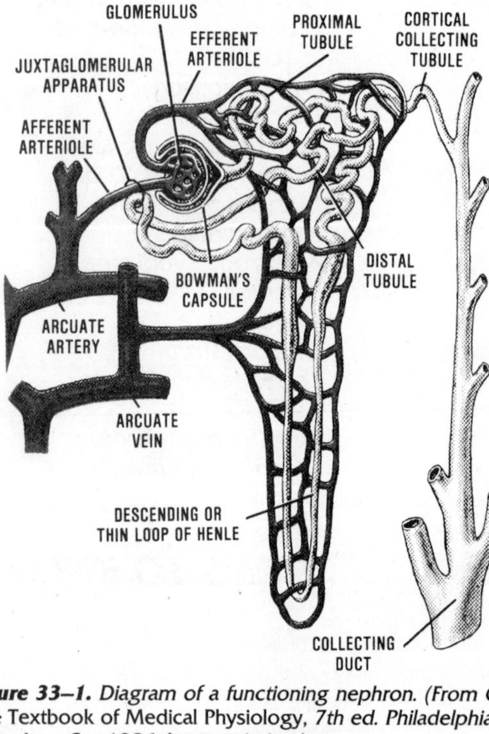

Functions of the kidneys include:
1. Filtering and excreting waste products to avoid toxicity.
2. Secreting substances to maintain the acid-base, electrolyte, and fluid balance.
3. Reabsorbing nutrients, e.g., amino acids, glucose, sodium, and others.
4. Secreting hormones, e.g., renin, erythropoietin, prostaglandin for endocrine activity, and conversion of vitamin D into an active form.
5. Concentrating filtrate.

Renal Disorders

Renal disease affects approximately eight million people in the United States (Burge et al, 1984). Interferences with normal kidney functions may result from infections, inflammation, or blockages such as those from cysts, renal calculi, injuries, or tumors. Renal disease can affect the entire nephron or different parts of it: Nephritis (an inflammatory disorder) can affect the glomerulus, tubules, or interstitial renal tissue; glomerulonephritis is the result of damage in the glomeruli; nephrosis is the result of very permeable renal tubules; and renal failure is severe loss of renal function resulting from glomerular or tubular insufficiency. Since various parts of the kidney have different functions, therapy for each disease varies. Cardiovascular disease may affect the kidneys by the change in blood flow, sustained hypertension (which may be caused either by the heart or kidneys), and/or degenerative tissue changes in the kidney.

URINARY TRACT INFECTIONS

Pathophysiology. The simplest and most common kidney abnormality is urinary tract infection. It is usually caused by bacteria but may result from an injury or obstruction, such as kidney stones. If untreated, chronic pyelonephritis and renal failure may develop.

Nutritional Care. Increased fluid intake is the main dietary goal. Previously, an acidic urine ash via diet or vitamin C was prescribed. Cranberry

Figure 33–1. Diagram of a functioning nephron. (From Guyton AC: Textbook of Medical Physiology, 7th ed. Philadelphia, W. B. Saunders, Co, 1986, by permission.)

juice has been used for preventing and treating urinary tract infection and calculi. While most fruits metabolize to alkaline residues, cranberries, prunes, and plums increase urinary acidity. However, the end results of their intake is not predictable; variations of urinary acidification result, but some subjects still manifest progressive increases in urinary calcium (Kahn et al, 1967). Current pharmacological agents are more dependable, provide explicit results, and curb infection.

ACUTE GLOMERULONEPHRITIS

Pathophysiology. Inflammation or injury of glomeruli is called glomerulonephritis. One to two weeks after an infection, particularly a streptococcal infection, acute glomerulonephritis may develop. Most children recover completely, but a large number of adults may develop a chronic disorder, which can be inactive for long periods of time, and do not fully recover. The inflammation may lead to scarring and loss of filtering surface within the glomeruli. Initially, hematuria (blood in the urine) occurs followed by oliguria (reduced urine secretion) and then anuria (no urine secretion). Weakness, lethargy, and anorexia may be present. Hypertension with edema, particularly of the face, may develop.

Principles of Nutritional Care. The goal of diet therapy is to provide adequate nutritional support. Serum chemistry values that indicate accumulation of metabolic wastes dictate the appropriate therapy: Protein is restricted for uremia, potassium for hyperkalemia, and sodium for edema. Adequate replacement fluid is provided for diuresis.

CHRONIC GLOMERULONEPHRITIS

Pathophysiology. Each recurrence of nephritis destroys renal tissue and decreases renal function. However, most patients may not have had the acute glomerulonephritis. Since the disease may be asymptomatic for long periods of time and is of unknown etiology, clinical testing may be the only way of detecting it. Proteinuria and hematuria reflect damage to the glomeruli. As the disease progresses, hypertension, a lowered serum protein level, edema, and vascular changes occur.

Principles of Nutritional Care. Dietary changes are made to restore or maintain optimum nutritional status. Protein must be supplied to replace the amount lost, but at the same time, the waste products of protein metabolism should be mini-

mized. Electrolytes, sodium, and potassium are controlled in order to curtail edema and maintain potassium balance.

NEPHROTIC SYNDROME (NEPHROSIS)

Pathophysiology. This condition is characterized by heavy proteinuria. Degenerative lesions of the renal tubules result in increased capillary permeability in the glomeruli. The nephrotic syndrome is characterized by heavy proteinuria, hypoalbuminemia, edema, and hypercholesterolemia. Because of such large losses of proteins, some of which may include those that bind thyroxine and iron, hypothyroidism and/or anemia may result. Nephrosis is primarily a disease of young children.

Principles of Nutritional Care. The primary objectives of diet therapy are to control edema and replace protein losses. The presence of edema is usually treated with a reduction in sodium intake along with the use of diuretics. An appropriate level of sodium is 40 to 90 mEq (1000 to 2000 mg). Caution must be exercised to prevent hypokalemia.

The replacement of protein losses must be balanced with a sufficient intake of nonprotein calories. Protein requirements may be determined as follows (Moffitt, 1985):

1.1 gm of protein $\div$ kg of IBW + protein lost in urine = protein requirements/24 hours.

Protein requirement $\div$ 24 hours
  $\times$ 70% = high biological value protein
  $\times$ 30% = low biological value protein

Caloric requirements are between 40 to 60 kcal/kg/day. Carbohydrates and fats should be utilized in sufficient quantity to provide a kilocalorie-to-nitrogen ratio of approximately 150:1 in order to prevent nitrogen wasting.

Hypercholesterolemia is primarily a result of protein losses; cholesterol and fats are usually not restricted unless the hyperlipidemia is extremely elevated.

ACUTE RENAL FAILURE

Pathophysiology. Acute renal failure occurs abruptly, frequently after burns, injuries, shock, or sepsis. It occurs more frequently in adults than in infants or children; generally, renal function is restored when renal cells are regenerated.

Glomerular filtration rate is reduced and waste

products accumulate. Oliguria (less than 400 to 500 ml urine excretion in 24 hours) is the hallmark of acute renal failure. To eliminate solute metabolic wastes, at least 600 ml/day must be excreted.

There are two distinct phases of acute renal failure. The first is the oliguric phase, which may last about two days. The second, or diuretic, phase is a recovery period. The urinary output may double each day. While urine excretion may approach a normal level, kidney function is still poor, and uremia is present. Dialysis may be the major form of treatment during both of these phases. Renal function gradually improves, but it may take up to one year before full recovery.

Principles of Nutritional Care. Nutritional support must be concerned with supplying adequate energy, which is increased owing to the catabolic stress. This is accomplished by controlling the protein intake (because of the uremia) and by correcting the metabolic acidosis and fluid and electrolyte imbalances. It is indeed a complicated and delicate task. Many patients are critically ill and cannot take food orally; intravenous feedings may be used alone or in combination with tube or oral feedings, as necessary.

Energy. The energy needs are high, ranging from 2000 to 5000 kcal/day. Since protein intake is restricted, energy must be supplied from carbohydrates and fats. Even these must be low in electrolytes. In addition to refined sweets and fats, low-protein, high-energy, low-electrolyte commercial preparations may supplement kilocalories with minimum amounts of fluid. Some of these are Hy-Cal (Beecham Laboratories), Cal Power (General Mills), Polycose (Ross), and Lipomul Oral (Upjohn). If patients are unable to ingest and adequate amount of calories, intravenous glucose feedings may be used.

Protein. Even though the by-products of protein metabolism are accumulating, and thus enhancing the onset of uremia, it is important that the patient receive some protein to establish nitrogen balance. While the optimal amount of protein given initially is controversial, 0.5 gm/kg of IBW per day (20 to 40 gm of high-biological-value protein) is usually recommended if the patient is not on dialysis. For the dialyzed patient, the protein intake is liberalized accordingly. As the kidney function improves, as evidenced by the glomerular filtration rate (GFR), the protein intake is increased to at least the RDA.

When the protein intake is as low as 20 to 40 gm, 80 percent of that protein should be the high-biological-value protein found in meat, fish, poultry, eggs, and milk. This leaves only 8 gm of protein from other protein-containing foods, such as breads, cereals, and vegetables. Therefore, low-protein bread is used.

Glucose intravenous feedings only *reduce* protein catabolism. Intravenous feedings should be supplemented with special formulations that contain essential amino acids (EAA) for a positive nitrogen balance in renal patients. Such commercial products include Amin-aid (McGaw) and Travasorb Renal (Travenol). As a part of total parenteral nutrition (TPN), the total daily dosage is 20 to 40 gm of EAA.

Supplementation of EAA may be required in severely uremic patients for a positive nitrogen balance. These products discussed above are also available as oral tablets and powders. They can be used in an oral diet or tube feeding and are frequently advisable not only because the total protein of the diet is limited, but because the specific amino acid patterns are different from regular foods. As the restriction for protein is lowered to 20 gm, only milk and egg proteins or EAA formulas are used. When 35 to 40 gm of protein are allowed, perhaps 20 gm from EAA formulations with the remaining from any source would be permitted.

Fluid and Sodium Balance. In both phases of the disease, fluid intake, which is extremely important, is regulated according to fluid output. Initially, fluids are restricted in the oliguric phase to the previous day's output plus a hypothetical allowance for insensible water losses and any losses from vomitus or diarrhea (Table 33–1). Dehydration and fluid overload are both potential problems that should be guarded against by careful monitoring of the patient's weight and serum sodium. During the diuretic phase, fluid intake is increased to offset losses; normal saline intravenous feedings may be necessary.

Sodium is also dependent on the level of urinary excretion. During the oliguric phase, sodium restriction may be 20 to 40 mEq (500 to 1000 mg).

Table 33–1. Calculation of Fluid Requirements for Acute Renal Failure

Measured urine output of previous 24 hours	−250 ml
Insensible water loss in 24 hours (Depends on room temperature, humidity, and body temperature)	−900 ml
Water loss in vomitus	−100 ml
Total water loss in 24 hours	−1250 ml
Water produced by metabolism in 24 hours (Not allowing for catabolism and weight loss)	+350 ml
Water requirements for 24 hours	900 ml
Water in usual diet in 24 hours	−500 ml
Additional fluid intake needed in 24 hours	400 ml

Potassium. During the oliguric phase, potassium levels are closely monitored and intake is restricted accordingly. Hyperkalemia (<5 mEq/L) is a potential problem because potassium excretion is decreased when the urine volume is decreased, and tissue breakdown causes the release of potassium from the damaged cells. Because acute renal failure is usually sudden, hyperkalemia is a life-threatening situation and may be the main reason for initiating dialysis.

Oral feedings may be restricted to 1.0 to 1.5 gm of potassium until urine output increases and the serum potassium levels are normalized.

Other methods of reducing serum potassium levels may be used. Intravenous glucose and insulin forces potassium from the serum into the cell. Cation exchange resin drugs (such as Kayexalate) exchange sodium for potassium. However, these drugs are unpleasant and could aggravate the edema already present.

Clinical Implications:

- Sorbitol may be given to increase fluid loss from diarrhea.
- When energy intake is limited, a weight loss of 0.2 to 0.3 kg/day may be expected; failure to lose 0.2 during the oliguric phase indicates fluid retention.
- Anemia may be a result of complications during acute renal failure. Patients should be assessed for this.
- After acute renal failure, fluid and electrolytes may require hourly adjustments.

CHRONIC RENAL FAILURE

Pathophysiology. Failure of kidney function to return to normal after acute renal failure or progressive deterioration of the nephrons results in chronic renal failure. Metabolic wastes in the blood, specifically urea and other nitrogenous products, are not removed, and the blood urea nitrogen (BUN) rises. The excessive retention of byproducts from protein metabolism in the blood produces a toxic condition called uremia. Azotemia refers to nitrogenous products from protein catabolism in the blood without the clinical symptoms of uremia being present. The uremic syndrome includes: (1) azotemia (retention of urea, creatinine, and other products of protein metabolism), (2) progressive acidosis, (3) oliguria (decreased urine formation), and (4) various electrolyte disturbances.

In the first stage of chronic renal failure, approximately one half to two thirds of the nephrons are not functioning, which results in decreased renal reserve or renal impairment. In the second stage, the kidneys cannot maintain homeostasis and mild azotemia develops, which is reflected in slight elevations of BUN, creatinine, and uric acid and a mild anemia. The third stage, referred to as renal failure, is characterized by moderate to severe azotemia. There is a marked elevation of BUN and creatinine and pronounced anemia. In the final stage, 90 percent of kidney function has been lost and uremia is present. Damage is irreversible; dialysis or transplantation is essential.

Related Complications. Because the disease progresses over a long period of time, many other conditions are frequently observed.

Both hypertriglyceridemia and hypercholesterolemia are characteristic of massive proteinuria and chronic renal failure. Even though the regular dietary restrictions pertaining to cardiovascular disease may have meaning for the renal patient, these additional restrictions have been difficult to incorporate and may not be effective (Green et al, 1985). The imbalance of sodium and potassium may produce hypertension and edema.

Increased phosphorus levels cause hyperparathyroid activity, which elevates plasma calcium and results in calcium deposits in the soft tissues as well as skeletal disorders, unless corrected. Vitamin D metabolism is disturbed as renal function becomes impaired. This relates directly to the calcium absorbed and leads to renal osteodystrophy, e.g., a combination of various changes in bones associated with renal failure. Moderate dietary restriction of protein and control of serum calcium and phosphate should begin early in patients with renal failure to prevent secondary hyperparathyroidism and renal osteodystrophy from developing as well as to delay the progression of chronic renal failure (Maschio et al, 1982).

Decreased taste perception in uremic patients may affect appetite. As renal failure advances, thresholds for both sour and sweet tastes progressively increase (the ability to detect sour tastes deteriorates first) (Burge et al, 1984). Most children with renal disease need extremely high concentrations of sweetness or sourness to identify flavors (Spinozzi, 1979). Zinc supplementations with adequate protein intake for nitrogen balance may improve this condition if depletion is present (Burge et al, 1984).

Anemia may be attributed to decreased production and survival of red blood cells. The severity of anemia is roughly related to the degree of azotemia. Each increment of 10 mg/dl of serum urea nitrogen correlates to a hemoglobin decrement of 1 gm/dl (Moore & Maher, 1984). This relationship is useful in determining when anemia is disproportionately severe for the degree of renal failure.

Other possible causes of anemia besides renal disease (such as iron deficiency from gastrointestinal bleeding, folate or vitamin B_{12} deficiency, and drug-induced hemolysis) must be carefully assessed and treated. Specific treatments for anemia include curtailing blood loss, judicious treatment of acidosis and phosphate retention, and transfusions in symptomatic patients (Moore & Maher, 1984).

Nutritional Assessment. An energetic and enthusiastic health care team is vital for monitoring and promoting a nutritional program for the renal patient. In no other illness is an individualized diet plan as important as in renal disease. The professional responsible for prescribing the diet must rely on frequent laboratory tests, anthropometric measurements, and feedback from the patient. Monitoring food intake or analyzing food diaries as well as information from anthropometric and biochemical laboratory tests reflect dietary compliance. These assessment tools can also be used to encourage the patient to continue the diet.

Principles of Nutritional Care. In chronic renal failure, early dietary restrictions result in a more optimistic outcome. The rate of renal failure depends to a large extent on how early the dietary prescription is begun. Higher protein intake requires more work for the kidneys to excrete waste products. Dialysis and even death can be postponed for many months by rational diet therapy to protect the residual renal function and to reduce azotemia and uremia (Burton & Hirschman, 1983).

Patients with chronic renal failure are frequently malnourished. Increased protein breakdown is compounded by poor appetite that results in inadequate nutrient management of malnutrition; anemia; abnormalities of calcium, phosphorus, and vitamin D metabolism; hypertension and salt balance; and potassium and acid-base balance.

Objectives of the dietary regimen are to:
1. Maintain optimal nutritional status and stimulate patient well-being.
2. Provide adequate kilocaloric intake.
3. Regulate protein intake in order to: (a) minimize uremic toxicity, (b) prevent net protein catabolism, (c) provide for continuous growth in children, and (d) retard progression of renal failure and postpone the initiation of dialysis.

4. Regulate fluid intake to balance fluid output by the regulation of sodium and the restriction of potassium.
5. Provide supplements of appropriate vitamins and minerals.

In the first stage of chronic renal failure, diet restrictions are not indicated unless hypertension is present, in which case sodium and kilocalories (for weight loss) would be limited. Adequate calories should be provided so that protein is not utilized for energy, thereby increasing the work load of the kidney.

In the second stage, restrictions may be necessary in electrolyte intake, especially sodium and potassium as well as phosphorus. The degree of restriction depends on the state of hydration and hypertension. Fluid intake is dictated by the urine output and degree of hydration. If urinary excretion is reduced, potassium and phosphate are restricted. Protein and caloric restrictions are usually not necessary.

In the third stage, strict diet modifications are usually necessary. Protein is limited to 0.6 to 1.0 gm/kg of IBW (40 to 60 gm) with 50 to 60 percent of this amount from high-biological-value proteins. Sodium, potassium, and phosphorus are dependent on individual body signs: degree of hydration (sodium), serum potassium levels, and serum phosphate levels. Fluid is determined by the amount of insensible losses plus the urine volume from the previous day or the amount needed to maintain the desired weight. Energy intake is not restricted in order to prevent catabolism.

In the last stage of renal failure, many nutrients are closely monitored. Appropriate exchange lists have been developed for the complicated renal diet (see Appendix D–7). Sample meal patterns are in Appendix D–8.

Protein. For chronic renal failure, there is a fine line between avoiding uremic toxicity from excessive protein intake while preventing malnutrition due to inadequate amounts of protein. Moderate protein restriction is an acceptable and effective way of delaying functional renal deterioration. Low-protein diets may result in reduced quality of life but are necessary (Table 33–2). A low-protein diet decreases nausea, vomiting, and fatigue. These restrictions are difficult for many patients to become accustomed to.

Protein restriction is usually initiated when the glomerular filtration rate (GFR) is below 25 mg/minute. Protein intake can be determined by using the GFR formulations in Table 33–3.

Women and small men may be restricted to about 35 gm/day of protein with at least 20 to 24

Table 33–2. Low-Protein Products and Their Sources*

Product	Source
Aproten Low-Protein Pasta, Rusks, Porridge Dietetic Paygel Baking Mix Dietetic Paygel Wheat Starch Low-Protein Canned Bread Prono Imitation Jello	Dietary Specialties, Inc. P.O. Box 227 Rochester, NY 14601
Cellu Wheat Starch Lo Pro Pastas Low-Protein Baking Mix and Bread	Chicago Dietetic Supply, Inc. 405 East Shawnut Avenue La Grange, IL 60525
Controlyte	D.M. Doyle Pharmaceutical Co. Highway 100 at West 23rd Street Minneapolis, MN 55416
Low-Protein Bread and Mix Potato Mix Egg Replacer	Ener-G Foods, Inc. 1526 Utah Avenue, South Seattle, WA 98134
Welplan Bread Welplan Golden Raisin Cookies Welplan Savory (Cheese) Cookies	Anglo-Dietetics LTD. 641 Lancaster Pike Frazer, PA 19355

Low-Protein Chocolate-Flavored Chip Cookies; Low-Protein
   Butterscotch Chip Cookies
Low-Protein Bread
Baking Mix
Wheat Starch
Anellini (Ring Macaroni)
Ditalini (Short-Ribbed Macaroni)
Rigatoni (Long-Ribbed Macaroni)
Tagliatelle (Fat Noodles)
Rusks
Prono (low-protein gelatin—lime, cherry, orange, and
   strawberry)
Cal Plus (powdered high-calorie supplement)
	Dietary Specialties, Inc.
	P.O. Box 227
	Rochester, NY 14601

Product 80056	Mead Johnson Laboratories Evansville, IN 47721

*From Walser, M; Imbembo, AL; Margolis, S; et al: *Nutritional Management: The Johns Hopkins Handbook.* Philadelphia, W. B. Saunders Co, 1984, with permission.

gm of high-quality protein. The goal is to maintain nitrogen balance on the reduced intake using as little as 37 to 40 gm/day of protein without synthetic amino acid supplements.

Supplementation of essential amino acids (EAA) (discussed in the section on acute renal failure) may be required in severely uremic patients for positive nitrogen balance. Since this diet is highly restrictive, patient adherence is not too successful. The use of EAA supplements with 20 gm of unrestricted proteins is a more popular regimen.

It is not clear whether the low-protein diet is beneficial because of its low-protein content or its low-phosphorus content (Giordano, 1982). Therefore, a low-phosphorus, low-nitrogen (LPLN) diet is often selected. The LPLN diet supplies for each kilogram of body weight, approximately 0.5 gm of high-biological-value protein, 0.7 mg of phosphorus, and 35 kcal/day (Barsotti et al, 1983).

Energy Intake. With severe protein restrictions, higher levels of carbohydrates (particularly those with little or no protein) and fats are increased to utilize the minimal protein intake for growth and maintenance of tissues. Renal patients require more energy than the RDA to increase body weight. Very high energy levels are required, which can be calculated utilizing the guidelines in Table 33–3.

Carbohydrate intake probably will be about 1500 to 2000 kcal with 750 to 800 kcal from fat to provide the total intake of 2000 to 2500 kcal/day.

Table 33–3. Dietary Guidelines for Chronic Renal Failure

Daily *protein intake* is restricted as the GFR falls according to these guidelines:*

> 20 to 25 ml/minute = 60 to 90 gm
> 15 to 20 ml/minute = 50 to 70 gm
> 10 to 15 ml/minute = 40 to 55 gm
> 4 to 10 ml/minute = about 40 gm (0.55 to 0.60 gm/kg/day)

Caloric intake can be determined as follows:†

Adults:	over 17 years of age—35 to 40 kcal/kg of body weight
Children:	1 to 3 years of age—100 kcal/kg of body weight
	4 to 6 years of age—90 kcal/kg of body weight
	7 to 10 years of age—80 kcal/kg of body weight
Adolescents:	11 to 17 years of age—40 to 50 kcal/kg of body weight

Sodium and Fluid Intake:*
  Normal restriction: 1 to 3 gm sodium; 1500 to 3000 ml fluid
  Polyuria: 6 to 8 gm sodium; fluid unlimited
  Oliguria or anuria: 1 to 1.5 gm sodium; 750 to 1500 ml (determined by previous day's output + 500 ml)

Potassium:
  Oliguria or anuria: 70 mEq

Calcium and Phosphorus Intake:*
  Reduce to achieve a normal serum phosphorus level; then supplement calcium (1 gm)

Vitamins:
  Daily supplement necessary; be sure it does not contain too much vitamin A and D. Vitamin D is usually supplemented in the form of calcitriol.

*From Kopple, JD: Nutritional therapy in kidney failure. *Nutrition Review* 39(5):193, 1981.
  †From Chicago Dietetic Association and South Surburban Dietetic Association of Cook and Will Counties: *Manual of Clinical Dietetics*, 2nd ed. Philadelphia, W. B. Saunders Co, 1981.

Carbohydrates, whether cereals, grains, or vegetables, must be evaluated by their protein content. Low-protein bread is used to increase the caloric content and to allow the patient to have more protein from sources of high biological value.

Hard candies, gumdrops, jellies, honey, sugar, marshmallows, and Popsicles can be utilized to increase kilocalories. However, even with urging, it is often impossible to motivate patients with renal disease to eat hard candy and other simple sugars because of their anorexia. Commercial preparations discussed in the section on acute renal failure can be used to increase caloric intake.

Clinical Implications:

- After severe protein depletion, anabolic steroids may assist in reversing a negative nitrogen balance (Brundage, 1980).
- For patients with heavy proteinuria or those receiving steroids, an allowance of protein is added to the diet for protein lost in the urine (Giordano, 1982).
- Carbohydrate intolerance may occur in severe renal failure and may require avoidance of concentrated sources of sugar (Brundage, 1980).
- Rigid protein restriction (less than 0.5 mg/kg/day) may lower plasma urea nitrogen concentration but does not warrant the associated malnutrition; it should be used only as a temporary measure until more definitive therapy—dialysis or transplantation—is available.

Calcium and Phosphorus. Renal failure causes phosphate retention, which reduces the plasma calcium concentration. One of the goals of dietary management is to achieve acceptable levels of calcium and phosphorus without elevating concentrations of parathyroid hormone.

When the serum creatinine exceeds 3 mg/dl, phosphate will be retained, and intake of phosphorus should be restricted. To maintain a low to normal level of 2.0 to 3.0 mg/dl of serum phosphorus often requires reducing phosphorus intake to 600 to 1200 mg/day (Kopple, 1981). Since calcium intake is restricted, phosphorus is automatically limited because they are present in many of the same foods (see Appendix D–4).

Protein restriction aids the low-phosphorus diet. A protein intake of 0.5 gm/day/kg of body weight would supply about 800 mg of phosphorus if the types of animal product were not specified. However, by choosing animal and vegetable foodstuffs containing the lowest amount of phosphorus (e.g., egg whites and vegetables) instead of dairy products, egg yolks, and liver, the daily phosphorus intake can be reduced to about 500 mg, which is about one third the intake of an unrestricted mixed diet. Meat and fish may even be boiled to further remove phosphate (Barsotti et al, 1983).

When the serum calcium and phosphorus product is greater than 70 (see Chapter 12), calcium is severely restricted and dietary phosphorus is decreased; phosphate-binding antacids or aluminum hydroxide gels are given (Brundage, 1980). They should be taken with meals to bind dietary phosphorus efficiently (Moore & Maher, 1984).

Calcium supplements (usually calcium carbonate, 1 gm/day) are started after a normal serum phosphorus level is achieved. Small amounts of calcitriol (Rocaltrol), the active form of vitamin D, will induce normal serum calcium levels with an adequate calcium intake (Moore & Maher, 1984) and improve phosphorus metabolism and osteodystrophy.

Clinical Implications:

- Serum calcium and phosphorus should be monitored to achieve normal concentrations.
- Large quantities of phosphate binders are needed. Since they are unpalatable, switching preparations may be useful; they may also be incorporated into recipes for cookies or breads.
- Excessive absorption of aluminum from the use of phosphate binders may result in osteomalacia and/or dementia (Moore & Maher, 1984).
- Since there are no satisfactory alternatives to phosphate binders at this date, prompt control of these dietary factors is desired.
- Hypercalcemia may result from the supplementation of calcitriol; close monitoring is essential. The selection of calcitriol is preferred because it has a shorter half-life than vitamin D (Moore & Maher, 1984). Vitamin D analogues may decrease daily calcium requirements by increasing intestinal calcium absorption (Kopple, 1981).

Fluids and Sodium. Fluid overload or dehydration must be controlled by balancing the intake against the output. For each 24 hours, a fluid intake level that totals 500 to 800 ml plus the previous 24-hour urine volume is recommended, as shown in Table 33–1. Anephric patients are limited to 800 ml/24-hr (Brundage, 1980). Overhydration is a danger when the glomerular filtration rate (GFR) falls below 2 to 5 ml/minute.

Fluids low in protein, sodium, and potassium are chosen. Water, cranberry juice, and sugar-sweetened, fruit-flavored drink mixes contain minimal amounts of these nutrients, so they are allowed liberally with fluid volume limitation. Grape and apple juices are also permissible. Some thirst-quenching suggestions for patients on fluid restrictions are listed in Chapter 5.

The amount of sodium reabsorbed decreases as renal insufficiency progresses. Moderate sodium intake is usually acceptable until end-stage renal disease occurs. At that time, patients may develop edema, hypertension, or congestive heart failure unless sodium and water are restricted.

As renal failure advances, patients may be unable to conserve sodium. With low-sodium intake, sodium depletion may develop. Therefore, patients with chronic renal failure who have no symptoms of fluid overload, hypertension, or heart failure should cautiously be given increased amounts of sodium to determine their tolerance (Kopple, 1981). A daily intake of 1.0 to 3.0 gm (40 to 130 mEq) of sodium and 1500 to 3000 ml of fluid should maintain sodium and water balance in most patients with advanced renal failure.

Sodium restriction may be as low as 400 mg in order to decrease edema and lower blood pressure. Patients who lose excessive amounts of sodium in their urine may require 6000 to 8000 mg/day of sodium to prevent hypotension and dehydration (Rodriquez & Hunter, 1981). When oliguria or anuria is present, limitations of 1.0 to 1.5 gm/day of sodium and 750 to 1500 ml/day of fluid are recommended (Kopple, 1981). (See Chapter 32.)

Potassium. Since foods low in potassium are often high in sodium and vice versa, both potassium and sodium allowances must be carefully planned. Even though the kidney is the major route for potassium excretion, patients do not usually become hyperkalemic until the latter stages of renal failure, unless there is: (1) excessive intake of potassium, (2) acidosis, oliguria, or hypoaldosteronism, or (3) catabolic stress. For the patient with oliguria or anuria, a restriction of 0.5 mEq/day of potassium per kg of body weight (about 35 to 40 mEq of potassium) is advised (Kopple, 1981).

Restriction of protein automatically limits potassium, since meat, whole grains, and legumes contain large amounts. However, a diet can easily contain 3 to 8 gm/day of potassium without careful selection since fruits and vegetables contain appreciable amounts.

Clinical Implications:

- Since the diurnal pattern of normal kidney function is lost, the time span for liquid intake is increased to require intake during the night.
- An excess or depletion of potassium can cause cardiac arrhythmias. Hyperkalemia can occur quickly and without warning causing cardiac depression, arrhythmias, and eventually, cardiac arrest. Therapeutic measures must be promptly initiated for hyperkalemia.
- Helping the renal patient understand the importance of controlling fluids cannot be overemphasized. If excessive fluids are removed by aggressive dialysis, severe muscle cramps, headache, nausea, vomiting, and a sudden drop in blood pressure may follow.
- If the sodium content of the community water supply is high, locally-bottled carbonated beverages and wine, or other alcoholic beverages may contribute appreciably to the sodium content of the diet. Drinking water may have to be either restricted or distilled.
- Rapid weight gain (with constant kilocalorie intake) plus increased blood pressure indicate the sodium intake is too high. On the other hand, weight loss and decreased blood pressure imply too little sodium intake. Body weight must be monitored daily with serum sodium levels and blood pressure in order to estimate the most suitable sodium allowance.
- Nutrition and nursing services must cooperate closely to prevent serious errors in fluid and electrolyte balance among renal patients. Strict fluid limitations must allow enough water for medications.
- Hypermagnesemia may occur with the additional intake from, for example, antacids, laxatives, or enemas—all of which may contain large amounts of magnesium.
- Patients with significant renal disease should be cautioned against eating foods rich in potassium, such as dried fruits.

Trace Elements. Patients with chronic uremia or those who are on dialysis may need oral ferrous sulfate supplements or intramuscular or intravenous injections of iron.

A zinc deficiency may be a major cause of impaired cellular immunity in chronic renal failure (Antoniou et al, 1981). Zinc supplements (0.5 mg/kg of body weight are often given to uremic patients to improve the hypogeusia (decreased taste acuity) and appetites (Rodriquez & Hunter, 1981; Decreased taste acuity, 1981). Results vary among different patients.

Vitamins. Frequently, water-soluble vitamins are deficient in uremic patients because of (1) poor intake of nutrient-dense food sources and dietary restrictions, (2) losses during dialysis, and (3) altered metabolism due to drugs and/or uremia (Kopple, 1981). To insure adequate intake, daily vitamin supplements are recommended for uremic patients. Usually, vitamin supplements do not include biotin, so 10 mg/day of biotin has been given to treat neurological disorders related to uremia such as dialysis dementia, encephalopathy, and peripheral neuropathy (Yatzidis et al, 1981).

Vitamin D conversion to its active form occurs in the kidney; renal failure may result in a deficiency. Myopathy, such as severe weakness in the proximal muscles of the limbs, may result from vitamin D deficiency. Supplementation is usually in the form of calcitriol, the activated form of vitamin D, because its conversion in the kidney is limited.

Clinical Implications:

- The requirements and tolerances for vitamin D supplements may decrease over time; patients must be monitored carefully (Kopple, 1981).
- Most regular multivitamin pills are not advisable because they contain an excess of vitamins A and D for the renal patient (Burton & Hirschman, 1983).

Acid-Base Balance. As renal failure advances, acidosis increases. This phenomenon demineralizes bone, retards growth in children, and exacerbates the fatigue, nausea, and vomiting of uremia and, if severe, can cause cardiovascular collapse. Acidosis should usually be treated when the serum bicarbonate falls below 18 mEq/L. Either sodium bicarbonate or Shohl's solution (Bicitra) can be given. Tablets of sodium bicarbonate cause excessive eructation (belching) in some patients and are poorly tolerated (Moore & Maher, 1984).

Menu Planning. Creativity is necessary to avoid monotony and boredom in the severely restricted renal diet. The more restrictions, the more difficult it is to please the patient and maintain desired goals. Searching for variety, changing the diet daily, and avoiding the same meal on the same day of the week can improve compliance.

NUTRITION FOR CHILDREN WITH RENAL DISEASE

Achieving normal growth in the first two years and catch-up growth in the older, growth-retarded uremic child is a true challenge. Catch-up growth is most difficult. Children whose chronic renal failure (CRF) started at birth are especially small and have marked retardation in skeletal maturation. EAA supplements are used to provide sufficient protein, but the child must be closely monitored because malnutrition and the metabolic disturbances of uremia appear to be more severe in prepubertal children than in adults. Their growth rate is generally poor (Chantler et al, 1980).

Therapeutic diets for the child are composed of ordinary foods, but the amounts are modified and measured, particularly with exactness for total fluid intake. Children must learn to measure all fluids precisely rather than estimating intake. They usually become quite adept at taking medications with little fluid. Also, the child who carefully follows sodium restriction experiences a decrease in thirst.

Protein usually is less restricted for children than adults. Instead of the usual RDA of 2 to 2.5 gm/kg, the minimum protein restriction for children is more often 1 to 1.3 gm/kg of body weight. At least 75 percent of the total protein should be of high biological value (eggs, milk, or meat) to assure an adequate intake of the essential amino acids (Walser et al, 1984).

Even with the recommended intake of 60 to 100 kcal/kg of body weight, the potential growth in height is never achieved. This large amount of kilocalories is often difficult for children to consume.

Stressing allowances rather than restrictions is more optimistic, particularly for children. The child and his/her family should eat meals together with only a slightly modified diet for the child (Hetrick et al, 1979). Preparation of fresh or frozen vegetables with no added sodium or potassium salt allows others to season their food at the table.

Nondairy creamers and whipped toppings may be substituted for dairy products. Candies and cookies made with margarine and honey are more appealing than the early diets of sugar with rice or in butter balls.

Few infants in renal failure need to be placed on fluid restrictions; sodium, potassium, and protein are usually the only problem nutrients. Breast milk is ideal because of the low solute load (Hetrick et al, 1979).

As the child progresses to finger foods, the usual finger foods are often unacceptable. For the young renal failure patient, dry cereals, flavored gelatin cubes, fresh green beans or carrots, marshmallows, salt-free crackers with jelly or honey and margarine, julienne meat, and sticky rice are suitable (Hetrick et al, 1979).

Clinical Implications:

- Children must be taught adequate oral hygiene and dental care to prevent dental caries from the high-carbohydrate intake.
- Avoid all-you-can-eat situations to prevent overindulgence, but do not avoid special occasions entirely.
- Small, hard candies are surprisingly easy to aspirate and should not be offered to young children.
- Particularly for children, an unusually high BUN value may not necessarily indicate an excessively high intake of protein but rather an inadequate dietary intake of nonprotein kilocalories. An unusually low BUN may denote poor nutritional intake, including inadequate protein and nonprotein kilocalories. Complete clinical assessment is required (Spinozzi, 1979).

Dialysis

When kidney function fails, dialysis (removal of toxic substances from the blood and body fluids) must be employed. Peritoneal dialysis uses the peritoneal membrane as the semipermeable membrane and was the only choice of dialysis for some time. More recently, hemodialysis (i.e., extracorporeal dialysis using an artificial kidney employing a synthetic semipermeable membrane) became available. Continuous ambulatory peritoneal dialysis (CAPD) is the newest technical development. This type as well as peritoneal dialysis may be used at home or in centers.

The long-term prognosis for survival on maintenance dialysis is encouraging. Young adults without extrarenal systemic disease and using outpatient dialysis face an annual mortality of less than two percent (Manis & Friedman, 1979). Even with dialysis and/or transplantation, nutritional care is still important for these patients.

HEMODIALYSIS

The treatment of choice for end-stage renal disease is hemodialysis because it is more efficient than peritoneal dialysis. The patient must have a cannula implanted in the wrist; blood passes through a thin membrane in an artificial kidney to the dialyzing fluid to remove unwanted substances (Figure 33–2). The artificial kidney can function about twice as rapidly as two normal kidneys together, but it can be used for no more than 12 hours every three to four days because of the danger from excess heparin (which is added to prevent coagulation), hemolysis, and infection (Guyton, 1986).

PERITONEAL DIALYSIS

Some persons prefer peritoneal dialysis because it is less drastic. It can be more quickly initiated than hemodialysis because a dialyzing machine is not needed, anticoagulants are not necessary, and there is no need for vascular cannulization.

The feeling of fullness that patients experience with the dialysis solution in the peritoneal cavity often causes anorexia, but this disappears within the first few months (Sorrels, 1981).

Fluid restriction is one of the most important aspects of the diet for the dialysis patient. Weight gain between dialysis treatments should not exceed 1 lb. (Burton & Hirschman, 1983). Weight should be measured daily to determine the fluid and sodium regimen. Excess fluid increases weight, results in edema and dyspnea, and may

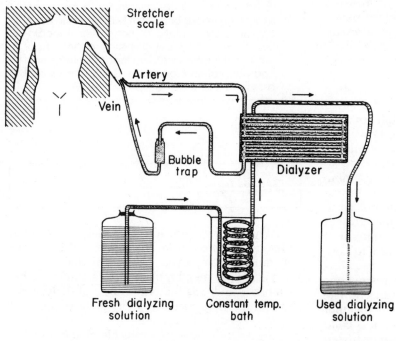

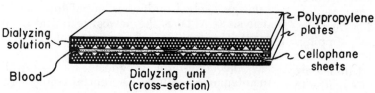

Figure 33–2. Diagram of the artificial kidney. (From Guyton AC: Textbook of Medical Physiology, 7th ed. Philadelphia, W. B. Saunders Co, 1986, by permission.)

cause hypertension. On the other hand, too little fluid results in a decreased GFR. Losses from nausea, vomiting, or diarrhea must be replaced promptly to avoid electrolyte imbalances.

In peritoneal dialysis, sodium intake is restricted to 2 to 3 gm/day because sodium exchange is less effective in peritoneal dialysis than in hemodialysis (Rodriquez & Hunter, 1981). Since peritoneal dialysis is of longer duration and is necessary more frequently than hemodialysis, potassium intake is not as restricted as in hemodialysis. The low-potassium recommendations are difficult to attain because the high-protein foods recommended are also high in potassium (Rodriquez & Hunter, 1981).

Clinical Implications:

- Patients receiving maintenance hemodialysis should receive a calcium supplement.
- The risk of infection is greatly increased during maintenance hemodialysis treatment. This impaired immune function may be reversed by improvement in the nutritional status (Hak et al, 1982).
- A major complication of long-term peritoneal dialysis is peritonitis, which increases protein losses (Rodriquez & Hunter, 1981). Protein depletion also increases the chances of peritonitis.
- Anorexia in peritoneal dialysis may be due to fluid depletion and can be resolved with proper use of dialysis solutions (Sorrels, 1981).
- Diabetic patients are more sensitive to potassium excesses from dialysis than others (ADA, 1981).
- Excessive aluminum in dialysis patients causes a progressive syndrome called dialysis dementia and osteomalacia. The aluminum from the dialysate is the major source of excess aluminum (Kopple, 1981).
- Hemodialysis patients with protein catabolic rates below 0.8 gm/kg/day should be considered high-risk patients; morbidity and mortality are high among these patients with low-protein intake (Acchiardo et al, 1983).

CONTINUOUS AMBULATORY PERITONEAL DIALYSIS

Continuous ambulatory peritoneal dialysis (CAPD) is a new technical development in which the dialysate is left in the peritoneum and exchanged manually four or five times daily.

Because this form of peritoneal dialysis is continuous, sodium and potassium need not be restricted. In fact, approximately 250 mEq (11 gm) of sodium is required to prevent hypotension. This is an average intake, but if the patient has been on sodium restriction, such an allowance may be undesirably salty (Rodriquez & Hunter, 1981). Since phosphate restriction is not necessary, milk products may be included in the diet. Phosphate binders are usually not needed as in hemodialysis.

Protein requirements of 1.2 gm/kg of body weight are similar to those with intermittent peritoneal dialysis (Kopple & Blumenkrantz, 1983).

Water-soluble vitamin supplements include the RDAs for each of the water-soluble vitamins except as follows: pyridoxine hydrochloride, 5 to 10 mg/day; ascorbic acid, 70 to 100 mg/day; and folic acid, 1 mg/day (Kopple & Blumenkrantz, 1983).

Transplantation

Protein intake should be increased to 1.5 to 2 gm/kg of body weight per day for efficient healing. Corticosteroids affect the patient in several ways: (1) Protein catabolism is increased; (2) water and sodium (restricted to 2 gm/day) are retained; (3) appetite is stimulated; and (4) potassium excretion is increased. An antidiuretic drug may be required for hypertension. Dietary suggestions include low-calorie snacks and avoidance of high-carbohydrate and high-potassium foods (Rodriquez & Hunter, 1981).

Dietary Compliance

It is indeed naive when the physician, dietitian, and nurse assume that a patient will accept a diet prescription even in the face of lethal consequences. The strict diet, fluid restrictions, and medication regimen facing the person dependent upon dialysis top the list of psychological, social, and physical problems. About half of the persons on dialysis adhere fairly well to the restrictions. Most abuse comes in the form of weight gain between dialysis sessions (Agashua et al, 1981).

A thorough understanding of the causes of noncompliance has important prophylactic implications for staff and patients. The psychological state of patients, their personality, attitudes, beliefs, and orientations can make the difference between rehabilitation and chronic invalidism.

Dependence on dialysis compounds the problem of diminished self-esteem, particularly with men. Apathy and helplessness may contribute to the patient's feeling that deprivation is fruitless since eating may be his/her main enjoyable activity. The assault on the patient's independence, self-esteem, body image, and physical sense of well-being is significant; all of these factors influence dietary compliance.

Dietary compliance can be more successful with a number of interventionist programs, e.g., patient education, psychotherapy, behavioral strategies, and relaxation therapy. Behavioral therapy can have a significant impact by dealing with recurrent episodes of dietary abuse, sexual dysfunction, and marital conflicts as well as providing opportunities for developing new skills, eating habits, interests, and social roles. Most of all, the individual gains the satisfaction of being in control of his/her own affairs (internal orientation), which enhances compliance with the regimen and increases the pleasure of life (Agashua et al, 1981).

Praise and contingencies, such as tokens for preferred meals or access to early dialysis sessions, increase compliance. Immediate reinforcements are more beneficial than the anticipation of completing long-range goals (Keane et al, 1981).

Urinary Calculi

Another serious problem occurring in the renal system is that of urinary calculi, or stone formation.

NEPHROLITHIASIS (RENAL CALCULI)

In industrialized nations, the incidence of urolithiasis (the formation of urinary calculi and its associated illness) continues to increase significantly. More stones occur among affluent populations, as defined by the mean annual salary and by food expenditures. In fact, the only dietary factor that correlates consistently with the occurrence of stones is the intake of animal protein, particularly meat, fish, and poultry. Conversely, there is a very low incidence of upper urinary tract stones among those with a relatively high intake of vegetable protein (Robertson et al, 1979).

The higher the intake of animal protein, the more likely the individual will have an episode with multiple stones rather than a single stone. With decreased intake of animal protein, the excretion of calcium, oxalate, and uric acid decreases, and the risk of stone formation falls significantly (Robertson et al, 1979). Additionally, a high-calcium, low-phosphorus diet imbalance or increased production of a vitamin D analogue promotes renal lithiasis (Pemberton & Gastineau, 1981, Kark & Oyama, 1980).

These renal stones may be anywhere in the urinary tract but are usually in the kidney. "Sand" or "gravel" is the term used for tiny stone particles, but other types of stones, such as giant staghorn calculi, can fill the entire renal pelvis. This calculus is called a stone because of its crystallization formation with a nucleation of crystallites developing from supersaturated urine and growth by aggregation to form larger particles. Small stones can pass out of the body, but some become trapped in the urinary tract.

Normally, citrate, magnesium, and sodium act as solubilizers to inhibit crystallization. Other substances such as aluminum, ferric iron, and silicone may have the reverse effect. Silicones may come from drinking water or magnesium trisilicate.

RENAL CALCULI AND URINARY STASIS

Gravity plays an important part in kidney functions first by the thrust of the blood into the nephrons, and later by the urine flowing freely from the renal pelvis into the ureter. When the patient is lying down, gravity no longer helps the flow, and urine stagnates in the renal pelvis. If the urine is not excreted, the tiny particles and crystals that ordinarily would be passed out, stay in the renal pelvis. They form the nuclei for renal "recumbency" stones that develop within 14 to 21 days among 15 to 30 percent of all immobilized patients (Fig. 33–3). For this reason, patients are encouraged to become ambulatory as soon as possible and to drink as much fluid as appropriate for the stage of kidney disorder. For immobilized patients, the calcium intake should be limited to about 800 mg/day during the first three to six months or until there is weight-bearing activity (Pemberton & Gastineau, 1981).

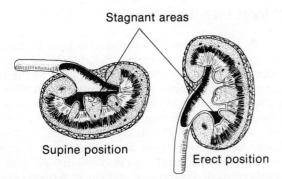

Figure 33–3. The effect of gravity upon renal flow out of the renal pelvis. (From Luckmann J, Sorensen KC: Medical-Surgical Nursing: A Psychophysiologic Approach. Philadelphia, W. B. Saunders Co, 1980, by permission. After Olsen EU, Schroeder LM: The hazards of immobility: Effects on urinary function. American Journal of Nursing, 67(4):791, 1967.)

Other factors that contribute to recumbency stones include: (1) a slightly alkaline urine (common during bed rest), (2) urinary tract infection, (3) elevated calcium concentrations in the urine (urinary calcium can triple after only two weeks of immobilization), and (4) elevated phosphorus due to osteoporosis of disuse.

TYPES OF RENAL STONES

Calcium. Calcium stones are far more common in Caucasian men than in any other population, and the peak incidence is during the third to fifth decades of life (Broadus & Thier, 1979). Excessive absorption of dietary calcium (absorptive hypercalciuria) is responsible for about one fourth of urinary tract stones (Marwick, 1983).

Stones may contain only one substance or a combination of substances, but calcium is found in 75 percent of all urinary tract stones. Yet, many individuals with hypercalciuria have normal calcium intake. If hyperuricosuria is associated with calcium stones, but the stones contain no uric acid, reducing uric acid excretion will diminish the chances of forming new calcium stones.

Calcium-oxalate, the prevalent stone composition, is directly correlated with increased consumption of calcium, sugar, and animal protein by accelerating the urinary excretion of calcium, oxalate, and uric acid. Restriction of calcium and refined carbohydrates and substituting fiber, especially whole-grain bread or unprocessed bran for part of the high animal protein intake, can reduce urinary calcium excretion (Rao et al, 1982).

Oxalate. The next most frequent type of renal stones is composed of oxalate. Oxalic acid is an end product of ascorbic acid and metabolism in man; therefore, high ascorbic acid supplements should be avoided (Metheny, 1982). Moderate to large quantities of oxalic acid are present in spinach and other green leafy vegetables, sweet potatoes, rhubarb, parsley, peppers, oranges, and cranberries as well as grape juice, nuts, cocoa, tea, and cola beverages. Although the mechanism is unknown, oxalate stones are prevalent in areas where cereals are a major part of the diet and least often in dairy farming regions.

Pyridoxine is given to patients with oxalate stones because its deficiency may increase oxalate crystal formation. Pharmacological doses during infancy may not only prevent but also reverse the course of renal failure induced by Type I primary hyperoxaluria (Alinei et al, 1984).

Struvite, or Triple Phosphate. Patients with chronic urinary tract infections from bacterial organisms tend to develop struvite stones. Paraplegics are the largest group at risk from this type of kidney stone since they often have a neurogenic bladder. The prevalence of struvite stones is estimated at 15 to 25 percent of all renal stones with high morbidity and mortality (Marwick, 1983).

Ingestion of cranberry juice is sometimes recommended to acidify the urine. However, commercially-prepared cranberry juices contain only about 26 percent cranberry juice and are not thought to be consistently effective (Metheny, 1982). Most physicians rely on pharmacological agents.

These stones are particularly difficult to eradicate because they form around a nucleus of bacteria, which is thereby protected from antibiotics. In fact, even after surgical removal of the stones, any small fragment that might be left will start a new cycle. The recent development of removing kidney stones by lithotripsy means that surgery is unnecessary and, more important, no fragments remain for new stone formation. This procedure of using extracorporeal shock-wave lithotripsy is continued until the stones are crushed small enough to be passed out of the body.

Uric Acid. Uric acid stone disease (gout) accounts for approximately 10 percent of the renal stones in the United States. Although there is no obvious abnormality of uric acid metabolism in most patients with uric acid stones, patients with abnormal metabolism are at much higher risk for stone formation. In patients with gout and overproduction of uric acid, the incidence may be as high as 40 percent (Broadus & Thier, 1979).

The primary cause of uric acid stones is a high-purine diet. Acidic urine aids the formation of these stones, so an alkaline-ash diet is recommended (see Appendix D–6). Milk, fruits (except cranberries, plums, and prunes), rhubarb, vegetables (especially legumes and green vegetables), and small amounts of ham, beef, halibut, trout, and salmon are recommended. Prevention of dehydration is most important for these patients as is weight reduction since excessive weight usually accompanies gout.

When patients with calcium stones are found to be hyperuricosuric, the usual reason is an abnormally large intake of meat, fish, and poultry or other high-purine foods. Meat, fish, and poultry intake should be limited to 6 or 7 oz./day, mainly by using those items low in fat. A calcium-restricted diet is not needed as much as lowering the dietary purine intake. Organ meats (liver, heart, etc.), anchovies, sardines, meat extracts, gravy, broth, and bouillon are high in purine content. Alcohol interferes with uric acid excretion and should be eliminated or restricted. Reducing the purine intake is ideal, but allopurinol treatment is the current preferred treatment to lower the urinary uric acid level (Coe, 1981).

GENERAL DIET THERAPY

About 90 percent of the stones pass through the urinary tract. No matter what type of renal stone, fluid intake should be increased to dilute urine. Patients should drink one glass (8 to 10 oz. or 250 to 300 ml) of water (or fluid) every hour during the day with two large glasses before bedtime or at least 3000 ml/day. Nocturnal voiding should be followed with another glass of water. At least half the fluid ingested should be water (Pemberton & Gastineau, 1981). If nausea and vomiting are present, intravenous fluids may be needed. At least 25 percent of these patients have recurrences unless high-fluid intakes are continued.

Acid-ash or alkaline-ash diets have been recommended for various renal calculi according to the type of stone. However, there is some controversy currently over these concepts (Dwyer et al, 1985).

Advice for patients with kidney stones is offered in Table 33–4.

Table 33–4. Nutritional Principles for Patients with Kidney Stones*

(Outline used as a basis for discussion with patient with kidney stones.)

It has been shown that eating excessive sugar and animal protein, e.g., meat, milk, can cause changes in the chemical composition of the urine that leads to formation of stones.

On the other hand if people eat plenty of cereal fibre this may protect them from these effects.

If you have a tendency to form renal stones try to change your eating habits in the following way:

1. Eat plenty of cereal fibre *with each meal.* This can be done by eating foods in their natural unrefined form—e.g. *wholemeal* bread or bread with added bran. High Bran breakfast cereal—All Bran, Weetabix, Shredded Wheat, Bran Flakes.
   Use *wholemeal* flour in baking.
   High Bran crispbread and biscuits.
   Wholegrain or brown rice.
   Wholewheat spaghetti and lasagne.
   By adding bran to food. Two teaspoons of bran can be added to each helping of soup, stew, mince, scrambled eggs, etc.
   Eating plenty of fruit and vegetables will also help to increase your fibre intake.
   Eat potatoes with their *skins* (just scrub them to remove dirt!).
2. Cut down on animal protein, particularly meat. On average we eat about *twice* as much protein as we need. Do not eat more than two items from the following list each day.
   1 egg
   2 oz. cheese
   1 Yogurt
   3 oz. cooked meat
   Do not drink more than ⅔ pint of milk a day.
3. Avoid refined foods, e.g. sugar and sugary foods.
   Cut out sugar in drinks.
   Avoid sweets, chocolates, soft drinks, tinned fruit, sweet cakes and biscuits.
4. Drink plenty—aim for 5 pints per day at least.
   Remember, clear water is better than sweetened drinks.
   If you have been advised to avoid high oxalate foods—avoid excessive consumption of tea—especially strong tea and coffee.
   Avoid chocolate, peanuts, spinach, rhubarb, and beetroot.

This advice is *not* a special diet. Many nutritionists would agree that it is a very healthy eating pattern and is therefore suitable for all the family.

---

*From Rao, PN; Prendiville, V; Buxton, A; et al: Dietary management of urinary risk factors in renal stone formers. *British Journal of Urology* 54:578, 1982.

Clinical Implications:

- Bleeding (hematuria), severe pain (renal colic), backache, nausea, and vomiting can result from renal calculi.
- For immobilized patients, the diet may be changed to acid-ash to lower the pH and to prevent urinary infection.
- Catheterization should be avoided if at all possible to prevent infection (Sorensen & Luckmann, 1986).
- Frequently the adult who has consumed excessive amounts of calcium (more than three servings per day) and has the tendency toward urolithiasis, overreacts when stones form. The admonition to consume less calcium does not mean to eliminate calcium intake. Calcium should not be reduced to less than 600 mg/day. If it is, negative calcium and increased oxalate excretion may result (Pemberton & Gastineau, 1981). Increased fluid intake and increased weight-bearing exercises are advised.
- Calcium restriction is beneficial for patients when hypercalciuria is caused by exaggerated intakes of calcium. Since calcium restriction is always associated with an increase in oxalate excretion, oxalate restriction should also be limited to decrease the risk of stones (Bataille et al, 1983).
- Since oxalic acid or oxalate result from the metabolism of vitamin C, long-term, excessive intakes (about 4 gm or less over a longer period of time) may precipitate oxalic acid stones (Pemberton & Gastineau, 1981). Acidic urine caused by high vitamin C intake promotes uric acid stone formation.

• FALLACIES and FACTS

FALLACY: Severe or total restriction of protein is prescribed for renal failure.

- **FACT:** Formerly, this was the practice. Today, protein restriction is less severe, and the amount may even be considered high for patients on dialysis. A diet high in kilocalories, protein, and water-soluble vitamins is recommended to lessen muscle-wasting and to improve clinical status. Patients undergoing hemodialysis three times weekly should receive at least 1.0 gm of protein per kilogram of body weight daily. An additional 0.2 gm/kg/day either as protein or as essential amino acids may also be recommended (Kopple et al, 1978).

FALLACY: Sodium restriction is one of the first steps in treating renal disease.

- **FACT:** Sodium restriction should never be prescribed in uncomplicated renal disease without hypertension and edema. Patients with tubular involvement, such as pyelonephritis or interstitial nephritis, polycystic renal disease, or bilateral hydronephrosis, will lose more sodium than patients with glomerulonephritis (Anderson et al, 1973). If normotension or hypotension is present, sodium intake may need to be increased rather than decreased (Berglund et al, 1976). Furthermore, treatment of renal disease with oral calcium carbonate may be associated with an increased urinary sodium excretion (Papovtzer & Robinette, 1974).

FALLACY: Drink as little fluid as possible to make less work for the kidneys and to prevent kidney disease.

- **FACT:** Normally, at least six to eight glasses of water or fluid should be included daily. The kidneys require fluid to function. In some kidney conditions, fluid intake may be restricted, but the prevention of renal stones requires large intakes of fluids. Proteins, not fluids, are responsible for most of the extra work of the kidneys.

Summary

The kidneys may be called the master chemists of the body. They reabsorb sodium, potassium, glucose, and amino acids and remove foreign toxic substances from the body as well as the waste products from protein metabolism (urea, nitrogen, uric acid, and creatinine). They can also make a wide range of adjustments for balancing fluid intake and output.

When irreversible kidney disorders occur, the dietary prescription is one of the most significant tools to delay the course of illness. Protein is immediately restricted in order to avoid the extra work of excreting the metabolic waste products and to minimize uremic toxicity. Carbohydrates and fats are carefully selected to provide the necessary protein-sparing kilocalories for energy needs. Metabolism and requirements for many nutrients may change frequently in renal failure. Maintaining electrolyte levels within normal limits, treating hypertension, preventing protein catabolism while restricting protein intake to lessen the work of the kidneys, and avoiding dehydration and overhydration are goals of dietary intervention. Finally, maintenance of optimal nutritional status for as normal growth and health as possible is imperative.

Nephrolithiasis, or kidney stones, may cause excruciating pain. Excessive calcium, oxalate, and/or uric acid with inadequate fluid intake are among the main causes. Immobilization is a strong conducive factor; bacterial infections may precipitate stones. Diet and fluid intake are effective in both preventing and treating urolithiasis.

Review Questions

1. Why is a high-potency vitamin pill undesirable for the renal patient?
2. What nutrients are usually supplemented in chronic renal failure?
3. How are the diets modified for kidney disorders?
4. Plan a diet for one day for 40 gm of protein, 1500 mg of potassium, and 1000 mg of sodium.

Case Study: Mr. G.M. woke suddenly in the middle of the night with excruciating pain just below his rib cage. After entering the hospital emergency room, a diagnosis of calcium renal stones was made. What are the next steps in his medical care plan? What can he do to prevent recurrences of kidney stones?

Case Study: Mr. G.J., a 57-year-old business executive, has been treated for hypertension and hypertensive renal disease for the past 23 years. He is now in end-stage renal failure and being treated with hemodialysis three times per week. A 2000 kcal diet with 60 gm of protein, 2000 mg of sodium, 1500 mg of potassium, and 800 ml of fluid is ordered.

1. Why is the protein intake not restricted to less than 40 gm in order to decrease the BUN?
2. What is the desirable weight gain between dialysis treatments?
3. If the protein intake were increased by 20 gm, why would the potassium intake have to be decreased?
4. What foods have high potassium levels?
5. Write a sample menu plan for Mr. G.J.
6. If a 2000 kcal diet is prescribed, are vitamin supplements necessary?

REFERENCE LIST

Acchiardo, SF; Moore, LW; Latour, PA: Malnutrition as the main factor in morbidity and mortality of hemodialysis patients. *Kidney Inter* 24(suppl 16):S199, 1983.

Agashua, PA; Lyle, RC; Livesley, WJ; et al: Predicting dietary non-compliance of patients on intermittent haemodialysis. *J Psychosomatic Research* 25(4):289, 1981.

American Dietetic Association (ADA): *Handbook of Clinical Dietetics*. New Haven, Yale University Press, 1981.

Alinei, P; Guignard, JP; Jaeger, PH: Pyridoxine treatment of type I hyperoxuria. *N Engl J Med* 311(12):798, 1984.

Anderson, CF; Nelson, RA; Margie, JD; et al: Nutritional therapy for adults with renal disease. *JAMA* 223(1):68, 1973.

Antoniou, LD; Shalhoub, RJ; Schecter, GP: The effect of zinc on cellular immunity in chronic uremia. *Am J Clin Nutr* 34(9):1912, 1981.

Barsotti, G; Morelli, E; Giannoni, A; et al: Restricted phosphorus and nitrogen intake to slow the progression of chronic renal failure: A controlled trial. *Kidney Int* 24(suppl 16):278, 1983.

Bataille, P; Charransol, G; Gregorie, I; et al: Effect of calcium restriction on renal excretion of oxalate and the probability of stones in the various pathophysiological groups with calcium stones. *J Urol* 130(2):218, 1983.

Berglund, G; Wallentin, I; Wikstrand, J; et al: Sodium excretion and sympathetic activity in relation to the severity of hypertensive disease. *Lancet* 1 (February 14):324, 1976.

Broadus, AE; Their, SO: Metabolic basis of renal-stone disease. *N Engl J Med* 300(15):839, 1979.

Brundage, DJ: *Nursing Management of Renal Problems*. St. Louis, C.V. Mosby Co, 1980.

Burge, JC; Schemmel, RA; Park, HS: Taste acuity and zinc status in chronic renal disease. *J Am Diet Assoc* 84(10):1203, 1984.

Burton, BT; Hirschman, GH: Current concepts of nutritional therapy in chronic renal failure: An update. *J Am Diet Assoc* 82(4):359, 1983.

Chantler, C; Bishti, ME; Caunahan, R: Nutritional therapy in children with chronic renal failure. *Am J Clin Nutr* 33(7):1689, 1980.

Chicago Dietetic Association and South Suburban Dietetic Association of Cook and Will Counties (CDA): *Manual of Clinical Dietetics*, 2nd ed. Philadelphia, W.B. Saunders Co, 1981.

Coe, FL: Calcium stones. *JAMA* 246(21):2500, 1981.

Decreased taste acuity in chronic renal patients. *Nutr Rev* 39(5):207, 1981.

Dwyer, J; Foulkes, E; Evans, M; et al: Acid/alkaline ash diets: Time for assessment and change. *J Am Diet Assoc* 85(7):841, 1985.

Giordano, C: Protein restriction in chronic renal failure. *Kidney Inter* 22(4):401, 1982.

Green, EM; Perez, GO; Hsia, SL; et al: Effect of egg supplements on serum lipid in uremic patients. *J Am Diet Assoc* 85(3):355, 1985.

Guyton, AC: *Textbook of Medical Physiology*, 7th ed. Philadelphia, W.B. Saunders Co, 1986.

Hak, LJ; Leffel, MS; Lamanna, RW; et al: Reversal of skin test anergy during maintenance hemodialysis by protein and calorie supplementation. *Am J Clin Nutr* 36(6):1089, 1982.

Hetrick, A; Frauman, AC; Gilman, CM: Nutrition in renal disease: When the patient is a child. *Am J Nurs* 79(12):2152, 1979.

Kahn, HD; Panariello, VW; Saeli, J: Effect of cranberry juice on urine. *J Am Diet Assoc* 51(2):251, 1967.

Kark, RM; Oyama, JH: Nutrition, hypertension and kidney diseases. In *Modern Nutrition in Health and Disease*, 6th ed. Edited by RS Goodhart; ME Shils. Philadelphia, Lea & Febiger, 1980, p 998.

Keane, TM; Prue, DM; Collins, FL: Behavioral contracting to improve dietary compliance in chronic renal dialysis patients. *Br Ther Exp Psychiat* 12(1):63, 1981.

Kopple, JD: Nutritional therapy in kidney failure. *Nutr Rev* 39(5):193, 1981.

Kopple, JD; Blumenkrantz, MJ: Nutritional requirements for patients undergoing continuous ambulatory peritoneal dialysis. *Kidney Int* 24(suppl 16):S295, 1983.

Kopple, JD; Jones, M; Fakuda, S; et al: Amino acid and protein metabolism in renal failure. *Am J Clin Nutr* 31(11):1532, 1978.

Manis, T; Friedman, EA: Dialytic therapy for irreversible uremia. *N Engl J Med* 301(23):1260, 1979.

Marwick, C: New drugs selectively inhibit kidney stone formation. *Med News* 250(3):321, 1983.

Maschio, G; Oldrizzi, L; Tessitore, N; et al: Effect of dietary protein and phosphorus restriction on the progression of early renal failure. *Kidney Inter* 22(4):371, 1982.

Metheny, N: Renal stones and urinary pH. *Am J Nurs* 82(9):1372, 1982.

Moffitt, KS: Personal communication, September 25, 1985.

Moore, J; Maher, JF: Management of chronic renal failure. *Am Fam Physician* 30(2):204, 1984.

O'Hare, JA; Murnaghan, DJ: Reversal of aluminum-induced hemodialysis anemia by a low-aluminum dialysate. *N Engl J Med* 306(11):654, 1982.

Papovtzer, MM; Robinette, JB: Effect of oral calcium carbonate on urinary excretion of Ca, Na, and Mg in advanced renal disease. *Proc Soc Exp Biol Med* 145:222, 1974.

Pemberton, CM; Gastineau, CF (eds): *Mayo Clinic Diet Manual*. Philadelphia, W.B. Saunders Co, 1981.

Rao, PN; Prendiville, V; Buxton, A; et al: Dietary management of urinary risk factors in renal stone formers. *Br J Urol* 54(6):578, 1982.

Robertson, WG, Peacock, M; Heyburn, PJ; et al: Should recurrent calcium oxalate stone formers become vegetarians? *Br J Urol* 51(6):427, 1979.

Rodriquez, DJ; Hunter, VM: Nutritional intervention in the treatment of chronic renal failure. *Nurs Clin North Am* 16(3):573, 1981.

Rosman, JB; ter Wee, PM; Meijer, S; et al: Prospective randomized trial of early dietary protein restriction in chronic renal failure. *Lancet* 2(December 8):1291, 1984.

Sorensen, KC; Luckmann, J: *Basic Nursing: A Psychophysiologic Approach*, 2nd ed. Philadelphia, W.B. Saunders Co, 1986.

Sorrels, AJ: Peritoneal dialysis: A rediscovery. *Nurs Clin North Am* 16(3):515, 1981.

Spinozzi, NS: Teaching nutritional management to children on chronic hemodialysis. *J Am Diet Assoc* 75(8):157, 1979.

Walser, M; Mullan, HD; Walker, JZ; et al: Modifications in protein. Nutritional aspects of renal failure. In *Nutritional Management: The Johns Hopkins Handbook*. Edited by M Walser; AL Imbembo; S Margolis; et al. Philadelphia, W.B. Saunders Co, 1984.

Yatzidis, H; Koutsicos, D; Alaveras, AG; et al: Biotin for neurologic disorders of uremia. *N Engl J Med* 305(13):764, 1981.

Further Study

Berkelhammer, CH; Leiter, LA; Jeejeebhoy, KN; et al: Skeletal muscle function in chronic renal failure: An index of nutrition status. *Am J Clin Nutr* 42(5):845, 1985.

Bonomini, V; Feletti, C; Scolari, MP; et al: Atherosclerosis in uremia. *Am J Clin Nutr* 33(7):1493, 1980.

Broyer, M; Guillot, M; Niaudet, P; et al: Comparison of three low-nitrogen diets containing essential amino acids and their alpha analogues for severely uremic children. *Kidney Inter* 24(suppl 16):290, 1983.

Cook, LS: Renal trauma a challenging assessment, a cause for cautious care. *RN* 46(2):58, 1983.

Dubin, S; Jackson, A: Automatic calculation for the renal failure diet. *J Am Diet Assoc* 84(5):568, 1984.

Harum, P: Renal nutrition for the renal nurse. *ANNA J* 11(5):38, 1984.

Hetrick, A; Frauman, AC; Gilman, CM: Nutrition in renal disease: When the patient is a child. *Am J Nurs* 79(12):2152, 1979.

Mitch, WE; Sapir, DG: Evaluation of reduced dialysis frequency using nutritional therapy. *Kidney Int* 20(1):122, 1981.

Procci, WR: Psychological factors associated with severe abuse of the hemodialysis diet. *Gen Hosp Psychiatry* 3(2):111, 1981.

Roberts, SG: Cooking demonstration workshops as teaching technique for dialysis dietitians. *CRN Quarterly* 8(fall):13, 1984.

Salusky, IB; Fine, RN; Nelson, P; et al: Nutritional status of children undergoing continuous ambulatory peritoneal dialysis (CAPD). *Am J Clin Nutr* 38(4):599, 1983.

Smith, LH; Van Der Berg, CG; Wilson, DM: Nutrition and urolithiasis. *N Engl J Med* 298(2):87, 1978.

Cookbooks

Association of Michigan Nephrology Dietitians: *Diet Instruction Manual*. Ann Arbor, MI, Kidney Foundation of Michigan, 1975.

General Clinical Research Center: *The Low Oxalate Diet Book* (1981). University of California, San Diego Medical Center University Hospital, 225 Dickinson St, San Diego, CA 92103.

Jones, O: *Diet Guide for Patients on Chronic Dialysis*. DHEW Pub. No. (NIH) 75-685. Bethesda, MD, Artificial Kidney-Chronic Uremia Program, National Institute of Arthritis, Metabolism and Digestive Diseases, National Institute of Health, 1976.

Kidney Foundation of Illinois: *Fun with Food for Dialysis Patients* (1977). Illinois Council on Renal Nutrition, 127 N. Dearborn, Chicago, IL 60602.

Menu Magic. National Kidney Foundation of Texas, 13500 Midway Road, Suite 101, Dallas, TX 75244.

US Public Health Service: *Living with End-Stage Renal Failure. A Book for Patients*. Washington, DC, US Government Printing Office, 1976.

Wilkens, K (ed): *Suggested Guidelines for Nutrition Care of Renal Patients*. Chicago, American Dietetic Association, 1986.

Dietary Management of Disorders of the Hematopoietic System

34

THE STUDENT WILL BE ABLE TO:

- *Describe the various types of nutritional anemia.*
- *Discuss the differences between folic acid dificiency and pernicious anemia.*
- *Recommend dietary prescriptions for each of the nutritional anemias.*

OBJECTIVES

TERMS TO KNOW

Anemia

ETIOLOGY AND DIAGNOSIS

Anemia describes a decrease in the quantity of hemoglobin, the number of red cells, the volume of packed cells (hematocrit), or a combination of these. Nutritional anemias may be caused by a lack of dietary iron, vitamin B$_{12}$, or folic acid; other factors may also be responsible. The three main causes of anemia are: (1) loss of blood from external or internal hemorrhage, (2) hemolysis or increased destruction of red blood cells (RBC), also called erythrocytes, or (3) reduced production of RBC and hemoglobin (dyshematopoiesis).

Microcytic hypochromic anemia is caused most often by iron deficiency, lead intoxication, and/or thalassemia. Macrocytic normochromic anemia is usually caused by liver diseases. Megaloblastic anemia may be caused by either a deficiency of folic acid or vitamin B$_{12}$, though folic acid is more frequently the cause (Carpentieri et al, 1983). Both nutrients are necessary in the development of RBC. Determination of the type of anemia and the extent of the pathophysiology must include a thorough medical history, laboratory assessments, and physical examination.

Medical History. The diagnosis of anemia should involve questions about diet, pica, environment, use of drugs, fever, fatigability, bleeding episodes (particularly of the gastrointestinal tract), susceptibility to bruising, and infections.

Laboratory Assessments. One of the simplest and first steps in identification of anemia is a hemoglobin (Hb) value two standard deviations or more below the mean. Venous specimens are more accurate than capillary samples obtained by skin prick (Carpentieri et al, 1983). The marked decrease in Hb concentration caused by anemia reduces maximal work performance (Finch & Cook, 1984).

Mean corpuscular volume (MCV) provides a useful morphological differential diagnosis of microcytic and macrocytic anemia. MCV is a readily-available but frequently-overlooked diagnostic aid in pernicious anemia. An elevated MCV may also be an initial clue to the diagnosis of hemolytic anemia. This MCV information is part of a routine order for hemoglobin values but is often treated as throwaway information (Schmidt, 1981). Two other red blood cell indexes—mean corpuscular hemoglobin concentration (MCHC) and mean corpuscular hemoglobin (MCH)—are of questionable

value (Fischer & Fischer, 1983). Table 34–1 lists laboratory values for anemia and iron deficiency by race and age. Table 34–2 lists erythrocyte values for infants and children.

Hematological values are consistently lower in blacks than in whites without any apparent reason. For the time being, the new values for sex and age may be applied to black subjects by subtracting 0.73 gm/dl uniformly from sets of values for whites (Garn et al, 1981). With such an adjustment, fair evaluations may be determined.

Pathophysiology. All anemias reduce the oxygen-carrying capacity of the blood, which in turn, causes tissues to become relatively oxygen-starved. Therefore, pallor and lethargy are common signs. In severe cases, there may be a hunger or gasping for air. A small child may breathe rapidly and actually appear to be fighting for air (Winick, 1984). Irritability, malaise, and decreased attention span are typical signs. Petechiae (pinpoint subcutaneous hemorrhage), ecchymoses (small hemorrhagic spots larger than petechiae), jaundice, lymphadenopathy, heart murmur, and organomegaly are the most common helpful findings in the physical examination of children. Clinical manifestations common to all chronic anemias include reduction of capacity for hard physical work, fatigability, headache, anorexia or capricious appetite, heartburn, palpitation, dyspnea, ankle edema, vasomotor disturbances, and numbness or tingling. Abnormalities in epithelial tissues include sore tongue and mouth, angular stomatitis, and thinning or spooning of nails, as shown in Figure 34–1 (Gardner et al, 1977). Conditions that indicate anemia may include hypertension and other specific signs of renal, endocrine, or collagen-vascular diseases (Carpentieri et al, 1983).

ESSENTIAL NUTRIENTS

While treatments vary for different anemias, the three nutrients absolutely essential for the accelerated cell repletion during anemia are folic acid, vitamin B$_{12}$, and zinc. Zinc is necessary for cell division. Since it is not a structural element in hemoglobin or any other major blood protein, blood loss is not accompanied by the loss of large quantities of zinc. However, when blood loss occurs, more RBC have to be made, for which more zinc is needed. Anemia is not likely from zinc deficiency alone, but zinc deficiency usually accompanies iron anemia because they are found in the same food sources.

Table 34—1. Laboratory Values by Race and Age for Diagnosis of Anemia and Iron Deficiency*

Sex	Age	Race	n	Hb	MCV	Fe/TIBC	EP
	yr			gm/dl	μ	%	gm/dl RBC
Males and females	3–5	AR	587	12.5	81	23	54
		W	496	12.5	81	24	54
		B	71	12.1	82	22*	56
	6–8	AR	315	12.8	82	24	53
		W	267	12.8	82	24	53
		B	39	12.6	83	24	51
	9–11	AR	430	13.2	84	24	53
		W	369	13.3	84	25	53
		B	53	12.4*	83	22*	51
Males	12–14	AR	278	14.0	85	24	50
		W	242	14.0	85	24	50
		B	31	13.1*	85	25	44*
	15–17	AR	371	14.8	87	28	46
		W	308	14.9	87	28	46
		B	52	13.9*	87	27	42*
	18–44	AR	2195	15.3	89	29	45
		W	1914	15.3	89	29	45
		B	227	14.5*	89	30	43
	45–64	AR	1433	15.2	90	28	46
		W	1295	15.2	90	28	46
		B	117	14.2*	90	24*	48
	65–74	AR	884	14.9	91	29	48
		W	795	14.9	91	29	48
		B	68	13.8*	88	25*	50
Females	12–14	AR	299	13.4	86	25	52
		W	253	13.4	86	25	52
		B	42	13.0*	88	25	47*
	15–17	AR	260	13.5	88	25	51
		W	229	13.5	88	25	51
		B	26	12.8*	89	26	51
	18–44	AR	1999	13.5	90	26	51
		W	1745	13.6	90	26	51
		B	216	12.8*	90	24	53
	45–64	AR	1400	13.7	90	26	51
		W	1273	13.8	90	26	51
		B	110	13.0*	88	22*	47
	65–74	AR	974	13.8	90	26	53
		W	884	13.9	90	26	53
		B	80	13.0*	88	26	53

*From Yip, R; Johnson, C; Dallman, PR: Age-related changes in laboratory values used in the diagnosis of anemia and iron deficiency. *American Journal of Clinical Nutrition* 39(3):427, 1984, with permission. Laboratory values by race: median values are shown for Hb, MCV, Fe/TIBC, and EP in all races (AR), whites (W) and blacks (B). Values in blacks that differ significantly (p<0.05) *and* by more than 5% from those in whites are marked with an asterisk.

Table 34–2. *Erythrocyte Values (mean − 2SD) for Pediatric Patients**

Age	Hb (gm/dL)†	MCV (fL)	MCH (pg)
1 month	14 (−3)	105 (−20)	34 (−5)
2 months	11 (−2)	95 (−20)	30 (−4)
6 months	12 (−2)	85 (−10)	28 (−5)
1 year	12 (−2)	80 (−10)	27 (−4)
2 years	13 (−2)	80 (− 5)	28 (−3)
6 years	13 (−2)	85 (−10)	29 (−4)
12 years	14 (−2)	85 (−10)	31 (−5)

*From Carpentieri, U; Smith, LR; Daeschner, CW; et al: Why is my child so pale? Evaluation of anemia in children. *Texas Medicine* 79 (March):71, 1983.

†Hematocrit values are usually three times the hemoglobin values. All hemoglobin values have been rounded to the next unit. Reticulocyte count is 3%–5% in the first three days of life; 1%–3% thereafter. MCV (mean corpuscular volume), until recently expressed in μ^3, is now more correctly expressed in femtoliters, or 10^{-15}L. MCH (mean corpuscular hemoglobin) was given in $\mu\mu$g but now is stated in picograms, or 10^{-12}g.

The nutrient crucial to the synthesis of hemoglobin is iron. Without sufficient iron, the synthesis of hemoglobin is reduced within the maturing red cell, resulting in anemia.

Clinical Implications:

- Capillary blood samples obtained by skin prick have a higher hemoglobin concentration than venous samples (up to 3 to 4 gm/dl during the first few hours of life). A capillary hematocrit is higher than a venous hematocrit (from 15 to 20 percent at birth to five to eight percent in older infants) (Carpentieri et al, 1983).
- Anemic children have more illnesses, more feeding difficulties, and more behavioral problems. They are usually irritable and unresponsive. Iron deficiency anemia is believed to re-

duce a child's ability to concentrate (Finch & Cook, 1984).

- Anemia develops very slowly; the person continues activities but gradually slows down without recognizing the condition.
- Persons who have had malabsorption syndromes or gastrointestinal operations are prone to develop anemia months or even years later.
- Evaluations of anemia utilizing laboratory assessments must be deliberate; individual interpretations allowing variance in cutoff points lead to inadequate evaluations (Woo et al, 1981).

Loss of Blood

ACUTE HEMORRHAGE

The most immediate cause of anemia is sudden blood loss. The abrupt loss of one L or more of blood from trauma can produce shock. Acute hemorrhage can result in death if 2 to 3 L of blood are lost rapidly, but if this amount is lost over a period of 24 to 48 hours, survival is possible. Acute loss of blood requires transfusions for immediate replacement.

Each milliliter of whole blood contains an average of 0.7 mg of iron. For 500 ml of blood loss, about 350 mg or about ⅓ gm of iron is lost. The average adult has about 2.5 gm of iron.

A blood transfusion can replace the immediate blood loss; however, the original blood supply still must be restored by an increase in the pro-

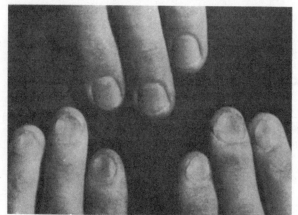

Figure 34–1. *Fingernails of an iron-deficient adult (below) compared with those of a normal subject. Reproduced, with permission, from: Rosenbaum, E; Leonard, JW: Nutritional iron deficiency anemia in an adult male. Annals of Internal Medicine, 60:683, 1964.*

duction of RBC and Hb. RBC are replenished rapidly, but the restoration of Hb and the replacement of body stores for the future depend largely on the diet following a transfusion.

CHRONIC HEMORRHAGE

Gastric ulcer, colitis, untreated hemorrhoids, or long-term aspirin consumption can be responsible for chronic hemorrhage. Chronic infections, such as lung abscess, tuberculosis, pyelonephritis, and rheumatoid arthritis, can cause anemia by defective RBC production and decreased RBC lifespan. Neither responds to typical treatments for anemia until the infection has subsided.

Iron Deficiency Anemia

The estimated worldwide prevalence of iron deficiency is exceedingly high—in the hundreds of millions (Finch & Cook, 1984). At least 20 percent of the U.S. population is estimated to be iron deficient. Highest prevalences for anemia occur in infants, teenage girls, young women, and elderly men (Dallman et al, 1984). Iron deficiency anemia in women of childbearing age is a recognized public health concern in the United States; more than 400,000 women suffer from preventable anemia (Meyers et al, 1983).

DIAGNOSIS

Initially, the person with iron deficiency tires easily, and the iron stores in the bone marrow are reduced. There is less resistance to infections. Only when the stores are nearly exhausted does the Hb concentration begin to decline, which causes mild and then increasingly severe anemia. In iron deficiency anemia, the HB is low; therefore, RBC contain less color (hypochromia) than normal (Fig. 34–2).

IRON LOSSES AND REQUIREMENTS

Daily basal physiological losses of iron from the body result from sweating and gastrointestinal bleeding. For a 70 kg man, this loss is about 1 mg; for a 55 kg woman, it is about 0.8 mg. Additionally, the iron requirement may be increased during various stages of life, which can result in negative iron balance. An inadequate dietary supply

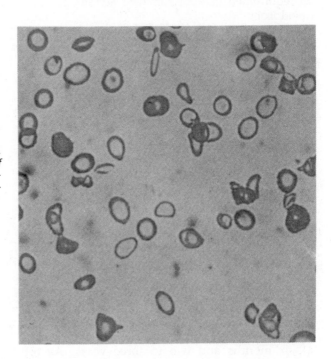

Figure 34–2. *Blood from a patient with iron-deficiency anemia. Note that the red blood cells are hypochromic (due to lack of hemoglobin) and microcytic (approximately × 500). (From Solomon, EP, Davis, PW: Human Anatomy and Physiology. Philadelphia, Saunders College Publishing, 1983, with permission.)*

of iron is usually the cause, but poor absorption may also be responsible.

Menstrual Losses. Menstrual blood losses result in increased iron requirements. These losses are very constant in a particular woman, yet they vary markedly between different women. An average daily iron menstrual blood loss is 0.6 mg. However, in 25 percent of women weighing an average of 55 kg, losses exceed 0.9 mg/day; in 10 percent, they exceed 1.4 mg/day, with a *total* iron requirement of more than 2.2 mg/day. A larger or smaller woman will have varying iron requirements because the size of the uterus is proportional to the total body weight and size. Oral contraceptives reduce menstrual losses by half and intrauterine contraceptive devices increase losses by about 50 percent (Hallberg, 1982).

Pregnancy and Lactation. Iron deficiency anemia in women of childbearing age is a recognized public health concern in the United States; the prevalence of iron deficiency anemia for these women ranges from five to 15 percent (Meyers et al, 1983). Not only is iron deficiency a problem in these young women before conception, but the demands for additional iron during pregnancy become very difficult to meet. The total iron requirements for pregnancy may be estimated at 1000 mg for the fetus, placenta, blood loss during delivery, and basal losses (see Table 15–6). If the mother weighs 55 kg and has the maximum of 200 mg of iron stored at the beginning of pregnancy, the total requirement is approximately 800 mg of additional iron.

Most of the iron is needed during the last trimester at the rate of 7 to 8 mg/day. Even with the enhanced absorption rate commonly associated with increased needs, the diet seldom can meet this demand, so supplementation early during the pregnancy is recommended. A reasonable expectation for iron absorption from supplementation is about 2 mg/day.

Lactation offers the mother a chance to recover some of the iron lost during pregnancy since only about 1 mg/day is required with none required for menses (Hallberg, 1982).

Growth. Adequate stores of iron provide the newborn's supply for the first four to six months of life. Since the small amounts of iron provided in breast milk are extremely well absorbed, additional sources may not be required until approximately six months of age. Iron-fortified foods such as cereal may be used at that time. Formulas are usually fortified.

The period of highest risk for iron deficiency to develop in early childhood is between the ages of six months and two to three years. As the growth rate slows, the iron requirement decreases. The growth spurt of adolescence requires about 0.5 to 1 mg/day (Hallberg, 1982). At that time, male and female requirements begin to vary.

The peak in Hb concentration for both sexes is in the early twenties, then gradually declining with age except for an increase in postmenopausal women (Dallman et al, 1984). Generally, males maintain higher Hb levels throughout life (Yip et al, 1984).

Adult males store 500 to 1000 mg of iron, but adult females store much less, seldom exceeding 500 mg. The male not only stores more iron but needs less. After the male body is mature, only 1 mg or less of iron is required daily to replace physiological blood losses (Finch & Cook, 1984). The mean iron intake of the average American male and postmenopausal female is usually adequate until age 75, when iron derived from meat sources decreases and cereal sources increase (Lynch et al, 1982). Table 34–3 shows estimated daily iron requirements.

Other Iron Losses. About 200 mg of iron is lost for each blood donation of 400 to 450 ml, representing an increased requirement of 0.5 mg/day of iron for one year (Hallberg, 1982).

Other conditions that increase iron requirements include parasite infestations (especially hookworms), gastrointestinal lesions (both malignant and nonmalignant) in the elderly (Stuckey, 1983), and chronic illnesses that cause poor absorption in the gastrointestinal tract (gluten-sensitive enteropathy or Crohn's disease).

NUTRITIONAL CARE

When iron utilization by the body is considered, it has more unusual characteristics than those of most other nutrients. The type of iron, other food intake, and method of food preparation plus the physical status of the digestive tract are influential factors (see Chapter 12). When discussing food intake with the patient, the combinations of foods eaten and method of preparation are as important as the individual foods. Increasing consumption of iron-containing foods will also increase zinc intake (Winick, 1984).

SUPPLEMENTAL IRON TREATMENT

When anemia occurs, the diet alone cannot supply adequate amounts of iron, so iron supple-

Table 34–3. Estimated Iron Requirements in mg/day*

	External Loss†	Menses	Pregnancy "Cost"	Growth	Fe Requirement	Daily Food Intake Requirement§
Adult males (50–100 kg)	0.65 – 1.3				0.65 – 1.3	6.5 – 13
Nonmenstruating women (45–70 kg)	0.6 – 0.9				0.6 – 0.9	6 – 9
Menstruating women (45–70 kg)	0.6 – 0.9	0.1 – 1.4			0.7 – 2.3	7 – 23
Pregnancy (50–80 kg)	0.65 – 1.0		1.0 – 2.5		1.65 – 3.5	16.5 – 35
Adolescent boys (50–100 kg)	0.65 – 1.3			0.35 – 0.7	1 – 2	10 – 20
Adolescent girls (45–70 kg)	0.6 – 0.9	0.1 – 1.4		0.3 – 0.45	1 – 2.7	10 – 27
Children‡					0.4 – 1.0	4 – 10
Infants‡					0.5 – 1.5	5 – 15

*From Beutler, E: Iron. In *Modern Nutrition in Health and Disease*, 6th ed. Edited by RS Goodhart; ME Shils. Philadelphia, Lea & Febiger, 1980.

†0.013 mg/kg.

‡Estimates taken from Finch, CA; Beutler, E; Brown, EB; et al: Iron Deficiency in the United States. *Journal of American Medical Association* 203(6):407, 1968.

§Assuming 10 per cent absorption.

mentation is necessary. Zinc supplementation should be implemented also if iron anemia is treated with iron supplementation.

Ferrous sulfate tablets are usually given. Ferrous sulfate, ferrous gluconate, or ferrous fumarate in oral doses provide about 200 mg of elemental iron daily, which is usually considered optimal treatment. If oral iron supplements are not tolerated well, they may be taken with meals or the dose reduced to 110 to 120 mg of elemental iron. The hemoglobin commonly rises 1 to 2 gm/dl/week. As the hemoglobin reaches normal levels, iron absorption declines. Initially, a hemoglobin response of less than 2 gm/dl in three weeks is inadequate and should be investigated (Stuckey, 1983).

Clinical Implications:

- Hemoglobin and hematocrit measurements are not suitable screening tests for iron deficiency in the elderly, particularly older blacks, unless the tables are adjusted for race and age. If the criteria for anemia is based on young adult males, a very large percentage of elderly males will be anemic (Yip et al, 1984). The same problems exist for infants one to two years of age; their laboratory values can only be a rough estimate.
- Iron deficiency in the elderly may be due to gastrointestinal blood loss, frequently caused by gastrointestinal cancer. An intensive search for the cause of iron deficiency in the elderly is recommended.
- RBC transfusions are not specific therapy but only temporary treatment for anemia.
- In conditions with low gastric acidity, iron deficiency results because an acid medium enhances iron absorption.

- Enteric-coated iron tablets may not be dissolved rapidly enough to be effective for individuals with achlorhydria, previous surgical procedures, or rapid transit times.
- When iron supplementation is required, the presence of riboflavin and vitamin C in the supplement increases absorption (Powers et al, 1983). Additional zinc is also required (Winick, 1984).
- If excess iron is administered, hemosiderosis or iron overload may result in long-term pulmonary, hepatic, and myocardial problems.
- Hemosiderosis may occur from multiple blood transfusions or a failure to regulate absorption as well as excessive iron intake.
- Competitive long-distance running induces gastrointestinal blood loss and may contribute to iron deficiency (Stewart et al, 1984).
- Healing is adversely affected in patients who are severely anemic (a Hb level below 6 mg/100 ml of blood), but mild or moderate degrees of anemia have no effect on the healing process (Chaudhary & Sarkar, 1982).

Megaloblastic Anemia: Folic Acid Deficiency

Megaloblastic anemia refers to extra large RBC, but fewer in number. The erythroblastic cells of the bone marrow (precursors of mature erythrocytes) do not proliferate rapidly, and they become larger than usual with hemoglobin synthesis continuing at a normal rate. These abnormally large adult erythrocytes (macrocytes) have flimsy membranes, are irregular and oval in shape, and fragile. Anemia results from their decreased numbers and shorter lives. Diagnosis is complicated because distinguishing the various types of megaloblastic anemias is difficult.

Close interrelationships exist between vitamin B_{12} and folic acid. At one stage of RBC maturation, every red cell requires vitamin B_{12}—at another stage, folic acid. Folic acid was previously thought to cure pernicious anemia, but the nervous system deteriorated relentlessly with only folic acid supplementation. For this reason, unsuspected pernicious anemia caused by vitamin B_{12} deficiency may be hidden by folic acid doses; therefore, only very small amounts are allowed in multivitamin mixtures.

ETIOLOGY

The RDA for folate is 400 mcg, but a minimum of about 200 mcg/day of folate is sufficient to maintain folate nutriture of healthy males (Milne et al, 1983). During periods of increased erythrocyte turnover or in sickle cell anemia, folate requirements are increased. Any increase in the metabolic rate (e.g., from infection or hyperthyroidism) or anything that increases cell turnover (e.g., hemolytic anemia, rapid fetal tissue growth, or malignant tumors) increases the daily folate requirement (Herbert et al, 1980).

PATHOPHYSIOLOGICAL SYMPTOMS

Macrocytic anemia caused by folic acid deficiency is very common in pregnant women, infants, senior citizens, and alcoholics. Alcohol increases the requirement for folic acid (Walser et al, 1984); almost half of the alcoholics who are hospitalized have this anemia. Symptoms include weakness, shortness of breath, sore mouth and tongue, diarrhea, and edema. Achlorhydria, which is often present in vitamin B_{12} deficiency, is seldom present. Degenerative changes in the nervous system are not as severe either.

NUTRITIONAL CARE

A daily intake of *raw* fruits and green leafy vegetables is especially useful to maintain folic

Table 34—4. *Folic Acid Content of Foods in Micrograms (mcg) per Serving**

5–20 mcg/serving		20–50 mcg/serving	
Carrot	1 medium	Green beans	1 cup
Ear of corn	1 medium	Cucumber	1 small
Mushrooms	3 large	Squash	2/3 cup
Potato	1 medium	Strawberries	1 cup
Apple	1 medium	Egg	1 large
Hard cheese	1 oz.	Kidney	3 oz.
Grapefruit	1/2 medium	Shell fish	6 oz.
Milk	8 oz.	Yogurt	8 oz.
Bread	1 slice		
Sesame seeds	1 Tbsp.		
Lean beef, veal or pork	6 oz.		

100–150 mcg/serving		200–300 mcg/serving	
Liver (all)	3 oz.	Brewer's yeast	1 Tbsp.
Broccoli	2 stalks	Spinach	4 oz.
Orange juice	6 oz.		

*Winick, M: Nutritional anemias. *Nutrition & Health* 6(2), 1984, with permission.

acid intake (Table 34–4). Folic acid is not stored by the body in any appreciable amount, so adequate amounts must be consumed daily (Winick, 1984). The patient recovering from folate deficiency should maintain a well-balanced diet high in fruits and vegetables with appropriate supplementation and should be frequently monitored by laboratory assessments to prevent relapse (see Chapter 11).

Clinical Implications:

- Treatment with folates must not be initiated until vitamin B_{12} status has been assessed. Folate improves the anemic symptoms without curing the neurological problems of pernicious anemia. If neurological symptoms continue long enough, they may become irreversible.
- Infants fed only goat's milk require supplementation because it is exceptionally low in folic acid.
- Both folate and iron are necessary for hematopoiesis. When folate is deficient, iron supplements are usually needed, too.
- High concentrations of folic acid can have a convulsant effect (Herbert et al, 1980).
- The adverse gastrointestinal effects of iron ingestion may be decreased if taken with folate (Herbert et al, 1980).
- Oral contraceptive pills may decrease the absorption and increase the excretion of folic acid (Winick, 1984).

- Especially for the diagnosis of macrocytic anemia, laboratory tests should be obtained as soon as possible to avoid the possibility of changes induced by the hospital diet, medication, or RBC transfusions (Stuckey, 1983).

Megaloblastic Pernicious Anemia: Vitamin B$_{12}$ Deficiency

Pernicious (meaning harmful or fatal) anemia was so named because, at one time, its progressive deterioration led to death within about three years. Today, however, the prognosis is excellent; the neurological complications can be prevented or cured with vitamin B$_{12}$ treatment.

Pernicious anemia is more common among women than men. It is most common among vegetarians who avoid eating dairy products and eggs.

ETIOLOGY

Normal human gastric juice contains an intrinsic factor (IF) that combines with an extrinsic factor (EF) contained in animal protein for vitamin B$_{12}$ absorption. Pernicious anemia, also called megaloblastic anemia, occurs when vitamin B$_{12}$ is not absorbed in a normal manner because of inadequate ingestion, absorption, or utilization and/or increased requirements, excretion, or destruction (Herbert et al, 1980). Alcohol increases the requirement for vitamin B$_{12}$, which frequently results in anemia (Walser, 1984).

PATHOPHYSIOLOGICAL SYMPTOMS

Nonspecific symptoms are typical of pernicious anemia. Anorexia, weight loss, weakness, palpitations, light-headedness, syncope, and headache are observed. Among the elderly, angina pectoris and mild ankle edema from fluid retention is present. Sore tongue, parethesias in the extremities, disturbances of gait, bladder and bowel disorders, paranoia, hallucinations, and disturbances of memory or affect (e.g., forgetfulness, irritability) may be present. Symptoms include pale, flabby, yellowish skin; a glazed, red, sore tongue; or rapid pulse with slight cardiac enlargement. Loss of vibratory sense and incoordination in lower extremities, loss of finer coordination of the fingers, and evidence of peripheral nerve degeneration are common neurological findings (Wintrobe et al, 1974).

With vitamin B$_{12}$ malabsorption or no dietary source (as in strict vegetarianism), normal stores of vitamin B$_{12}$ are usually sufficient for three to four years. Deficiency signs are not observed until total body content drops to less than 500 mcg. The total body vitamin B$_{12}$ content is normally about 5000 mcg with about one third of it stored in the liver.

Elderly people with undiagnosed pernicious anemia are frequently labeled "old age casualties" and placed in mental or custodial institutions without any further treatment. Pernicious anemia rarely occurs early in life; the average age is 60 years. Elderly individuals need not have intramuscular injections for the treatment of pernicious anemia (Crosby, 1980). The cost of the liquid vitamin is much less than an injection and is more accessible.

Clinical Implications:

- For individuals who have recently been diagnosed with pernicious anemia, inquire about supplemental use of vitamin C, which enhances the absorption of vitamin B$_{12}$.
- Sound nutritional information is particularly important to patients with pernicious anemia since it usually occurs in those who are not eating a well-balanced diet.
- Vitamin B$_{12}$ is extremely potent; only small amounts are required. A therapeutic dose ranges from 6 to 150 mcg.
- Patients who have permanent gastric or ileal damage should understand that monthly injections of vitamin B$_{12}$ will be necessary for life (Herbert et al, 1980).
- Measurement of cobalamin levels in all patients with Lhermitte's sign (an electric-shock–like dysesthesia produced by neck flexion) seems justified because the neuropathy of cobalamin deficiency may precede hematological changes in some patients (Butler et al, 1981).
- An increase in mean corpuscular volume (MCV) is a clue to the possibility of vitamin B$_{12}$ deficiency of any type (including pernicious anemia) or of folate deficiency. It is not a sign of vitamin deficiency but can lead to an ear-

lier diagnosis of these vitamin deficiencies (Hall, 1981).

Sickle Cell Anemia

Most cases of sickle cell anemia occur among blacks and Hispanics of Caribbean ancestry; however, persons from the Mediterranean area or southern Asian ancestry may also inherit this condition. About one in every 400 to 600 blacks and one in every 1000 to 1500 Hispanics have sickle cell disease (March of Dimes, 1985).

One in ten black Americans carries the gene. With a couple who both carry a sickle cell gene, the chances are two in four that each child will have the trait and that one in four will develop sickle cell disease; this same ratio is present with each pregnancy.

In sickle cell anemia, the oxygen-carrying RBC changes into a crescent or sickle shape in-stead of the usual round shape (Fig. 34–3). Then, sickle cells may become stuck in tiny blood vessels causing bouts of pain and damage to vital organs, such as the brain, lungs, and kidneys, leading to disability or even death. Patients tire easily and may often be short of breath and prone to infections. Hematuria and urinary tract infections are more frequent in those with the sickle cell trait (Serjeant, 1983).

A diagnosis of iron deficiency in sickle cell disease is difficult because usual iron values for blacks differ from the norms. Surprisingly, data show men in this group to be iron deficient more often than women (Rao et al, 1984). Individual monitoring is essential before any iron supplements are prescribed because that may reduce the amount of zinc absorption and utilization. In fact, zinc supplementation is more in order.

Zinc deficiency may exist in adults with sickle cell anemia (Prasad, 1981). Supplementation in these patients significantly increases weight, growth of pubic hair, serum testosterone level, and zinc levels. The unusual condition of hyperzincuria found in patients with sickle cell anemia appears to increase requirements of zinc. If intake

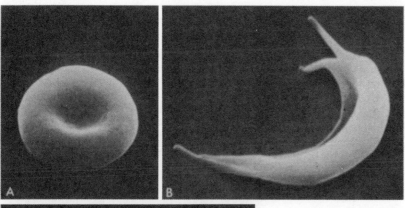
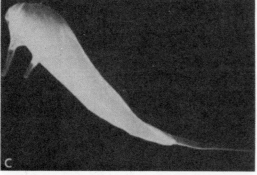

Figure 34–3. Scanning electron micrograph of erythrocytes. Comparison of a normal cell (A) and deoxygenated sickled cells (B and C). (Courtesy of Dr. James White, from Bunn, HG, Forget, BG, Ranney HM: Human Hemoglobins. Philadelphia, W. B. Saunders Co, 1977, with permission.)

is decreased, zinc deficiency results (Prasad, 1985).

Even though mild folate deficiency is routinely found in children with sickle cell disease, folate supplementation should be reviewed on an individual basis.

Other Anemic Conditions

One of the most common inherited diseases of the blood in the United States is thalessemia; some 2500 people are hospitalized every year for treatment. Usually, they are of Mediterranean, southern Asian, or African ancestry (March of Dimes, 1984). Nutrient supplementation is of no benefit to these patients. Blood transfusions lessen the effects of thalassemia, but a major problem is the buildup of iron in the heart and other organs.

Sideroblastic anemia is caused by drugs (isoniazid alcohol), dietary abuse, or genetic factors. Pyridoxine hydrochloride is often used to treat hereditary sideroblastic anemia. Idiopathic and preleukemic sideroblastic anemias rarely respond fully to therapy, but partial responses have been seen with pharmacological dosages of pyridoxine, liver extract, tryptophan, and oxymetholone. Folic acid always is prescribed (Bateman, 1980).

There are other conditions causing anemia, but most of these are treated by transfusions and/or medications. Diet therapy for these patients involves maintaining an optimal nutritional balance. Some examples of these types are aplastic anemia and leukemia. In some of these cases, iron, zinc, folate, and/or vitamin B_{12} are periodically used as supplements.

In cases of malnutrition where protein intake is too low, as in kwashiorkor, anemia will result. Even with adequate iron intake, if protein is lacking, anemia results. A well-balanced diet is essential for all of these conditions.

• FALLACIES and FACTS

FALLACY: *Pale individuals are anemic.*
  • **FACT:** *Skin color may be pale with or without anemia present. Pallor may be masked by skin pigmentation. Laboratory test-*

ing is appropriate for individuals who look very pale and have other anemic symptoms (Carpentieri et al, 1983).

FALLACY: *All older people have "iron-poor blood" and should take iron supplements.*
  • **FACT:** *Some elderly persons self-medicate with iron supplements, which may cause iron overload, especially in males. While iron deficiency does not appear to be a general consequence of aging, each person should be screened for anemia.*

FALLACY: *Individuals who feel tired all the time should be given vitamin B_{12} injections to perk them up.*
  • **FACT:** *Vitamin B_{12} deficiency is only one factor related to specific types of anemia. There are even more causes for persons to feel tired. Self-medication is not advised.*

FALLACY: *A particular iron supplement at a reduced price contains 10 times the RDA for iron and is the best buy.*
  • **FACT:** *The price of the iron tablet is not the main consideration. Only the amount prescribed by the physician should be purchased. That may, or may not be, the most economical one available.*

FALLACY: *High doses of oral zinc can be used to treat many illnesses.*
  • **FACT:** *Large quantities of zinc may interfere with copper absorption causing sideroblastic anemia (Patterson et al, 1985). Self-medication is rarely useful and almost always harmful.*

Summary

Nutritional anemias may be caused by deficiencies of iron, vitamin B_{12}, and/or folic acid. Laboratory assessments are important to determine whether one, two, or even all three of these nutrients are significantly low in the patient. Folic acid supplementation should never be initiated without analysis of the vitamin B_{12} condition; it may mask the symptoms of pernicious anemia allowing harmful progression of neurological deterioration.

The prevalence of anemias caused by nutritional deficiencies worldwide demands the attention of health professionals. The strong inverse relationship between economic development and prevalence of iron deficiency makes it easy to predict where major problems are likely to exist and where major efforts should be directed.

For all anemias, effective therapy is dependent upon correctly identifying the basic underlying pathology as soon as possible to avoid the delay of appropriate treatment.

Review Questions

1. Why must pernicious anemia be identified and treated before folic acid deficiency treatment is started?
2. List the symptoms and causes of iron deficiency anemia.
3. Why is additional zinc necessary for successful iron supplementation?
4. What recommendations could you offer to assure the availability of folic acid?

Case Study: Mrs. I.H. is a 74-year-old widow. She has lived alone since her husband's death 12 years ago. She has complained of fatigue for the past two years. The clinic determines that her hemoglobin is 8.6 gm/dl and hematocrit 25.8 percent. On questioning by the nurse, Mrs. I.H. states, "Cooking isn't any fun anymore." Although she lives close to the market, she buys mostly prepackaged meals. She also has dentures that "never did fit tight" and so chooses foods that are soft and require minimal chewing.

1. What additional data do you need?
2. List at least one possible nursing diagnosis and goal.
3. To increase the possibility of achieving the goal, what lifestyle factors must you take into consideration?
4. The desirable level of Mrs. I.H.'s hemoglobin is _____.

REFERENCE LIST

Bateman, CJ: Sideroblastic anemia. *Arch Intern Med* 140(10): 1278, 1980.

Butler, WM; Taylor, HG; Diehl, LF: Lhermitte's sign in cobalamin (vitamin B₁₂) deficiency. *JAMA* 245(10):1059, 1981.

Carpentieri, U; Smith, LR; Daeschner, CW; et al: Why is my child so pale? Evaluation of anemia in children. *Tex Med* 79(3):71, 1983.

Chaudhary, VK; Sarkar, SK: A study of wound healing in iron deficiency anemia. *J. Indian Med Assoc* 79(12):160, 1982.

Crosby, WH: Improvisation revisited. Oral cyanocobalamin without intrinsic factor for pernicious anemia. *Arch Intern Med* 140(12):1582, 1980.

Dallman, PR; Yip, R; Johnson, C: Prevalence and causes of anemia in the United States, 1976 to 1980. *Am J Clin Nutr* 39(3):437, 1984.

Fischer, SL; Fischer, SP: Mean corpuscular volume. *Arch Intern Med* 143(1):282, 1983.

Finch, CA; Cook, JD: Iron deficiency. *Am J Clin Nutr* 39(3):471, 1984.

Gardner, GW; Edgerton, VR; Senewiratne, B; et al: Physical work capacity and metabolic stress. *Am J Clin Nutr* 30(6):910, 1977.

Garn, SM; Ryan, AS; Abraham, S; et al: Suggested sex and age appropriate values for "low" and "deficient" hemoglobin levels. *Am J Clin Nutr* 34(9):1648, 1981.

Hall, CA: Vitamin B₁₂ deficiency and early rise in mean corpuscular volume. *JAMA* 245(11):1144, 1981.

Hallberg, I: Iron absorption and iron deficiency. *Hum Nutr Clin Nutr* 36C(4):259, 1982.

Herbert, V; Colman, N; Jacob E: Folic acid and vitamin B₁₂. In *Modern Nutrition in Health and Disease*, 6th ed. Edited by RS Goodhart; ME Shils. Philadelphia, Lea & Febiger, 1980, p 229.

Lynch, SR; Finch, CA; Monsen, ER; et al: Iron status of elderly American. *Am J Clin Nutr* 36(5):1032, 1982.

March of Dimes: *Sickle Cell Anemia. Public Health Education Information Sheet*. New York, Birth Defects Foundation, July 1985.

March of Dimes: *Thalassemia. Public Health Education Information Sheet*. New York, Birth Defects Foundation, November 1984.

Meyers, LD; Habicht, J; Johnson, CL; et al: Prevalences of anemia and iron deficiency anemia in black and white women in the United States estimated by two methods. *Am J Public Health* 73(9):1042, 1983.

Milne, DB; Johnson, LK; Mahalko, JR; et al: Folate status of adult males living in a metabolic unit: Possible relationships with iron nutriture. *Am J Clin Nutr* 37(5):768, 1983.

Patterson, WP; Winkelmann, M; Perry, MC: Zinc-induced copper deficiency: Megamineral sideroblastic anemia. *Ann Intern Med* 103(3):385, 1985.

Powers, HJ; Bates, CJ; Prentice, AM; et al: The relative effectiveness of iron and iron with riboflavin in correcting a microcytic anaemia in men and children in rural Gambia. *Hum Nutr Clin Nutr* 37C(6):413, 1983.

Prasad, AS: Nutritional zinc today. *Nutr Today* 16(2):4, 1981.

Prasad, AS: Clinical manifestations of zinc deficiency. *Ann Rev Nutr* 5:341, 1985.

Rao, KRP; Patel, AR; McGinnis, P; et al: Iron stores in adults with sickle cell anemia. *J Lab Clin Med* 103(5):792, 1984.

Schmidt, PJ: Mean corpuscular volume and anemia. *JAMA* 246(17):1899, 1981.

Serjeant, GR: Sickle haemoglobin and pregnancy. *Br Med J* 287(September 3):628, 1983.

Stewart, JG; Ahlquist, DA; McGill, DB; et al: Gastrointestinal blood loss and anemia in runners. *Ann Intern Med* 100(6):834, 1984.

Stuckey, WJ: Common anemias: A practical guide to diagnosis and management. *Geriatrics* 38(8):42, 1983.

Walser, M: Iron. In *Nutritional Management: the Johns Hopkins Handbook*. Edited by M Walser; Al Imbembo; S Margolis; et al. Philadelphia, W.B. Saunders Co, 1984.

Winick, M: Nutritional anemia. *Nutr Health* 6(2), 1984.

Wintrobe, MM; Thorn, GW; Adams, RD; et al (eds): *Harrison's Principles of Internal Medicine*, 7th ed. New York, McGraw-Hill Book Co, 1974.

Woo, B; Jen, P; Rosenthal, PE; et al: Anemic inpatients. Correlates of house officer performance. *Arch Intern Med* 141(8):1199, 1981.

Yip, R; Johnson, C; Dallman, PR: Age-related changes in laboratory values used in the diagnosis of anemia and iron deficiency. *Am J Clin Nutr* 39(3):427, 1984.

Further Study

Crosby, WH: Iron deficiency: Seven rules for corrective therapy. *Consultant* 20(1):49, 1980.
Crosby, WH: Pernicious anemia. JAMA 250(24):3336, 1983.

Gordon-Smith, EC: Management of aplastic anaemia. *Br J Haematol* 53(2):185, 1983.
Minot, GR; Murphy, WP: Treatment of pernicious anemia by a special diet. *JAMA* 250(24):3328, 1983.
Serjeant, GR: Sickle haemoglobin and pregnancy. *Br Med J* 287(September 3):628, 1983.
White, WB; Reik, L Jr; Cutlip, DE: Pernicious anemia seen initially as orthostatic hypotension. *Arch Intern Med* 141(10):1543, 1981.

Dietary Management of Allergies and Adverse Reactions

35

OBJECTIVES

THE STUDENT WILL BE ABLE TO:

- **Define allergy and discuss the problems of identifying food allergies.**
- **Identify various allergic reactions.**
- **Plan a rotation diet for two weeks.**
- **List the foods that are most often allergenic.**

TERMS TO KNOW

Allergen
Allergy
Anaphylaxis
Antibodies
Antigen
Atopic
Elimination diets
Food challenge
Food hypersensitivity
Food intolerance
Gamma E immunoglobulin (IgE)
Histamine
Oligoantigenic
Rotation diet

Although adverse reactions to food have been blamed for symptoms involving virtually every organ system, the concept of food allergies is controversial. Adverse reactions to foods do occur, but the pathophysiological basis is sometimes unknown. A change both in lifestyle and food intake may be the only method of treatment.

Etiology

Adverse reactions to foods may be due to immunological, biochemical, or psychological factors. Food allergy (or food hypersensitivity) refers to an immunologically-mediated adverse reaction occurring reproducibly after the ingestion of a particular food. Emotional factors or stress may accentuate an allergic response by aggravating the sensitivities produced and by decreasing the absorption of nutrients, which combat the incidence.

Food intolerances should not be confused with food allergies. Food intolerances include genetically determined adverse reactions, e.g., phenylketonuria caused by the inability to metabolize phenylalanine. Food intolerances due to biochemical reactions may result from benzoate, tartrazine, salicylates, and sulfites (Atkins, 1983).

Mechanism of the Immunological Allergic Response

The body's immunological system is designed to defend the body from invading foreign substances, or antigens. This system, which is useful when protecting the body from disease and infection, may create an undesirable allergic reaction to natural substances, such as protein. Antibodies, or immunoglobulins, are produced by the body to combat the invading antigen. One type, gamma E immunoglobulin (IgE), is produced excessively in the allergic person. Instead of protecting the body, it causes an antigen-antibody reaction, or allergy. Since IgE is present especially in the nose, bronchial tubes, and mucosa of the gastrointestinal tract, these places are affected most often.

Once an antigen-antibody reaction sets off the immune reaction, the response may range from a localized reaction to a fatal systemic anaphylactic response. This exaggerated allergic reaction to an antigen is brought about by large quantities of IgE antibodies and the release of histamine. Widespread peripheral vasodilation as well as increased permeability of the capillaries and marked loss of plasma from the circulation follow. The slow-reacting substance of anaphylaxis (SRS-A) is also released from the cells, and this can cause smooth muscle spasms of the bronchioles, resulting in an attack of asthma and possible death by suffocation. Because of SRS-A, the administration of an antihistamine has little effect upon the asthma attack, since histamine is not the main factor (Guyton, 1986). The person can die of circulatory shock within a few minutes unless treated with adrenergic agents to counteract the effect of histamine.

Pathophysiological Symptoms

One of the main reasons for lack of identification of food allergies is the unlimited number of symptoms that may appear. A hypersensitive person usually has one predominant condition but may encounter others on different occasions.

Food reactions may begin at the initial site exposed to the antigen (the mouth) with itching, burning, and swelling of the lips, tongue, gums, buccal mucosa, and pharynx. Other symptoms may include flushing, a sensation of warmth or cold, tiredness, headache, and palpitations. Or, these direct symptoms may be bypassed, and reactions in the skin (e.g., urticaria, angioedema, or atopic eczema), atopic rhinitis, or asthma may occur instead.

Allergic reactions can resemble almost any other type of physical problem or illness, e.g., ulcers, gallbladder attacks, or heart disease. It is actually referred to as "the great masquerader" (Breneman, 1978). Types of food allergy reactions are listed in Table 35–1.

ASTHMA

This chronic pulmonary disease is characterized by increased irritability of the airways and manifested by recurrent episodes of generalized

Table 35–1. *Possible Clinical Manifestations of Food Allergy*

System	Symptoms
Respiratory System	Chronic rhinitis Asthma Croup Cough Serous otitis media Bronchitis
Gastrointestinal System	Nausea, vomiting Diarrhea Colic Protein-losing enteropathy Cheilitis Constipation Failure to thrive Gastrointestinal blood loss Iron deficiency anemia Malabsorption
Skin Reactions	Urticaria Eczema Pruritus Angioedema Atopic dermatitis Rashes
Central Nervous System	Headaches (sinus, migraine, tension or cluster) Tension fatigue syndrome Drowsiness, listlessness Irritability Excessive sweating Attention deficit disorder with hyperactivity Depression

airway obstruction that resolve spontaneously or after appropriate therapy. Possible prevention of the allergic reaction is a critical part of the treatment. Even though other precipitating factors, e.g., pollens, molds, weather changes, and exercise, may be stronger influences, food is usually a factor. Table 35–2 shows these offending factors and their relative importance.

Acute asthma attacks may resemble systemic anaphylactic reactions. However, clinical severity does not seem to be an indicator of mortality since more than half of the deaths are among cases considered to be mild (Rubinstein et al, 1984).

Patients with endogenous asthma may have abnormal tryptophan metabolism. The product of its metabolism, serotonin, interferes with the body's use of tryptophan. By limiting the diet of endogenous asthmatics to a tryptophan content of 200 to 350 mg/day, symptoms improve (Unge et al, 1984).

RHINITIS

For those who have never experienced one, an allergic reaction may be difficult to understand. A person with rhinitis can be completely exhausted after a brief, intense round of sneezing (Fig. 35–1).

Rhinitis is caused by the histamines released, so antihistamines are used to treat the condition. In rhinitis, the reaction is mainly in the nose with local vascular dilation and resultant increased capillary pressure and permeability. This causes rapid fluid leakage into the tissues of the nose with nasal linings becoming swollen and secretory. In time, polyps may result from this irritation. Itching of the eyes and nose or coughing may be part of the attack.

ATOPIC ALLERGIES

This hypersensitivity is often genetically transmitted, even though the specific reaction may be diverse. Production of IgE antibodies is increased to such allergens as pollen, dust, foods, insect bites, and environmental inhalants.

URTICARIA

When an antigen enters a specific area on the skin, a localized anaphylactoid reaction may result with an increased permeability of the capillaries that leads to swelling of the skin (hives) in only a few minutes. If exposure is anticipated, an antihistamine may be taken beforehand to ward off or lessen the attack.

MIGRAINE

Some foods are more likely to precipitate migraine headaches. A positive family history exists in 70 percent of the individuals with migraines (Perkin & Hartje, 1983). Vasoconstriction from the migraine causes disturbances in the sensory areas of the posterior half of the cerebral cortex. If the patient does not understand that these bizarre manifestations are caused by migraine, s/he may

Table 35–2. Precipitants of Asthmatic Symptoms in Various Age Groups*

Relative Importance Overall	Precipitating Factors†	Age Group			
		Infancy	Early Childhood	Later Childhood	Adulthood
1.	Infections (viral)	+ + + +	+ + +	+(+)	+ + +
2.	Weather changes	+ +	+ + + +	+ + + +	+ +
3.	Exercise	(+)	+ +	+ + +	+ +
4.	Indoor inhalants	+(+)	+ + +	+ + +	+ + +
5.	Pollens and molds	0	+ +	+ + +	+ + +
6.	Irritants	(+)	+(+)	+ +	+ + +
7.	Foods	+ +	+	(+)	(+)
8.	Emotions	(+)	(+)	(+)	(+)

*American Academy of Allergy and Immunology: *Adverse Reactions to Foods.* NIH Publication No. 84-2442, July 1984.
† + + + + = Most important precipitating factor; (+) = questionable importance.

confuse them with potential mental illness. Even though they last only a few minutes, they can be frightening.

Scintillating scotoma (flashes of light, multi-colored streaks, and even total loss of vision) may occur for a few seconds. Blurred vision and difficulty in depth perception can continue longer. Tactile sensations such as tingling or numbness in the face, tongue, fingers, hands, or arm can occur. Dizziness, loss of balance and body position may be associated with the headache. Hearing complaints include high-pitched ringing or buzzing or a rushing noise like water or wind coming from the middle of the head rather than from the ears (Speer, 1982). Some of these symptoms may occur without the severe migraine headache, which makes them even more mysterious.

URINARY TRACT

Women with lower urinary tract symptoms such as dysuria, frequency, urgency, and recurrent pyuria have been shown to have a history of food allergies. Certain foods are directly implicated: citrus fruits, tomatoes, condiments (particularly pepper), and chocolate (Speer, 1982) as well as grapes, apples, and watermelon (Powell & Powell, 1954). Elimination of the offending foodstuffs relieves urinary tract symptoms.

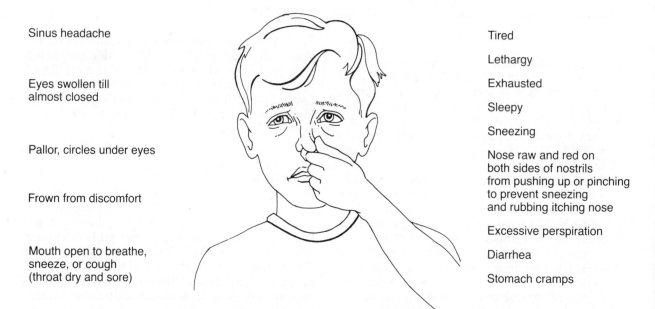

Sinus headache

Eyes swollen till almost closed

Pallor, circles under eyes

Frown from discomfort

Mouth open to breathe, sneeze, or cough (throat dry and sore)

Tired

Lethargy

Exhausted

Sleepy

Sneezing

Nose raw and red on both sides of nostrils from pushing up or pinching to prevent sneezing and rubbing itching nose

Excessive perspiration

Diarrhea

Stomach cramps

Figure 35–1. Progression of rhinitis symptoms in a child or adult with food hypersensitivity.

Factors Contributing to Allergic Reactions

ANTIGEN PENETRATION

Food antigens are normally handled without unusual reactions by the gastrointestinal tract. Gamma A immunoglobulin (IgA) present in the mucous coat of the intestine may prevent antigen penetration. An immature gastrointestinal tract is more susceptible to allergic reactions because of a lack of IgA, allowing antigen absorption. This is more likely to occur in premature infants and in infants up to six months of age.

Gastrointestinal disorders may also lead to excessive antigen uptake. In this case, gastrointestinal cells are damaged and the mucus destroyed, which may cause increased permeability and permit increased antigen penetration.

Proteins are the most frequent penetrating antigen because of their large molecular structure. Incompletely-digested food (and consequently more antigens or food allergens) enter the mucosa and the bloodstream, stimulating antibody production and causing allergic reactions.

HEREDITY

Allergies are frequently inherited. If one parent is allergic, a child has a 50 percent chance of having food allergies; if both parents have allergies, the child has a 75 percent chance (Frazier, 1980). Allergies may also occur without a family history.

FOOD ALLERGENS

A patient may be allergic to only one food or to many. Some of the foods that are most often allergenic include eggs, peanuts, milk, wheat,

Table 35–3. Frequency of Sensitivity To Foods

Most often	Least often
Beef	Apples
Citrus fruits, especially oranges	Apricots
	Barley
Chocolate	Beets
Cola	Carrots
Corn	Chicken
Egg whites	Cranberries
Fermented cheeses	Grapes
Fish	Green beans
Shellfish	Honey
Milk	Lamb
Peanuts/nuts	Oats
Pork	Peas
Strawberries	Peaches
Tomatoes	Pineapple
Wheat	Rice
Wines	Rye
	Squash
	Sweet potatoes
	Tapioca
	Tea

pork, chocolate, soy, and tomatoes, which are used in so many recipes and sauces (Table 35–3).

Different foods are more likely to cause specific reactions. Ingestion of fish or fresh fruit by a patient allergic to them results in urticaria more often than eczema, asthma, or migraine. Chocolate induces symptoms of nasal allergy or of migraine (Tuft & Mueller, 1970).

ALLERGIC LOAD

Several combined allergenic factors, such as stress, decreased health status, or high-pollen counts, may make an individual unable to tolerate a particular food (Table 35–4). Yet, at another time, without these other factors present, the food may be acceptable. For example, avoiding milk only during ragweed season may relieve allergic symptoms. If a food is eaten often or in large quantities, the possibility of developing allergic reactions is increased.

Foods within botanic families sometimes share antigenic and biological similarities. For example, a person who is allergic to peanuts may also be allergic to peas and other legumes in that family. Some food families are more likely to produce allergic reactions from all the individual constituents than others. Sensitivity to one type of fish may mean sensitivity to similar fish. However, sensitivity to shellfish generally does not imply sensitivity to bony fish, even though both

Table 35–4. Combined Effects of Allergenic Factors

Points		Degree of Symptoms
27	- -	
26	- -	
25	- -	
24	- -	Severe
23	- -	
22	- -	
21	- -	
20	- - - - - - - - - anxiety - - - - - - - - - -	
19	- -	
18	- -	
17	- -	Moderate
16	- -	
15	- - - - - - - - - milk - - - - - - - - - -	
14	- -	
13	- -	
12	- -	
11	- - - - - - - - - sweet roll - - - - - - - - -	
10	- -	Mild
9	- -	
8	- - - - - - - - - dust - - - - - - - - -	
7	- -	
6	- -	
5	- -	None
4	- -	
3	- -	
2	- -	
1	- -	

Allergenic Factors: Foods, pollen: temperature exposure (hot, cold); pets, animals; environment: dust, mold, grass; stress: emotions, pressure.

Example: Points for exposure to allergens and the quantity or time period:

Cleaning house (dust) 1 hour	8
Eating sweet roll (wheat)	3
Drinking 1 glass milk	4
Anxiety (rushing to meet deadline)	5
Total accumulated points	20

may occur (Galant, 1980). Sensitivity to cow's milk rarely implies sensitivity to beef. Table 35–5 arranges different foods according to biological families.

Food Intolerances

Many adverse food responses are intolerances because they do not involve an immune reaction. They may be caused by abnormal chemical reactions, food contamination, gastrointestinal disorders, or enzyme deficiencies. Symptoms may be any of those typical of an immunologically-mediated reaction, although other responses may also be seen. Lactose intolerance is relatively common and is usually caused by an inherited lactase deficiency (see Chapter 4).

PHARMACOLOGICAL AGENTS IN FOODS

Naturally-occurring chemicals in some foods are pharmacological agents. They may cause adverse reactions even in persons without a history of allergies. The degree of reaction varies, but the offending ingredient may affect anyone.

Phenylethylamine. Phenylethylamine is principally found in red wine, chocolate, and aged cheese. This substance is especially offensive for individuals susceptible to migraine headaches.

Histamine. Since rhinitis is caused by the release of histamines, foods containing large amounts of histamine should be suspected offenders, especially fermented cheeses, sauerkraut, and wine. Canned foods vary, but salted fish (sardines and anchovies) are usually highest (Lessof, 1983).

Salicylate. Foods with a high content of natural salicylate include dried fruits, oranges, berries, apricots, pineapples, cucumbers, gherkins, endive, olives, grapes, almonds, licorice, peppermint, honey, tomato sauce, tea, wines, and liqueurs. Several herbs and spices contain salicylate, e.g., thyme, mint, paprika, rosemary, oregano, and curry (Truswell, 1985). Salicylates have been accused of causing hyperactivity, although this has not been scientifically proven. Although 10 to 20 percent of asthmatics react negatively to aspirin, it is rarely necessary to restrict salicylate-containing foods.

Methylxanthines. Caffeine, theobromine, and theophylline are methylxanthines found in many medications, foods, and especially tea, coffee, and chocolate (see Chapter 22). When large quantities are consumed, central nervous system stimulation may cause neurological and/or hypertensive symptoms.

Tyramine. Vasoactive amines, including tyramine, epinephrine, norepinephrine, dopamine, histamine, and 5-hydroxytryptamine, mainly affect the gastrointestinal tract and central nervous system and have been associated with migraine headaches. Although the subject is controversial, some physicians recommend omitting the following foods for patients with migraines: most cheese, brewer's yeast, Chianti, and canned fish. Although chocolate does not contain tyramine, it does contain large amounts of phenylalanine,

Text continued on page 691

Table 35–5. *Foods Classified According to Biological Relationship**

Animal Groups	Animal Groups
1. Amphibians	Pleuronectidae
frog	flounder
	halibut
2. Birds (flesh and organs)	Salmonidae
chicken	grayling
Cornish hen	salmon
duck	trout
goose	whitefish
grouse	Scienidae
guinea hen (fowl)	croaker
partridge	drum
pheasant	redfish
pigeon (squab)	sea trout
quail	weakfish
turkey	Scombridae
	bonito
3. Crustaceans	mackerel
crab	tuna
crayfish	Serranidae
lobster	grouper
prawn	rockfish
shrimp	white bass
	Siluridae
4. Eggs	bullhead
ovomucoid	catfish
ovovitellin	Soleidae
white	sole
whole	Sparidae
yolk	porgy
	red snapper
5. Fish (representative families)	Stolephoridae
Acipenseridae	anchovy
sturgeon (caviar)	Xyphidae
Anguillidae	swordfish
eel	
Argentinidae	**6. Red meats (flesh and internal organs)**
smelt	Cow
Carangidae	beef
pompano	veal
Centrarchidae	Gelatin
black bass	Goat
crappie	Sheep
sunfish	lamb
herring	mutton
sardine	Sweetbread
shad	bacon
sprat	ham
Cyprinidae	pork
carp	sausage
Esocidae	scrapple
muscallonge	
pickerel	**7. Milk products (cow, goat)**
pike	butter
Gadidae	buttermilk
cod	casein
haddock	cheese
hake	cream
pollack	sour
scrod	whipped
Mugilidae	ice cream
mullet	lactalbumin
Percidae	milk
perch	condensed

Table continued on following page

Table 35–5. Foods Classified According to Biological Relationship* Continued

Animal Groups (continued)

7. Milk products (cow, goat) (continued)
      evaporated
      homogenized
      powdered
      raw
      skimmed
   selected infant formulas
   yogurt

8. Mollusks
      abalone
      clam
      cockle
      mussel
      octopus
      oyster
      quahog
      scallop
      snail (escargot)
      squid

9. Reptiles
      alligator
      crocodile
      rattlesnake
      terrapin
      turtle

Plant Groups

10. Apple family
      apple
         cider
         vinegar
      crab apple
      pear
      quince
      quince seed

11. Banana family
      banana*
      plantain

12. Beech family
      beechnut
      chestnut
      chinquapin

13. Birch family
      filbert
      hazelnut
      wintergreen (*Betula* spp.)

14. Buckwheat family
      buckwheat
      rhubarb
      sorrel

15. Cashew family
      cashew
      mango
      pistachio

16. Citrus family
      citron
      grapefruit
      kumquat
      lemon
      lime
      orange
      tangelo
      tangerine

17. Cola nut family
      chocolate (cocoa)
      cola (kola) nut

18. Fungi
      mushroom
      truffle
      yeast
         baker's
         brewer's
         distiller's
         Fleischmann's
         lactose-fermenting
         lager beer

19. Ginger family
      cardamon
      East Indian arrowroot
      ginger
      turmeric

20. Goosefoot family
      beet
      lamb's-quarters
      spinach
      Swiss chard

21. Gourd (melon) family
      cantaloupe (muskmelon)†
      casaba (winter melon)
      Chinese watermelon
      citron melon
      cucumber
      gherkin
      honeydew melon
      Persian melon
      pumpkin
      summer squash
      watermelon†
      winter squash

22. Grape family
      champagne
      grape
      raisin
      vinegar (wine)
      wine (grape)

23. Grass (cereal) family
      bamboo
      barley
      corn (maize)
      hominy

Table 35–5. Foods Classified According to Biological Relationship* Continued

Plant Groups (continued)

malt (germinated grain)
millet
oats
popcorn
rice
rye
sorghum
sugar cane
wheat
  bran
  germ
  gliadin
  globulin
  glutenin
  leucosin
  proteose
  whole

24. Heath family
  black huckleberry
  blueberry
  cranberry
  wintergreen (*Pyrola* spp.)

25. Laurel family
  avocado
  bay leaf
  cinnamon
  sassafras

26. Lecythis family
  Brazil nut

27. Lily family
  aloe
  asparagus
  chives
  garlic
  leek
  onion
  sarsaparilla
  shallot

28. Madder family
  coffee

29. Mallow family
  cottonseed
  marshmallow
  okra (gumbo)

30. Mint family
  balm
  basil
  catnip
  horehound
  Japanese artichoke
  lavender
  marjoram
  mint
  oregano
  peppermint
  rosemary

sage
savory
spearmint
thyme

31. Morning glory family
  sweet potato
  yam

32. Mulberry family
  breadfruit
  breadnut
  fig
  hops

33. Mustard family
  broccoli
  Brussels sprouts
  cabbage
  cauliflower
  collards
  garden cress
  horseradish
  kale
  kohlrabi
  mustard
  radish
  rutabaga
  turnip
  watercress

34. Myrtle family
  allspice
  clove
  guava
  myrtle
  pimento

35. Nightshade family
  bell pepper
  cayenne pepper
  chili (paprika) (red pepper)
  eggplant
  ground-cherry
  melon pear
  potato (white)
  strawberry tomato
  tobacco
  tomato

36. Nutmeg family
  mace
  nutmeg

37. Olive family
  jasmine
  olive

38. Orchid family
  vanilla

39. Palm family
  cabbage palm

Table continued on following page

Table 35–5. Foods Classified According to Biological Relationship* Continued

Plant Groups (continued)

39. Palm family (continued)
    coconut
    dates

40. Papaya family
    papain
    papaya

41. Parsley family
    anise
    caraway
    carrot
    celeriac
    celery
    coriander
    dill
    fennel
    parsley
    parsnip

42. Pea (legume) family
    acacia
    alfalfa
    black-eyed pea (cowpea)
    broad bean (fava bean)
    carob bean (St. John's bread)
    chick-pea (garbanzo)
    kidney bean
    navy bean
    pinto bean
    string bean
    Jack bean
    lentil
    licorice
    lima bean
    mesquite
    pea
    peanut
    soybean
    tamarind
    tragacanth

43. Pepper family
    black pepper

44. Pine family
    juniper
    pine nut (Pignolia)

45. Pineapple family
    pineapple

46. Plum family
    almond
    apricot
    cherry
    peach
    nectarine
    plum
    prune

47. Poppy family
    poppyseed

48. Rose family
    black raspberry
    blackberry
    boysenberry
    dewberry
    loganberry
    red raspberry
    strawberry

49. Saxifrage family
    currant
    gooseberry

50. Sunflower (composite‡, aster) family
    absinthe (sagebrush, wormwood)
    artichoke
    chamomile
    chicory
    dandelion
    endive
    escarole
    Jerusalem artichoke
    lettuce
    oyster plant (salsify)
    safflower
    sunflower seed
    tansy
    tarragon

51. Tea family
    tea

52. Walnut family
    black walnut
    butternut
    English walnut
    hickory nut
    pecan

*Adapted from American Academy of Allergy and Immunology: *Adverse Reactions to Foods.* NIH Publication No. 84-2442, July 1984.

†Reported palatal itching and swelling in ragweed-sensitive patients after ingestion of melons and bananas has no basis in similarity of food groups, nor do these fruits have antigens that cross-react with ragweed antigen E.

‡Members of the *Compositae* family have cross-reacting antigens with members of the family *Ambrosiaceae,* of which ragweed is a member. This shared property explains reactions, for example, to ingestion of chamomile tea in ragweed-sensitive individuals. (Similarly, ragweed-sensitive patients may react to pyrethrum, an insecticide made from chrysanthemums, members of the *Compositae* family. This reaction is not food related, however.)

which has also been associated with migraine attacks (Galant, 1980). Shellfish, strawberries, tomatoes, peanuts, pork, and pineapple naturally contain vasoactive amines associated with urticaria, eczema, and pruritus.

REACTIONS TO FOOD ADDITIVES

To add to the confusion of discovering offending foods, many substances are added to foods. Just two examples are cottonseed oil, which may be used to polish fruits, and ethylene gas used to hasten the ripening of bananas.

Sulfites. Sulfites (any salt of sulfurous acid) are often added to products, such as salad greens, vegetables, and fruits, in order to maintain freshness. They are also used in wines, some beers, and dried fruits (Truswell, 1985).

Sulfites particularly affect asthmatic individuals; in fact, so many people are affected that their use has been curtailed or banned in many products (Taylor, 1986). Food labels should declare the presence of sulfites to protect the food-sensitive consumer.

The degree of sensitivity determines the amount of food that can be safely consumed. For example, a patient with a 200 mg threshold for sulfites would be unlikely to have a severe reaction to most sulfited foods because very few contain this amount (except sulfited lettuce or greens from salad bars, dried fruit, guacamole, and heavily sulfited hash-brown potatoes). Of course, the quantity of food consumed as well as the amount of sulfite is an influential factor (Taylor, 1986).

Monosodium Glutamate (MSG). MSG is frequently used as a flavor enhancer, especially in oriental foods. Severe attacks of asthma and dizziness have been associated with ingestion of MSG.

Nitrates. Sodium nitrate is used as a preservative in many breakfast and luncheon meats and cheeses. In susceptible individuals, nitrates have caused gastrointestinal disorders, headaches, and urticaria.

Tartrazine (FD&C Yellow No. 5). Tartrazine gives a lemon yellow color to foods and some medicines. It is found in pickles, cake mixes and cakes, packaged soup, custard, instant puddings, colored candies, jelly, ice cream, mustard, and yogurt (Truswell, 1985). Allergic reactions to tartrazine include asthma, rhinitis, and urticaria. Individuals who are sensitive to aspirin are frequently sensitive to tartrazine.

TOXINS IN FOODS

Many individuals are especially sensitive to other substances found in foods. Mold is usually an offensive substance for persons with rhinitis. Patients with airborne mold sensitivity will usually benefit from a mold-free diet.

CONTAMINANTS

One of the complicating factors involves contaminants. For example, a person may react to beef one time and not another. Upon thorough examination the streptomycin used to treat cattle may cause a reaction in a person who might have had a streptomycin injection very early in life resulting in hypersensitivity to it.

Even packaging for the food may be the cause. The contamination may also come from insects, molds, antibiotics, or bacteria if the food is improperly handled.

Clinical Implications:

- With improper handling, food may become contaminated from insects, molds, antibiotics, or bacteria.
- The aspirin-sensitive person must be wary of foods that contain natural salicylates as well as those to which salicylates have been added.
- Severe sensitivity to eggs, fish, or shellfish can be a life-threatening situation.
- Sulfite-induced asthma can also be life-threatening (Taylor, 1986).
- Advise patients with a history of migraines to use monosodium glutamate sparingly.
- Fresh meats are more advisable than cured meats; hot dogs, bacon, ham, and salami, for example, have been demonstrated to cause vascular headache in some individuals.
- Three well-balanced meals a day are recommended. Skipped meals, prolonged fasting or excessive amounts of carbohydrates at any single meal are associated with headache.

Health Application: Prevention of Allergies

A hypersensitive mother could protect her fetus against allergies by avoiding foods to which she is hypersensitive and/or those most likely to cause allergic reactions, e.g., eggs or peanuts. In addition, intakes of wheat, fish, and citrus should be reduced during the last trimester of pregnancy and during lactation (Bellanti, 1984).

Avoidance of highly allergenic foods during the first 12 to 18 months of life can be one of the primary steps to prevent or lessen allergies later in life. The ideal food for the infant is breast milk because it is hypoallergenic. Breast-feeding is encouraged for at least six months to avoid antigens from formula. If a formula is chosen, special hypoallergenic formulas are available (see Chapter 16).

Foods that are relatively nonallergenic may be added slowly after six months. Whole cow's milk should not be added until the infant is at least one year old. The introduction of solid foods should be delayed: vegetables, rice, meat, fruit at 6 to 12 months of age; milk, wheat, corn, citrus, and soy at 12 to 18 months; egg at 24 months; and peanuts and fish at 36 months (Schatz & Zeiger, 1986).

As a general rule, if food allergy is discovered and abstinence begun in a very young child, tolerances to the food will return quickly. A patient who is six weeks old may develop a tolerance in about three months; if six months old, it takes about six months; if six years old, about one year; and if fifteen years old, it may take as long as two years to develop a tolerance (Breneman, 1978).

Diagnosis of Food Allergies

Suspecting food allergies is the main factor in their diagnosis. Failure to recognize and control food allergy throughout life accounts for unnecessary morbidity, invalidism, and even mortality. If physical examinations, laboratory tests, x-ray films, and other assessments are negative and a food allergy is not considered, the patient may be incorrectly labeled as psychoneurotic, which may lead to the inappropriate use of tranquilizers, sedatives, or psychotherapy without successful results.

CHILDHOOD

The easiest age to evaluate allergies is infancy. Even then, the diversity of symptoms can complicate a proper diagnosis. In infancy, allergy to cow's milk is nearly always the cause of nasobronchial symptoms (including croup), colic and other digestive symptoms, dermatitis, eczema, unusual restlessness, irritability, and discomfort (Rowe & Rowe, 1972).

Occasionally, breast-fed infants develop an allergy to foods ingested by the mother and present in her milk. When the mother eliminates this food in her diet, the symptoms disappear. Most of these infants can tolerate the offending food when it is introduced cautiously at a later age (Bahna, 1984).

ADULTS

Food allergies become extremely difficult to identify in adults because so many different foods (and food additives) are consumed, which may be further complicated by over-the-counter and prescription drugs. The allergic person can also have clear-cut reactions to other substances, e.g., cats, dust, and mold. After discovering some clearly identified allergic responses, further testing may not be used to determine if the patient is allergic to other substances. Another complicating factor is the change in allergic reactions. While some allergens continue to be aggravating, others may cease to offend and allergic responses to new allergens may develop. An accurate assessment is often difficult because the reaction may occur even days later.

SKIN TESTS

For a number of substances, e.g., dust, mold, and pollen, skin tests can clearly identify the potential offenders. However, skin testing for foods is not reliable. False-positives prevent accurate diagnosis unless combined with other data. Different foods vary in their predictability. For example, skin test reactions to peas are more clinically meaningful than those to wheat (Galant, 1980).

RAST

The radioallergosorbent test (RAST) detects specific antibodies against foods and indicates the presence of the Type I (or IgE-mediated) allergic reaction (Perkin & Hartje, 1983). The RAST by itself cannot be regarded as reliable for detecting food allergies. Although no more sensitive than the skin test, it is more expensive and causes a delay in obtaining results. However, it is used in the rare patient with skin disease so extensive as to preclude appropriate skin testing. The major advantage to this test is the lack of risk to the patient (Atkins, 1983).

However, neither test is recommended for food items for two reasons: (1) They may cause extreme reactions, or (2) they may not cause any reaction because of changes to the food in the digestive tract. None of the other biochemical tests are recommended for food.

FOOD DIARIES AND HISTORIES

By maintaining a complete list of foods eaten, the manner of preparation, and resulting reactions, a food not previously suspected may be implicated. Certain antigens may be denatured by heating, whereas others may become more allergenic. For example, proteins from cow's milk are heat-labile, but mild heating in the presence of lactose may enhance its allergenicity (Atkins, 1983). The frequencies and amounts of foods consumed may determine the reaction. Medications, even antihistamines, must be reported to give accuracy to these interpretations. Emotional and environmental factors, such as current pollen count, are significant to this background report.

Ingestion of even a minute amount of an allergenic food may cause a reaction that lasts seven to ten days (Rowe & Rowe, 1972). This implies continued detailed scrutiny of the diary to determine the offending substance.

FOOD ELIMINATION AND CHALLENGE

The only reliable method of diagnosing food allergy is by observing cessation of symptoms when the specific food is eliminated from the diet and return of symptoms following oral challenge (Dannaeus, 1983). A food diary should be kept to note the occurrence of adverse symptoms.

Elimination Phase. A simple type of elimination diet restricts only one food at a time. If symptoms disappear, this simple restriction can be continued without further testing. However, identification of food allergies is rarely this simple.

Most elimination diets require far greater restriction. Rowe (1972) has been the main pioneer in prescribing these. His technique uses a cereal-free (gluten-free) diet first for about three weeks, and if that does not produce the desired results, a fruit-free, cereal-free elimination diet is tried. These are continued until the desired effects are achieved with different foods being eliminated each time.

Ordinarily, suspected allergenic foods, as identified by skin prick tests and food history or diary, are eliminated from the diet for 14 days or until symptoms are gone. All products containing the suspected food and its derivatives must be eliminated. Identifying specific foods in commercial products can be difficult. Label reading is imperative. But even when the label includes all the ingredients, a person may not know that milk products include caseinate, casein, or whey and that egg products may be listed as ovomucoid or ovomucin (Bahna, 1984). Even more frustrating, however, is the fact that ingredient labeling can be omitted if the government has established standards of product identity.

In the past, fasting has been employed during this elimination period for extremely sensitive patients (Hughes, 1978). This is especially dangerous for children and should be carefully supervised even in adults.

Nutritionally adequate hypoallergenic monomeric formulas (see Appendix A–2) can be used during this phase. Vivonex (Norwich-Eaton), Pregestimil, or Nutramigen (Mead Johnson) are suitable. Flavored formulas are necessary if consumption is to be accepted. The monomeric formula with water is utilized for a minimum of seven days or up to three weeks. When symptoms subside, suspected foods can be introduced.

Sometimes, a basic elimination diet may be used to start the investigation. Such a diet is listed in Table 35–6. Foods that are the least likely to cause allergic reactions are used as the basis for this initial diet (Focus on Guidelines for Following an Elimination Diet).

Older children with slow reactions, such as migraine to many foods, require an oligoantigenic diet based on lamb, potatoes, beans, peas, soya milk, apples, sugar, color-free vitamins and minerals, and water for two weeks. Then, one food may be introduced at a time to observe reactions. Children usually outgrow their allergies, so the restricted food may be reintroduced after one year for further observation (Soothill, 1984).

During this elimination phase, diets may not be nutritionally adequate. Efforts should be made to make the diet as adequate as possible, using hypoallergenic protein and vitamin and mineral supplements. These nutritionally inadequate diets should be well planned and continued only as long as is necessary.

Challenge Phase. When the individual is symptom-free, one food at a time is added to the diet as a food challenge. If the item has been eliminated for 14 days or more, reintroduction may

Table 35—6. *Basic Elimination Diet**

Foods and Beverages Allowed	Items to Be Avoided
Apricots	Tea
Cranberries	Coffee
Grapes	Colas
Peaches	Soft drinks
Pears	Chewing gum
Pineapple	All medications except those prescribed by a physician
Asparagus	All foods not listed under first column
Beets	
Carrots	
Green beans	
Lettuce and other greens (except spinach)	
Squash	
Sweet potato	
Lamb, beef (well done)	
Rice (brown, whole-grain)	
Plain rice products without added ingredients	
Rye Krisps	
Tapioca	
Kosher pareve oleomargarine (i.e., made without milk)	
Safflower oil	
White vinegar	
Iodized salt	
Sugar (cane or beet)	
Water	

Sample
Form: *Format for Physician's Instructions*

Stay on basic diet for ___ days.
Then, on ___ , add ___ , alone, first thing in a.m.   Result
Next, on ___ , add ___ , alone, first thing in a.m.   _____
Next, on ___ , add ___ , alone, first thing in a.m.   _____
                         KEEP A DIET DIARY AS INSTRUCTED

*Only foods on this list are allowed. Even with this limited list, try to use as much variety as possible. All fruits and vegetables, except lettuce, must be cooked. Lettuce must be thoroughly washed and *not* have sulfites added to it.

enhance the response. For safety reasons, the doses may start as low as 10 to 100 mg of the suspected food.

Ideally, a food challenge is performed in a manner that eliminates the bias of the patient and observer. A double-blind procedure in which neither the patient nor the observer are aware of the food being given is best; however, a single-blind food challenge (i.e., the patient does not know the food being given) is informative and used more frequently.

Disguising foods for blind testing is challenging and often impossible. Capsules may contain small amounts of the dehydrated food. Some food can be incorporated into special recipes to mask their identity. If no symptoms appear, the dose is increased two to ten times. Patients are always closely observed following testing, and those with a history of life-threatening anaphylactic reactions are never tested in this manner (Atkins, 1983).

Open food challenges are sometimes used (the patient knows the food being tested). Standard-sized portions of the suspected food are given and symptoms are monitored. If symptoms appear, the food should be eliminated for one to two weeks, and then reintroduced to confirm the symptom.

When more than one food is suspected, food challenges are carried out one at a time, allowing time between challenges for symptoms to develop and to disappear before trying another food. Usually, foods most likely to elicit an allergic response are introduced first to minimize the testing period. Table 35–7 summarizes the diagnostic management of food allergies along with the advantages and disadvantages of each method.

FOCUS ON GUIDELINES FOLLOWING AN ELIMINATION DIET

1. Appropriate menus and recipes for bakery products are necessary.

2. Sources to purchase unusual foods should be supplied. Soy- or lima-potato bakery products sold in health food stores and supermarkets nearly always contain wheat or gluten and sometimes contain milk and other forbidden foods not listed on their labels. (One good source for milk-free products such as bread and crackers is a Kosher food store.) If a milk-free butter substitute is to be used, Willow Run Margarine (Shedd-Bartush Foods, Inc., Detroit, MI) may be chosen.

3. Do not include even a trace of any food unless it is allowed.

4. Utensils must be absolutely clean to avoid cross-contamination.

5. Foods assumed to be the least offensive are introduced first to allow more variety as soon as possible, e.g., fruits and vegetables (except tomatoes and citrus fruits, which are frequently allergenic).

6. If allergic responses occur, the fruit or vegetable should be removed for at least one month before being introduced again.

7. Seasons must be considered. Some foods may be tolerated in summer but not in winter and vice versa (probably due to the allergic load). After foods causing seasonal reactions are eliminated, the patient must remember that it may be as long as three weeks before such foods are entirely eliminated from the body with resultant relief of symptoms.

Clinical Implications:

- Intradermal skin testing to foods is generally avoided because it is associated with a greater danger of systemic reactions and local nonspecific reactions (Atkins, 1983).
- Prick skin tests (with a wheal 3 mm larger than the negative control) and the RAST (a Phadebas score of 3 to 4) were both found to have marginal value in accurately predicting clinical hypersensitivity, but the negative results are excellent predictors of the absence of clinical hypersensitivity (Sampson, 1984).
- Extreme caution with close supervision must be practiced in treating infants because limited diets may be dangerously inadequate (Soothill, 1984).

- Elimination diets should be used only for short periods (not more than 14 days) with careful substitution of foods with similar nutrient value.

Treatment

Because allergic reactions can be as varied as their sources, this mysterious puzzle requires all the attention it can muster from the medical team of physician, nurse, dietitian, patient, and family. Death is a very real possibility that may result directly from asthma, from intake of a gastrointestinal allergen, or as a devious complication that occurs from living with the more "simple" allergies daily. Convulsive coughing and sneezing from rhinitis may cause hiatus hernias, improper food intake, malnutrition with its many ramifications, or death from choking.

DESENSITIZATION

Subcutaneous injections are effective in desensitizing individuals for most environmental allergens (except for some animals). However, this technique is *not* useful for food allergies.

FOOD AVOIDANCE

Eliminating the allergen from the body is the ideal way to stop the allergic reaction, but this is more difficult than it might seem. The rotation diets may offer enough relief for the patient to manage a more normal lifestyle, even though the allergy is still present.

PHARMACOLOGICAL TREATMENT

Antihistamines are probably the most common chemical mediator of hypersensitivity reactions to foods. However, they are most effective if taken 20 to 60 minutes before exposure to the offending food.

Cromolyn sodium (disodium cromoglycate) is a prophylactic drug used 30 to 60 minutes before food intake. Doses are initially very high, but gradually are reduced to the smallest effective

Table 35–7. Diagnostic Dietary Management for the Patient With Suspected Food Allergy*

Description	Advantages	Disadvantages	Usual Use
		I. Diet Diary	
Patient or parent of patient keeps running account of all foods eaten by patient over a given period. Patient or parent of patient describes results and physician interprets them.	Simple Cheap Can be done at home under "natural" conditions	"Fishing in the dark" Not safe if adverse reaction is serious Subjective description of signs of reaction by patient or parent Subjective interpretation of results by physician	When an intermittent problem involving an unknown foodstuff is suspected
		II. Random Single Food Elimination and Probability Single or Multiple Food Elimination	
On the basis of allergy history, a single food or multiple foods are eliminated from diet, generally for 3 days to 3 weeks. The food is then usually restored to diet. The process of single food elimination and rechallenge is repeated two or three times to confirm relationship between symptoms and food ingestion. Single or multiple foods may be tried in this fashion on a rotating schedule.	Simple Cheap Can be done at home under "natural" conditions	"Fishing in the dark" Not safe if the adverse reaction to food is serious Trial is open, and attention is brought to the patient and his problem Subjective description of signs and symptoms by patient or parent of patient. Subjective interpretation of results by physician	
		III. Elimination Diet	
Patient is placed on a standard "Rowe" type of diet for 2 or more weeks at home; then foods, usually in large amounts, are added at 3- to 7-day intervals. Patient or parent of patient describes results and physician interprets them.	Simple Cheap Can be done at home under "natural" conditions Late reactions to foods can be screened by altering intervals between individual food challenges Multiple foods and food combinations can be screened	Study is not blind nor does it involve placebo Not safe if adverse reaction is serious Subjective description of signs of reaction by patient or parent of patient Subjective interpretation of results by physician	When chronic, continuous, or frequent recurrent signs and symptoms are suspected of being related to an unknown foodstuff

quantity. It has been used successfully in patients with milk-induced asthma (Bahna, 1984).

Caffeine opens the airways for asthmatics through bronchodilation. Three cups of coffee (averaging a total of 433 mg caffeine) can produce a 20 percent increase in forced expiratory volume, the equivalent of 200 mg of aminophylline, a bronchodilator (Caffeine, 1984).

For a severe food reaction, the attending physician or allergist would meet the patient at the hospital emergency room. For minor reactions, one of the following measures may be useful:

1. Take regularly prescribed medication for the individual or Alka-Seltzer Effervescent Antacid without aspirin (wrapped in gold foil not blue) in half of a glass of water to neutralize the reaction. Dosage is half of a tablet for children and two tablets for adults. (Infants should be taken to the physician.)

2. One fourth to 1 tsp. of baking soda in a glass of water may be substituted for Alka Seltzer.

3. If a food can be identified immediately after consumption, vomiting can remove some of the allergen.

___

Clinical Implications:

- Since oral cromolyn sodium contains lactose, it may cause gastrointestinal symptoms in lactose-intolerant individuals (Bahna, 1984).
- Caffeine is partly metabolized to theophylline. A large intake of caffeine in conjunction with large doses of the drug theophylline might lead to a degree of toxicity not expected from

Table 35–7. Diagnostic Dietary Management for the Patient With Suspected Food Allergy* Continued

Description	Advantages	Disadvantages	Usual Use
IV. Individual Blind Food Challenges in the Hospital			
Patient is usually placed under controlled conditions for a short period of time. Results of blind challenge are compared with placebo challenge. Results of study are observed by physician.	Blind placebo test Objective description of results by physician Objective interpretation of results by physician Other natural environmental factors partially controlled Safe; early treatment of adverse reaction to foods possible while patient is under direct observation Patient or family of patient more easily convinced to eliminate suspicious food from regular diet	Complicated Expensive Challenge not done under "natural" conditions "Late" food reactions difficult to uncover because of length of time patient must be under controlled conditions May involve informed consent Positive reaction does not classify cause of reaction Negative reaction does not imply that patient never had or never will have an adverse reaction to specific food used as challenge	Only in clinical studies
V. Blind Food Challenge Following Fast or Synthetic Diet in Environmental Control Unit			
As in III; results are compared with placebo and objectively interpreted by physician	As in IV, except that all natural environmental factors are controlled as much as possible Late food reactions and combinations can be studied because patient is usually confined for longer period of time	As in IV	In chronic disease studies

*From American Academy of Allergy and Immunology: *Adverse Reactions to Foods.* NIH Publication No. 84-2442, July 1984.

the prescribed theophylline alone. (Caffeine, 1984).

• A warning tag or bracelet, such as Medic Alert, is an excellent idea for severely allergic individuals (Frazier, 1980).

• Patients with a history of potentially life-threatening allergic reactions are advised to carry antihistamines and an epinephrine-containing syringe at all times; they should be instructed about their appropriate use (Atkins, 1983).

Nutritional Care

NUTRIENT REQUIREMENTS

Apparently, children with severe allergic and inflammatory reactions have an increased need for nutrients. Of course, restricted diets can place strains on food intake, but even when the intakes are satisfactory, some children show subnormal levels of iron, prealbumin, and albumin. Losses of protein may occur in children with widespread eczema or a gastrointestinal allergy (Dannaeus, 1983).

Linear growth is below normal in many children with asthma, even with supplemented diets. Instead, only increased weight results. The cause of growth retardation in asthmatic children is unknown (Cogswell & El-Bishti, 1982).

ELIMINATION DIET

The ideal and simplest treatment for allergies is to eliminate the offending food from the diet. However, this can rarely be accomplished totally because of the difficulty in accurate identification, multiplicity of food allergens, and addition of the food into many varied products (masked identity). Still, part of the total treatment program probably will attempt to eliminate some foods.

The importance of replacing eliminated foods with those of similar nutrient value is critical. For example, a child who must avoid milk needs a food replacement for the nutrients normally provided by milk, especially calcium, protein, and riboflavin.

ROTATION DIETS

Rotary diversified diets were proposed by Rinkel in 1934 (Rowe & Rowe, 1972). Modifications of this original plan are most useful today to reduce food allergy loads.

For some people, a diet that rotates the various food families over a period of four to five days allows the potentially allergenic food to be acceptable (see Table 35–5). A four-day rotation is used since two to four days is the approximate gastrointestinal transit time. In patients who have mild to moderate sensitivity to several foods that cannot be completely avoided, rotation diets may be both effective and more convenient than strict elimination of these foods. This does not mean that the allergy disappears, but the total allergy load may be better tolerated because the immune system is not continually challenged with offending foods. Many persons have so many allergens that this is the only feasible way to handle their diets (*Focus on Guidelines for a Rotation Diet*).

Clinical Implications:

- Obviously, patients must be experiencing allergic symptoms when any dietary program is instigated to be able to define the degree of improvement.
- A low or moderate level of allergic reactions on a rotation diet may actually indicate a delayed "out-growing" of the food sensitivity or it may indicate a lower initial sensitivity (Bahna, 1984).
- An egg-sensitive baby should not be vaccinated against flu, German measles, or mumps because all of these vaccines use eggs to culture the virus. If vaccination is imperative, the pediatrician should be informed of existing allergies. No immunization of any kind should be given to atopic babies unless they look and feel healthy. Inoculation and vaccination should be postponed as long as possible, even one or two years, to protect the child. A vial of epinephrine must be on hand for emergencies. Combined injections of DPT (diphtheria, pertussis, and tetanus) may be given separately for reduced reactions.
- Choose seasons for vaccinations when the child is least affected by allergies (Somekh, 1974).

- Persons may react to an alcoholic beverage if they are allergic to the substance from which it is made, e.g., corn or wheat. Alcohol is not the allergen, but it may hasten absorption from the gastrointestinal mucosa increasing the adverse effects.
- For the severely allergic person, extreme caution must be used when preparing and storing foods in order to avoid cross-contamination, e.g., foods should be tightly covered in the refrigerator and the same spoon should not be used to stir different foods.

FOCUS ON GUIDELINES FOR A ROTATION DIET

1. Initially the diet may consist of the foods listed in Table 35–6 to test for relief of allergic reactions. Do not start food challenges until all symptoms subside. After a period of at least two weeks, other foods may be individually added. If symptoms do not subside within one week, one food at a time may have to be consumed.

2. Each family of foods may be used only every fifth day and then only one food from the particular family. Small portions may even be advantageous.

3. After one food from a family is accepted (after being tested on at least three different occasions), introduce one from another family. Later, a second food from the first family may be introduced. But, the first food cannot be served with it. It is not necessarily true that if one food is acceptable, the other foods from that same family will be, too.

4. If allergic reactions occur from one food, do not try it again for at least three months.

5. Do not introduce any of the highly allergenic foods into the diet until other foods have been accepted. This increases the variety in the diet faster.

6. When adding new foods, it is better to eat it alone rather than with other foods. It should be cooked, if possible, to reduce the possibility of an allergic reaction; it should be served plain without additional seasonings.

7. Do not eat any questionable food until the reaction subsides.

8. Keep complete records of food intake with the time and descriptions of reactions. (Reactions may appear 48 hours or longer after the test.)

• FALLACIES and FACTS

FALLACY: *When testing foods to be accepted into the diet, ice cream can be eaten to check for milk tolerance.*

• **FACT:** *Ice cream is not acceptable as a test for milk tolerance because it contains many other substances, any one of which might be offenders.*

FALLACY: *People with allergies should drink decaffeinated coffee.*

• **FACT:** *Whether decaffeinated or not, coffee gives the same reaction, except for the pharmacological effect of caffeine. Allergic sensitivity to caffeine is rare, but sensitivity to coffee is common.*

FALLACY: *Honey cures allergies if it comes from the area where the patient lives.*

• **FACT:** *There is no evidence that this is true. The theory is that honey contains local pollens that can help build resistance in the patient to these allergens. In fact, the person may react to honey if the bees have fed on flowers or plants to which s/he is allergic. However, honey rarely causes clinical symptoms of allergy (Tuft & Mueller, 1970).*

FALLACY: *If a person is listed as specializing in allergies, the patient should choose him/her for treatment.*

• **FACT:** *Unfortunately everyone treating allergies is not qualified to do so. S/he must be a physician who belongs to the American Academy of Allergy and Immunology (AAAI). This was formerly known as the American Academy of Allergy (AAA).*

Summary

A dietary history, including symptoms and environmental factors, can be a useful starting point in the treatment of food allergies; a food diary is very important during treatment. In spite of several laboratory tests that can provide additional information, the most valuable as well as the least expensive procedure for diagnosis is the elimination diet followed by food challenge testing. However, when food avoidance does not produce the desired results, a rotation diet may allow some foods to be consumed with less severe allergic reactions.

Basic principles to prevent as well as to treat allergies include (Chase & Dupont, 1980):

1. Eat a varied diet; avoid excessive quantities of any one food.

2. Replace each food that is omitted from the diet with one of similar nutrient value.

3. Know what the patient is actually eating.

The identification and treatment of allergies is a complex problem facing the public and the medical profession. In spite of all the frustrations, however, the rewards are worthwhile.

Review Questions

1. Plan meals for one day for a wheat-free diet.
2. Why is a food diary important?
3. What are some reactions that might occur with a migraine headache?
4. How can an infant be protected from potential allergies?
5. Name five of the most common foods that cause allergic reactions.
6. Plan a rotation diet for two weeks.

Case Study: Susan P. is a college freshman who has had asthma since she was four years old. During her first semester, she lived in the dormitory and ate in the university's cafeteria.The second semester she moved into her own apartment. Since she dislikes cooking and wants to lose 5 lbs., she's been eating salads at a local restaurant frequently. She has noted a dramatic increase in asthmatic episodes this semester.

1. What changes in Susan's life have taken place in the past year?

2. Differentiate between food intolerance and food allergies.

3. List the procedures that might be used to diagnose a food allergy.

4. What food allergies are the least likely to resolve with age?

REFERENCE LIST

American Academy of Allergy: Position statements: Controversial techniques. *J Allergy Clin Immunol* 67(5):333, 1981.

American Academy of Allergy and Immunology Committee on Adverse Reactions to Foods. *Adverse Reactions to Foods.* NIH Pub. No. 84-02442, July 1984.

Atkins, FM: The basis of immediate hypersensitivity reactions to foods. *Nutr Reviews* 41(8):229, 1983.

Bahna, SL: Management of food allergies. *Ann Allergy* 53(6):678, 1984.

Bellanti, JA: Prevention of food allergies. *Ann Allergy* 53(6):683, 1984.

Breneman, JC: *Basics of Food Allergy.* Springfield, IL, Charles C. Thomas Co, 1978.

Caffeine opens airways for asthmatics. *JAMA* 251(4):441, 1984.

Chase, HP; Dupont, J: General nutritional considerations. In *Allergic Diseases of Infancy, Childhood, and Adolescence*. Edited by CW Bierman; DS Pearlman. Philadelphia, W. B. Saunders Co, 1980.

Cogswell, JJ; El-Bishti, MM: Growth retardation in asthma: Role of calorie deficiency. *Arch Dis Child* 57(6):473, 1982.

Dannaeus, A: Management of food allergy in infancy. *Ann Allergy* 51(2, Part 2):303, 1983.

Frazier, CA: *Basics of Food Allergy*. New York, The New York Times Book Co, 1980.

Galant, SP: Common food allergens. In *Allergic Diseases of Infancy, Childhood and Adolescence*. Edited by CW Bierman; DS Pearlman. Philadelphia, W. B. Saunders Co, 1980.

Guyton, AC: *Textbook of Medical Physiology*, 7th ed. Philadelphia, W. B. Saunders Co, 1986.

Lessof, MH (ed): *Clinical Reactions to Food*. New York, John Wiley & Sons, 1983.

Parcker, C: Food allergies. *Am J Nurs* 80(2):262, 1980.

Patterson, R (ed): *Allergic Diseases: Diagnosis and Management*. Philadelphia, J. B. Lippincott Co, 1985.

Perkin, JE; Hartje, J: Diet and migraine: A review of the literature. *J Am Diet Assoc* 83(4):459, 1983.

Powell, NB; Powell, ER: Vesical allergy in females. *South Med J* 47:841, 1954.

Rowe, AH; Rowe, A, Jr: *Food Allergy in its Manifestations and Control and the Elimination Diets*. Springfield, Charles C. Thomas Co, 1972.

Rubinstein, S; Hindi, RD; Moss, RB; et al: Sudden death in adolescent asthma. *Ann Allergy* 53(4):311, 1984.

Sampson, HA: Immunologically-mediated adverse reactions to foods: Role of T cells and cutaneous reactions. *Ann Allergy* 53(6):472, 1984.

Schatz, M; Zeiger, RS: The prevention of allergic disease in infants from atopic families. Presented at the annual American Dietetic Association, Las Vegas, NE, October, 1986.

Somekh, E: *Allergy and Your Child*. New York, Harper & Row, 1974.

Soothill, JF: Prevention of food allergic disease. *Ann Allergy* 53(6):689, 1984.

Speer, F: *Food Allergy*. Boston, John Wright-PSG Inc, 1982.

Taylor, SL: Food allergies and sensitivities. *J Am Diet Assoc* 86(5):599, 1986.

Truswell, AS: Food sensitivity. *Br Med J* 291(October 5):949, 1985.

Tuft, L; Mueller, HL: Allergy in Children. Philadelphia, W. B. Saunders Co, 1970.

Unge, G; Tornling, G; Malmgren, R; et al: Tryptophan and endogenous asthma. *Eur J Respir Dis* 65(suppl 136):175, 1984.

Further Study

American Dietetic Association: *Food Sensitivity*. Chicago, American Dietetic Association, 1985.

Atkins, FM; Metcalfe, DD: The diagnosis and treatment of food allergy. *Ann Rev Nutr* 4:233, 1984.

Denman, AM; Mitchell, B; Ansel, BM: Joint complaints and food allergic disorders. *Ann Allergy* 51(2):260, 1983.

Egger, J; Carter, CM; Wilson, J; et al: Is migraine food allergy? *Lancet* 2(October 15):865, 1983.

Foucard, T: Developmental aspects of food sensitivity in childhood. *Nutr Rev* 42(3):98, 1984.

Hannuksela, M: Food allergy and skin disease. *Ann Allergy* 51(2):269, 1983.

Huang, As; Fraser, WM: Are sulfite additives really safe? *N Engl J Med* 31(8):542, 1984.

Hughes, EC; Gott, PS; Weinstein, RC; et al: Migraine: A diagnostic test for etiology of food sensitivity by a nutritionally supported fast and confirmed by long-term report. *Ann Allergy* 55(1):28, 1985.

Johansson, SG: Immunological mechanisms of food sensitivity. *Nutr Rev* 42(3):79, 1984.

May, CD: Food sensitivity: Facts and fancies. *Nutr Rev* 42(3):72, 1984.

Metcalfe, DD: Diagnostic procedures for immunologically-mediated food sensitivity. *Nutr Rev* 42(3):92, 1984.

Petitpierre, M; Gumowski, P; Girard, J-P: Irritable bowel syndrome and hypersensitivity to food. *Ann Allergy* 54(6):538, 1985.

Schultz, CM: Sulfite sensitivity. *Am J Nurs* 86(8):914, 1986.

Resources

Allergy Foundation of America
801 Second Avenue
New York, NY 10017

Milk-free products:
Borden's Prescription Products Division
350 Madison Avenue
New York, NY 10017

Milk- and wheat-free products:
Chicago Dietetic Supply
405 E. Shawmut Avenue
LaGrange, IL 60525

For a list of dietetic products that can be ordered as well as a list of distributors:
Chicago Dietetic Supply House, Inc.
1750 West Van Buren Street
Chicago, IL 60612

Milk-, egg-, and wheat-free products:
General Mills
9200 Wayzata Boulevard
Minneapolis, MN 55440

Milk- and wheat-free products:
Gerber Baby Foods Co.
Professional Communications Department
Freemont, MI 49412

Good Housekeeping Institute
959 Eighth Avenue
New York, NY 10019

Loma Linda Foods
Riverside, Ca 92505

Mead Johnson & Company
  (Presgestimil or Nutramigen)
Evansville, IN 47221

Ross Laboratories (Vivonex)
625 Cleveland Avenue
Columbus, OH 43216

Appendices

Appendix A–1. Nutritive Values of Food*

	Approximate Measure	Weight (gm)	Kilocalories	Protein (gm)	Fat (gm)	Saturated fat (gm)	Mono-unsaturated fat (gm)
Dairy Products (Cheese, Cream, Imitation Cream, Milk, and Related Products)							
Cheese							
Blue	1 oz.	28	101	6.0	8.0	5.0	1.0
Camembert	1 oz.	28	85	5.0	6.0	4.0	1.0
Cheddar	1 oz.	28	114	7.0	9.0	5.0	2.0
Cheddar, shredded	1 cup	113	455	28.0	37.0	23.0	8.0
Cottage, creamed (4% fat)	1 cup	210	217	26.0	9.0	5.0	2.0
Cottage, low-fat (2%)	1 cup	226	203	31.0	4.0	2.0	1.0
Cottage, low-fat (1%)	1 cup	226	164	28.0	2.0	1.0	0.50
Uncreamed (dry curd, >½%)	1 cup	145	123	25.0	0.61	0.40	0.10
Cream	1 oz.	28	100	2.0	10.0	6.0	2.0
Mozzarella (with whole milk)	1 oz.	28	81	5.0	6.0	3.0	1.0
Mozzarella (with part skim milk)	1 oz.	28	72	6.0	4.0	2.0	1.0
Parmesan, grated	1 Tbsp.	6	28	2.0	1.0	1.0	0.48
Provolone	1 oz.	28	101	7.0	7.0	4.0	1.0
Ricotta (with whole milk)	1 oz.	28	49	3.0	3.0	2.0	0.82
Ricotta (with part skim milk)	1 oz.	28	39	3.0	2.0	1.0	0.54
Romano	1 oz.	28	111	9.0	7.0	—	—
Swiss	1 oz.	28	108	8.0	7.0	5.0	1.0
Pasteurized process							
American	1 oz.	28	107	6.0	8.0	5.0	2.0
Swiss	1 oz.	28	96	7.0	7.0	4.0	1.0
Pasteurized process cheese food (American)	1 oz.	28	94	5.0	7.0	4.0	1.0
Pasteurized process cheese spread (American)	1 oz.	28	83	4.0	6.0	3.0	1.0
Cream, sweet							
Half-and-half	1 Tbsp.	15	29	0.41	2.0	1.0	0.73
Light, coffee, or table	1 Tbsp.	14	43	0.32	4.0	2.0	1.0
Cream, whipping, unwhipped							
Light	1 Tbsp.	14	51	0.31	5.0	3.0	1.0
Heavy	1 Tbsp.	3	9	0.12	0.83	0.52	0.21
Cream, whipped topping (pressurized)	1 cup	14	30	0.45	3.0	1.0	0.76
Cream products, imitation							
Sweet creamer, liquid (frozen)	1 Tbsp.	15	20	0.15	1.0	0.30	0.02
Sweet creamer, powdered	1 tsp.	1	10	0.09	0.70	0.64	0.02
Whipped topping, frozen	1 Tbsp.	4	14	0.06	1.0	1.0	0.06
Whipped topping, powdered	1 Tbsp.	5	9	0.18	0.62	0.53	0.04
Whipped topping, pressurized	1 Tbsp.	4	11	0.04	0.98	0.83	0.09
Sour dressing (imitation sour cream)	1 Tbsp.	14	25	0.50	2.0	1.0	0.28
Milk							
Whole (3.3% fat)	1 cup	244	150	8.0	8.0	5.0	2.0
Low-fat (2%)	1 cup	244	121	8.0	4.0	2.0	1.0
Low-fat (2%), with added protein	1 cup	245	125	8.0	4.0	2.0	1.0
Low-fat (2%), protein fortified	1 cup	246	137	9.0	4.0	3.0	1.0
Low-fat (1%)	1 cup	244	102	8.0	2.0	1.0	0.70
Low-fat (1%), with added protein	1 cup	245	104	8.0	2.0	1.0	0.60
Low-fat (1%), protein fortified	1 cup	246	119	9.0	2.0	1.0	0.70
Nonfat (skim)	1 cup	245	86	8.0	0.44	0.29	0.10
Nonfat (skim, with added protein solids)	1 cup	245	90	8.0	0.61	0.40	0.10
Nonfat (skim, protein-fortified)	1 cup	246	100	9.0	0.62	0.40	0.1

Appendix A–1. Nutritive Values of Food* (Continued)

Poly-unsaturated fat (gm)	Cholesterol (mg)	Dietary fiber (gm)	Carbo-hydrate (gm)	Calcium (mg)	Iron (mg)	Zinc (mg)	Vitamin A (IU)	Thiamin (mg)	Riboflavin (mg)	Niacin (mg)	Ascorbic acid (mg)
0.2	21.0	—	0.67	151.0	0.1	0.8	206	0.01	0.1	0.3	—
0.1	20.0	—	0.13	109.0	0.1	0.7	261	0.01	0.1	0.2	—
0.2	29.0	—	0.36	204.0	0.2	0.9	299	0.01	0.1	0	—
0.7	119.0	—	1.0	815.0	0.8	3.5	1197	0.03	0.4	0.1	—
0.2	31.0	—	5.0	126.0	0.3	0.8	342	0.04	0.3	0.3	—
0.1	19.0	—	8.0	155.0	0.4	0.9	158	0.05	0.4	0.3	—
0.1	10.0	—	6.0	138.0	0.3	0.9	84	0.05	0.4	0.3	—
0.0	10.0	—	2.0	46.0	0.3	0.7	44	0.04	0.2	0.2	—
0.2	31.0	—	0.76	23.0	0.3	0.2	410	0.01	0.1	0	—
0.2	22.0	—	0.64	148.0	0.1	0.6	227	0.0	0.1	—	—
0.1	16.0	—	0.79	185.0	0.1	0.8	168	0.01	0.1	—	—
0.0	4.0	—	0.23	86.0	0.1	0.2	43	0.0	0.0	—	—
0.1	20.0	—	0.62	216.0	0.2	0.9	233	0.01	0.1	—	—
0.1	14.0	—	0.86	58.0	0.1	0.3	138	0.0	0.1	—	—
0.1	8.0	—	1.0	77.0	0.1	0.4	122	0.01	0.1	—	—
—	29.0	—	1.0	305.0	—	—	164	—	0.1	—	—
0.2	26.0	—	0.97	275.0	0.1	1.1	243	0.01	0.1	—	—
0.2	27.0	—	0.46	176.0	0.1	0.9	347	0.01	0.1	—	—
0.1	24.0	—	0.61	221.0	0.2	1.0	231	—	0.1	—	—
0.1	18.0	—	2.0	165.0	0.2	0.9	262	0.01	0.1	—	—
0.1	16.0	—	2.0	160.0	0.1	0.7	225	0.01	0.1	—	—
0.1	9.0	—	0.55	14.0	0.0	—	108	0.0	—	—	0.1
0.1	16.0	—	0.44	10.0	0.0	—	168	0.0	—	—	0.1
0.1	20.0	—	0.42	9.0	—	—	218	—	—	—	0.1
—	2.0	—	0.47	3.0	—	—	34	—	—	—	—
0.1	6.0	—	0.61	16.0	—	—	113	0.01	—	—	0.1
—	—	—	1.0	1.0	—	—	13	—	—	—	—
—	—	—	1.0	0.44	—	—	3	—	—	—	—
—	—	—	1.0	0.31	—	—	40	—	—	—	—
—	0.50	—	0.83	4.0	—	—	18	—	—	—	—
—	—	—	0.71	0.25	—	—	20	—	—	—	—
0.1	—	—	0.69	16.0	—	—	1	0.01	—	—	0.1
0.2	33.0	—	11.0	291.0	0.1	0.9	307	0.09	0.4	0.2	2.3
0.1	18.0	—	11.0	297.0	0.1	0.9	500	0.10	0.4	0.2	2.3
0.1	18.0	—	12.0	313.0	0.1	—	500	0.10	0.4	0.2	2.5
0.1	19.0	—	13.0	352.0	0.1	1.1	500	0.11	0.5	0.2	2.8
0.1	10.0	—	11.0	300.0	0.1	0.9	500	0.10	0.4	0.2	2.4
0.1	10.0	—	12.0	313.0	0.1	—	500	0.10	0.4	0.2	2.5
0.1	10.0	—	13.0	349.0	0.1	1.1	500	0.11	0.5	0.2	2.8
—	4.0	—	11.0	302.0	0.1	—	500	0.09	0.3	0.2	2.4
—	5.0	—	12.0	316.0	0.1	1.0	500	0.10	0.4	0.2	2.5
—	5.0	—	13.0	352.0	0.1	1.1	500	0.11	0.5	0.2	2.8

Appendix continued on following page

Appendix A–1. Nutritive Values of Food* (Continued)

	Approximate Measure	Weight (gm)	Kilocalories	Protein (gm)	Fat (gm)	Saturated fat (gm)	Mono-unsaturated fat (gm)
Buttermilk	1 cup	245	99	8.0	2.0	1.0	0.5
Canned, evaporated, whole	1 cup	252	338	17.0	19.0	11.0	5.0
Canned, evaporated, skim	1 cup	255	199	19.0	0.51	0.31	0.10
Canned, sweetened, condensed	1 cup	306	982	24.0	26.0	16.0	6.0
Dried, nonfat, instant	1 cup	68	244	23.0	0.49	0.32	0.10
Milk beverages							
Chocolate milk, regular	1 cup	250	208	7.0	8.0	5.0	2.0
Chocolate milk, low-fat (2%)	1 cup	250	179	8.0	5.0	3.0	1.0
Chocolate milk, low-fat (1%)	1 cup	250	158	8.0	2.0	1.0	0.70
Eggnog (commercial)	1 cup	254	342	9.0	19.0	11.0	5.0
Malted milk, home-prepared, chocolate	1 cup	265	233	9.0	9.0	5.0	—
Malted milk, natural, home-prepared	1 cup	265	236	10.0	9.0	5.0	—
Shake, thick, chocolate	10.6 oz.	300	356	9.0	8.0	5.0	2.0
Shake, thick, vanilla	11 oz.	313	350	12.0	9.0	5.0	2.0
Milk desserts, frozen							
Ice cream, regular (11% fat)	1 cup	133	269	4.0	14.0	8.0	3.0
Ice cream, soft serve	1 cup	173	377	7.0	22.0	13.0	5.0
Ice cream, rich (16% fat)	1 cup	148	349	4.0	23.0	14.0	6.0
Ice milk (about 4.3% fat)	1 cup	131	184	5.0	5.0	3.0	1.0
Ice milk, soft serve (2.6% fat)	1 cup	175	223	8.0	4.0	2.0	1.0
Sherbet (about 2% fat)	1 cup	193	270	2.0	3.0	2.0	1.0
Milk desserts, other							
Custard, baked	1 cup	265	305	14.0	15.0	6.0	5.0
Pudding, vanilla (blancmange)	1 cup	255	285	9.0	10.0	6.0	2.0
Pudding, Tapioca cream	1 cup	165	220	8.0	8.0	4.0	2.0
Pudding, regular (cooked)	1 cup	260	320	9.0	8.0	4.0	2.0
Pudding, instant	1 cup	227	231	9.0	2.0	1.0	0.60
Yogurt							
Made with low-fat milk, fruit-flavored	8 oz.	227	144	11.0	3.0	2.0	0.80
Made with low-fat milk, plain	8 oz.	227	127	13.0	0.41	0.26	0.10
Made with whole milk	8 oz.	227	139	7.0	7.0	4.0	1.0
Eggs, large (24 oz. per dozen):							
Raw, whole	1	50	79	6.1	5.0	1.7	2.0
Raw, white	1	33	16	3.3	—	—	—
Raw, yolk	1	17	63	2.8	5.0	1.7	2.1
Cooked, fried in butter	1	46	83	5.4	6.0	2.4	2.2
Cooked, hard-boiled	1	50	79	6.1	5.0	2.0	2.0
Cooked, poached	1	50	79	6.0	5.0	1.7	2.0
Cooked, scrambled with milk and butter	1	64	95	5.0	7.0	2.8	2.3
Fats, oils, and Related Products							
Butter							
Regular	1 Tbsp.	14	100	0.1	11.0	7.1	2.9
Regular, pat	1 pat	5	36	—	4.0	2.5	1.0
Whipped	1 Tbsp.	9	64	0.1	7.0	4.5	1.9
Whipped, pat	1 pat	3	27	—	3.0	1.9	0.8
Fat, cooking	1 Tbsp.	12	113	—	12.0	3.2	5.7
Lard	1 Tbsp.	12	115	—	12.0	5.0	5.2
Margarine							
Regular	1 Tbsp.	14	101	0.1	11.0	2.2	5.3
Regular, pat	1 pat	5	35	—	4.0	0.8	1.9
Soft	1 Tbsp.	14	100	0.1	11.0	1.9	4.5
Whipped	1 Tbsp.	9	70	—	8.0	1.4	3.6

Appendix A–1. Nutritive Values of Food* (Continued)

Poly-unsaturated fat (gm)	Cholesterol (mg)	Dietary fiber (gm)	Carbo-hydrate (gm)	Calcium (mg)	Iron (mg)	Zinc (mg)	Vitamin A (IU)	Thiamin (mg)	Riboflavin (mg)	Niacin (mg)	Ascorbic acid (mg)
—	9.0	—	11.0	285.0	0.1	1.0	81	0.08	0.4	0.1	2.4
0.4	73.0	—	25.0	658.0	0.5	1.9	612	0.12	0.8	0.5	4.7
—	10.0	—	28.0	740.0	0.7	2.3	1000	0.12	0.8	0.4	3.2
0.7	104.0	—	166.0	868.0	0.6	2.9	1004	0.28	1.3	0.6	7.0
—	12.0	—	35.0	837.0	0.2	3.0	1612	0.28	1.2	0.6	3.8
0.2	30.0	—	25.0	280.0	0.6	1.0	302	0.09	0.4	0.3	2.3
0.1	17.0	—	26.0	284.0	0.6	1.0	500	0.09	0.4	0.3	2.3
0.1	7.0	—	26.0	287.0	0.6	1.0	500	0.10	0.4	0.3	2.3
0.6	149.0	—	34.0	330.0	0.5	1.2	894	0.09	0.5	0.3	3.8
—	34.0	—	29.0	304.0	0.5	1.1	326	0.14	0.4	0.7	2.3
—	37.0	—	26.0	347.0	0.3	1.1	376	0.20	0.5	1.3	2.3
0.2	32.0	—	63.0	396.0	0.9	1.4	258	0.14	0.7	0.4	—
0.2	37.0	—	55.0	457.0	0.3	1.2	357	0.09	0.6	0.5	—
0.3	59.0	—	31.0	176.0	0.1	1.4	543	0.05	0.3	0.1	0.7
0.6	153.0	—	38.0	236.0	0.4	1.0	794	0.08	0.4	0.2	0.9
0.5	88.0	—	32.0	151.0	0.1	1.2	897	0.04	0.3	0.1	0.6
0.1	18.0	—	29.0	176.0	0.2	0.5	214	0.08	0.3	0.1	0.8
0.1	13.0	—	38.0	274.0	0.3	0.9	175	0.12	0.5	0.2	1.2
0.1	14.0	—	58.0	103.0	0.3	1.3	185	0.03	0.1	0.1	3.9
0.7	278.0	—	29.0	297.0	1.1	—	930	0.11	0.5	0.3	1.0
.2	36.0	—	41.0	298.0	0.0	—	410	0.08	0.4	0.3	2.0
0.5	80.0	—	28.0	173.0	0.7	—	480	0.07	0.3	0.2	2.0
2.0	32.0	—	59.0	265.0	0.8	—	340	0.05	0.4	0.3	2.0
0.1	10.0	—	43.0	345.0	0.2	1.7	104	0.08	0.4	0.2	1.5
0.1	14.0	—	16.0	415.0	0.2	2.0	150	0.10	0.5	0.3	1.8
—	4.0	—	17.0	452.0	0.2	2.2	16	0.11	0.5	0.3	1.0
0.1	29.0	—	10.0	274.0	0.1	1.3	279	0.07	0.3	0.2	1.2
0.6	274.0	—	0.6	28.0	1.04	0.72	260	0.044	0.150	0.031	—
—	—	—	0.4	4.0	0.01	0.01	—	0.002	0.094	0.029	—
0.6	272.0	—	—	26.0	0.95	0.58	313	0.043	0.074	0.012	—
0.6	246.0	—	0.5	26.0	0.92	0.64	286	0.033	0.126	0.026	—
0.6	274.0	—	0.6	28.0	1.04	0.72	260	0.037	0.143	0.030	—
0.6	273.0	—	0.6	28.0	1.04	0.72	259	0.035	0.127	0.026	—
0.6	248.0	—	1.4	47.0	0.93	0.70	311	0.039	0.156	0.042	0.130
0.3	30.0	—	—	3.0	0.02	0.01	428	0.001	0.005	0.006	—
0.1	11.0	—	—	1.0	0.01	—	153	—	0.002	0.002	—
0.2	19.0	—	—	2.0	0.01	0.01	275	—	0.003	0.004	—
0.1	8.0	—	—	1.0	0.01	—	116	—	0.001	0.002	—
3.1	—	—	—	—	—	—	—	—	—	—	—
1.3	12.0	—	—	0.01	—	0.01	—	—	—	—	—
3.1	—	—	0.1	4.0	0.01	—	463	0.001	0.005	0.003	0.022
1.1	—	—	—	1.0	—	—	165	0.001	0.002	0.001	0.008
4.1	—	—	0.1	3.0	—	—	463	0.001	0.004	0.003	0.020
2.1	—	—	—	2.0	—	—	310	—	—	—	—

Appendix continued on following page

Appendix A–1. *Nutritive Values of Food* (Continued)

	Approximate Measure	Weight (gm)	Kilocalories	Protein (gm)	Fat (gm)	Saturated fat (gm)	Mono-unsaturated fat (gm)
Oil, salad or cooking							
Corn	1 Tbsp.	13	120	—	13.0	1.7	3.4
Olive	1 Tbsp.	13	119	—	13.0	1.9	9.6
Peanut	1 Tbsp.	13	119	—	13.0	2.3	6.2
Safflower	1 Tbsp.	13	120	—	13.0	1.3	1.6
Soybean oil, hydrogenated	1 Tbsp.	13	120	—	13.0	1.0	5.8
Soybean-cottonseed blend, hydrogenated	1 Tbsp.	13	120	—	13.0	2.4	3.9
Salad dressings, commercial							
Mayonnaise	1 Tbsp.	14	98	0.2	11.0	1.6	2.4
Mayonnaise-type, regular	1 Tbsp.	14	57	0.1	4.0	0.7	1.4
Mayonnaise-type, low-calorie	1 Tbsp.	16	20	—	2.0	0.4	0.4
Tartar sauce, regular	1 Tbsp.	14	75	—	8.0	1.5	1.8
Thousand Island, regular	1 Tbsp.	15	58	0.1	5.0	0.9	1.7
Thousand Island, low-calorie	1 Tbsp.	15	24	0.1	1.0	0.2	0.4
Fish, Shellfish, Meat, Poultry, and Related Products							
Fish and shellfish							
Bluefish, baked with butter	3 oz.	85	134	22.0	4.0	—	—
Clams, raw, meat only	3 oz.	85	65	11.0	1.0	0.30	—
Clams, canned, solids and liquid	3 oz.	85	44	6.0	1.0	0.20	—
Crabmeat (white or king), canned	1 cup	135	135	24.0	3.0	0.60	0.40
Fish sticks, breaded, frozen	1 oz.	28	50	5.0	3.0	—	—
Haddock, breaded, fried	3 oz.	85	140	17.0	5.0	1.00	2.0
Ocean perch, breaded, fried	1 fillet	85	195	16.0	11.0	2.00	4.0
Oysters, raw, meat only	1 cup	240	160	20.0	4.0	1.00	0.20
Salmon, pink, canned	3 oz.	85	120	17.0	5.0	0.90	0.80
Sardines, Atlantic, canned in oil	3 oz.	85	175	20.0	9.0	2.00	2.0
Scallops, frozen, breaded and fried	6	30	58	5.0	2.0	—	—
Shrimp, canned, meat only	3 oz.	85	100	21.0	1.0	0.20	0.10
Shrimp, french fried	3 oz.	85	190	17.0	9.0	2.00	3.0
Tuna, canned in oil	3 oz.	85	170	24.0	7.0	1.00	1.0
Tuna salad	1 cup	205	350	30.0	22.0	4.00	6.0
Meat and meat products							
Bacon (20 slices/lb, raw)	2 slices	12	72	3.0	6.0	2.00	3.0
Beef, cooked:							
Cuts, braised, simmered							
Lean and fat	3 oz.	85	245	21.0	23.0	9.50	6.50
Lean only	2.5 oz.	71	158	21.6	7.3	2.00	1.77
Ground beef, broiled							
Lean with 10% fat	3 oz.	85	217	21.6	13.9	5.50	3.90
Lean with 21% fat	3 oz.	85	240	21.8	16.2	6.40	6.95
Roast, oven-cooked, relatively fat, as rib							
Lean and fat	3 oz.	85	308	18.3	25.5	10.80	13.61
Lean only	2 oz.	57	136	15.6	7.8	3.30	2.78
Roast, oven-cooked, as lean as heel of round							
Lean and fat	3 oz.	85	222	25.3	12.6	4.80	2.70
Lean only	2.8 oz.	79	127	24.4	7.7	2.70	1.02
Steak, relatively fat (sirloin):							
Lean and fat	3 oz.	85	271	22.7	19.4	8.13	11.11
Lean only	2 oz.	57	135	17.2	6.7	2.7	1.62
Steak, relatively lean (round)							
Lean and fat	3 oz.	85	179	26.2	7.5	2.8	1.80
Lean only	2.4 oz.	68	130	21.5	4.2	1.5	1.50
Beef, canned corned beef	3 oz.	85	213	23.0	12.7	5.3	4.5

Appendix A–1. Nutritive Values of Food* (Continued)

Poly-unsaturated fat (gm)	Cholesterol (mg)	Dietary fiber (gm)	Carbo-hydrate (gm)	Calcium (mg)	Iron (mg)	Zinc (mg)	Vitamin A (IU)	Thiamin (mg)	Riboflavin (mg)	Niacin (mg)	Ascorbic acid (mg)
7.8	—	—	—	—	—	—	—	—	—	—	—
1.1	—	—	—	0.02	0.05	0.01	—	—	—	—	—
4.2	—	—	—	0.01	—	—	—	—	—	—	—
10.0	—	—	—	—	—	—	—	—	—	—	—
4.7	—	—	—	—	—	—	—	—	—	—	—
6.2	—	—	—	—	—	—	—	—	—	—	—
5.6	8.0	—	0.4	2.0	0.10	0.02	39	—	—	—	—
3.1	4.0	—	3.5	2.0	—	—	32	—	—	—	—
1.0	2.0	—	2.0	3.0	—	—	40	—	—	—	—
4.1	9.0	—	1.0	3.0	0.10	—	30	—	—	—	—
3.9	4.0	—	2.4	2.0	0.10	0.02	50	—	—	—	—
1.0	2.0	—	2.5	2.0	0.10	—	49	—	—	—	—
—	59.0	—	—	24.0	0.60	—	43	0.09	0.1	1.0	—
—	42.0	—	2.0	59.0	2.0	1.0	90	0.08	0.2	1.0	8.0
—	53.0	—	1.0	47.0	3.0	1.0	—	0.01	0.1	0.90	—
0.1	135.0	—	1.0	61.0	1.0	5.0	—	0.11	0.1	2.0	—
—	14.0	—	2.0	3.0	0.10	—	—	0.01	—	0.5	—
1.2	42.0	—	5.0	34.0	1.0	—	—	0.03	0.1	2.0	2.0
2.3	32.0	—	6.0	28.0	1.0	—	—	0.10	0.1	1.0	—
0.1	118.0	—	8.0	226.0	15.0	21.0	740	0.34	0.4	6.0	—
0.1	33.0	—	—	167.0	0.70	0.81	60	0.03	0.2	6.0	—
0.5	85.0	—	—	372.0	2.0	—	190	0.02	0.2	4.0	—
—	19.0	—	3.0	—	—	0.39	—	—	—	—	—
—	128.0	—	1.00	98.0	1.0	1.0	50	0.01	—	1.0	—
2.0	105.0	—	9.0	61.0	1.0	—	—	0.03	0.1	2.0	—
0.7	54.0	—	—	7.0	1.0	0.98	70	0.04	0.1	10.0	—
6.7	68.0	—	7.0	41.0	2.0	—	590	0.08	0.2	10.0	2.0
0.7	10.0	—	0.07	1.0	0.21	0.41	—	0.09	—	0.93	4.0
0.4	78.0	—	—	8.0	2.21	4.67	30	—	0.179	2.94	—
0.2	64.0	—	—	9.8	2.66	6.21	10	—	0.167	3.25	—
0.3	71.0	—	—	6.0	2.3	3.0	20	—	0.2	5.10	—
0.41	77.0	—	—	9.3	2.28	3.0	31	—	0.176	4.56	—
0.8	73.0	—	—	10.0	2.20	3.0	70	—	0.130	3.10	—
0.33	46.0	—	—	5.6	1.66	5.0	11	—	0.128	2.33	—
0.2	81.0	—	—	5.0	2.73	4.0	10	—	0.213	3.30	—
0.1	78.0	—	—	10.2	3.05	3.05	—	—	0.183	4.38	—
0.6	77.0	—	—	9.0	2.50	3.5	50	—	0.150	4.0	—
0.2	51.0	—	—	4.5	1.42	3.01	10	—	0.112	2.68	—
0.4	72.0	—	—	5.0	2.3	3.50	20	—	0.190	4.80	—
0.2	55.0	—	—	4.0	1.96	3.79	10	—	0.184	3.72	—
0.2	73.0	—	—	17.0	1.77	3.03	—	—	0.200	2.90	1.28

Appendix continued on following page

Appendix A–1. Nutritive Values of Food* (Continued)

	Approximate Measure	Weight (gm)	Kilocalories	Protein (gm)	Fat (gm)	Saturated fat (gm)	Mono-unsaturated fat (gm)
Beef, corned beef hash	1 cup	220	400	19.0	25.0	11.9	10.9
Beef, dried, chipped	2 ½ oz. jar	71	117	20.7	2.8	1.1	2.2
Beef and vegetable stew	1 cup	245	220	16.0	11.0	4.9	4.5
Beef potpie (1/3 of 9″ diam. pie)	1 piece	210	515	21.0	30.0	7.9	12.8
Chili con carne with beans, canned	1 cup	255	340	19.0	16.0	7.5	6.8
Heart, beef, lean, braised	3 oz.	85	148	24.5	4.8	1.4	1.1
Lamb, cooked							
Chop, rib, lean and fat	3.1 oz.	85	344	17.0	30.0	14.0	11.0
Chop, rib, lean only	2 oz.	56	119	15.0	5.0	2.0	2.0
Leg, roasted, lean and fat	3 oz.	85	235	22.0	16.0	7.0	6.0
Leg, roasted, lean only	2 oz.	70	129	19.0	4.0	2.0	1.0
Shoulder, roasted, lean and fat	3 oz.	85	285	18.0	23.0	10.0	8.0
Shoulder, roasted, lean only	2.3 oz.	65	132	17.0	6.0	3.0	2.0
Liver, beef, fried	3 oz.	85	195	22.0	9.0	2.0	3.0
Pork, cured, cooked							
Ham, light-cure, lean and fat	3 oz.	85	151	19.0	7.0	2.0	—
Luncheon meat, boiled ham	1 oz.	28	51	4.0	2.0	0.96	1.0
Luncheon meat, canned	2 oz.	56	135	9.0	10.0	3.0	6.0
Pork, fresh, cooked							
Chop, loin, lean and fat	2.7 oz.	76	265	18.0	20.0	7.0	9.0
Chop, loin, lean only	2 oz.	56	145	15.0	8.0	2.0	3.0
Roast, oven-cooked, lean and fat	3 oz.	85	258	21.0	18.0	6.0	10.0
Roast, lean only	2.4 oz.	68	162	19.0	8.0	3.0	4.0
Shoulder cut, lean and fat	3 oz.	85	140	24.0	4.0	1.0	3.0
Shoulder cut, lean only	2.2 oz.	62	151	15.0	9.0	3.0	3.0
Sausages							
Bologna	1 oz.	28	70	4.0	5.0	1.0	3.0
Braunschweiger	1 oz.	28	102	3.0	9.0	3.0	3.0
Deviled ham, canned	1 Tbsp.	13	45	2.0	4.0	1.0	1.0
Frankfurter (8 per 1 lb. pkg.)	1	57	183	6.0	16.0	6.0	6.0
Meat, potted, canned	1 Tbsp.	13	30	2.0	2.0	—	—
Pork link (16 per 1 lb. pkg.)	1 link	13	48	2.0	4.0	1.0	2.0
Salami, dry type	1 slice	10	41	2.0	3.0	1.0	1.0
Salami, cooked type	1 slice	28	71	4.0	5.0	2.0	3.0
Vienna sausage (7 per 4 oz. can)	1	16	45	1.0	4.0	1.0	1.0
Veal, medium fat, cooked, boneless							
Cutlet	3 oz.	85	185	23.0	9.0	4.0	3.0
Rib	3 oz.	85	230	23.0	14.0	6.0	5.0
Chicken, cooked							
Breast, fried, boneless	2.8 oz.	79	176	25.0	7.0	1.0	1.0
Drumstick, fried, boneless	1.3 oz.	36	90	9.0	5.0	1.0	1.0
Chicken, canned, boneless	3 oz.	85	140	18.0	6.0	1.0	3.0
Chicken and noodles, (home recipe)	1 cup	240	365	22.0	18.0	5.0	7.0
Chicken chow mein, canned	1 cup	250	95	7.0	—	—	—
Chicken chow mein (home recipe)	1 cup	250	255	31.0	10.0	2.0	3.0
Chicken potpie (⅓ of 9″ diam.)	1 piece	232	545	23.0	31.0	11.0	10.0
Turkey, roasted, without skin:							
Dark meat	3 oz.	85	159	24.0	6.0	2.0	3.0
Light meat	3 oz.	85	133	25.5	2.7	0.9	1.5
Light and dark meat, chopped	3 oz.	85	144	24.9	4.2	1.4	2.2

Fruits and Fruit Products

Apple, raw, unpeeled, 2¾″ diam.	1	138	81	0.3	0.5	0.1	2.2

Appendix A–1. Nutritive Values of Food* (Continued)

Poly-unsaturated fat (gm)	Cholesterol (mg)	Dietary fiber (gm)	Carbo-hydrate (gm)	Calcium (mg)	Iron (mg)	Zinc (mg)	Vitamin A (IU)	Thiamin (mg)	Riboflavin (mg)	Niacin (mg)	Ascorbic acid (mg)
0.5	50.0	–	24.0	29.0	4.4	–	–	–	0.2	4.6	–
0.1	650.0	–	1.1	14.0	3.6	3.72	–	–	0.230	2.70	–
0.2	72.0	3.190	15.0	29.0	2.9	–	2400	–	0.170	4.7	17.0
6.7	44.0	–	39.0	29.0	3.8	–	1720	–	0.3	5.0	6.0
0.3	38.0	5.000	31.0	82.0	4.3	–	150	–	0.180	3.3	–
0.6	164.0	–	0.4	5.0	6.38	2.66	–	–	1.311	3.46	1.20
1.1	82.0	–	–	7.0	0.96	3.0	–	0.11	0.2	3.0	–
0.2	55.0	–	–	5.0	1.0	2.0	–	0.09	0.1	3.0	–
0.6	82.0	–	–	9.0	1.0	3.0	–	0.13	0.2	4.0	–
0.2	66.0	–	–	8.0	1.0	3.0	–	0.12	0.2	4.0	–
0.9	82.0	–	–	9.0	1.0	3.0	–	0.11	0.2	4.0	–
0.2	68.0	–	–	8.0	1.0	3.0	–	0.10	0.2	3.0	–
0.9	372.0	–	5.0	9.0	7.0	3.0	45,416	0.22	3.6	14.0	23.0
–	50.0	–	–	7.0	1.0	2.0	–	0.62	0.3	5.0	19.0
0.4	15.0	–	0.88	1.0	0.28	0.61	–	0.24	0.1	1.0	7.0
0.9	27.0	–	0.16	2.0	0.54	1.0	–	0.30	0.1	1.0	–
2.1	71.0	–	–	4.0	0.62	1.0	6	0.64	0.3	4.0	0.19
0.7	54.0	–	–	4.0	0.52	1.0	4	0.55	0.2	3.0	0.17
2.2	77.0	–	–	5.0	0.84	1.0	6	0.70	0.2	4.0	0.30
0.8	62.0	–	–	4.0	0.74	1.0	4	0.62	0.2	3.0	0.24
0.8	78.0	–	–	6.0	1.0	2.0	5	0.80	0.3	3.0	0.30
0.8	60.0	–	–	4.0	0.95	2.0	4	0.36	0.2	2.0	0.18
0.5	17.0	–	0.21	3.0	0.22	0.58	–	0.15	–	1.0	9.0
0.8	44.0	–	0.88	3.0	2.0	0.80	3983	0.07	0.4	2.0	2.0
0.4	10.0	–	–	1.0	0.30	0.24	–	0.02	–	0.20	–
1.2	29.0	–	1.0	6.0	0.66	1.0	–	0.11	0.1	1.0	15.0
–	15.0	–	–	–	–	–	–	–	–	0.20	–
0.5	11.0	–	0.13	4.0	0.16	0.33	–	0.10	–	0.59	–
0.1	8.0	–	0.16	1.0	0.13	0.42	–	0.09	–	0.56	–
0.2	17.0	–	0.70	2.0	0.57	0.60	–	0.04	0.1	0.97	3.0
0.2	8.0	–	0.33	2.0	0.14	0.26	–	0.01	–	0.26	–
0.4	87.0	–	–	9.0	2.0	3.0	–	0.06	0.2	4.0	–
0.6	87.0	–	–	10.0	2.0	3.0	–	0.11	0.3	6.0	–
0.9	71.0	–	1.0	12.0	0.95	0.87	39	0.06	0.1	10.0	–
0.9	33.0	–	0.60	4.0	0.50	1.0	30	0.03	0.1	2.0	–
1.0	46.0	–	–	11.0	1.0	–	200	0.01	0.1	5.0	1.0
3.5	96.0	–	26.0	26.0	2.0	–	430	0.05	0.2	4.0	–
–	98.0	–	18.0	45.0	1.0	–	150	0.05	0.1	1.0	13.0
3.1	98.0	–	10.0	58.0	2.0	–	280	0.08	0.2	4.0	10.0
5.6	72.0	–	42.0	70.0	3.0	–	3090	0.34	0.3	5.0	5.0
1.5	72.0	–	–	27.0	1.0	3.0	–	0.05	0.2	3.0	–
0.7	58.0	–	–	16.0	1.1	1.7	–	0.05	0.11	5.8	–
1.1	65.0	–	–	21.0	1.5	2.6	–	0.05	0.15	4.6	–
–	–	2.8	21.0	10.0	0.2	–	74	0.02	0.02	0.1	7.0

Appendix continued on following page

Appendix A–1. *Nutritive Values of Food* (Continued)*

	Approximate Measure	Weight (gm)	Kilocalories	Protein (gm)	Fat (gm)	Saturated fat (gm)	Mono-unsaturated fat (gm)
Apple, raw, unpeeled, 3¼″ diam.	1	212	123	0.4	0.8	0.1	—
Apple juice, bottle or canned	1 cup	248	116	0.1	0.3	—	—
Applesauce, canned, sweetened	1 cup	255	194	0.5	0.5	0.1	—
Applesauce, canned, unsweetened	1 cup	244	106	0.4	0.1	—	—
Apricot, raw	1	35	17	0.5	0.1	—	—
Apricots, canned in heavy syrup	1 cup	258	214	1.4	0.2	—	—
Apricots, dried, uncooked	1 cup	130	310	4.8	0.6	—	—
Apricot nectar, canned	1 cup	251	141	0.9	0.2	—	—
Avocado, California	1	216	382	4.6	37.4	5.6	22.0
Avocado, Florida	1	304	339	4.8	27.0	5.3	15.7
Banana without peel	1	119	109	1.2	0.6	0.2	—
Banana flakes	1 Tbsp.	6	21	0.2	0.1	—	—
Blackberries, fresh	1 cup	144	74	1.0	0.6	—	—
Blueberries, fresh	1 cup	145	82	—	0.5	—	—
Cherries, sour, pitted, canned	1 cup	256	232	1.9	0.2	0.1	—
Cherries, sweet, fresh	10	68	49	0.8	0.6	0.1	—
Cranberry juice cocktail, bottled, sweetened	1 cup	253	147	0.1	0.1	—	—
Cranberry sauce, sweetened, canned	1 Tbsp.	17	26	—	—	—	—
Dates, whole, without pits	10	83	228	1.6	0.4	—	—
Fruit cocktail, canned in heavy syrup	1 cup	255	186	1.0	0.2	—	—
Grapefruit, pink or red	½	246	73	1.4	0.2	—	—
Grapefruit, white	½	236	77	1.6	0.2	—	—
Grapefruit, canned, sections	1 cup	254	152	1.4	0.2	—	—
Grapefruit juice, canned, unsweetened	1 cup	247	93	1.3	0.2	—	—
Grapefruit juice, canned, sweetened	1 cup	250	116	1.5	0.2	—	—
Grapefruit juice, frozen, diluted	1 cup	247	102	1.4	0.3	—	—
Grapes, Thompson, seedless	10	50	31	0.3	0.2	—	—
Grapes, Tokay or Emperor	10	60	42	0.4	0.3	0.1	—
Grape juice, canned or bottled	1 cup	253	155	1.4	0.2	0.1	—
Grape juice, frozen, diluted	1 cup	250	128	0.5	0.2	0.1	—
Grape drink, canned	1 cup	250	135	—	—	—	—
Lemon, fresh, size 165	1	74	21	0.8	0.2	—	—
Lemon juice, fresh	1 cup	244	60	0.9	—	—	—
Lemon juice, canned or bottled, un-sweetened	1 cup	244	52	—	0.7	0.1	—
Lemonade, frozen, diluted	1 cup	248	105	—	—	—	—
Limeade, frozen, diluted	1 cup	247	100	—	—	—	—
Lime juice, fresh	1 cup	246	66	1.1	0.2	—	—
Lime juice, canned, unsweetened	1 cup	246	51	0.6	0.6	0.1	—
Melon, cantaloupe, fresh	1 cup	160	57	1.4	0.4	—	—
Melon, honeydew, fresh	1 cup	170	60	0.8	0.2	—	—
Orange, whole, 2⅝″ diam.	1	131	62	1.2	0.2	0.02	—
Orange sections without membranes	1 cup	180	85	1.7	0.2	0.03	—
Orange juice, fresh	1 cup	248	111	1.7	0.5	0.06	—
Orange juice, canned, un-sweetened	1 cup	249	104	1.5	0.4	0.05	—
Orange juice, frozen, diluted	1 cup	249	112	1.7	0.1	0.02	—
Papayas, fresh, 1/2″ cubes	1 cup	140	54	0.9	0.2	0.06	—

Appendix A–1. *Nutritive Values of Food* (Continued)*

Poly-unsaturated fat (gm)	Cholesterol (mg)	Dietary fiber (gm)	Carbo-hydrate (gm)	Calcium (mg)	Iron (mg)	Zinc (mg)	Vitamin A (IU)	Thiamin (mg)	Riboflavin (mg)	Niacin (mg)	Ascorbic acid (mg)
—	—	4.3	32.0	15.0	0.4	0.1	113	0.04	0.03	0.2	11.0
—	—	—	29.0	16.0	0.9	0.1	2	0.05	0.04	0.2	2.0
—	—	2.8	50.0	9.0	0.9	0.1	28	0.03	0.07	0.5	4.0
—	—	1.9	27.0	7.0	0.3	0.1	70	0.03	0.06	0.5	2.0
—	—	0.5	3.0	4.0	0.2	0.1	930	0.01	0.01	0.2	3.0
—	—	—	55.0	22.0	0.8	0.3	3174	0.05	0.06	—	8.0
—	—	—	80.0	59.0	6.1	—	9412	0.01	0.20	3.9	3.0
—	—	0.8	36.0	17.0	—	0.2	3304	0.02	0.04	0.7	1.0
3.7	—	5.8	14.0	23.0	2.5	0.9	1322	0.23	0.26	4.2	17.0
5.3	—	8.3	27.0	33.0	1.6	1.3	1860	0.33	0.37	5.8	24.0
—	—	1.7	27.0	7.0	0.4	0.2	96	0.05	0.12	0.6	10.0
—	—	—	5.0	1.0	0.1	—	19	0.01	0.02	0.2	0.40
—	—	6.5	18.0	46.0	0.8	0.4	237	0.04	0.06	0.6	30.0
—	—	4.3	20.0	9.0	0.2	0.2	145	0.07	0.07	0.5	18.0
—	—	0.6	59.0	26.0	3.3	0.2	1827	0.04	0.10	0.4	5.0
—	—	1.0	11.0	10.0	0.3	—	146	0.03	0.04	0.3	4.0
—	—	—	37.0	8.0	0.4	—	—	0.01	0.04	0.1	108.0
—	—	—	6.0	0.63	—	—	3	—	—	—	0.34
—	—	4.2	61.0	27.0	—	0.2	42	0.08	0.08	1.8	—
—	—	1.6	48.0	16.0	0.7	0.2	522	0.05	0.05	—	4.0
—	—	—	18.0	36.0	0.3	0.2	637	0.10	0.05	0.5	91.0
—	—	—	19.0	28.0	0.1	0.2	23	0.09	0.05	0.6	78.0
—	—	0.6	39.0	36.0	1.0	0.2	—	0.10	0.05	0.6	54.0
—	—	—	22.0	18.0	0.5	0.2	18	0.10	0.05	0.6	72.0
—	—	—	27.0	20.0	0.9	0.1	—	0.10	0.06	0.8	67.0
—	—	—	24.0	19.0	0.3	0.1	22	0.10	0.05	0.5	83.0
—	—	0.8	8.0	7.0	0.1	—	50	0.05	0.03	0.2	2.0
—	—	—	10.0	6.0	0.2	—	43	0.06	0.03	0.2	6.0
—	—	—	37.0	22.0	0.6	0.1	20	0.07	0.09	0.7	0.20
—	—	—	31.0	9.0	0.3	0.1	19	0.04	0.07	0.3	59.0
—	—	—	35.0	8.0	0.3	—	—	0.03	0.03	0.3	—
—	—	—	6.0	19.0	0.4	—	21	0.03	0.02	0.1	39.0
—	—	—	21.0	18.0	0.1	0.1	49	0.07	0.02	0.2	112.0
—	—	—	15.0	26.0	0.3	0.1	37	0.10	0.02	0.5	60.0
—	—	—	28.0	2.0	0.1	—	10	0.01	0.02	0.2	17.0
—	—	—	27.0	3.0	—	—	—	—	—	—	6.0
—	—	—	22.0	22.0	0.1	0.1	25	0.05	0.03	0.2	72.0
—	—	—	16.0	30.0	0.6	0.1	40	0.08	0.01	0.4	15.0
—	—	0.5	13.0	17.0	0.3	0.2	5158	0.06	0.03	0.9	67.0
—	—	—	15.0	10.0	0.1	—	68	0.13	0.03	1.0	42.0
—	—	—	15.0	52.0	0.1	0.09	269	0.11	0.05	0.4	69.0
—	—	—	21.0	72.0	0.2	0.13	369	0.16	0.07	0.5	95.0
—	—	—	25.0	27.0	0.5	0.13	496	0.22	0.07	—	124.0
—	—	—	24.0	21.0	1.1	0.17	437	0.15	0.07	0.8	85.0
—	—	—	26.0	22.0	0.2	0.13	194	0.20	0.05	0.5	96.0
—	—	1.3	13.0	33.0	0.1	0.10	2819	0.04	0.05	0.5	86.0

Appendix continued on following page

Appendix A–1. *Nutritive Values of Food* (Continued)*

	Approximate Measure	Weight (gm)	Kilocalories	Protein (gm)	Fat (gm)	Saturated fat (gm)	Mono-unsaturated fat (gm)
Peach, whole, 1½" diam., peeled	1	87	37	0.6	0.1	0.01	—
Peach, sliced, fresh	1 cup	170	73	1.2	0.2	0.02	—
Peaches, canned in syrup	1 cup	256	190	1.2	0.2	0.03	—
Peaches, canned in water	1 cup	244	58	1.1	0.1	0.02	—
Peaches, dried, uncooked	1 cup	160	383	5.8	1.2	0.13	—
Peaches, frozen, sliced, sweetened	1 cup	250	235	1.6	0.3	0.04	—
Pears, Bartlett, 2½" diam.	1	166	98	0.6	0.7	0.04	—
Pear, Bosc, 2½" diam.	1	141	83	0.5	0.6	0.03	—
Pear, Anjou, 3" diam.	1	200	118	0.8	0.8	0.04	—
Pear, canned in syrup	1 cup	255	188	0.5	0.3	0.02	—
Pineapple, fresh, diced	1 cup	155	77	0.6	0.7	0.05	—
Pineapple, canned in heavy syrup— crushed, chunks, or tidbits	1 cup	255	131	0.9	0.3	0.02	—
Pineapple juice, unsweetened, canned	1 cup	250	139	0.8	0.2	0.01	—
Plums, fresh, Japanese	1	66	36	0.5	0.4	0.03	—
Plums, canned in heavy syrup	1 cup	258	230	0.9	0.3	0.02	—
Prunes, dried, uncooked	4	49	117	1.3	0.3	0.02	—
Prune juice, canned or bottled	1 cup	256	181	1.5	0.1	0.01	—
Raisins, seedless	1 cup	145	434	4.7	0.7	0.22	—
Raisins, packet (½ oz)	1	14	42	0.5	0.1	0.02	—
Raspberries, red, fresh	1 cup	123	61	1.1	0.7	0.02	—
Raspberries, red, frozen, sweetened	1 cup	250	256	1.7	0.4	0.01	—
Rhubarb, cooked, fresh, added sugar	1 cup	270	380	1.0	—	—	—
Rhubarb, cooked, frozen, sweetened	1 cup	240	279	0.9	0.1	—	—
Strawberries, fresh, whole	1 cup	149	45	0.9	0.5	0.03	—
Strawberries, frozen, sweetened, sliced	1 cup	255	245	1.4	0.3	0.02	—
Strawberries, frozen, sweetened, whole	1 cup	255	200	1.3	0.3	0.02	—
Tangerine, raw, 2⅜" diam.	1	84	37	0.5	0.2	0.02	—
Tangerine juice, canned, sweetened	1 cup	249	125	1.3	0.5	0.03	—
Watermelon, fresh	1 cup	160	50	—	0.7	—	—
Grain Products							
Bagel, 3" diam., egg	1	55	163	6.0	1.4	0.50	0.9
Bagel, 3" diam., water	1	55	163	6.0	1.4	0.20	0.4
Barley, pearled, light, uncooked	1 cup	200	700	16.0	2.0	0.30	0.2
Biscuit, baking powder (home recipe)	1	28	105	2.0	5.0	1.20	2.0
Biscuit, baking powder (mix)	1	28	93	2.0	3.3	0.60	1.1
Breadcrumbs, enriched, dry, grated	1 cup	100	390	13.0	5.0	1.00	1.6
Breads							
Boston brown, canned	1 slice	45	95	2.0	1.0	0.10	0.2
Cracked-wheat (18 slices/loaf)	1 slice	25	65	2.0	0.9	0.10	0.2
French	1 slice	35	98	3.0	1.4	0.20	0.4
Vienna	1 slice	25	70	2.0	—	0.20	0.3
Italian, enriched	1 slice	30	85	3.0	—	—	—
Raisin, enriched (18 slices/loaf)	1 slice	25	69	2.0	—	0.20	0.3
Rye, American, light	1 slice	25	65	2.0	0.9	—	—
Rye, Pumpernickel	1 slice	32	81	2.0	1.1	0.10	—

Appendix A–1. Nutritive Values of Food* (Continued)

Poly-unsaturated fat (gm)	Cholesterol (mg)	Dietary fiber (gm)	Carbo-hydrate (gm)	Calcium (mg)	Iron (mg)	Zinc (mg)	Vitamin A (IU)	Thiamin (mg)	Riboflavin (mg)	Niacin (mg)	Ascorbic acid (mg)
—	—	0.5	9.0	5.0	0.1	0.12	465	0.02	0.04	0.9	5.0
—	—	1.0	18.0	9.0	0.2	0.23	910	0.03	0.07	1.7	11.0
—	—	1.1	51.0	8.0	0.7	0.22	849	0.03	0.06	1.6	7.0
—	—	1.1	14.0	6.0	0.8	0.22	1298	0.02	0.05	1.3	7.0
—	—	—	98.0	45.0	6.5	0.92	3461	—	0.34	7.0	7.0
—	—	—	59.0	6.0	0.9	0.13	709	0.03	0.09	1.6	235.0
—	—	4.1	25.0	19.0	0.4	0.20	33	0.03	0.07	0.2	6.0
—	—	3.5	21.0	15.0	0.4	0.17	28	0.03	0.06	0.1	5.0
—	—	4.9	30.0	22.0	0.5	0.24	39	0.04	0.08	0.2	7.0
—	—	2.3	48.0	12.0	0.6	0.21	—	0.03	0.06	0.6	2.0
—	—	2.4	19.0	11.0	0.6	0.12	35	0.14	0.06	0.7	23.0
—	—	1.9	33.0	36.0	—	0.29	37	0.23	0.06	0.7	19.0
—	—	—	34.0	42.0	0.6	0.29	12	0.14	0.06	0.6	26.0
—	—	—	8.0	2.0	0.1	0.06	213	0.03	0.06	0.3	6.0
—	—	1.1	60.0	24.0	2.2	0.19	668	0.04	0.10	0.8	1.0
—	—	—	30.0	24.0	1.2	0.26	973	0.04	0.08	—	1.0
—	—	—	44.0	30.0	3.0	0.52	9	0.04	0.18	2.0	10.0
—	—	—	115.0	71.0	3.0	0.38	11	0.23	0.13	1.2	4.0
—	—	—	11.0	6.0	0.3	0.04	1	0.02	0.01	0.1	0.46
—	—	5.8	14.0	27.0	0.7	0.57	160	0.04	0.11	1.1	30.0
—	—	11.7	65.0	38.0	1.6	0.45	149	0.05	0.11	0.6	41.0
—	—	—	97.0	211.0	1.6	0.22	220	0.05	0.14	0.8	16.0
—	—	—	74.0	348.0	0.5	0.20	166	0.04	0.06	0.5	7.0
—	—	2.8	10.0	21.0	0.6	0.19	41	0.03	0.10	0.3	84.0
—	—	7.1	66.0	28.0	1.5	0.14	61	0.04	0.13	1.0	106.0
—	—	7.1	53.0	29.0	1.2	0.14	70	0.04	0.20	0.7	101.0
—	—	—	9.0	12.0	0.1	—	773	0.09	0.02	0.1	25.0
—	—	—	29.0	45.0	0.5	0.06	1046	0.15	0.05	0.2	54.0
—	—	0.3	11.0	13.0	0.3	0.11	585	0.13	0.03	0.3	15.0
0.8	8.00	—	30.0	23.0	1.5	0.3	17	0.21	0.16	1.0	—
0.6	—	—	30.0	23.0	1.5	0.3	—	0.21	0.16	1.0	—
0.8	—	—	158.0	32.0	4.2	—	—	0.24	0.10	6.0	—
1.2	—	—	13.0	34.0	0.4	—	—	0.08	0.08	0.70	—
0.7	—	—	13.0	58.0	0.6	0.2	15	0.12	0.11	0.84	—
1.4	—	—	73.0	122.0	3.6	—	—	0.35	0.35	4.0	—
0.2	—	—	21.0	41.0	0.9	—	—	0.08	0.04	0.70	—
0.2	—	—	12.0	16.0	0.7	—	—	0.10	0.10	0.84	—
0.4	—	—	17.0	38.0	1.1	0.2	—	0.16	0.12	1.0	—
0.3	—	—	12.0	27.0	0.8	0.2	—	0.12	0.09	1.0	—
0.1	—	—	17.0	5.0	0.7	—	—	0.12	0.07	1.0	—
0.2	—	—	13.0	25.0	0.8	0.2	—	0.08	0.16	1.0	—
0.1	—	—	12.0	20.0	0.7	0.3	—	0.10	0.08	0.83	—
0.2	—	—	15.0	22.0	0.9	0.4	—	0.11	0.17	1.0	—

Appendix continued on following page

Appendix A–1. Nutritive Values of Food* (Continued)

	Approximate Measure	Weight (gm)	Kilocalories	Protein (gm)	Fat (gm)	Saturated fat (gm)	Mono-unsaturated fat (gm)
White bread, enriched							
Soft-crumb type (18 slices/loaf)	1 slice	25	66	2.0	—	0.20	0.3
Soft-crumb type, toasted	1 slice	22	67	2.0	—	0.20	0.3
Firm-crumb type (20 slices/loaf)	1 slice	23	61	1.0	0.9	0.20	0.3
Firm-crumb type, toasted	1 slice	20	65	2.0	1.0	0.20	0.3
Whole-wheat bread							
Soft-crumb type (16 slices/loaf)	1 slice	28	68	2.0	1.2	0.10	0.2
Soft-crumb type, toasted	1 slice	24	67	2.0	1.2	0.10	0.2
Firm-crumb type (18 slices/loaf)	1 slice	25	61	2.0	1.1	0.10	0.2
Firm-crumb type, toasted	1 slice	21	59	2.0	1.0	0.10	0.2
Breakfast cereals							
Cooked							
Corn (hominy) grits, enriched	1 cup	242	146	3.0	0.5	—	—
Corn (hominy) grits, unenriched	1 cup	242	146	3.0	0.5	—	—
Farina, quick cooking, enriched	1 cup	233	116	3.0	0.2	—	—
Oatmeal or rolled oats	1 cup	234	145	6.0	2.4	0.44	0.8
Wheat, rolled	1 cup	240	180	5.0	1.0	—	—
Wheat, whole-meal	1 cup	245	110	4.0	1.0	—	—
Ready-to-eat							
Bran flakes	1 cup	49	159	5.0	0.7	—	—
Bran flakes with raisins	1 cup	56	178	4.0	0.3	—	—
Cornflakes	1 cup	25	98	1.0	0.1	—	—
Cornflakes, sugar-coated	1 cup	35	133	1.0	0.1	—	—
Corn-oat flour, puffed	1 cup	38	149	2.0	0.5	—	—
Corn, shredded	1 cup	25	95	2.0	—	—	—
Oats, puffed	1 cup	25	100	3.0	1.0	—	—
Rice, puffed	1 cup	14	56	0.90	0.1	—	—
Rice, puffed, presweetened	1 cup	28	115	1.0	—	—	—
Wheat flakes	1 cup	30	105	3.0	—	—	—
Wheat, puffed	1 cup	12	44	1.0	0.1	—	—
Wheat, puffed, presweetened	1 cup	38	140	3.0	—	—	—
Wheat, shredded (oblong biscuit)	1	23	83	2.0	0.3	—	—
Wheat germ	1 Tbsp.	113	431	32.0	12.1	2.09	3.7
Buckwheat flour, light	1 cup	98	340	6.0	1.0	0.20	0.4
Bulgur, canned, seasoned	1 cup	135	245	8.0	4.0	—	—*
Cakes made from cake mixes with enriched flour							
Angelfood (¹⁄₁₂ of cake)	1 piece	53	142	4.0	0.12	—	—
Coffeecake (¹⁄₆ of cake)	1 piece	72	230	5.0	7.0	2.0	2.7
Cupcake (2½″ diam.), no icing	1	25	90	1.0	3.0	0.8	1.2
Cupcake with chocolate icing	1	36	130	2.0	5.0	2.0	1.6
Devil's food with chocolate icing (¹⁄₁₆ of cake)	1 piece	69	235	3.0	8.0	3.1	2.8
Gingerbread (¹⁄₉ of cake)	1 piece	63	175	2.0	4.0	1.1	1.8
White (¹⁄₁₆ of cake)	1 piece	71	271	3.0	11.0	3.0	2.9
Cakes made from home recipes using enriched flour							
Boston cream pie with custard filling (¹⁄₁₂ of cake)	1 piece	69	210	3.0	6.0	1.9	2.5
Fruit cake, dark (¹⁄₃₀ of cake)	1 piece	15	55	1.0	2.0	0.5	1.1
Plain, sheet cake (¹⁄₉ of cake)	1 piece	86	315	4.0	12.0	3.3	4.9

Appendix A–1. *Nutritive Values of Food* (Continued)*

Poly-unsaturated fat (gm)	Cholesterol (mg)	Dietary fiber (gm)	Carbo-hydrate (gm)	Calcium (mg)	Iron (mg)	Zinc (mg)	Vitamin A (IU)	Thiamin (mg)	Riboflavin (mg)	Niacin (mg)	Ascorbic acid (mg)
0.3	–	–	12.0	31.0	0.7	0.2	–	0.12	0.08	0.94	–
0.3	–	–	12.0	31.0	0.7	0.2	–	0.10	0.08	0.94	–
0.3	–	–	11.0	29.0	0.7	0.1	–	0.11	0.07	0.86	–
0.3	–	–	12.0	22.0	0.6	0.1	–	0.07	0.06	0.80	–
0.2	–	–	12.0	20.0	–	0.5	–	0.10	0.06	1.0	–
0.2	–	–	12.0	19.0	0.9	0.5	–	0.08	0.06	1.0	–
0.3	–	–	11.0	18.0	0.9	0.4	–	0.09	0.05	0.96	–
0.3	–	–	10.0	17.0	0.8	0.4	–	0.07	0.05	0.92	–
0.1	–	0.6	31.0	1.0	1.6	0.2	–	0.24	0.15	1.0	–
0.1	–	0.6	31.0	1.0	0.5	0.2	–	0.05	0.02	0.48	–
0.1	–	–	24.0	4.0	1.2	0.2	–	0.19	0.12	1.0	–
0.9	–	2.1	25.0	20.0	1.6	1.1	38	0.26	0.05	0.30	–
–	–	–	41.0	19.0	1.7	1.1	–	0.17	0.07	2.0	–
–	–	–	23.0	17.0	1.2	1.2	–	0.15	0.05	1.0	–
–	–	6.0	39.0	26.0	7.8	2.0	2160	0.60	0.70	8.0	26.0
–	–	7.1	46.0	27.0	6.7	1.7	1852	0.60	0.60	7.0	2.0
–	–	0.5	21.0	2.0	0.6	0.1	95	0.10	–	1.0	13.0
–	–	0.4	31.0	1.0	2.2	–	1543	0.50	0.50	6.0	19.0
–	–	0.5	34.0	4.0	1.0	0.8	1675	0.50	0.60	6.0	20.0
–	–	–	22.0	1.0	0.6	0.1	–	0.33	0.05	4.0	13.0
–	–	0.1	19.0	44.0	4.0	0.7	1100	0.33	0.38	4.0	13.0
–	–	0.1	12.0	1.0	0.1	0.1	–	0.02	0.01	0.42	–
–	–	0.2	26.0	3.0	–	1.5	1240	–	–	–	15.0
–	–	2.0	24.0	12.0	4.8	0.7	1320	0.40	0.45	5.0	16.0
–	–	0.4	9.0	3.0	0.6	0.3	–	0.02	0.03	1.0	–
–	–	0.4	33.0	7.0	–	2.0	1680	0.50	0.57	6.0	20.0
–	–	2.2	18.0	10.0	0.7	0.6	–	0.07	0.06	1.0	–
5.6	–	–	56.0	50.0	10.3	18.8	188	1.89	0.93	6.0	7.0
0.4	–	–	78.0	11.0	1.0	–	–	0.08	0.04	0.40	–
–	–	–	44.0	27.0	1.9	–	–	0.08	0.05	4.0	–
–	–	–	31.0	50.0	0.5	0.1	–	0.06	0.12	0.6	–
1.5	–	–	38.0	44.0	1.2	–	120	0.14	0.15	1.3	–
0.7	–	–	14.0	40.0	0.3	–	40	0.05	0.05	0.4	–
0.6	15.0	–	21.0	47.0	0.4	–	60	0.05	0.06	0.4	–
1.1	33.0	–	40.0	41.0	1.0	–	100	0.07	0.10	0.6	–
1.1	1.0	–	32.0	57.0	0.9	0.3	–	0.09	0.11	0.8	–
1.2	3.0	–	41.0	70.0	0.7	0.3	21	0.07	0.11	0.7	–
1.3	–	–	34.0	46.0	0.7	–	140	0.09	0.11	0.8	–
0.5	7.0	–	9.0	11.0	0.4	–	20	0.02	0.02	0.2	–
2.6	1.0	–	48.0	55.0	0.9	0.3	150	0.13	0.15	1.1	–

Appendix continued on following page

Appendix A–1. *Nutritive Values of Food* (Continued)*

	Approximate Measure	Weight (gm)	Kilocalories	Protein (gm)	Fat (gm)	Saturated fat (gm)	Mono-unsaturated fat (gm)
Plain, sheet cake with uncooked white icing	1 piece	121	445	4.0	14.0	4.7	5.5
Sponge cake (¹⁄₁₂ of cake)	1 piece	66	188	4.0	3.0	1.1	1.3
Cookies made with enriched flour							
Brownie with nuts (from mix)	1	20	85	1.0	4.0	0.9	1.4
Chocolate chip, commercial	4	42	200	1.0	9.0	2.8	2.9
Chocolate chip, from home recipe	4	40	185	1.0	10.0	3.5	4.5
Fig bars, square	4	56	211	2.0	3.0	0.8	1.2
Gingersnaps, 2″ diam.	4	28	137	1.0	6.0	0.7	1.0
Macaroons, 2¾″ diam.	2	38	180	2.0	9.0	—	—
Oatmeal with raisins, 2⅝″ diam.	4	52	246	2.0	10.0	2.0	3.3
Plain, from commercial dough	1	12	60	0.50	3.0	0.7	1.3
Sandwich type (chocolate or vanilla)	4	40	200	1.0	9.0	2.2	3.9
Vanilla wafers	10	40	185	1.0	5.0	1.7	—
Cornmeal							
Whole-ground, unbolted, dry	1 cup	122	435	11.0	5.0	0.5	1.0
Bolted (nearly whole-grain), dry	1 cup	122	440	11.0	4.0	0.5	0.9
Degermed, enriched, dry	1 cup	138	500	11.0	2.0	0.2	0.4
Degermed, enriched, cooked	1 cup	240	120	3.0	—	—	0.1
Degermed, unenriched, dry	1 cup	138	500	11.0	2.0	0.2	0.4
Degermed, unenriched, cooked	1 cup	240	120	3.0	—	—	0.1
Crackers							
Graham, plain, 2½″ square	2	14	55	1.0	1.0	0.3	0.5
Rye wafers, whole grain	2	13	45	2.0	—	—	—
Saltines, made with enriched flour	4	11	50	1.0	1.0	0.4	0.5
Danish pastry (about 4¼″ diam.)	1	65	250	4.0	13.0	4.7	6.1
Doughnuts made with enriched flour							
Cake type, plain	1	25	104	1.0	5.0	1.2	2.0
Yeast-leavened, glazed	1	50	205	3.0	11.0	3.3	5.8
Macaroni, enriched, cooked, firm	1 cup	130	190	7.0	1.0	—	—
Macaroni, enriched, tender	1 cup	140	155	5.0	1.0	—	—
Macaroni, enriched, with cheese, canned	1 cup	240	230	9.0	10.0	4.2	3.1
Macaroni and cheese (home recipe)	1 cup	200	430	17.0	22.0	8.9	8.8
Muffins made with enriched flour							
Blueberry (home recipe)	1	40	110	3.0	4.0	1.1	1.4
Bran (home recipe)	1	40	112	2.0	5.0	1.2	1.4
Corn (home recipe)	1	40	125	3.0	4.0	1.2	1.6
Plain (home recipe)	1	40	120	3.0	4.0	1.0	1.7
Corn (from mix)	1	40	130	3.0	4.0	1.2	1.7
Noodles, egg, enriched, cooked	1 cup	160	200	7.0	2.0	—	—
Noodles, chow mein, canned	1 cup	45	220	6.0	11.0	—	—
Pancakes (4″ diam.), buckwheat	1	27	55	2.0	2.0	0.8	0.90
Pancakes (4″ diam.), plain (home recipe)	1	27	60	2.0	2.0	0.5	0.80
Pancakes, plain (mix)	1	27	58	1.0	2.0	0.7	0.70
Pies, piecrust made with enriched flour and vegetable shortening							

Appendix A–1. Nutritive Values of Food* (Continued)

Poly-unsaturated fat (gm)	Cholesterol (mg)	Dietary fiber (gm)	Carbo-hydrate (gm)	Calcium (mg)	Iron (mg)	Zinc (mg)	Vitamin A (IU)	Thiamin (mg)	Riboflavin (mg)	Niacin (mg)	Ascorbic acid (mg)
2.7	1.0	—	77.0	61.0	0.8	—	240	0.14	0.16	1.1	—
0.5	162.0	—	35.0	25.0	1.1	0.8	125	0.09	0.13	0.7	—
1.3	—	—	13.0	9.0	0.4	—	20	0.03	0.02	0.2	—
2.2	22.0	—	27.0	11.0	0.9	0.2	24	0.06	0.09	0.8	—
2.9	21.0	—	25.0	13.0	1.0	0.2	17	0.06	0.06	0.6	—
0.7	—	—	42.0	40.0	1.4	0.4	62	0.08	0.07	0.7	—
0.6	—	—	18.0	10.0	0.6	0.1	10	0.06	0.05	0.5	—
—	—	—	25.0	10.0	0.3	—	—	0.02	0.06	0.2	—
2.0	—	—	35.0	17.0	1.1	0.3	41	0.09	0.08	—	—
0.7	—	—	7.0	4.0	0.1	—	7	0.03	0.02	0.2	—
2.2	—	—	28.0	10.0	0.7	0.3	—	0.06	0.10	0.7	—
—	25.0	—	30.0	16.0	0.6	—	50	0.10	0.09	0.8	—
2.5	—	—	90.0	24.0	2.2	—	620	0.46	0.13	2.4	—
2.1	—	—	91.0	21.0	2.2	—	590	0.37	0.10	2.3	—
0.9	—	—	108.0	8.0	5.9	2.0	610	0.61	0.36	4.8	—
0.2	—	—	26.0	2.0	1.0	—	140	0.14	0.10	1.2	—
0.9	—	—	108.0	8.0	1.5	2.0	610	0.19	0.07	1.4	—
0.2	—	—	26.0	2.0	0.5	—	140	0.05	0.02	0.2	—
0.3	—	0.40	10.0	6.0	0.5	0.1	—	0.02	0.08	0.5	—
—	—	1.73	10.0	7.0	0.5	—	—	0.04	0.03	0.2	—
0.4	2.0	0.16	8.0	1.0	0.5	0.1	—	0.50	0.05	0.4	—
3.2	—	—	29.0	68.0	1.2	0.5	69	0.16	0.15	1.5	—
1.1	10.0	—	12.0	11.0	0.4	0.1	14	0.06	0.05	0.4	—
3.3	13.0	—	22.0	16.0	0.6	—	25	0.10	0.10	0.8	—
—	—	—	39.0	14.0	1.4	0.7	—	0.23	0.13	1.8	—
—	—	—	32.0	11.0	1.3	0.7	—	0.20	0.11	1.5	—
1.4	42.0	—	26.0	199.0	1.0	—	260	0.12	0.24	1.0	—
2.9	42.0	—	40.0	362.0	1.8	—	860	0.20	0.40	1.8	—
0.7	21.0	—	17.0	34.0	0.6	—	90	0.09	0.10	0.7	—
0.8	21.0	—	16.0	53.0	1.3	1.1	206	0.10	0.11	1.3	2.48
0.9	21.0	—	19.0	42.0	0.7	—	120	0.10	0.10	0.7	—
1.0	21.0	—	17.0	42.0	0.6	—	40	0.09	0.12	0.9	—
0.9	21.0	—	20.0	96.0	0.6	—	100	0.08	0.09	0.7	—
—	50.0	—	37.0	16.0	1.4	—	110	0.22	0.13	1.9	—
—	5.0	—	26.0	—	—	—	—	—	—	—	—
0.4	20.0	—	6.0	59.0	0.4	0.2	60	0.04	0.05	0.2	—
0.5	20.0	—	9.0	27.0	0.4	0.2	30	0.06	0.07	0.5	—
0.3	20.0	—	19.0	35.0	0.3	0.2	38	0.04	0.06	0.3	—

Appendix continued on following page

Appendix A–1. *Nutritive Values of Food* (Continued)*

	Approximate Measure	Weight (gm)	Kilocalories	Protein (gm)	Fat (gm)	Saturated fat (gm)	Mono-unsaturated fat (gm)
Apple (⅐ of pie)	1	135	323	2.0	13.0	3.9	6.0
Banana (⅐ of pie)	1	130	285	6.0	12.0	3.8	4.0
Blueberry (⅐ of pie)	1	135	325	3.0	15.0	3.5	6.0
Cherry (⅐ of pie)	1	135	350	4.0	15.0	4.0	6.0
Custard (⅐ of pie)	1	130	285	8.0	14.0	4.8	5.0
Lemon meringue (⅐ of pie)	1	120	300	3.0	11.0	3.7	4.0
Mincemeat (⅐ of pie)	1	135	365	3.0	16.0	4.0	6.0
Peach, (⅐ of pie)	1	135	345	3.0	14.0	3.5	6.0
Pecan (⅐ of pie)	1	118	495	6.0	27.0	4.0	14.0
Pumpkin (⅐ of pie)	1	130	275	5.0	15.0	5.4	5.0
Piecrust (home recipe) made with enriched flour and vegetable shortening, baked (9″ diam.)	1	180	900	11.0	60.0	14.8	26.0
Pizza, with cheese, baked ⅛ of 12″ diam.	2	120	290	39.0	8.0	3.4	3.0
Popcorn, popped, plain	1 cup	6	25	1.0	—	—	0.10
Popcorn, popped with oil and salt	1 cup	9	40	1.0	2.0	1.5	0.20
Popcorn, sugar-coated	1 cup	35	135	2.0	1.0	0.5	0.20
Pretzel, Dutch, twisted	1	16	60	2.0	1.0	—	—
Pretzels, thin, stick, 1¼″ long	10	2	11	0.28	0.11	—	—
Rice, brown, long-cooked	1 cup	195	232	4.0	1.0	—	5.0
Rice, brown, Uncle Ben's	1 cup	146	220	5.0	1.0	—	—
Rice, white, enriched, long-grain, cooked	1 cup	205	225	4.0	—	0.1	0.10
Rice, parboiled, cooked	1 cup	175	185	4.0	—	0.1	0.10
Rolls, enriched, commercial							
Brown-and-serve	1	26	85	2.0	2.0	0.4	0.70
Cloverleaf	1	28	85	2.0	2.0	0.4	0.60
Frankfurter or hamburger	1	40	114	3.0	2.0	0.5	0.80
Hard (3¾″ diam.)	1	50	155	5.0	2.0	0.4	0.60
Hoagie or submarine	1	135	390	12.0	4.0	0.9	1.0
Spaghetti, enriched, cooked firm	1 cup	130	190	7.0	1.0	—	—
Spaghetti, enriched, cooked tender	1 cup	140	155	5.0	1.0	—	—
Spaghetti, enriched, in tomato sauce with cheese, canned	1 cup	250	190	6.0	2.0	0.5	0.30
Spaghetti with meat balls and tomato sauce (home recipe)	1 cup	248	330	19.0	12.0	3.3	6.0
Spaghetti with meat balls and tomato sauce (canned)	1 cup	250	260	12.0	10.0	2.2	3.0
Toaster pastry	1	50	196	1.0	5.0	—	—
Waffles made with enriched flour (7″ diam.), home recipe	1	75	245	6.0	12.0	2.3	2.0
Waffles made with enriched flour (7″ diam.), from mix	1	75	205	7.0	8.0	2.8	2.0
Wheat flour, all-purpose							
Sifted, spooned	1 cup	115	420	12.0	1.0	0.2	0.10
Unsifted, spooned	1 cup	125	455	13.0	1.0	0.2	0.10
Wheat flour, self-rising, enriched	1 cup	125	440	12.0	1.0	0.2	0.10

Legumes (Dry), Nuts, Seeds, and Related Products

Almonds, chopped	1 cup	130	766	25.0	67.0	6.4	47.0
Beans, dry, cooked and drained							
Great Northern	1 cup	180	210	14.0	1.0	—	—
Lima	1 cup	170	208	11.0	0.54	0.1	—
Pea (navy)	1 cup	190	225	15.0	1.0	—	—

Appendix A–1. Nutritive Values of Food* (Continued)

Poly-unsaturated fat (gm)	Cholesterol (mg)	Dietary fiber (gm)	Carbo-hydrate (gm)	Calcium (mg)	Iron (mg)	Zinc (mg)	Vitamin A (IU)	Thiamin (mg)	Riboflavin (mg)	Niacin (mg)	Ascorbic acid (mg)
3.6	—	—	49.0	12.0	1.2	0.2	25	0.15	0.11	1.2	2.0
2.3	40.0	—	40.0	86.0	1.0	—	330	0.11	0.22	1.0	1.0
3.6	—	—	47.0	15.0	1.4	—	40	0.15	0.11	1.4	4.0
3.6	—	—	52.0	19.0	0.9	—	590	0.16	0.12	1.4	—
2.5	—	—	30.0	125.0	1.2	—	300	0.11	0.27	0.8	—
2.3	—	—	47.0	15.0	0.9	0.3	167	0.10	0.12	0.7	3.7
3.6	—	—	56.0	38.0	1.9	—	—	0.14	0.12	1.4	1.0
3.6	—	—	52.0	14.0	1.2	—	990	0.15	0.14	2.0	4.0
6.3	—	—	61.0	55.0	3.7	—	190	0.26	0.14	1.0	—
2.4	—	—	32.0	66.0	1.0	—	3210	0.11	0.18	1.0	—
14.9	—	—	79.0	25.0	3.1	—	—	0.47	0.40	5.0	—
1.2	56.0	—	39.0	220.0	1.6	1.7	750	0.34	0.29	4.2	2.4
0.2	—	—	5.0	1.0	0.2	0.5	—	—	0.01	0.1	—
0.2	—	—	5.0	1.0	0.2	0.4	—	—	0.01	0.2	—
0.4	—	—	30.0	2.0	0.5	—	—	—	0.02	0.4	—
—	—	—	12.0	4.0	0.2	0.2	—	0.05	0.04	0.7	—
—	—	—	2.0	0.78	0.1	—	—	0.01	0.01	0.1	—
—	—	—	49.0	23.0	1.0	—	—	0.18	0.04	2.7	—
—	—	—	46.0	16.0	0.9	—	—	0.18	0.04	4.2	—
0.1	—	—	50.0	21.0	1.8	0.7	—	0.23	0.02	2.1	—
0.1	—	—	41.0	33.0	1.4	0.7	—	0.19	0.02	2.1	—
0.5	—	—	14.0	20.0	0.8	0.2	—	0.10	0.06	0.9	—
0.4	—	—	15.0	21.0	0.8	0.2	—	0.11	0.07	0.9	—
0.6	—	—	20.0	53.0	1.2	0.2	—	0.20	0.13	1.6	—
0.5	—	—	30.0	24.0	1.2	0.3	—	0.20	0.12	1.7	—
1.4	—	—	75.0	58.0	3.0	—	—	0.54	0.32	4.5	—
—	—	—	39.0	14.0	1.4	0.7	—	0.23	0.13	1.8	—
—	—	—	32.0	11.0	1.3	0.7	—	0.20	0.11	1.5	—
0.4	4.0	—	39.0	40.0	2.8	—	930	0.35	0.28	4.5	10.0
0.9	75.0	—	39.0	124.0	3.7	—	1590	0.25	0.30	4.0	22.0
3.9	39.0	—	29.0	53.0	3.3	—	1000	0.15	0.18	2.3	5.0
—	—	—	35.0	96.0	2.0	0.3	482	0.16	0.17	2.1	—
1.4	45.0	—	25.0	154.0	1.5	0.7	140	0.18	0.24	1.5	—
1.2	45.0	—	27.0	179.0	1.0	—	170	0.14	0.22	0.9	—
0.5	—	—	88.0	18.0	3.3	0.8	—	0.74	0.46	6.1	—
0.5	—	—	95.0	20.0	3.6	0.8	—	0.80	0.50	6.6	—
0.5	—	—	93.0	331.0	3.6	—	—	0.80	0.50	6.6	—
12.8	—	6.1	26.0	346.0	4.8	3.8	—	0.27	1.01	4.4	0.8
—	—	—	38.0	90.0	4.9	1.8	—	0.25	0.13	1.3	—
—	—	7.1	40.0	54.0	4.2	1.3	630	0.24	0.16	1.8	17.2
—	—	—	40.0	95.0	5.1	1.8	—	0.27	0.13	1.3	—

Appendix continued on following page

Appendix A–1. Nutritive Values of Food* (Continued)

	Approximate Measure	Weight (gm)	Kilocalories	Protein (gm)	Fat (gm)	Saturated fat (gm)	Mono-unsaturated fat (gm)
Beans, dry, canned							
White with frankfurters	1 cup	255	365	19.0	18.0	–	–
White with pork and tomato sauce	1 cup	255	310	16.0	7.0	2.4	2.0
White with pork and sweet sauce	1 cup	255	385	16.0	12.0	4.3	5.0
Red kidney	1 cup	255	230	15.0	1.0	–	–
Brazil nuts, shelled	1 oz.	28	186	4.0	18.0	4.6	6.0
Cashew nuts, roasted in oil	1 oz.	28	163	4.0	13.0	2.7	7.0
Coconut, shredded or grated	1 cup	80	283	2.0	26.0	23.8	1.0
Filberts (hazelnuts), chopped	1 oz.	28	179	3.0	17.0	1.3	13.0
Lentils, whole, cooked	1 cup	200	210	16.0	–	–	–
Peanuts, roasted in oil, salted	1 oz.	28	165	7.0	14.0	1.9	6.0
Peanut butter	1 Tbsp.	16	95	4.0	8.0	1.4	3.0
Peas, split, dry, cooked	1 cup	200	230	16.0	1.0	–	–
Pecans, chopped or pieces	1 oz.	28	189	2.0	19.0	1.5	12.0
Pumpkin and squash kernels, dry	1 oz.	28	153	6.0	13.0	2.5	4.0
Sunflower seeds, dry, hulled	1 oz.	28	161	6.0	14.0	1.5	2.0
Walnuts, black, chopped or broken	1 oz.	28	172	6.0	16.0	1.0	3.0
Walnuts, ground (finely)	1 oz.	28	172	6.0	16.0	1.0	3.0
Walnuts, Persian or English, chopped	1 oz.	28	181	4.0	17.0	1.6	2.0
Sugars and Sweets							
Cake icings							
Boiled, white, plain	1 cup	94	295	1.0	–	–	–
Uncooked, chocolate	1 cup	275	1035	9.0	38.0	23.4	11.7
Uncooked, creamy fudge (mix)	1 cup	245	830	7.0	16.0	5.1	6.7
Uncooked, white	1 cup	319	1200	2.0	21.0	12.7	5.1
Candy							
Caramels, plain or chocolate	1 oz.	28	115	1.0	3.0	1.6	1.1
Chocolate, milk, plain	1 oz.	28	146	2.0	9.0	5.6	3.0
Chocolate, semisweet, small pieces	1 cup	170	860	7.0	61.0	36.2	19.8
Chocolate-coated peanuts	1 oz.	28	161	5.1	12.0	4.0	4.8
Fondant, uncoated	1 oz.	28	106	–	1.0	0.1	0.3
Fudge, chocolate, plain	1 oz.	28	116	1.0	3.0	1.3	1.4
Gumdrops	1 oz.	28	101	–	–	–	–
Hard	1 oz.	28	111	–	–	–	–
Marshmallows	1 oz.	28	91	1.0	–	–	–
Chocolate-flavored beverage powders							
With nonfat dry milk	1 oz.	28	101	5.1	1.0	0.5	0.3
Without milk	1 oz.	28	101	1.0	1.0	0.4	0.2
Honey, strained or extracted	1 Tbsp.	21	65	–	–	–	–
Jams and preserves	1 Tbsp.	20	55	–	–	–	–
Jams and preserves	1 packet	14	40	–	–	–	–
Jellies	1 Tbsp.	18	50	–	–	–	–
Jellies	1 packet	14	40	–	–	–	–
Syrups							
Chocolate-flavored, thin-type	1 fl. oz.	38	90	1.0	1.0	0.5	0.3
Chocolate-flavored, fudge-type	1 fl. oz.	38	125	2.0	5.0	3.1	1.6
Molasses, cane, light	1 Tbsp.	20	50	–	–	–	–
Molasses, cane, blackstrap	1 Tbsp.	20	45	–	–	–	–
Sorghum	1 Tbsp.	21	55	–	–	–	–
Table blends, chiefly corn	1 Tbsp.	21	60	–	–	–	–

Appendix A-1. Nutritive Values of Food* (Continued)

Poly-unsaturated fat (gm)	Cholesterol (mg)	Dietary fiber (gm)	Carbo-hydrate (gm)	Calcium (mg)	Iron (mg)	Zinc (mg)	Vitamin A (IU)	Thiamin (mg)	Riboflavin (mg)	Niacin (mg)	Ascorbic acid (mg)
–	4.0	–	32.0	94.0	4.8	–	330	0.18	0.15	3.3	–
0.6	4.0	–	48.0	138.0	4.6	–	330	0.20	0.08	1.5	5.0
1.1	4.0	–	54.0	161.0	5.9	–	–	0.15	0.10	1.3	–
–	–	–	42.0	74.0	4.6	1.9	10	0.13	0.10	1.5	7.7
7.1	–	–	3.0	49.0	–	1.3	–	0.28	0.03	0.5	0.2
2.1	–	–	8.0	11.0	1.2	1.3	–	0.12	0.05	0.5	–
0.5	–	–	12.0	12.0	1.9	0.9	–	0.05	0.02	0.4	2.6
1.8	–	–	4.0	53.0	0.9	0.7	18	0.14	0.03	0.3	0.3
–	–	–	39.0	50.0	4.2	2.0	40	0.14	0.12	1.2	–
4.1	–	–	5.0	24.0	0.5	1.9	–	0.08	0.03	4.2	–
2.3	–	–	2.0	5.0	0.3	0.5	–	0.02	0.02	2.2	–
–	–	–	42.0	22.0	3.4	2.1	80	0.30	0.18	1.8	–
4.8	–	–	5.0	10.0	0.6	1.6	36	0.24	0.04	0.3	0.6
5.6	–	–	5.0	12.0	4.3	2.1	107	0.06	0.09	0.5	–
8.5	–	–	5.0	33.0	1.9	1.4	14	0.65	0.07	1.3	–
10.4	–	–	3.0	16.0	0.9	–	83	0.06	0.03	0.2	–
10.3	–	–	3.0	16.0	0.9	–	83	0.06	0.03	0.2	–
9.0	–	–	5.0	26.0	0.7	0.8	34	0.11	0.04	0.3	0.9
–	–	–	75.0	2.0	–	–	–	–	0.03	–	–
1.0	–	–	185.0	165.0	3.3	–	580	0.060	0.28	0.60	1.0
3.10	–	–	183.0	96.0	2.7	–	–	0.050	0.20	0.70	–
0.50	–	–	260.0	48.0	–	–	860	–	0.06	–	–
0.10	–	–	22.0	42.0	0.4	–	–	0.010	0.05	0.10	–
0.30	–	–	16.0	65.0	0.3	–	80	0.020	0.10	0.10	–
1.70	–	–	97.0	51.0	4.4	–	30	0.020	0.14	0.90	–
2.13	–	–	11.0	33.0	0.4	–	–	0.101	0.05	2.13	–
0.10	–	–	25.0	4.0	0.3	–	–	–	–	–	–
0.61	–	–	21.0	22.0	0.3	–	–	0.01	0.03	0.10	–
–	25.3	–	25.0	2.0	0.1	–	–	–	–	–	–
–	–	–	28.0	6.0	0.5	–	–	–	–	–	–
–	–	–	23.0	5.0	0.5	0.01	–	–	–	–	–
–	2.0	–	20.0	169.0	0.5	0.35	10	0.04	0.21	0.20	1.01
–	–	–	25.0	9.0	0.6	0.35	5	0.01	0.03	0.10	–
–	–	–	17.0	1.0	0.1	0.02	–	–	0.01	0.10	–
–	–	–	14.0	4.0	0.2	–	–	–	0.01	–	–
–	–	–	10.0	3.0	0.1	–	–	–	–	–	–
–	–	–	13.0	4.0	0.3	–	–	–	0.01	–	1.0
–	–	–	10.0	3.0	0.2	–	–	–	–	–	1.0
–	–	–	24.0	6.0	0.6	0.30	–	–	0.03	0.20	–
0.10	–	–	20.0	48.0	0.5	0.30	60	0.01	0.08	0.20	–
–	–	–	13.0	33.0	0.9	–	–	0.01	0.01	–	–
–	–	–	11.0	137.0	3.2	–	–	0.02	0.04	0.40	–
–	–	–	14.0	35.0	2.6	–	–	–	0.02	–	–
–	–	–	15.0	9.0	0.8	0.01	–	–	–	–	–

Appendix continued on following page

Appendix A–1. *Nutritive Values of Food* (Continued)*

	Approximate Measure	Weight (gm)	Kilocalories	Protein (gm)	Fat (gm)	Saturated fat (gm)	Mono-unsaturated fat (gm)
Sugars							
Brown, pressed-down	1 cup	220	820	—	—	—	—
White, granulated	1 cup	192	720	—	—	—	—
White, granulated	1 Tbsp.	12	45	—	—	—	—
White, powdered, sifted	1 cup	100	385	—	—	—	—
Vegetables and Vegetable Products							
Asparagus, green, cooked, drained							
Cuts and tips, fresh	1 cup	180	44	4.0	0.6	0.13	—
Cuts and tips, frozen	1 cup	180	50	5.0	0.8	0.17	—
Spears, fresh	4	60	14	1.0	0.2	0.04	—
Spears, frozen	4	60	16	1.0	0.3	0.06	—
Asparagus, green, canned, spears	4	80	15	1.0	0.5	0.12	—
Beans, cooked							
Lima, immature seeds, frozen							
Fordhooks	1 cup	170	170	10.0	0.6	0.13	—
Baby	1 cup	180	188	12.0	0.5	0.12	—
Snaps, green:							
Fresh	1 cup	125	44	2.0	0.4	0.08	—
Frozen cuts	1 cup	135	36	1.0	0.2	0.04	—
Frozen, French style	1 cup	135	36	1.0	0.2	0.04	—
Canned cuts	1 cup	135	27	1.0	0.1	0.03	—
Snaps, yellow or wax:							
Fresh cuts, French style	1 cup	125	44	2.0	0.4	0.08	—
Frozen cuts	1 cup	135	36	1.0	0.2	0.04	—
Canned cuts	1 cup	136	26	1.0	0.1	0.03	—
Bean sprouts, mung, raw	1 cup	104	32	3.0	0.2	0.15	—
Bean sprouts, cooked drained	1 cup	125	26	2.0	0.1	0.03	—
Beets, cooked, diced or sliced	1 cup	170	52	1.0	0.1	0.01	—
Beets, canned, whole, small	1 cup	246	71	2.0	0.2	0.03	—
Beets, canned, diced or sliced	1 cup	170	54	1.0	0.2	0.04	—
Beet greens, leaves and stems, cooked	1 cup	145	40	3.0	0.3	0.05	—
Blackeyed peas, immature seeds, cooked							
Fresh	1 cup	165	179	13.0	1.3	0.35	—
Frozen	1 cup	170	224	14.0	1.1	0.30	—
Broccoli, cooked, drained							
Fresh stalk, medium	1 stalk	88	24	2.0	0.3	0.05	—
Fresh, stalks cut	1 cup	155	46	4.0	0.4	0.07	—
Frozen, stalk	1 stalk	185	51	5.0	0.2	0.03	—
Brussels sprouts, cooked:							
Fresh (7–8 sprouts)	1 cup	156	60	3.0	0.8	0.16	—
Frozen	1 cup	155	65	5.0	0.6	0.13	—
Cabbage							
Fresh, finely shredded or chopped	1 cup	90	21	1.0	0.2	0.02	—
Fresh, cooked	1 cup	145	30	1.0	0.4	0.05	—
Red, fresh	1 cup	70	19	0.97	0.2	0.02	—
Savoy, fresh	1 cup	70	19	1.0	0.1	0.01	—
Cabbage, celery, fresh (also called pe-tsai or bok choy)	1 cup	76	12	0.91	0.1	0.03	—
Carrots, raw							
Whole	1	72	31	0.74	0.1	0.02	—
Grated	1 cup	110	48	1.0	0.2	0.03	—
Carrots, cooked	1 cup	156	70	1.0	0.3	0.05	—
canned, sliced	1 cup	146	34	0.94	0.3	0.05	—

Appendix A–1. Nutritive Values of Food* (Continued)

Poly-unsaturated fat (gm)	Cholesterol (mg)	Dietary fiber (gm)	Carbo-hydrate (gm)	Calcium (mg)	Iron (mg)	Zinc (mg)	Vitamin A (IU)	Thiamin (mg)	Riboflavin (mg)	Niacin (mg)	Ascorbic acid (mg)
—	—	—	212.0	187.0	7.5	—	—	0.02	0.07	0.40	—
—	—	—	192.0	—	—	0.10	—	—	—	—	—
—	—	—	12.0	—	—	0.01	—	—	—	—	—
—	—	—	100.0	—	0.1	—	—	—	—	—	—
—	—	—	7.0	44.0	1.2	0.9	1492	0.18	0.22	1.9	36.0
—	—	—	8.0	41.0	1.1	1.0	1472	0.12	0.19	1.9	43.0
—	—	—	2.0	14.0	0.4	0.3	497	0.06	0.07	0.6	12.0
—	—	—	2.0	13.0	0.4	0.3	490	0.04	0.06	0.6	14.0
—	—	—	1.0	15.0	1.5	0.3	640	0.05	0.08	0.6	12.0
—	—	—	32.0	38.0	2.3	0.7	324	0.12	0.10	1.8	21.0
—	—	—	35.0	50.0	3.5	1.0	300	0.13	0.10	1.4	10.0
—	—	2.3	9.0	58.0	1.6	0.4	833	0.09	0.12	0.8	12.0
—	—	2.2	8.0	61.0	1.1	0.8	713	0.07	0.10	0.6	11.0
—	—	2.2	8.0	61.0	1.1	0.8	713	0.07	0.10	0.6	11.0
—	—	1.8	6.0	35.0	1.2	0.4	471	0.02	0.08	0.3	6.0
—	—	2.3	9.0	58.0	1.6	0.4	833	0.09	0.12	0.8	12.0
—	—	2.2	8.0	61.0	1.1	0.8	713	0.07	0.10	0.6	11.0
—	—	1.8	6.0	36.0	1.2	0.4	474	0.02	0.08	0.3	6.0
—	—	1.1	6.0	14.0	0.9	0.4	22	0.09	0.13	0.8	13.0
—	—	—	5.0	15.0	0.8	0.6	17	0.06	0.13	1.0	14.0
—	—	—	11.0	18.0	1.0	0.4	22	0.05	0.02	0.5	9.0
—	—	—	16.0	34.0	1.6	0.6	28	0.03	0.09	0.4	9.0
—	—	—	12.0	32.0	3.1	0.4	30	0.02	0.05	0.2	5.0
—	—	—	7.0	165.0	2.7	0.7	7344	0.17	0.42	0.7	35.0
—	—	—	29.0	46.0	2.4	1.3	1051	0.11	0.18	1.8	2.0
—	—	—	40.0	40.0	3.6	2.4	128	0.44	0.11	1.2	4.0
—	—	1.2	4.0	42.0	0.8	0.4	1356	0.06	0.10	0.6	82.0
—	—	—	8.0	178.0	1.8	0.2	2198	0.13	0.32	1.2	98.0
—	—	4.1	9.0	94.0	1.1	0.6	3482	0.10	0.15	0.8	73.0
—	—	2.2	13.0	56.0	1.9	0.5	1122	0.17	0.12	0.9	96.0
—	—	2.8	12.0	38.0	1.1	0.5	912	0.16	0.18	0.8	70.0
—	—	—	4.0	42.0	0.5	0.2	113	0.05	0.03	0.3	42.0
—	—	—	6.0	47.0	0.6	0.2	125	0.08	0.08	0.3	35.0
—	—	0.8	4.0	36.0	0.3	0.1	28	0.04	0.02	0.2	39.0
—	—	—	4.0	25.0	0.3	—	700	0.05	0.02	0.2	21.0
—	—	—	2.0	58.0	0.2	0.2	912	0.03	0.04	0.3	20.0
—	—	1.1	7.0	19.0	0.4	0.1	20,250	0.07	0.04	0.7	6.0
—	—	1.6	11.0	30.0	0.5	0.2	30,940	0.11	0.06	1.0	10.0
—	—	2.0	16.0	48.0	—	0.5	38,300	0.05	0.09	0.8	3.0
—	—	1.8	8.0	38.0	0.9	0.4	20,110	0.03	0.04	0.8	4.0

Appendix continued on following page

Appendix A–1. *Nutritive Values of Food* (Continued)*

	Approximate Measure	Weight (gm)	Kilocalories	Protein (gm)	Fat (gm)	Saturated fat (gm)	Mono-unsaturated fat (gm)
Cauliflower							
Fresh, chopped	1 cup	100	24	1.0	0.2	0.03	—
Cooked, fresh (flower buds)	1 cup	124	30	2.0	0.2	0.05	—
Cooked, frozen (flowerets)	1 cup	180	34	2.0	0.4	0.06	—
Celery, Pascal, raw							
Stalk, large outer	1	40	6	0.26	—	0.01	—
Pieces, diced	1 cup	120	18	0.80	0.1	0.04	—
Collards							
Cooked, fresh	1 cup	190	27	2.0	0.3	—	—
Cooked, frozen	1 cup	170	61	5.0	0.7	—	—
Corn, sweet, cooked							
Fresh ear, 5″ by 1¾″	1	140	83	2.0	—	0.15	—
Frozen ear, 5″ long	1	229	118	3.0	0.9	0.14	—
Frozen, kernels	1 cup	165	134	4.0	0.1	0.02	—
Canned, cream style	1 cup	256	186	4.0	1.1	0.17	—
Canned, whole kernel, vacuum pack	1 cup	210	166	5.0	1.1	0.16	—
Canned, whole kernel, wet pack	1 cup	165	132	4.0	1.6	0.25	—
Cucumber slices, without peel	6–8 slices	28	3	0.15	—	0.01	—
Dandelion greens, cooked	1 cup	105	35	2.0	0.6	—	—
Endive, curly, fresh	1 cup	50	8	0.62	0.1	0.02	—
Kale, cooked, fresh	1 cup	130	41	2.0	0.5	0.07	—
Kale, cooked, frozen	1 cup	130	39	3.0	0.6	0.08	—
Lettuce, fresh							
Butterhead, leaves	2–3	15	1	0.19	—	—	—
Crisphead (iceberg), shredded	1 cup	55	7	0.56	0.1	—	—
Looseleaf, chopped or shredded	1 cup	55	9	0.72	0.2	—	—
Mushrooms (raw, sliced, or chopped)	1 cup	70	18	1.0	0.3	—	—
Mustard greens, cooked	1 cup	140	21	3.0	0.3	—	—
Okra pods, cooked, 3″ by ⅝″	1 cup	160	50	2.0	0.3	0.1	—
Onions							
Mature, fresh, chopped	1 cup	170	57	2.0	0.4	0.1	—
Mature, cooked	1 cup	210	58	1.0	0.3	0.1	—
Young green, bulb	6	30	7	0.52	—	—	—
Parsley, raw, chopped	1 Tbsp.	4	1	0.09	—	—	—
Parsnips, cooked	1 cup	155	126	2.0	0.5	0.1	—
Peas							
Green, canned	1 cup	170	118	7.0	0.6	0.1	—
Green, frozen, cooked	1 cup	160	126	8.0	0.4	0.1	—
Peppers, hot, red, seedless	1 tsp.	2	5	—	—	—	—
Peppers, sweet							
Raw	1 pod	74	18	0.63	0.3	—	—
Cooked	1 pod	73	13	0.45	0.2	—	—
Potatoes, cooked							
Baked, peeled after baking	1	156	145	3.0	0.2	—	—
Boiled, peeled after boiling	1	137	119	2.0	0.1	—	—
Boiled, peeled before boiling	1	135	116	2.0	0.1	—	—
French fried, frozen	10	50	111	1.0	4.4	2.1	0.8
Hash brown, frozen	1 cup	155	340	4.0	17.9	7.0	3.2
Mashed, fresh, with milk and butter	1 cup	210	222	3.0	8.9	2.2	2.3
Mashed, dehydrated flakes	1 cup	210	166	4.0	4.6	1.4	2.1
Potato chips	10	20	105	1.0	7.1	1.8	1.4
Potato salad with cooked salad dressing	1 cup	250	358	6.0	20.5	3.6	2.7
Pumpkin, canned	1 cup	245	83	2.0	0.7	0.4	—
Radishes, fresh	4	18	2	0.11	0.1	—	—

Appendix A–1. *Nutritive Values of Food* (Continued)*

Poly-unsaturated fat (gm)	Cholesterol (mg)	Dietary fiber (gm)	Carbohydrate (gm)	Calcium (mg)	Iron (mg)	Zinc (mg)	Vitamin A (IU)	Thiamin (mg)	Riboflavin (mg)	Niacin (mg)	Ascorbic acid (mg)
—	—	—	4.0	29.0	0.6	0.2	16	0.08	0.06	0.6	71.0
—	—	1.0	5.0	34.0	0.5	0.3	18	0.08	0.06	0.7	68.0
—	—	—	6.0	30.0	0.7	0.2	40	0.07	0.10	0.6	56.0
—	—	0.4	1.0	14.0	0.2	0.1	51	0.01	0.01	0.1	2.0
—	—	1.1	4.0	44.0	0.6	0.2	152	0.04	0.04	0.4	7.0
—	—	—	5.0	148.0	0.8	1.2	4218	0.03	0.08	0.4	18.0
—	—	—	12.0	357.0	1.9	0.5	10,170	0.08	0.20	1.1	44.0
—	—	—	19.0	2.0	0.5	0.4	167	0.17	0.06	1.2	4.0
—	—	2.7	28.0	4.0	0.8	0.8	266	0.22	0.09	1.9	6.0
—	—	3.5	33.0	4.0	0.5	0.6	408	0.11	0.12	2.1	4.0
—	—	—	46.0	8.0	—	1.4	248	0.06	0.14	2.5	11.0
—	—	—	40.0	10.0	0.9	—	506	0.09	0.15	2.5	17.0
—	—	2.2	30.0	8.0	1.4	0.6	256	0.05	0.08	1.5	7.0
—	—	0.1	0.81	3.0	0.1	0.1	12	0.01	0.01	0.1	1.0
—	—	—	6.0	147.0	1.9	—	12,290	0.14	0.18	—	18.0
—	—	—	1.0	26.0	0.4	0.4	1026	0.04	0.04	0.2	3.0
—	—	—	7.0	94.0	1.2	0.3	9620	0.07	0.09	0.6	53.0
—	—	—	6.0	179.0	1.2	0.2	8260	0.06	0.15	0.9	32.0
—	—	0.1	0.35	4.0	—	—	145	0.01	0.01	—	1.0
—	—	0.5	1.0	10.0	0.3	0.1	182	0.03	0.02	0.1	2.0
—	—	—	1.0	37.0	0.8	0.1	1045	0.03	0.04	0.2	9.0
—	—	—	3.0	4.0	0.9	0.3	—	0.07	0.31	2.9	2.0
—	—	—	2.0	103.0	—	—	4244	0.06	0.09	0.6	35.0
—	—	—	11.0	100.0	0.7	0.9	920	0.21	0.09	1.4	26.0
—	—	1.4	12.0	42.0	0.6	0.3	—	0.10	0.02	0.2	14.0
—	—	—	13.0	58.0	0.4	0.4	—	0.09	0.02	0.2	12.0
—	—	—	1.0	18.0	0.6	0.1	1500	0.02	0.04	—	13.0
—	—	—	0.28	5.0	0.2	—	208	—	—	—	3.0
—	—	4.2	30.0	58.0	0.9	—	—	0.13	0.08	1.1	20.0
—	—	6.0	21.0	34.0	1.6	1.2	1306	0.21	0.13	1.2	16.0
—	—	6.1	22.0	38.0	2.5	1.5	1068	0.45	0.16	2.4	15.0
—	—	—	1.0	5.0	0.3	0.1	1300	—	0.02	0.2	—
—	—	0.8	3.0	4.0	0.9	0.1	392	0.06	0.04	0.4	94.0
—	—	—	2.0	3.0	0.6	0.1	283	0.04	0.03	0.3	81.0
—	—	—	33.0	8.0	0.5	0.4	—	0.16	0.03	2.2	20.0
—	—	—	27.0	7.0	0.4	0.4	—	0.14	0.03	1.0	17.0
—	—	—	27.0	10.0	0.4	0.4	—	0.13	0.03	1.8	10.0
2.1	—	—	17.0	3.0	0.7	0.2	—	0.06	0.02	1.1	5.0
9.0	—	—	43.0	24.0	2.3	0.5	—	0.17	0.03	3.8	9.0
0.2	4	—	35.0	54.0	0.5	0.6	355	0.18	0.08	2.3	12.0
0.2	4	—	27.0	65.0	1.3	—	189	0.06	0.11	1.7	6.0
4.0	—	—	10.0	4.0	0.2	0.2	—	0.03	—	0.8	8.0
1.3	171	—	27.0	48.0	1.6	0.8	523	0.19	0.15	2.2	24.0
—	—	—	19.0	64.0	3.4	0.4	54,040	0.06	0.13	0.9	10.0
—	—	—	0.64	3.0	0.1	0.1	1	—	0.01	0.1	4.0

Appendix continued on following page

Appendix A–1. *Nutritive Values of Food* (Continued)*

	Approximate Measure	Weight (gm)	Kilocalories	Protein (gm)	Fat (gm)	Saturated fat (gm)	Mono-unsaturated fat (gm)
Sauerkraut, canned	1 cup	235	44	2.0	0.3	0.1	—
Spinach							
Fresh, chopped	1 cup	55	12	1.0	0.2	—	—
Cooked, fresh	1 cup	180	41	5.0	0.5	0.1	—
Cooked, frozen	1 cup	190	53	5.0	0.4	0.1	—
Canned	1 cup	205	47	5.0	1.0	0.2	—
Squash, cooked							
Summer, diced	1 cup	180	36	1.0	0.6	0.1	—
Winter, baked, mashed	1 cup	205	79	1.0	1.3	0.3	—
Sweet potatoes:							
Cooked, baked in skin, peeled	1	114	118	1.0	0.1	—	—
Candied, 2½ by 2″ piece	1	105	144	0.91	3.4	1.4	0.8
Canned, solid pack, mashed	1 cup	255	258	5.0	0.5	0.1	—
Canned, vacuum pack	1 piece	40	36	0.66	0.1	—	—
Tomatoes							
Fresh, 2⅗″ diam.	1	135	26	1.0	0.3	—	—
Canned, solids and liquid	1 cup	241	47	2.0	0.6	0.1	—
Tomato catsup	1 Tbsp.	15	15	—	—	—	—
Tomato juice, canned	1 cup	243	41	1.0	0.1	—	—
Turnips, cooked	1 cup	156	28	1.0	0.1	—	—
Turnip greens, cooked, fresh	1 cup	144	29	1.0	0.3	0.1	—
Turnip greens, cooked, frozen	1 cup	165	49	5.0	0.7	0.2	—
Vegetables, mixed, cooked frozen	1 cup	182	108	5.0	0.3	0.1	—
Miscellaneous Items							
Baking powders (for home use)							
Sodium aluminum sulfate							
With monocalcium phosphate monohydrate	1 tsp.	3	5	—	—	—	—
With monocalcium phosphate monohydrate and calcium sulfate	1 tsp.	2	5	—	—	—	—
Straight phosphate	1 tsp.	3	5	—	—	—	—
Low sodium	1 tsp.	4	5	—	—	—	—
Barbecue sauce	1 Tbsp.	15	11	0.28	0.28	—	0.3
Beverages, alcoholic							
Beer	12 oz.	360	150	1.0	—	—	—
Gin, rum, vodka, or whisky							
80-proof	1 oz.	28	65	—	—	—	—
86-proof	1 oz.	28	70	—	—	—	—
90-proof	1 oz.	28	74	—	—	—	—
Beverages, carbonated, sweetened							
Club soda	12 oz.	355	—	—	—	—	—
Cola	12 oz.	369	159	—	—	—	—
Fruit-flavored sodas	12 oz.	372	178	—	—	—	—
Ginger ale	12 oz.	366	113	—	—	—	—
Root beer	12 oz.	369	163	—	—	—	—
Chocolate, bitter or baking	1 oz.	28	146	3.0	15.0	9.0	4.0
Gelatin, dry, from envelope	1.7 gm	7	25	6.0	—	—	—
Gelatin dessert	1 cup	240	140	4.0	—	—	—
Mustard, prepared, yellow	1 tsp.	5	5	—	—	—	—
Olives, green, canned, medium	4	16	15	—	1.0	0.2	1.2
Olives, ripe, mission, small	3	9	15	—	2.0	0.2	1.2
Pickles, cucumber							
Dill, medium, whole	1	65	5	—	—	—	—
Fresh-pack, slices	2 slices	15	10	—	—	—	—
Sweet, gherkin, small, whole	1	15	20	—	—	—	—

Appendix A–1. Nutritive Values of Food* (Continued)

Poly-unsaturated fat (gm)	Cholesterol (mg)	Dietary fiber (gm)	Carbo-hydrate (gm)	Calcium (mg)	Iron (mg)	Zinc (mg)	Vitamin A (IU)	Thiamin (mg)	Riboflavin (mg)	Niacin (mg)	Ascorbic acid (mg)
—	—	—	10.0	72.0	3.5	0.4	42	0.05	0.05	0.3	34.0
—	—	1.8	1.0	56.0	1.5	0.3	3760	0.04	0.11	0.4	15.0
—	—	3.4	6.0	244.0	6.4	1.4	14,740	0.17	0.43	0.9	17.0
—	—	3.0	10.0	277.0	2.9	1.3	14,790	0.11	0.32	0.8	23.0
—	—	5.7	6.0	260.0	4.7	0.9	17,990	0.03	0.28	0.8	29.0
—	—	1.0	7.0	48.0	0.6	0.7	517	0.08	0.07	0.9	10.0
—	—	2.5	17.0	28.0	0.7	0.5	7292	0.17	0.05	1.4	19.0
—	—	2.0	27.0	32.0	0.5	0.3	24,880	0.08	0.15	0.7	28.0
0.1	—	—	29.0	27.0	1.2	0.2	4399	0.02	0.04	0.4	7.0
—	—	—	59.0	76.0	3.4	0.5	38,570	0.07	0.23	2.4	13.0
—	—	—	8.0	8.0	0.4	0.1	3194	0.01	0.02	0.3	10.0
—	—	1.1	5.0	9.0	0.6	0.1	1530	0.08	0.07	0.8	23.0
—	—	1.7	10.0	63.0	1.5	0.4	1450	0.11	0.07	1.8	36.0
—	—	—	4.0	3.0	0.1	—	210	0.01	0.01	0.2	2.0
—	—	—	10.0	21.0	1.4	0.3	1351	0.11	0.08	1.6	44.0
—	—	—	7.0	34.0	0.3	—	—	0.04	0.04	0.5	18.0
—	—	—	6.0	198.0	1.1	0.2	7917	0.07	0.10	0.6	39.0
—	—	—	8.0	251.0	3.2	0.7	13,160	0.09	0.12	0.8	36.0
—	—	4.2	21.0	44.0	1.5	0.9	7784	0.13	0.22	1.5	5.0
—	—	—	1.0	58.0	—	—	—	—	—	—	—
—	—	—	1.0	183.0	—	—	—	—	—	—	—
—	—	—	1.0	239.0	—	—	—	—	—	—	—
—	—	—	2.0	207.0	—	—	—	—	—	—	—
0.6	—	—	2.0	3.0	0.1	—	135	—	—	0.1	1.0
—	—	—	14.0	18.0	0.1	0.2	—	0.01	0.11	2.2	—
—	—	—	—	30.0	—	—	—	—	—	—	—
—	—	—	—	30.0	—	—	—	—	—	—	—
—	—	—	—	30.0	—	—	—	—	—	—	—
—	—	—	—	18.0	—	—	—	—	—	—	—
—	—	—	40.0	11.0	0.2	0.2	—	—	—	—	—
—	—	—	45.0	15.0	0.4	0.3	—	—	—	—	—
—	—	—	28.0	11.0	0.2	—	—	—	—	—	—
—	—	—	42.0	15.0	0.2	0.2	—	—	—	—	—
0.4	—	—	8.0	22.0	1.9	—	20	0.01	0.07	0.4	—
—	—	—	—	—	0.4	—	—	—	—	—	4.0
—	—	—	34.0	—	—	—	—	—	—	—	—
—	—	—	—	4.0	0.1	—	—	—	—	—	—
0.1	—	—	—	8.0	0.2	—	40	—	—	—	—
0.1	—	—	—	9.0	0.1	—	9	—	—	—	—
—	—	—	1.0	17.0	0.7	0.2	70	—	0.01	—	4.0
—	—	—	3.0	5.0	0.3	—	20	—	—	—	1.0
—	—	—	5.0	2.0	0.2	—	10	—	—	—	1.0

Appendix continued on following page

Appendix A–1. Nutritive Values of Food* (Continued)

	Approximate Measure	Weight (gm)	Kilocalories	Protein (gm)	Fat (gm)	Saturated fat (gm)	Mono-unsaturated fat (gm)
Relish, finely chopped	1 Tbsp.	15	20	–	–	–	–
Popsicle	1	95	70	–	–	–	–
Soups, canned, condensed							
Cream of chicken							
with milk	1 cup	248	191	7.0	11.0	4.6	3.6
with water	1 cup	244	116	3.0	7.0	2.1	2.3
Cream of mushroom							
with milk	1 cup	248	203	6.0	13.0	5.1	2.9
with water	1 cup	244	129	2.0	8.0	2.4	1.7
Tomato							
with milk	1 cup	248	160	6.0	6.0	2.9	1.7
with water	1 cup	244	86	2.0	1.0	0.4	0.5
Bean with pork, with water	1 cup	250	173	7.0	5.0	1.5	1.8
Beef broth, bouillon, or consommé	1 cup	240	16	2.0	0.53	0.3	–
Beef noodle, with water	1 cup	244	84	4.0	3.0	1.1	0.7
Clam chowder, Manhattan style	1 cup	245	78	4.0	2.0	0.4	0.4
Minestrone, with water	1 cup	241	83	4.0	2.0	0.5	0.9
Split pea, with water	1 cup	253	189	10.0	4.0	1.8	1.2
Vegetable beef, with water	1 cup	245	79	5.0	1.0	0.8	–
Vegetarian, with water	1 cup	241	72	2.0	1.0	0.3	–
Dehydrated							
Bouillon cube, ½"	1	4	6	0.62	0.14	0.1	–
Mix, unprepared, onion	1½ oz.	42	125	4.0	2.0	0.6	2.5
Mix, chicken noodle, with water	1 cup	252	53	2.0	1.0	0.3	–
Mix, onion, with water	1 cup	246	28	1.0	0.57	0.1	–
Mix, tomato vegetable with noodles, with water	1 cup	253	55	2.0	0.87	0.4	–
Vinegar, cider	1 Tbsp.	15	–	–	–	–	–
White sauce, medium	1 cup	250	405	10.0	31.0	19.3	7.8
Yeast, Baker's, dry, active	1 pkg.	7	20	3.0	–	–	–
Yeast, Brewer's, dry	1 Tbsp.	8	25	3.0	–	–	–

*Data from Nutritionist III Software, Silverton, OR, utilizing the following sources: *Agriculture Handbooks* No. 8-1 through 8-12. USDA, 1977–1985; *Nutritive Value of American Foods in Common Units,* USDA No. 456, 1975; *Provisional Table on the Nutrient Content of Bakery Foods and Related Items,* USDA, May 1981; *Nutrient Content of Beverages,* USDA, September 1982; *Provisional Table on the Nutrient Content of Frozen and Canned Vegetables,* USDA, April 1979; *Vitamin E Content of Foods,* USDA, December 1979; *Folacin in Selected Foods,* USDA, December 1979; and Pennington, JA; Church, HN: *Food Values of Portions Commonly Used,* 14th ed. New York, Harper & Row, 1985.

Appendix A–1. Nutritive Values of Food* (Continued)

Poly-unsaturated fat (gm)	Cholesterol (mg)	Dietary fiber (gm)	Carbo-hydrate (gm)	Calcium (mg)	Iron (mg)	Zinc (mg)	Vitamin A (IU)	Thiamin (mg)	Riboflavin (mg)	Niacin (mg)	Ascorbic acid (mg)
–	–	–	5.0	3.0	0.1	–	–	–	–	–	–
–	–	–	18.0	–	–	–	–	–	–	–	–
1.3	27	–	15.0	180.0	0.7	0.7	715	0.07	0.26	0.9	1.0
1.1	10	–	9.0	34.0	0.6	0.6	560	0.03	0.06	0.8	0.2
4.6	20	–	15.0	178.0	0.6	0.6	154	0.08	0.28	0.9	2.0
4.5	2	–	9.0	46.0	0.5	0.6	–	0.05	0.09	0.7	1.0
1.0	17	–	22.0	159.0	1.8	0.3	849	0.13	0.25	1.5	67.0
1.0	–	–	16.0	13.0	1.8	0.2	688	0.09	0.05	1.4	66.0
2.4	3	–	22.0	81.0	2.0	1.0	889	0.09	0.03	0.6	1.0
–	–	–	0.1	15.0	0.4	–	–	0.01	0.05	1.9	–
0.8	5	–	8.0	15.0	1.1	1.5	629	0.07	0.06	1.1	0.3
1.3	2	–	12.0	34.0	1.9	0.9	920	0.06	0.05	1.3	3.0
1.3	2	–	11.0	34.0	0.9	0.7	2337	0.05	0.04	0.9	1.0
0.4	8	–	28.0	22.0	2.3	1.3	444	0.15	0.08	1.5	1.0
–	5	–	10.0	17.0	1.1	1.5	1891	0.04	0.05	1.0	2.0
–	–	–	12.0	21.0	1.1	0.5	3005	0.05	0.05	0.9	1.0
–	0.14	–	0.58	–	0.1	–	–	0.01	0.01	0.1	–
1.1	2.0	–	22.0	59.0	0.6	0.3	8	0.12	0.26	2.2	0.98
–	3.0	–	7.0	32.0	0.5	0.2	63	0.07	0.06	0.9	0.30
–	–	–	5.0	13.0	0.1	0.1	2	0.03	0.06	0.5	0.20
–	–	–	10.0	8.0	0.6	0.2	190	0.06	0.05	0.8	6.0
–	–	–	1.0	1.0	0.1	–	–	–	–	–	–
0.8	33.0	–	22.0	288.0	0.5	0.5	1150	0.12	0.43	0.7	2.0
–	–	–	3.0	3.0	1.1	–	–	0.16	0.38	2.6	–
–	–	–	3.0	17.0	1.4	–	–	1.25	0.34	3.0	–

Appendix A–2. Nutritional Analysis of Enteral Formulas

Product	Manu-facturer	Kcal/ml	mOsm/kg H$_2$O	Nonprotein Kcal/gm: Nitrogen	Protein gm	Protein Kcal% total	Protein Source	Fat gm	Fat Kcal% total	Fat Source
Amin-Aid	American McGaw	1.9	1095	800	19	4	ESS AA	46	21	SO LEC M/D GLY
Casec	Mead Johnson	370 per 100 gm	–	–	88 per 100 gm	95	CAS	2 per 100 gm	5	–
Citrotein	Doyle	0.66	495	–	44	25	Egg white solids	2	2	SO M/D GLY
Compleat-B	Doyle	1.07	405	131	43	16	Beef NF dry milk Veg	43	36	CO, Beef, M/D GLY
Compleat Modified	Doyle	1.07	300	131	43	16	Beef Cas Veg	37	31	CO, Beef
Controlyte	Doyle	2.0	598		0.16	0.03	–	96	43	SO
Criticare HN	Mead Johnson	1.06	650	148	38	14	HCAS	3	3	SAF O
Enrich	Ross	1.1	480	148	39	15	CAS Soy	37	30	CO
Ensure	Ross	1.06	450	153	37	14	CAS Soy	37	31.5	CO
Ensure HN	Ross	1.06	470	124	44	17	CAS Soy	35	30	CO
Ensure Plus	Ross	1.5	600	146	55	15	CAS Soy	53	32	CO
Ensure Plus HN	Ross	1.5	650	125	63	17	CAS Soy	49	30	CO
Entri-pak with Entrition	Biosearch	1	300	153.5	35	14	CAS	35	31.5	CO M/D GLY
Hepatic-Acid II	American McGaw	1.1	560	148	37.5	15	AA	31	28	SO M/D GLY
High Nitrogen Vivonex	Norwich Eaton	1	810	127	44	18	AA	1	1	SAF O
Instant Breakfast	Carnation	1.06	677–715	88	58	22	Milk CAS Soy	31	26	W
Instant Breakfast	Delmark	1.2	N/A	96	62.5	21	Milk CAS NF dry milk	37.5	28	W M/D GLY
Isocal	Mead Johnson	1.06	300	167	34	13	CAS Soy	44	37	SO MCT
Isocal HCN	Mead Johnson	2	740	145	75	15	CAS	91	40	SO MCT
Isotein HN	Doyle	1.2	300	86	68	23	D LAC CAS	34	25	SO MCT
Magnacal	Biosearch	2.0	590	154	70	14	CAS	80	36	SO
MCT Oil	Mead Johnson	7.7	–	–	–	–	–	933	100	MCT
Meritene Liquid	Doyle	0.96	505	79	58	24	CONC SW+S milk CAS	32	30	CO M/D GLY
Meritene Powder	Doyle	1.06	690	71	69	26	Milk CAS	34	29	W
Micro Lipid	Biosearch	4.5	80	–	–	–	–	500	100	SAF O
Moducal	Mead Johnson	380 per 100 gm	variable	–	–	–	–	–	–	–

Appendix A–2. Nutritional Analysis of Enteral Formulas (*Continued*)

Composition/liter

Carbohydrate

gm	Kcal%	Source	Na mEq	K mEq	Form	Kcal to meet U.S. RDA	Feature
366	75	MAL SUC	<14	<6	Powder	—	Renal disease
—		—	150 per 100 gm	<1 per 100 gm	Powder	—	Modular protein
130	73	SUC MAL	30	18	Powder	1028.5	Minimal residue
128	48	H CER S Veg NF dry milk, MAL, fruit	56	36	Liquid	1600	Standard milk containing
140	53	H CER S Fruit Veg	29.5	36	Liquid	1600	Isotonic tube feeding
286	57	HCS	0.8	0.4	Powder	—	Modular CHO-Fat
222	83	MAL HCS	27.5	34	Liquid	2120	Oligomeric
160	55	HCS SUC SP	37	40	Liquid	1530	High fiber
145	54.5	HCS SUC	37	40	Liquid and Powder	2000	Standard tube/oral feeding
139	53	HCS SUC	40.5	40	Liquid	1400	High nitrogen tube/oral feeding
200	53	HCS SUC	50	59./5	Liquid	3000	Caloric dense
197	53	HCS SUC	51.5	46.5	Liquid	1420	Caloric dense High nitrogen
136	54.5	MAL	31	31	Liquid in Entri-pak	2000	Isotonic tube feeding
143	57	MAL SUC	<15	<6	Powder	—	Hepatic disease
210	81	GO	23	30	Powder	3000	Oligomeric High nitrogen
135	51	SUC CS LACT	41	70	Powder	1480	20% protein milk containing
154	51	LACT DEX SUC	39	67	Powder	850	>20% protein milk containing
132	50	MAL	23	34	Liquid	2120	Standard tube feeding
225	45	CSS	35	36	Liquid	3000	Caloric dense
156	52.5	MAL FRUC	30	22	Powder	2100	Isotonic >20% protein
250	50	MAL SUC	44	32	Liquid	2000	Caloric dense
—	—	—	—	—	Liquid	—	Modular fat
110	46	CSS SUC	38	41	Liquid	1200	Milk containing >20% protein
119	45	LACT SUC CS FRUC	44	68	Powder	1100	Milk containing >20% protein
—	—	—	—	—	Liquid	—	Modular fat
95 per 100 g	100	MAL	70 per 100 gm	<1 per 100 gm	Powder	—	Modular CHO

Appendix continued on following page

Appendix A–2. Nutritional Analysis of Enteral Formulas (*Continued*)

					Composition/liter					
					Protein			**Fat**		
Product	Manu-facturer	Kcal/ml	mOsm/kg H₂O	Nonprotein Kcal/gm: Nitrogen	gm	Kcal% total	Source	gm	Kcal% total	Source
Nutri-Aid	American McGaw	1.1	290	142	37	15	CAS	35	31.5	CO M/D GLY
Nutrisource Amino acids	Sandoz	390 per 100 gm	—	—	97 per 100 gm	100	AA	—	—	—
Nutrisource Amino acids High-branched chain	Sandoz	390 per 100 gm	—	—	97 per 100 gm	100	AA	—	—	—
Nutrisource Carbohydrate	Sandoz	3.2	—	—	—	—	—	—	—	—
Nutrisource Lipid LCT	Sandoz	2.2	—	—	—	—	—	24 gm per 100 ml	100	SO
Nutrisource Lipid MCT	Sandoz	2.0	—	—	—	—	—	24 gm per 100 ml	100	MCT
Nutrisource Protein	Sandoz	402 per 100 gm	—	—	76 per 100 gm	76	lactalbumin; egg white solids	71 per 100 gm	16	M/D GLY
Osmolite	Ross	1.06	300	153	37	14	CAS SOY	38.5	31	MCT CO SO
Osmolite HN	Ross	1.06	310	124	44	17	CAS SOY	37.0	30	MCT CO SO
Polycose Liquid	Ross	2.0	—	—	—	—	—	—	—	—
Polycose Powder	Ross	380 per 100 gm	—	—	—	—	—	—	—	—
Portagen	Mead Johnson	1.0	320	153	35	14	CAS	48.0	31	MCT CO
Precision High Nitrogen	Doyle	1.05	525	125	44	17	Egg white solids	1.3	1.1	MCT SO M/D GLY
Precision Isotonic	Doyle	1.0	300	183	29	12	Egg white solids	30	28	SO M/D GLY
Precision LR	Doyle	1.1	510	239	26	9.5	Egg white solids	1.6	1.3	MCT SO M/D GLY
Pro-Mix	Navaco	4 cal/gm	—	—	80 gm per 100 gm	100	Whey protein	—	—	—
Propak	Biosearch	4 cal/gm	—	—	77 gm per 100 gm	100	Whey protein	—	—	—
Pulmocare	Ross	1.5	490	125	63	17	CAS	92	55	CO
Renu	Biosearch	1.0	300	154	35	14	CAS	40	36	SO
Ross SLD	Ross	0.70	—	92	37.5	21	Egg white solids	0.5	0.6	—
Standard Vivonex	Norwich Eaton	1.0	550	286	22	8	AA	1.0	1.0	SAF O
Stresstein	Doyle	1.2	910	97	70	23	AA	28	20	MCT SO

Appendix A–2. Nutritional Analysis of Enteral Formulas (*Continued*)

Composition/liter

Carbohydrate

gm	Kcal%	Source	Na mEq	K mEq	Form	Kcal to meet U.S. RDA	Feature
135	54	CSS SUC	33	32	Liquid	2075	Isotonic tube/oral feeding
—	—	—	—	—	Powder	—	Modular amino acids
—	—	—	—	—	Powder	—	Modular high branched chain amino acids
80 per 100 ml	100	CSS	2 per 100 ml	<1 per 100 ml	Liquid	—	Modular carbohydrate
—	—	—	—	—	Liquid	—	Modular fat LCT
—	—	—	—	—	Liquid	—	Modular fat MCT
8.5	8	Polysorbate 80	270 per 100 gm	29 per 100 gm	Powder	—	Modular protein
145	55	HCS	24	26	Liquid	2000	Isotonic tube feeding
141	53	HCS	40.5	40	Liquid	1400	Isotonic tube feeding
50 gm per 100 ml	100	Glucose polymers	70 mg per 100 ml	<1 mEq per 100 ml	Liquid	—	Modular carbohydrate
94 gm per 100 gm	100	Glucose polymers	100 mg per 100 ml	<3 mEq per 100 mg	Powder	—	Modular carbohydrate
115	45	CSS SUC	21	32	Powder	—	Fat malabsorption
216	82	MAL SUC	61	33	Powder	3000	Standard tube oral feeding MCT oil
144	60	MAL SUC	35	26	Powder	1500	Isotonic tube feeding
248	89	MAL SUC	30	22	Powder	1900	Standard tube/oral feeding MCT oil
—	—	—	246 per 100 gm	22 per 100 gm	Powder	—	Modular protein
—	—	—	230 per 100 mg	13 per 100 gm	Powder	—	Modular protein
106	28	SUC HCS	57	49	Liquid	1420	Pulmonary disease
125	50	MAL SUC	22	32	Liquid	2000	Isotonic standard tube/ oral feeding
136.5	78	SUC HCS	36	21	Powder	840	Minimal residue
231	91	GO	20	30	Powder	1800	Oligomeric
170	57	MAL	28	28	Powder	2400	High branched chain AA

Appendix continued on following page

Appendix A–2. Nutritional Analysis of Enteral Formulas (*Continued*)

Product	Manu-facturer	Kcal/ml	mOsm/kg H₂O	Nonprotein Kcal/gm: Nitrogen	Protein gm	Protein Kcal% total	Protein Source	Fat gm	Fat Kcal% total	Fat Source
Sumacal	Biosearch	3.8/gm	–	–	–	–	–	–	–	–
Sustacal HC	Mead Johnson	1.5	650	134	61	16	CAS	57.5	34	SO
Sustacal Liquid	Mead Johnson	1.0	625	79	61	24	CAS SOY	23	21	SO
Sustacal Powder	Mead Johnson	1.33	1010	80	20.5	23	Non fat milk whole milk	9.2	23	Whole milk
Sustagen	Mead Johnson	1.7	—	72	109	24	Milk CAS	16	8	P W Milk
TraumaCal	Mead Johnson	1.5	550	89	83	22	CAS	68	41	SO MCT
Traum-Aid HBC	American McGaw	1.0	675	102	56	22	AA	12	11	SO MCT
Travasorb Hepatic	Travenol	1.1	690	218	29	11	AA	14	12	MCT SUN O
Travasorb HN	Travenol	1.0	560	126	45	18	H LACT	13	12	MCT SUN O
Travasorb Liquid Nutrition	Travenol	1.0	450	144	37	15	CAS SOY	37	33	CO SO
Travasorb MCT	Travenol	1.5	420	102	74	20	CAS Whey	50	30	MCT SUN O M/D GLY
Travasorb Renal	Travenol	1.35	590	362	23	7	ESS AA	18	12	MCT SUN O
Travasorb Std	Travenol	1.0	560	202	30	12	H LACT	13	12	MCT SUN O
TwoCal HN	Ross	2	–	125	83	17	CAS SOY	90.5	40.0	CO MCT
Vital High Nitrogen	Ross	1	460	125	42	17	H Whey meat, soy AA	11.0	9.0	SAF O MCT
Vitaneed	Biosearch	1	375	154	35	14	Beef CAS Veg	40.0	36.0	SO Beef
Vivonex Ten	Norwich Eaton	1	630	139	38	15	AA	5.0	4.5	SAF O

Courtesy of Fort Worth Dietetic Association: *Enteral Nutrition Formula Handbook.* Fort Worth, TX, 1984.

KEY TO ABBREVIATIONS:
AA = amino acids, CAS = casein, CHO = carbohydrate, CO = corn oil, CONC SW + S = concentrated sweet skim milk, CS = corn syrup, CSS = corn syrup solids, DEX = dextrose, D LAC = delactosed lactalbumin, ESS AA = essential amino acids, FRUC = fructose, GO = glucose oligosaccharides, H = hydrolyzed, H CER S = hydrolyzed cereal solids, HCS = hydrolyzed corn starch, LACT = lactose, LCT = long-chain triglycerides, LEC = lecithin, MAL = maltodextrin, MCS = modified corn starch, MCT = medium-chain triglycerides, M/D GLY = mono- and diglycerides, NF = nonfat milk, P = powdered whole milk, SAF O = safflower oil, SO = soy oil, SP = soy polysaccharide, SUC = sucrose, SUN O = sunflower oil, VEG = vegetables, W = whole milk.

NOTE: Nutritional analysis is listed for comparison and is based on current product information. Product availability and product formulation subject to change. The most current and complete information may be obtained from product labels. New products are introduced periodically. List of current product lines may be obtained from manufacturers.

Appendix A–2. Nutritional Analysis of Enteral Formulas (*Continued*)

Composition/liter

Carbohydrate

gm	Kcal%	Source	Na mEq	K mEq	Form	Kcal to meet U.S. RDA	Feature
95 per 100 gm	100	MAL	4	<1 per 100 gm	Powder	—	Modular carbohydrate
190	50	CSS SUC	36	37	Liquid	1800	Caloric dense
140	55	SUC CSS	40.5	52	Liquid	1080	Standard tube oral feeding >20% protein
48	54	SUC CSS LACT	53	86.0	Powder	1080	Milk containing >20% protein
312	68	CS LACT SUC	50	79.5	Powder	1750	Milk containing caloric dense >20% protein
143	38	CSS SUC	52	36	Liquid	3000	Caloric dense >20% protein
166	67	MAL	23	30	Powder	3000	High branched chain AA
209	77	GO SUC	19	29	Powder	2270	Heptatic disease
175	70	GO	40	30	Powder	2000	Oligomeric High nitrogen
145	58	SUC CSS	30	31	Liquid	2000	Standard tube/ oral feeding
185	50	MAL	23	67	Powder	2000	>20% protein caloric dense with MCT oil
271	81	GO SUC	—	—	Powder	—	Renal disease
190	76	GO	40	30	Powder	2000	Oligomeric
216	43	HCS	46	59	Liquid	1900	Caloric dense
188	74	HCS SUC	20	34	Powder	1500	Oligomeric High nitrogen
125	50	MAL fruit veg	22	32	Liquid	2000	Standard tube feeding
206	82	GO	20	20	Powder	2000	Oligomeric High BCAA

Appendix A–3 *Nutritional Analysis of Fast Foods*

	Weight (gm)	Energy (Kcal)	Protein (gm)	Carbohydrate (gm)	Fat (gm)	Cholesterol (mg)	Sodium (mg)	Potassium (mg)
Arby's[1]								
Junior Roast Beef	86	218	12	22	8.0	20.0	345	—
Regular Roast Beef	147	353	22	32	15.0	39.0	590	—
Beef 'N Cheddar	190	490	24	51	21.0	51.0	1520	—
Bacon 'N Cheddar Deluxe	225	561	28	36	34.0	78.0	1385	—
King Roast Beef	192	467	27	44	19.0	49.0	765	—
Super Roast Beef	234	501	25	50	22.0	40.0	800	—
Chicken Breast Sandwich	210	592	28	56	27.0	57.0	1340	—
Hot Ham 'N Cheese Sandwich	161	353	26	33	13.0	50.0	1655	—
Turkey Deluxe	197	375	24	32	17.0	39.0	850	—
Baked Potato, Plain	312	290	8	66	0.5	—	12	—
Superstuffed Potato—Deluxe	312	648	18	59	38.0	72.0	475	—
Superstuffed Potato—Broccoli and Cheddar	340	541	13	72	22.0	24.0	475	—
Superstuffed Potato—Mushroom and Cheese	300	506	16	61	22.0	21.0	635	—
Superstuffed Potato—Taco	425	619	23	73	27.0	145.0	1065	—
Vanilla Shake	250	295	8	44	10.0	30.0	245	—
Chocolate Shake	300	384	9	62	11.0	32.0	300	—
Jamocha Shake	305	424	8	76	10.0	31.0	280	—
French Fries	71	211	2	33	8.0	6.0	30	—
Potato Cakes	85	201	2	22	14.0	13.0	425	—
Burger King[2]								
Whopper Sandwich	281	628	27	46	36	90	880	545
Whopper with Cheese	306	711	33	47	43	113	1164	568
Whopper Jr. Sandwich	150	322	15	30	17	41	486	275
Whopper Jr. with Cheese	161	364	27	31	20	52	628	287
Bacon Double Cheeseburger	202	510	27	31	33	104	728	363
Hamburger	122	275	15	29	12	37	509	235
Cheeseburger	133	317	17	30	15	48	651	247
Chicken Tenders		204	20	10	10	47	636	200
Regular French Fries	68	227	3	24	13	14	160	360
Regular Onion Rings	76	274	4	28	16	—	665	173
Apple Pie	128	305	3	44	12	4	412	122
Chocolate Shake	282	320	8	46	12	NA	205	505
Vanilla Shake	282	321	9	49	10	NA	202	567
Whaler Fish Sandwich	205	488	19	45	27	77	592	369
Chicken Specialty Sandwich	207	688	26	56	40	82	1423	375
Specialty Ham and Cheese Sandwich	220	471	23	44	24	70	1534	419
French Toast Sticks		499	9	49	29	74	498	126
Great Danish		500	5	40	36	6	288	116
Church's Fried Chicken[3]								
Chicken Breast Portion	121	278	21	9.4	17.3	—	560	—
Chicken Wing-Breast Portion	136	303	22	8.9	19.7	—	583	—
Chicken Thigh	120	306	19	9.2	21.6	—	448	—
Chicken Leg	83.3	147	13	4.5	8.6	—	286	—
Chicken Nuggets (Regular)	18	55	3	3.7	3.1	—	125	—
Chicken Nuggets (Spicy)	18	52	3	3.4	2.9	—	91	—
Catfish	21.3	67	4	3.8	4.0	—	151	—
Hushpuppy (one)	23	78	1	11.6	2.9	—	55	—
Dairy Queen[4]								
Cone—Small	85	140	3	22	4	10.0	45	—
Cone—Regular	142	240	6	38	7	15.0	80	—
Cone—Large	213	340	9	57	10	25.0	115	—

Appendix A–3 Nutritional Analysis of Fast Foods (Continued)

Percent of U.S. Recommended Daily Allowances (U.S. RDAs)

Protein	Vitamin A	Vitamin C	Vitamin B_1	Vitamin B_2	Niacin	Calcium	Iron	Vitamin B_{12}	Phosphorus
20	*	*	10	15	20	4	10	—	—
35	*	2	15	25	38	8	20	—	—
40	*	*	8	20	25	8	30	—	—
45	*	6	10	15	30	10	15	—	—
45	2	4	20	35	50	10	25	—	—
40	15	60	25	35	45	10	25	—	—
45	*	*	15	15	50	10	20	—	—
40	4	40	65	30	30	20	10	—	—
35	6	8	15	25	60	8	15	—	—
10	*	105	20	8	25	2	10	—	—
30	20	4	15	25	30	30	15	—	—
20	10	6	20	20	30	15	15	—	—
25	15	4	15	25	35	30	15	—	—
35	60	8	25	15	40	45	20	—	—
10	8	4	8	35	*	30	4	—	—
15	8	4	8	35	2	30	6	—	—
15	6	*	6	30	15	30	6	—	—
4	*	10	6	*	10	*	6	—	—
4	*	6	6	*	8	*	4	—	—
42	14	19	25	25	35	8	28	—	24
49	21	19	25	29	35	21	28	—	36
23	6	10	16	15	20	4	16	—	13
27	10	10	16	17	20	11	16	—	19
49	8	*	20	25	31	17	21	—	33
23	3	5	16	15	20	4	16	—	12
27	7	5	16	17	20	10	16	—	19
31	2	*	5	5	35	2	7	—	24
5	*	NA	7	2	11	*	7	—	11
6	*	*	*	*	*	12	7	—	20
5	*	8	18	9	6	*	7	—	3
13	*	*	8	32	*	26	9	—	26
14	*	*	7	34	*	27	9	*	28
29	*	*	18	12	20	5	9	—	25
40	3	*	30	18	52	8	16	—	27
37	15	12	58	25	31	19	16	—	38
14	*	*	16	15	16	8	16	—	12
8	NA	NA	18	12	16	9	9	—	NA
—	—	—	—	—	—	—	—	—	—
—	—	—	—	—	—	—	—	—	—
—	—	—	—	—	—	—	—	—	—
—	—	—	—	—	—	—	—	—	—
—	—	—	—	—	—	—	—	—	—
—	—	—	—	—	—	—	—	—	—
—	—	—	—	—	—	—	—	—	—
6	2	*	2	10	*	10	2	6	10
10	4	*	4	20	*	15	4	10	20
20	8	*	8	30	*	25	8	15	30

Appendix continued on following page

Appendix A–3 Nutritional Analysis of Fast Foods (Continued)

	Weight (gm)	Energy (Kcal)	Protein (gm)	Carbohydrate (gm)	Fat (gm)	Cholesterol (mg)	Sodium (mg)	Potassium (mg)
Dipped Cone—Small	92	190	3	25	9	10.0	55	—
Dipped Cone—Regular	156	340	6	42	16	20.0	100	—
Dipped Cone—Large	234	510	9	64	24	30.0	145	—
Sundae—Small	106	190	3	33	4	10.0	75	—
Sundae—Regular	177	310	5	56	8	20.0	120	—
Sundae—Large	248	440	8	78	10	30.0	165	—
Shake—Small	241	409	8	69	11	30.0	150	—
Shake—Regular	418	710	14	120	19	50.0	260	—
Shake—Large	489	831	16	140	22	60.0	304	—
Malt—Small	241	438	8	77	10	30.0	150	—
Malt—Regular	418	760	14	134	18	50.0	260	—
Malt—Large	489	889	16	157	21	60.0	304	—
Float	397	410	5	82	7	20.0	85	—
Banana Split	383	540	9	103	11	30.0	150	—
Parfait	283	430	8	76	8	30.0	140	—
Hot Fudge Brownie Delight	266	600	9	85	25	20.0	225	—
Strawberry Shortcake	312	540	10	100	11	25.0	215	—
Freeze	397	500	9	89	12	30.0	180	—
Mr. Misty—Small	248	190	0	48	0	0	<10	—
Mr. Misty—Regular	330	250	0	63	0	0	<10	—
Mr. Misty—Large	439	340	0	84	0	0	<10	—
Mr. Misty Kiss	89	70	0	17	0	0	<10	—
Mr. Misty Freeze	411	500	9	91	12	30	140	—
Mr. Misty Float	411	390	5	74	7	20	95	—
Buster Bar	149	448	10	41	29	10	175	—
Dilly Bar	85	210	3	21	13	10	50	—
DQ Sandwich	60	140	3	24	4	5	40	—
Single Hamburger	148	360	21	33	16	45	630	—
Double Hamburger	210	530	36	33	28	85	660	—
Triple Hamburger	272	710	51	33	45	135	690	—
Single with Cheese	162	410	24	33	20	50	790	—
Double with Cheese	239	650	43	34	37	95	980	—
Triple with Cheese	301	820	58	34	50	145	1010	—
Hot Dog	100	280	11	21	16	45	830	—
Hot Dog with Chili	128	320	13	23	20	55	985	—
Hot Dog with Cheese	114	330	15	21	21	55	990	—
Super Hot Dog	175	520	17	44	27	80	1365	—
Super Hot Dog with Chili	218	570	21	47	32	100	1595	—
Super Hot Dog with Cheese	196	580	22	45	34	100	1605	—
Fish Fillet	177	430	20	45	18	40	674	—
Fish Fillet with Cheese	191	483	23	46	22	49	870	—
Chicken Breast Fillet	202	608	27	46	34	78	725	—
French Fries	71	200	2	25	10	10	115	—
French Fries—Large	113	320	3	40	16	15	185	—
Onion Rings	85	280	4	31	16	15	140	—
Jack in the Box Restaurants[5]								
Breakfast Jack		307	18	30	13	203	871	—
Supreme Crescent		547	20	27	40	178	1053	—
Sausage Crescent		584	22	28	43	187	1012	—
Canadian Crescent		452	19	25	31	226	851	—
Scrambled Eggs Breakfast		720	26	55	44	260	1110	—
Pancake Breakfast		630	16	79	27	85	1670	—
Hamburger		276	13	30	12	29	521	—
Cheeseburger		323	16	32	15	42	749	—
Mushroom Burger		477	28	30	27	87	906	—
Jumbo Jack		485	26	38	26	64	905	—
Jumbo Jack with Cheese		630	32	45	35	110	1665	—
Bacon Cheeseburger Supreme		724	34	44	46	70	1307	—
Swiss and Bacon Burger		643	33	31	43	99	1354	—

Appendix A–3 Nutritional Analysis of Fast Foods (Continued)

Percent of U.S. Recommended Daily Allowances (U.S. RDAs)

Protein	Vitamin A	Vitamin C	Vitamin B_1	Vitamin B_2	Niacin	Calcium	Iron	Vitamin B_{12}	Phosphorus
6	2	*	2	10	*	10	2	6	10
10	4	*	4	20	*	15	4	10	20
20	8	*	8	30	*	25	8	15	30
6	2	*	2	10	*	10	2	6	15
10	4	*	4	20	*	20	6	10	20
15	8	*	6	25	*	25	8	15	30
15	10	*	10	30	*	30	10	20	30
30	15	*	15	45	2	45	15	30	50
25	20	*	20	55	2	55	20	35	60
15	10	*	15	35	2	30	15	20	35
30	15	*	20	50	4	45	25	35	60
25	20	*	25	60	4	55	30	45	70
10	4	*	4	15	*	20	6	10	20
15	15	25	10	30	2	25	10	15	35
15	8	6	6	25	*	25	8	15	30
20	6	*	8	20	*	20	10	10	30
15	8	20	15	30	*	25	10	4	30
20	8	*	10	30	*	30	10	15	35
*	*	*	*	*	*	*	*	*	*
*	*	*	*	*	*	*	*	*	*
*	*	*	*	*	*	*	*	*	*
*	*	*	*	*	*	*	*	*	*
20	8	*	8	30	*	30	8	10	20
10	4	*	4	15	*	20	4	10	20
15	2	*	8	10	10	10	6	6	25
6	2	*	2	10	*	10	2	4	10
6	*	*	2	4	2	6	*	2	6
30	2	*	20	10	25	10	20	25	15
60	2	*	30	20	45	10	35	45	30
80	4	*	40	30	70	10	50	70	45
35	4	*	20	10	25	20	20	30	25
70	8	*	30	25	45	35	35	50	50
90	8	*	40	35	70	35	50	80	70
15	*	*	8	8	15	8	8	15	8
20	*	*	10	15	20	8	10	20	15
20	2	*	8	10	15	15	8	20	20
25	*	*	15	15	25	15	15	25	15
30	*	*	15	25	30	15	15	30	25
35	2	*	15	15	25	25	8	30	30
30	*	*	40	25	40	15	20	15	15
35	10	*	45	30	40	25	20	20	20
45	2	4	40	35	40	15	30	10	25
2	*	15	4	7	4	*	2	*	6
5	*	25	6	2	6	*	6	*	10
45	*	*	20	20	50	10	25	6	25
29	9	*	31	24	15	17	17	—	—
31	11	*	43	32	21	15	15	—	—
34	11	*	40	30	23	17	16	—	—
29	10	5	33	24	18	13	19	—	—
40	15	20	45	35	25	25	30	—	—
25	10	45	40	25	25	10	15	—	—
20	1	2	24	14	16	7	15	—	—
24	6	2	24	16	17	16	15	—	—
43	8	5	29	17	38	22	30	—	—
39	7	9	34	13	35	10	38	—	—
50	15	8	35	20	60	25	25	—	—
52	12	5	37	30	44	31	27	—	—
51	8	5	30	24	34	23	26	—	—

Appendix continued on following page

Appendix A–3 Nutritional Analysis of Fast Foods (Continued)

	Weight (gm)	Energy (Kcal)	Protein (gm)	Carbohydrate (gm)	Fat (gm)	Cholesterol (mg)	Sodium (mg)	Potassium (mg)
Ham and Swiss Burger		638	36	37	39	117	1330	—
Chicken Supreme		601	31	39	36	60	1582	—
Club Pita		284	22	30	8	43	953	—
Moby Jack		444	16	39	25	47	820	—
Regular Taco		191	8	16	11	21	406	—
Super Taco		288	12	21	17	37	765	—
Taco Salad		377	31	10	24	102	1436	—
Pasta Seafood Salad		394	15	32	22	48	1570	—
Chicken Strips Dinner		689	40	65	30	100	1213	—
Shrimp Dinner		731	22	77	37	157	1510	—
Sirloin Steak Dinner		699	38	75	27	75	969	—
Regular French Fries		221	2	27	12	8	164	—
Onion Rings		382	5	39	23	27	407	—
Cheese Nachos		571	15	49	35	37	1154	—
Supreme Nachos		718	23	66	40	55	1782	—
Apple Turnover		410	4	45	24	15	350	—
Vanilla Shake		320	10	57	6	25	230	—
Chocolate Shake		330	11	55	7	25	270	—
Strawberry Shake		320	10	55	7	25	240	—

Kentucky Fried Chicken[6]

	Weight (gm)	Energy (Kcal)	Protein (gm)	Carbohydrate (gm)	Fat (gm)	Cholesterol (mg)	Sodium (mg)	Potassium (mg)
Original Recipe Chicken Wing (edible portion)	56	181	11.8	5.77	12.3	67.0	387	—
Side Breast (edible portion)	95	276	20.0	10.1	17.3	96.0	654	
Center Breast (edible portion)	107	257	25.5	8.0	13.7	93.0	532	—
Drumstick (edible portion)	58	147	13.6	3.4	8.82	81.0	269	—
Thigh (edible portion)	96	278	18.0	8.4	19.2	122.0	517	—
Extra Crispy Chicken Wing (edible portion)	57	218	11.5	7.81	15.6	63.0	437	—
Side Breast (edible portion)	98	354	17.7	17.3	23.7	66.0	797	—
Center Breast (edible portion)	120	353	26.9	14.4	20.9	93.0	842	—
Drumstick (edible portion)	60	173	12.7	5.9	10.9	65.0	346	—
Thigh (edible portion)	112	371	19.6	13.8	26.3	121.0	766	—
Kentucky Nuggets (one)	16	46	2.82	2.2	2.88	11.9	140	—
Kentucky Nugget Sauces								
Barbeque	1 oz.	35	0.3	7.1	0.57	<1.0	450	—
Sweet and Sour	1 oz.	58	0.1	13.0	0.56	<1.0	148	—
Honey	0.5 oz.	49	—	12.1	< 0.01	<1.0	15	—
Mustard	1 oz.	36	0.88	6.04	0.91	<1.0	346	—
Buttermilk Biscuit (one)	75	269	5.1	31.6	13.6	<1.0	521	—
Mashed Potatoes with Gravy	86	62	2.1	10.3	1.4	<1.0	297	—
Mashed Potatoes	80	59	1.9	11.6	0.6	<1.0	228	—
Chicken Gravy	78	59	2.0	4.4	3.7	2.0	398	—
Kentucky Fries	119	268	4.8	33.3	12.8	1.8	81	—
Corn-on-the-Cob	143	176	5.1	31.9	3.1	<1.0	<21	—
Cole Slaw	79	103	1.3	11.5	5.7	4.0	171	—
Potato Salad	90	141	1.8	12.6	9.27	11.0	396	—
Baked Beans	89	105	5.1	18.4	1.2	<1.0	387	—

McDonald's[7]

	Weight (gm)	Energy (Kcal)	Protein (gm)	Carbohydrate (gm)	Fat (gm)	Cholesterol (mg)	Sodium (mg)	Potassium (mg)
Egg McMuffin	138	340	18.5	31.0	15.8	259.0	885	—
Hotcakes with Butter and Syrup	214	500	7.9	93.9	10.3	47.1	1070	—
Scrambled Eggs	98	180	13.2	2.5	13.0	514.2	205	—
Sausage	53	210	9.8	0.6	18.6	38.8	423	—
English Muffin with Butter	63	186	5.0	29.5	5.3	15.4	310	—
Hash Brown Potatoes	55	125	1.4	14.6	8.9	3.6	325	—

Appendix A–3 Nutritional Analysis of Fast Foods (Continued)

Percent of U.S. Recommended Daily Allowances (U.S. RDAs)

Protein	Vitamin A	Vitamin C	Vitamin B_1	Vitamin B_2	Niacin	Calcium	Iron	Vitamin B_{12}	Phosphorus
55	9	16	51	28	38	27	34	–	–
47	9	7	35	22	53	24	17	–	–
35	5	7	52	19	39	8	14	–	–
25	6	*	27	15	14	16	12	–	–
12	8	*	5	10	5	10	6	–	–
19	12	3	8	5	7	15	9	–	–
47	23	11	12	31	30	28	24	–	–
24	47	35	25	14	9	21	33	–	–
61	8	20	30	17	93	11	22	–	–
34	8	20	26	10	35	37	27	–	–
59	3	13	45	30	62	22	53	–	–
4	*	5	5	2	6	1	3	–	–
8	*	5	14	7	9	3	8	–	–
22	10	5	7	11	5	37	8	–	–
35	20	14	10	15	16	41	18	–	–
6	*	*	15	6	10	*	8	–	–
20	*	*	10	20	2	35	*	–	–
25	*	*	10	35	2	35	4	–	–
25	*	*	10	25	2	35	2	–	–
26.13	1.12	*	2.24	3.62	15.96	3.77	2.52	–	–
44.54	*	*	4.43	10.62	34.2	4.84	4.38	–	–
56.59	*	*	5.71	8.18	50.82	3.93	3.51	–	–
30.16	*	*	3.87	7.85	14.5	1.28	3.32	–	–
39.89	2.88	*	5.12	16.38	23.04	2.76	5.81	–	–
25.59	*	*	2.28	4.36	14.25	2.14	2.88	–	–
39.42	*	*	5.23	7.49	32.34	3.19	4.79	–	–
59.73	*	*	6.4	9.18	50.4	3.49	4.8	–	–
28.13	*	*	3.2	8.47	14.1	1.52	3.37	–	–
43.56	*	*	5.97	15.81	25.76	4.61	6.72	–	–
6.26	*	*	1.3	1.81	5.18	0.24	0.73	–	–
0.46	7.4	0.59	0.76	0.86	0.95	0.61	1.38	–	–
0.17	1.19	0.52	0.38	*	0.19	0.46	0.92	–	–
0.06	*	*	*	0.18	0.18	0.06	0.59	–	–
1.35	*	*	1.32	0.48	0.79	1.02	1.42	–	–
7.85	*	*	19.0	7.5	9.0	7.65	6.79	–	–
3.18	*	*	*	2.12	5.16	1.91	1.96	–	–
2.95	*	*	*	2.21	4.8	2.06	1.56	–	–
3.0	*	*	*	1.65	2.34	0.86	2.69	–	–
7.32	*	4.56	11.11	3.36	13.68	2.43	5.22	–	–
7.92	5.43	3.81	9.53	6.64	9.3	0.72	4.37	–	–
1.94	5.37	31.2	2.11	1.53	1.03	2.85	1.05	–	–
2.77	1.8	4.5	4.8	1.38	3.02	1.04	1.75	–	–
7.8	*	3.56	4.15	2.3	2.49	5.36	7.96	–	–
28.5	11.8	–	31.3	26.0	18.8	22.6	16.3	–	–
12.2	5.1	7.9	17.1	21.4	11.3	10.3	12.4	–	–
29.4	13.0	2.0	5.2	27.7	1.0	6.1	14.1	–	–
19.5	–	–	18.0	6.2	10.4	1.6	4.6	–	–
7.7	3.3	1.4	18.9	28.9	13.1	11.7	8.4	–	–
2.5	–	6.9	0.06	–	4.1	0.5	2.2	–	–

Appendix continued on following page

Appendix A–3 Nutritional Analysis of Fast Foods (Continued)

	Weight (gm)	Energy (Kcal)	Protein (gm)	Carbohydrate (gm)	Fat (gm)	Cholesterol (mg)	Sodium (mg)	Potassium (mg)
Biscuit with Sausage	121	467	12.1	35.3	30.9	48.0	1147	—
Biscuit with Bacon, Egg, and Cheese	145	483	16.5	33.2	31.6	262.5	1269	—
Sausage McMuffin with Egg	165	517	22.9	32.2	32.9	287.0	1044	—
Hamburger	100	263	12.4	28.3	11.3	29.1	506	—
Cheeseburger	114	318	15.0	28.5	16.0	40.6	743	—
Quarter Pounder	160	427	24.6	29.3	23.5	81.0	718	—
Quarter Pounder with Cheese	186	525	29.6	30.5	31.6	107.0	1220	—
Big Mac	200	570	24.6	39.2	35.0	83.0	979	—
Filet-O-Fish	143	435	14.7	35.9	25.7	46.6	799	—
McD.L.T.	254	680	30.0	40.0	44.0	101.0	1030	—
Chicken McNuggets	109	323	19.1	13.7	20.2	62.5	512	—
French Fries	68	220	3.0	26.1	11.5	8.57	109	—
Apple Pie	85	253	1.87	29.3	14.0	12.4	398	—
Vanilla Shake	291	352	9.3	59.6	8.4	30.6	201	—
Chocolate Shake	291	383	9.9	65.5	9.0	29.7	300	—
Strawberry Shake	290	362	9.0	62.1	8.7	32.2	207	—
Soft-Serve Cones	115.0	189	4.3	31.2	5.2	23.5	109.0	—
Strawberry Sundae	164.0	320	6.0	54.0	8.7	24.6	90.0	—
Hot Fudge Sundae	164.0	357	7.0	58.0	10.8	26.6	170.0	—
Caramel Sundae	165.0	361	7.2	60.8	10.0	31.4	145.0	—
McDonaldland Cookies	67.0	308	4.0	49.0	11.0	10.0	358.0	—
Chocolaty Chip Cookies	69.0	342	4.0	45.0	16.0	18.0	313.0	—
Chef Salad	273.0	226	21.0	5.7	13.0	125.0	853.0	—
Shrimp Salad	236.0	102	14.0	4.5	2.6	187.0	571.0	—
Garden Salad	204.0	91	6.1	4.3	5.5	110.0	102.0	—
Chicken Oriental Salad	280.0	146	23.0	4.0	3.9	91.5	266.0	—
Side Salad	114.0	48	3.4	2.6	2.6	41.5	43.1	—
Bleu Cheese Dressing	2.5	342	2.6	5.4	34.4	31.3	760.0	—
French Dressing	2.5	285	0.4	12.7	25.8	<1.0	852.0	—
House Dressing	2.0	326	1.0	3.6	34.2	13.7	502.0	—
Thousand Island Dressing	2.5	396	1.1	9.64	39.3	48.4	599.0	—
Lite Vinaigrette Dressing	2.0	50	0.79	6.58	2.3	<1.0	300.0	—
Oriental Salad Dressing	2.0	103	1.1	23.8	—	<1.0	551.0	—
Pizza Inn[8]								
Pan Pizza with:								
Pepperoni	—	418	17	43	18	25	1087	—
Canadian Bacon	—	380	17	43	14	22	991	—
Black Olives	—	395	15	43	16	17	997	—
Green Olives	—	385	16	43	15	17	1220	—
Onions	—	371	15	43	14	17	884	—
Green Peppers	—	370	15	43	14	17	884	—
Mushrooms	—	371	15	43	14	17	940	—
Cheese		368	15	43	14	17	883	
Thin Crust Pizza with:	—							
Pepperoni	—	276	11	28	13	17	846	—
Canadian Bacon	—	237	11	28	9	14	749	—
Black Olives	—	252	9	28	11	10	756	—
Green Olives	—	242	9	28	10	10	978	—
Onions	—	228	9	28	9	10	642	—
Green Peppers	—	228	9	28	9	10	642	—
Mushrooms	—	229	9	28	9	10	698	—
Cheese	—	226	9	28	9	10	641	—
Wendy's[9]								
¼ lb. Single Hamburger on Multigrain Wheat Bun	119	340	25	20	17	67	290	310

Appendix A–3 Nutritional Analysis of Fast Foods (Continued)

Percent of U.S. Recommended Daily Allowances (U.S. RDAs)

Protein	Vitamin A	Vitamin C	Vitamin B_1	Vitamin B_2	Niacin	Calcium	Iron	Vitamin B_{12}	Phosphorus
18.6	1.2	—	37.1	12.8	17.0	8.2	11.4	—	—
25.4	13.1	2.7	20.3	25.6	11.6	0.2	14.3	—	—
33.7	13.1	—	56.1	29.1	22.3	19.6	19.3	—	—
19.0	2.0	3.0	20.6	12.9	20.4	8.4	15.8	—	—
23.2	7.1	3.4	19.8	14.1	21.7	16.9	15.8	—	—
37.9	2.6	4.3	23.5	18.8	36.0	9.8	23.9	—	—
45.5	12.3	4.7	24.8	24.1	35.3	25.5	26.9	—	—
37.9	7.6	5.0	32.0	22.4	36.0	20.3	27.2	—	—
22.7	3.7	—	23.8	13.5	15.0	13.3	13.7	—	—
45.0	10.0	15.0	35.0	25.0	40.0	25.0	35.0	—	—
29.4	—	3.5	10.9	8.3	37.6	1.1	7.0	—	—
4.6	—	20.9	8.1	1.2	11.3	0.9	3.4	—	—
2.9	—	—	1.3	1.2	0.9	1.4	3.5	—	—
20.7	7.0	5.3	7.7	41.1	1.7	32.9	1.0	—	—
22.0	7.0	—	7.8	25.7	2.5	32.0	4.7	—	—
20.0	7.5	6.8	7.7	25.6	1.7	32.2	1.0	—	—
6.6	4.4	—	8.1	1.2	2.2	0.9	3.4	—	—
10.1	5.5	4.7	4.4	17.4	5.2	17.4	2.1	—	—
10.8	4.6	4.1	4.4	18.4	5.6	21.5	3.4	—	—
11.1	5.6	6.0	4.4	18.4	5.0	20.0	1.3	—	—
7.0	—	2.0	15.0	14.0	14.0	1.0	8.0	—	—
7.0	2.0	2.0	8.0	12.0	9.0	3.0	9.0	—	—
32.7	25.07	33.5	23.62	19.24	25.89	22.15	7.12	—	—
21.97	14.8	16.75	8.82	7.78	8.6	6.35	4.83	—	—
9.39	13.02	16.75	5.42	9.57	4.7	10.4	3.5	—	—
35.31	24.07	36.3	9.33	9.88	37.79	4.73	7.62	—	—
5.25	10.0	7.77	3.79	5.35	2.16	4.73	2.0	—	—
3.92	—	—	1.89	6.67	0.28	7.31	0.72	—	—
0.65	10.63	—	0.94	—	0.85	0.4	0.61	—	—
1.5	—	—	1.51	4.0	0.31	2.08	0.94	—	—
1.74	3.83	—	1.42	2.5	0.85	1.34	1.44	—	—
1.22	—	—	1.13	1.0	0.4	0.53	0.88	—	—
1.66	—	3.31	1.13	2.0	1.39	1.47	3.06	—	—
—	—	—	—	—	—	—	—	—	—
—	—	—	—	—	—	—	—	—	—
—	—	—	—	—	—	—	—	—	—
—	—	—	—	—	—	—	—	—	—
—	—	—	—	—	—	—	—	—	—
—	—	—	—	—	—	—	—	—	—
—	—	—	—	—	—	—	—	—	—
—	—	—	—	—	—	—	—	—	—
—	—	—	—	—	—	—	—	—	—
—	—	—	—	—	—	—	—	—	—
—	—	—	—	—	—	—	—	—	—
—	—	—	—	—	—	—	—	—	—
—	—	—	—	—	—	—	—	—	—
—	—	—	—	—	—	—	—	—	—
—	—	—	—	—	—	—	—	—	—
35	*	*	15	10	25	2	15	—	—

Appendix continued on following page

Appendix A–3 Nutritional Analysis of Fast Foods (Continued)

	Weight	Energy	Protein	Carbohydrate	Fat	Cholesterol	Sodium	Potassium
	(gm)	(Kcal)	(gm)	(gm)	(gm)	(mg)	(mg)	(mg)
¼ lb. Single Hamburger on White Bun	117	350	21	27	18	65	410	275
½ lb. Double Hamburger on White Bun	197	560	41	24	34	125	575	485
¼ lb. Bacon Cheeseburger on White Bun	147	460	29	23	28	65	860	330
Chicken Sandwich on Multigrain Wheat Bun	128	320	25	31	10	59	500	320
2 oz. Kids' Meal Hamburger	75	220	13	11	8	20	265	150
8 oz. Chili	256	260	21	26	8	30	1070	585
French Fries (Salted)	98	280	4	35	14	15	95	635
Taco Salad	357	390	23	36	18	40	1100	790
Frosty Dairy Dessert	243	400	8	59	14	50	220	585
Hot Stuffed Baked Potatoes								
Plain (8.8 oz.)	250	250	6	52	2	trace	60	1360
Sour Cream and Chives	310	460	6	53	24	15	230	1420
Cheese	350	590	17	55	34	22	450	1380
Chili and Cheese	400	510	22	63	20	22	610	1590
Bacon and Cheese	350	570	19	57	30	22	1180	1380
Broccoli and Cheese	365	500	13	54	25	22	430	1550
Stroganoff and Sour Cream	406	490	14	60	21	43	910	1920
Chicken a la King	358	350	15	59	6	20	820	1550

* Contains less than 2 percent of the RDA.
[1] Nutrient data from Arby's and independent laboratories.
[2] From Burger King Corp., 7360 N. Kendall Dr., Miami, FL.
[3] Nutrient data based on Texas Testing Laboratories, Inc., Dallas, TX. Averaged analysis of products (May 1985).
[4] These figures are for Dairy Queen products and portions as specified by American Dairy Queen Corporation using Dairy Queen authorized products. Nutrient data reviewed and edited by Dr. David J. Aulik in cooperation with Raltech Scientific Services (formerly WARF Institute, Madison, WI).
[5] Nutritional analysis provided by Foodmaker, Inc., San Diego, CA 92123.
[6] Analytical testing conducted by Hazleton Laboratories America, Inc.
[7] From McDonald's Corp., Oak Brook, IL. Nutrient analysis by Hazleton Laboratories America, Inc., Chemical and Biomedical Sciences Division.
[8] Values for pizza are based on one slice (⅛ of a 13-inch pizza). Calculations from USDA Handbook No. 8.
[9] From Wendy's International, Inc., Dublin, OH. Nutrient data based on studies by Hazleton Laboratories America, Inc.

Appendix A–3 Nutritional Analysis of Fast Foods (Continued)

Percent of U.S. Recommended Daily Allowances (U.S. RDAs)

Protein	Vitamin A	Vitamin C	Vitamin B_1	Vitamin B_2	Niacin	Calcium	Iron	Vitamin B_{12}	Phosphorus
35	N/A	N/A	15	15	25	4	25	–	–
60	N/A	N/A	15	25	45	4	35	–	–
45	8	*	20	15	30	15	20	–	–
35	*	*	15	8	50	2	8	–	–
20	N/A	N/A	10	10	15	2	10	–	–
30	20	10	6	10	15	8	25	–	–
6	N/A	20	10	2	15	*	6	–	–
35	35	35	10	20	15	20	25	–	–
20	10	*	8	30	*	30	6	–	–
8	*	60	15	6	15	2	15	–	–
8	10	60	15	8	15	4	15	–	–
35	20	60	15	15	15	35	15	–	–
40	15	60	20	15	20	25	20	–	–
35	15	60	15	10	15	20	15	–	–
20	35	150	20	15	20	25	15	–	–
15	6	60	15	15	20	8	20	–	–
15	2	60	20	10	30	6	15	–	–

Appendix B–1. *Mean Heights and Weights and Recommended Energy Intake**

Category	Age (years)	Weight (kg)	Weight (lb.)	Height (cm)	Height (in.)	Energy Needs (with range) (kcal)		Energy Needs (with range) (MJ)
Infants	0.0–0.5	6	13	60	24	kg × 115	(95–145)	kg × 0.48
	0.5–1.0	9	20	71	28	kg × 105	(80–135)	kg × 0.44
Children	1–3	13	29	90	35	1300	(900–1800)	5.5
	4–6	20	44	112	44	1700	(1300–2300)	7.1
	7–10	28	62	132	52	2400	(1650–3300)	10.1
Males	11–14	45	99	157	62	2700	(2000–3700)	11.3
	15–18	66	145	176	69	2800	(2100–3900)	11.8
	19–22	70	154	177	70	2900	(2500–3300)	12.2
	23–50	70	154	178	70	2700	(2300–3100)	11.3
	51–75	70	154	178	70	2400	(2000–2800)	10.1
	76+	70	154	178	70	2050	(1650–2450)	8.6
Females	11–14	46	101	157	62	2200	(1500–3000)	9.2
	15–18	55	120	163	64	2100	(1200–3000)	8.8
	19–22	55	120	163	64	2100	(1700–2500)	8.8
	23–50	55	120	163	64	2000	(1600–2400)	8.4
	51–75	55	120	163	64	1800	(1400–2200)	7.6
	76+	55	120	163	64	1600	(1200–2000)	6.7
Pregnancy						+300		
Lactation						+500		

*The data in this table have been assembled from the observed median heights and weights of children together with desirable weights for adults with mean heights of men (70 in.) and women (64 in.) between the ages of 18 and 34 years as surveyed in the U.S. population.

The energy allowances for the young adults are for men and women doing light work. The allowances for the two older age groups represent mean energy needs over these age spans, allowing for a 2-percent decrease in basal (resting) metabolic rate per decade and reduction in activity of 200 kcal/day for men and women between 51 and 75 years, 500 kcal for men over 75 years, and 400 kcal for women over 75 years. The customary range of daily energy output is shown in parentheses for adults and is based on a variation in energy needs of ±400 kcal at any one age, emphasizing the wide range of energy intakes appropriate for any group of people.

Energy allowances for children through age 18 are based on median energy intakes of children of these ages followed in longitudinal growth studies. The values in parentheses are 10th and 90th percentiles of energy intake, to indicate the range of energy consumption among children of these ages.

From Food and Nutrition Board, National Academy of Sciences-National Research Council: *Recommended Dietary Allowances,* 9th ed., Washington, D.C., 1980.

Appendix B–2. *Estimated Safe and Adequate Daily Dietary Intakes of Additional Selected Vitamins and Minerals**

	Age (years)	Vitamins			Trace Elements†						Electrolytes		
		Vitamin K (μg)	Biotin (μg)	Pantothenic Acid (mg)	Copper (mg)	Manganese (mg)	Fluoride (mg)	Chromium (mg)	Selenium (mg)	Molybdenum (mg)	Sodium (mg)	Potassium (mg)	Chloride (mg)
Infants	0–0.5	12	35	2	0.5–0.7	0.5–0.7	0.1–0.5	0.01–0.04	0.01–0.04	0.03–0.06	115–350	350–925	275–700
	0.5–1	10–20	50	3	0.7–1.0	0.7–1.0	0.2–1.0	0.02–0.06	0.02–0.06	0.04–0.08	250–750	425–1275	400–1200
Children and	1–3	15–30	65	3	1.0–1.5	1.0–1.5	0.5–1.5	0.02–0.08	0.02–0.08	0.05–0.1	325–975	550–1650	500–1500
	4–6	20–40	85	3–4	1.5–2.0	1.5–2.0	1.0–2.5	0.03–0.12	0.03–0.12	0.06–0.15	450–1350	775–2325	700–2100
Adolescents	7–10	30–60	120	4–5	2.0–2.5	2.0–3.0	1.5–2.5	0.05–0.2	0.05–0.2	0.1–0.3	600–1800	1000–3000	925–2775
	11+	50–100	100–200	4–7	2.0–3.0	2.5–5.0	1.5–2.5	0.05–0.2	0.05–0.2	0.15–0.5	900–2700	1525–4575	1400–4200
Adults		70–140	100–200	4–7	2.0–3.0	2.5–5.0	1.5–4.0	0.05–0.2	0.05–0.2	0.15–0.5	1100–3300	1875–5625	1700–5100

*From Food and Nutrition Board, National Academy of Sciences–National Research Council: *Recommended Dietary Allowances*, 9th ed. Washington, DC, 1980. Because there is less information on which to base allowances, these figures are not given in the main table of the RDA and are provided here in the form of ranges of recommended intakes.

†Since the toxic levels for many trace elements may be only several times usual intakes, the upper levels for the trace elements given in this table should not be habitually exceeded.

Appendix B–3. U.S. Recommended Daily Allowance (U.S. RDA)*

	Adults and Children Over 4 yrs.†	Children Under 4 yrs.	Infants Under 13 months	Pregnant or Lactating Women
Protein	65 g‡	28 g‡	25 g‡	65 g‡
Vitamin A	5,000 IU	2,500 IU	2,500 IU	8,000 IU
Vitamin C	60 mg	40 mg	40 mg	60 mg
Thiamin	1.5 mg	0.7 mg	0.7 mg	1.7 mg
Riboflavin	1.7 mg	0.8 mg	0.8 mg	2.0 mg
Niacin	20 mg	9.0 mg	9.0 mg	20 mg
Calcium	1.0 g	0.8 g	0.8 g	1.3 g
Iron	18 mg	10 mg	10 mg	18 mg
Vitamin D	400 IU	400 IU	400 IU	400 IU
Vitamin E	30 IU	10 IU	10 IU	30 IU
Vitamin B_6	2.0 mg	0.7 mg	0.7 mg	2.5 mg
Folacin	0.4 mg	0.2 mg	0.2 mg	0.8 mg
Vitamin B_{12}	6 mcg	3 mcg	3 mcg	8 mcg
Phosphorus	1.0 g	0.8 g	0.8 g	1.3 g
Iodine	150 mcg	70 mcg	70 mcg	150 mcg
Magnesium	400 mg	200 mg	200 mg	450 mg
Zinc	15 mg	8 mg	8 mg	15 mg
Copper	2 mg	1 mg	1 mg	2 mg
Biotin	0.3 mg	0.15 mg	0.15 mg	0.3 mg
Pantothenic acid	10 mg	5 mg	5 mg	10 mg

*For use in nutrition labeling of foods, including foods that are vitamin and mineral supplements.
†These values are on most nutrition labels.
‡If protein efficiency ratio of protein is equal to or better than that of casein U.S. RDA is 45 g for adults and pregnant or lactating women, 20 g for children under 4 years of age and 18 g for infants.

Appendix C–1 1983 Metropolitan Life Insurance Company Height and Weight Tables*

Men					Women				
Height Feet	Height Inches	Small Frame	Medium Frame	Large Frame	Height Feet	Height Inches	Small Frame	Medium Frame	Large Frame
5	2	128–134	131–141	138–150	4	10	102–111	109–121	118–131
5	3	130–136	133–143	140–153	4	11	103–113	111–123	120–134
5	4	132–138	135–145	142–156	5	0	104–115	113–126	122–137
5	5	134–140	137–148	144–160	5	1	106–118	115–129	125–140
5	6	136–142	139–151	146–164	5	2	108–121	118–132	128–143
5	7	138–145	142–154	149–168	5	3	111–124	121–135	131–147
5	8	140–148	145–157	152–172	5	4	114–127	124–138	134–151
5	9	142–151	148–160	155–176	5	5	117–130	127–141	137–155
5	10	144–154	151–163	158–180	5	6	120–133	130–144	140–159
5	11	146–157	154–166	161–184	5	7	123–136	133–147	143–163
6	0	149–160	157–170	164–188	5	8	126–139	136–150	146–167
6	1	152–164	160–174	168–192	5	9	129–142	139–153	149–170
6	2	155–168	164–178	172–197	5	10	132–145	142–156	152–173
6	3	158–172	167–182	176–202	5	11	135–148	145–159	155–176
6	4	162–176	171–187	181–207	6	0	138–151	148–162	158–179

*Weights for adults age 25 to 59 years based on lowest mortality. For determination of frame size see Appendix C–2. Weight in pounds according to frame size in indoor clothing (5 pounds for men and 3 pounds for women) wearing shoes with 1-inch heels.
Source of basic data *1979 Build Study*, Society of Actuaries and Association of Life Insurance Medical Directors of America. Courtesy of the Metropolitan Life Insurance Company, 1983.

Appendix C–2. Determination of Body Frame Size From Wrist Circumference*

Body Frame Size May Be Calculated Using the Formula:

$$r = \frac{\text{Height (cm)}}{\text{Wrist circumference (cm)}}$$

Frame Size Can Be Determined as Follows:

Males	Females
r > 10.4 = small frame	r > 11.0 = small frame
r = 9.6 to 10.4 = medium frame	r = 10.1 to 11.0 = medium frame
r < 9.6 = large frame	r < 10.1 = large frame

*From Grant, J: *Handbook of Total Parenteral Nutrition.* Philadelphia, W. B. Saunders Co, 1980, with permission.

Appendix C–3. Percentiles for Triceps Skinfold for Whites of the United States Health and Nutrition Examination Survey I of 1971 to 1974*

Age group	Triceps skinfold percentiles (mm²)															
	n	5	10	25	50	75	90	95	n	5	10	25	50	75	90	95
	Males								**Females**							
1–1.9	228	6	7	8	10	12	14	16	204	6	7	8	10	12	14	16
2–2.9	223	6	7	8	10	12	14	15	208	6	8	9	10	12	15	16
3–3.9	220	6	7	8	10	11	14	15	208	7	8	9	11	12	14	15
4–4.9	230	6	6	8	9	11	12	14	208	7	8	8	10	12	14	16
5–5.9	214	6	6	8	9	11	14	15	219	6	7	8	10	12	15	18
6–6.9	117	5	6	7	8	10	13	16	118	6	6	8	10	12	14	16
7–7.9	122	5	6	7	9	12	15	17	126	6	7	9	11	13	16	18
8–8.9	117	5	6	7	8	10	13	16	118	6	8	9	12	15	18	24
9–9.9	121	6	6	7	10	13	17	18	125	8	8	10	13	16	20	22
10–10.9	146	6	6	8	10	14	18	21	152	7	8	10	12	17	23	27
11–11.9	122	6	6	8	11	16	20	24	117	7	8	10	13	18	24	28
12–12.9	153	6	6	8	11	14	22	28	129	8	9	11	14	18	23	27
13–13.9	134	5	5	7	10	14	22	26	151	8	8	12	15	21	26	30
14–14.9	131	4	5	7	9	14	21	24	141	9	10	13	16	21	26	28
15–15.9	128	4	5	6	8	11	18	24	117	8	10	12	17	21	25	32
16–16.9	131	4	5	6	8	12	16	22	142	10	12	15	18	22	26	31
17–17.9	133	5	5	6	8	12	16	19	114	10	12	13	19	24	30	37
18–18.9	91	4	5	6	9	13	20	24	109	10	12	15	18	22	26	30
19–24.9	531	4	5	7	10	15	20	22	1060	10	11	14	18	24	30	34
25–34.9	971	5	6	8	12	16	20	24	1987	10	12	16	21	27	34	37
35–44.9	806	5	6	8	12	16	20	23	1614	12	14	18	23	29	35	38
45–54.9	898	6	6	8	12	15	20	25	1047	12	16	20	25	30	36	40
55–64.9	734	5	6	8	11	14	19	22	809	12	16	20	25	31	36	38
65–74.9	1503	4	6	8	11	15	19	22	1670	12	14	18	24	29	34	36

*From Frisancho, AR: New norms of upper limb fat and muscle areas for assessment of nutritional status. *American Journal of Clinical Nutrition* 34(11):2530, 1981, with permission.

Appendix C–4. *Percentiles of Upper Arm Circumference (mm) and Estimated Upper Arm Muscle Circumference (mm) for Whites of the United States Health and Nutrition Examination Survey I of 1971 to 1974**

Age group	Arm circumference (mm)								Arm muscle circumference (mm)						
	5	10	25	50	75	90	95		5	10	25	50	75	90	95
Males															
1–1.9	142	146	150	159	170	176	183		110	113	119	127	135	144	147
2–2.9	141	145	153	162	170	178	185		111	114	122	130	140	146	150
3–3.9	150	153	160	167	175	184	190		117	123	131	137	143	148	153
4–4.9	149	154	162	171	180	186	192		123	126	133	141	148	156	159
5–5.9	153	160	167	175	185	195	204		128	133	140	147	154	162	169
6–6.9	155	159	167	179	188	209	228		131	135	142	151	161	170	177
7–7.9	162	167	177	187	201	223	230		137	139	151	160	168	177	190
8–8.9	162	170	177	190	202	220	245		140	145	154	162	170	182	187
9–9.9	175	178	187	200	217	249	257		151	154	161	170	183	196	202
10–10.9	181	184	196	210	231	262	274		156	160	166	180	191	209	221
11–11.9	186	190	202	223	244	261	280		159	165	173	183	195	205	230
12–12.9	193	200	214	232	254	282	303		167	171	182	195	210	223	241
13–13.9	194	211	228	247	263	286	301		172	179	196	211	226	238	245
14–14.9	220	226	237	253	283	303	322		189	199	212	223	240	260	264
15–15.9	222	229	244	264	284	311	320		199	204	218	237	254	266	272
16–16.9	244	248	262	278	303	324	343		213	225	234	249	269	287	296
17–17.9	246	253	267	285	308	336	347		224	231	245	258	273	294	312
18–18.9	245	260	276	297	321	353	379		226	237	252	264	283	298	324
19–24.9	262	272	288	308	331	355	372		238	245	257	273	289	309	321
25–34.9	271	282	300	319	342	362	375		243	250	264	279	298	314	326
35–44.9	278	287	305	326	345	363	374		247	255	269	286	302	318	327
45–54.9	267	281	301	322	342	362	376		239	249	265	281	300	315	326
55–64.9	258	273	296	317	336	355	369		236	245	260	278	295	310	320
65–74.9	248	263	285	307	325	344	355		223	235	251	268	284	298	306
Females															
1–1.9	138	142	148	156	164	172	177		105	111	117	124	132	139	143
2–2.9	142	145	152	160	167	176	184		111	114	119	126	133	142	147
3–3.9	143	150	158	167	175	183	189		113	119	124	132	140	146	152
4–4.9	149	154	160	169	177	184	191		115	121	128	136	144	152	157
5–5.9	153	157	165	175	185	203	211		125	128	134	142	151	159	165
6–6.9	156	162	170	176	187	204	211		130	133	138	145	154	166	171
7–7.9	164	167	174	183	199	216	231		129	135	142	151	160	171	176
8–8.9	168	172	183	195	214	247	261		138	140	151	160	171	183	194
9–9.9	178	182	194	211	224	251	260		147	150	158	167	180	194	198
10–10.9	174	182	193	210	228	251	265		148	150	159	170	180	190	197
11–11.9	185	194	208	224	248	276	303		150	158	171	181	196	217	223
12–12.9	194	203	216	237	256	282	294		162	166	180	191	201	214	220
13–13.9	202	211	223	243	271	301	338		169	175	183	198	211	226	240
14–14.9	214	223	237	252	272	304	322		174	179	190	201	216	232	247
15–15.9	208	221	239	254	279	300	322		175	178	189	202	215	228	244
16–16.9	218	224	241	258	283	318	334		170	180	190	202	216	234	249
17–17.9	220	227	241	264	295	324	350		175	183	194	205	221	239	257
18–18.9	222	227	241	258	281	312	325		174	179	191	202	215	237	245
19–24.9	221	230	247	265	290	319	345		179	185	195	207	221	236	249
25–34.9	233	240	256	277	304	342	368		183	188	199	212	228	246	264
35–44.9	241	251	267	290	317	356	378		186	192	205	218	236	257	272
45–54.9	242	256	274	299	328	362	384		187	193	206	220	238	260	274
55–64.9	243	257	280	303	335	367	385		187	196	209	225	244	266	280
65–74.9	240	252	274	299	326	356	373		185	195	208	225	244	264	279

*From Frisancho, AR: New norms of upper limb fat and muscle areas for assessment of nutritional status. American Journal of Clinical Nutrition 34(11):2530, 1981, with permission.

Appendix C–5a. Arm Anthropometry Nomogram for Adults*

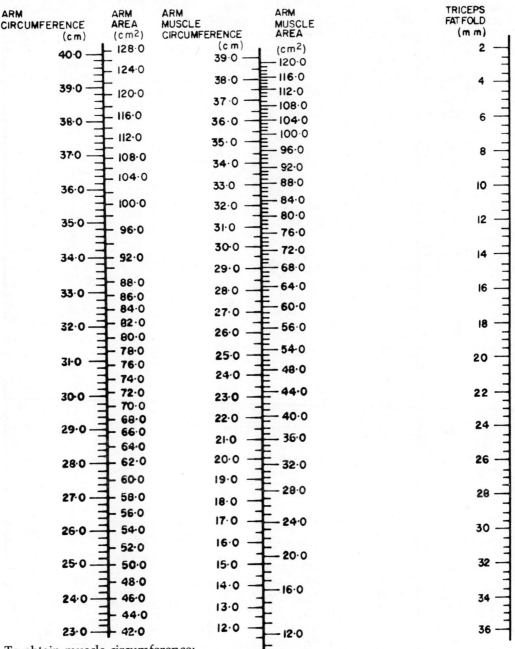

To obtain muscle circumference:
1. Lay ruler between values of arm circumference and fatfold.
2. Read off muscle circumference on middle line.

To obtain tissue areas:
1. The arm areas and muscle areas are alongside their respective circumferences.
2. Fat area = arm area − muscle area.

*From Gurney, JM; Jelliffe, DB: Arm anthropometry in nutritional assessment: Nomogram for rapid calculation of muscle circumference and cross-sectional muscle fat areas. *American Journal of Clinical Nutrition* 26(9):912, 1973, with permission.

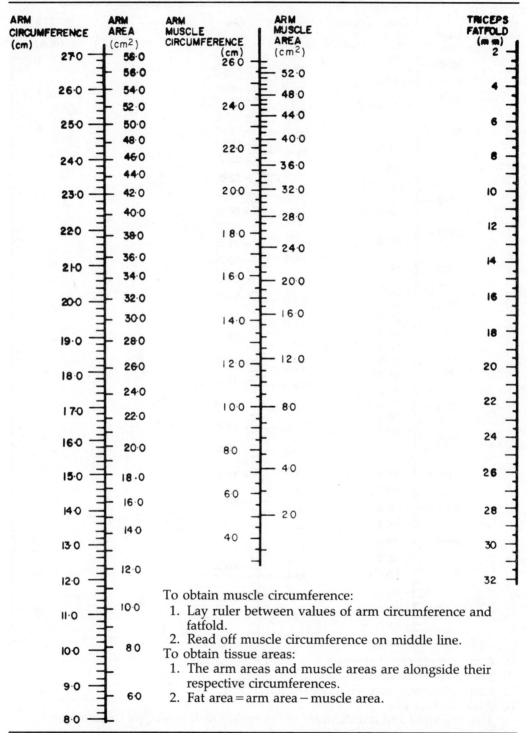

To obtain muscle circumference:
1. Lay ruler between values of arm circumference and fatfold.
2. Read off muscle circumference on middle line.

To obtain tissue areas:
1. The arm areas and muscle areas are alongside their respective circumferences.
2. Fat area = arm area − muscle area.

*From Gurney, JM; Jelliffe, DB: Arm anthropometry in nutritional assessment: Nomogram for rapid calculation of muscle circumference and cross-sectional muscle fat areas. *American Journal of Clinical Nutrition* 26(9):912, 1973, with permission.

NAME _____ RECORD # _____

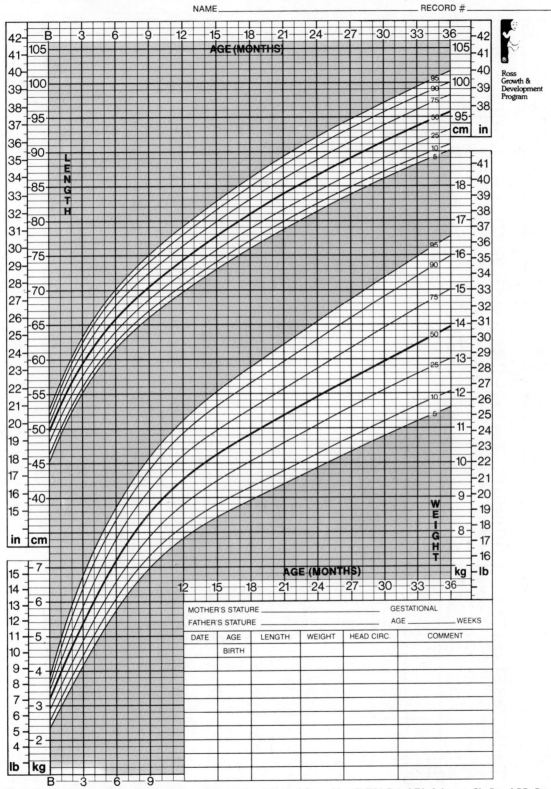

Appendix C–6a. *Physical growth of girls: Birth to 36 months. Adapted from: Hamill PVV, Drizd TA, Johnson CL, Reed RB, Roche AF, Moore WM: Physical growth : National Center for Health Statistics percentiles. AM J CLIN NUTR 32:607-629, 1979. Data from the Fels Longitudinal Study, Wright State University School of Medicine, Yellow Springs, Ohio, by permission.*
© 1982 Ross Laboratories

NAME_____ RECORD #_____

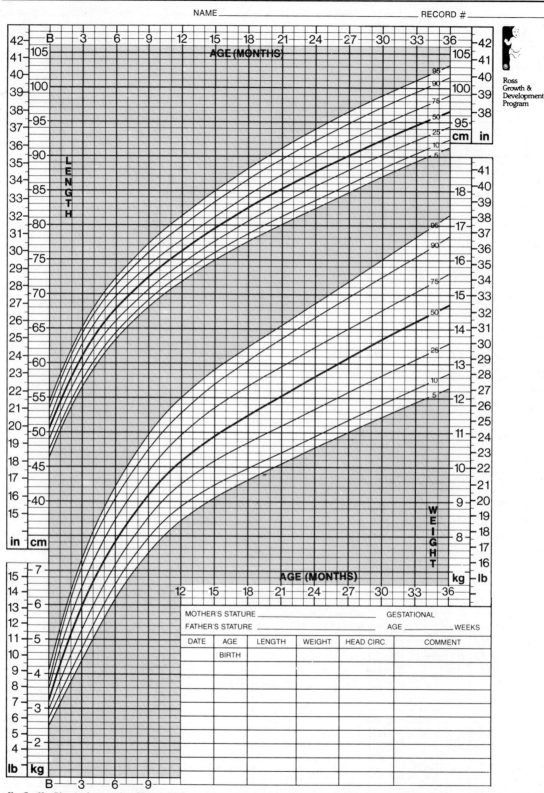

Ross
Growth &
Development
Program

MOTHER'S STATURE_____ GESTATIONAL
FATHER'S STATURE_____ AGE_____WEEKS

DATE	AGE	LENGTH	WEIGHT	HEAD CIRC.	COMMENT
	BIRTH				

Appendix C–6b. Physical growth of boys: Birth to 36 months. Adapted from: Hamill PVV, Drizd TA, Johnson CL, Reed RB, Roche AF, Moore WM: Physical growth : National Center for Health Statistics percentiles. AM J CLIN NUTR 32:607-629, 1979. Data from the Fels Longitudinal Study, Wright State University School of Medicine, Yellow Springs, Ohio, by permission.

Appendix C–6c. Girls: 2 to 18 Years Physical Growth NCHS Percentiles*

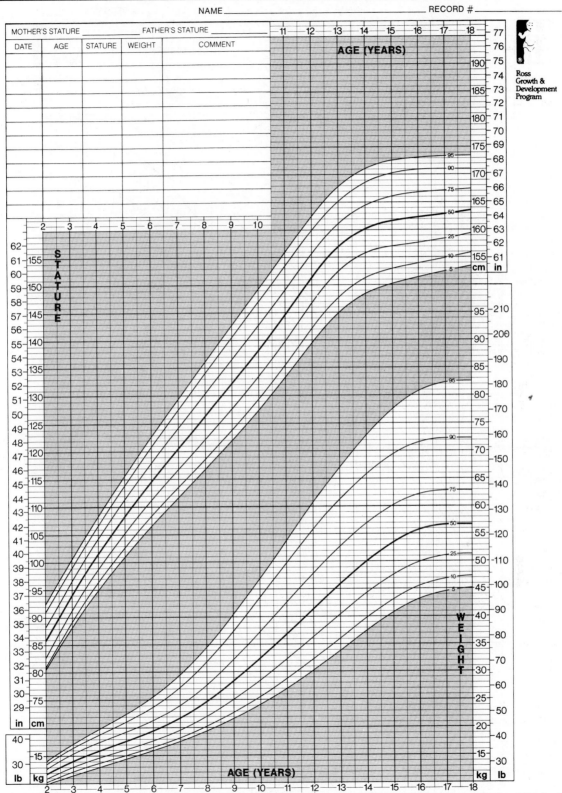

Appendix C–6c. Physical growth of girls: 2 to 18 years old. Adapted from: Hamill PVV, Drizd TA, Johnson CL, Reed RB, Roche AF, Moore WM: Physical growth: National Center for Health Statistics percentiles. AM J CLIN NUTR 32:607-629, 1979. Data from the National Center for Health Statistics (NCHS), Hyattsville, Maryland.

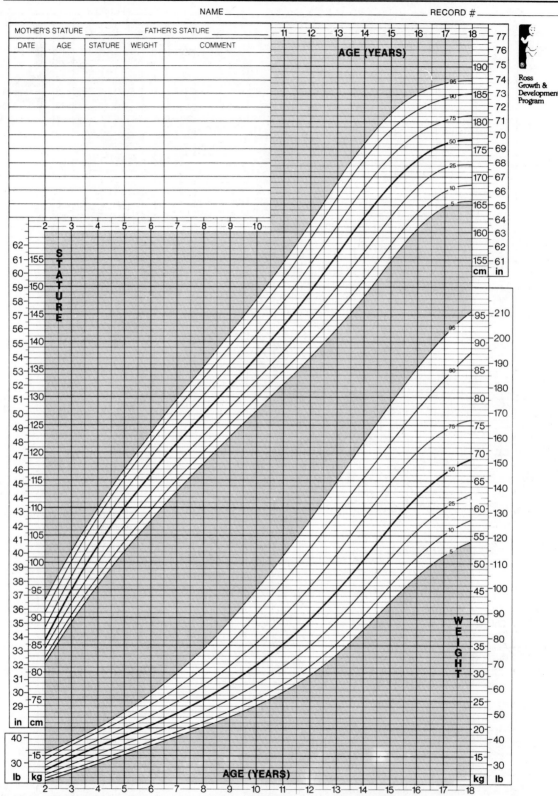

Appendix C–6d. Physical growth of boys: 2 to 18 years old. Adapted from: Hamill PVV, Drizd TA, Johnson CL, Reed RB, Roche AF, Moore WM: Physical growth: National Center for Health Statistics percentiles. AM J CLIN NUTR 32:607-629, 1979. Data from the National Center for Health Statistics (NCHS), Hyattsville, Maryland. © 1982 Ross Laboratories

Appendix C–7. Physiological Values for Evaluating Nutritional Status

Blood or Serum Values

Physical Measurements	Normal Ranges
Osmolality	275–297 mOsm/kg
pH	
Arterial blood	7.35–7.45
Venous blood	7.34–7.41
Specific gravity	1.025–1.030
Viscosity	4.5–5.0
Protein	
Protein, total	6.6–7.5 gm/dl
Albumin	4.0–5.5 gm/dl
Globulin	1.5–3.0 gm/dl
Albumin/globulin ratio	1.2–2.5
Fibrinogen	0.2–0.4 gm/100 ml
Hemoglobin	
Men	14–18 gm/dl
Women	12–16 gm/dl
Children	10–18 gm/dl
Hematology	
Cell volume	39–50%
Erythrocytes	
Men	4.2–5.4 million/mm^3
Women	3.6–5.0 million/mm^3
Hematocrit (Vol % red cells or packed cell volume)	
Men	40–54%
Women	37–47%
Leukocytes	5000–10,000/mm^3
Platelets (thrombocytes)	125,000–350,000/mm^3
Whole blood volume	55–80 ml/kg
White blood count	5000–10,000/mm^3
Basophils	0–1.0%
Eosinophils	0.5–4%
Lymphocytes	20–40%
Monocytes	4–8%
Neutrophils	50–65%
Nitrogenous substances	
Amino acid nitrogen	4–8 mg/100 ml
Ammonia, blood	40–110 mg/dl
Creatinine	0.2–1.5 mg/dl
Nonprotein nitrogen, blood	25–35 mg/dl
Blood urea nitrogen (BUN)	8–18 mg/100 dl
Urea, blood	20–45 mg/dl
Uric acid, blood	2.5–7 mg/dl
Minerals	
Base, total fixed (serum)	142–155 mEq/L
Calcium, serum	4.5–5.3 mEq/L
Chlorides, serum	95–105 mEq/L
Copper	0.75–1.45 mcg/ml
Iodine, protein-bound	4.0–8.0 mcg/dl
Iron	
Men	75–175 mcg/dl
Women	65–165 mcg/dl
Iron-binding capacity, total or transferrin test	250–450 mg/dl
Magnesium	1.5–2.5 mEq/L
Phosphorus, inorganic (serum)	2.5–4.5 mg/dl
Potassium (serum)	3.5–5.0 mEq/L
Sodium (serum)	136–142 mEq/L (<65 years old)
	132–140 mEq/L (>65 years old)
Sulfates, inorganic (serum)	0.5–1.0 mEq/L
Zinc	0.75–1.4 mcg/ml
Carbohydrates	
Glucose (fasting blood sugar, FBS)	
Serum	70–110 mg/dl
Whole blood	60–100 mg/dl

Appendix continued on following page

Appendix C–7. *Physiological Values for Evaluating Nutritional Status* (*Continued*)

Blood or Serum Values (*Continued*)

Physical Measurements	*Normal Ranges*
Lipids	
Fats, neutral	140–300 mg/dl
Fatty acids, serum (total)	350–450 mg/dl
Vitamins	
Ascorbic acid	
Serum	0.3–2.0 mg/dl
White blood cells	25–40 mg/dl
Carotene	48–200 mcg/dl
Folate (serum)	2–20 ng/ml
Riboflavin	15–25 mcg/dl
Thiamin	2–5 mcg/dl
Vitamin A	50–125 IU/dl
Vitamin B_{12}	300–8000 mcg/dl
Blood Gases	
Carbon dioxide content	
Serum	45–75 vol%
Whole blood	40–60 vol%
Oxygen content	
Arterial blood	5–22 vol%
Venous blood	11–16 vol%
Oxygen saturation	
Arterial blood	≥95%
Venous blood	70–80%

Appendix C–7. *Physiological Values for Evaluating Nutritional Status (Continued)*

Urine Values

Physical Measurements	Normal Ranges
pH	5.5–8.0
Osmolality	<100, dehydration >800
Specific gravity	1.001–1.035
Volume	800–1600 ml/24 hr
Constituents	
Total solids	50–70 gm/24 hr
Acetone bodies	0.003–0.015 gm/24 hr
Calcium	males <275 mg/24 hr
	females <250 mg/24 hr
Chloride (as NaCl)	10–20 gm/24 hr
Glucose	trace
Iron	0.001–0.006 gm/24 hr
Nitrogenous constituents	
Total nitrogen	10–18 gm/24 hr
Amino acids	50–200 mg/24 hr
Ammonia	0.5–1.0 gm/24 hr
Creatinine clearance	0.7–1.5 mg/ml
Protein (albumin)	10–100 mg/24 hr
Uric Acid	0.4–1.0 gm/24 hr (normal diet)
Oxalate	30–90 mEq/24 hr
Potassium	40–80 mEq/24 hr
Sodium	130–200 mEq/24 hr
Vanillylmandelic acid (VMA)	Up to 9 mg/24 hr

Appendix C–8. Nutrients Detrimentally Affected by Drugs*

Drugs by Classification	GI Disturbances	Anorexia	Protein Metabolism	Carbohydrate Metabolism	Fat Metabolism	Vitamin A	Vitamin D	Vitamin K	Thiamin	Riboflavin	Niacin	Vitamin B₁₂	Vitamin B₆	Folate	Vitamin C	Calcium	Phosphorus	Iron	Sodium	Potassium	Magnesium	Zinc	Remarks
Analgesics																							
Alcohol			X						X			X		X							X		
Aspirin								X						X	X			X		X		X	
Antacids																							
Aluminum hydroxide									X								X						
Magnesium hydroxide (and others)									X									X					
Sodium bicarbonate														X	X								Can cause alkalosis if taken with milk.
Anticoagulants																							
Coumarin derivatives		X						X															Antagonized by high levels of vitamins K and E.
Anticonvulsants																							
Phenobarbital							X					X	X	X		X					X		
Phenytoin							X					X	X	X		X					X		Supplement with less than 5 mg/day folic acid.
Primidone		X					X					X	X	X		X							
Antidepressants																							
Lithium carbonate	X																						Force fluids.
MAO inhibitors				X																			Avoid foods high in tyramine.
Antigout																							
Colchicine	X		X		X	X						X				X			X	X	X		Decreased serum cholesterol.
Antimicrobials																							
Chloramphenicol			X							X		X	X	X				X					
Penicillin																				X			Do not take with acidic beverages.
Tetracycline	X	X	X			X		X							X	X		X			X		Do not take with milk products, iron, or antacids.
Neomycin		X	X	X	X	X	X	X				X				X		X	X	X			Can lead to deficiency of fat-soluble vitamins.
Erythromycin	X																						Do not take with acidic beverages.
Sulfonamides	X	X												X									
Griseofulvin	X	X																X		X			Optimal absorption with high-fat meal.
Antineoplastic																							
Methotrexate	X	X	X	X	X							X		X									
5-Fluorouracil	X	X	X	X	X							X											Force fluids; avoid alcohol.

760

Drug	Dietary Consideration
Antiparkinsonian	
Levodopa	Antagonized by high-protein, B$_6$-rich foods.
Antitubercular	
Para-aminosalicylic acid	Force fluids.
Isonicotinic acid hydrazide	Avoid foods high in tyramine.
Cycloserine	
Cathartics	
Bisacodyl	Alkaline foods will dissolve coating, causing GI irritation.
Mineral oil	
Phenolphthalein	
Chelating Agents	
Penicillamine	Force fluids (16 oz. at bedtime).
Corticosteroids	Food may protect stomach against ulceration.
Diuretics	
Furosemide	Encourage foods high in potassium and calcium.
Thiazides	Avoid imported licorice; encourage high-potassium foods.
Triamterene	Avoid high-potassium foods.
Spironolactone	
Hypocholesterolemics	
Cholestyramine resin	
Clofibrate	
Hypotensive Agents	
Hydralazine	
Methyldopa	Take with food to increase bioavailability.
Oral Contraceptives	
Sedatives/Hypnotics	
Glutethimide	
Barbiturates	
Uricosuric	
Allopurinol	Force fluids.
Probenecid	Force fluids.

*Adapted from Roe, DA: Handbook: Interaction of Selected Drugs and Nutrients in Patients. Chicago, American Dietetic Association, 1982.

Appendix C–9. Possible Interrelationships Among the Four Parameters of Nutritional Assessment*

	Anthropometry	Laboratory	Physical Signs	Dietary Intake
Calories	Underweight (weight for height less than 80% of usual)		Muscular system—muscle wasting Skin—loss of subcutaneous fat, delayed wound healing	Inadequate food intake for caloric requirement, including fat, CHO, and protein
Protein	Underweight (weight for height less than 80% of usual)	Low serum albumin Low T-lymphocyte count Low Hgb–normocytic anemia Low Hct–normocytic anemia Low serum creatinine Unreactivity to skin tests (PPD, *Candida,* DNCB)† Low serum vitamin	Hair—lack of natural shine, dull, dry, sparse, shedding, dyspigmented, loss of curl, easily pluckable Muscular system—muscular wasting Skin—pressure sores, edematous, delayed wound healing	Inadequate intake from meat/protein group (meat, poultry, fish, dried beans and peas, eggs) and/or milk group (cheese, milk)
Fat	Underweight (weight for height less than 80% of usual)		Skin—sandpaper feel, dry and flaky, loss of subcutaneous fat	Insufficient butter, fat, margarine, oils, salad dressing
Vitamins A		Low serum vitamin A† Low serum carotene†	Eyes—Bitot's spots, dryness of eye membranes, soft cornea Skin—sandpaper feel, dry and flaky	Insufficient intake of green leafy or yellow vegetables (carrots, spinach, broccoli)
Riboflavin		Low urinary riboflavin excretion†	Face—scaling of skin around nostrils Eyes—redness and fissuring of eyelid corners Lips—redness and swelling, cracks at sides of mouth Tongue—magenta color	Insufficient intake from milk group (milk, cheese, yogurt)
Niacin		Low urinary niacin metabolite excretion†	Lips—cracks at sides of mouth Tongue—abnormally red Skin—red, swollen, pigmentation, scaling around nostrils Eyes—redness and fissuring of eyelid corners	Inadequate intake from bread and cereal group (enriched and whole grain products) and/or meat group (meat, poultry, fish, liver)

Appendix C–9. *Possible Interrelationships Among the Four Parameters of Nutritional Assessment* * (*Continued*)

	Anthropometry	Laboratory	Physical Signs	Dietary Intake
Thiamin		Low urinary thiamin excretion		Inadequate intake from bread and cereal group (enriched and whole-grain products) and/or meat group (pork)
B_6		Low Hgb—microcytic anemia Low Hct—microcytic anemia Low urinary B_6 level†	Eyes—redness and fissuring of eyelid corners Lips—cracks at sides of mouth Tongue—abnormally red	Inadequate intake of meat, vegetables, whole-grain cereals
Folate		Low Hgb—macrocytic anemia Low Hct—macrocytic anemia Low serum folic acid†	Tongue—abnormally red, raw, fissured, swollen, pale, atrophic, smooth Skin—excessive darkness	Inadequate intake of green, leafy vegetables, liver, wheat germ, whole-grain products
B_{12}		Low Hgb—macrocytic anemia Low Hct—macrocytic anemia Low serum B_{12}†	Tongue—abnormally red, pale, atrophic, smooth Skin—excessive darkness	Inadequate intake of animal products
C		Low serum vitamin C†	Gums—spongy, bleeding, abnormally red Skin—petechiae, delayed wound healing	Inadequate intake of citrus fruits or juices (orange, grapefruit)
D		Low serum calcium† Low serum phosphate†		Inadequate intake from milk group (milk, cheese, yogurt)
K		Prothrombin deficiency†		
Minerals				
Iron		Low Hgb—microcytic anemia Low Hct—microcytic anemia	Eyes—pale eye membranes Tongue—pale, atrophic, smooth Nails—spoon-shaped, brittle, ridged Skin—pale	Inadequate intake of meat group (red meats, liver, dried beans, peas), bread and cereal group (enriched cereal products), dried fruits
Zinc		Low serum zinc†		

*From *A Guide to Nutritional Care*. Mead Johnson Nutritional Division, Mead Johnson & Co, Evansville, IN 47721.
†These tests are recommended in this nutritional assessment program (see Sauerblich, HE; Dowdy, RP; Skala, H: *Laboratory Tests for the Assessment of Nutritional Status.* Cleveland, CRC Press, Inc, 1974, for further details).

Appendix D–1. *Dietary Fiber and Carbohydrate Content of Foods*
*per 100 gm Edible Portion**

FOOD	Carbohydrate			Dietary Fiber (gm)
	Total (gm)	Sugar† (gm)	Starch (gm)	
Cereals and breads				
Arrowroot	94.0	Trace	94.0	—
Barley (pearl), raw	83.6	Trace	83.6	6.5
Barley, boiled	27.6	Trace	27.6	2.2
Bemax	44.7	16.0	28.7	—
Bran (wheat)	26.8	3.8	23.0	44.0
Corn flour	92.0	Trace	92.0	—
Custard powder	92.0	Trace	92.0	—
Flour (whole meal 100%)	65.8	2.3	63.5	9.6
Flour, brown (85%)	68.8	1.9	66.9	7.5
Flour, white (72%)	74.8	1.5	73.3	3.0
Flour, household, plain	80.1	1.7	78.4	3.4
Flour, self-rising	77.5	1.4	76.1	3.7
Patent (40%)	78.0	1.4	76.6	—
Macaroni, raw	79.2	Trace	79.2	—
Macaroni, boiled	25.2	Trace	25.2	—
Oatmeal, raw	72.8	Trace	72.8	7.0
Porridge	8.2	Trace	8.2	0.8
Rice, polished, raw	86.8	Trace	86.8	2.4
Rice, boiled	29.6	Trace	26.9	0.8
Rye flour (100%)	75.9	Trace	15.9	—
Sago, raw	94.0	Trace	94.0	—
Semolina, raw	77.5	Trace	77.5	—
Soya flour, full fat	23.5	11.2	12.3	11.9
Soya flour, low fat	28.2	13.4	14.8	14.3
Spaghetti, raw	84.0	2.7	81.3	—
Spaghetti, boiled	26.0	0.8	25.2	—
Spaghetti, canned, in tomato sauce	12.2	3.4	8.8	—
Tapioca, raw	95.0	Trace	95.0	—
Bread				
Whole meal	41.8	2.1	39.7	8.5
Brown	44.7	1.8	42.9	5.1
Hovis	45.1	2.4	42.7	4.6
White	49.7	1.8	47.9	2.7
White, fried	51.3	1.7	49.6	(2.2)‡
Toasted	64.9	2.1	62.8	(2.8)
Dried crumbs	77.5	2.6	74.9	(3.4)
Currant	51.8	13.0	38.8	(1.7)
Malt	49.4	18.6	30.8	—
Soda	56.3	3.0	53.3	2.3
Rolls, brown, crusty	57.2	2.1	55.1	(5.9)
Rolls, brown, soft	47.9	1.9	46.0	(5.4)
Rolls, white, crusty	57.2	2.1	55.1	(3.1)
Rolls, white, soft	53.6	1.9	51.7	(2.9)
Rolls, starch reduced	45.7	1.6	44.1	(2.0)
Chapatis with fat	50.2	1.8	46.5	3.7
Chapatis without fat	43.7	1.6	42.1	(3.4)
Breakfast cereals				
All-Bran	43.0	15.4	27.6	26.7
Corn Flakes	85.1	7.4	77.7	11.0
Grape Nuts	75.9	9.5	66.4	7.0
Muesli	66.2	26.2	40.0	7.4
Puffed Wheat	68.5	1.5	67.0	15.4
Ready Brek	69.9	2.2	67.7	7.6
Rice Krispies	88.1	9.0	79.1	4.5
Shredded Wheat	67.9	0.4	67.5	12.3
Special K	78.2	9.6	68.6	5.5
Sugar Puffs	84.5	56.5	28.0	6.1
Weeta Bix	70.3	6.1	66.5	12.7
Biscuits				
Chocolate, full coated	67.4	43.4	24.0	3.1

Appendix D–1. Dietary Fiber and Carbohydrate Content of Foods
per 100 gm Edible Portion* (Continued)

| | Carbohydrate | | | Dietary |
FOOD	Total (gm)	Sugar† (gm)	Starch (gm)	Fiber (gm)
Cream crackers	68.3	Trace	68.3	(3.0)
Crisp bread, rye	70.6	3.2	67.4	11.7
Crisp wheat, starch reduced	36.9	7.4	29.5	4.9
Digestive, plain	66.0	16.4	49.6	(5.5)
Digestive, chocolate	66.5	28.5	38.0	3.5
Ginger nuts	79.1	35.8	43.3	2.0
Homemade	65.5	26.8	38.7	1.7
Matzo	86.6	4.2	82.4	3.9
Oatcakes	63.0	3.1	59.9	4.0
Sandwich	69.2	30.2	39.0	1.2
Semisweet	74.8	22.3	52.5	2.3
Short-sweet	62.2	24.1	38.1	1.7
Shortbread	65.5	17.2	48.3	2.1
Wafers, filled	66.0	44.7	21.3	1.6
Water biscuits	75.8	2.3	73.5	(3.2)
Fruits				
Apples, just flesh	11.9	11.8	0.1	2.0
Apples, flesh, skin, core	9.2	9.1	0.1	1.5
Apples, cooking, raw	9.6	9.2	0.4	2.4
Apples, stewed, no sugar	8.2	7.9	0.3	2.1
Apples, stewed, with sugar	17.3	17.0	0.3	1.9
Apricots, fresh, raw	6.7	6.7	0	2.1
Apricots, stewed, no sugar	5.7	5.6	0	1.7
Apricots, stewed, with sugar	15.6	15.6	0	1.6
Apricots, dried, raw	43.4	43.4	0	24.0
Apricots, dried, stewed, without sugar	16.1	16.1	0	8.9
Apricots, dried, stewed, with sugar	19.9	19.9	0	8.5
Apricots, canned	27.7	27.7	0	1.3
Avocados	1.8	1.8	Trace	2.0
Bananas, raw	19.2	16.2	3.0	3.4
Blackberries, raw	6.4	6.4	0	7.3
Blackberries, stewed, no sugar	5.5	5.5	0	6.3
Blackberries, stewed, with sugar	14.8	14.8	0	5.7
Cherries, eating, raw	11.9	11.9	0	1.7
Cherries, cooking, raw	11.6	11.6	0	1.7
Cherries, stewed, no sugar	9.8	9.7	0	1.4
Cherries, stewed, with sugar	20.1	19.7	0	1.2
Cranberries, raw	3.5	3.5	0	4.2
Currants, black, raw	6.6	6.6	0	8.7
Currants, black, stewed, no sugar	5.6	5.6	0	7.4
Currants, black, stewed, with sugar	15.0	15.0	0	6.8
Currants, red, raw	4.4	4.4	0	8.2
Currants, red, stewed, no sugar	3.8	3.8	0	7.0
Currants, red, stewed, with sugar	13.3	13.3	0	6.4
Currants, white, raw	5.6	5.6	0	6.8
Currants, stewed, no sugar	4.8	4.8	0	5.8
Currants, stewed, with sugar	14.2	14.2	0	5.3
Currants, dried	63.1	63.1	0	6.5
Dates, dried	63.9	63.9	0	8.7
Dates, dried, with pits	54.9	54.9	0	7.5
Figs, green, raw	9.5	9.5	0	2.5
Figs, dried, raw	52.9	52.9	0	18.5
Figs, stewed, no sugar	29.4	29.4	0	10.3
Figs, stewed, with sugar	34.3	34.3	0	9.7
Fruit pie filling, canned	25.1	23.2	1.9	(1.8)
Fruit salad, canned	25.0	25.0	0	1.1
Gooseberries, green raw	3.4	3.4	0	3.2
Gooseberries, stewed, no sugar	2.9	2.9	0	2.7
Gooseberries, stewed, with sugar	12.5	12.5	0	2.5
Gooseberries, ripe, raw	9.2	9.2	0	3.5
Grapes, black, raw	15.5	15.5	0	0.4

Appendix continued on following page

Appendix D–1. Dietary Fiber and Carbohydrate Content of Foods
per 100 gm Edible Portion* (Continued)

| | Carbohydrate | | | Dietary |
FOOD	Total (gm)	Sugar† (gm)	Starch (gm)	Fiber (gm)
Grapes, white, raw	16.1	16.1	0	0.9
Grapefruit, raw	5.3	5.3	0	0.6
Grapefruit, canned	15.5	15.5	0	0.4
Green gages	11.8	11.8	0	2.6
Green gages, stewed, no sugar	10.0	10.0	0	2.2
Green gages, stewed, with sugar	19.4	19.2	0	2.1
Guavas, canned	15.7	15.7	Trace	3.6
Lemons, whole	3.2	3.2	0	5.2
Lemon juice, fresh	1.6	1.6	0	0
Loganberries, raw	3.4	3.4	0	6.2
Loganberries, stewed, no sugar	3.1	3.1	0	5.7
Loganberries, stewed, with sugar	13.4	13.4	0	5.2
Loganberries, canned	26.2	26.2	0	3.3
Lychees, raw	16.0	16.0	0	(0.5)
Lychees, canned	17.7	17.7	0	0.4
Mandarin oranges, canned	14.2	14.2	0	0.3
Mangoes, raw	15.3	15.3	Trace	(1.5)
Mangoes, canned	20.3	20.2	0.1	1.0
Melons				
Cantaloupe, raw	5.3	5.3	0	1.0
Yellow honeydew, raw	5.0	5.0	0	0.9
Watermelon, raw	5.3	5.3	0	—
Mulberries, raw	8.1	8.1	0	1.7
Nectarines, raw	12.4	12.4	0	2.4
Olives, in brine	Trace	Trace	0	4.4
Oranges, raw	8.5	8.5	0	2.0
Orange juice, fresh	9.4	9.4	0	0
Passion fruit, raw	6.2	6.2	0	15.9
Pawpaw, canned	17.0	17.0	0	0.5
Peaches, fresh, raw	9.1	9.1	0	1.4
Peaches, dried, raw	53.0	53.0	0	14.3
Peaches, stewed, no sugar	19.6	19.6	0	5.3
Peaches, stewed, with sugar	23.3	23.3	0	5.1
Peaches, canned	22.9	22.9	0	1.0
Pears, eating	10.6	10.6	0	2.3
Pears, cooking, raw	9.3	9.3	Trace	2.9
Pears, stewed, no sugar	7.9	7.9	Trace	2.5
Pears, stewed, with sugar	17.1	17.1	Trace	2.3
Pears, canned	20.0	20.0	0	1.7
Pineapple, fresh	11.6	11.6	0	1.2
Pineapple, canned	20.2	20.2	0	0.9
Plums, Victoria dessert, raw	9.6	9.6	0	2.1
Plums, cooking, raw	6.2	6.2	0	2.5
Plums, stewed, no sugar	5.2	5.2	0	2.2
Plums, stewed, with sugar	15.3	15.1	0	1.9
Pomegranate juice	11.6	11.6	0	0
Prunes, dried, raw	40.3	40.3	0	16.1
Prunes, stewed, no sugar	20.4	20.4	0	8.1
Prunes, stewed, with sugar	26.5	26.5	0	7.7
Raisins, dried	64.4	64.4	0	6.8
Raspberries, raw	5.6	5.6	0	7.4
Raspberries, stewed, no sugar	5.9	5.9	0	7.8
Raspberries, stewed, with sugar	17.3	17.3	0	7.0
Raspberries, canned	22.5	22.5	0	(5.0)
Rhubarb, raw	1.0	1.0	0	2.6
Rhubarb, stewed, no sugar	0.9	0.9	0	2.4
Rhubarb, stewed, with sugar	11.4	11.4	0	2.2
Strawberries, raw	6.2	6.2	0	2.3
Strawberries, canned	21.1	21.1	0	1.0
Sultanas, dried	64.7	64.7	0	7.0
Tangerines, raw	8.0	8.0	0	1.9

Appendix D–1. Dietary Fiber and Carbohydrate Content of Foods
per 100 gm Edible Portion* (Continued)

FOOD	Carbohydrate			Dietary Fiber (gm)
	Total (gm)	Sugar† (gm)	Starch (gm)	
Nuts				
Almonds	4.3	4.3	0	14.3
Barcelona nuts	5.2	3.4	1.8	10.3
Brazil nuts	4.1	1.7	2.4	9.0
Chestnuts	36.6	7.0	29.6	6.8
Cob or hazelnuts	6.8	4.7	2.1	6.1
Coconut, fresh	3.7	3.7	0	13.6
Coconut, milk	4.9	4.9	0	(Trace)
Coconut, desiccated	6.4	6.4	0	23.5
Peanuts, fresh	8.6	3.1	5.5	8.1
Peanuts, roasted, salted	8.6	3.1	5.5	8.1
Peanut butter, smooth	13.1	6.7	6.4	7.6
Walnuts	5.0	3.2	1.8	5.2
Vegetables				
Artichokes, globe, boiled	2.7	—	0	—
Asparagus, boiled	1.1	1.1	0	1.5
Aubergine, raw	3.1	2.9	0.2	2.5
Beans, French, boiled	1.1	0.8	0.3	3.2
Beans, runner, raw	3.9	2.8	1.1	2.9
Beans, broad, boiled	7.1	0.6	6.5	4.2
Beans, red kidney, raw	45.0	(3.0)	(42.0)	(25.0)
Bean sprouts, canned	0.8	0.4	0.4	3.0
Broccoli, tops, raw	2.5	2.5	Trace	3.6
Broccoli, boiled	1.6	1.5	0.1	4.1
Brussels sprouts, raw	2.7	2.6	0.1	4.2
Brussels sprouts, boiled	1.7	1.6	0.1	2.9
Cabbage, red, raw	3.5	3.5	Trace	3.4
Cabbage, white, raw	3.5	3.7	0.1	2.7
Carrots, old, raw	5.4	5.4	0	2.9
Carrots, boiled	4.3	4.2	0.1	3.1
Carrots, young, boiled	4.5	4.4	0.1	3.0
Carrots, canned	4.4	4.4	Trace	3.7
Cauliflower, raw	1.5	1.5	Trace	2.1
Cauliflower, boiled	0.8	0.8	Trace	1.8
Celery, raw	1.3	1.2	0.1	1.8
Celery, boiled	0.7	0.7	0	2.2
Chicory, raw	1.5	—	0	—
Corn, sweet, on-the-cob, raw	23.7	1.7	22.0	3.7
Corn, sweet, on-the-cob, boiled	22.8	1.7	21.1	4.7
Corn, sweet, canned, kernels	16.1	8.9	7.2	5.7
Cucumber, raw	1.8	1.8	0	0.4
Endive, raw	1.0	1.0	0	2.2
Horseradish, raw	11.0	7.3	3.7	8.3
Leeks, raw	6.0	6.0	0	3.1
Leeks, boiled	4.6	4.6	0	3.9
Lentils, raw	53.2	2.4	50.8	11.7
Lentils, split, boiled	17.0	0.8	16.2	3.7
Lettuce, raw	1.2	1.2	Trace	1.5
Mushrooms, raw	0	0	0	2.5
Mustard and cress, raw	0.9	0.9	0	3.7
Okra, raw	2.3	2.3	Trace	(3.2)
Onions, raw	5.2	5.2	0	1.3
Onions, boiled	2.7	2.7	0	1.3
Parsley, raw	Trace	Trace	0	9.1
Parsnips, raw	11.3	8.8	2.5	4.0
Parsnips, boiled	13.5	2.7	10.8	2.5
Peas, fresh, raw	10.6	4.0	6.6	5.2
Peas, fresh, boiled	7.7	1.8	5.9	5.2
Peas, frozen, raw	7.2	4.1	3.4	7.8
Peas, frozen, boiled	4.3	1.0	3.3	12.0
Peas, canned, garden	7.0	3.6	3.4	6.3

Appendix continued on following page

Appendix D–1. Dietary Fiber and Carbohydrate Content of Foods per 100 gm Edible Portion* (Continued)

FOOD	Carbohydrate			Dietary Fiber (gm)
	Total (gm)	Sugar† (gm)	Starch (gm)	
Peas, processed	13.7	1.3	12.4	7.9
Peas, dried, raw	50.0	2.4	47.6	16.7
Peas, dried, boiled	19.1	0.9	18.2	4.8
Peas, split, dried, raw	56.6	1.9	54.7	11.9
Peas, split, dried, boiled	21.9	0.9	21.0	5.1
Peas, chick Bengal gram, raw	50.0	(10.0)	(40.0)	(15.0)
Peas, red pigeon, raw	54.0	(9.0)	(45.0)	(15.0)
Peppers, green raw	2.2	2.2	Trace	0.9
Peppers, green, boiled	1.8	1.7	0.1	0.9
Plantain, green, raw	28.3	0.8	27.5	(5.8)
Plantain, green, boiled	31.1	0.9	30.2	6.4
Potatoes, old, raw	20.8	0.5	20.3	2.1
Potatoes, boiled	19.7	0.4	19.3	1.0
Potatoes, mashed, with margarine and milk	18.0	0.6	17.4	0.9
Potatoes, baked	25.0	0.6	24.4	2.5
Potatoes, new, boiled	18.3	0.7	17.6	2.0
Potatoes, new, canned	12.6	0.4	12.2	2.5
Potatoes, instant powder	73.2	2.2	71.0	16.5
Potatoes, instant powder, made up	16.1	0.5	15.6	3.6
Potato chips	49.3	0.7	48.6	11.9
Pumpkin, raw	3.4	2.7	0.7	0.5
Radishes, raw	2.8	2.8	0	1.0
Spinach, boiled	1.4	1.2	0.2	6.3
Spring greens, boiled	0.9	0.9	0	3.8
Sweet potatoes, raw	21.5	(9.7)	(11.8)	(2.5)
Sweet potatoes, boiled	20.1	9.1	11.0	2.3
Tomatoes, raw	2.8	2.8	Trace	1.5
Tomatoes, canned	2.0	2.0	Trace	0.9
Turnips, raw	3.8	3.8	0	2.8
Turnips, boiled	2.8	2.3	0	2.2
Turnip tops, boiled	0.1	0	0.1	3.9
Watercress, raw	0.7	0.6	0.1	3.3
Yams, raw	32.4	1.0	31.4	(4.1)
Yams, boiled	29.8	0.2	29.6	3.9

*Adapted from Floch, M.H.: *Nutrition and Diet Therapy in Gastrointestinal Disease.* New York, Plenum Medical Book Company, 1981. Data from Paul, A.A., and Southgate, D.A.T.: *McCance and Widdowson's The Composition of Foods.* 4th ed. New York, Elsevier/North Holland Biomedical Press, 1978.

†Sugar includes all free monosaccharides and disaccharides.

‡Values in parentheses are taken from the literature.

Appendix D–2. Cholesterol and Fat Content of Foods*

Food	Amount	Cholesterol (mg)	Total Fat (g)	Saturated Fat (g)	Polyunsaturated Fat (g)
Meat, Fish, Poultry (cooked)					
LOW-FAT, LESS THAN 3 G/OZ					
Beef					
Brisket, lean only	28 g (1 oz.)	25.5	2.9	1.3	0.2
Flank steak	28 g (1 oz.)	25.5	2.0	0.9	0.1
T-bone steak, lean	28 g (1 oz.)	25.5	2.9	1.2	0.2
Sirloin steak, lean	28 g (1 oz.)	25.5	2.2	0.9	0.1
Short plate, lean	28 g (1 oz.)	25.5	2.9	1.3	0.2
Round steak, lean	28 g (1 oz.)	25.5	1.8	0.8	0.1
Rump, lean	28 g (1 oz.)	25.5	2.6	1.1	0.2
Pork					
Leg, lean only	28 g (1 oz.)	25.0	2.5	0.9	0.1
Leg, cured lean	28 g (1 oz.)	25.0	2.5	0.8	0.3
Lamb					
Leg, lean only	28 g (1 oz.)	27.0	2.7	1.1	0.2
Loin, lean only	28 g (1 oz.)	27.0	1.7	0.7	0.1
Rib, lean only	28 g (1 oz.)	27.0	2.0	0.8	0.1
Shoulder, lean only	28 g (1 oz.)	27.0	1.6	0.7	0.1
Veal					
All cuts, separable lean	28 g (1 oz.)	25.2	0.7	0.2	0.1
Foreshank, total edible	28 g (1 oz.)	25.2	2.9	1.2	0.1
Fish (fillet)					
Anchovies	28 g (1 oz.)	—	1.8	0.5	0.6
Bass, striped	28 g (1 oz.)	—	0.6	0.1	0.2
Cod, Atlantic	28 g (1 oz.)	14.0	0.2	tr	0.1
Flounder	28 g (1 oz.)	14.0	0.3	0.1	0.1
Haddock	28 g (1 oz.)	17.0	0.2	tr	0.1
Halibut, Atlantic	28 g (1 oz.)	14.0	0.3	0.1	0.1
Herring, Atlantic	28 g (1 oz.)	24.0	1.7	0.5	0.4
Mackerel, Atlantic	28 g (1 oz.)	27.0	2.7	0.7	0.7
Perch (ocean)	28 g (1 oz.)	—	0.7	0.1	0.2
Pike, northern	28 g (1 oz.)	—	0.2	tr	0.1
Rockfish	28 g (1 oz.)	—	0.4	0.1	0.2
Salmon, pink	28 g (1 oz.)	9.8	1.5	0.2	0.6
Salmon, sockeye	28 g (1 oz.)	9.8	2.5	0.5	1.3
Sole, lemon	28 g (1 oz.)	—	0.2	tr	0.1
Sturgeon, common	28 g (1 oz.)	—	0.9	0.2	0.1
Trout, rainbow	28 g (1 oz.)	15.4	1.3	0.3	0.4
Tuna, albacore, water-canned, light	28 g (1 oz.)	17.6	1.9	0.6	0.5
Whitefish	28 g (1 oz.)	—	1.5	0.2	0.4
Clam (ark shell)	28 g (1 oz.)	14.0	0.4	0.1	0.1
Crab, blue	28 g (1 oz.)	28.0	0.4	0.1	0.2
Crab, Alaskan King	28 g (1 oz.)	—	0.4	0.1	0.2
Oyster, Eastern	28 g (1 oz.)	56.0	0.6	0.1	0.2
Oyster, Pacific	28 g (1 oz.)	56.0	0.6	0.1	0.3
Mussel, California	28 g (1 oz.)	42.0	0.5	0.1	0.2
Scallop	28 g (1 oz.)	15.0	0.2	tr	0.1
Lobster	28 g (1 oz.)	56.0	0.3	tr	0.2
Shrimp	28 g (1 oz.)	42.0	0.3	tr	0.2
Lobster tail	28 g (1 oz.)	56.0	0.3	tr	0.1
Poultry (roasted)					
Chicken, dark (no skin)	28 g (1 oz.)	25.0	2.7	0.7	0.7
Chicken, light (no skin)	28 g (1 oz.)	22.0	1.3	0.4	0.3
Turkey, dark (no skin)	28 g (1 oz.)	28.0	2.2	0.7	0.7

Appendix continued on following page

Appendix D–2. Cholesterol and Fat Content of Foods* (Continued)

Food	Amount	Cholesterol (mg)	Total Fat (g)	Saturated Fat (g)	Polyunsaturated Fat (g)
Turkey, light (no skin)	28 g (1 oz.)	22.0	1.0	0.3	0.3
MEDIUM-FAT, LESS THAN 5 G/OZ					
Beef					
Chuck, lean	28 g (1 oz.)	25.0	3.9	1.7	0.2
Rib, lean	28 g (1 oz.)	25.0	3.9	1.7	0.2
Ground beef, 15%	28 g (1 oz.)	25.0	4.2	1.8	0.3
Pork					
Loin, lean only	28 g (1 oz.)	25.0	3.9	1.3	0.4
Loin, cured	28 g (1 oz.)	25.0	4.9	1.7	0.5
Veal					
Leg, total edible	28 g (1 oz.)	25.2	3.1	1.3	0.2
Loin, total edible	28 g (1 oz.)	25.2	3.8	1.6	0.2
Shoulder, total edible	28 g (1 oz.)	25.2	3.6	1.5	0.2
Rib, total edible	28 g (1 oz.)	25.2	4.7	2.0	0.3
HIGH-FAT, MORE THAN 5 G/OZ					
Beef					
Brisket, total edible	28 g (1 oz.)	25.0	9.7	4.1	0.4
Chuck, total edible	28 g (1 oz.)	25.0	10.3	4.3	0.4
Rib, whole	28 g (1 oz.)	25.0	11.0	4.6	0.4
Ground beef, 20%	28 g (1 oz.)	25.0	6.3	2.7	0.3
Pork					
Boston blade	28 g (1 oz.)	25.0	9.2	3.3	1.0
Spareribs	28 g (1 oz.)	25.0	10.9	3.8	1.2
Leg, fresh	28 g (1 oz.)	25.0	5.7	2.0	0.6
Leg, cured	28 g (1 oz.)	25.0	6.2	2.2	0.8
Boston blade, cured	28 g (1 oz.)	25.0	7.2	2.5	0.8
Lamb					
Leg, total edible	28 g (1 oz.)	28.0	5.9	2.7	0.3
Loin	28 g (1 oz.)	28.0	9.1	4.2	0.5
Rib	28 g (1 oz.)	28.0	10.1	4.7	0.6
Shoulder	28 g (1 oz.)	28.0	7.5	3.5	0.4
Veal					
Breast, total edible	28 g (1 oz.)	25.2	5.9	2.6	0.4
MISCELLANEOUS MEATS					
Organ Meats					
Brains	28 g (1 oz.)	560.0	2.4	0.6	0.3
Kidneys	28 g (1 oz.)	225.0	3.4	1.3	0.5
Liver, chicken	28 g (1 oz.)	208.0	1.2	0.5	0.3
Liver, beef or veal	28 g (1 oz.)	122.0	1.1	0.4	0.2
Sweetbreads	28 g (1 oz.)	130.0	6.5	2.7	0.3
Heart	28 g (1 oz.)	77.0	1.6	0.5	0.2
Giblets	28 g (1 oz.)	60.0	0.9	0.3	0.2
Gizzard	28 g (1 oz.)	55.0	0.9	0.3	0.2
Tongue	28 g (1 oz.)	25.0	4.7	1.6	0.6
Variety Meats					
Cold cuts (average)	28 g (1 oz.)	25.0	7.6	2.7	0.9
Frankfurter (sample)	45 g (1 avg)	18.0	13.0	4.9	1.6
Sausage, pork, cooked	28 g (1 oz.)	18.2	9.1	3.3	1.1
Bacon, cooked	5 g	3.0	3.4	1.3	0.4
Egg					
Whole, one	50 g	274.0	5.6	1.7	0.7
Yolk	17 g	274.0	5.6	1.7	0.7
White	33 g	0.0	0.0	0.0	0.0

Appendix D–2. Cholesterol and Fat Content of Foods* (Continued)

Food	Amount	Cholesterol (mg)	Total Fat (g)	Saturated Fat (g)	Polyunsaturated Fat (g)
Cheese					
LOW-FAT, LESS THAN 3 G/OZ					
Cottage cheese, dry	28 g (1 oz.)	1.9	0.1	0.1	tr
Cottage cheese, 1% fat	28 g (1 oz.)	1.1	0.3	0.2	tr
Cottage cheese, 2% fat	28 g (1 oz.)	2.2	0.5	0.3	tr
Cottage cheese, regular	28 g (1 oz.)	4.2	1.3	0.8	tr
Ricotta, part-skim	28 g (1 oz.)	8.7	2.2	1.4	0.1
MEDIUM-FAT, LESS THAN 5 G/OZ					
Mozzarella, low moisture, part skim	28 g (1 oz.)	16.2	4.5	2.8	0.1
Mozzarella, part skim	28 g (1 oz.)	15.1	4.8	3.0	0.1
Ricotta, whole milk	28 g (1 oz.)	14.3	3.6	2.3	0.1
HIGH-FAT, MORE THAN 5 G/OZ					
American, processed	28 g (1 oz.)	26.3	8.8	5.5	0.3
Blue	28 g (1 oz.)	21.0	8.0	5.2	0.2
Camembert	28 g (1 oz.)	20.0	6.8	4.3	0.2
Cheddar	28 g (1 oz.)	29.4	9.3	5.9	0.3
Cheese food, American, cold-pack	28 g (1 oz.)	17.9	6.4	4.3	0.2
Cheese food, American, processed	28 g (1 oz.)	17.9	6.9	4.3	0.2
Cheese spread	28 g (1 oz.)	15.4	5.9	3.7	0.2
Colby	28 g (1 oz.)	26.6	9.0	5.7	0.3
Cream	28 g (1 oz.)	30.8	9.8	6.2	0.4
Edam	28 g (1 oz.)	24.9	7.8	4.9	0.2
Feta	28 g (1 oz.)	24.9	6.0	4.2	0.2
Fontina	28 g (1 oz.)	32.5	8.7	5.4	0.5
Gouda	28 g (1 oz.)	31.9	7.7	4.9	0.2
Gruyère	28 g (1 oz.)	30.8	9.1	5.3	0.5
Limburger	28 g (1 oz.)	25.2	7.6	4.7	0.1
Mozzarella, whole milk	28 g (1 oz.)	21.8	6.0	3.7	0.2
Mozzarella, whole milk, low-moisture	28 g (1 oz.)	24.9	6.9	4.4	0.2
Muenster	28 g (1 oz.)	26.9	8.4	5.4	0.2
Neufchâtel	28 g (1 oz.)	21.3	6.6	4.1	0.2
Parmesan (hard)	28 g (1 oz)	19.0	7.2	4.6	0.2
Port du Salut	28 g (1 oz)	34.4	7.9	4.7	0.2
Provolone	28 g (1 oz)	19.3	7.5	4.8	0.2
Roquefort	28 g (1 oz)	25.2	8.6	5.4	0.4
Swiss, natural	28 g (1 oz)	25.8	7.7	5.0	0.3
Swiss, process	28 g (1 oz)	23.8	7.0	4.5	0.2
Tilsit, whole milk	28 g (1 oz)	28.6	7.3	4.7	0.2
Other Dairy Products					
Butter	5 g (1 tsp)	11.0	4.1	2.5	0.2
Milk, low-fat, 2%	244 g (1 cup)	18.0	4.7	2.9	0.2
low-fat, 1%	244 g (1 cup)	10.0	2.6	1.6	0.1
nonfat	245 g (1 cup)	4.0	0.4	0.3	tr
evaporated, skim	32 g (1 oz)	1.0	0.1	tr	tr
evaporated, whole	32 g (1 oz)	9.0	2.4	1.5	0.1
whole	244 g (1 cup)	33.0	8.2	5.1	0.3
low-sodium	244 g (1 cup)	33.0	8.4	5.3	0.3
dry, nonfat	30 g (¼ cup)	6.0	0.2	0.2	tr
condensed	38 g (1 oz)	13.0	3.0	2.1	0.1
chocolate, whole	250 g (1 cup)	30.0	8.5	5.3	0.3
chocolate, 1%	250 g (1 cup)	7.0	2.5	1.5	0.1
Yogurt, plain, whole	227 g (1 cup)	29.0	7.4	4.8	0.2

Appendix continued on following page

Appendix D–2. Cholesterol and Fat Content of Foods* (Continued)

Food	Amount	Cholesterol (mg)	Total Fat (g)	Saturated Fat (g)	Polyunsaturated Fat (g)
Yogurt, plain, 2% milk	227 g (1 cup)	14.0	3.5	2.3	0.1
Yogurt, fruited, 2%	227 g (1 cup)	10.0	2.6	1.7	0.1
Half and half cream, 11% fat	15 g (1 tbs)	6.0	1.7	1.1	0.1
Coffee cream, 20% fat	15 g (1 tbs)	10.0	2.9	1.8	0.1
Medium cream, 25% fat	15 g (1 tbs)	13.0	3.8	2.3	0.1
Light whipping cream, 30% fat	15 g (1 tbs)	17.0	4.6	2.9	0.1
Heavy whipping cream, 37% fat	15 g (1 tbs)	21.0	5.6	3.5	0.2
Pressurized whipping cream	3 g (1 tbs)	2.0	0.7	0.4	tr
Eggnog	254 g (1 cup)	149.0	19.0	11.3	0.9
Ice cream, vanilla, regular, 10% fat	133 g (1 cup)	59.0	14.3	8.9	0.5
Ice cream, vanilla rich, 16% fat	148 g (1 cup)	88.0	23.7	14.7	0.9
Ice milk, vanilla, 4% fat	131 g (1 cup)	18.0	5.6	3.5	0.2
Ice milk, soft, vanilla	175 g (1 cup)	13.0	4.6	2.9	0.2
Sherbet	193 g (1 cup)	14.0	3.8	2.4	0.1
Sour cream, regular	24 g (2 tbs)	10.0	5.0	3.1	0.2

Nondairy Products

Food	Amount	Cholesterol (mg)	Total Fat (g)	Saturated Fat (g)	Polyunsaturated Fat (g)
Coffee whitener	15 g (½ oz)	0.0	1.5	0.3	tr
Coffee whitener, powder	2 g (1 tbs)	0.0	0.7	0.7	tr
Dessert topping, powder	1.3 g (1 tbs)	0.0	0.5	0.5	tr
Pressurized dessert topping	4 g	0.0	0.9	0.8	tr
Frozen dessert topping	4 g (1 tbs)	0.0	1.0	0.9	tr
Sour cream, imitation	28 g (2 tbs)	0.0	5.5	5.0	tr

Fats

Food	Amount	Cholesterol (mg)	Total Fat (g)	Saturated Fat (g)	Polyunsaturated Fat (g)
Butter	5 g (1 pat)	11.0	4.1	2.5	0.2
Coconut oil	14 g (1 tbs)	–··	13.6	11.8	0.2
Corn oil	14 g (1 tbs)	—	13.6	1.7	8.0
Cottonseed oil	14 g (1 tbs)	—	13.6	3.5	7.1
Olive oil	14 g (1 tbs)	—	13.5	1.8	1.1
Palm oil	14 g (1 tbs)	—	13.6	6.7	1.3
Peanut oil	14 g (1 tbs)	—	13.5	2.3	4.3
Poppyseed oil	14 g (1 tbs)	—	13.6	1.8	8.5
Safflower, linoleic	14 g (1 tbs)	—	13.6	1.2	10.1
oleic	14 g (1 tbs)	—	13.6	0.8	1.9
Sesame oil	14 g (1 tbs)	—	13.6	1.9	5.7
Soybean oil	14 g (1 tbs)	—	13.6	2.0	7.9
Sunflower oil, less than 60% linoleic	14 g (1 tbs)	—	13.6	1.4	5.5
Sunflower oil, more than 60% linoleic	14 g (1 tbs)	—	13.6	1.4	8.9

Margarines

STICK

Food	Amount	Cholesterol (mg)	Total Fat (g)	Saturated Fat (g)	Polyunsaturated Fat (g)
Coconut, safflower (liquid) coconut and palm (hydrogenated)	5 g (1 tsp)	—	3.8	2.7	0.6
Corn, hydrogenated	5 g (1 tsp)	—	3.8	0.6	0.8
liquid and hydrogenated	5 g (1 tsp)	—	3.8	0.7	1.1
Lard	5 g (1 tsp)	—	3.8	1.5	0.4
Soybean, liquid and hydrogenated	5 g (1 tsp)	—	3.8	0.6	1.2
Sunflower (liquid), soybean, cottonseed (hydrogenated)	5 g (1 tsp)	—	3.8	0.6	1.9

SOFT

Food	Amount	Cholesterol (mg)	Total Fat (g)	Saturated Fat (g)	Polyunsaturated Fat (g)
Corn, liquid and hydrogenated	5 g (1 tsp)	—	3.8	0.7	1.5
Safflower, liquid and hydrogenated	5 g (1 tsp)	—	3.8	0.4	2.1
Soybean (liquid) and soybean and cottonseed (hydrogenated)	5 g (1 tsp)	—	3.8	0.8	1.4

Appendix D–2. Cholesterol and Fat Content of Foods* (Continued)

Food	Amount	Cholesterol (mg)	Total Fat (g)	Saturated Fat (g)	Polyunsaturated Fat (g)
Soybean, hydrogenated	5 g (1 tsp)	–	3.8	0.6	1.3
Sunflower (liquid) and cottonseed and peanut (hydrogenated)	5 g (1 tsp)	–	3.8	0.6	2.3
LIQUID					
Soybean (hydrogenated) and soybean and cottonseed (liquid)	5 g (1 tsp)	–	3.8	0.6	1.7
Salad Dressing					
Blue cheese	15 g (1 tbs)	–	8.0	1.5	4.3
Italian, low calorie	15 g (1 tbs)	1.0	1.5	0.2	0.9
regular	15 g (1 tbs)	–	7.1	1.0	4.1
Mayonnaise, sunflower and soybean	14 g (1 tbs)	–	11.0	1.2	7.6
soybean	14 g (1 tbs)	8.0	11.0	1.6	5.7
Mayonnaise, imitation (soybean)	15 g (1 tbs)	4.0	2.9	0.5	1.6
Mayonnaise-type	15 g (1 tbs)	4.0	4.9	0.7	2.6
Russian, low calorie	16 g (1 tbs)	1.0	0.7	0.1	0.4
regular	15 g (1 tbs)	–	7.8	1.1	4.5
Thousand Island, low-calorie	15 g (1 tbs)	2.0	1.6	0.2	1.0
regular	16 g (1 tbs)	–	5.6	0.9	3.1
French (clear)	14 g (1 tbs)	–	9.8	1.8	4.7
Sandwich spread	15 g (1 tbs)	12.0	5.2	0.8	3.1
Shortenings-Solid					
Soybean and cottonseed	13 g (1 tbs)	–	12.8	3.2	3.3
Soybean and palm	13 g (1 tbs)	–	12.8	3.9	1.8
Lard and vegetable oil	13 g (1 tbs)	–	12.8	5.2	1.4
Nuts					
Almonds	15 g (½ oz)	–	8.1	0.6	1.5
Brazil nuts	15 g (½ oz)	–	10.2	2.6	3.8
Cashews	15 g (½ oz)	–	6.8	1.4	1.1
Chestnuts	15 g (½ oz)	–	0.4	tr	0.2
Filberts	15 g (½ oz)	–	9.7	0.7	1.0
Macadamia	15 g (½ oz)	–	11.4	1.6	0.3
Peanuts (average)	15 g (½ oz)	–	7.5	1.4	2.2
Pecans	15 g (½ oz)	–	10.7	0.9	2.7
Pistachio	15 g (½ oz)	–	8.0	1.1	1.1
Walnuts, English	15 g (½ oz)	–	9.5	1.0	6.3
Walnuts, black	15 g (½ oz)	–	8.9	0.8	6.1
Peanut butter, unhydrogenated	60 g (2 tbs)	–	13.8	2.5	4.1
Peanut butter, hydrogenated	60 g (2 tbs)	–	14.4	2.9	4.2
Miscellaneous					
Avocado	50 g (¼)	–	8.2	1.2	0.9
Coconut, shredded	7.5 g (1 tbs)	–	5.3	4.7	1.0
Olives, black	15 g (½)	–	3.9	0.5	0.3
Olives, green	15 g (½)	–	3.6	0.5	0.3
Cereal Products					
Bread, all varieties	25 g (1 slice)	0	0.8	0.2	0.3
Bagel	28 g (½ bagel)	0	2.0	0.3	0.9
English muffin	28 g (½ muffin)	0	0.0	0.2	tr
Roll, dinner type	28 g (1 roll)	0	1.6	0.4	0.4
Bun, frankfurter or hamburger	30 g (1 roll)	0	3.0	1.2	0.4

Appendix continued on following page

Appendix D–2. *Cholesterol and Fat Content of Foods** *(Continued)*

Food	Amount	Cholesterol (mg)	Total Fat (g)	Saturated Fat (g)	Polyunsaturated Fat (g)
Crackers: saltine-type	11 g (4 crackers)	0	1.3	0.3	0.3
butter-type	16 g (5 crackers)	3.0	2.9	1.0	0.5
Cereals, hot and cold		tr	tr	tr	tr
Pasta products, plain		tr	tr	tr	tr
Wheat germ	10 g (1 Tbsp.)	0	1.1	0.2	0.7
Specialty Products					
Cheezola (Fisher)	28 g (1 oz.)	5.0	6.0	1.0	4.0
Golden Image, Mild Imitation Cheddar (Kraft)	28 g (1 oz.)	10.0	9.0	2.0	4.0
Golden Image American Flavored Imitation					
Pasteurized Process cheese Food (Kraft)	28 g (1 oz.)	5.0	6.0	1.0	2.0
Count Down, 99% fat-free	28 g (1 oz.)	1.4	0.3	—	—
Egg Substitutes					
Egg Beaters	60 g (¼ cup)	0	0	0	0
Scramblers	57 g (¼ cup)	0	3.0	1.0	2.0

*From Walser, M; Imbembo, A L; Margolis, S; et al: Nutritional Management: The Johns Hopkins Handbook. Philadelphia, W. B. Saunders Co, 1984, with permission.

Appendix D–3. *Sodium and Potassium Content of Foods**

Food	Approximate Measurement	Weight (gm)	Sodium (mg)	Potassium (mg)
Breads				
Biscuit, baking powder	1	28	262.0	56.0
Bread				
Cornbread	1	45	126.0	42.0
White	1 slice	45	231.0	50.0
Muffin, bran	1	40	168.0	98.0
Roll				
Brown & serve	1	26	144.0	25.0
Hamburger or hotdog	1	40	241.0	36.0
Breakfast Cereals				
Corn flakes	1 cup	22	281.0	20.0
Oatmeal, cooked	1 cup	234	1.0	132.0
Puffed rice	1 cup	28	21.0	43.0
Shredded wheat biscuit	1	23	0.47	77.0
Combination Foods				
Beef potpie	1 cup	210	596.0	334.0
Beef stew with vegetables	1 cup	245	1006.0	613.0
Chili con carne with beans (canned)	1 cup	255	1354.0	594.0
Pizza, pepperoni	1 slice	120	817.0	216.0
Spaghetti with tomato sauce and cheese	1 cup	250	955.0	408.0
Taco	1	81	456.0	263.0
Dairy Products				
Cheese				
American processed	1 oz.	28	411.0	46.0
Cheddar	1 oz.	28	178.0	28.0

Appendix D–3. Sodium and Potassium Content of Foods* (Continued)

Food	Approximate Measurement	Weight (gm)	Sodium (mg)	Potassium (mg)
Cottage, uncreamed	1 cup	145	19.0	47.0
Cream	1 oz.	28	85.0	34.0
Swiss	1 oz.	28	74.0	31.0
Cheese food, American processed	1 oz.	28	341.0	79.0
Cheese spread, processor	1 oz.	28	385.0	69.0
Cream				
Half-and-half	1 Tbsp.	15	6.0	19.0
Sour	1 Tbsp.	14	7.0	20.0
Whipped topping, frozen	1 Tbsp.	4	1.0	0.88
Milk				
Buttermilk	1 cup	245	257.0	371.0
Evaporated (can)	1 cup	252	267.0	764.0
Low fat (1%)	1 cup	244	123.0	381.0
Low fat (2%)	1 cup	244	122.0	377.0
Whole (3.3%)	1 cup	244	120.0	370.0
Yogurt, plain, from whole milk	1 cup	227	105.0	351.0
Desserts				
Cake				
Coffee (1/6 of cake)	1 piece	72	310.0	78.0
White with chocolate icing (1/16th)	1	71	200.0	76.0
Cookie				
Oatmeal with raisins	4	52	148.0	90.0
Vanilla wafer	4	16	40.0	11.0
Ice cream, vanilla (10% fat)	1 cup	133	116.0	257.0
Pie, banana cream (1/7 of pie)	1	130	252.0	264.0
Pudding, butterscotch, instant	1 cup	28	244.0	1.0
Sherbet, orange (2% fat)	1 cup	193	88.0	198.0
Eggs				
Egg, hard cooked, large	1	50	69.0	65.0
Fats, Oils, Salad Dressings				
Margarine				
Regular hard stick, unsalted	1 tsp.	4	0.10	1.0
Regular hard stick	1 tsp.	4	47.0	2.0
Salad dressing				
French, commercial	1 Tbsp.	15	214.0	12.0
French, low-calorie, commercial	1 Tbsp.	16	128.0	13.0
Mayonnaise type	1 Tbsp.	14	104.0	1.0
Vegetable oil, corn	1 Tbsp.	218	0	0
Fish				
Clams, raw, meat only	3 oz.	85	102.0	154.0
Lobster, with butter	3 oz.	85	212.0	45.0
Oysters, raw	3 oz.	85	113.0	102.0
Salmon				
Fresh, broiled with butter	3 oz.	28	32.0	125.0
Pink, canned	3 oz.	85	441.0	306.0
Sardines, canned in oil	3 oz.	85	552.0	501.0
Scallops, steamed	3 oz.	85	225.0	404.0
Tuna, canned in water, low-sodium	3 oz.	85	34.0	221.0
Fruits and Fruit Juices				
Apple, raw (2¾″ diameter)	1	138	1.0	159.0
Apple juice	1 cup	248	7.0	296.0
Applesauce, canned, sweetened	1 cup	255	8.0	156.0
Apricots				
Canned in water	1 cup	243	7.0	465.0

Appendix continued on following page

Appendix D–3. *Sodium and Potassium Content of Foods* (Continued)*

Food	Approximate Measurement	Weight (gm)	Sodium (mg)	Potassium (mg)
Dried, uncooked	1 cup	130	13.0	1791.0
Fresh	1	35	0.36	105.0
Avocado	1	216	25.0	1369.0
Banana	1	119	1.0	471.0
Banana flakes	1 Tbsp.	6	0	92.0
Blackberries, fresh	1 cup	144	0	282.0
Blueberries	1 cup	145	9.0	129.0
Cherries				
Sour, canned in water	1 cup	244	17.0	240.0
Sweet, fresh	10	68	0	152.0
Dates, dried	10	80	2.0	541.0
Figs				
Canned in heavy syrup	1 cup	259	3.0	258.0
Dried, uncooked	1 cup	199	22.0	1418.0
Fresh	1	50	1.0	116.0
Fruit cocktail	1 cup	248	9.0	235.0
Grapefruit				
Canned in water	1 cup	244	5.0	322.0
Fresh	1/2	246	0	312.0
Grapefruit juice, canned, unsweetened	1 cup	247	3.0	378.0
Grapes				
Fresh, American type	10	92	2.0	176.0
Fresh, European type	10	160	3.0	296.0
Grape juice, canned or bottled	1 cup	253	7.0	334.0
Mangos, fresh	1	207	4.0	322.0
Melon, cantaloupe, fresh	1 cup	160	14.0	494.0
Nectarine	1	136	0	288.0
Oranges				
Fresh	1	131	0	237.0
Sections	1 cup	180	0	326.0
Orange juice, frozen, diluted	1 cup	249	2.0	474.0
Papaya, fresh	1	140	4.0	359.0
Peaches				
Canned in water	1 cup	244	8.0	241.0
Dried	1 cup	160	12.0	1594.0
Fresh	1	87	0	171.0
Peach nectar, canned	1 cup	249	17.0	101.0
Pears				
Canned in juice	1 cup	248	10.0	238.0
Dried	1 cup	180	10.0	959.0
Fresh, Bartlett	1	166	1.0	208.0
Pear nectar, canned	1 cup	250	9.0	33.0
Pineapple				
Canned in juice	1 cup	250	4.0	304.0
Fresh	1 cup	155	1.0	175.0
Juice	1 cup	250	2.0	334.0
Plums				
Purple, canned in water	1 cup	249	2.0	314.0
Fresh	1	66	0	113.0
Prunes, dried	1 cup	161	6.0	1200.0
Prune juice, canned or bottled	1 cup	256	11.0	706.0
Raisins, seedless	1 cup	145	17.0	1089.0
Rhubarb, fresh, cooked with sugar	1 cup	270	5.0	548.0
Strawberries, fresh	1 cup	149	2.0	247.0
Tangerines, fresh	1	84	1.0	132.0
Tangerine juice, canned	1 cup	249	2.0	443.0
Watermelon	1 cup	160	3.0	186.0
Grains and Grain Products				
Cornstarch	1 cup	128	0	0
Crackers				
Cheese	10	10	120.0	18.0
Graham	2	14	66.0	55.0

Appendix D—3. *Sodium and Potassium Content of Foods** *(Continued)*

Food	Approximate Measurement	Weight (gm)	Sodium (mg)	Potassium (mg)
Oyster	10	4	53.0	5.0
Ry Krisp	4	8	74.0	40.0
Saltines	4	11	147.0	13.0
Wheat Thins	10	18	—	—
Macaroni, cooked	1 cup	105	1.0	64.0
Noodles, egg, enriched, cooked	1 cup	160	3.0	70.0
Pancakes, from mix	1	27	160.0	43.0
Popcorn				
Popped plain	1 cup	6	0	—
Popped with oil and salt	1 cup	9	174.0	—
Pretzel, thin-stick	10	2	48.0	3.0
Rice, white, long-grain	1 cup	185	5.0	170.0
Spaghetti, cooked	1 cup	140	1.0	85.0
Waffles, enriched (home recipe)	1	75	445.0	129.0
Meats and Luncheon Meats				
Bacon, cooked	2	12	202.0	61.0
Beef				
Lean and fat, cooked	3 oz.	85	58.0	184.0
Dried chipped (2½ oz. jar)	1	71	3052.0	142.0
Liver, cooked	3 oz.	85	156.0	323.0
Bologna, pork	1 oz.	28	335.0	80.0
Corned beef, canned	3 oz.	85	1105.0	—
Frankfurter	1	57	639.0	95.0
Ham, lean only	3 oz.	85	1128.0	269.0
Lamb chop	3 oz.	85	58.0	259.0
Pork chop, lean, cooked	3 oz.	85	63.0	355.0
Sausage link, cooked	1	13	168.0	47.0
Sausage patty, cooked	1 oz.	27	349.0	97.0
Veal, cooked	3 oz.	85	68.0	259.0
Miscellaneous				
Baking powder	1 tsp.	3	339.0	5.0
Baking soda	1 tsp.	3	821.0	—
Olives, green	4	4	80.0	1.0
Pickle, dill, cucumber	1	65	928.0	130.0
Nuts				
Slivered almonds	1 oz.	28	3.0	207.0
Coconut, shredded	1 cup	80	16.0	285.0
Peanuts, roasted in oil	1 oz.	28	4.0	200.0
Pecans	1 oz.	28	0.26	111.0
Peanut butter				
Low-sodium	1 Tbsp.	16	5.0	1
Smooth type	1 Tbsp.	16	75.0	110.0
Poultry				
Chicken breast, no skin, cooked	3 oz.	85	62.0	217.0
Chicken leg, no skin, cooked	1	95	87.0	230.0
Duck, cooked	3 oz.	85	55.0	214.0
Turkey, light and dark meat	3 oz.	85	60.0	253.0
Sauces, Gravies, Dips				
Gravy, brown, dehydrated	1 cup	16	7.0	0.44
Mustard, yellow, prepared	1 tsp.	5	65.0	7.0
Sauces				
Barbecue	1 Tbsp.	15	127.0	27.0
Cheese (mix)	1 cup	279	1566.0	554.0
Spaghetti (canned)	1 cup	249	1236.0	957.0
Soy	1 Tbsp.	18	1029.0	64.0
Tomato, canned, low-sodium	1 cup	226	65.0	—

Appendix continued on following page

Appendix D–3. *Sodium and Potassium Content of Foods* (Continued)*

Food	Approximate Measurement	Weight (gm)	Sodium (mg)	Potassium (mg)
Tomato, canned	1 cup	245	1481.0	908.0
Tomato catsup				
Regular	1 Tbsp.	15	156.0	54.0
Low-sodium	1 Tbsp.	15	90.0	54.0
Soup				
Beef broth with water	1 cup	240	782.0	130.0
Chicken noodle	1 cup	241	1107.0	55.0
Cream of mushroom with water	1 cup	244	1031.0	101.0
Salt	1 tsp.	5	1955.0	0.30
Vegetables and Vegetable Juices				
Artichokes, cooked	1 cup	120	79.0	316.0
Asparagus				
Canned spears	1 cup	242	903.0	403.0
Frozen spears	1 cup	180	7.0	392.0
Fresh, cooked	1 cup	180	8.0	558.0
Beans				
Limas, frozen, cooked	1 cup	170	90.0	694.0
Snap, green, cuts	1 cup	135	17.0	151.0
Snap, yellow or wax, canned	1 cup	136	340.0	148.0
Beets, sliced, cooked	1 cup	170	84.0	532.0
Beet greens, cooked	1 cup	145	346.0	1308.0
Broccoli, cooked	1 cup	155	16.0	254.0
Brussels sprouts, cooked	1 cup	156	34.0	494.0
Cabbage				
Cooked	1 cup	145	27.0	297.0
Fresh, shredded	1 cup	90	16.0	221.0
Carrots				
Cooked	1 cup	156	104.0	354.0
Raw, grated	1 cup	72	25.0	233.0
Cauliflower, cooked	1 cup	124	8.0	400.0
Celery, fresh	1 stalk	40	35.0	114.0
Chard, Swiss	1 cup	175	313.0	961.0
Corn				
Sweet, boiled, ear	1	140	13.0	192.0
Sweet, canned kernels	1 cup	165	470.0	160.0
Frozen kernels	1 cup	165	8.0	228.0
Cucumber, raw, peeled	6–9 pieces	28	0.5	42.0
Dandelion greens, cooked	1 cup	105	46.0	244.0
Eggplant, cooked	1 cup	96	3.0	238.0
Kale				
Cooked from frozen	1 cup	130	20.0	417.0
From fresh	1 cup	130	30.0	296.0
Kohlrabi, cooked	1 cup	165	34.0	561.0
Leeks, raw		124	25.0	223.0
Lettuce, iceberg, chopped	1 cup	55	4.0	86.0
Mushrooms, raw, chopped	1 cup	70	2.0	260.0
Mustard greens, cooked	1 cup	140	22.0	283.0
Okra, cooked	1 cup	160	8.0	514.0
Onions, cooked	1 cup	210	16.0	318.0
Parsnips, cooked	1 cup	155	16.0	574.0
Peas				
Cowpeas, cooked	1 cup	165	7.0	693.0
Green, fresh	1 cup	145	6.0	290.0
Green, canned	1 cup	170	372.0	294.0
Green, frozen	1 cup	160	140.0	268.0
Peppers				
Sweet, cooked	1	73	2.0	94.0
Sweet, raw	1 cup	74	2.0	144.0
Potato				
Baked	1	156	8.0	610.0
Boiled	1	137	6.0	515.0

Appendix D–3. Sodium and Potassium Content of Foods* (Continued)

Food	Approximate Measurement	Weight (gm)	Sodium (mg)	Potassium (mg)
Chips	10	20	18.0	52.0
Pumpkin	1 cup	245	12.0	504.0
Radishes, raw	4	4	1.0	10.0
Rutabagas, cooked	1 cup	170	30.0	488.0
Sauerkraut	1 cup	235	1561.0	401.0
Spinach				
Cooked, fresh	1 cup	180	126.0	838.0
Canned	1 cup	205	55.0	709.0
From frozen	1 cup	190	163.0	566.0
Squash				
Acorn, baked	1 cup	205	9.0	896.0
Hubbard, mashed	1 cup	236	12.0	504.0
Winter, mashed	1 cup	205	3.0	895.0
Zucchini, canned	1 cup	227	850.0	622.0
Sweet potato, baked	1	114	12.0	397.0
Tomato	1	135	10.0	279.0
Tomato juice				
Canned, regular	1 cup	243	877.0	535.0
Canned, low-sodium	1 cup	244	24.0	536.0
Tomato paste				
Canned, regular	1 cup	262	2070.0	2442.0
Canned, low-sodium	1 cup	262	170.0	2442.0
Turnips, cooked	1 cup	156	78.0	211.0
Turnip greens, cooked	1 cup	144	41.0	293.0

*Data from Nutritionist III Software, Silverton, OR.

Appendix D–4. Calcium and Phosphorus Content of Foods*

	Amount	Gm/serving	Calcium (mg)	Phosphorus (mg)
Beverages				
Beer, regular	12 oz.	360	18	108
Chocolate-flavored beverage powder, nonfat dry milk added	1 oz.	28	167	155
Chocolate-flavored beverage powder, without milk added	1 oz.	28	9	48
Coffee	8 oz.	240	17	5
Grape soda	12 oz.	372	15	0
Root beer	12 oz.	369	15	2
Tang, instant breakfast drink (dry)	1 oz.	28	71	75
Breads				
Biscuit, baking powder	1	28	58	128
Corn, with enriched cornmeal	1	45	48	43
White, enriched	1	45	56	48
Whole-wheat, with enriched flour	1	25	18	65
Breakfast Cereals				
Kellogg's Corn Flakes	1 cup	22	0.68	14
Oatmeal	1 cup	234	20	178
Shredded wheat (large biscuit)	1	23	10	86

Appendix continued on following page

Appendix D—4. Calcium and Phosphorus Content of Foods* (Continued)

	Amount	Gm/serving	Calcium (mg)	Phosphorus (mg)
Dairy Products				
Cheddar cheese	1 oz.	28	206	146
Cottage cheese, dry curd	1 cup	145	46	151
Swiss cheese	1 oz.	28	275	173
Cheese food, American, pasteurized, process cheese	1 oz.	28	165	131
Cheese spread, American, pasteurized, process cheese	1 oz.	28	160	204
Half-and-half	1 Tbsp.	15	15	14
Whipped topping (imitation), powdered, made with whole milk	1 Tbsp.	1	1	1
Buttermilk	8 oz.	245	285	219
Milk, chocolate	8 oz.	250	280	251
Milk, low-fat (1% fat)	8 oz.	244	300	235
Milk, low-fat (2% fat)	8 oz.	244	297	232
Milk, whole	8 oz.	244	291	228
Yogurt, plain	8 oz.	227	274	215
Desserts				
Sheet cake, with uncooked icing (⅑ of cake)	1	121	61	91
Cookie, oatmeal with raisins	4	52	17	57
Cookie, vanilla wafer	4	16	6	10
Custard, baked	1 cup	265	297	310
Doughnut, cake type	1	25	11	55
Doughnut, yeast	1	50	16	33
Frozen yogurt, fruit varieties	8 oz.	226	200	200
Granola bar	1	24	14	66
Ice cream, vanilla	1 cup	133	176	134
Pie, cherry (½ of pie)	1	135	19	34
Pie, custard (⅐ of pie)	1	130	125	147
Pudding, butterscotch	1 cup	28	1	102
Sherbet, orange	1 cup	193	103	74
Eggs				
Egg, whole, hard cooked	1	50	28	90
Egg white, raw, large	1	33	4	4
Egg yolk, raw, large	1	17	26	86
Fats/Oils, Salad Dressings				
Butter	1 pat	5	1	1
Margarine	1 pat	5	1	1
Salad dressing, French	1 Tbsp.	15	1	2
Salad dressing, mayonnaise type	1 Tbsp.	14	2	4
Fish				
Ocean perch	3 oz.	85	28	192
Salmon, fresh	3 oz.	85	352	355
Salmon, canned	3 oz.	85	167	243
Sardines, canned	3 oz.	85	372	423
Tuna, canned in water	3 oz.	85	4	187
Fruits, Fruit Juices				
Blackberries, fresh	1 cup	144	46	30
Orange, fresh	1	131	52	18
Orange juice	1 cup	249	22	40
Peaches, dried	1 cup	160	45	191
Peach, fresh	1	87	5	11
Raspberries, canned	1 cup	256	27	23
Rhubarb, fresh, cooked with sugar	1 cup	270	211	41
Tangerine, fresh	1	84	12	8

Appendix D—4. Calcium and Phosphorus Content of Foods* (Continued)

	Amount	Gm/ serving	Calcium (mg)	Phosphorus (mg)
Grains, Grain Products				
Crackers, graham	2	14	6	21
Crackers, saltines	4	11	1	10
Macaroni, enriched, cooked	1 cup	105	8	53
Noodles, egg, enriched, cooked	1 cup	160	16	94
Pancakes	1	27	35	70
Popcorn, popped, plain	1 cup	6	1	17
Rice, brown, long-grain, cooked	1 cup	195	23	—
Rice, white, long-grain, enriched	1 cup	185	44	174
Spaghetti, enriched, cooked	1 cup	140	11	70
Waffles	1	75	154	135
Meats, Luncheon Meats				
Bacon, cured pork	2	12	1	42
Beef cuts	3 oz.	85	10	114
Beef liver	3 oz.	85	9	405
Bologna	1 oz.	28	3	39
Pork chop, loin	3 oz.	85	6	237
Nuts, Seeds, Nut Products				
Peanuts, oil-roasted	1 oz.	28	24	144
Peanut butter, smooth type	1 Tbsp.	16	5	60
Poultry				
Chicken breast, roasted, no skin	3 oz.	85	12	193
Chicken leg, roasted, no skin	3 oz.	85	10	155
Sugars/Sweets				
Milky Way Bar	1	60	—	—
Honey, strained	1 Tbsp.	21	1	1
Jelly	1 Tbsp.	18	4	1
Molasses, cane, light	1 Tbsp.	20	33	9
Sugar, brown	1 Tbsp.	13	11	2
Sugar, white	1 Tbsp.	12	0	0
Vegetables, vegetable juices				
Artichokes, boiled, drained	1 cup	120	47	72
Asparagus, frozen, boiled	1 cup	180	41	99
Beans, Fordhook lima	1 cup	170	38	153
Beans, pinto	1 cup	28	14	—
Beet greens, boiled	1 cup	145	165	58
Broccoli, fresh, boiled	1 cup	155	178	74
Brussels sprouts, fresh, boiled	1 cup	156	56	88
Cabbage, raw	1 cup	90	42	20
Collards, boiled	1 cup	190	148	19
Corn, boiled	1 cup	140	2	79
Kale, boiled	1 cup	130	94	36
Mushrooms, raw	1 cup	70	4	72
Mustard greens, boiled	1 cup	140	103	58
Okra, boiled	1 cup	160	100	90
Peas, green, frozen and boiled	1 cup	160	38	144
Potato, baked, flesh only	1	156	8	78
Potato chips	10	20	8	28
Spinach, boiled	1 cup	180	244	100
Squash, acorn, baked	1 cup	205	90	93
Turnip greens, boiled	1 cup	144	198	41

*Data from Nutritionist III Software, Silverton, OR.

Appendix D–5 *Caffeine Content of Foods*

Product	Amount	Caffeine Content	
		Average (mg)	Range (mg)
Coffee*			
Brewed, drip method	5 oz.	115	60–180
Brewed, percolator	5 oz.	80	40–170
Instant	5 oz.	65	30–120
Brewed decaffeinated	5 oz.	3	2–5
Instant decaffeinated	5 oz.	2	1–5
Tea*			
Brewed, major U.S. brands	5 oz.	40	20–90
Brewed, imported brands	5 oz.	60	25–110
Instant	5 oz.	30	25–50
Iced	12 oz.	70	67–76
Cocoa beverage*	5 oz.	4	2–20
Chocolate milk beverage*	8 oz.	5	2–7
Milk chocolate*	1 oz.	6	1–15
Dark chocolate, semisweet*	1 oz.	20	5–35
Baker's chocolate*	1 oz.	26	26
Chocolate-flavored syrup*	1 oz.	4	4
Soft drinks†			
Regular colas	12 oz.	—	30–46
Decaffeinated colas	12 oz.	—	trace
Diet colas	12 oz.	—	0–59
Decaffeinated diet colas	12 oz.	—	0–trace
Orange, lemon-lime, root beer, tonic, ginger ale, club soda	12 oz.	—	0
Other regular	12 oz.	—	0–93

*From Lecos, C: The latest caffeine scorecard. Reprinted from *FDA Consumer,* March 1984. (Data from FDA, Food Additive Chemistry Evaluation Branch, based on evaluations of existing literature on caffeine levels.)

†Data from *What's in Soft Drinks.* Washington, DC, National Soft Drink Association, July 1985.

Appendix D—6. *Acid-Base Ash Resulting from Metabolism of Foods*

Acid Ash	Alkaline Ash	Neutral
Meats	Milk products	Butter and margarine
Beef	Milk	Sugars and syrups
Fish	Cream	Fats and oils
Fowl	Buttermilk	Beverages
Shellfish	Nuts	Coffee
Eggs	Almonds	Tea
Cheese	Chestnuts	Starches
Peanut butter	Coconut	
Vegetables	Vegetables	
Corn	All types	
Lentils	Fruit	
Fat	Citrus	
Bacon	All others	
Nuts	Jams and jellies	
Brazil	Honey	
Filberts		
Peanuts		
Walnuts		
Fruit		
Cranberries		
Plums		
Prunes		
Bread		
Bread (all types)		
Crackers		
Macaroni		
Spaghetti		
Noodles		
Dessert		
Cakes		
Cookies		

Appendix D–7. Exchange Lists for Renal Diets*

Milk Exchanges

AVERAGE ANALYSIS:		
Protein	4.0 g	
Sodium	60.0 mg	
Potassium	170.0 mg	
Phosphorus	110.0 mg	
Calcium	140.0 mg	
Calories	varies	

Chocolate milk (whole milk)	½ cup	Ice milk, hard	¾ cup
Cream, half and half	½ cup	Skim milk	½ cup
Evaporated whole milk, canned	¼ cup	Whole milk	½ cup

Meat Exchanges

AVERAGE ANALYSIS:		
Protein	6.9 g	
Sodium	30.0 mg	
Potassium	95.0 mg	
Phosphorus	75.0 mg	
Calcium	15.0 mg	
Calories	75	

SEAFOOD		MEAT	
Bluefish, cooked	1 oz.	Beef, lean, cooked, rump	1 oz.
Clams, soft, raw, fresh	¼ cup	Chicken, cooked	1 oz.
Cod, fresh, cooked	1 oz.	Lamb, lean, cooked, shoulder	1 oz.
Flounder, cooked	1 oz.	Liver (chicken), cooked	1 oz.
Haddock, cooked	1 oz.	Pork, lean, cooked, loin	1 oz.
Halibut, cooked	1 oz.	Turkey, cooked	1 oz.
Lobster, cooked	1 oz.	Veal, cooked, loin	1 oz.
Ocean perch, cooked	1 oz.		
Oysters, raw	1 oz.		
Salmon, canned, cooked	1 oz.	Egg	2 oz.
Shrimp, cooked	1 oz.		
Tuna, canned, low sodium	1 oz.		

Fruit Exchanges

GROUP A†

AVERAGE ANALYSIS:		
Protein	0.5 g	
Sodium	1.5 mg	
Potassium	115.0 mg	
Phosphorus	12.0 mg	
Calcium	15.0 mg	
Calories	40–80	

Apple, fresh (2½" diam.)	1	Raspberries, red, fresh, canned or frozen	½ cup
Applesauce, sweetened	½ cup	Strawberries, fresh, canned, unsweetened	½ cup
Apricot, fresh	1 cup		
Blackberries, fresh or frozen	½ cup	Strawberries, frozen, whole, sweetened	½ cup
Blueberries, fresh or frozen	½ cup		
Cherries, fresh	½ cup	Tangerine, fresh, medium	1
Figs, fresh, medium	1 cup		
Grapefruit, fresh, sections	½ cup	JUICES	
Mandarin orange sections	½ cup	Apple juice	½ cup
Pears, canned, sweetened	½ cup	Birdseye Awake	½ cup
Pineapple, fresh or canned, sweetened	½ cup	Grape juice	½ cup
Plum, fresh, prune type	2 cups	Peach nectar	½ cup
Watermelon, diced	½	Pear nectar	½ cup

GROUP B†

AVERAGE ANALYSIS:		
Protein	0.7 g	
Sodium	3.5 mg	
Potassium	215.0 mg	

Appendix D–7. Exchange Lists for Renal Diets* (Continued)

Fruit Exchanges (*Continued*)

Phosphorus	18.0 mg
Calcium	18.0 mg
Calories	40–80

Apricots, canned, halves, sweetened	½ cup	Peach, fresh	1 medium
Banana, sliced	½ cup	Peach, canned, sweetened	½ cup
Cantaloupe, cubed, fresh	½ cup	Pear, fresh, Bartlett	1 medium
Casaba, cubed, fresh	½ cup	Plums, canned, sweetened	½ cup
Cherries, red, canned	½ cup	Rhubarb, cooked, sweetened	½ cup
Figs, canned, sweetened	½ cup		
Fruit cocktail, canned, sweetened	½ cup	JUICES	
		Apricot nectar	½ cup
Grapefruit sections, canned, unsweetened	½ cup	Blackberry juice	½ cup
		Grapefruit juice	½ cup
Grapes, fresh	1 cup	Orange juice	½ cup
Honeydew, cubed, fresh	½ cup	Pineapple juice	½ cup
Melon balls, frozen	½ cup	Prune juice	½ cup
Orange sections, fresh	½ cup	Tomato juice, low-sodium	½ cup
Papaya, fresh, cubed	½ cup		

Bread/Cereals Exchanges

GROUP A[†]

AVERAGE ANALYSIS:		
Protein	2.0 g	
Sodium	1.0 mg	
Potassium	38.0 mg	
Phosphorus	27.0 mg	
Calcium	5.0 mg	
Calories	70	

Bread, salt-free	1 slice	Cornflakes, salt-free	1 cup
Grits	½ cup	Oatmeal, regular, cooked	½ cup
Flour, wheat	2 tbs.	Puffed Rice (Quaker Oats)	1 cup
Matzo	1 piece	Cream of Wheat, regular, enriched	½ cup
Pasta, macaroni, spaghetti, noodles, etc.	½ cup	Puffed wheat (Quaker Oats)	1 cup
Popcorn, popped in oil	1 cup	Shredded Wheat, Spoon Size, (Kellogg's)	½ cup
Rice, white enriched, cooked	½ cup		

GROUP B[†]

AVERAGE ANALYSIS:		
Protein	2.0 g	
Sodium	125.0 mg	
Potassium	35.0 mg	
Phosphorus	31.0 mg	
Calcium	16.0 mg	
Calories	70 or more	

Biscuit, homemade (2″ diameter—¼″ high)	1	Bran flakes, 40% (Kellogg's)	¾ cup
Bread, white, whole wheat, rye, or raisin	1 slice	Cap'n Crunch (Quaker Oats)	¾ cup
		Cocoa Krispies (Kellogg's)	¾ cup
Bread, French	¾ slice	Rice Chex (Ralston)	¾ cup
Doughnut, raised	1 small	Special K (Kellogg's)	¾ cup
Muffin, plain	1	Sugar Corn Pops (Kellogg's)	1½ cup
English muffin (Thomas)	½	Sugar Smacks (Kellogg's)	1 cup
Pancake, homemade 1–4″ diam	1	Crackers, animal	10
Roll, dinner 1–2½″ diam	1	Cracker, graham, plain (5″ × 2½″)	1
Roll, hamburger, hot dog, or kaiser	1 or ½	Crackers, unsalted (Nabisco)	4

Appendix continued on following page

Appendix D–7. *Exchange Lists for Renal Diets* (Continued)*

Fat Exchanges

AVERAGE ANALYSIS:		
Protein	trace	
Sodium	50.0 mg	
Potassium	1.0 mg	
Phosphorus	1.0 mg	
Calcium	1.0 mg	
Calories	45	

Butter	1 tsp	Mayonnaise	1 tsp
Margarine	1 tsp	Salad dressing (mayonnaise type)	1 tsp

Vegetable Exchanges

GROUP A[†]

AVERAGE ANALYSIS:	
Protein	1.0 g
Sodium	9.0 mg
Potassium	113.0 mg
Phosphorus	25.0 mg
Calcium	29.0 mg
Calories	25

Beans, cooked, green, fresh or frozen, or low sodium, canned	½ cup	Cucumber, fresh peeled	½ cup
Beans, cooked wax, fresh, or low sodium, canned	½ cup	Eggplant, cooked diced	½ cup
		Endive/Escarole, fresh, cut	½ cup
Beans, French cut, frozen, cooked	½ cup	Kale, fresh or frozen, cooked	½ cup
		Lettuce, iceberg, chopped	½ cup
Beets, canned, low sodium	½ cup	Mushrooms, fresh	½ cup
Cabbage, fresh or cooked	½ cup	Mustard greens, frozen, cooked	½ cup
Carrots, raw	½ cup	Okra, fresh, cooked, sliced	½ cup
Carrots, canned, low sodium	½ cup	Onions, fresh, or cooked	½ cup
Cauliflower, raw or fresh, cooked	½ cup	Peppers, green, fresh, cooked	½ cup
		Spinach, fresh, chopped, raw	½ cup
Celery, raw or cooked	¼ cup	Squash, summer, fresh, cooked	½ cup
Corn, kernels, fresh, cooked	½ cup	Tomato, medium, fresh	1 slice
Corn on cob, fresh, cooked	5″ cob	Turnips, fresh, cooked, diced	½ cup
Corn, canned, low sodium	½ cup	Turnip greens, frozen, cooked	½ cup

GROUP B[†]

AVERAGE ANALYSIS:	
Protein	1.7 g
Sodium	18.0 mg
Potassium	196.0 mg
Phosphorus	34.0 mg
Calcium	35.0 mg
Calories	35

Asparagus, fresh, frozen or low sodium canned, cooked	½ cup	Kohlrabi, fresh, raw or cooked	½ cup
Beets, fresh, sliced, cooked	½ cup	Mustard greens, fresh, cooked	½ cup
Broccoli, fresh or frozen, cooked	½ cup	Peppers, green, fresh, cooked	½ cup
Brussels sprouts, fresh or frozen	½ cup	Potato, boiled without skin, diced	½ cup
Carrots, fresh, cooked	½ cup	Radishes, sliced	½ cup
Cauliflower, frozen, cooked	½ cup	Squash, winter, frozen, cooked	½ cup
Chard, Swiss, cooked	½ cup	Sweet potato, canned	½ cup
Collards, fresh, cooked	½ cup	Tomato, fresh, 2″ diameter	1 slice
Corn, frozen, cooked	½ cup	Tomato, canned, low sodium	½ cup
Dandelion greens, fresh, cooked	½ cup	Vegetables, mixed, frozen	½ cup
French-fried potatoes	5 sticks		

Appendix D–7. Exchange Lists for Renal Diets* (Continued)

Calorie Supplements

Each of the foods listed in the amounts indicated yields approximately 100 calories.

CARBOHYDRATES—GROUP A

AVERAGE ANALYSIS:	Protein	0.1 g
	Sodium	9.0 mg
	Potassium	9.0 mg
	Phosphorus	4.0 mg
	Calcium	4.0 mg
	Calories	100

Low-protein porridge	¾ cup	Hard candy	1 oz
Low-protein noodles:		Table syrup	2 tbs
anellini, cooked	½ cup	Marshmallows	4 large
rigatoni, cooked	½ cup	Fruit ice	½ cup
tagliatelle, cooked	½ cup	Bright 'N' Early	8 oz
Low-protein bread	1 slice	Cranberry juice	8 oz
Cranberry sauce	¼ cup	Hi-C	8 oz
Honey	1½ tsp	Ginger ale	10 oz
Jelly	2 tbs	Grape soda	8 oz
Jam	3 tbs	Root beer	8 oz
Mints	37 pcs	Orange soda	8 oz
Jelly beans	1 oz		

MALTODEXTRIN SUPPLEMENTS (3 TBS)—GROUP B

AVERAGE ANALYSIS:	Protein	0.0 g
	Sodium	19.0 mg
	Potassium	trace
	Phosphorus	trace
	Calcium	trace
	Calories	93

Polycose liquid	Controlyte
Polycose powder	Moducal liquid
Hy-Cal	Moducal powder
Cal Plus	Sumacal

DAIRY SUBSTITUTES—GROUP C

AVERAGE ANALYSIS:	Protein	0.3 g
	Sodium	24.0 mg
	Potassium	23.0 mg
	Phosphorus	24.0 mg
	Calcium	17.0 mg
	Calories	100

Dessert topping, pressurized can	¾ cup	Powdered dessert topping	1 cup
Frozen dessert topping	½ cup	Rich's liquid	3 tbs

FAT—SALT-FREE (1 TBS)—GROUP D

AVERAGE ANALYSIS:	Protein	trace
	Sodium	trace
	Potassium	trace
	Phosphorus	trace
	Calcium	trace
	Calories	115

Unsalted butter	Vegetable oils
Unsalted margarine	Vegetable shortenings

*From Walser, M; Imbembo, AL; Margolis, S; et al: *Nutritional Management: The Johns Hopkins Handbook.* Philadelphia, W B Saunders Co, 1985, with permission.

†Foods in the B group contain more of the restricted nutrients (sodium, potassium, phosphorus, and calcium) than those in the A group, which are used less frequently.

Appendix D–8. *Sample Meal Patterns for Predialysis, Hemodialysis, and Peritoneal Dialysis[a,b] (Based on 70-kg Person)*

Foods	25 g Protein; 500 mg Phosphorus[c]	40 g Protein; 600 mg Phosphorus	70 g Protein; 2 g Sodium	105 g Protein; 2 g Sodium
BREAKFAST				
Meat Exchanges	—	1	1	2
Bread Exchange A or B	2	2	2	2
Fruit Exchange A or B	1	1	1	1
Fat Exchanges	2	3	3	3
Milk Exchanges	—	—	2	2
Calorie Supplements				
Group A	2	1	1	—
Group B	1	1	1	1
Group C	2	2	—	—
Group D	d	d	d	d
LUNCH				
Meat Exchanges	1	1	2	3
Bread Exchanges A or B	2	2	2	2
Vegetable Exchange A or B	—	1	1	1
Fruit Exchange A or B	1	1	1	1
Fat Exchanges	3	3	3	3
Calorie Supplements				
Group A	1	1	1	—
Group B	1	1	1	½
Group D	d	d	d	d
MIDAFTERNOON SNACK				
Calorie Supplement				
Group A	1	2	1	—
Fruit Exchange A or B	1	—	—	—
DINNER				
Meat Exchanges	—	1	2	4
Bread Exchanges A or B	—	1	2	2
Vegetable Exchange A or B	2	1	1	1
Fruit Exchange A or B	1	1	1	1
Milk Exchanges	—	—	2	—
Fat Exchanges	4	3	3	3
Calorie Supplements				
Group A	2	1	1	—
Group B	1	1	1	½
Group D	d	d	d	d
EVENING SNACK				
Milk Exchange	—	—	—	1
Meat Exchange	—	—	—	1
Bread Exchanges A or B	1	1	—	2
Fruit Exchange A or B	—	—	1	1
EVENING SNACK				
Fat Exchange	1	—	—	1
Calorie Supplements				
Group A	1	1	2	—
Group B	1	1	—	—
Group D	d	d	d	d

[a]From Walser, M; Imbembo, AL; Margolis, S; et al: *Nutritional Management: The Johns Hopkins Handbook.* Philadelphia, WB Saunders Co, 1984, with permission.

[b]Exchanges are given in Appendix D–7.

[c]To be used only with supplemental essential amino acids and/or ketoacids.

[d]As desired.

Appendix E–1. *Nutrition Resources*

Allergy Foundation of America
801 Second Avenue
New York, NY 10017

American Cancer Society
Unproven Methods Committee
90 Park Avenue
New York, NY 10017

American Cancer Society
Montgomery County Unit
344 University Blvd, West
Silver Spring, MD 20910

American Council on Science & Health
1995 Broadway, 18th Floor
New York, NY 10023
(212) 362–7044

American Diabetes Assoc.
Two Park Avenue
New York, NY 10018

American Dietetic Assoc.
620 North Michigan Avenue
Chicago, IL 60611

American Heart Assoc.
7320 Greenville Avenue
Dallas, TX 75231

American Home Economics Assoc.
2010 Massachusetts Avenue, NW
Washington, DC 20036

American Institute for Cancer Research
803 West Broad Street
Falls Church, VA 22046

American Institute of Nutrition
9650 Rockville Pike
Bethesda, MD 20014

American Medical Association
Department of Foods and Nutrition
535 North Dearborn Street
Chicago, IL 60610

American National Red Cross
Food and Nutrition Consultant
National Headquarters
Washington, DC 20006

American Public Health Assoc.
1015 Fifteenth Street, NW
Washington, DC 20005

American Society for Clinical Nutrition
9650 Rockville Pike
Bethesda, MD 20014

Arthritis Foundation National Office
3400 Peachtree Road, NE
Atlanta, GA

Cereal Institute, Inc.
1111 Plaza Drive
Schaumburg, IL 60195

Consumer Reports
256 Washington Street
Mount Vernon, NY 10553

Council of Better Business Bureaus
Standards and Practices
1515 Wilson Blvd.
Arlington, VA 22209
(703) 276–0100

Food and Nutrition Board
National Academy of Sciences–
    National Research Council
2102 Constitution Avenue
Washington, DC 20418

General Foods Corporation
250 North Street
White Plains, NY 10602

General Mills, Inc.
9200 Wayzata Blvd.
Minneapolis, MN 55426

Gerber Products
Department of Nutrition
Fremont, MI 49412

Leukemia Society of America, Inc.
National Headquarters
800 Second Avenue
New York, NY 10017
(212) 573–8484

Mead Johnson & Company
2404 West Pennsylvania Street
Evansville, IN 47721

Metropolitan Life Insurance Company
Health and Welfare Division
One Madison Avenue
New York, NY 10010

National Assoc. of Anorexia Nervosa
    and Associated Disorders
P.O. Box 271
Highland Park, IL 60035
(312) 831–3438

National Cancer Institute
Office of Cancer Communications
Bldg. 31, Rm 10A18
9000 Rockville Pike
Bethesda, MD 20205

National Dairy Council
11 North Canal Street
Chicago, IL 60606

National Health Information Clearing House
P.O. Box 1133
Washington, DC 20013

Appendix continued on following page

Appendix E–1. *Nutrition Resources (Continued)*

National Council Against Health Fraud
P.O. Box 1276
Loma Linda, California 92354
(714) 796–3067

National Council on Alcoholism
733 Third Avenue
New York, NY 10017

National Nutrition Consortium
1635 "P" Street, Suite 1
Washington, DC 20036

National Dairy Council
6300 North River Road
Rosemont, IL 60018

National Foundation/March of Dimes
P.O. Box 2000
White Plains, NY 10605

National Live Stock and Meat Board
Nutrition Research Department
444 North Michigan Avenue
Chicago, Il 60611

National Patient Education Library
S.S.M. Family Medicine Center
2900 Baltimore
Kansas City, MO 64108
(800) 821–6671

The Nutrition Foundation, Inc.
Office of Education and Public Affairs
888 Seventeenth Street, NW
Washington, DC 20006

Nutrition Forum Newsletter
P.O. Box 1747
Allentown, PA 18105
(215) 437–1795

Ross Laboratories
Columbus, OH 43216

Society for Nutrition Education
2140 Shattuck Avenue, Suite 1110
Berkeley, California 94704

United Fresh Fruit and Vegetable Assoc.
1019 Nineteenth Street, NW
Washington, DC 20006

Appendix E–2. *Governmental Agencies*

Federal Trade Commission
Sixth Street & Pennsylvania Ave, NW
Washington, DC 20580
(202) 523–3598

Food and Drug Administration
Office of Consumer Affairs
5600 Fishers Lane
Rockville, MD 20857
(301) 443–3170
(Or contact the Regional
   FDA Office in your area)

Food and Nutrition Information
Education Resources Center
National Agricultural Library
10301 Baltimore Blvd, Rm 304
Beltsville, MD 20705

U.S. Postal Service
Postal Inspector's Office
475 L'Enfant Plaza, SW
Washington, DC 20260
(202) 523–2557
(Or contact your local
   postal authority)

U.S. Department of Agriculture
Washington, DC 20250
   Agricultural Research Service
   Extension Service
   Food and Nutrition Service
   Office of Information

U.S. Department of Health and Human Services
Office of Child Development
200 Independence Ave, SW
Washington, DC 20201

U.S. Department of Health and Human Services
Food and Drug Administration
5600 Fishers Lane
Rockville, MD 20857

Appendix E–3. Recommended Journals

American Journal of Clinical Nutrition
American Journal of Nursing
American Journal of Public Health
Contemporary Nutrition (General Mills)
Dietetic Currents (Ross Laboratories)
Dairy Council Digest (National Dairy Council)
The Diabetes Educator
Journal of the American Dietetic Association
Journal of the American Medical Association

Journal of Nutrition
Journal of Nutrition Education
Journal of Parenteral and Enteral Nutrition
Nutrition and the MD
Nutrition Reviews
Nutrition Today
Nutrition Support Services
RD (Norwich Eaton)

Appendix F–1. Commonly Used Equivalents

Measure	Equivalent
60 drops	1 tsp., 5 cc, 5gm
1 gm	1 ml
1 cc	1 gm
1 tsp.	5 gm
3 tsp.	1 Tbsp.
1 Tbsp.	15 gm
1 Tbsp.	1 oz.
1 oz. (fluid)	30 gm
4 oz.	120 gm
8 oz.	240 gm
16 Tbsp.	1 cup
1 qt.	960 gm
1 lb.	454 gm
1.06 qt.	1 L
1 L	1000 ml

Appendix F–2. *Conversions to and from Metric Measures*

Known	Multiply by	To Know
Length		
inches	25.4	millimeters
inches	2.54	centimeters
feet	30.48	centimeters
meters	3.281	feet
Weight		
grains	64.7999	milligrams
ounces (Av.)	28.35	grams
pounds (Av.)	454.0	grams
pounds	0.454	kilograms
kilograms	2.205	pounds
Capacity (Liquid)		
teaspoons	4.7	milliliters
tablespoons	14.1	milliliters
fluid ounces	29.573	milliliters
cups (8 oz.)	238.0	milliliters
pints	0.473	liters
quarts	0.946	liters
Energy Units		
kilocalories	4.184	kilojoules
kilojoules	0.239	kilocalories

Temperature

To convert Celsium degrees into Fahrenheit, multiply by $\frac{9}{5}$ and add 32:

$$25°C = (25 \times \frac{9}{5}) + 32° = (45 + 32) = 77°F$$

To convert Fahrenheit degrees into Celsius, subtract 32 and multiply by $\frac{5}{9}$:

$$95°F = (95 - 32) \times \frac{5}{9} = 63 \times \frac{5}{9} = 35°C$$

Frequently used temperatures:

Boiling point of water	100°C	212°F
Body temperature	37°C	98.6°F
Freezing point of water	0°C	32°F

Weight

To convert pounds to kilograms, divide the pounds by 2.2:

$$\frac{160 \text{ lb.}}{2.2} = 72.72 \text{ kg}$$

Height

To convert feet and inches to centimeters, multiply the inches by 2.54:

$$6 \text{ feet} = 72 \text{ inches}$$
$$72 \times 2.54 = 182.8 \text{ cm}$$

Appendix F–3. *Conversion of Milligrams to Milliequivalents**

To convert milligrams (mg) to milliequivalents (mEq):

$$\frac{\text{Milligrams}}{\text{Atomic weight}} \times \text{Valence} = \text{Milliequivalents}$$

Mineral Element	Chemical Symbol	Atomic Weight	Valence
Chlorine	Cl	35.4	1
Potassium	K	39	1
Sodium	Na	23	1
Calcium	Ca	40	2
Magnesium	Mg	24.3	2
Sulfur	S	32	
Sulfate	SO$_4$	96	2

To convert specific weight of sodium to sodium chloride:

Milligrams of sodium $\times 2.54 =$ Milligrams of sodium chloride

To convert specific weight of sodium chloride to sodium:

Milligrams of sodium chloride $\times 0.393 =$ Milligrams of sodium

Sodium Milligrams	Sodium Milliequivalents	Sodium Chloride Grams
500	21.8	1.3
1,000	43.5	2.5
1,500	75.3	3.8
2,000	87.0	5.0

*From Pemberton, CD; Gastineau, CF (eds.): *Mayo Clinic Diet Manual,* 5th ed. Philadelphia, W B Saunders Co, 1981, with permission.

INDEX and GLOSSARY

Note: Page numbers in *italics* refer to illustrations; page numbers followed by t refer to tables.

Appestat (*Continued*)
    system in each individual determining the
      preferred body weight, 455
Appetite The natural desire for food, 16
  drug effect on, 415, 416–417t
  illness and, 355
Arachidonic acid, 125
Ariboflavinosis, 181
Arm circumference, 370, *370*
  nomogram for, for adults, 751t
    for children, 752t
  percentiles for, 750t
Arthritis, rheumatoid, 617
  joint pathology in, *617*
Ascites, due to cirrhosis, 551
-ase Suffix frequently used in naming an enzyme;
    it is usually attached to a stem word designat-
    ing the substrate, the nature of the substrate,
    or the type of reaction, 534
Aseptic Sterile; free from disease-producing
    germs.
Aspartame, 238, 240–241t
  diabetic use of, 589
Asphyxiation, food-related, of infants and chil-
    dren, 298
Aspirate To remove fluid using negative pres-
    sure, usually by inhaling.
Assessment The act of critically analyzing and
    evaluating the status of a particular condition
    or individual, 6, *7*
  nutritional. See *Nutritional assessment.*
Asthenia Weakness; loss of strength.
  due to insulin deficiency, 570
Asthma, 682
  precipitating factors of, according to age group,
    684t
Atherosclerosis, 624, *625*
Athletic competition, energy requirements for,
    145–150, 147t
Atopy Clinical hypersensitivity with a genetic or-
    igin, 683
ATP (adenosine triphosphate) High-energy phos-
    phate bond that is the major source of energy
    for the cell, 53, 137
Atrophy Wasting; reduced size of organ or
    tissue.
Attention deficit disorder (ADD), 305
Avitaminosis Deficiency disease due to a lack or
    deficiency of a vitamin in the diet or malab-
    sorption.
Azotemia The occurrence of nitrogen compounds
    in the blood, 651

B vitamins. See also *Vitamin B₆* and *Vitamin B₁₂.*
  for stressed patient, 504
  in pregnancy, 263
Bacteria, intestinal, 104
Bactericidal Lethal to bacteria, 221
Bacteriostatic Hindering the growth of bacteria,
    221
Balloon procedure, for weight reduction, 471
Basal energy expenditure (BEE) Term used in ref-
    erence to the basal metabolic rate (BMR), 141
Basal metabolic rate (BMR) The least amount of
    energy required for the involuntary work of
    the body in order to maintain life, including

Basal metabolic rate (BMR) (*Continued*)
    respiration, circulation, and maintenance of
    muscle tone and body temperature, 138
  determination of, 141
  factors affecting, 138–140
  of adult, 315
  weight control and, 455
Basal metabolism, 138–140
Base Substance that combines with an acid to
    form a salt; also called alkali, 69
  as food additive, 226t
Behavior modification, for weight control, 467
  of alcoholic with cirrhosis, 550
Beikost Food other than milk; first solid food
    eaten by infants, 294
Beriberi, 177, *180*
Beta-carotene, 157
Beta oxidation, 123
Beverage, alcoholic. See *Alcohol.*
  for athletic competition, 147
BHA Butylated hydroxyanisole, 119
BHT Butylated hydroxytoluene, 119
Bifidus factor Group of nitrogen-containing poly-
    saccharides present in mammalian milk that
    inhibits growth of harmful bacteria in the in-
    testinal tract.
Bile Secretion produced by the liver, which is
    stored and concentrated in the gallbladder,
    that aids in the digestion of fats, 46
  absence of, 46
Bile salts, fat emulsification and, 120
Biliary cirrhosis, primary, vitamin A deficiency
    with, 161
Bioavailability The degree to which a nutrient is
    available for use to the body.
  food-drug interactions affecting, 416–423
Biochemical indicators, of nutritional status, 372
Bioflavonoids Naturally occurring substances that
    have biological activity; originally called vita-
    min P; widely distributed in plants, 190
Biological activity Processes among living organ-
    isms.
Biological value A measurement of protein to as-
    sess its ability to support growth, i.e., the ex-
    tent to which a protein contains the proper
    proportions of essential amino acids needed
    by the body, 76
Biotin, 179t, 185
Black American food pattern, 332–333
Bland diet, in ulcer management, 520
Blended tube feedings, 387, 388t
Blindness, taste, of cancer patient, 520
Blood
  sugar level in, 99–101
    fasting, 100, *100*
    hormonal maintenance of, 101, *102*
    in diabetes mellitus, 584–586
  values of, for evaluating nutritional status,
    757–758t
Blood loss, anemia due to, 670–671
Blood pressure, age variations of, 637t
Body fluids, distribution of, 58, *59*
  electrolytes in, 62, *63*
  osmolality of, 63
Body frame, determination of, from wrist circum-
    ference, 749t

Cancer (*Continued*)
  supplemental feedings for patient with, 490-491
  therapy for, types of, 485–487
CAPD Continuous ambulatory peritoneal dialysis, 659
Carbohydrate, 92–111
  absorption of, 99
  as energy source, 138
  body compounds containing, 103t
  classification of, 94–98, 97
  complex, increasing in diet, 238
  dental caries and, 109
  dietary, functions of, 104–105
    nutritional classification of, 97
  digestion of, 98, 99
  exchange system use of, 435
    determining amount for, 446, 448
  foods containing, 106, 106t, 764–768t
  health issues involving, 108–109
  intake of, 98
  malabsorption of, 107
  metabolism of, 99–104, 103
  obesity and, 109
  parenteral solutions of, 398, 399t
  requirements for, dietary, 105
    for diabetic, 573t, 574
    for elderly, 316
  10 grams, foods to provide, 586t
Carbohydrate loading Consumption of controlled carbohydrate diet to increase glycogen stores for increased endurance, 148–150
Carcinogenesis, food additives and, 228
Cardiovascular disease, 624
Caries, dental, 305
    carbohydrates and, 109
Cariogenic Tending to cause dental caries.
Carnitine, 190
Carotene Precursor of vitamin A; found in yellow and dark green leafy plants, 157
  sources of, 159
Carrier (1) A person who harbors and transmits a communicable disease without showing symptoms; (2) a substance that transports another compound, 47
Catabolism Process of converting larger complex substances into simpler substances, thereby releasing energy, 52
  classification of, 503t
  energy requirements for, 502, 503t
  protein, 79
  timing of response of, to infection, *505*
Catecholamines A group of adrenergic compounds (dopamine, epinephrine, and norepinephrine) released at the sympathetic nerve endings that are secreted in response to a physiological stress, 498
Cation An ion that carries a positive charge, 62
cc Cubic centimeter.
Cellulose Polysaccharide found in plant tissues; provides bulk or roughage for humans since it is an indigestible carbohydrate, 98
  food sources of, 106t, 107t
Cephalin, 126
Cereal. See *Bread/cereal group.*
Cerebrosides, 127

Charting, 8, *9*
CHD. See *Coronary heart disease.*
Cheilosis Cracking and soreness at the corners of the mouth, usually a symptom of riboflavin deficiency, 181
Chemotherapy Treatment of a disease or illness using medication.
  cancer, 486
    alimentary tract effects of, 486t
Chenodeoxycholic acid (CDCA), for gallstone therapy, 554
Children
  basal caloric requirements for, calculation of, 295t
  breakfast requirements for, 302
  eating behavior of, parental guidance for, 302
  feeding, 299–301
    preschool, 299–300
      food pattern for, 300t
    school-age, 301
    toddler, 299
  fluid requirements of, 294t
  fluoride supplementation for, 295t
  healthy diet for, 303
  hyperactivity of, 305
  illness of, nutritional needs during, 306
  lead toxicity in, 306
  renal disease of, nutrition for, 657
  school lunch for, 303, *304*
Chinese food pattern, 335–336
Chloride, requirements for, with parenteral nutrition, 401, 401t
Chlorine, 201
Cholecystectomy, postoperative diet for, 554
Cholecystitis, 553
  nutritional care of, 554
Cholecystokinin, 46, 553
Cholelithiasis, 553
  nutritional care for, 554
Cholesterol Fat-like substance present in all body cells and synthesized by the liver; found only in animal products, 119
  avoiding excessive, for optimal health, 237
  chemical structure of, *120*
  dietary factors affecting, 627
  foods containing, 128, 129–130t, 769–774t
  functions of, in body, 127
  metabolism of, essential fatty acids and, 125
  normal limits for, 627t
Cholesterol/saturated-fat index (CSI), 629, 630t
  of Western diet vs. low-fat diet, 631t
Choline A chemical synthesized in the body that functions along with vitamins; deficiencies have not been observed, and no recommendations for supplementation are advised, 190
Chromium, 209–210
  supplementation of, with parenteral nutrition, 402t
Chronic Long-lasting.
Chronic obstructive pulmonary disease (COPD) Long-lasting obstruction of bronchial air flow, 504–506
Chylomicron A lipoprotein that transports fat, mainly triglycerides, from the gastrointestinal tract through the lymphatic system after